Science and Application of High-Intensity Interval Training

Editors

Paul Laursen, PhD

Martin Buchheit, PhD

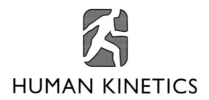

HUMAN KINETICS

Library of Congress Cataloging-in-Publication Data

Names: Laursen, Paul, 1971- editor. | Buchheit, Martin, 1978- editor.
Title: Science and application of high-intensity interval training : solutions to the programming
    puzzle / Paul Laursen, Martin Buchheit, editors.
Description: Champaign, IL : Human Kinetics, [2018] | Includes bibliographical references
    and index.
Identifiers: LCCN 2018030511 (print) | LCCN 2018044768 (ebook) | ISBN 9781492586890
    (ebook) | ISBN 9781492552123 (print)
Subjects: LCSH: Interval training. | Athletes—Training of.
Classification: LCC GV481 (ebook) | LCC GV481 .S333 2018 (print) | DDC 613.7/04—dc23
LC record available at https://lccn.loc.gov/2018030511

ISBN: 978-1-4925-5212-3 (print)

The web addresses cited in this text were current as of October 2018, unless otherwise noted.

Senior Acquisitions Editor: Roger W. Earle
Senior Developmental Editor: Cynthia McEntire
Indexer: Rebecca McCorkle
Permissions Manager: Martha Gullo
Graphic Designer: Whitney Milburn
Cover Designer: Keri Evans
Cover Design Associate: Susan Rothermel Allen
Photo Asset Manager: Laura Fitch
Photo Production Manager: Jason Allen
Senior Art Manager: Kelly Hendren
Art Style Development: Joanne Brummett
Illustrations: © Human Kinetics
Production: Westchester Publishing Services
Printer: Walsworth

Human Kinetics books are available at special discounts for bulk purchase. Special editions or book excerpts can
also be created to specification. For details, contact the Special Sales Manager at Human Kinetics.

Printed in the United States of America   10 9 8 7 6 5 4 3

The paper in this book was manufactured using responsible forestry methods.

Human Kinetics
1607 N. Market Street
Champaign, IL 61820
USA

United States and International
Website: **US.HumanKinetics.com**
Email: info@hkusa.com
Phone: 1-800-747-4457

Canada
Website: **Canada.HumanKinetics.com**
Email: info@hkcanada.com

E7078

Tell us what you think!
Human Kinetics would love to hear what we
can do to improve the customer experience.
Use this QR code to take our brief survey.

Contents

PART I

Understanding High-Intensity Interval Training

1

Genesis and Evolution of High-Intensity Interval Training

Paul Laursen and Martin Buchheit with contributions
from Jean Claude Vollmer

Of all the factors related to sport performance that you'll ever read about, coaches and sport professionals will unequivocally agree that it is the preparatory training completed that has the greatest impact on sport performance. The preparatory training includes the highly important mental aspect, but additionally skill or technique development, tactical intelligence, and, of course, physical development. With training, we're preparing the body for war on the battlefield: the pitch, the court, the field, the road, the track, or in the water. So for athletes, coaches, and practitioners passionate about maximizing performance, investing thought and time toward planning in this area is worthwhile.

To prepare physically, varying amounts of different types of training will be important, depending on the context of the sport or event that is attempting to be optimized for, and this important component of the performance enhancement puzzle will be expanded on shortly. For now, we can say generally that varying appropriate amounts of both high-intensity training as well as continuous low-intensity training are critical ingredients needed to maximize performance in nearly all athletes who need a blend of prolonged endurance and high-intensity speed or power (16, 24). While there is little doubt that varying amounts of both types of training can effectively improve different aspects of performance-related

physiological function and physical development, the focus of this book of course will be on high-intensity interval training (HIIT) and how it can help to solve important aspects of an athlete's complex training program puzzle. When we consider the relatively simple adjustments to training programs that focus on submaximal aerobic endurance design, it's easy to see that the modification task involved (i.e., progressively increasing exercise duration) pales in comparison to that of HIIT format selection, where multiple moving parts within the format (intensity, duration, recovery, etc.) create immense complexity in design possibility and related physiological outcomes.

Defining HIIT

Let's begin with a simple definition. HIIT is usually defined as exercise consisting of repeated bouts of high-intensity work performed above the lactate threshold (a perceived effort of "hard" or greater) or critical speed/power, interspersed by periods of low-intensity exercise or complete rest. As we will outline, there are many ways that definition can be achieved, however, figure 1.1 provides a broad illustration of the concept. The general basis of high-intensity interval training can be described simply as follows: Imagine performing a bout of exercise at an intensity

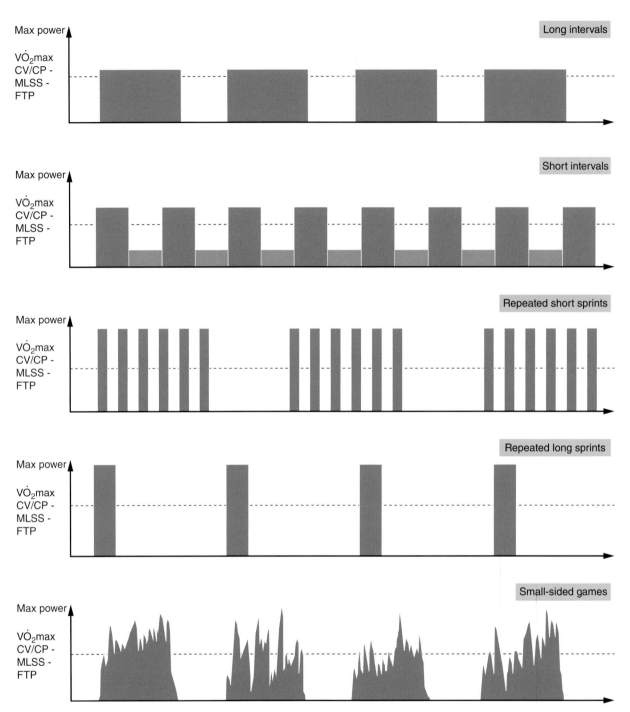

Figure 1.1 Schematic diagram illustrating the general concept of high-intensity interval training (HIIT) defined as repeated bouts of high-intensity exercise performed above the lactate threshold or critical speed/power, interspersed by periods of low-intensity exercise or complete rest. The five main HIIT formats, including long intervals, short intervals, repeated sprints of short and long and game-based training durations, are shown. Blue bars = effort intervals, green = relief intervals.

above your lactate threshold, or critical velocity/ power (refer to chapter 4). To be clear here, this is an exercise intensity that is unsustainable, and one at which your brain would eventually force you to lower your intensity if you were to sustain it for as long as you could. It feels hard, and you know that fatigue would be inevitable at this pace if you were to hold on. Higher levels of sugar-burning glycolysis are needed generally to sustain the energy demand, and lactate accumulates to high levels typically at the point of fatigue. Now, if we took that same high-intensity effort and separated it with pauses that included periods of complete rest or lower levels of active recovery, that glycolytic energy rate is eased so that lactate production is more in check, whilst the cardiovascular strain remains high, and perceived effort, although still high, is reduced and manageable. This is one of the features of HIIT that absolutely fascinated us when we first started research into the topic. As shown early by Per-Olof Åstrand and colleagues who worked with him (2, 10), metabolic rate can be as high as the maximal rate of oxygen uptake ($\dot{V}O_2$max), yet reasonably tolerated at relatively low concentrations of blood lactate (i.e., <4mM). From this work and others in the field, interval training was originally proposed as a method that allowed athletes to do greater volumes of conditioning work with less physiological strain. Ultimately, this broken exercise format of HIIT enables either a more manageable training session with the same training stress, or alternatively, the accumulation of a greater total amount of a high-intensity exercise stimulus if the sequence continues to be repeated. To be clear, by performing such high-intensity work intermittently instead of continuously, a person can maintain a high-intensity stimulus for longer, with less accumulated physical strain, and with beneficial adaptations that can be specific to sport demands. While interval training can be associated with a high degree of physical effort, fatigue, and acute discomfort, when applied properly with adequate recovery, it clearly has been shown to elicit rapid improvements in various aspects of performance and physiology.

History of HIIT

With Jean Claude Vollmer

Interval training has a relatively long tradition. Rumor has it that it may have started sometime around the year 1912. Based on advice received in letters from his brother, another professional runner living in the United States, Hannes Kolehmainen of Finland, was seen preparing for races using 5 to 10 repetitions at his specific 10 km race pace of 3:05/ km (19 km/h), before winning the 10,000 m event at the Olympics. In the 1920s and 1930s, coach Lauri Pihkala continued the development of these earlier HIIT forms with Paavo Nurmi (figure 1.2), one of the best middle- and long-distance runners in the world at that time. Nurmi was known as the "Flying Finn" and set 22 official world records at distances between 1500 m and 20 km, winning nine gold and three silver medals in his 12 Olympic Games events. His daily routines (26) were as follows:

- Early morning: 10 to 12 km walk interspersed with a few sprints, followed by generic gym exercises and a bath.
- One hour later, main training as: 4 to 5 × 80 to 120 m sprints, then 400 to 1000 m high-speed running, and finally 3000 to 4000 m high-speed running.
- Evening training: 4000 to 7000 m cross-country run, followed by 4 to 5 × 120 m sprints.

In the 1930s, Swedish coach Gösta Holmé is said to have invented Fartlek, meaning speed play

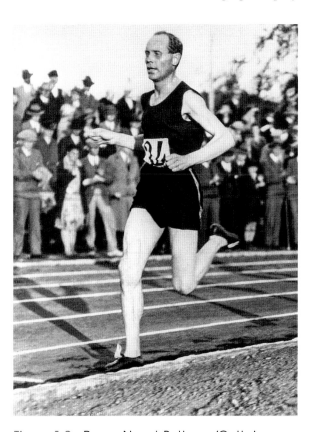

Figure 1.2 Paavo Nurmi. Bettmen/Getty Images

running, in Swedish. Such training is documented as being used often, from then into the early 1940s, to prepare a number of Swedish endurance runners and cross-country skiers, including modifying this type of training across various terrain types, termed *natural interval training*.

An example of a Fartlek session at that time might include the following:

1. Easy run for 5 to 10 min
2. 1200 to 2400 m fast run at a regular tempo
3. 5 min fast walk
4. Repeated 50 to 60 m sprints (separated by a recovery jog until the athlete feels ready to start again with the same quality). As many as needed to "feel" fatigue, before a 5 min walk
5. Acceleration starts over 3 to 4 strides, as explosive as possible
6. 160 to 180 m uphill running
7. Recovery jog

Athletes were allowed to repeat these seven points as they wished, but were instructed to ensure that they always felt fresh. When perceived fatigue approached a high level, they were requested to stop the session, which could be performed up to five times a week.

Following these earlier developments in Finland and Sweden, the German coach Woldemar Gerschler continued to popularize the use of intervals with the runner Rudolf Harbig, who established an astonishing 800 m world record in 1939 (1:46.6). Some sample sessions from that runner are shown in table 1.1.

HIIT became popularized further in the 1950s after triple gold Olympic (1952 Helsinki) champion in the 5000 m, 10,000 m, and marathon events, Emil Zátopek from Czechoslovakia (figure 1.3), described his training. According to Ettema (13), from early 1943, with his coach Josef Hron, Zátopek performed short interval training, running at paces near his critical velocity, calculated from his personal best

Table 1.1 Sample Session Prescribed by German Coach Woldemar Gerschler to Runner Rudolf Harbig to Establish His 800 m World Record in 1939

Date	Session
April 13	Jog 30 min 4×200 m in 23.8, 23.8, 24.3, 24.0 s (recovery 5 min walk) Jog 10 min 600 m in 1:25.3
April 23	Jog 30 min 800 m in 2:11 Jog 15 min 800 m in 2:02 Jog 10 min 600 m in 1:28
May 2	Jog 20 min 5×200 m in 23.2, 23.8, 24.6, 24.7, 24.2 s (recovery 5 min walk)
June 1	Jog 20 min Crouch sprint starts: 2×30 m, 2×50 m, 2×80 m, 1×150 m, 1×200 m, 1×400 m
June 7	Jog 25 min 2×300 m in 38.2 s (recovery 5 min jog) Jog 10 min 500 m in 1:11 Jog 15 min 200 m in 24.0 s
July 13*	Jog 20 min 600 m in 1:27 Jog 10 min 300 m in 36.9 s Jog 10 min 500 m in 1:06.7

* Last session before 800 m world record on July 15.

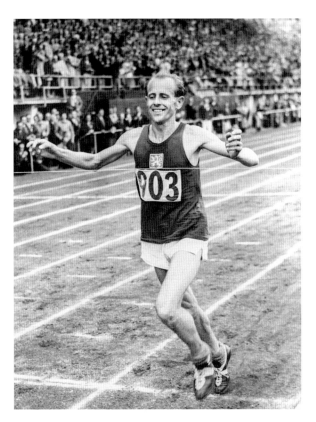

Figure 1.3   Emil Zátopek. Bettmen/Getty Images

in 3 to 10 km events. This was estimated to be 85% of his velocity at $\dot{V}O_2$max ($v\dot{V}O_2$max; 20 km/h, or 1:12 per 400m), with daily training that included 5×200 m + 20×400 m + 2×200 m (for a total of 10 km), or the famous 100×400 m interspersed by 200 m recovery runs (45 s to 1:30). Remarkably, it was reported that Zátopek was already playing with some of the HIIT variables we will expand on in chapter 4, to modify the physiological responses during his winter build-up phase. That is, he would lower the intensity of the exercise runs and increase the intensity of his recovery jog (i.e., decreasing the amplitude), which would increase and decrease reliance on aerobic and anaerobic systems, respectively. At this point in time, Zátopek and Hron were already shaping their HIIT sessions to solve their performance puzzle.

From 1952 to 1956 in Hungary, coach Mihály Igloi and his runners Sándor Iharos (one of only two athletes with Paavo Nurmi to have held outdoor world records over 1500 m, 5000 m, and 10,000 m), István Rózsavölgyi (world record holder over 1000 m, 1500 m, and 2000 m in 1956), and László Tabori (on September 6, 1956, he equaled the 1500 m world record—set only a month earlier by

Iharos—with a time of 3:40.8), pushed world records further using forms of HIIT repeated twice a day, extending the volume of repetitions run at high-intensity. After the 1956 Melbourne Olympics, Igloi immigrated to the United States and spread further his methods at the Los Angeles Track Club. Among other runners, he coached Bob Schul, who won Olympic Gold in Tokyo (1964) in the 5000 m. An example of a weekly microcycle for Rózsavölgyi in April is shown in table 1.2.

Around the same time, Franz Stampfl, an Austrian who left the German Nazi regime, helped promote repetition work in England with his followers Chris Chataway (5000 m record holder in 1954; 13:51.6) and Chris Brasher (Olympic Gold Medalist in the 3,000 m steeplechase in 1956 in Melbourne; 8:41.2) and Roger Bannister; the former men paced Bannister to break the 4 min mile record in 1954.

While Kolehmainen, Nurmi, Harbig, Rózsavölgyi, and Stampfl had reportedly used sets of high-speed repetition runs (called "repetition work"), none, with the exception of Zátopek, were yet training using actual HIIT sequences that incorporate much shorter recovery periods between repetitions and larger series volumes. It was only later into the 1950s when physiologists made suggestions to coaches and their athletes to shorten recovery intervals. These recommendations were based on heart radiographies and ECG data from hundreds of athletes. Their combined goal was to increase the level of acute physiological response during training.

At that time in fact, the main physiological benefits of HIIT were thought to arise during processes occurring within the recovery periods, a phenomenon we will highlight in chapters 3 and 4. According to Billat (4), interval training was first described, in a scientific journal, by physiologists Reindell and Roskamm (23), who were inspired through discussions with coach Woldemar Gerschler, and together created the Fribourg interval training method. Different HIIT formats (that in our book we will begin to term *weapons*), were presented at various coaching conferences (1), which tended to be either long (e.g., $6\text{-}10 \times 600$ m in 1:38-1:42 with recovery periods of 1:30-2:00, or $6\text{-}8 \times 1200$ m in 3:24-3:30 with recoveries of 1:30-2:00) or short intervals (e.g., up to 100 reps of 100-200 m runs in 14-16 s and 30-33 s interspersed with 30 to 60 s rest periods). In 1960, the pioneering Swedish physiologist Per-Olof Åstrand described the cardiorespiratory responses to long interval training (3 min efforts) at a velocity

Table 1.2 Sample Weekly Microcycle Used by István Rózsavölgyi in His Lead-Up to the 1956 Olympics

Day	Training
1	2×4×300 m in 45.0 s (recovery 100 m jog) 10×100 m in 15.0 to 18.0 s (recovery 50 m jog) 6×300 m in 45.0 s (recovery 5 min jog) 10×100 m alternatively in either 16.0 to 18.0 s or 14.0 to 15.0 s (recovery 50 m jog)
2	5×5×200 m in 27.0 to 28.0 s (recovery 100 m jog) 6×100 m in 15.0 s (recovery 50 m jog)
3	10 to 15 km fartlek 15×100 m (recovery 50 m jog)
4	5×300 m easy, 5×300 m fast, 5×300 m very fast, 5×300 m easy 10×100 m in 16.0 s (recovery 50 m jog) 6×300 m at 80% personal best 10×100 m fast, 10×100 m easy
5	10×10×100 m (alternatively high and moderate speed between series)
6	10×150 m moderate pace 2×3×400 m in 55.0 to 56.0 s (recovery 300 m jog between reps and 400 m walk between series) 10×100 m (recovery 50 m jog) 10×100 m high tempo (recovery 50 m jog between reps and 400 m walk between series)
7	Cross-country race

of 90% to 95% v$\dot{V}O_2$max, known already to elicit $\dot{V}O_2$max in the last repetitions, despite complete passive rest intervals. Åstrand et al. (2) considered that this was one of the best forms of interval training to improve $\dot{V}O_2$max, since all cardiorespiratory parameters were at their maximum. Remarkably, Christensen and colleagues (10) showed that very short interval training, consisting of 10 s runs at 100% of v$\dot{V}O_2$max interspersed with 10 s of complete rest, could elicit $\dot{V}O_2$max under low blood lactate levels (<4 mmol).

In the late 1960s, the American group of Fox, Robinson, and Wiegman (14) were one of the first to compare metabolic energy use during continuous and interval running at the same exercise rate, and like others, showed a slower accumulation of lactic acid, and delayed fatigue with interval training, speculated to be due likely to the replenishment and subsequent reutilization of phosphagen reserves via the muscle's oxygen-storing myoglobin. As a result, athletes were shown to be able to accomplish larger quantities of work at very high intensities.

In the field, the 1960s saw a large development of HIIT methodology and especially its use within block periodization approaches, thanks to, among others, Australian Percy Wells Cerutty, coach of Herb Elliott (1500 m Olympic Gold in Rome 1960 in 3:35.6) and New Zealander Sir Arthur Lydiard (coach of Peter Snell, triple Olympic Gold medalist, and only male since 1920 to win both the 800 m (world

record in 1962 on a grass track, 1:44.3) and 1500 m at the same Olympic Games, in Tokyo 1964 (18).

The 1970s and 1980s saw more athletes using interval training in the field. More thought and reflection appeared to spread, as the preparation of training began to be considered more and more like a puzzle that needed solving. Different forms of training were trialed and tested, including long slow running of great distance (24), as well as various specific paces thought to enhance physiology or prepare optimally for competition. These philosophies, inspired largely by Lydiard (18), evolved today into what is more commonly referred to as "polarized training" (24). Here, roughly 80% of an athlete's training volume is performed at an intensity below his so-called aerobic threshold (elaborated on in chapter 3), while the remaining 20% of the training, including HIIT, is performed above this intensity. The integration of HIIT into an athlete's complete training system gathered momentum and acceptance throughout the world, with Franck Horwill implementing a five-speed system with Sebastian Coe, who won four Olympic medals, including 1500 m gold at the 1980 and 1984 Olympic Games. Paul Schmidt in Germany and Moniz Pereira from Portugal continued to develop the idea in the 1980s that HIIT was a necessary part of a runner's training program puzzle. Commercialization and professionalization within running led to further improvements in understanding HIIT responses and the effect of variable manipulation, with anecdotal reports from coaches on the different effects of manipulating training intensity, duration, repetitions, series, inter-reps and inter-series recovery modalities, as well as terrain (hill, grass, sand). It was not until the 1990s that more detailed work on interval training was published for the masses by Tim Noakes, in his famous book *The Lore of Running* (21) and Jack Daniels with *Jack Daniels' Formula* (12). Subsequently, most other individual athlete sports naturally followed the lead of running and adopted similar training tactics, including cycling, swimming, rowing, cross-country skiing, and triathlon (see related chapters).

The year 2000 began an explosion of work in the area of interval training research, beginning with Billat's work that focused on aerobic (4) and anaerobic (5) interval training for runners, and Laursen and Jenkins (17) reviewed the physiological basis for interval training across individual athlete-based endurance sports. An outpouring of academic research followed (literally thousands of papers on HIIT) from both areas of sport application (6, 7) and exercise science (19) thereafter.

Team Sports

While research performed across traditional individual Olympic-based sports shows direct correlations between various levels of physical capacity and performance, the relationship for team and racket-based sports outcomes (i.e., winning a match or scoring a goal) is not as straightforward. Nevertheless, a rigorous preparation of physical capacities has always been believed to be of high importance for successful outcomes. Historically, team sport coaches often had backgrounds as physical education teachers and were therefore well versed in the physical preparation principles that they borrowed from track-and-field coaches. For this reason, HIIT has nearly always been incorporated into team training schedules. Examples include run-based formats directly taken from track-and-field practices (series of 100 and 200 m efforts, up to 1 km repetitions, or using 15 s on/off formats), or even using more sport-specific approaches, namely game-based HIIT (figure 1.1), with athletes practicing their sports at high-metabolic work intensities alongside specific rules and typical sport constraints, often termed small-sided games in the team sport context (22).

In the 1970s in the United Kingdom, Tom Reilly, who some have termed "the father of football

(soccer) science," alongside his pioneering work in monitoring, training-load quantification, and player education, showed additionally that HIIT may be important for some aspects of team sport performance (22). Around the same time in Italy, a strong athletic culture led by Enrico Arcelli used modifications of the track-and-field HIIT approach in their practice. This work, which used HIIT, paved the way for others within the Italian Association of Fitness coaches. Also in Italy, the famous Milanello training center, the Milan Lab, was the first institution fully devoted to sports science in football, embracing innovation and technology. Following Reilly, the Scandinavian group of Bjorn Ekblom, Jens Bangsbo, and Paul Balsom published much work in the area, summarized in Bangsbo's 1994 book, *Fitness Training in Soccer: A Scientific Approach* (3), which led the basis of interval training for soccer. Subsequently, most other team sport codes followed the lead of football and adopted similar training tactics.

The progressive development of team sports into the mass entertainment entities they now are came with an explosion of staff employed to maximize performance and outcomes (see, for example, Part II). Team sports, and more especially top football (soccer) clubs (e.g., Manchester United, Arsenal, Liverpool, and Paris SG), youth academies (e.g., Aspire in Qatar), as well as other football codes including AFL and Rugby and, more recently, various U.S.-based sports (basketball, American football, baseball, and ice hockey), today employ physical conditioning specialists alongside sport science research specialists, including physiologists, biomechanists, statisticians, and technology support experts. Similar teams of experts are amassed in today's leading country institutes and academies focused on individual athlete performance (cycling, track and field, swimming, rowing, triathlon, cross-country skiing, etc.), preparing for Olympic games and world championship performances. These physical preparation teams' combined roles are to establish noninvasive monitoring systems and advise on areas of potential performance enhancement. As a result of both our increased knowledge and the explosion of human resources, HIIT practices at the elite level may now be less empirical, but pursuant of specificity and individualization, replaced by monitored and tailored sequences across the most relevant HIIT formats (8, 9, 15).

In 2013, we published a two-part review (6, 7) that combined our applied work as embedded practitioners in high-performance sport, along with our academic research experience. It was an expansion of the ideas outlined in these publications alongside the assistance of Dr. Jackson Fyfe to navigate us through the complexities of the strength training interference phenomenon (chapter 6), Dr. Phillip Maffetone to ensure we understand HIIT's effect from a holistic standpoint (chapter 7), in addition to outlining methods we can use to program the load of HIIT (chapter 8) and monitor its response (chapter 9), that form part I of this book. The second half of our book is dedicated to the application of these principles for, give or take, the world's top 20 sports that typically apply HIIT in their practice. Each application chapter in part II, generously contributed by some of the best practitioners and coaches in the field today, additionally provide tools you can use to maximize athletic performance in these sports. Combined, both science and application sections expose opportunities for future investigation by today's students and researchers in academic institutions throughout the world. We hope that you, the reader, enjoy its contents and find it useful.

Performance Enhancement Puzzle

While the focus of our book is on high-intensity interval training, we're mostly all here to learn how we can use HIIT to improve the physiology that maximizes performance. From a physical preparation standpoint, what can be gained with HIIT that could enhance performance? Perhaps before we go there, we need to pause for a moment to gain clarity around an important question. That question is: What is performance? Performance probably means something a little different for everyone. For MB, in his home environment, performance might mean that his team is able to recover quicker between high-intensity actions while maintaining a higher playing tempo and better tactical alertness during a football match, alongside more goals scored over his opposition. For PL, performance might mean he's seeing an already high cycling power output and running speed enhanced in training alongside improved finish time in his triathletes. You'll have your own point of view depending on where you're coming from, and what's meaningful to you, as will all the sport-specific contributing experts in the application chapters that accompany the second half of our book. Typically, however, if we want to put a general definition on performance in the context of most sports, we refer to the ability to carry out or accomplish an action, task, or function. To do so, we must usually keep fatigue at bay. In this regard, HIIT is an important component of most sports' training programs, as it's a training format that allows specific preparation toward meeting the physical demands of performance. Thus, when we're referring to how HIIT fits into the programming puzzle, we mean that we're trying our best to select the HIIT sequence that best enhances physiological adaptation or outcome. These adaptations or outcomes from an HIIT session should be preparing athletes or teams optimally, placing them in the best possible physiological state they can be in before they perform in their event or match.

Before moving forward with HIIT design and shaping the puzzle piece, we need to take a step back first and ask a few more questions. First of all: How important is physical preparation in the big picture of our sport? We need to ask this question, as it provides us clarity as to where we should be focusing our time and energy. If you're reading this book, then it's likely that physical preparation is your specialty and of high interest. Regardless, it's important to appreciate that physical preparation might not actually be the critical thing that is necessary to maximize your sport's outcome (hard to believe, we know). In the context of some sports, in order to be a valued member of your team, it's important to have clarity in this regard, so that appropriate focus can be made toward the things that matter. The important first question then is: How important is physical preparation relevant to other critical factors that relate to sporting success, such as skills and tactics? Figure 1.4 provides an example of how this differs throughout the sports presented in our book.

Once we are clear on the level of importance of physical preparation, it's now time to begin exploring where HIIT fits into the physical preparation puzzle matrix. Here again, HIIT is a critical weapon we can use to shape the puzzle piece, but it can't be considered the only form of preparation. HIIT is one of a number of different components of the programming puzzle that we must consider, with different emphases varying dependent on the nuances of the sport. Skill development, technique, match intelligence, tactics, coordination, pacing, agility, recovery, strength, explosive power, endurance, repeated sprint ability, anaerobic speed reserve, tempo training, and others, must also be considered alongside HIIT.

But sport requires energy and various forms of fatigue resistance. Having these features in an athlete is critical in so many sports and is the hallmark of

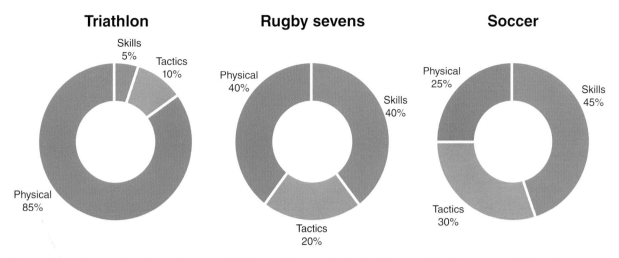

Figure 1.4 Respective importance of skills, tactics, and physical capacities for successful performance in three competitive sports. Overall estimation for all field positions pooled.

successful athletes. Thus, HIIT is often the critical tool or weapon we can use to shape the puzzle piece to achieve optimal physiological state and subsequent performance probability for a number of sports that are of interest on the world stage. In this book, our aim is to outline the science that explains how the weapons work and how they can be manipulated to hit our physiological targets. Our expert sport practitioners will guide us toward their use of HIIT at the coalface of elite sport in our application chapters.

HIIT is highly complicated, and to solve the puzzle, you need to shape the puzzle piece appropriately to solve the fit. Our aim is to provide you, the reader, with the tools to shape this important piece of your programming puzzle.

There are many ways that we can shape an HIIT puzzle piece (see chapter 4), but only so many options we have to solve the fit appropriately. Consider the analogy of baking a cake. For any cake, the ingredients are pretty simple and largely the same: flour, butter, sugar, eggs, and a bit of baking powder. But are all cakes the same? Clearly not. Preparing for a sport isn't that different in this context. Getting the raw ingredients together, like athletes, tactics, and skills, is relatively straightforward. But when we look to physical preparation, the number of moving parts can make programming rather daunting. Thus, the challenging aspect of baking a cake for many sports is how best to prepare athletes physically, using intelligent programming and rapid adjustment in line with forever-changing circumstances.

Switching analogies, and back to the programming puzzle. Where does one begin? Figure 1.5 illustrates the main considerations we need to make

before designing our HIIT sessions. Once we're clear of the importance of physical preparation for our sport (figure 1.4), we next need to look at:

1. the sport's physical demands,
2. athlete profile(s),
3. long-term adaptation targets, and
4. training periodization or how the training plan fluctuates daily, weekly, and season long, depending on our aims and the sport/event schedule.

All these factors merge to establish the desired physiological objectives of the HIIT session. Once we're clear on our physiological aims, which establish which of the five physiological targets we're aiming to hit (HIIT types), we can then appropriately choose from five broad HIIT formats (weapons) and their manipulations (figure 1.5), which we will expand on throughout part I of the book.

Consideration 1: Sport Demands

First and foremost, we need to understand the required systems to enhance relevant to the sport in question. What are the sport demands? How does meeting these demands enhance probability toward hitting our performance target?

Do we need a good level of aerobic power/endurance due to the duration of the activity? Does the sport involve high-intensity supramaximal anaerobic efforts? High-level strength? Speed? Repeated intermittent high-intensity efforts? Combinations of many of these features? Every sport is different, but we first

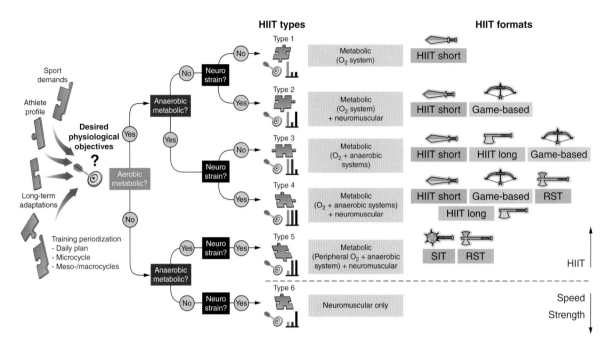

Figure 1.5 Factors to consider to appropriately choose an HIIT session type include the sport demands, the athletes the training is being applied to, the desired long-term adaptations, as well as the periodization aspects. Together, these determine the desired physiological response (aerobic metabolic, anaerobic metabolic, neuromuscular) to target. These six physiological response targets are divided into the following categories (used throughout): type 1, aerobic metabolic, with large demands placed on the oxygen (O_2) transport and utilization systems (cardiopulmonary system and oxidative muscle fibers); type 2, metabolic as type 1 but with a greater degree of neuromuscular strain; type 3, metabolic as type 1 with a large anaerobic glycolytic energy contribution but limited neuromuscular strain; type 4, metabolic as type 3 but a high neuromuscular strain; type 5, a session with limited aerobic response but with a large anaerobic glycolytic energy contribution and high neuromuscular strain; and type 6 (not considered HIIT) involving a high neuromuscular strain only, referring typically to speed and strength training. The HIIT formats (weapons) that can be selected to appropriately hit the HIIT target–type responses include short intervals, long intervals, repeated sprint training, sprint interval training, and game-based HIIT, described in detail in chapters 4 and 5.

Adapted from M. Buchheit and P.B. Laursen, "High-Intensity Interval Training, Solutions to the Programming Puzzle: Part I: Cardiopulmonary Emphasis," *Sports Medicine* 43, no. 5 (2013): 313-338.

must gain clarity around what it is we're trying to create in our athletes before we design the program. As one example, consider that an 800 m runner would likely favor a greater proportion of "anaerobic-based" HIIT compared to a marathon runner.

Making observations relative to how the ideal athlete looks from a physical standpoint, in addition to reading literature in the area, may be a prudent starting point.

Figure 1.6 shows the key sports described in our book and how the importance of the three main physical capacities (speed, strength, and endurance) may vary with respect to each other from sport to sport. Thus, HIIT type, volume, and programming should be made appropriately in line with its impor-

tance. HIIT in its various formats (figure 1.5), provides weapons we can use to hit the physiological targets of importance for each athlete and their sport (figure 1.6).

Consideration 2: Athlete Profiles

We humans are all unique. We all have our strengths and weaknesses. This makes us interesting. But this individuality creates an important consideration when we're trying to build performance, either for single sport performers or especially when we have a team of athletes. Each athlete we come across may require a different HIIT strategy to affect her individual physiology targets. While all players may be of the same age, playing on the same

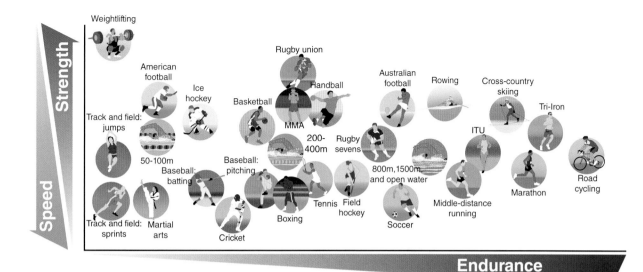

Figure 1.6 Various sports, their physical demands relative to needed speed, strength, and endurance.

Adapted from G.A. Nader, "Concurrent Strength and Endurance Training: From Molecules to Man," *Medicine & Science in Sports & Exercise* 38, no. 11 (2006): 1965-1970.

team, their physical capacities are notably dissimilar. As a result, the best HIIT type to select for each athlete would ideally be very different (figure 1.5). An added layer of complexity that practitioners must consider is that not only do differing athlete profiles create distinct individual needs but also that individual athletes encounter unique responses to the same HIIT format (11).

Considerations 3 and 4: Long-Term Adaptation Targets and Periodization

As mentioned, choosing the appropriate HIIT session to achieve the necessary physiological response for a given training cycle is no simple task, and some call this the art of good programming. This is ultimately what we hope you will learn most from this book. We want to teach the art and science of HIIT programming. Why should a short interval session go here, and repeated sprint training go there, and not the other way around? Where does strength training fit into the mix, and how does that impair or complement adjacent HIIT programming? What is the best way to shape the HIIT puzzle piece and its associated physiological response so that it appropriately fits into your weekly or monthly training block? Figure 1.7 provides an illustration of the concept from the world of elite football and road running using two different typical weekly patterns.

For both scenarios, the problems are clearly depicted. How do we best place HIIT across other important aspects of training throughout the week, such as endurance, strength, and speed sessions. How do we consider the impact of one session against the other, so that physiological outcomes of importance for our sport are maximized? Importantly, the physiological consequences from the appropriately selected HIIT session should provide the proper acute signaling response to elicit the optimal adaptations needed.

The general rules that guide HIIT selection for a given day/session include selecting:

1. the session's likely acute metabolic and neuromuscular response,

2. the associated cellular signaling that will target long-term adaptations,

3. the accumulated training load arising from other sessions that constrain/dictate the HIIT type,

4. the time needed to recover from the session (including the added HIIT sequence), and

5. its impact on the quality and ability to perform in subsequent sessions.

For these reasons, on a short-term basis, training periodization has a large impact on the HIIT prescription. Thus, many of the desired training adaptations are often considered as being training cycle

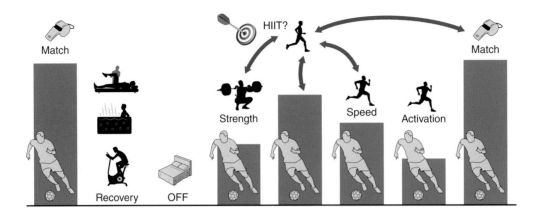

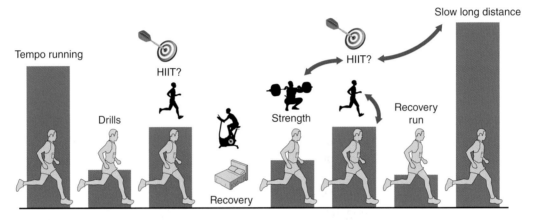

Figure 1.7 Two different typical weekly patterns (Team sports, with endurance, strength, and speed sessions on different days) and road running: day-to-day planning to shape the puzzle piece on a microcycle level, where the physiological objectives of the HIIT session must be considered in relation to the programming of other sessions. Vertical axis and blue shading illustrates the predicted training load (intensity×volume; see chapter 8).

dependent. To illustrate, within the team sport setting, generic aerobic power development might be emphasized in the initial phase of the preseason compared to more sport-specific and anaerobic-like HIIT sessions emphasized toward the start of the competitive season. Additionally, for athletes training twice a day, and/or in team sport players aiming to enhance metabolic and neuromuscular systems simultaneously, the physiological strain associated with a given HIIT session needs to be considered in relation to the demands of other physical and technical/tactical sessions so as to avoid overload and enable appropriate adaptation. Specifically here, our aim is to maximize a given training stimulus and minimize musculoskeletal injury risk. Thus, there are likely several approaches (i.e., HIIT formats) that, considered in isolation, will achieve a similar metabolic and/or neuromuscular training adaptation outcome. However, the ability of the coach and practitioner to

understand the isolated effects of various HIIT variables may assist with selection of the most appropriate HIIT session to apply to help solve the puzzle, at the right place and time.

Choosing the best solution to such a puzzle might be analogous to how an admiral goes about deciding which operation is best suited to take out a given military target, and we'll come back to this analogy throughout the text. While mass destruction weapons might hit all targets at once (e.g., training systematically very hard, "no pain, no gain approach," HIIT format type 4), collateral damage often occurs (analogous to added stress, extra fatigue, more injury/illness). Sometimes then, the best solution might involve specific "Navy SEAL–type" operations (John Rambo), for more specific targeting of the required physiological capacities, but with less risk of collateral damage. Along these lines, HIIT sessions should first be specific to the physiological adaptations desired (figure 1.5) and not necessarily compulsory to the sport itself.

Summary

High-intensity interval training is usually defined as exercise consisting of repeated bouts of high-intensity work performed above the lactate threshold (a perceived effort of "hard" or greater) or critical speed/power, interspersed by periods of low-intensity exercise or complete rest.

The five main HIIT formats tend to involve long intervals, short intervals, as well as repeated sprints of short and long durations, as well as game-based HIIT.

To use HIIT appropriately, practitioners should:

1. Understand the context, including the sport, individual athlete needs and unique responses, phase of the training cycle, and the possible interference effects.

2. Define the target (desired physiological response/adaptation and, in turn, one of the six target types).

3. Choose (one of the) appropriate HIIT formats (HIIT short intervals, HIIT long intervals, game-based HIIT, RST, and SIT).

4. Manipulate the HIIT variables to shape the piece (described in chapters 4 and 5).

5. Monitor the load (chapter 8) and its response (chapter 9).

From its early beginnings on the track at the start of the 19th century, HIIT has reached exponential growth in popularity in academic research, high-performance sport, and the health-and-fitness sector, where today it is now considered the highest interest topic (25). Notwithstanding its high importance, HIIT is one of a number of tools in the coach's and practitioner's toolbox that they can use to enhance physical performance. Understanding the sport demands, individual athlete profile, and periodization phase is needed before we put pen to paper and prescribe the session. Here, we begin our journey into HIIT by describing its traditional methods of programming (chapter 2), the underlying physiological targets it affects (chapter 3), the factors we can manipulate to form HIIT weapons (chapter 4), and how to fine-tune them (chapter 5). But we are not finished there, as other factors of the training program puzzle that complement HIIT must be considered. To this end, Dr. Jackson Fyfe will navigate us through the complexities of strength training (chapter 6) and Dr. Phillip Maffetone will ensure we understand HIIT's effect from a holistic health standpoint (chapter 7) before we outline methods we can use to program HIIT load (chapter 8) and monitor its response (chapter 9). Once the science is outlined, we'll pass the baton to practitioners embedded in 20 of the world's most popular sports, and learn how they effectively apply these concepts in their practices at the coalface of the world's leading sports. We hope you enjoy the journey of understanding HIIT and its application as much as we have.

Traditional Methods of HIIT Programming

• • • • • •

Martin Buchheit and Paul Laursen

Several approaches for prescribing high-intensity interval training (HIIT) have been developed, with the aim directed at ensuring athletes reach the required exercise intensity of their training sessions in a somewhat controlled and individualized way. While incremental laboratory-based test parameters may be the most accurate way to calibrate an HIIT session, a number of field-based maximal-critical speed and power analysis tools and methods may be more practical, objective, and effective for achieving the desired training and performance outcome. In this chapter, we describe the various traditional approaches used by coaches, scientists, and practitioners to calibrate interval training intensity. Procedures may include a rating of perceived exertion (RPE)-based prescription, the maximal aerobic speed and power-based method, the 30-15 intermittent fitness test, anaerobic speed reserve measures, all-out sprint training, the track-and-field or team sport approaches, and also heart rate and power meter-based approaches.

RPE-Based Prescription

Prescribing the intensity of an HIIT session using the RPE method (55) is highly attractive due to its simplicity. This method does not require the monitoring of heart rate, speed, or power. A coach can just instruct, "You're running 4×4 min hard, with 2 min walk recovery intervals." It's a versatile method that can be used anywhere. Coaches have used this method more than any other for the last century to prescribe independent variables such as the duration or distance of work and relief intervals (105). Importantly, the athlete can self-regulate his exercise intensity based on how the exercise feels, the athlete's brain being the best sensor globally of how in balance his body is (95). In the laboratory, the intensity selected is typically the maximal sustainable exercise intensity perceived as hard to very hard (i.e., ≥6 on a CR-10 Borg scale and ≥15 on a 6-20 scale) and is based on the athlete's experience in the session, the session goal, and external considerations related to training periodization. While the specific roles (or contributions) played by varying biological afferents and other neurocognitive processes involved with the selection of an exercise intensity based on effort are debated (see viewpoint/counterpoint (81)), RPE responses may reflect "a conscious sensation of how hard, heavy, and strenuous the exercise is" (82), relative to the combined physiological (44), biomechanical, and psychological (83) stress or fatigue imposed on the body during exercise (110).

In practice, the first benefit of RPE-guided HIIT sessions (105, 106) is that they do not require any knowledge of the athletes' fitness level, making them highly convenient to use. Test results are not required. Therefore the RPE method is considered a universal exercise regulator, irrespective of the exercise mode and variations in terrain and environmental conditions. Interestingly, the RPE-based prescription method has been shown to promote the same physiological outcomes as a heart rate–calibrated program over 6 wk in young women (41).

However, the method does not allow for the precise manipulation of the physiological response to a given HIIT session, which could limit the ability to target a specific adaptation. For example, Seiler and Sylta (107) compared the physiological and RPE responses in 63 well-trained cyclists performing three different maximal-effort HIIT sessions differing only in work bout and accumulated duration. Sessions were prescribed as 4×16 min, 4×8 min, or 4×4 min, all separated by 2 min recovery periods. Sessions (mean(SD)) were performed at 95(5), 106(5), and 117(6)% of 40 min time trial power during 4×16, 4×8, and 4×4 min sessions, respectively. Percent peak heart rate of the efforts were 89(2)%, 91(2)%, and 94(2)%, with blood lactate concentration at 4.7(1.6), 9.2(2.4), and 12.7(2.7) mM, respectively. While all sessions were instructed to be maximal efforts, RPE increased with lowered volumes of accumulated work duration and with higher intensity. This highlights a limitation of the RPE method, with the duration of the prescribed effort influencing the physiological outcome or effect. While the RPE method is popular and often used with objective monitoring, use of the RPE method solely without other markers of performance (i.e., speed, power) and its related physiological response (i.e., HR, lactate) can present a level of uncertainty within a coach's and practitioner's programming puzzle.

Maximal Aerobic Speed and Power

The speed and/or power associated with the body's maximal oxygen uptake ($\dot{V}O_2max$; so-called v/p$\dot{V}O_2$max or maximal aerobic speed/power [MAS/MAP] (8, 69)) has been shown to be a useful reference intensity for programming HIIT (6, 7, 76). To be clear, $\dot{V}O_2max$ is described as the greatest amount of oxygen that can be used at the cellular level for the entire body, and is related primarily to the ability of the heart and circulatory system to transport oxygen and the ability of body tissues to use it

(expanded on in chapter 3). It makes intuitive sense to be mindful of the performance level associated with this factor, as $\dot{V}O_2max$ has been consistently correlated with distance running (94) and cycling performance (63). The attractiveness of the v/p$\dot{V}O_2$max method is that it represents an integrated measure of both $\dot{V}O_2max$ and the energetic cost of running/cycling into a single factor, and might represent an athlete's peak locomotor ability (figures 2.1 and 2.2) (8). Since v/p$\dot{V}O_2$max is theoretically the lowest speed/power needed to elicit $\dot{V}O_2max$, it makes intuitive sense for this marker to represent an ideal reference for training (8, 76, 90).

The v/p$\dot{V}O_2$max can be determined, or estimated, using a number of different ways. Some of these include the following:

1. For running, the linear relationship between $\dot{V}O_2$ and running speed established at a submaximal speed (46) or the individual cost of running is used to calculate a theoretical running speed for a given $\dot{V}O_2max$, either with (53) or without (74) resting $\dot{V}O_2$ values.

2. Direct measurement (i.e., pulmonary gas exchange (9)) during ramp-like incremental running or cycling tests to exhaustion is used, either on a track or treadmill or by using an ergometer (78). On the track, the University of Montreal track test (UM-TT (79)) is the protocol most commonly used with team sport athletes (16, 56), although the Vam-Eval has also been used (40) and differs from the UM-TT in that it has smoother speed increments and shorter inter-cone distances. The Vam-Eval has received growing interest since it may be easier to administer in young populations and non-distance running specialists (25, 89). For cyclists, progressive tests to exhaustion on a cycle ergometer using fast ramp step increases (i.e., 30 W/min) that elicit $\dot{V}O_2max$ and its associated power output (78) can be used. Similar methods can be used for evaluation with other modes of exercise, including rowing (43) and cross-country skiing (114).

Since the true v/p$\dot{V}O_2$max during incremental tests requires $\dot{V}O_2$ measures to determine the lowest speed/power that elicits $\dot{V}O_2max$ (generally defined as a plateau in $\dot{V}O_2$ or an increase less than 2.1 mL·min^{-1}·kg^{-1} despite an increase in running speed of 1 km/h (9) or power output increase of 30 W (78)), the final (peak) incremental test speed/power reached at the end of these tests (V/P$_{IncTest}$)

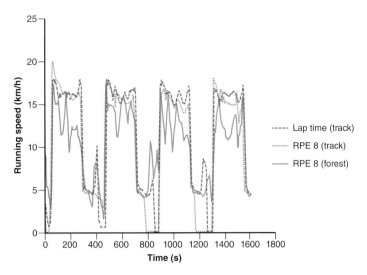

Figure 2.1 Running speed during long-interval HIIT with pace dictated through audio feedback (blue line), where beeps sound at appropriate time intervals to guide pace in a team sport athlete running at 95% of $V_{IncTest}$, or RPE on either a track (orange line) or in a forest (green line). Note that running at an RPE of 8 (10 pt scale) results in very similar speed patterns compared to using the more controlled audio feedback on the track. Interestingly, running speed shows large variations in relation to changes in running terrain in the forest, likely to be independent of metabolic strain (RPE 8). Thus, RPE can allow athletes to regulate running speed at the required level of exertion relative to more controlled means.

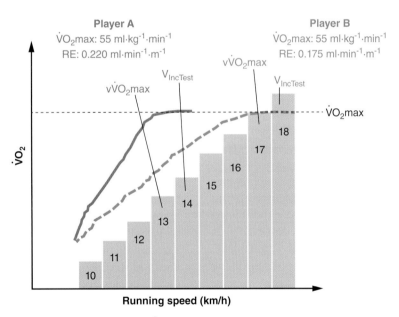

Figure 2.2 Time course of oxygen uptake ($\dot{V}O_2$) during an incremental test for two players with similar $\dot{V}O_2$max but with different running economy. Player A (blue) presents a poor economy, while player B (green) a very good running economy. The energetic cost of running being greater for player A, the velocity at which he reaches $\dot{V}O_2$max ($v\dot{V}O_2$max) and therefore the final velocity ($V_{IncTest}$) of the test are both substantially lower than for player B.

Adapted from M. Buchheit, "The 30-15 Intermittent Fitness Test: 10 Year Review," *Myorobie Journal* 1 (2010): 1-19.

is only an approximation of v/p$\dot{V}O_2$max. These two distinct speeds/powers are strongly correlated (r >0.90 (79)), but V/P$_{IncTest}$ can be 5% to 10% greater than v/p$\dot{V}O_2$max, with individuals possessing greater anaerobic reserves presenting generally a greater v/p$\dot{V}O_2$max – V/P$_{IncTest}$ difference (discussed subsequently).

Despite the subtleties, a number of indirect methods can be used to predict v/p$\dot{V}O_2$max that may be more practical for field testing, including:

1. Running: A 5 min exhaustive run (5), since the average time to exhaustion at v$\dot{V}O_2$max has been reported to range from 4 to 8 min (8, 70). The v$\dot{V}O_2$max calculated from this test has been shown to be largely correlated with the V$_{IncTest}$ reached in the UM-TT (r = 0.94) and on a ramp treadmill test (r = 0.97) (5), while being slightly (i.e., 1 km/h range) slower and faster than these velocities, respectively. However, the v$\dot{V}O_2$max estimated via the 5 min test may be influenced by pacing strategies and likely is most applicable to use with trained runners able to run at v$\dot{V}O_2$max for approximately 5 min. However, this 5 min test is used more in the research setting, and a comparable test in the field, as used with Australian rules football teams, might involve 2 km time trials (typically about 6 to 7 min) that are far easier to administer (see chapter 25).

2. Cycling: A 4 min all-out cycling power test in either the laboratory or in the field using a power meter, since the power output sustainable over 4 min, or the maximal mean power output (MMP), tends to be within close range of the p$\dot{V}O_2$max (99) (75, 77). Practically speaking for cycling coaches and practitioners, the simple process of monitoring cycling performance with a power meter and related software programs enables the detection of p$\dot{V}O_2$max or V/P$_{IncTest}$, simply called 4 min MMP, and is assessed either in the field or specifically using a power profile test (99) (see chapter 15).

3. Rowing: A 2 km rowing time trial (about 6 to 7 min) on a Concept II ergometer, which is also performance specific as most rowing events are determined over this competition distance (39) (see chapter 16).

Technically speaking, it's important to remember that V/P$_{IncTest}$ or v/p$\dot{V}O_2$max can be method (69) and protocol dependent (91). An estimated v$\dot{V}O_2$max (47, 53) has been shown to be lower than a measured v$\dot{V}O_2$max (9) and V/P$_{IncTest}$ (8, 62). Additionally, irrespective of the method used to determine v/p$\dot{V}O_2$max, protocols with longer stage durations tend to elicit lower speed/power values (91), while larger speed/power increments (resulting in shorter tests) may result in higher speed/power values, the anaerobic capacity of the individual being the confounding variable in the assessment. Similarly, v/p$\dot{V}O_2$max can be inversely related to the terrain or treadmill slope (98). Endurance-trained athletes are likely able to tolerate longer stages and, therefore, less likely to present impairments in v/p$\dot{V}O_2$max with variations in protocol (3).

Nevertheless, Manoel et al. (80) compared the effects of 4 wk of training prescribed using the time limit associated with either V$_{IncTest}$ or v$\dot{V}O_2$max in moderately trained endurance runners. The authors showed similar improvements in both groups, suggesting that use of V$_{IncTest}$ can be recommended in the field, as it can be easily self-administered on a treadmill. V$_{IncTest}$ can be determined in the field with the UM-TT (79) or the Vam-Eval (40), since, in addition to not requiring sophisticated apparatus (i.e., metabolic carts), the tests conform with the incremental rate of 0.5 km/h per minute recommended for accurate v$\dot{V}O_2$max determination (4) and account for the anaerobic contribution necessary to elicit $\dot{V}O_2$max.

Global positioning system (GPS) technology, though not without its limitations, is becoming more reliable and is certainly the most practical method for remote monitoring. As with cycling power meters, GPS systems can be integrated with online software platforms to enable seamless integration and calculation of V$_{IncTest}$ in the field. For cycling training prescription without access to sophisticated equipment such as metabolic carts, p$\dot{V}O_2$max and P$_{IncTest}$ may be most practically estimated in the field using a calibrated power meter to enable determination of 4 min MMP (99).

The reliability of v/p$\dot{V}O_2$max and V/P$_{IncTest}$ (as examined using coefficients of variation, CV) has been shown to be good: 3% for v$\dot{V}O_2$max in moderately trained middle- and long-distance runners (92); 3.5% for UM-TT V$_{IncTest}$ in moderately trained athletes (79); 3.5% (90% confidence limits: 3.0;4.1 (Buchheit, unpublished results)) for Vam-Eval V$_{IncTest}$ in 65 highly trained young football players; 2.5% and 3% for treadmill V$_{IncTest}$ in well-trained male distance (104) and recreational runners (62), respectively; 1%-2% for the 5 min test in a heterogeneous sporting population (45); and about 2% in well-trained cyclists (77).

However, it is worth noting that using v/pV̇O$_2$max or V/P$_{IncTest}$ as the reference running speed or power output is essentially suitable for long (2 to 6 min) intervals performed around v/pV̇O$_2$max (90% to 105%). For sub- and supramaximal training intensities, however, the importance of other physiological attributes should be considered. For instance, endurance capacity (the so-called anaerobic threshold, or capacity to sustain a given percentage of v/pV̇O$_2$max over time (11)) and anaerobic power/capacity (10) are likely to influence time to exhaustion, and in turn, the physiological responses.

Heart Rate-Based Prescription

Today the monitoring of an athlete's heart rate is probably the most commonly measured physiological marker used to control or measure exercise intensity in the field (19). Setting an exercise intensity using HR zones is well suited to prolonged and submaximal exercise bouts; however, its effectiveness for controlling or adjusting the intensity of an HIIT session may be limited. Indeed, HR alone cannot inform on the intensity of physical work performed above v/pV̇O$_2$max, which represents a large proportion of HIIT prescriptions (6, 7, 76). Additionally, while HR is expected to reach maximal values (>90%-95% HR$_{max}$) for exercise at or below v/pV̇O$_2$max, this is not always the case, especially for very short (<30 s) (92) and medium-long (i.e., 1-2 min) (106) intervals. This is related to the well-known HR lag at exercise onset, where HR is much slower to respond compared with the V̇O$_2$ response (figure 2.3) (42). Further, HR inertia at exercise cessation (i.e., HR recovery) can also be problematic for prescribing in this context, since this can create an overestimation of the actual work or physiological load that occurs during recovery periods (106). It has been shown that substantially different exercise sessions, as assessed by accumulated blood lactate levels during run-based HIIT (105) or by running speed during matches (SSG) (86), can have relatively similar overall average HR responses (figure 2.4). Thus, the temporal dissociation between HR, V̇O$_2$, blood lactate levels, and work output during HIIT limits our ability to accurately

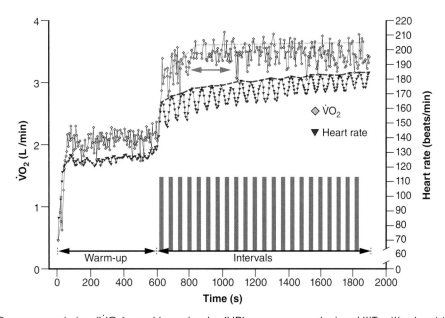

Figure 2.3 Oxygen uptake (V̇O$_2$) and heart rate (HR) responses during HIIT with short intervals (30 s at 105% vV̇O$_2$max interspersed with 30 s at 60%). Note the dissociation between V̇O$_2$ and HR responses at the start of the exercise, i.e., HR adapts much slower than V̇O$_2$, revealing its poor value to inform directly on metabolic demands.

Adapted by permission from A.W. Midgley, L.R. McNaughton, and S. Carroll, "Reproducibility of Time at or Near V̇O$_2$max during Intermittent Treadmill Running," *International Journal of Sports Medicine* 28 no. 1 (2007): 40-47. © Georg Thieme Verlag KG

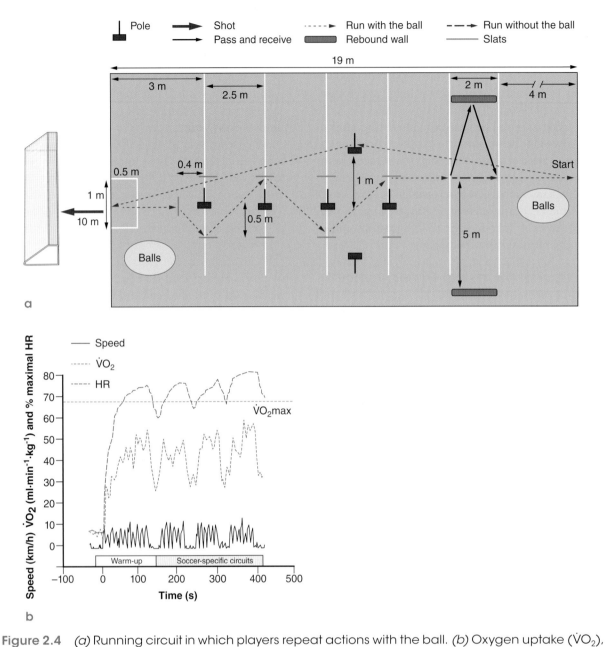

Figure 2.4 *(a)* Running circuit in which players repeat actions with the ball. *(b)* Oxygen uptake ($\dot{V}O_2$), heart rate (HR), and speed during the warm-up and the three exercise bouts in a representative player.

Adapted by permission from M. Buchheit, C. Manouvrier, J. Cassirame, and J.B. Morin, "Monitoring Locomotor Load in Soccer: Is Metabolic Power, Powerful?" *International Journal of Sports Medicine* 36 no. 14 (2015): 1149-1155.

estimate intensity during HIIT sessions using HR alone. Instead it should be used as one of a number of markers in assessment (see chapters 8 and 9). Further, it is difficult to imagine how an athlete would practically control or adjust exercise intensity *during* an interval, especially for athletes running at high speed, where viewing HR from a watch is difficult. To investigate this directly, Rabbini and Buchheit (100) compared HIIT prescription over 4 to 5 wk in two groups of young soccer

players, one using HR-based prescription (HIIT using 90%-95% HR_{max}) and the other using the speed reached at the end of the 30-15 intermittent fitness test (V_{IFT}) as the reference for running intensity (expanded on shortly). All tactical and technical training remained the same in both groups, and all HIIT sessions were completed twice per week, involving 3 sets of 3:30 duration. Results showed that using the V_{IFT} as a reference speed for HIIT programming produced greater high-intensity intermittent running performance improvements compared with HR-based methods. Thus, HR *monitoring* over prescription per se is what occurs in practical settings in most sports. For example, in endurance sports, a session might be prescribed as a level 5 (L5) workout (5-zone intensity model), and in either case, the athlete will know from experience to perform these sessions at the appropriate pace or power output (RPE method). In this case, HR is simply monitored to observe the response. Similarly in team sports, it is common to use HR responses to standardized HIIT (with individual target running distances prescribed) as monitoring points throughout the season (i.e., fitness testing without formal testing, per se) (30). For example, Buchheit et al. (30) used this strategy with an Australian rules football team during a 4 min 15″15″ HIIT session, revealing that fitness and the HR response to HIIT was maintained during their 2 wk Christmas break.

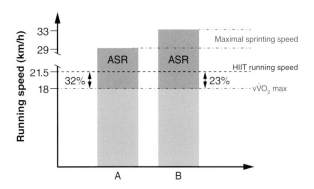

Figure 2.6 The anaerobic speed reserve (ASR) of two players having a similar $v\dot{V}O_2$max but different maximal sprinting speed. During an HIIT session, player B with the greater ASR will work at a lower percentage of his ASR and will therefore present a lower exercise load compared to player A.

Reprinted by permission of Springer Nature from M. Buchheit and P.B. Laursen, "High-Intensity Interval Training, Solutions to the Programming Puzzle: Part I: Cardiopulmonary Emphasis," *Sports Medicine* 43 no. 5 (2013): 313-338.

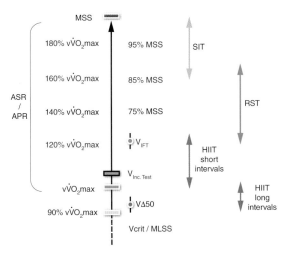

Figure 2.5 Intensity range used for the various HIIT formats. ASR: anaerobic speed reserve; APR: anaerobic power reserve; MLSS: maximal lactate steady state; MSS: maximal sprinting speed; RST: repeated-sprint training; SIT: sprint interval training; $\dot{V}O_2$max: maximal oxygen uptake; $v\dot{V}O_2$max: minimal running speed required to elicit $\dot{V}O_2$max, VΔ50: speed halfway between $v\dot{V}O_2$max and MLSS; Vcrit: critical velocity; V_{IFT}: peak speed reached at the end of the 30-15 intermittent fitness test; $V_{IncTest}$: peak incremental test speed.

Adapted by permission of Springer Nature from M. Buchheit and P.B. Laursen, "High-Intensity Interval Training, Solutions to the Programming Puzzle: Part I: Cardiopulmonary Emphasis," *Sports Medicine* 43 no. 5 (2013): 313-338.

Thus far we have been largely discussing HIIT programming methods that more or less apply to exercise performed above critical power but below $v/p\dot{V}O_2$max. The following sections highlight the different options available for the prescription of supramaximal training (i.e., training at intensities greater than $v/p\dot{V}O_2$max).

Anaerobic Speed Reserve

Anaerobic speed reserve (ASR) describes the exercise capacity between one's $v/p\dot{V}O_2$max and his maximal sprinting speed (MSS) or anaerobic peak power (i.e., MMP_{5s}; figure 2.5). Consideration for an individual's ASR is often not fully taken into account by coaches and scientists in their training prescription. While track-and-field (running) coaches have indirectly used this concept for years to set the work interval intensity (see chapter 13), its scientific basis and interest was brought forth only two decades ago, when Blondel and coworkers (10) showed that time to exhaustion at intensities above $v\dot{V}O_2$max were better related to the ASR and MSS than to $v\dot{V}O_2$max. Subsequently, research (35, 111, 112) showed using an empirical prediction model that the proportion of ASR used could determine performance during all-out efforts lasting between a few seconds and several minutes. While these studies have used continuous exercise, ASR

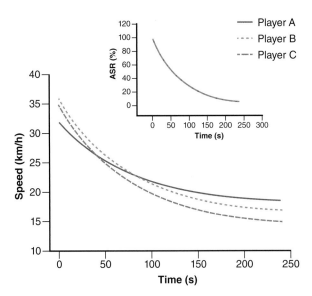

Figure 2.7 Predicted speed/duration relationship in three soccer players with different maximal sprinting (MSS) and aerobic (MAS) speeds and peak speed reached in the 30-15 intermittent fitness test (V_{IFT}). Player A: 32, 18, and 21 km/h for MSS, MAS, and V_{IFT}, respectively; player B: 36, 16, and 20.5 km/h; and player C: 35, 14, and 18.5 km/h.

Reprinted by permission of Springer Nature from M. Buchheit and P.B. Laursen, "Dr. Boullosa's Forgotten Pieces Don't Fit the Puzzle," *Sports Medicine* 44 no. 5 (2014): 1171-1175.

has only recently been considered in relation to high-intensity intermittent running (20, 24) and repeated-sprint performance (23, 26, 85, 109). In practice, two athletes can present with clearly different MSS ability, despite a similar $v\dot{V}O_2$max (figure 2.6 (17)). If during an HIIT session they exercise at a similar percentage of $v\dot{V}O_2$max, as is generally implemented in the field (e.g., Dupont et al. (57)), the exercise will actually involve a different proportion of their ASR (figure 2.7), which results in a different physiological demand, and in turn, a different exercise tolerance (17). Therefore, it appears that, in addition to $v\dot{V}O_2$max, the measurement of MSS and ASR should be considered for individualizing training intensity during supramaximal HIIT (i.e., figure 2.6) (10, 17).

A limited number of methods for determining MSS and peak power are known, but these methods are unlikely to produce differences as great as those seen with $v/p\dot{V}O_2$max or $V/P_{IncTest}$ measurement (21). For MSS determination, the use of a flying 10 (27) or 20 m (12, 96) time is probably the most common

method of determination, although peak instantaneous speed can also be measured now with radar gun technology (73) or GPS (2). The difference between these methods is generally less than 2%, which is substantially lower than the possible 20% difference that can be observed for $v\dot{V}O_2$max or $V_{IncTest}$ determination (21). Moreover, the typical error of measurement for MSS (1%) is clearly lower than that of $V_{IncTest}$ (3.5%) (22). Taken together, this suggests that determination of ASR is less likely to be affected by variations in MSS compared to $v\dot{V}O_2$max and $V_{IncTest}$ estimation (21).

For peak cycling power, all-out cycling power output over 6 s can be reliably assessed in the laboratory (84), and in practice also can be carefully monitored in the field in cyclists using power meters (99). Doing so enables estimate of the anaerobic work capacity, or W'. The concept of W' is expanded on in chapter 4.

30-15 Intermittent Fitness Test (30-15 IFT) (https://30-15ift.com)

While using the ASR to individualize exercise intensity for supramaximal runs might represent an improvement over that of $v\dot{V}O_2$max or $V_{IncTest}$, it still does not capture the overall picture of the different physiological variables of importance during team- or racket-based specific HIIT sessions or middle-distance running (103). In many sports, HIIT is performed indoors and includes repeated very short work intervals (<45 s). This implies that, in addition to the proportion of the ASR used, the responses to these forms of HIIT appear related to an individual's metabolic inertia (e.g., $\dot{V}O_2$ kinetics) at the onset of each short interval, physiological recovery capacities during each rest interval, and change of direction ability since indoor HIIT is often performed using shuttles (16, 17). Programming HIIT without taking these variables into consideration may result in sessions with different aerobic and anaerobic/neuromuscular demands, which prevents the standardization of training load, and may limit the ability to target specific physiological/neuromuscular adaptations (16). To overcome the limitations inherent with the measurement of $v\dot{V}O_2$max and ASR, the 30-15 intermittent fitness test (30-15 IFT; figure 2.8) was developed for intermittent exercise and change of direction (COD)-based HIIT prescription (13, 16, 17).

THE 30-15 INTERMITTENT FITNESS TEST

Martin Buchheit

Everything started during the summer of 1999. As a strength and conditioning coach—and player—in a French handball team in Strasbourg (performing at the 4th French level), I was at this time using the University of Montreal track test (29) to evaluate the cardiovascular fitness of our players, and using the final velocity attained in this test (V_{UMTT}) to individualize running distances during interval training sessions (3, 24). For long intervals, this worked fine. Each player could cover a known distance based on their own capacity. This saw us performing well at 85%-90% of V_{UMTT} for 10–12 or even 15 min. However, later during the preparatory phase, when we started to work at higher intensities indoors (i.e., shuttle runs at intensity above V_{UMTT}), things became more complex. Some players were struggling, while for others the work was easy. That surprised me, since I was still individualizing running distance based on a player's physiological capacity (i.e., 120% of V_{UMTT}).

Across the team, players had different athletic and anthropometric profiles: some were tall, some were short, some were quick, and some were slow. This made me realize that the players' responses to HIIT with changes of direction (COD) were clearly related to many factors other than those evaluated with the UMTT track test (e.g., COD ability, inter-effort recovery abilities, anaerobic capacity, and speed). A new field test was clearly needed—one that could assess, in addition to maximal cardiorespiratory fitness, these additional factors. The idea of an intermittent incremental field test that included COD, taxing as well the anaerobic glycolytic system, and allowing higher maximal running speeds than the usual protocols, was conceived.

It took me more than a year of reading, attending talks, and experimenting with trials before the actual 30-15 IFT protocol was finished (7). Across different surfaces and in different venues, I have personally trialed more than 30 different versions of the test, based on different increments, stage durations, recovery periods, etc. Eventually, the 30-15 IFT was "born" in July 2000, using the following formula:

> Repeated 40 m shuttle runs over 30 s, interspersed with 15 s of active (walking) recovery, with speed increments of 0.5 km/h per stage.

Today, the test is used all over the world in almost every possible sport. Due to the daily requests received from users running the test in their setting, I produced an app that anyone can use in their own setting. The 30-15 IFT App was released in August 2018 and received more than 2000 downloads in its first week. This continued high interest in the test from practitioners all around the world is the most rewarding gift I could have ever dreamed of 18 years ago.

The 30-15 IFT was designed to elicit maximal HR and $\dot{V}O_2$, but additionally provide measures of ASR, inter-effort recovery capacity, acceleration, deceleration, and COD abilities (15, 16, 32). The final speed reached during the test, V_{IFT}, is therefore a product of those abilities. In other words, the 30-15 IFT is highly specific, not to a sport, but to the training sessions commonly performed in intermittent sports (17). While the peak speeds reached in the different Yo-Yo tests (1) (e.g., vYo-YoIR1 for the Yo-Yo intermittent recovery level) (1) have similar physiological requirements, only the V_{IFT} can be used accurately for training prescription. For instance, vYo-YoIR1 cannot be directly used for

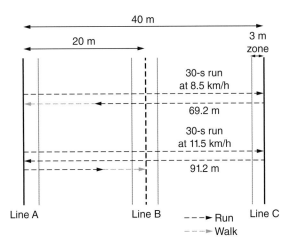

Figure 2.8 Area prepared for the 30-15 IFT and example of two intermittent runs. For the run at 8.5 km/h (about 69.2 m in 30 s), subjects start at line A, run to line C crossing line B and then return. After crossing line B again, they stop after 8.5 m and walk to line A during the 15 s recovery to be ready for the next stage. For the run at 11.5 km/h (about 91.2 m in 30 s), subjects start at line A, make one complete round trip, and stop after 9.5 m when going toward line B, then walk to line B during the 15 s of recovery for the next start. Note that calculation of targeted distances takes into account the time needed for the direction changes (for more, see https://30-15ift.com).

Reprinted from M. Buchheit, "The 30-15 Intermittent Fitness Test: 10 Year Review," *Myorobie Journal* 1 (2010): 1-19.

training prescription since, in contrast to V_{IFT} (13), its relationship with $V_{IncTest}$ (and $v\dot{V}O_2$ max) is speed dependent (58). When running at vYo-YoIR1, slow and less-fit athletes use a greater proportion of their ASR, while fitter athletes run below their $v\dot{V}O_2$max (figure 2.9). Finally, V_{IFT} has been shown to be more accurate than $V_{IncTest}$ for individualizing HIIT with COD in well-trained team sport players (16), and its reliability is good, with the typical error of measurement (expressed as CV) shown to be 1.6% (95% CL, 1.4 to 1.8) (14). Also of note, since V_{IFT} is 2 to 5 km/h (15%-25%) faster than $v\dot{V}O_2$max or $V_{IncTest}$ (13, 17, 32), it is necessary to adjust the percentage of V_{IFT} used when programming. While HIIT is generally performed around $v\dot{V}O_2$max (i.e., 100%-120% (6, 7)), V_{IFT} constitutes the upper limit for these exercises (i.e., 100% except for very short intervals and all-out repeated-sprint training). Thus, the 30-15 IFT permits improved precision of programming by individualizing the intensity and duration of the prescribed interval bouts around

intensities ranging from 85% to 105% of V_{IFT} (28, 31, 33, 51, 93).

To offer a real-life example, if we had a player with a V_{IFT} of 19 km/h performing a 15 s/15 s HIIT run at 95% of V_{IFT} (rest interval: passive), his target distance would be $(19/3.6) \times 0.95 \times 15 = 75$ m (19 is divided by 3.6 to convert km/h to m/s, for convenience) (18). When it comes to implementing HIIT in the field using targeted shuttle run distances, in addition to the fraction of V_{IFT} used, additional time needed to implement changes of direction must also be considered to equalize to the straight-line run cardiorespiratory load equivalent. Indeed, adding CODs over the same shuttle distances and durations have been shown to substantially increase relative exercise intensity (52) (more related to the number of CODs and its effect on running speed) (29). Thus, the COD correction factor can vary between 3% and 30%. While robust scientific evidence may be lacking, in practice a player's height and training volume can be considered for individual adjustments, with smaller and more-trained athletes typically presenting better COD ability (29), thereby requiring a lower correction factor. Presently the correction factor lacks direct individualization and is based more on a player's average profile. As the adjusted difference is typically not greater than 1 to 2 m, the shuttle distance can be modified a posteriori, as needed, so splitting hairs worrying about precision here is not required. Figure 2.10 shows normal values for the 30-15 IFT test across various sports and playing standards (for more, see https://30-15ift.com).

All-Out Sprint Training

Repeated all-out sprinting efforts or repeated sprint training (RST; figure 2.11) are exactly that—all-out sprints performed over a given distance or duration (61, 72). In practical terms, such sessions can be divided into either short (3-10 s; RST) or long (30-45 s; sprints) duration sprints, the latter termed sprint interval training (SIT). Since such exercise is consistently performed all-out, it can be prescribed without the need to pretest the individual (i.e., $v/p\dot{V}O_2$max is not specifically needed to calibrate the intensity).

We described the cardiorespiratory and muscle oxygenation responses to all-out sprint interval training (26; figure 2.11). In this study, well-trained cyclists performed 6×30 s all-out cycling sprints, each separated by 2 min of passive recovery. Despite a 21% decline in power output, we showed a progressive increase in muscle O_2 extraction with each suc-

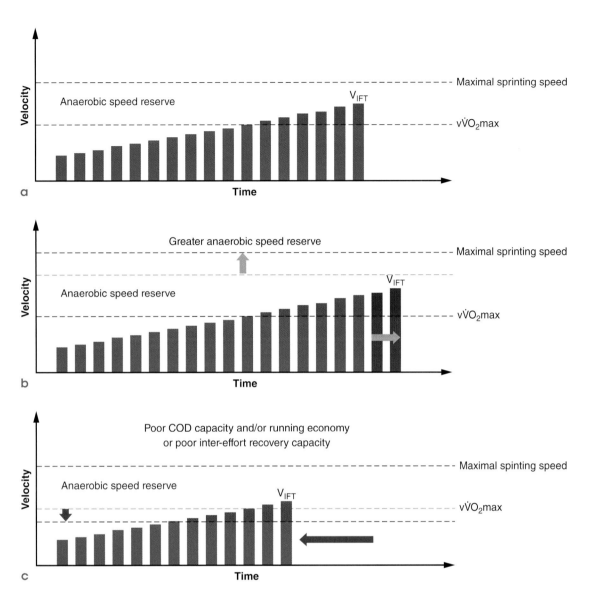

Figure 2.9 The importance of the anaerobic speed reserve (ASR) contribution toward reaching the final speed during the 30-15 intermittent fitness test (V_{IFT}). *(a)* Once the minimum speed required to elicit maximal oxygen uptake ($v\dot{V}O_2max$) is reached, the additional energy provided during the remaining stages is derived mostly from anaerobic sources. Therefore, for a given $v\dot{V}O_2max$, the greater maximal sprinting speed (MSS), and hence the ASR (or at least the greater the proportion used), the greater the number of supra-$v\dot{V}O_2max$ stages that will be completed and the faster the V_{IFT}. *(b)* This player has a greater ASR and is able to reach, for a similar $v\dot{V}O_2max$, two further stages during the 30-15 IFT (1 km/h). Since the ASR (or the proportion used) also influences what can be achieved during high-intensity intermittent runs, the use of the V_{IFT}, and not $v\dot{V}O_2max$, enables the programming of similar (anaerobic and neuromuscular) training loads in workouts for each player. *(c)* The importance of change of direction (COD) abilities and/or inter-effort recovery abilities on the V_{IFT} reached, since both directly influence the energetic cost of running during the test. As running economy determines the speed reached for a given $\dot{V}O_2max$ (and also ASR), a player with a poor COD will have a greater energetic cost of running and will present a lower $v\dot{V}O_2max$ and, therefore, a slower V_{IFT}. Similarly, poor inter-effort recovery ability will be associated with a steeper $\dot{V}O_2$/velocity relationship and/or premature muscular fatigue, resulting in slower running velocities. As for ASR, V_{IFT} takes into account COD and inter-effort recovery abilities and enables a more accurate tool to adjust training distances for these individual qualities.

Adapted from M. Buchheit, "The 30-15 Intermittent Fitness Test: 10 Year Review," *Myorobie Journal* 1 (2010): 1-19.

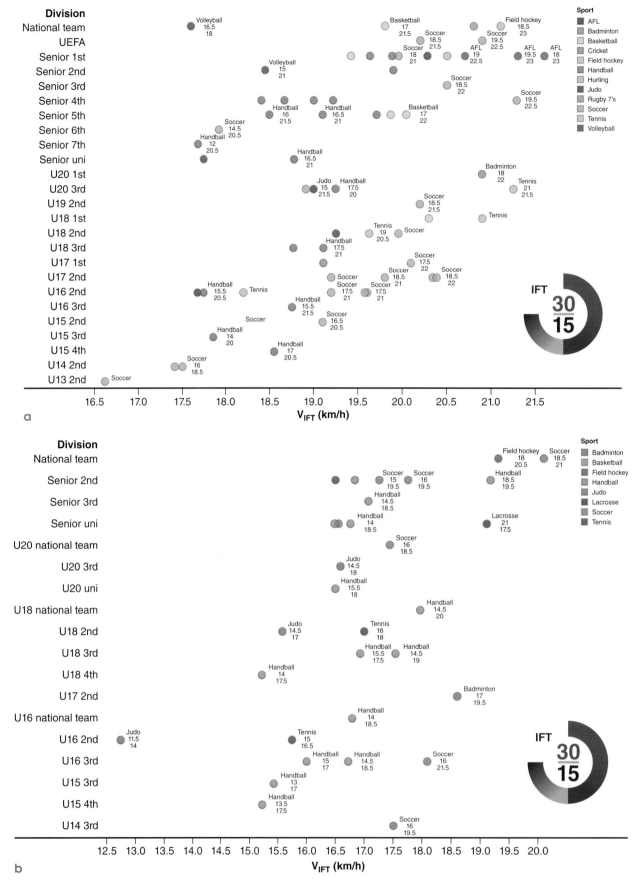

Figure 2.10 30-15 IFT performances across a selection of sports and playing standards for (a) men (n = 891) and (b) women (n = 542). Handball and soccer were chosen as the most complete samples, which were complemented with select group examples from different sports and standards. Contributions to the dataset provided by Cesar Meylan, Morgan Landrain, Daniel Peso, Alberto Pérez de Ciria, Andy Murray, Marcus Urban, Nick Poulos, Jack Nayler, Pat Sweeney, Shane Malone, Sebastian Knapić, Giacomo Schillaci, Antonio Dello Iacono, Simon Eustace, Heddy Arab, Thorsten Völler, Janeth Miranda, Francisco Javier Santos-Rosa Runao, Jamie Cook, Jaime Fernandez, Franck Kuhn, and David Hamilton.

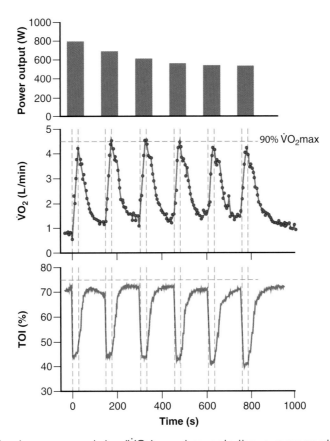

Figure 2.11 Power output, oxygen uptake ($\dot{V}O_2$), and muscle tissue oxygenation index (TOI) during a sprint interval training session (6×30 s all-out cycling sprints, 2 min passive recovery) completed by a well-trained cyclist. Note from this study that there was a progressive increase in muscle O_2 extraction with successive sprint repetitions, despite the decline in cycling power output, hence highlighting the increased reliance on aerobic metabolism as an interval training progresses in duration.

Data from M. Buchheit, C.R. Abbiss, J.J. Peiffer, and P.B. Laursen, "Performance and Physiological Responses During a Sprint Interval Training Session: Relationships With Muscle Oxygenation and Pulmonary Oxygen Uptake Kinetics," *European Journal of Applied Physiology* 112 no. 2 (2011): 767-779.

cessive sprint repetition (as shown by near-infrared spectroscopy), highlighting the progressive increase in aerobic energy system involvement that occurs as an all-out sprint interval training session progresses. This greater aerobic involvement drives fatigue-resistant adaptations that enhance subsequent all-out sprint performance.

Track-and-Field Approach

To program HIIT for endurance runners, coaches have traditionally used specific running speeds based on individual set times for distances ranging from 800 to 5000 m, but without using physiological markers such as heart rate, speeds associated with $\dot{V}O_2$max, or lactate turnpoints (7). Coaches and athletes have been, and still are, highly successful using this approach (see for example chapter 13). The attraction

of this method is that the entire locomotor profile (i.e., both maximal sprinting and aerobic speeds of the athlete) can be used to shape the HIIT session, so that each run can be performed in accordance with the athlete's (maximal) potential. While for short intervals (i.e., 10-60 s) the reference running time will be a percentage of the time measured over a maximal 100 to 400 m sprint, the speed maintained over 800-1500 m to 2000-3000 m can be used to calibrate longer intervals (e.g., 2-4 to 6-8 min). To illustrate this empirical programming approach, Pirie (97) provides session examples in athletes across different locomotor profiles for us. A sprinter capable of running 100 m inside 11 s might reasonably take 12 to 13 s for his 100 m training runs. A 400 m man under 50 s might cover 100 m in 14 to 15 s; the 800 m man under 1:53 and a 1500 m runner under 3:50 in 14 to 15 s; the longer-distance runner inside 14:30 or 10,000 m inside

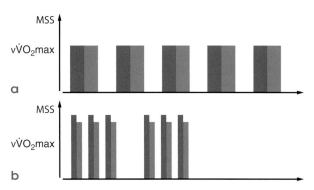

Figure 2.12 Running objectives during two track sessions for two athletes with different locomotor profiles. Runner A: $V_{IncTest}$ 21.5 km/h, MSS 33.5 km/h; runner B: $V_{IncTest}$ 21.5 km/h, MSS 29 km/h. (a) 12 × 400 m (only the first 5 repetitions are shown). As runs are performed around the $V_{IncTest}$, they perform the same work in 65 s. (b) 2 × 3 × 200 m. As runs are performed at a speed close to MSS, runner A (blue) performs these in 25 s, while runner B (green) performs these in 29 s.

31:00 in 16 to 17 s. For training at 200 m, the sprinter might run that distance in 25 to 26 s, the quarter miler in 28 to 30 s, 800 and 1500 m men in about 30 s, and long-distance runners in 33 to 34 s. The intervals between repetitions will, like those for the 100 m training, depend on the athlete's ability: if in the intermediate stage, 60 s; if a beginner, 75 s. After 3 or 4 mo, 40 repetitions should be reached (97). The disadvantage of this approach, however, is that it may be a bit harder for the coach to consciously manipulate the acute physiological load of the HIIT session and precisely target a specific adaptation (i.e., figure 2.12). Additionally, this approach tends to be reserved for highly experienced coaches and well-trained athletes, for whom target running times on several set distances are known. The translation and application of the track-and-field method to other sports is difficult. For example, how might a coach determine the expected 800 m run time for a 2.10 m tall basketball player who has never run more than 40 s continuously on a court before? Thus, using the track-and-field approach for nontrack-and-field athletes is unlikely to be appropriate, practical, or effective.

Game-Based HIIT or Small-Sided Games

Due to the technical and tactical requirements of team sports, and following the important principle of training specificity, game-based conditioning (i.e.,

so-called small-sided games, SSGs) (31, 37, 59, 73) or skill-based conditioning (60, 108) have received an exponential growth in interest (68). While understanding of the $\dot{V}O_2$ responses to game-based HIIT or SSG is limited (33, 37, 38), T (time) at $\dot{V}O_2$max during an SSG in national-level handball players was achieved for 70% of the session (i.e., 5:30 of the 8 min game) (33). Although the training effectiveness of such an approach has been shown (31, 49, 67, 73), SSGs have limitations that still support the use of less-specific (i.e., run-based) but more-controlled HIIT formats at certain times of the season or for specific player needs (figure 2.13). The acute physiological load of an SSG session can be manipulated by changing the technical rules (50), the number of players and pitch size (101), but the overall load cannot, by default, be precisely standardized. Within-player responses to SSGs are highly variable (poor reproducibility for blood lactate [coefficient of variation (CV): 15%-30%] and high-intensity running responses [CV: 30%-50%] (65, 66)), and the between-player variability in the (cardiovascular) responses is higher than more-specific run-based HIIT (68). During SSG in handball, average $\dot{V}O_2$ was shown to be inversely related to $\dot{V}O_2$max (33), suggesting a possible ceiling effect for $\dot{V}O_2$max development in fitter players. Additionally, reaching and maintaining an elevated cardiac filling pressure is believed to be necessary to improve maximal cardiac function (chapter 3) (48, 64). The repeated changes in movement patterns and the alternating work and rest periods during SSGs might therefore induce variations in muscular venous pump action, which can, in turn, limit the maintenance of a high stroke volume (SV) throughout the exercise and compromise long-term adaptations (71). Compared with generic run-based exercises, the $\dot{V}O_2$ to heart rate (HR) ratio, which can be used with caution as a surrogate of changes in SV during constant exercise when the arteriovenous O_2 difference is deemed constant (113), is also likely lower during SSGs (33, 37, 38). While this ratio is generally close to 1 during run-based long intervals (i.e., $\dot{V}O_2$ at 95% $\dot{V}O_2$max for HR at 95% of maximal HR_{max} (34, 102)), some have reported values at 79% $\dot{V}O_2$max and 92% HR_{max} during basketball drills (37) and at 52% $\dot{V}O_2$max and 72% HR_{max} during a 5-a-side indoor soccer game (38). This confirms the aforementioned possible limitations with respect to SV enlargement, and suggests that assessment of cardiopulmonary responses during SSGs (and competitive games) using HR may be misleading (87). Finally, the $\dot{V}O_2$

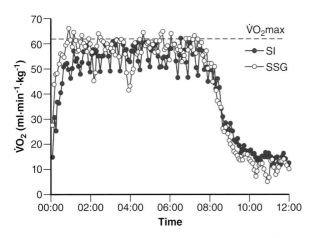

Figure 2.13 Example of the oxygen uptake ($\dot{V}O_2$) response obtained in the same player during an 8 min small-sided game (SSG) and a short-interval HIIT session (SI, 15 s at 95% of VIFT and 15 s passive). $\dot{V}O_2$max refers to the maximal oxygen uptake measured during an incremental test (31).

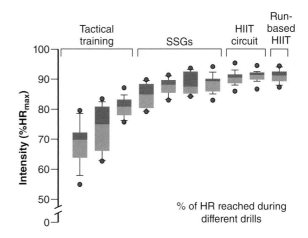

Figure 2.14 HR responses during tactical training, small-sided games (SSGs), circuit training and run-based HIIT.

Reprinted by permission of Springer Customer Service Centre GmbH from S.V. Hill-Haas, B. Dawson, F.M. Impellizzeri, and A.J. Coutts, "Physiology of Small-Sided Games Training in Football," *Sports Medicine* 41 no. 3 (2011): 199-220.

vs. speed (33) and HR vs. speed (87) relationships also tend to be higher during SSGs compared with generic running, possibly due to higher muscle mass involvement. While this method of training is often considered to be highly specific, this is not always the case, since during competitive games players often have more space to run and reach higher running speeds (up to 85%-90% of maximal sprinting speed (36, 54, 88)) for likely similar metabolic demands. Finally, there is a very important aspect of such sport-specific HIIT that should not be overlooked. That is, in contrast with run-based exercises, the likely greater occurring neuromuscular load due to the frequently repeated accelerations, decelerations, and changes of direction is very difficult to predict and needs to be accounted for in terms of neuromuscular load programing (chapter 3). Game-based HIIT and SSG intricacies are expanded on in chapters 4 and 5.

As shown nicely by Hill-Haas et al. (68), the heart rate responses to various football training activities, including SSGs, are shown in figure 2.14. Notwithstanding the limitations of inferring metabolic demands with HR measurement, SSGs achieve high workloads (near 90% HR$_{max}$), only slightly less than circuit and HIIT efforts. Thus, SSGs are an effective tool in the practitioner's programming puzzle toolbox, so long as their advantages and limitations are realized. The efficacy of SSGs may be revealed by

the fact that they tend to be used within nearly all team and racket sport practitioner application chapters in part II.

Summary

In summary, this chapter has highlighted the varying ways that HIIT is traditionally prescribed in practice by coaches to solve their performance puzzles. Using RPE-based prescription would be considered the universal HIIT practice, and is still used by most coaches today. Intervals calibrated with reference to the maximal aerobic speed and power are thought to be critical prescription components for many sports, and the upcoming chapter explains to us why that might be the case. Additionally, HR-based monitoring as opposed to prescription per se was shown to be the more efficacious method of use across HIIT. The somewhat forgotten anaerobic speed reserve, or upper capacity for high-intensity exercise above v/p$\dot{V}O_2$max, is an important factor to consider when calibrating supramaximal efforts, and the 30-15 intermittent fitness test was shown to be an effective means of measuring its capacity for appropriate HIIT prescription in team sports to target specific adaptations. Other methods of HIIT prescription that may be specific to the sport in general include the track-and-field approach and small-sided games for team sports.

Physiological Targets of HIIT

• • • • • •

Martin Buchheit and Paul Laursen

A well-known exercise training principle is that of progressive overload. The overload principle states that by working harder than is typically done in practice and creating stress, there will be a subsequent rebound adaptation in various physiological systems so that future stress is better tolerated (19). Thus, a general purpose of HIIT is to stress specific physiological systems used in sport to an equal or greater extent than that required during competition so that new levels of performance can be reached.

While a key focus of preparation for many sports must involve a high level of specific skill practice, the physical component of sport performance, such as that involved with completing a match, race, or competition, is often difficult to directly replicate day in and day out without running into major issues in preparation. As we alluded to in the opening chapter, replication of precise event stress at or above that which is occurring in an event or match is analogous to the mass destruction weapon approach, which in addition to being less specific to the adaptations required, also can run us toward problems that fall under the umbrella of overtraining, resulting in fatigue, injury, or some of the health aspects that will be emphasized in chapter 7. Thus, we need to go deeper into the science to help us solve our training program puzzle.

High-intensity interval training (HIIT) and its effects are complex. In general the scientific basis of HIIT is to produce a high-intensity overload stimulus that offers the best signal to enhance the physiological capacity of certain systems of importance for the performance target in question. The next logical step therefore is to break down the HIIT response into distinct physiological categories that can become targets for our programming. The purpose of this chapter, then, is to understand the general physiological targets of importance for exercise performance, alongside the varying acute responses and potential adaptations to various forms of HIIT.

General Physiological Responses to HIIT

It is commonly accepted that many of the biochemical and physiological adaptations that accompany training occur in response to an increase in target cell energy demands (43, 73). Any exercise training session will challenge, at different respective levels relative to the training content, both the metabolic and the neuromuscular/musculoskeletal systems (34, 163). The metabolic system refers to three distinct yet closely related integrated processes, including

1. the splitting of the stored phosphagens (ATP and PCr),

2. the nonaerobic breakdown of carbohydrate (anaerobic glycolytic energy production), and

3. the combustion of carbohydrates and fats in the presence of oxygen (oxidative metabolism, or aerobic system) (64).

It is therefore possible to precisely characterize the acute physiological responses of any HIIT session based on the respective contribution of these three metabolic processes and the neuromuscular load and musculoskeletal strain.

As will be outlined in detail in chapters 4 and 5, the intensity, duration, number, and series of work and rest intervals that form a given HIIT session can be altered to tax particular metabolic pathways within muscle cells, as well as neuromuscular features. HIIT provides the signal to enhance oxygen delivery to target cells (muscle and nerve cells) for aerobic respiration in addition to its effect on altering the oxidative and glycolytic function of muscle cells. A more effectual locomotor profile then arises from training adaptations at both the cellular and systemic levels.

In this chapter, we will outline the general physiological responses that occur with HIIT. For simplicity and practicality, we have reduced the number of systems of focus to three of key importance and made specific reference to the aerobic oxidative system, the anaerobic glycolytic system, and the neuromuscular system (figure 3.1). As shown in figure 3.1, the anatomy and physiology of the human body involves a number of key metabolic systems and structures of importance. Any of these areas may be of prominence for specific aspects of sport performance in question; however, the degree of involvement of these may depend on the associated sport's demands, the sport's weekly training pattern, or the individual athlete (chapter 1, figure 1.5). These important structures and systems, their function, and potential for adaptation will be elaborated on in this chapter.

Aerobic Oxidative System

Fundamentally, life, including sport performance, requires energy. Chemically speaking, this comes from the production and breakdown, or phosphorylation and rephosphorylation, of the energy molecule adenosine triphosphate (ATP). *Aerobic respiration* is the term we give to the generation of ATP via oxidative phosphorylation. As the name implies, oxidative phosphorylation requires large quantities of oxygen to nourish the cells of the body. Efficiency of this oxygen delivery is of particular importance to achieve peak-level exercise performance in most sports.

The cardiopulmonary system, made up of the lungs, heart, blood, and vessels, is the system that facilitates uptake of oxygen from the environment and its transport to the working cells of the body, primarily skeletal muscle, but additionally cardiac muscle and neural tissue, including the brain. Understanding the system and additionally methods of maximizing its function has been a focused research area for exercise physiologists over the last century.

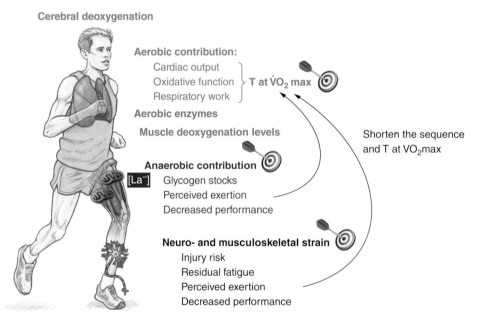

Figure 3.1 Key structural and metabolic targets of importance with HIIT, including the aerobic oxidative system, the anaerobic glycolytic system, and the neuromuscular system.

Integration of Maximal Cardio-pulmonary and Cellular Oxidative Function: Time at V̇O₂max

At first blush, the perspective taken when one views the aerobic energy system is that it is the system responsible for life activities at rest and during steady-state submaximal activities. While that is true, what is less appreciated may be its importance at high metabolic rates. At the upper end of the spectrum, elite endurance athletes, such as runners, cyclists, and cross-country skiers, report maximal oxygen uptake (V̇O₂max) values that range from 70 to 85 mL·kg⁻¹·min⁻¹ (96). Achieving high rates of aerobic function, in both slow- and fast-twitch motor units, is critical for achieving high rates of energy production without fatigue. Thus, locomotor performance associated with V̇O₂max, and the duration of training time amounted at V̇O₂max, may be important. Indeed, V̇O₂max might represent the integration of maximal cardiovascular and muscle metabolic (oxidative) function (26, 96).

HIIT protocols that elicit V̇O₂max, or at least a very high percentage of V̇O₂max, may provide the most effective stimulus for enhancing V̇O₂max. While evidence to justify the need to exercise at such an intensity remains unclear, it can be argued that only exercise intensities near V̇O₂max allow for both the large motor unit recruitment (i.e., type II muscle fibers) (2, 68) and attainment of near-maximal ventilatory rates (89) and cardiac output, which, in turn, jointly signal for oxidative muscle fiber adaptation (including respiratory muscle) and myocardium enlargement (113) (and hence, V̇O₂max). For an optimal stimulus (and forthcoming cardiovascular and peripheral adaptations), it is believed that athletes should spend at least several minutes per HIIT session in their red zone, which generally means attaining an intensity of greater than 90% of V̇O₂max (12, 103, 118, 119). Consequently, despite our limited understanding of the dose-response relationship between the training load and training-induced changes in physical capacities and performance (which generally shows large interindividual responses (21, 162)), there has been a growing interest from the sport science community to characterize training protocols that allow athletes to maintain the longest time above 90% V̇O₂max (T at V̇O₂max, see Midgley and McNaughton (117) for review).

Manipulating parameters to maximize T at V̇O₂max is complicated, and a more comprehensive analysis of the V̇O₂ responses to different forms of HIIT, from long intervals to SIT sessions through to short intervals and repeated-sprint sequences, will be the focus of chapter 5. Generally, both short (less than 60 s effort above v/pV̇O₂max) and long intervals (greater than 60 s effort at about v/pV̇O₂max) described in that chapter are effective methods of accumulating effective quantities (more than 10 min) of time at 90% to 95% V̇O₂max. While T at V̇O₂max may be an important marker to observe when attempting to maximize performance potential, other physiological factors in isolation should also be examined.

Respiratory Function During HIIT

In addition to T at V̇O₂max, other targets in the cardiopulmonary system should also be considered to fully characterize the training stimulus when programming HIIT. The lungs as an organ are generally considered to be overbuilt structures, and in the healthy condition will typically not pose any real limitation to oxygen delivery (49). However, it has been reported that up to 50% of elite endurance athletes display a desaturation of arterial oxygen saturation at high exercise intensities near V̇O₂max, a phenomenon known as exercise-induced arterial hypoxemia (EIH) (133). The mechanisms describing EIH are variable and include a number of relatively unalterable factors including a ventilation-perfusion mismatch, transit time diffusion limitation, pulmonary edema, and a relative hypoventilation (49). In fact, there is some evidence that EIH develops as a natural consequence of gains in V̇O₂max and endurance running ability following HIIT (122). Unfortunately, this occurrence, which may be due to a number of genetically derived factors creating individual differences in anatomy and physiology, is relatively unalterable. However, supplementation with blood buffers, such as sodium bicarbonate, may improve arterial saturation due to the Bohr effect and a right shift in the oxyhemoglobin desaturation curve (124). Furthermore, the occurrence of EIH in an athlete might also highlight an opportunity to attempt a legal blood volume enhancement strategy, such as using heat or altitude training (chapter 4). Thus, oxyhemoglobin saturation at V̇O₂max, alongside a hematological profile, can be measured in the elite endurance athlete to assess the potential for performance enhancement due to respiratory function limitations.

Cardiac Function During HIIT

A variable that is substantially more malleable, and the key facilitator of aerobic function, is the heart's cardiac output, or the volume of blood that the heart can pump over a given time period. Cardiac output is typically expressed in liters per minute and has been reported to be as high as 40 L/min in elite athletes (53). As most sporting events are prolonged and require repeated high-intensity movement, it's not surprising that this key oxygen delivery system is considered by most as a fundamental variable of importance related to sport performance (96).

As maximal heart rate tends to be more or less fixed in athletes, not varying by more than 1 or 2 beats per minute each year (109), the main variable that adapts and changes with training tends to be the heart's stroke volume, or the volume of blood pumped with each beat (96). Stroke volume can be improved via two means. The first is through an increase in left-ventricular contractile force, while the other is through an increase in cardiac filling pressure (113), which increases end diastolic volume and resultant stroke volume via Starling's law (142). Improved cardiac filling pressure occurs with exercise, but also when the blood or plasma volume of the cardiovascular system is increased, as is the case following either exercise training or heat exposure, in which dehydration causes the kidney to retain salt and water in the cardiovascular system in the presence of raised serum aldosterone levels (42). However, the key signal

for making the chronic adaptations necessary, and the one we will focus on here, is the heightened cardiac filling pressure attained with HIIT.

Since reaching and maintaining an elevated cardiac filling pressure is believed to be necessary for improving maximal cardiac function (41, 46, 79), training at the intensity associated with maximal stroke volume may be warranted (104). Defining the key intensity accompanying maximal stroke volume is difficult, however, since this requires the continuous monitoring of the variable during exercise (70, 104, 106, 121, 135). Whether stroke volume is maximal at v/p$\dot{V}O_2$max, or prior to its occurrence, is still debated (see figure 3.2) (44, 69, 166). Stroke volume behavior during exercise is likely protocol dependent (115) and affected by training status (166), although this is not always the case (44). Moreover, there is only limited data available on cardiac function during exercise that resembles field-based HIIT sessions (70, 106, 121, 135). Studies have shown that maximal stroke volume is reached within ≈1 min (see figure 3.3) (121), ≈2 min (56, 70, 106), and ≈4 min (135), before decreasing (56, 70, 121) or remaining stable (106, 135) prior to fatigue. Nevertheless, inconsistencies with exercise intensity, individual training background, and particular hemodynamic behaviors (e.g., presence of a heart

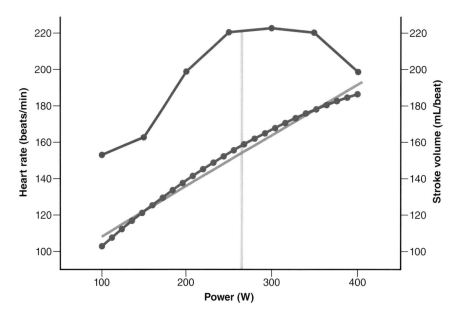

Figure 3.2 Time course of heart rate (HR; blue) and stroke volume (SV; red) during an incremental test in a subject presenting a typical break point in the HR-power curve. The orange line represents the HR responses if the relationship between HR and power output was linear.

Reprinted by permission from P.M. Lepretre, C. Foster, J.P. Koralsztein, and V.L. Billat, "Heart Rate Deflection Point as a Strategy to Defend Stroke Volume During Incremental Exercise," *Journal of Applied Physiology* 98 no. 5 (2005): 1660-1665.

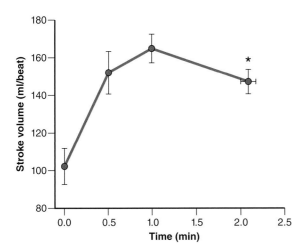

Figure 3.3 Stroke volume changes during constant load supramaximal cycling to exhaustion. Data are means +/– S.E.M. for 8 subjects; (*: p<0.05).

Reprinted by permission from S.P. Mortensen, R. Damsgaard, E.A. Dawson, N.H. Secher, and J. Gonzalez-Alonso, "Restrictions in Systemic and Locomotor Skeletal Muscle Perfusion, Oxygen Supply and VO2 During High-Intensity Whole-Body Exercise in Humans," *Journal of Physiology* 586 no. 10 (2008): 2621-2635.

rate deflection at high intensity (105)), as well as methodological considerations involved with measuring stroke volume, may contribute to these reported differences (44, 69, 166).

Based on the aforementioned studies measuring the time course of maximal stroke volume, it would appear, at least initially, that HIIT protocols involving long intervals (i.e., efforts greater than 60 s) should be applied in training when the goal is to enhance an athlete's maximal cardiac output (stroke volume). Based on this logic, short-interval HIIT (i.e., repeated 15 to 60 s bouts) would be assumed initially as a poor strategy unlikely to be effective for reaching maximal stroke volume and associated cardiac filling pressure, the short time course unable to trigger maximal stroke volume rates. Additionally, the alternating work and rest periods inherent with short-interval HIIT have been reported to induce variations in the action of the venous muscle pump, which may, in turn, limit the maintenance of a high stroke volume during the recovery period between intervals (84). Thus, logic to this point tells us that short-interval HIIT provides us with limited value if the goal of HIIT is to enhance maximal cardiac output. However, there are other aspects of HIIT sessions that we need to explore to confirm short-interval effectiveness, or lack thereof.

Particularly, we need to examine what happens to cardiac function during the rest or recovery periods

between HIIT bouts. In the 1970s, Cumming reported in fact that maximal stroke volume values were reached during the exercise *recovery* phase, and not during the exercise period itself, irrespective of the exercise intensity (45). While these results were measured during supine exercise in untrained patients, and despite contradictory claims (4), they contributed to the widespread belief that the repeated recovery periods and their associated high stroke volume accounted for the effectiveness of HIIT for improving cardiocirculatory function (59). In support of this, Takahashi et al. (157) found that stroke volume was 10% higher during the first 80 s of an active recovery (20% $\dot{V}O_2$max) following a preceding submaximal cycling bout (60% $\dot{V}O_2$max) in untrained males. Surprisingly, however, these hypothetical changes in stroke volume during recovery had never before been examined during typical HIIT sessions in athletes, and limited data is available examining the recovery intensity between HIIT work bouts.

To address some of these limitations, Buchheit, Racinais, and Girard (reported in Buchheit and Laursen (27)) measured hemodynamics during short-interval HIIT in a well-trained cyclist. Interestingly, their findings (figure 3.4) partly confirmed Cumming's results. Irrespective of the exercise chosen, i.e., incremental test, 3 min at p$\dot{V}O_2$max, or repeated 15 s sprints (30% of the anaerobic power reserve, APR), stroke volume in a well-trained cyclist (PPO = 450 W, $\dot{V}O_2$max = 69 mL·min^{-1}·kg^{-1}) showed its highest values consistently during the recovery periods in his natural upright position on the bike. While acknowledging the limitations inherent to the impedance method used (PhysioFlow, Manaetec, France (38, 136)), these data suggest that despite its supramaximal nature, HIIT sessions may elicit cardiovascular adaptations via activity occurring specifically during the recovery periods.

Another uncertainty challenging the programming thoughts of practitioners and scientists surrounds the recovery intensity between HIIT bouts and what is best to maximize stroke volume. Should recovery be active and, if so, how active? Should it be passive? To examine this, Stanley and Buchheit (154) again used the PhysioFlow device to measure the effect of the recovery interval intensity on maximal stroke volume during 3 × 3 min work periods at 90% p$\dot{V}O_2$max followed by 2 min recovery intervals at either 0%, 30%, or 60% p$\dot{V}O_2$max in well-trained cyclists. Interestingly, stroke volume was equal across the three recovery intensities, including a passive recovery trial (figure 3.5). This important

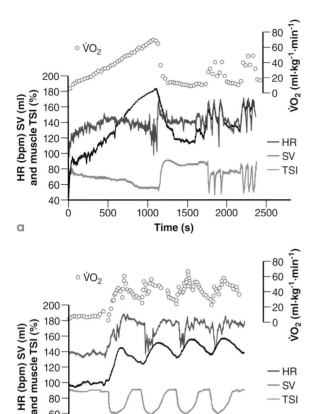

a

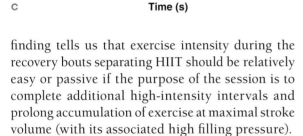

c

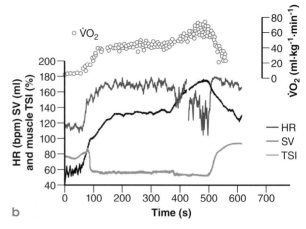

b

Figure 3.4 Oxygen uptake ($\dot{V}O_2$), heart rate (HR), stroke volume (SV), and muscle oxygenation (tissue saturation index, TSI) during an incremental test followed by (a) 2 sets of 3 supramaximal 15 s sprints (35% anaerobic power reserve, APR); (b) a 5 min bout at 50% of the power associated with $\dot{V}O_2$max (p$\dot{V}O_2$max) immediately followed by 3 min at p$\dot{V}O_2$max; and (c) the early phase of an HIIT session (i.e., first four exercise bouts (15 s at 35% APR/45 s passive) in a well-trained cyclist. Note the reductions in SV for intensities above 50% of $\dot{V}O_2$max during both the incremental and constant power tests. In contrast, maximal SV values are consistently observed during the post-exercise periods, either following incremental, maximal, or supramaximal exercises.

Reprinted by permission of Springer Nature from M. Buchheit and P.B. Laursen, "High-Intensity Interval Training, Solutions to the Programming Puzzle: Part I: Cardiopulmonary Emphasis," *Sports Medicine* 43, no. 5 (2013): 313-338.

finding tells us that exercise intensity during the recovery bouts separating HIIT should be relatively easy or passive if the purpose of the session is to complete additional high-intensity intervals and prolong accumulation of exercise at maximal stroke volume (with its associated high filling pressure).

The key takeaway messages from these data are that stroke volume can actually increase during the recovery bouts between HIIT work efforts, irrespective of the HIIT format (long or short), and the recovery intensity (degree of active versus passive recovery exercise) does not appear to add to the degree of maximal stroke volume attainment. As a result, recovery should be near passive to allow for work output during the HIIT effort phases to be maximized. To illustrate the effectiveness of short-interval HIIT for maximal stroke volume engagement, take for example an HIIT session involving 3 sets of 8 × 15 s sprint repetitions (30% of anaerobic power reserve, APR) interspaced with 45 s of passive recovery (long enough for peak stroke volume to be reached). Such a format would in theory allow an athlete to maintain his peak stroke volume for 24 × 20 s = 480 s, which is similar to the effort that

can be sustained during a constant-power exercise to exhaustion (106).

As a final note on the cardiovascular aspect of training, many authors, including yours truly (PL; (103)), have attempted to individualize and optimize between-work bout recovery duration using the return of HR to either a fixed value or percentage of its HR_max (1, 149). The present understanding of the determinants of HR recovery suggests, however, that this practice is not very relevant (145). During recovery, HR is neither related to systemic O_2 demand nor muscular energy turnover (32, 168) but rather to the magnitude of the central command and metaboreflex stimulations (142). That is, its response is complex and unlikely to be relevant within the context of achieving heightened levels of performance on subsequent HIIT work bouts. While it may be an important marker to monitor (chapters 8 and 9), its

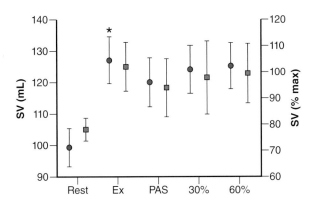

Figure 3.5 Stroke volume (SV) during different intensities during the HIIT session: preexercise rest (Rest), 3 min work periods at 90% pVO₂max (Ex), passive recovery (PAS), low-intensity recovery (30%), and moderate-intensity recovery (60%). Data are presented as mean (n = 14; red circles) and percentage of incremental test peak values (n = 5; blue squares). * indicates a small difference versus PAS. For clarity, the statistical symbols have been omitted for differences between rest and all other intensities as all differences are clear and large. Data, as a percentage of incremental test peaks, was provided to indicate the relative load and demonstrated similar trends to raw values.

Reprinted by permission from J. Stanley and M. Buchheit, "Moderate Recovery Unnecessary to Sustain High Stroke Volume During Interval Training: A Brief Report," *Journal of Sports Science and Medicine* 13 no. 2 (2014): 393-396.

use for optimizing recovery during an HIIT session is currently not relevant.

In summary, reaching and maintaining an elevated cardiac filling pressure via maximizing time at high stroke volume may be a key stimulus for improving maximal cardiac function, and this appears to occur during both long and short intervals. As between-bout recovery intensity appears to have little to no effect on cardiovascular responses, athletes should be encouraged to reduce recovery intensity, toward very easy work or passive rest, when the aim is to increase work intensity or work duration at high intensity through a greater number of HIIT repetitions. Based on the information presented to this point, prescribing a variety of HIIT types to gain the stroke volume adaptation advantages of each exercise format might be best practice. HIIT sessions including near-to-maximal long intervals with long recovery durations (e.g., 3 to 4 min intervals and greater than 2 min recovery) might allow athletes to reach a high stroke volume during the work and

relief intervals. Even longer 4 min intervals at about 90% to 95% v/pVO₂max are also very popular (78, 79, 90). Alternatively, repeated short supramaximal work intervals (e.g., 15 to 30 s) with long recovery periods (greater than 45 s) might also be effective for reaching high values both during exercise (58) and in recovery. However, whether maximal cardiac output adaptations also occur following long- and short-interval sessions (i.e., continuous versus intermittent), or whether achieving a certain quantity of time at maximal cardiac output (T at Qcmax) is needed to maximize its adaptation, is still unknown. In the only longitudinal study we are aware of comparing the effect of short versus long HIIT on maximal cardiovascular function (79), there was a *small* trend for greater improvement in maximal cardiac output for the long-interval protocol (ES = +1 versus +0.7 for 4 × 4 min versus 15/15, respectively). Nevertheless, when the aim of the HIIT session is to maximize cardiac function, data to date suggests that prescribing a variety of short- and long-HIIT formats may fall under the category of best practice in most sports where this physiological component is important.

Muscle and Cerebral Oxygenation During HIIT

The repeated fluctuation of O₂ concentration in working muscle and brain during exercise training is likely to be one of a number of critical signals responsible for the improved muscular oxidative capacities and performance improvement shown following training (47, 48, 87). Such low levels of oxygenation during training are known to promote an improved energy state in working muscle, as indicated by a more-protected high-energy phosphate potential. By way of illustration, when Kilding and colleagues supplemented athletes with oxygen, so that they had likely improved tissue oxygenation during an HIIT session, it resulted in a *lowered* effect on improvements in physiological variables and subsequent performance compared with normoxic HIIT (97). To be clear, the participants improved less with the supplemental oxygen treatment during HIIT, as it likely lowered the local deoxygenation on the tissues of importance (muscle and nerve tissue), resulting in a lowered signal or stimulus for aerobic cellular adaptations (see below).

Strenuous and prolonged exercise additionally challenges brain oxygenation, both in normoxic (139) and hypoxic (160) conditions. Brain oxygenation is decreased at exhaustion at sea level during maximal (139) and supramaximal (120% to 150% VO₂max

(147, 148)) work. Low levels of brain oxygenation can trigger central fatigue in hypoxic environments (120), and may (152) or may not (15) be associated with impaired high-intensity exercise performance (160). Thus, manipulation of muscle and/or cerebral oxygenation to low levels are likely important features to consider when programming HIIT. To be clear, ensuring athletes are familiar with low levels of cerebral deoxygenation during training might help in delaying central fatigue and exhaustion during competition. Put another way, athletes must be comfortable with being uncomfortable. Whether training is achieved in a normoxic or hypoxic (i.e., at altitude) environment is typically not obligatory, unless of course competition occurs in such an environment, which is an entirely different topic. What does appear to be important, however, is that athletes achieve a certain degree of cerebral deoxygenation challenge during training. (See also environmental hypoxia section in chapter 4.)

Muscle oxygenation changes during exercise are clearly affected by different HIIT variables. Muscle oxygenation, as measured by near-infrared spectroscopy (NIRS), reflects the balance between O_2 demand and delivery. Therefore, the greater the mismatch between O_2 demand and delivery, the greater the deoxygenation (74, 75). Whether muscle $\dot{V}O_2$ during exercise is more related to metabolic inertia or reduced muscle blood flow and O_2 delivery is still debated (36, 72, 95). It is evident, however, that muscle deoxygenation levels increase in parallel with increases in exercise intensity during incremental testing (9), although direct comparisons between exercises of different intensities are limited (6, 125, 146). The rate of deoxygenation is likely exercise intensity dependent, with higher exercise intensity eliciting faster deoxygenation levels (6), but contrasting results have also been reported (146). One clear effect of supramaximal (all-out) work performed during HIIT, repeated-sprint sequences (RSS), and sprint interval training (SIT) sessions is that it enables large levels of muscle (23, 25, 33) and cerebral (147, 148) desaturation to be reached. For example, the absolute muscle deoxygenation reported during a SIT session (including 30 s sprints) is profound (Δ tissue oxygenation index, TOI = −27%), and similar to values observed during interventions known to produce near-to-maximal muscle desaturation (i.e., maximal voluntary leg contractions (37) or post 2 min upper-body limb occlusion (98)). Indeed, muscle deoxygenation during SIT (~30 s all out) may be two-fold greater than during shorter

(i.e., 4 s,) repeated maximal running sprints (ΔTOI = −12% (23)).

For a given supramaximal work intensity (i.e., 120% of v/p$\dot{V}O_2$max), the longer the work interval, the greater the deoxygenation (39, 40, 158). However, close inspection of the data presented by Turner et al. (figure 3.6 (158)) suggests that, with a work:relief ratio of 1:2 (and a 20 W relief intensity), the magnitude of muscle deoxygenation does not increase further after 30 s of exercise (i.e., Δ deoxyhemoglobin ≈ 6, 28, 32, and 32 μM for 10, 30, 60, and 90 s efforts at 120% p$\dot{V}O_2$max). In the studies by Christmass and colleagues, higher deoxygenation levels were reached after 40 s, compared with 12 (39) or 26 s (40) of exercise, while a trend toward a plateauing in deoxyhemoglobin was evident during the latter portion of the 40 s analysis (40). Taken together, these results suggest that to reach maximal muscle (and probably cerebral) deoxygenation levels, all-out efforts lasting 30 to 40 s may be preferred. A long between-sprint recovery (i.e., 4 min), as generally implemented during typical SIT sessions (35, 88), is probably not required to repeatedly reach these levels of deoxygenation. When such efforts are interspersed with 2 min of passive rest (25, 31), a complete reoxygenation can occur and the magnitude of (at least muscle) deoxygenation has been shown to increase with sprint repetitions (30), likely related to greater energy requirements from fatigued muscles per unit of external work (8, 172). Finally, if we consider that repeated fluctuations of muscular deoxygenation levels during training sessions are likely key signals for improving muscular oxidative capacities (47, 48), and with greater exercise intensities eliciting the greatest deoxygenation levels, it seems prudent to recommend periods of high-amplitude HIIT to achieve the necessary training adaptations (i.e., HIIT including near-to-maximal effort intensity interspersed with passive rest).

In summary, the key HIIT targets to maximize oxygen delivery and uptake often involve strategies that prolong T at $\dot{V}O_2$max, lengthen time under high cardiac filling pressure and maximal stroke volume, as well as strategies that cause large fluctuations in muscle and/or cerebral oxygenation levels. In chapter 5, we will further explore how different HIIT parameters can be manipulated to emphasize these specific physiological HIIT target types.

Metabolic Systems in Skeletal Muscle

Like all cells in the body, muscle cells require energy to do their job. Sport performances often exemplify

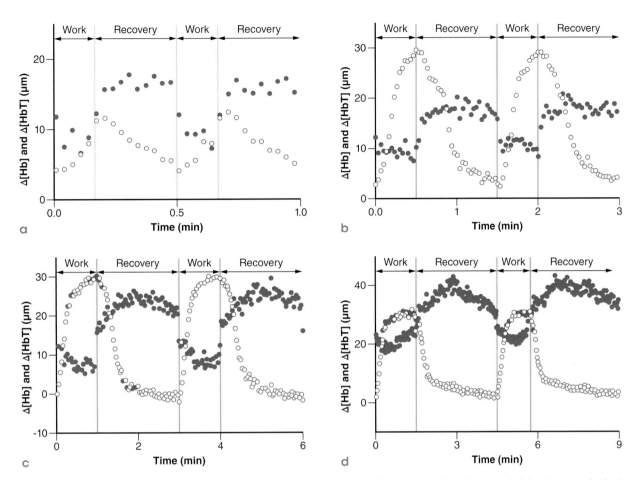

Figure 3.6 Representative responses in a single subject of deoxygenated hemoglobin (open circles) and total hemoglobin (filled circles) in the vastus lateralis muscle. Changes in hemoglobin and deoxygenated hemoglobin expressed as change from baseline to four intermittent exercises: *(a)* 10 s effort/20 s of rest; *(b)* 30 s/60 s; *(c)* 60 s/120 s; *(d)* 90 s/180 s. The exercise intensity was set at 120% of pVO₂ max for the four intermittent exercises.

Reprinted by permission from A.P. Turner, A.J. Cathcart, M.E. Parker, C. Butterworth, J. Wilson, and A.A. Ward, "Oxygen Uptake and Muscle Desaturation Kinetics during Intermittent Cycling," *Medicine & Science in Sports & Exercise* 38 no. 3 (2006): 492-503.

some of the highest rates of muscular metabolic energy transfer in modern life. The efficiency of energy production in skeletal muscle may be determined by an integration of the metabolic pathways supplying ATP (capacity of glycolytic and oxidative enzymes) and the excitation-contraction processes that utilize it (73). Following various forms of HIIT, both the oxidative enzyme pathways responsible for aerobic respiration, as well as the anaerobic glycolytic enzyme system important for generating ATP at rapid rates without oxygen, are typically upregulated (55, 76, 80, 107, 110, 130, 137, 167).

A well-functioning aerobic oxidative system, referring to the energy pathways involved with producing ATP aerobically in muscle, is often of great importance for sport performance. We just learned of the importance of oxygen delivery to cells via the

cardiopulmonary system for high-intensity exercise performance. Increased capillarization of those engaged muscle cells, a process termed *angiogenesis*, which increases the surface area of engagement between the cardiovascular system and the muscle cell, is also needed to facilitate efficient oxygen extraction (85). However, we have been more or less referring to these delivery systems in isolation, when in reality there must be a receiving end to that oxygen delivery, with fuel, predominantly glucose and fatty acids, able to be burned in those muscle cells in the presence of oxygen to generate energy for movement. The majority of this burning, or oxidation of fuel, happens specifically in the cell's mitochondria, via a number of metabolic pathways and enzyme reactions. Interestingly, current consensus holds that the functional condition and quantity of an organism's

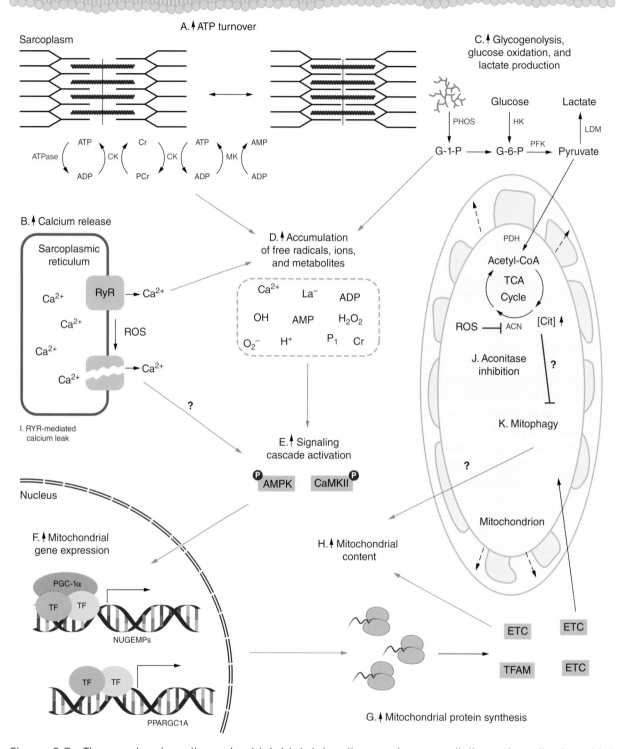

Figure 3.7 The mechanisms through which high-intensity exercise may elicit greater mitochondrial adaptations to aerobic training compared to lower intensities of exercise. Exercising at a higher intensity requires greater ATP turnover (A), increases calcium release (B), and involves greater use of carbohydrates for fuel (C), compared to exercising at a lower intensity. As a result, there is a greater accumulation of metabolites, ions, and free radicals (D), which increase the activation of signaling proteins (E), including Ca2+/calmodulin-dependent protein kinase II (CaMKII) and AMP-activated protein kinase (AMPK). The increased activity of these protein kinases causes greater rates of gene

mitochondria, the energy powerhouses of our body's cells, determines the health and longevity of a person (108), and may be one of many reasons to ensure that sport and/or exercise is part of a daily routine throughout the lifespan.

Figure 3.7, from MacInnis and Gibala (111), provides a schematic representation of a muscle cell and its key working parts impacted by HIIT, and provides an important foundation for the physiological HIIT targets that will be described throughout the book.

While figure 3.7 provides the microlevel perspective for the inner workings of a body's muscle cell when it receives the HIIT stimulus, figure 3.8 gives us a more macro whole-body perspective, and for this example, we present data from an elite Australian male road cyclist. During submaximal continuous exercise, there is a relatively stable and constant ATP turnover in the cell that is met by the oxygen source we've just described. Under this steady rate condition (i.e., 65% $\dot{V}O_2$max), there is a balanced level of carbohydrate and fat oxidation used to meet the ATP turnover needed. When higher energy demand is called on, as it is with high-intensity exercise, there are broadly two new conditions that can occur in the muscle based on the degree of intensity required by the nervous system. First, as intensity increases with continuous exercise, a point occurs above which the higher ATP turnover rate is usually met by a greater degree of carbohydrate over fat oxidation. This intensity is typically called the *aerobic threshold* and may represent the maximal rate of the body's fat oxidation. The first lactate threshold, or 1 mmol/L increase in blood lactate above baseline levels, or first *ventilatory threshold* (VT_1; first increase in minute ventilation relative to oxygen uptake), is the progressive exercise test marker of this point (figure 3.8; (123)). Second, under the con-

dition at which energy demand is greater than the ATP turnover that can be met aerobically with oxygen (i.e., critical speed/power intensity or anaerobic threshold; see chapter 4), the ATP turnover can be temporarily met via an increase in glycolytic rate without oxygen (anaerobic), with pyruvate accepting the protons needed to allow the chemical process to continue generating energy. Subsequently, lactate and hydrogen, or lactic acid, is formed and diffused into the bloodstream (figure 3.8). This maximal lactate steady state, or critical power, can also be seen as the point at which there is a substantial increase in the minute ventilation relative to the volume of carbon dioxide production (bicarbonate buffering of lactic acid).

Recall that above our critical power, VT_2 or maximal lactate steady state, is the exercise intensity that constitutes an HIIT session. Such high-intensity exercise induces a number of downstream actions in muscle cells as a consequence to the action that may be important to mention due to the adaptation signals they may induce. When a muscle's motor neuron initiates action to contract, the cell's sarcoplasmic reticulum increases calcium release in muscle to signal for the contraction process to occur, which causes actin-myosin filaments to move across one another and shorten (figure 3.7). When the energy demand across larger and larger motor units is initiated, as it is with various HIIT forms, and for longer durations, this demands a greater use of carbohydrates to be used as fuel compared to lower-intensity exercise. Thus, acutely, high-intensity exercise above critical speed/power, such as HIIT, specifically draws on greater rates of carbohydrate oxidation, predominantly from stored glycogen reserves. The high carbohydrate use with HIIT is important to appreciate, as with finite reserves of glycogen, HIIT programming

Figure 3.7 *(continued)*
expression for PGC-1α, which in turn acts as a transcriptional coactivator for nuclear genes encoding mitochondrial proteins (F). In turn, mitochondrial protein synthesis rates are greater for high-intensity exercise (G), leading to a greater increase in mitochondrial content (H) relative to exercise at a lower intensity. Two additional reactive oxygen species (ROS)-mediated mechanisms include fragmentation of the ryanodine receptor (RyR) of the sarcoplasmic reticulum and increased intracellular calcium concentrations (I), a signal for mitochondrial biogenesis. Inhibition of aconitase (J) in the tricarboxylic acid cycle (TCA) and an increase in intracellular citrate concentration has been suggested to increase mitochondrial content via a reduction in mitophagy with HIIT. ACN: aconitase; ATPase: adenosine triphosphatase; CK: creatine kinase; ETC: electron transport chain; PHOS: glycogen phosphorylase; HK: hexokinase; LDH: lactate dehydrogenase; MK: myosin kinase; PFK: phosphofructokinase; PDH: pyruvate dehydrogenase; TFAM: transcription factor A mitochondria.

Reprinted by permission from M.J. MacInnis and M.J. Gibala, "Physiological Adaptations to Interval Training and the Role of Exercise Intensity," *Journal of Physiology* 595 no. 9 (2017): 2915-2930.

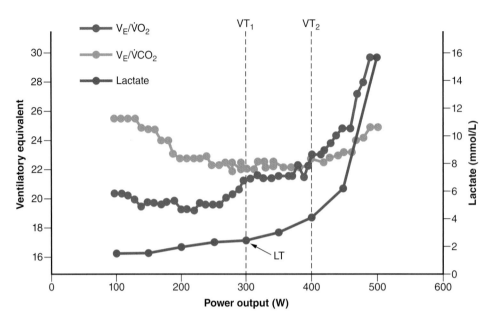

Figure 3.8 Various anaerobic threshold demarcation points during a progressive exercise test (100 W + 50 W/5 min) in an elite Australian cyclist ($\dot{V}O_2$max = 78.2 mL·kg^{-1}·min^{-1}). The first ventilatory threshold (VT$_1$) and lactate threshold (LT) occurred at 300 W, while the second ventilatory threshold (VT$_2$) and/or respiratory compensation point occurred at 400 W.

Adapted by permission from R.U. Newton, P.B. Laursen, and W. Young, "Clinical Exercise Testing and Assessment of Athletes," in *Olympic Textbook of Medicine in Sport,* edited by M.P. Schwellnus (Oxford, UK: Blackwell Publishing, 2008), 160-199.

needs to be appropriately managed with this in mind so as to solve the puzzle appropriately (see sections in chapters 1, 4, and 5).

In addition to the larger draw on energy reserves during high-intensity exercise, which lowers the ratio of ATP:ADP, metabolites, ions, and free radicals also accumulate in muscle. Together these acute demands increase the activation of signaling proteins, with the two most noteworthy including the kinases CaMKII and AMPK (111). The increased activity of these protein kinases causes far greater rates of gene expression from the so-called "master switch," the PGC-1α, which in turn acts as a transcriptional coactivator for nuclear genes encoding mitochondrial proteins (111). As a result, HIIT, in a variety of forms, has been shown to enhance mitochondrial protein synthesis rates, leading to a greater increase in mitochondrial content, fat oxidation rates, GLUT4 transporters, glycogen content, and oxidative fiber-type conversion (figure 3.9) (5, 102).

Indeed, the density of mitochondria in skeletal muscle may be the fundamental regulator of substrate metabolism during exercise, with increased mitochondrial content promoting a greater reliance on fat oxidation and a proportional decrease in carbohydrate oxidation (86). Following adaptation, compared to an equivalent bout of exercise done prior, glycogen degradation and lactate production at a given intensity will be reduced, with lactate threshold increased, thus allowing individuals to exercise for longer durations and at greater percentages of their $\dot{V}O_2$max (96). Practically speaking, exercise feels easier at the same work rate, amounting to less fatigue and faster recovery (161). As we described in chapter 1, practitioners must be mindful of the anaerobic training volume in their programs, due to its potential to create fatigue aspects that might carry over and interfere with subsequent training content (i.e., skill-based work or other high-intensity sessions, and potentially contributing to overtraining, chapter 7). Thus, training that emphasizes aerobic energy turnover, with limited anaerobic engagement, tends to be prioritized for most practitioners and coaches, whose aim is to instill a good level of fatigue resistance in their athletes. Generally, sessions with a large aerobic energy involvement and little neuromuscular stress elicit low overall fatigue, thereby permitting athletes to execute their tactical and skill-based training content appropriately. Aerobic-based metabolic sessions, in which the byproducts of energy production are for the most part simply CO_2 and water, should be emphasized

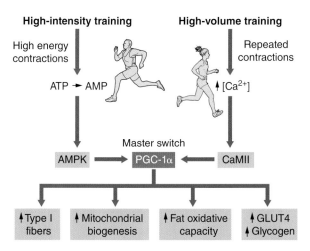

High-intensity training

High energy contractions

ATP → AMP

High-volume training

Repeated contractions

↑[Ca²⁺]

Master switch

AMPK → PGC-1α ← CaMII

↑Type I fibers   ↑Mitochondrial biogenesis   ↑Fat oxidative capacity   ↑GLUT4 ↑Glycogen

Figure 3.9 Simplified model of the adenosine monophosphate kinase (AMPK) and Ca²⁺ calmodulin-dependent protein kinase II signaling pathways, as well as their similar downstream target, the peroxisome proliferator-activated receptor-g coactivator-1α (PGC-1α). This "master switch" is thought to be involved in promoting the development of the aerobic muscle phenotype. High-intensity training appears more likely to signal via the AMPK pathway, while high-volume training appears more likely to operate through the CaMK pathway. Both signals, from a blend of distinct periods of high- and low-intensity exercise, may be important. ATP: adenosine triphosphate; AMP: adenosine monophosphate; GLUT4: glucose transporter 4; Ca²⁺: intramuscular calcium concentration.

Adapted by permission from P.B. Laursen, "Training for Intense Exercise Performance: High-Intensity or High-Volume Training?" *Scandinavian Journal of Medicine & Science in Sports* 20 Suppl 2 (2010): 1-10.

with a high level of implementation in nearly every sport's program (chapter 5; type 1, 2, 3, 4 targets).

Anaerobic Glycolytic System

While the cardiorespiratory and cellular aerobic oxidative systems, and to a lesser extent muscle deoxygenation, tend to be the main variables of interest of understanding HIIT format design, anaerobic glycolytic energy contribution (see (14, 34, 163)) is another important parameter to consider. Increases in ATP turnover rate via heightened rates of glycolytic capacity may facilitate important improvements in short-duration sport performance. Glycolytic enzyme activity, in particular that of lactate dehydrogenase, phosphofructokinase, and glycogen phosphorylase, has been shown to increase after both

short (less than 10 s) and long (greater than 10 s) duration sprint interval training (140), alongside improved physical work capacity (107, 110, 130, 137). While the plasticity or ability to change the capacity of the anaerobic energy system with HIIT appears less compared to the aerobic oxidative system, the anaerobic energy contribution to high-intensity exercise may change more due to the enhanced ability of the neuromuscular system to engage a greater number of larger motor units, including more fast-twitch muscle fibers (discussed subsequently).

While a noninvasive method of assessing anaerobic glycolytic energy contribution to high-intensity exercise has not been definitively established (116), the maximal accumulated oxygen deficit (MAOD) method (64) and muscle lactate concentration rate estimate (99) tend to be the preferred methods. The MAOD method, however, has a number of limitations (7, 12, 126) and such data have only been reported in a few HIIT-related studies (156, 163). Methods used to estimate MAOD are variable, but best practice is currently thought to involve using 10×4 min submaximal exercise bouts to establish the power output:$\dot{V}O_2$ relationship before solving for the y-intercept value based on the performance power output achieved using a sport-specific supramaximal exercise (figure 3.10) (126).

While the MAOD method has been referred to where possible, blood lactate accumulation can also be reported as a surrogate marker of anaerobic glycolytic capacity (28). The use of blood lactate concentration to assess anaerobic glycolytic energy contribution has a number of limitations, including large individual responses, prior nutritional substrate status (171), session timing in relation to prior exercise (92), timing of sampling post exercise (112), the effect of aerobic fitness (11), and its poor association with muscle lactate (93), especially following high-intensity intermittent exercise (99). Nevertheless, since all subjects would generally be expected to present with normal nutritional/substrate stores when involved in a study, the potential influence of these latter factors for the studies reviewed in our book is likely to be low. Therefore, with the aforementioned limitations in mind, we have used blood lactate changes during exercise to estimate anaerobic energy contribution for a given exercise (10). In an attempt to compare the anaerobic glycolytic energy contribution during different forms of HIIT, we will focus herein on post-HIIT values and on the initial rate of blood lactate accumulation in the first 5 min of exercise (134). This latter measure was selected

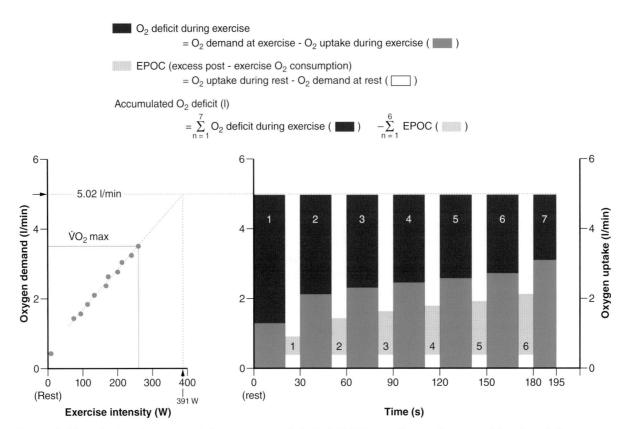

Figure 3.10 Maximal accumulated oxygen deficit (MAOD) method of anaerobic glycolytic energy measurement estimation. For the intermittent exercise, the oxygen demand was taken from the linear extrapolations of the oxygen demand versus power output relationship established during a pretest. The oxygen deficit during each bout of the exercise was taken as the difference between the oxygen demand and the oxygen uptake during the intermittent exercise. The excess post-exercise oxygen consumption (EPOC), which reflects a recovery of the body's oxygen stores and possibly some resynthesis of phosphocreatine during the rest periods, was calculated as the difference between measured oxygen uptake during the rest periods and the resting oxygen demand. The oxygen demand at rest between each bout of exercise was set equal to the resting oxygen uptake measured before the experiment. MAOD during exhaustive intermittent exercise was calculated to be the difference between the sum of the oxygen deficit during each bout of the intermittent exercises and the sum of the EPOC during the rest period between bouts of intermittent exercise.

Reprinted by permission from I. Tabata, K. Irisawa, M. Kouzaki, K. Nishimura, F. Ogita, and M. Miyachi, "Metabolic Profile of High Intensity Intermittent Exercises," *Medicine & Science in Sports & Exercise* 29 no. 3 (1997): 390-395.

due to the fact that blood lactate values collected after prolonged HIIT bouts do not permit discrimination between different HIIT sessions. For example, at exhaustion in any exercise bout, participants have already reached a plateau in their blood lactate accumulation (51, 52). The 5 min duration was chosen since it corresponds to the average time-to-exhaustion shown for continuous exercise at v$\dot{V}O_2$max (13, 82), is near the duration of long-interval bouts used with typical HIIT sessions, as well as being the duration of most RSS (chapters 4 and 5). Additionally, this duration approximates the time needed for blood

lactate levels to normalize as a function of the metabolic demand (10, 77). For reviewed studies in which blood lactate values were not provided ~5 min following exercise onset, the rate of blood lactate accumulation was linearly extrapolated to a predicted 5 min value using pre- and post- (immediate) exercise measures. (Only exercises lasting 2 to 6 min were included in this analysis.) Post-HIIT blood lactate values were categorized as very low (less than 3 mmol/L), low (3 to 6 mmol/L), moderate (greater than 6 mmol/L to 10 mmol/L), high (greater than 10 mmol/L to 14 mmol/L), and very high (greater than 14 mmol/L). HIIT sessions were also categorized based on the initial rate of blood lactate accumulation as follows:

strongly aerobic: less than 3 mmol·L·5 min^{-1};

aerobic: greater than 3 mmol·L·5 min^{-1};

mildly anaerobic: greater than 4 mmol·L·5 min^{-1};

anaerobic: greater than 5 mmol·L·5 min^{-1};

strongly anaerobic: greater than 6 mmol·L·5 min^{-1} (28).

Controlling the level of anaerobic glycolytic energy contribution during HIIT sessions is another important programming consideration we can use to optimize an athlete's preparation. There are likely two main scenarios to bear in mind when it comes to selecting the appropriate anaerobic contribution of an HIIT sequence: limiting or enhancing the anaerobic contribution, for various purposes. In the first scenario, such as during busy training schedules, when there is little time to recover between sessions (certain distance runners training twice a day, subsequently performing large volumes of HIIT, or in team sport players juggling field work, gym sessions, and matches), coaches may prefer a lower volume of lactic sessions to avoid overload, allowing players to be ready to perform during frequent competitions (100). In contrast, at some key moments during the team sport season, and for a number of sports in which a high glycolytic energy contribution and/or the ability to tolerate high levels of acidosis are required (e.g., track-and-field sprint athletes, some team sports), coaches may actually prefer to program these lactic sessions. As described by Iaia and Bangsbo (88), so-called *lactic training* is designed to stimulate the anaerobic glycolytic system and involves periods of exercise performed at intensities above v/pV̇O$_2$max. Lactic training may be further divided into a number of different formats, broadly defined as pure speed training, speed endurance training, or speed endurance maintenance training (88) (chapter 5; type 3, 4, 5 targets). Finally, the programming of HIIT with a high anaerobic contribution can also be viewed from the broader training perspective, where it's not the session response per se that matters most but rather its effect on glycogen stores and the subsequent training sequences that may occur. In fact, training low (169, 170) (i.e., when glycogen stores are low) is becoming more popular and has been shown to enhance aerobic adaptations in the muscle (mitochondrial biogenesis; figures 3.7 and 3.9) (94). While there are

many ways to induce glycogen depletion to allow athletes to train low, such as dietary manipulation and fasting (see chapters 4 and 7), using endurance training sessions (169) or more importantly, HIIT with high energy contributions, may be the more controllable options. The nuances of glycolytic energy contribution and adaptation following HIIT are complex, as a result of the various parameters that can be manipulated with HIIT, and these distinctions will be expanded on in chapter 4.

Neuromuscular System

Every movement made by athletes requires communication between the brain and the muscles. The neuromuscular system, which includes the muscles of the body and the nerves serving them, enables this coordination. The fundamental unit of the nervous system, the motor unit, includes the motor nerve and all of the fibers it innervates. The ratio of motor nerve to fiber number explains our fine versus gross motor movement (54).

When we refer to the musculoskeletal and neuromuscular load associated with HIIT, we mean the various physical stressors an athlete's anatomy encounters during a training session and the acute effects this has on both the neuromuscular and musculoskeletal systems. Such stresses could include, among others, the tension developed in locomotor muscles, tendons, joints, and bone; the muscle fiber recruitment and the associated changes in neuromuscular performance that may occur as a function of the potential neural adjustments; and changes in force-generating capacity that occur during training. Indeed, the high exercise intensities (i.e., ≥90% to 95% v/pV̇O$_2$max to 100% of maximal sprinting speed or power), the changes of directions for some types of HIIT performed in racket and team sports, and the large volumes (runners can cover 6 to 8 km at vV̇O$_2$max per session) of HIIT sessions lead naturally to high engagement of both neuromuscular and musculoskeletal systems. HIIT-induced neuromuscular fatigue is a critical component that can influence a multitude of other important training content, from the ability to complete in full or with high quality any number of training components that could be considered key in an athlete's preparation, including:

1. the HIIT session itself, which can subsequently reduce T at V̇O$_2$max and, in turn, limit the ability to reach the desired metabolic adaptations (see chapter 5),

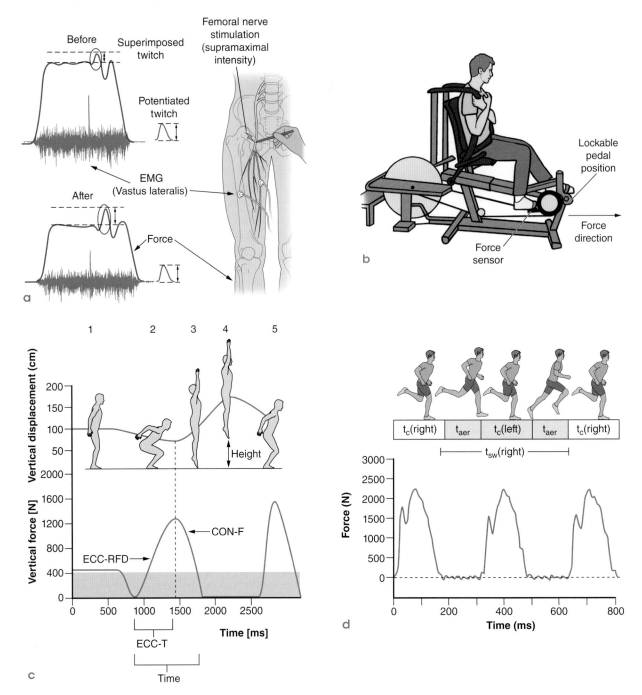

Figure 3.11 Tools used to measure the neuromuscular system response: (a) maximal voluntary contraction (MVC) on a classical leg-extension ergometer and the associated force and EMG responses, still considered the gold standard measurement of neuromuscular status, as additional neural stimulation allows the full characterization of muscle activation levels. This MVC was taken before and after a repeated-sprint cycling exercise (10×6 s with 30 s recovery). By comparing the twitch superimposed to an MVC and the twitch evoked on the relaxed muscle (i.e., femoral nerve supramaximal stimulation), the twitch interpolation technique in conjunction with surface EMG (i.e., root mean square [RMS] value normalized by the maximal muscle compound action potential [M-wave]) can noninvasively and reliably characterize muscle activation. Voluntary activation level (%) was estimated according to the following formula: (1 − [superimposed twitch/potentiated twitch] × 100). Note that both the voluntary activation level and the normalized RMS activity were depressed (−2.5% and −14.5%, respectively) compared with values obtained before exercise. (b) Innovative ergometer used to assess neuromuscular fatigue during cycling exercise (159). The pedal position is lockable and the transition from cycling to an isometric maximal voluntary contraction of the knee extensors at ~90 degree pedal position is lockable and the trans direction of applied force. (c) Countermovement jump (CMJ) and

2. a certain volume of low-intensity aerobic training due to HIIT-related locomotor fatigue (144), which would be expected to complement the overall training adaptations,

3. the execution of important skill training and associated learning (potential carryover effects from previous training sessions (19, 141)),

4. a resistance training session (chapter 6),

5. a carryover (20) or interference effect (60, 61), which can limit strength and explosive power development (chapter 6), and many other aspects related to injury risk, including traumatic-type injuries (127, 151) and overuse-type injuries both in runners (138) and team sport athletes (153).

The topic of interference is so important that we have an entire chapter devoted to it, written by a leader in the field, Dr. Jackson Fyfe (chapter 6), with specific reference to the complex integration of HIIT and resistance training.

In practice, coaches must choose between two main options: enhancing or limiting neuromuscular load during the HIIT sessions in their programs. At certain times they will seek to increase the neuromuscular characteristics of the HIIT sessions in an attempt to improve the athletes' locomotor function (i.e., running or movement economy) and, hypothetically, the fatigue resistance of the lower limbs (neuromuscular learning effect (20)). Many methods exist to stress the neuromuscular system specifically. Performing uphill HIIT sessions; climbing stairs in a stadium; running in the sand (12, 16, 62); introducing jumps, lunges, sit-ups; performing short shuttle runs or lateral running between work intervals (so-called Oregon circuits) (50); slowing cadence during cycling (131); adding eccentric cycling; and adding weights or bungees during rowing or kayak

training are all variations coaches have used to make gains and add stress to the neuromuscular system in varying sports. Nevertheless, neuromuscular strain, if maintained for several hours or days after the HIIT session, can have a direct effect on the quality of subsequent training sessions (both neuromuscular-oriented as strength or speed sessions), as well as lend to the possible interference phenomenon (60), or impact on technical and tactical sessions in team sports, not to mention the most important psychological component (see chapter 9).

In contrast to endurance athletes, team sport players generally tend to perform low-volume HIIT sessions with minimal acute neuromuscular strain or fatigue, so that athletes can gain freshness for upcoming tactical, strength, and speed sessions (24). In the final phase of team sport competition preparation, however, a high neuromuscular load during HIIT might also be needed in players to replicate specific game demands (81, 84). Finally, if we consider that a good athlete is first an injury-free healthy athlete, neuromuscular load also must be considered within the context of musculoskeletal pain and injury risk management. Running speed, time run at high intensity, as well as specific running patterns or ground surfaces, all known to influence the neuromuscular system, must also be considered when programming HIIT (28). HIIT type 2, 4, and 5 targets all involve neuromuscular engagement, and the refinements of the HIIT weapons to achieve these response types are elaborated on in chapter 5.

As we have just outlined, the impact that various forms of exercise training have on the neuromuscular system is important for a number of reasons. Despite the importance of controlling neuromuscular and musculoskeletal load during HIIT sessions, there has been limited data quantifying the effect of HIIT variable manipulation on neuromuscular

---

Figure 3.11 *(continued)*

associated force trace on a force plate that is used to calculate various indices such as fly time, peak power, velocity at takeoff, or rate of force development, all of which share various levels of association with neuromuscular fatigue (65). *(d)* Force trace during running, often used to assess stride parameters and leg stiffness, which is affected by neuromuscular fatigue.

Figure 3.11a: Reprinted by permission of Springer Nature from O. Girard, A. Mendez-Villanueva, and D. Bishop, "Repeated-Sprint Ability - Part I: Factors Contributing to Fatigue," *Sports Medicine* 41 no. 8 (2011): 673-694. Figure 3.11b: Adapted from R. Twomey, S.J. Aboodarda, R. Kruger, S.N. Culos-Reed, J. Temesi, and G.Y. Millet, "Neuromuscular Fatigue During Exercise: Methodological Considerations, Etiology and Potential Role in Chronic Fatigue," *Neurophysiologie Clinique/Clinical Neurophysiology* 47 no. 2 (2017): 95-110. (c) 2017 Elsevier Masson SAS. All rights reserved. Figure 3.11c: Adapted by permission from G. Laffaye, P.P. Wagner, and T.I.L. Tombleson, "Countermovement Jump Height: Gender and Sport-Specific Differences in the Force-Time Variables," *Journal of Strength and Conditioning Research* 28 no. 4 (2014): 1096-1105. Figure 3.11d: Reprinted by permission from P.G. Weyand, D.B. Sternlight, M.J. Bellizzi, and S. Wright, "Faster Top Running Speeds Are Achieved With Greater Ground Forces Not More Rapid Leg Movements," *Journal of Applied Physiology* 89 no. 5 (2000): 1991-1999.

function. Data on neural and muscular adjustments using force trace measures and motor nerve stimulation (101, 132, 150, 165) following high-intensity exercise suggests that fatigue induced by HIIT including either very short (less than 20 s) to short (≤1 min) or nonmaximal efforts (≤~120% vV̇O₂max) tends to be predominantly peripheral in origin (i.e., alterations to excitation-contraction coupling) (101, 132). In contrast, muscle fatigue during repeated long (i.e., ≥30 s) and all-out sprints may be more related to central mechanisms (57). However, few authors have investigated the neuromuscular responses to HIIT sessions using sport- and training-specific tasks, with maximal isometric voluntary contractions of the active musculature (i.e., maximal voluntary contractions, MVC) generally chosen as the laboratory-based task for assessment of neuromuscular changes (101, 132, 150, 165). This is problematic since (muscle) fatigue is task-specific (54). To partially overcome this task-related limitation (155), some researchers have developed a new ergocycle (figure 3.11b) that allows the measurement of maximal isometric force production during cycling-specific movements. In fact, in addition to the typical cycling mode, the pedals can be locked instantly in a fixed position, comparable to the standard position used during isometric evaluation. With this setup, participants' cycling can be brought to a complete stop within 1 s in the designated position for isometric evaluation. Isometric force can then be measured during voluntary and evoked contractions by a previously validated wireless pedal-force analysis system located between the pedal and the crank. For run-based sports, alternate and perhaps more-specific field-based measurements might include the assessment of changes in countermovement jump (CMJ) height and sprint speed (22, 128, 143), musculoskeletal stiffness regulation (50, 67), and stride parameters (66). While CMJ height reflects the efficiency of both muscle activation and muscle contractile properties (143), sprint speed can be a less-precise measurement of neuromuscular fatigue, as changes in inter- and intramuscular coordination factors, motor control, and/or stride parameters may limit the speed decrement during maximal sprints, so that fatigue appears to be less pronounced. For example, jump performance shows a much greater performance decrement (i.e., 3 times) than sprint performance during repeated sprint and jump sequences (29). This contrasts, however, with recent findings showing sprinting times and maximum theoretical horizontal velocity to be

more affected than CMJ performance following a fatiguing Rugby Sevens session (114). Differences may be related to the type of fatiguing exercise (repeated sprint and jump sequence versus full rugby session) and timing of the testing (during the sequence itself versus before and after a rugby session). Another limitation of these latter performance measures is that they are generally of maximal nature, while in practice HIIT with short and long intervals is often not performed at maximal intensity (i.e., less than maximal sprinting speed or peak power output; chapters 4 and 5). It is also worth noting that the acute effects of high-intensity running on leg muscle performance depend on the physiological characteristics and training history of the athlete (22, 71, 128). For example, while explosive athletes involved with speed events (i.e., track and field) or team sports generally show impairments in muscular performance following high-intensity exercises (63, 71, 128), endurance-trained athletes tend to show less impairment (71), no changes (63, 128), or even improvements (164) (possible postactivation potentiation (83)). During repeated-sprint exercises, similar findings have been reported, with endurance-trained athletes showing less fatigue than team sport athletes (18). Finally, with the exception of a very limited number of studies (17), post-exercise neuromuscular tests are generally performed either immediately after or 10 to 30 min following the HIIT sessions. Since residual fatigue is likely to be extended following such sessions, investigating the time course of muscular and neural responses to HIIT over a longer time course (i.e., hours/days (3, 91, 129)) is needed to assess potential carryover effects of HIIT on the subsequent training sessions (19). Figure 3.11 shows the tools used to measure the neuromuscular system response, including the MVC, cycling-MVC, CMJ, and stride parameters.

Summary

In summary, this chapter described the three key general physiological response targets involved with HIIT: the aerobic oxidative system, with particular reference to the delivery (cardiac output/stroke volume) and oxidative (mitochondrial) energy production components; the short-term anaerobic glycolytic energy system; and the various aspects affecting the neuromuscular and musculoskeletal systems. The next chapter details the intricacies of manipulating HIIT parameters and the ways these factors affect the acute physiological responses.

4

Manipulating HIIT Variables

• • • • • •

Martin Buchheit and Paul Laursen

This is a particularly important chapter in the book. Its contents may address questions that many students, coaches, scientists, and practitioners are likely to have. To introduce the content, we begin with our own personal stories of the journey we've taken to understanding high-intensity interval training (HIIT) variable manipulation. Ultimately, we probably have had many of the same questions about HIIT that you do. But we came at ours from somewhat different angles.

Paul Laursen's Experience

Following in my father's footsteps, I began running early as a child, which progressed into the sport of triathlon as the sport began to grow. I was good as an endurance athlete, but not the best. After an unsuccessful time trying to make a living from the sport of triathlon in my twenties, I developed a passion to try to understand endurance performance better. This was a selfish endeavor that stemmed directly from the frustration I felt with being unable to reach a certain standard in the sport.

When I began my doctoral studies in Australia at the beginning of the year 2000, there was a burning question I had at the time. If HIIT appeared so effective as a training strategy, what was the best type to use? Phrased another way, what was the best manipulation of exercise intensity, bout duration, and

recovery that elicits the most favorable adaptation and subsequent performance? How can you get the most bang for your buck out of a training session?

I personally found the related study by Dr. Nigel Stepto and colleagues (55) to be fascinating. In this study, the authors took 20 well-trained cyclists and divided them into five groups that performed vastly different interval sessions. While there were trends suggesting certain programs were better than others, what amazed me at the time was how nearly all programs were effective at least somehow at enhancing 40 km time trial performance, or related parameters, as well as the individual responses.

I distinctly recall asking for the thoughts of my PhD supervisor, Dr. David Jenkins. He replied, "Well, Paul, you know what they say, 'When it comes to training, there's more than one way to skin a cat.'" That was the first I'd ever heard the phrase, but it stuck with me, and I've since used it often. The old English proverb, "There's more than one way to skin a cat," meaning there's more than one way to do something, can sometimes be heard mentioned in the context of training chatter. As will be shown in this chapter, the number of moving parts within a high-intensity interval training (HIIT) session suggests this proverb well and truly does apply.

And that's when I began my own personal journey trying to examine the concept. For my PhD, I wanted to compare the effects of different forms of interval training on physiology and its subsequent performance response. Just like Stepto et al. (55) showed, I too found that there was indeed more than one way to skin a cat when it comes to HIIT and its associated physiological effects and performance outcomes (42).

How many ways you ask? We'll get to that. But before we do, we should hear from the man who has taught me much about skinning cats, Martin Buchheit. Around a similar time, Martin had related questions and was following his own journey toward discovering these.

Martin Buchheit's Experience

I was just 14 years old in the summer of September 1993 when I began my training in the Strasbourg talent center in the pursuit of becoming a professional handball player (which I never made). But I was highly motivated to train in the hopes of gaining fitness to make a good impression on the coach to be picked for the national junior handball team. At the time, I was used to spending my holidays in the French Alps, where my mother had a summer job.

In the Alps, I visited the guys at the local ski club. Given their good level of performance on the slopes, I expected their training to be well structured and that they might be eager to help me work on my leg strength in the gym. They allowed me to join their group of about 15 skiers, ranging in age from 12 to 18 yr. For my first strength session, I was able to lift about a third of what the others could squat, and they immediately started to take the piss out of me for wanting to become a pro handball player. I retorted enthusiastically, "I don't need the same quad strength as you guys, and I'll prove that to you tomorrow in the running session."

The next morning involved an HIIT session, consisting of 3 × 8 min blocks of 15 s/15 s runs over undulating rocky terrain. For me (and others) to better cope, they decided to drive the valley, so that the altitude wouldn't be an issue. This was a day I thought I might die. Even the 12-year-old girls outperformed me, and I felt like an idiot. I was destroyed. The skiers were flying, running everywhere, while I couldn't catch my breath. That was my first ever exposure to a 15 s/15 s short-interval session. From that day on, I knew I needed to understand better how the exercise format worked, and that I'd need to learn to train like these athletes in order to reach the professional standards needed for elite handball.

Fast forward to 1998 during my university studies, making my first steps into coaching, where I met Alain Quintallet, the strength and conditioning coach of the French national handball team, who shared my same interest in short HIIT. In fact, we had both independently come to appreciate through our own experimentation that prescribing short HIITs using only an exercise and rest interval duration (such as 15 s/15 s) resulted in highly variable exercise formats, and in turn, different physiological and performance responses. For example, in my 15 s/15 s short interval, I would advise my players to run 70 to 80 m over 40 m shuttles and have passive rest in between. Alain would have his players running straight lines outdoors more than 80 m, with an active jog in between repetitions. What option was best? Why would you use one over the other? Together, over many sleepless nights, we began experimenting and discussing the training intricacies of the different programming variables that we could use to better define HIIT formats, conceiving the best way to skin the cat. These dialogues led to the development of the 30-15 IFT in 2000 (12). From here, I met the great Veronique Billat at Evry University in the south of Paris. She indirectly introduced me to the Cosmed K4 device, which allowed me to gain great insight into the physiology of short intervals, such as the effect of varying exercise intensity and modality and the relevance of the 30-15 IFT (chapter 2).

How Many Ways Can You Skin a Cat?

From two different parts of the world, following two distinctly different failed pathways (both unable to reach the professional ranks in their respective sports), we both sought to answer similar questions. Whether it was how to train an elite cyclist on a bike, train a triathlete on the road, or to prepare a handball player to excel on the court, our goal was the same—what's the best way to skin the cat when it comes to training so that performance potential is maximized? Put another way, in the context of an athlete's training program puzzle, what's the best way to shape the puzzle piece—in terms of the HIIT duration, intensity, and format—to make it fit into the performance development puzzle, so that an athlete's future development and performance is optimized?

In 2007, we began our collaboration as young scientists at Edith Cowan University, in Perth, Australia, funded by the generous collaboration of our colleague, Professor Kazunori (Ken) Nosaka (figure 4.1). Over the subsequent decade, we worked on manipulating as many variables around HIIT as we could. Along with countless others who share our passion in this area, this chapter describes our interpretation of what we and others have found.

Manipulation of Interval Training Variables

Based on our stories, and as illustrated (figure 4.2), we feel there are 12 primary variables we can manipulate within a given HIIT session to skin the cat (11). The intensity and duration of work and relief intervals are the key influencing factors (4, 17). Then, the number of intervals, the number of series, and between-series recovery durations and intensities account for the total work performed. Exercise modality (i.e., running versus cycling or rowing, straight line versus uphill, change of direction running and ground surface) has to date received limited scientific interest, but it is clear that it represents a key variable to consider when programming HIIT, especially for team and racket sport athletes. Finally, both the environment (temperature, humidity, and partial pressure of oxygen) and nutritional factors are additional aspects that

can be manipulated to affect the acute physiological response. The manipulation of each variable in isolation likely has a direct impact on the metabolic, cardiopulmonary, and neuromuscular responses (chapter 3). When more than one variable is manipulated simultaneously, responses are more difficult to predict, since the factors are interrelated.

With these 12 moving parts, we had our colleague with expertise in mathematics, Dr Andrea Zignoli (CeRiSM Research Centre, Italy), work out for us using factorial analysis that in theory there could be 1,492,992 different combinations of HIIT sessions that could be created, and toward infinity. While there might be nearly 1.5 million ways to skin the cat with our HIIT programming, most of these would have no physiological meaning, so we'd best be more specific and purposeful than that toward achieving our objectives. Surely we can take this near infinite number of potential combinations and take a more useful approach to our programming. If we go back to where we began in chapter 1 with our individual athlete, alongside appreciating the important context of traditional approaches (chapter 2), how do we best adjust these 12 moving parts to achieve some of the desired physiological responses shown in chapter 3? The purpose of this chapter is to show some of the primary effects of these moving parts, so we can learn best how to go about manipulating

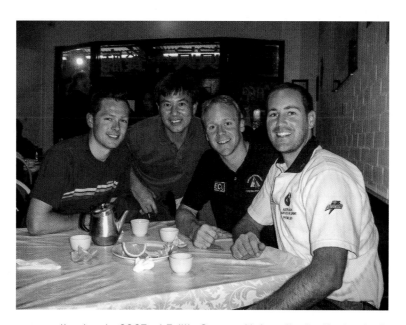

Figure 4.1 Colleagues gathering in 2007 at Edith Cowan University, Perth, Australia, to begin research into sport application of HIIT. Pictured left to right: Martin Buchheit, Kazunori (Ken) Nosaka, Paul Laursen, and Marc Quod.

Photo provided by Paul Laursen.

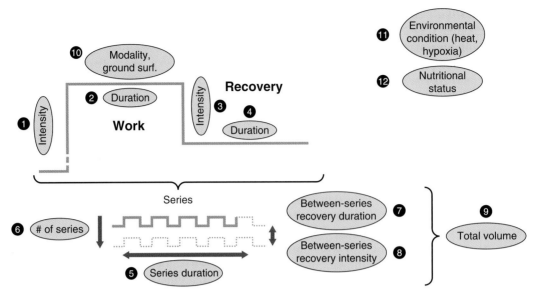

Figure 4.2 The 12 variables that can be manipulated to prescribe different HIIT sessions (11). These include (1) work bout intensity, (2) duration of the work bout, (3) recovery period intensity, (4) recovery period duration, (5) number of intervals or series duration, (6) number of interval bout series, and (7) the between-series recovery duration and (8) intensity. Variables 1 through 8 account for the (9) total work performed. Additionally, other factors that play a large role on the physiological outcome of an HIIT session are the (10) exercise mode and ground surface for run-based HIIT, (11) environment (heat and altitude), and (12) an athlete's nutrition practices.

a session's HIIT parameters to achieve our desired physiological targets.

Exercise Period Intensity

The first, and arguably most influential, characteristic of an HIIT session is the chosen intensity of the exercise period (figure 2.5). At the low end of the intensity spectrum is critical speed or maximal lactate steady state, an intensity largely maintainable for 30 to 60 min. At the high end, this intensity continuum consists of maximal sprinting speed or instantaneous peak power. This is the highest power the athlete can produce or fastest speed at which the athlete can move.

The determinants of all-out power or speed, from an absolute standpoint, relate to the phenotype of the individual in terms of his motor unit breakdown (slow- or fast-twitch muscle fiber predominance). While there is well-described variability of slow- and fast-twitch muscle proportions in human mixed muscle, the average human and athlete typically has about a 50% breakdown of each broad fiber type division (fast and slow twitch), acknowledging the fact that scientists have been able to take each of the broad-slow and fast-twitch categories and sub-

divide these even further. For argument's sake, and in the name of keeping things simple, we could say that we generally have slow (or type I), intermediate (or type IIa), and fast-twitch muscle fiber (or type IIb) groups. Additionally, the total numbers of motor units in a muscle group that can be engaged by the brain to produce the movement are influenced by the neuromuscular characteristics (chapter 3; (28)) and of course, training. Additionally, all-out maximal power or speed can relate to the individual's muscle mass or volume of motor units within a given functional muscle group, or cross-sectional area of muscle (39, 47).

When an individual motor unit of the millions in a working muscle group is stimulated by a nerve (called a motor neuron), it creates force and resulting movement until, bioenergetically or biochemically speaking, it fatigues. Fast-twitch motor units are fast to produce force, highly powerful, and predominantly glycolytic in nature; however, they fatigue rapidly. Alternatively, slow-twitch fibers produce less force slowly, but they are plentiful in mitochondria for ATP production and as a result are more resilient to fatigue. Intermediate muscle fibers are somewhere in between, having properties of both types. Throw an equal proportion of all these muscle fibers into mixed human muscle, and this maximal power and speed ability creates an interesting relationship with our second crucial HIIT variable, the exercise period duration.

Exercise Period Duration

The exercise period duration of an HIIT bout is clearly dependent on the exercise intensity, which, as we just learned, is reliant on the proportion of muscle fibers engaged, along with their varying twitch characteristics, and the absolute amount (volume or size) of these. The maximum period over which an exercise task can be sustained at a constant speed or power output is an inverse and curvilinear function of the exercise intensity, and is specific to the muscle fiber (or volume/proportion of engaged muscle fibers). The higher the exercise intensity, the shorter its duration, and conversely, within one's own individual limits. Thus, the power/speed time continuum describes the interplay and trade-off of exercise intensity and duration in a particular individual completing a specific movement task or exercise.

When we perform exercise at our maximal intensity for varying times, and we plot the power and or speed versus that duration, we see a classic power law distribution profile. This helps provide us with some relevant mathematical constructs and terms we can use to help us understand training and performance. One is called the critical power, whereas the other is termed the anaerobic work capacity, often termed W′ (W prime).

Critical Power (CP)

The critical power (CP) model describes the capacity to *sustain* a particular work rate as a function of time (*t*) for an individual. As first suggested by Hill in 1925 (38), when he plotted velocity versus time for world records in running and swimming over various distances, a hyperbolic relationship between work rate and time exists. The point at which the power curve intensity/duration distribution begins to level out, mathematically termed the *asymptote*, can be termed critical power (figure 4.3). Thus, critical power can be described as one's sustainable exercise intensity, roughly over 30 to 60 min. Physiologically speaking, this tends to correspond to an individual's maximal lactate steady state, or an exercise intensity at which blood lactate production appears balanced by its removal (see chapter 3).

Anaerobic Work Capacity (W′)

Anaerobic work capacity (W′), sometimes referred to as anaerobic speed or power reserve (ASR/APR), describes a theoretically finite or limited energy supply available above critical power. Figure 4.3 attempts to illustrate the W′/ASR/APR concept using a number of different-sized boxes across the various duration and intensity combinations above the critical power. Some boxes are tall and skinny, some are square and fat, and others are long and thin. What is interesting, however, is that the size or volume of each box is the same. The box size or box volume is our theoretical W′ and represents a finite source of stored energy, theoretically speaking, the stored anaerobic alactic (ATP/CP) and anaerobic glycolytic energy (chapter 3). What this tells us is that when we're performing exercise above our critical power, as we do with HIIT, we only have a finite amount of that energy to play with before we need to recover. While there are a number of different ways we might use that energy (i.e., boxes 1 to 4 in figure 4.3), we only have a limited amount.

We can equate W′ to a battery, which has a limited amount of stored energy (figure 4.4). When we exercise above our CP, we have to use some of this energy. Our battery runs down. However, if we allow a period of recovery, we can restore some of our W′ battery.

Recovery Period

The recovery period between intervals receives much discussion from sport commentators and coaches alike. The most common belief we have seen purported is that recovery from HIIT should be active to promote the removal of the noxious blood lactate that has accumulated in the muscle during the high-intensity work. But is that really the case?

The benefit of active recovery has often been assessed via changes in blood lactate concentration (3, 6), which has little to do with muscle lactate concentration (40). Additionally, neither blood (34, 58) nor muscle (40) lactate has any direct (or linear) relationship with performance capacity. Thus, there is little support from a scientific standpoint for the sport commentator's typical recommendation to keep recovery active so as to clear the noxious blood lactate. While long-held myths rarely change in a lifetime, this is an important concept to grasp as a student, coach, or practitioner going about your craft of solving the HIIT-performance puzzle.

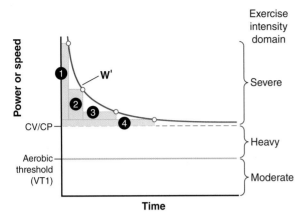

Figure 4.3 Critical power/velocity (CP/CV) and anaerobic work capacity (W'). The concept of W' is described further using the boxes numbered 1 through 4, which all show different usages of W' across varying intensity/duration combinations. Importantly, despite the different intensity/duration combinations, all W' boxes display the same total finite volume. VT$_1$: ventilatory threshold (aerobic threshold; see chapter 3).

Adapted by permission from A.M. Jones, A. Vanhatalo, M. Burnley, R.H. Morton, and D.C. Poole, "Critical Power: Implications for Determination of VO$_2$max and Exercise Tolerance," *Medicine & Science in Sports & Exercise* 42 no. 10 (2010): 1876-1890.

A better way to look at the recovery interval intensity and duration dynamics may be to consider it from the perspectives outlined in the HIIT work interval and duration description (figure 4.3). That is, we have a relatively finite energy source and need both time and certain conditions to optimize its repletion. A number of physiological aspects, such as those outlined in chapter 3, will influence this repletion of potential energy in muscle during the recovery period. One of the key factors is the quantity of a muscle's phosphocreatine (PCr) stores, sometimes called the short-term energy system. PCr is available in muscle to rapidly restore ATP levels. When PCr levels are high, so too is W', and vice versa.

Thus, a period of recovery allows our system to recharge our W' battery to perform more HIIT, which may provide important adaptation signals. The recovery dynamics are determined by the chosen recovery period intensity and duration.

The recovery period intensity and duration share a similar energetic relationship with the exercise period intensity and duration. That is, we'll recover quicker in a given time period when the intensity is lower, and additionally, we can recover further when the recovery duration is prolonged. Looked at from the other angle, we can increase the overall workload and metabolic rate of a given HIIT session when we

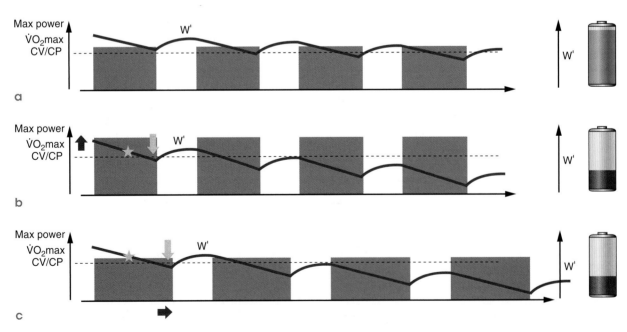

Figure 4.4 Finite W' being depleted with HIIT. The recovery period facilitates recovery of the W'. (a) An appropriate HIIT session for an individual in which W' is managed. (b) An HIIT session in which repeated bout intensity depletes W' toward a minimum (fatigue). (c) An HIIT session in which repeated bout duration depletes W' toward a minimum (fatigue).

either increase the recovery intensity (toward critical power) or lessen our recovery duration.

To illustrate the point, Dupont et al. (23) compared the effects of active (40% $\dot{V}O_2$max) versus passive recovery on how long subjects could repeat a 15 s/15 s intermittent high-intensity exercise sequence. Time to exhaustion for intermittent exercise with passive recovery (962 ± 314 s) was more than two times longer compared to the active recovery condition (427 ± 118 s). Thus, passive versus active recovery made a massive difference to the energy these subjects had available to perform their short-interval HIIT sessions. W′ was more protected. Looking at the flip side of the coin, average metabolic power during intermittent exercise with passive recovery was marginally lower compared to the active condition (48.9 ± 4.9 vs 52.6 ± 4.6 mL·kg⁻¹·min⁻¹). To explain these results, the authors measured oxyhemoglobin saturation (SaO_2) via near-infrared spectroscopy (NIRS) and showed that the mean rate of SaO_2 decrease was lower with passive recovery versus active recovery (figure 4.5). Thus, more available oxygen ultimately means better recovery of W′.

We also examined this concept using a repeated sprint training exercise format that is also in line with what team sport athletes in the field use, and compared the effect of active versus passive recovery on all-out running performance and physiological markers in male team sport athletes. Subjects performed six repeated maximal 4 s sprints interspersed with 21 s of either active (2 m/s) or passive (standing) recovery on a nonmotorized treadmill. Running speed was lower and speed decrement was greater when recovery was active versus passive. Additionally, oxygen uptake, blood lactate, and deoxyhemoglobin were higher, indicating a greater metabolic demand for active versus passive recovery with HIIT (15) (figure 4.6). Again, passive recovery clearly defended W′ better than active, allowing greater performance in subsequent bouts.

These studies highlight some opportunities where knowledge of the recovery intensity and duration kinetics can allow us to skin our cat optimally. For example, if we are after maximal recruitment (and likely adaptation signal) to our larger motor units, where engagement of such fibers is important, recovery should be maximal (i.e., exclusively passive over short durations) to allow for a higher reoxygenation of myoglobin, a higher PCr resynthesis, and a greater return of our W′. If practitioners still prefer the active recovery component (keeping athletes active or busy

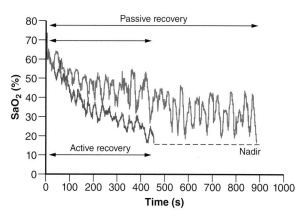

Figure 4.5 Effect of active versus passive recovery during a 15 s/15 s HIIT sequence to exhaustion. Passive recovery allowed subjects to double their exhaustion time, due in part to higher oxyhemoglobin saturation (SaO_2) and lower metabolic rates compared with the active recovery (40% $\dot{V}O_2$max) condition.

Reprinted by permission from G. Dupont, W. Moalla, C. Guinhouya, S. Ahmaidi, and S. Berthoin, "Passive Versus Active Recovery During High-Intensity Intermittent Exercises," *Medicine & Science in Sports & Exercise* 36 no. 2 (2004): 302-308.

alongside aerobic involvement), the detrimental effect of recovery exercise intensity on W′ can be compensated for by using a longer duration. Additionally, if we are time poor, or if a practitioner has a limited window to apply a metabolic stimulus, and total metabolic rate in a given time period is important, we can also use active recovery to raise the total metabolic work rate, depleting W′ faster and raising $\dot{V}O_2$ and lactate.

Figure 4.7 provides a theoretical framework for understanding the energetics of the recovery period. When the recovery intensity is low, the rate of W′ recovery is fast, and vice versa. Likewise, when the recovery duration is low, the repletion of our depleted W′ is limited.

As shown theoretically (figure 4.7), both the duration and intensity of the relief interval are important, and directly impact on the repletion of W′ and subsequent physiological effects of the HIIT session (45). Both the duration and intensity of the relief interval must be considered in light of:

1. Maximizing work capacity during subsequent intervals. Since active recovery can lower muscle oxygenation (15, 22), impair PCr resynthesis (O_2 competition), and trigger anaerobic system engagement during the following effort (50), it may be recommended to

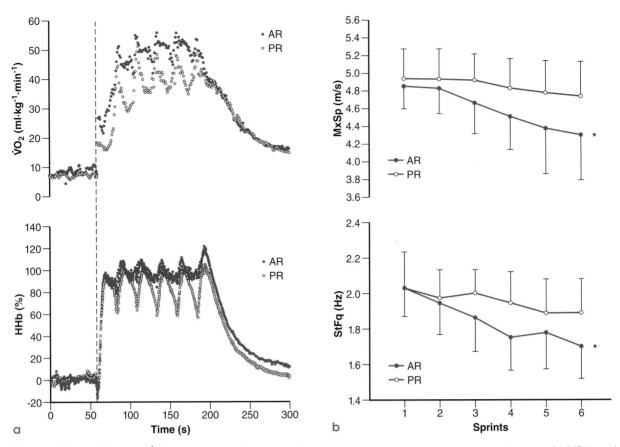

Figure 4.6 (a) Mean V̇O₂ and deoxyhemoglobin (HHb) expressed as a percentage of HHB level and (b) maximal speed (MxSp) and stride frequency (StFq) during six all-out sprints interspersed with 21 s of either active (AR) or passive recovery (PR). Values are means ± SD (n = 10).

Data from M. Buchheit, C. Cormie, C.R. Abbiss, S. Ahmaidi, K.K. Nosaka, and P.B. Laursen, "Muscle Deoxygenation During Repeated Sprint Running: Effect of Active vs. Passive Recovery," *International Journal of Sports Medicine* 30 no. 6 (2009): 418-425.

use passive recovery typically to allow the maintenance of work quality, and in turn, a longer T_{lim} (i.e., figure 4.7a).

2. Maintaining a minimal level of V̇O₂ to reduce T to V̇O₂max during subsequent intervals (i.e., starting from an elevated baseline) (7, 44). While performing active recovery between interval bouts is appealing to accelerate T to V̇O₂max and, in turn, induce a higher fractional contribution of aerobic metabolism to total energy turnover (21), its effects on performance capacity (T_{lim}, and hence, T at V̇O₂max) are not straightforward. In fact, during HIIT with short intervals, active recovery impairs W' recovery and, in turn, shortens T_{lim} and, in turn, T at V̇O₂max (figure 4.7c). While a beneficial performance effect on subsequent intervals can be expected

with long recovery periods (≥ 3 min) (8, 19, 21) when the possible washout effects overcome that of the likely reduced PCr resynthesis, active recovery performed during this period may also negate subsequent interval performance using both long periods at high intensities (>45% v/pV̇O₂max) (6) and short periods of varying intensity (22, 51). Again both may compromise T at V̇O₂max (figure 4.7, b and c). In the context of long-interval HIIT, passive recovery is therefore recommended when the relief interval is less than 2 or 3 min. If an active recovery is chosen for the above-mentioned reasons (7, 21, 44), relief intervals should last at least 3 or 4 min at a submaximal intensity (6) to allow the maintenance of high exercise intensity during the following interval.

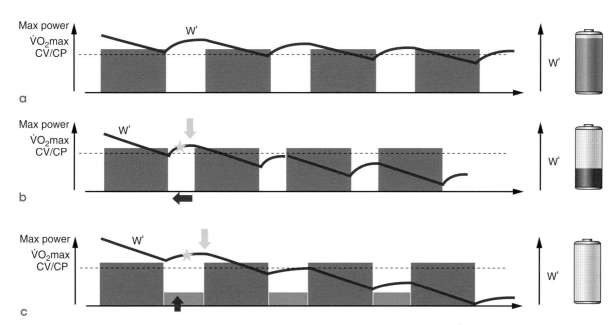

Figure 4.7 Influence of shortened duration and active recovery on W' repletion during HIIT. The recovery period facilitates recovery of W'. Blue represents the HIIT. Note that intensity is greater than the critical velocity/power (CV/CP). Purple line is W'. (a) In this HIIT session, W' is managed well. (b) The recovery duration is shortened and the time is not sufficient enough to recover W' substantially. (c) An active recovery condition, in which the heightened metabolic rate reduces even further the speed of W' recovery.

3. Maintenance of a high cardiovascular strain. As described in chapter 3 (figures 3.4 and 3.5), within the context of long-interval HIIT, stroke volume remains high with passive recovery, which may facilitate the signal to enhance cardiac output during HIIT (52). Recall too that the HR response during the recovery phase of HIIT is neither related to systemic O_2 demand nor muscular energy turnover (14, 59) but rather to central nervous system and metaboreflex responses (48). Thus, within any single HIIT session, the HR recovery response is somewhat irrelevant within the context of W'.

In summary, we have shown that the intensity and duration of the recovery phase has a substantial effect on both subsequent interval bouts and the HIIT session as a whole. If performance in repeated high-intensity bouts is important, recovery should be prolonged and passive (although recovery durations greater than 4 or 5 min make active recovery a good option also). If overall workload in a given time period is a priority, as it can be when a practitioner has only a short time window to work with, recovery intensity can be heightened or recovery

duration shortened to enhance overall work completed in a given time period and the associated physiological response.

In practice, active recovery is psychologically difficult to apply for the majority of athletes, especially for nonendurance athletes. When moderately trained runners ($v\dot{V}O_2max = 17.6$ km/h) were asked to self-select the nature of their relief intervals during an HIIT session (6×4 min running at 85% $v\dot{V}O_2max$ on a treadmill with 5% incline), they chose a *walking* recovery mode of about 2 min (49). Compared with 1 min recovery intervals, the 2 min recovery duration enabled runners to maintain higher running speeds; extending passive recovery to 4 min did not provide further benefits with respect to running speeds. Thus, best practice for the majority of long-interval HIIT appears to be 2 min of passive rest or easy walking.

Number of Intervals or Series Duration

When we refer to series duration, we're ultimately referring to the number of interval repetitions or HIIT bouts we're performing in a given training session (figure 4.2). In either case, the influence of these parameters relates to the total metabolic draw on the system. The more an HIIT session goes on, the larger the aerobic system draw is required, as the short-term systems (CP/glycolytic/W′) are taxed more and more, without adequate recovery time (unless recovery time is passive and prolonged; figure 4.7). Thus, the series duration is another way that we can skin the cat to affect the response of the training session. If we shorten the series duration (i.e., number of bouts), we generally enhance the metabolic rate or quality within a given time period, which might be appropriate in the context of allowing us to focus on other aspects of performance, such as for team sports where technical and tactical training may be prioritized. Alternatively, we can lengthen our series duration, drawing on aspects of endurance or fatigue resistance as per the needs of our more endurance-based athletes (figure 4.8).

Within the team sport context, we might use a number of shorter series, so that for a similar total number of repetitions, we achieve a higher volume of quality work. As illustrated in figure 4.8, for example, two periods of 4 min bouts separated by a longer recovery period (figure 4.8a) might be better than a single 8 min period of HIIT bouts in the context of achieving quality or intensity (figure 4.8c), as in this latter example, fatigue ensues, which can impact on the neuromuscular response (chapters 3 and 6). Finally, there is a lower limit we should place on our series duration in the context of targeting aerobic adaptations. Series duration should be no less than 3 or 4 min to enable athletes to reach a $\dot{V}O_2$ plateau (or near $\dot{V}O_2$max; see chapter 5). Generally, series durations are between 4 min (quality emphasis) and 14 min (endurance emphasis) (figure 4.8).

Number of Interval Bout Series (Total Volume)

As with our series duration (number of intervals; figure 4.2), the series number and total volume have a similar effect. The greater the number of series, the longer the overall session will be, and similarly, the greater the workload this creates (see again figure 4.8 a, b). The effect here again generally is to push the aerobic adaptation stimulus, unless recov-

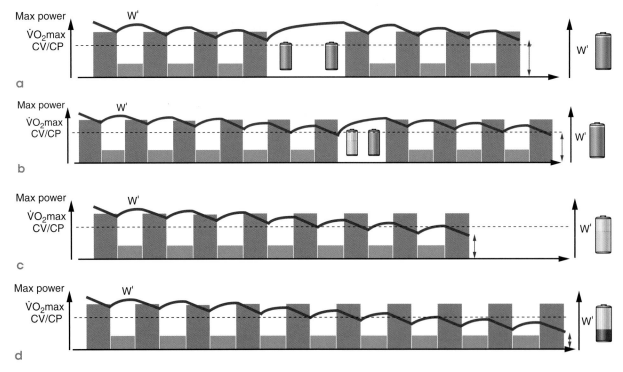

Figure 4.8 Theoretical impact of varying the series duration. (a) W′ is maintained in this 2×(4×4 min bouts) HIIT session separated by a single series recovery period. (b) Progression to a slightly more taxing session. (c) Alternate to session A, without the series recovery period (i.e., 8×4 min). (d) An excessively long series duration without adequate recovery.

ery duration is long and passive. Conversely, reducing the series number lowers the total volume of the training load.

This variable is essentially related to our training load, be that kilometers traveled or power produced for a given time, since the quantitative metabolic response can be equated between varying series durations depending on the recovery type (for elaboration, see chapter 8).

Between-Series Recovery Intensity and Duration

As per our recovery period intensity and duration (figure 4.2), the same rules apply. If we lower our between-series intensity, we'll speed the recovery of W′. Likewise again, if we lengthen the between-series recovery duration, we'll amplify W′ recovery. Conversely, a raised between-series recovery intensity or shorter duration will lower the W′ recovery rate and raise the metabolic rate within a given period of time (figure 4.9). Consequently, just as with our recovery period intensity and duration, we can facilitate either more quality work in a subsequent training series (with more passive and longer recovery) or achieve a higher metabolic rate in a given time period in the case where we are time starved and attempting to achieve a higher aerobic workload for a given period.

Total Work Performed (Volume)

To this point, variables 1 through 8 make up the ninth parameter, the total work performed in an HIIT session, or the session volume. This total amount of work or volume, a product of the session's overall intensity and duration, can be quantified in a number of ways (chapter 8) to enable appropriate progression of the training program parameters throughout a given training cycle. Knowledge of the total work performed can assist to prevent common pitfalls in which athletes perform too much HIIT work without appropriate recovery, which can lead to overtraining (chapter 7).

Exercise Modality

In general, when not specified, HIIT exercise modality tends to be that involved with the sport of interest, e.g., running for run-based sports, cycling for cyclists, boxing for boxers, rowing for rowers, etc. There are, however, many occasions when, for example, typical HIIT exercise modalities can be modified to adjust the acute metabolic or neuromuscular responses. In fact, when we refer to exercise modality in the context of an HIIT session (figure 4.2), we directly refer to the different ways we can manipulate the session to adjust the locomotor, neuromuscular, and musculoskeletal strain on the body. We originally

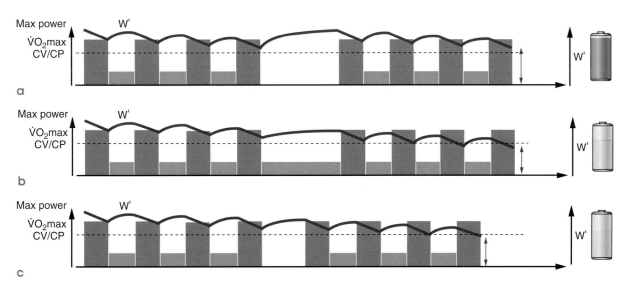

Figure 4.9 Between-series recovery intensity and duration effect. (a) Between-series recovery intensity is passive and prolonged, which enhances recovery and returns W′ adequately. (b) Between-series recovery intensity is higher (active), resulting in less recovery and associated W′ restoration. (c) Between-series recovery duration is shortened, which lowers between-series recovery and W′.

discussed this in chapter 3, and note that this can be implemented irrespective of the primary sport that the athlete participates in. On one end of the spectrum, we have the gross differences in mode, comparing across exercises like swimming, running, rowing, and cycling. However, other more subtle changes in exercise mode can be made to alter the training stress and stimulus: grass versus sand running; shuttle versus straight-line running; uphill versus downhill running; as well as cadence (cycling), bungy (rowing/kayak), and band, paddle, or sponge work (swimming).

Manipulations of the exercise mode can be used to target specific areas or regions of the body that need more or less locomotor, neuromuscular, or musculoskeletal strain versus (or in addition to) metabolic strain. In specific occasions for substitute soccer players, such as when increased neuromuscular load is required to compensate for the lack of on-field playing minutes, we may have them perform run-based sessions with more CODs than they'd usually encounter. Conversely, starting soccer players might perform treadmill HIIT sessions for the maintenance of central cardiovascular capacity alongside minimizing musculoskeletal strain that might be attained in matches. Heavy rugby players might perform low eccentric cycling HIIT sessions or even boxing-based HIIT to off-load their legs in the 2 to 4 d following a match, while cyclists might perform a swimming-based HIIT session as a means of achieving more whole-body aerobic exercise with

reduced lower leg involvement. For an 800 m runner showing evidence of low resiliency to musculoskeletal strain, a block of hill runs might be prescribed in the preparation phase to enhance this aspect, irrespective of the metabolic targets of the session (figure 4.10). Mode-specific effects (i.e., uphill versus straight-line running) on aerobic adaptation targets are expanded on throughout chapter 5, and a decision process flowchart to assist the practitioner with programming decisions is shown in figure 4.10.

Finally, it is also worth noting that many practitioners in team and racket sports use more sport-specific exercise modalities as alternatives to run-only efforts, e.g., tennis players hitting balls (chapter 18) or soccer players passing and shooting during short intervals (chapter 30). While the rationale for doing this still requires evidence-based support, the practice is believed to improve the magnitude of the HIIT-related physiological and locomotor gain transfer into the activity. Another benefit that is easy for everyone to appreciate is the greater motivation that athletes generally show when performing such HIIT sequences in a sport-specific fashion. In these particular drills, however, athletes are generally repeating closed skills with little decision-making and interactions with opponents, which questions its actual specificity and differentiates these HIIT exercises from proper game-based drills that involve aspects of playing, gaming, or puzzle solving (see chapter 2).

It is worth mentioning the widely used resistance-based HIIT circuit work that involves several different

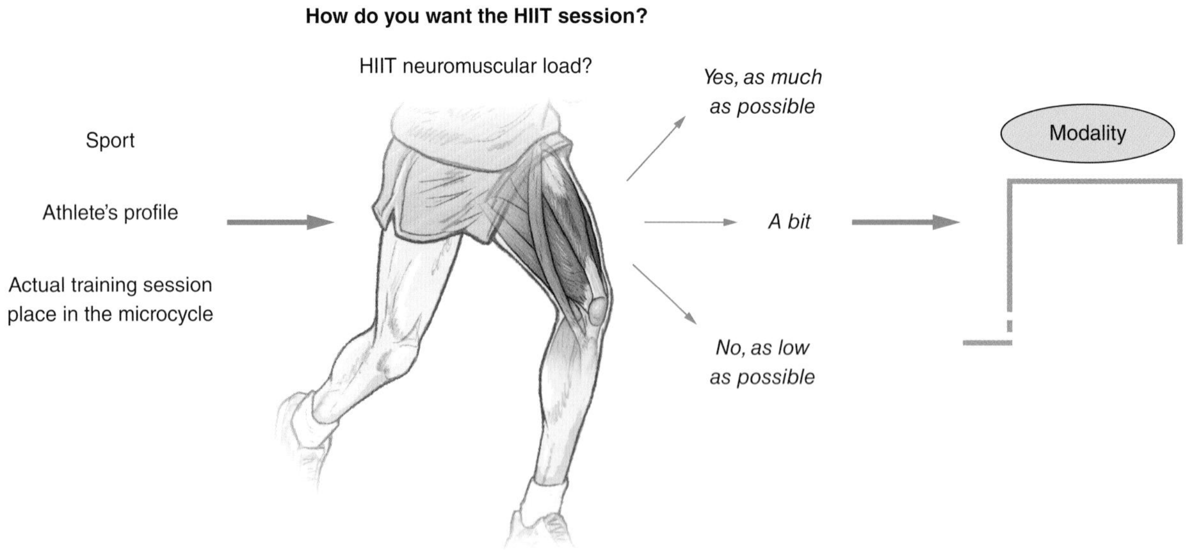

Figure 4.10 Ways to change modality, which likely affects musculoskeletal strain and neuromuscular load.

strength exercises during each exercise interval (e.g., generic exercises such as push-ups, squats, dips, crunches, lunges, etc.), repeated for 15 to 30 s, interspersed with passive rest (often with a 1:1 ratio), which might be considered as some of the most extreme forms of neuromuscular-oriented and demanding HIIT sequences known (type 4). Far from being specific to any sport, such exercise routines are believed to be a key component of a general physical preparation program, targeting both the cardiovascular and neuromuscular systems, especially during the initial stage of an athlete's program (e.g., preseason, building-up phases). Historically, these exercises were performed at a relatively low intensity (40% to 60% 1RM); however, the more recent explosion of circuit-training-related programs has extended to the use of heavy loading (>60% to 80% 1RM), which requires lower work:rest ratios. While research has shown that such HIIT sequences can be used to concurrently improve aerobic function (i.e., $\dot{V}O_2$max) and muscle strength (i.e., 1RM), benefits of such a training approach are likely to be exclusive only to individuals with limited initial fitness levels (i.e., the lower the initial fitness level, the greater the chance for $\dot{V}O_2$max and 1RM improvements). Our contrasting view today (46), in alignment with our philosophy set out in chapter 1 (figure 1.5), is that trained athletes need to be trained like Special Operation Navy Seals (13). Indeed, neither the metabolic nor the strength/power stimulus of such sequences would be considered intense enough to promote the desired adaptations for the elite athlete. We believe the toothpaste theory nicely illustrates the concept. The circuit-based approach can be likened to squeezing toothpaste only from the middle of the tube and is useful strategy for only a given period. Highly trained athletes require a more-focused target approach (i.e., separate HIIT and power, strength, and speed work) to get all the toothpaste out. While resistance-based HIIT circuits do a good job of squeezing from the middle of the tube, after some time they are an ineffective strategy for achieving any sort of outcome to get the toothpaste out, while squeezing strongly and consistently on just one side, and before the other, allows a much more efficient means of getting toothpaste on our brush.

Finally, we also feel that the practice of performing strength exercises during the work interval of an HIIT session may be at odds with the generic principles of strength exercise prescription. While the participation of the different energy system response targeted for metabolic conditioning is exercise duration dependent (which justifies the use of predefined work interval durations, see exercise period duration), strength exercises should be prescribed by a given number of repetitions in relation to the load and not by series duration (9).

Environment

The environment where HIIT is performed, namely the ambient temperature and humidity or atmospheric pressure, can create profoundly different physiological effects (30). Clearly we can push the envelope in this area by creating greater physiological stress in athletes over what they would typically have in normal training to enable them to be more fatigue resistant. Changes in environmental conditions can also be used to increase the internal:external load ratio, so that low mechanical work can be associated with high metabolic cost, which can be useful to limit neuromuscular load during an athlete's return to full training after an injury or a team's busy schedule. Of course, this is only if the training program is well managed. The two main environmental moderators include the environmental heat load (temperature and humidity) and the partial pressure of oxygen (altitude).

Heat Load

Heat load in the body can be altered in a number of ways. Heat load is a sum of heat gain and loss factors. Heat is gained via the body's own metabolic heat production (the breakdown of foodstuffs is relatively inefficient, and roughly 80% of the energetic process used to make energy is lost in the form of heat) along with the environmental heat load if greater than skin temperature. Heat is lost through the processes of convection, conduction, radiation, and sweat evaporation. In any condition where heat is gained, it becomes stored, and is stored largely in the core of the body (termed *core temperature*).

The rise in core temperature has a few effects that we'll all be very familiar with. First, we know it is uncomfortable, and the natural response is to lower exercise intensity in an attempt to control metabolic rate and lower the heat load (2). The heightened body temperature redistributes total body water to the skin for cooling via sweat evaporation, and heart rate is increased to maintain cardiac output and blood supply to working muscles (20).

While initially posing challenges to performance, the situation can create a number of positive effects that can be beneficial (30). First, the acutely lowered plasma volume creates a rebound effect and subsequently raises plasma volume in the recovery period (53), which can improve cardiovascular control and increase stroke volume. Additionally, the higher heat load creates increased energy demands that are initially met through increases in glycolysis during muscular contraction (26). This raised AMPk signaling increases the activity and amount of peroxisome proliferator-activated receptor gamma coactivator 1 alpha, a protein described in chapter 3 that can directly induce the primary adaptive responses to endurance exercise: mitochondrial biogenesis, angiogenesis, and increases in fat oxidation (5). Heat shock proteins (HSPs) are a group of proteins, the expression of which is increased when the cells are exposed to elevated temperatures. The increased activity of HSPs makes these cells more resilient to subsequent insult or heat exposure (36). Thus, environmental heat load can be manipulated a number of different ways that provide various potentially positive physiological effects (27).

Raised heat load also makes training feel harder and comes with added sympathetic nervous system stress. Rating of perceived exertion is increased alongside thermal discomfort. This all occurs without the need to increase the mechanical (neuromuscular and musculoskeletal) load in the body; in fact it can often be lower. Indeed, we typically find a downregulation of neural drive in such conditions, as HIIT becomes more difficult (1). This could be particularly the case with very hard efforts, such as sprint interval training, where achieving an all-out effort might be important (32, 33). Alternatively, warmer muscles from hotter temperatures can in some cases enable heightened levels of neuromuscular recruitment and associated physiological responses (16).

While we've highlighted the main adaptive benefits and opportunities, that is, heightened cardiometabolic responses, attention to tactical and technical aspects of sport and learning may be compromised and lowered central drive can also be problematic for training at certain times. Thus, appropriate timing of heat load before, during, and after HIIT is important and needs to be managed appropriately around context. One example often used across a number of sports is to perform an HIIT session in the heat to increase the metabolic load under low neuromuscular impact (HIIT type 1 response). Chapter 5 will expand on how we can use this factor to skin the cat appropriately to refine our weapons and hit our targets.

Hypoxia and Altitude

Another environmental factor that we might manipulate to skin the cat is the level of hypoxia an athlete's body is under. There are many ways this might be achieved, reviewed extensively by Girard and colleagues (31), including various forms of altitude training (both natural and simulated means), including local occlusion methods, as well as voluntary hypoventilation or breath holding (56). It's important for the reader to appreciate here that we are specifically only referring to the acute cardiometabolic responses that might be occurring in a single HIIT session, and not the chronic systemic responses that may occur with long-term training strategies at altitude where the aim is directed more toward achieving enhanced hematopoiesis (more red blood cells).

The main acute response of interest for hypoxic HIIT is that of its effect on enhancing enzymes of glycolysis, mediated by the oxygen-sensitive hypoxia-inducible factor (HIF)-1α (25) (figure 4.11). While the effects of hypoxic training on HIIT completed in hypoxic chambers has generated a number of impressive and insightful works of research from the laboratory of Professor Gregoire Millet and coworkers (10, 24), the practice of using artificial means of generating hypoxia is less common and typically reserved for athletes with access to specially designed facilities. Such altitude chambers (normobaric) are expensive and not always convenient to access for most athletes and teams. Moreover, accessing regions of true altitude (i.e., elevations between 1500 and 2200 m) is also not often convenient, and typically costly. Importantly, while there is evidence for a marginal benefit to training repeated sprint ability in hypoxic relative to normoxic conditions across studies (standard mean effect size = 0.46, 95% CI −0.02 to 0.93) (10), and although being used by many individual athletes and even some teams, the strategy of using hypoxic facilities has, in our opinion, a highly questionable cost:benefit ratio. Use of vascular occlusion methods, while perhaps used in certain individual cases, is also difficult for us to recommend based on the minor effects relative to the time and effort involved (relative to other factors in most athletes' performance puzzles). The one exception that has a certain level of practicality in our opinion might be sets of voluntary hypoventilation training, such as those sometimes performed in swimming HIIT for swimming and triathlon.

Heat

↑ Body temperature

↑ Sweat rate

↓ Plasma volume

↑ Heart rate

↑ Discomfort and RPE

↑ Glycolysis

↑ Muscle recruitment

↑ Internal/external load ratio

↓ Central drive

↑ Heat shock proteins

↓ Prolonged exercise and
   repeated sprint performance

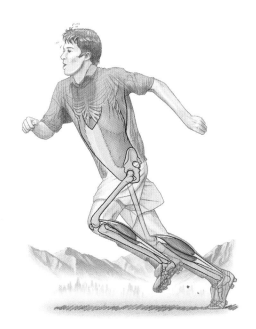

Hypoxia

↓ Muscle and cerebral oxygenation

↑ Heart rate

↑ Discomfort and RPE

↑ Glycolysis

↑ HIF-1α signaling

↑ Internal/external load ratio

↓ Central drive

↓ Prolonged exercise and
   repeated sprint performance

Figure 4.11 Acute impact of hot and hypoxic environments during HIIT.

Regardless, when athletes either reside in or travel to altitude and perform HIIT, there are similar physiological effects as those shown with heat training (30). For example, the lower partial pressure of oxygen in ambient air reduces the driving force of oxygen to bind to hemoglobin, lowering oxyhemoglobin saturation. The downstream effect is a lower partial pressure of oxygen in tissue, which targets the classic peripheral aerobic adaptations in muscle needed to provide enhanced energy needs, including increases in capillary density, myoglobin content, and oxidative enzymes. Additionally, heart rate is increased for the same absolute training intensity to facilitate the metabolic needs of tissues. Thus, we often observe reduced power and speed with prolonged efforts, and therefore enhanced acute metabolic responses relative to musculoskeletal and neuromuscular strain in normoxia. The effect on short-duration, high-intensity performance is unaffected, unless efforts are repeated (31). Thus, consideration for inter-bout and inter-series recovery intensity and duration is needed, depending on the training objectives. Additionally, as with heat stress, hypoxic stress can lower central drive, potentially diminishing training quality or influencing technical and tactical skill acquisition. On the one hand, this could potentially appear problematic due to the heightened cognitive challenge, while on the other hand, sometimes conditions made harder (through either altitude or heat) might facilitate heightened performance levels when the stress is removed. An

additional consideration for team sport players at altitude is the effect that the lower atmospheric pressure has on ball trajectory and associated task or skill performance. Thus, effects on skill or motor learning needed for team sport athletes need to be weighed against the possible physiological effects of training in such environments.

In summary, both heat and altitude can be used within the HIIT programming puzzle to affect the internal exercise cost to external power production ratio and the associated adaptive acute response to exercise training. Both heat and hypoxia are effective means of enhancing the acute metabolic response during exercise, which can be useful for enhancing the metabolic requirement of an exercise bout relative to the neuromuscular and musculoskeletal strain. As well, various means of creating hypoxic conditions during repeated sprinting appear effective at enhancing repeated sprint ability and glycolytic enzyme activity, although such training should be considered based on a cost:benefit ratio.

Nutrition

It's no secret that we all have to eat to survive. You wouldn't be reading this otherwise. Nutrition provides needed energy, the water that makes up the body, as well as everything we need to run our bodies (micronutrients, etc.). While this book is not about nutrition, nutrition clearly has an influence on the physiological effect of an HIIT bout, which is why we are covering it. While there are likely other subtle effects that can be caused by manipulating other dietary nutrients, including supplements, we will focus on what we believe are the key nutrient manipulations influencing physiological effects. These include the dietary carbohydrate availability, hydration status, and caffeine intake. Chapter 7 additionally explores some of the common pitfalls and detrimental effects a poor diet has on performance. Like environment, nutrition is an additional area that can help us make further benefits in training, if well manipulated.

Carbohydrate Availability

Carbohydrates are plant-derived sugars that come in a variety of forms. At the simplest level, and the level to which all carbohydrates are broken down eventually, is the compound glucose, a six-carbon molecule. Glucose is a primary metabolic fuel used by all cells to give us energy. Specifically it is the fuel of use for the process of anaerobic and aerobic glycolysis (chapter 3).

Notwithstanding the profound individual variance in the blood glucose response to the consumption of foodstuffs (64), there are some general principles we might appreciate around the topic of nutrition, acknowledging that refinement and optimization will exist at a monitored individual level. In the context of most athletes habituated to a mixed-Western diet high in carbohydrates, the act of lowering carbohydrate availability can create stress on (among others) muscle and nerve cells. The resultant lowered level of blood glucose, termed *hypoglycemia*, acutely creates a perceived feeling of fatigue and a reduced motivation to exercise. Ultimately this global effect of the lowered basal blood glucose level reduces systemic central nervous system activation. Under such conditions, acute high-intensity exercise capacity is typically reduced (35).

While high-intensity exercise capacity is typically lowered in the acute state, such a state can create an advantaged adaptive condition. Lower blood glucose concentrations reduce glycolytic capacity, which drives AMPk signaling for associated benefits (mitochondrial biogenesis and enhanced fat oxidation rates; chapter 3). The condition also makes training harder, without increasing mechanical (musculoskeletal and neuromuscular) load, which is something we often want during a training session. Alternatively, the condition can be nonoptimal in the context of the training condition, and could

acutely impair aspects such as mood, confidence, coordination, agility, judgment, game intelligence, learning, and so forth.

A number of methods can be used to lower carbohydrate availability. The most obvious is to lower carbohydrate consumption in the diet. This can be challenging for many athletes as it requires nutrition knowledge, and as mentioned, the individual response to foodstuffs is extremely variable. The social aspect of food (i.e., habits, eating what others eat, eating what someone serves you, etc.) and access to appropriate foods (low-carbohydrate foods can be difficult to source in many places) additionally make this intervention difficult. Typically, when lowering carbohydrate content from the diet, additional calories need to come from somewhere, and generally speaking this largely will come from fat, a concept that can be difficult for many to appreciate based on tradition, ingrained mind models, or instilled beliefs surrounding the effect of dietary fat on health. Regardless, a number of methods can be used to manipulate systemic levels of carbohydrate content or blood glucose, including eating low-carb high-fat (LCHF), fasting, and sleeping low.

Low-Carbohydrate High-Fat (LCHF) Diet

The low-carbohydrate high-fat diet is just what it sounds like. With protein levels similar to that of a typical mixed Western-based or high-carbohydrate diet (about 20%), fat calories are increased toward 70%, with carbohydrate content falling to 10%, or below 100 g in a given day (57). The LCHF diet has received considerable attention in social media, but few studies have assessed its effects. In most studies that have examined the impact of an LCHF diet on high-intensity performance, the time course has been relatively short (3 d to 3 wk). For example, when Havemann et al. (35) examined high- versus low-carbohydrate diets over 6 d in cyclists, overall 100 km performance time was not different; however, high-intensity 1 km sprint performance during the time trial was impaired on the high-fat relative to the high-carbohydrate diet. As well, the authors found significant increases in HR and effort perception with the LCHF diet after 6 d. However, as with training adaptation, which requires long periods of adaptation, dietary adaptation may follow a similar time course. To address this discrepancy in the literature, Cipryan et al. (18) recently had recreationally trained participants change from their habitual mixed Western-based diet to a ketogenic (<50 g CHO) diet over a 4 wk period. After this 4 wk period, performance and cardiorespiratory responses during a graded exercise test and HIIT were not impaired in the LCHF diet group. The LCHF group did, however, substantially increase their rates of fat oxidation. While more research is needed, it appears that short-duration time course adaptation periods can compromise HIIT performance, with adaptation requiring at least 4 wk. Additionally, LCHF diets substantially enhance fat oxidation, which is of importance for fatigue resistance and prolonged exercise performance (37).

Fasted Training

Fasted training is simply that—training in the fasted state. This can occur any time we decide not to eat for a given time period. Under the fasted condition, blood glucose and insulin levels drop and fat oxidation rates increase to meet the energetic demands. When we train under such a condition, we drive further the fat adaptations previously mentioned with the LCHF diet and with high-intensity training even more so (increased AMPk signaling (63)). Anecdotally speaking, this is a common approach to training for many athletes, especially endurance specialists (54).

Sleeping Low

When we feed in the evening (typical) and we go to sleep, we are in effect fasting. When we wake, still in the fasted state before breakfast, we can train without breakfast and we are in effect typically already 8 h fasted (54). Lowering carbohydrate content in the evening meal, which can subsequently lower muscle glycogen levels, termed *sleeping low*, can enhance the adaptations further. Indeed, Marquet et al. (43) have shown significant improvements in submaximal cycling economy, supramaximal cycling capacity, and 10 km running time in trained endurance athletes using such an approach.

Two-a-Day Training

We all know that athletes train, and many more than once in a day. When training occurs without refueling carbohydrate levels after the first session, muscle and liver glycogen levels may be only partially restored, and as a result, the same adaptations are driven in the subsequent session. As such, the signals for increased mitochondrial biogenesis (i.e., AMPk; chapter 3) and fat oxidation rates are enhanced (60, 62).

Hydration Status

When athletes train, specifically when they train in the heat, it's often emphasized that they need to maintain hydration status. While that might be true in some contexts, there are times in the healthy athlete context where exactly the opposite approach can enhance a physiological state. Indeed, a lowered hydration status, which acutely lowers plasma volume, creates stress in a number of different areas, including the heart and the kidneys (20). The endocrine system responds by retaining sodium at the level of the kidney (heightened aldosterone and arginine vasopressin levels), water follows, and plasma volume is increased. The enhanced plasma volume can be highly beneficial in a number of contexts, from creating partial heat acclimation to enhancing stroke volume through increased ejection fraction, thereby enabling cardiac stability. For example, Garrett et al. (29) showed that dehydration increased the desired adaptations from a short-term (5 d) heat acclimation protocol (90 min cycling in 35°C, 60% RH) in well-trained males. Aldosterone was enhanced more with dehydration, which was positively related to the plasma volume expansion, which tended to be larger in the dehydration condition. Thus, plasma volume expansion may be more pronounced with permissive dehydration and is one further factor that can be considered around HIIT to skin the cat. Of course, caution must be warranted when applying such maneuvers as physiological strain is likely to additionally be high, which could jeopardize other aspects of performance, such as skill development and tactical learning within the team sport context.

Caffeine

While there are, in our opinion, only a very small number of silver bullet solutions to solving the performance puzzle relative to the number of commercial claims, caffeine supplementation does show relatively consistent positive effects on exercise performance across a number of different conditions. In particular, caffeine couples well with train-low strategies to enhance acute HIIT performance. As described, under conditions of low-carbohydrate availability in athletes adapted to traditional Western diets (typical) or in any condition in which muscle glycogen content is substantially lowered (i.e., two-a-day training), HIIT performance (but not necessarily the acute signal/

response) is compromised (61). In any such condition (figure 4.11) when HIIT is planned, caffeine supplementation, typically taken in a variety of forms (including coffee and tea) approximately 1 h prior to the session, will enhance HIIT performance and potentially the acute metabolic signal in the larger motor units recruited. For example, Lane et al. (41) showed that caffeine ingestion (3 mg·kg·BM^{-1}) taken 1 h prior to an HIIT session (8×5 min maximal sustainable pace, 1 min recovery) conducted in a low-carbohydrate state enhanced power output by 3.5%. Thus, such a strategy may be particularly useful in athletes reluctant to train low for various reasons.

Figure 4.12 shows the main environmental and nutritional manipulations used to manipulate HIIT programming to assist practitioners to solve their programming puzzles.

In summary, we have outlined 12 different major ways that we can skin the cat around HIIT. With all those moving parts, how do we now take these and begin to make an impact on performance? How do we shape the puzzle piece so that it fits appropriately in the athlete's performance puzzle? How do we use this information to make useful weapons that will hit our physiological targets?

Skinning the Cat to Make Weapons

First, like soldiers going into battle, we need to make weapons if we are to take out our targets. Through trial and error and the experiences of many coaches, athletes, practitioners, scientists, and others who have gone before us, we feel there are five key weapons or formats we can form to induce the appropriate acute physiological response we are after to build our ultimate athletes. These formats include short intervals, long intervals, repeated-sprint training, sprint interval training, and game-based HIIT. These weapons can be used for different combat operations, depending on our physiological targets (figure 1.5).

Long Intervals

Long intervals are just that—long. In long intervals, we're using repeated bouts of the longer end of the intensity-time continuum around our v/p$\dot{V}O_2$max (95% to 105%) or 80% to 90% of V_{IFT}. The durations need to be longer than a minute to induce the acute metabolic and neuromuscular responses we are after, which we will allude to in the next chapter. For long intervals to be effective, they should be separated

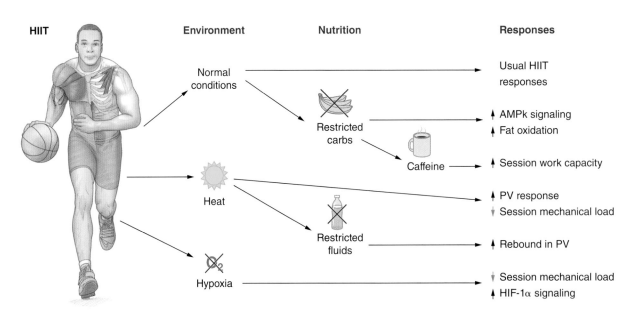

Figure 4.12 Impact of environment and nutrition and their associated acute responses.

by short durations (1 to 3 min) of passive recovery or longer durations of active recovery up to 45% of V_{IFT} or 60% of V/P$_{IncTest}$ (2 to 4 min; figure 4.13).

Short Intervals

Short intervals (figure 4.14) consist of interval bouts of less than 60 s repeated in a similarly short time duration. The dynamics of this format enable us to induce the acute metabolic and neuromuscular responses we are after, which we will allude to in the next chapter. For short intervals to form effective weapons we can use to hit our targets, they should be performed at between 90% and 105% of V_{IFT} (100% to 120% V/P$_{IncTest}$) for their repeated short duration (10 to 60 s), separated by less than a minute of recovery (passive to 45% V_{IFT} or 60% V/P$_{IncTest}$).

Repeated-Sprint Training

Repeated-sprint training is the first of our very high-intensity weapon formats we can use to target more high-end capacities or anaerobic speed/power reserve. These formats (figure 4.15) involve 3 to 10 s efforts of an all-out maximal intensity, with a variable recovery duration ranging from short and passive, to 45% V_{IFT} or 60% V/P$_{IncTest}$.

Sprint Interval Training

Sprint interval training is again all-out maximal sprinting efforts, only the duration is longer, in the 20 to 45 s range. Such efforts are exceptionally taxing, and recovery is passive and long (typically 1 to 4 min). Sprint interval training weapon formats are shown in figure 4.16.

Game-Based HIIT

Game-based HIIT (GBHIIT), including small-sided games (SSGs), discussed briefly in chapter 2 and expanded in detail in chapter 5, are ultimately sport-specific game-based forms of long intervals. Importantly, GBHIIT systematically includes decision-making and interactions with opponents (at least one in the case of racket sports) and teammates, which make these unique and different from typical sport-specific intervals (e.g., a tennis player hitting successive, but different, balls during a short interval). GBHIIT tends to run for 2 to 4 min at a sport-specific intensity of effort, which outside of the research setting can be difficult to quantify. Recovery durations are typically passive and range from 90 s to 4 min. Figure 4.17 illustrates a schematic representation of this weapon format.

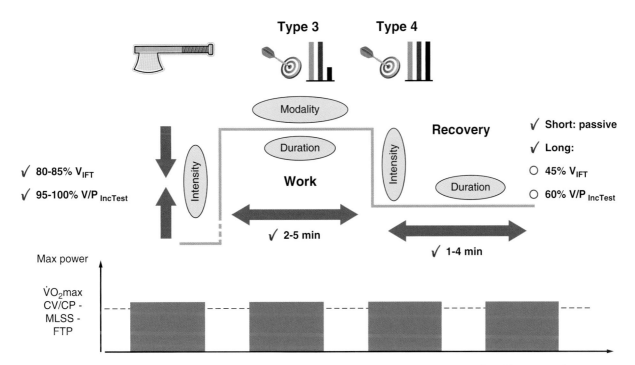

Figure 4.13 Long intervals and their recommended range of intensities, durations, and recovery characteristics.

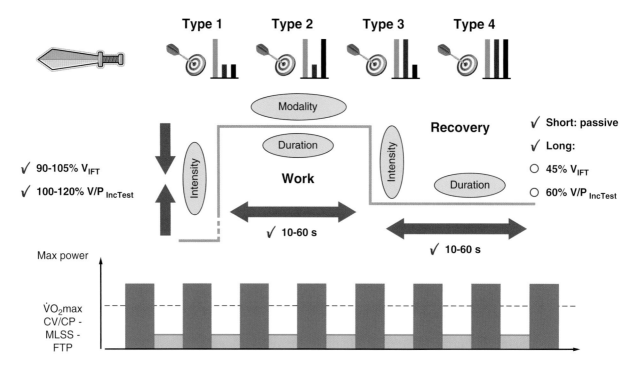

Figure 4.14 Short intervals and their recommended range of intensities, durations, and recovery characteristics.

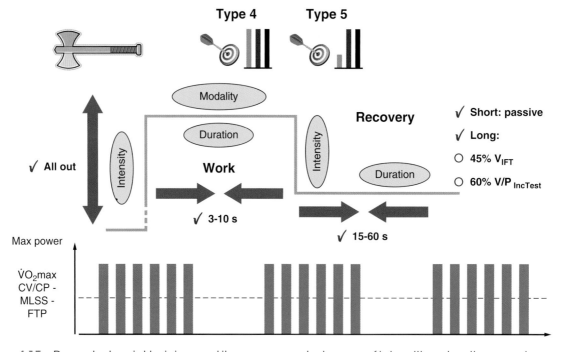

Figure 4.15 Repeated-sprint training and its recommended range of intensities, durations, and recovery characteristics.

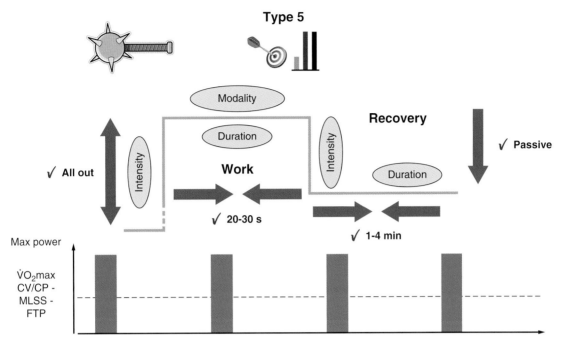

Figure 4.16   Sprint interval training.

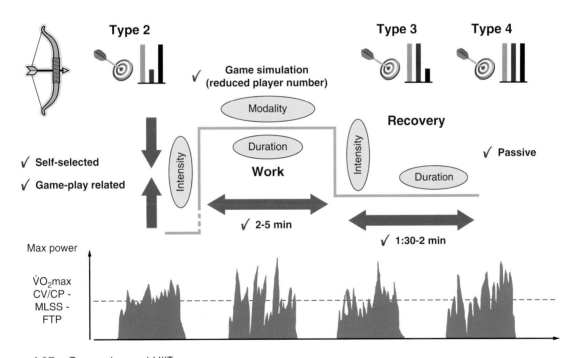

Figure 4.17   Game-based HIIT.

Summary

In summary, we have shown the 12 major factors we can manipulate when it comes to the development of an HIIT weapon. These were shown to be (1) the intensity of the work bout; (2) the duration of the work bout; (3) the intensity of the recovery period; (4) the duration of the recovery period; (5) the number of intervals or series duration; (6) the number of interval bout series; (7) the between-series recovery duration and (8) intensity; and, finally, (9) the total work performed. The other factors that play a large role on the physiological outcome of an HIIT session include (10) the exercise mode and ground surface for run-based HIIT; (11) the environment (heat and altitude); and (12) an athlete's nutrition practices shortly before (<24 h) and during the session.

While the foundations of our five key weapons are now formed, we need to go deeper with this information and further fine-tune these. Thus, in chapter 5 we will use our knowledge of how to skin a cat to refine and form more elaborate weapons that we can use to hit our military targets.

5

Using HIIT Weapons

• • • • • •

Martin Buchheit and Paul Laursen

To this point, we've described the history of high-intensity interval training (HIIT) (chapter 1), outlined traditional approaches coaches have used to calibrate their HIIT sessions (chapter 2), explained the general physiological responses (proxy adaptations) associated with HIIT (chapter 3), and broken down HIIT more specifically into the components we can use to form our five key weapons or formats (chapter 4). Recall that these weapons or formats include long intervals (figure 4.13), short intervals (figure 4.14), repeated-sprint training (figure 4.15), sprint interval training (figure 4.16), and game-based HIIT (figure 4.17).

Important components of any armed forces organization throughout history are the concepts of intelligence, tactics, and logistics. In this chapter, we're going to dive much deeper into the intelligence of our weapons so as to understand their intricacies. In doing so, we'll learn to use these weapons to hit the three main physiological targets we're after in our training, specifically the oxidative, anaerobic glycolytic, and neuromuscular responses (chapter 3).

As we've shown in chapter 4, the moving parts of HIIT can be manipulated to form different HIIT weapons or formats, as detailed initially in figure 1.5. These moving parts can be considered useful tools for adjusting HIIT to hit our physiological targets. Most practitioners think only how they'll use a chosen format, be that long intervals, repeated-sprint train-

ing, small-sided games, etc., within a given training program design. But as coaches and practitioners interested in maximizing performance further, we want to extend our thinking to a new level. Instead of thinking only about the format/weapon (what and when), the aim of this chapter is to learn to think more like a four-star practitioner, so as to learn how to fine-tune our high-performance weapon to get the most out of it. That's one of the main aims of this book. Instead of thinking format or weapon first, we'd like to challenge you to think target type first. Based on where we began in chapter 1 (figure 1.5), first we need to understand the sport demands and the context. When ultimately performance is the critical factor, how important is the physical preparation besides the context of the other factors integral to sport performance, such as skill and tactics (figure 1.4)? We need to prioritize our time and resources appropriately. After we're clear on the importance of HIIT, we next need to consider:

1. the sport's or player's physical demands;
2. athlete profiles, including athlete history, training age, and other individual characteristics;
3. long-term adaptation targets; and,
4. training periodization, or how the training plan fluctuates daily, weekly, and season long, depending on our aims and the sport or event schedule.

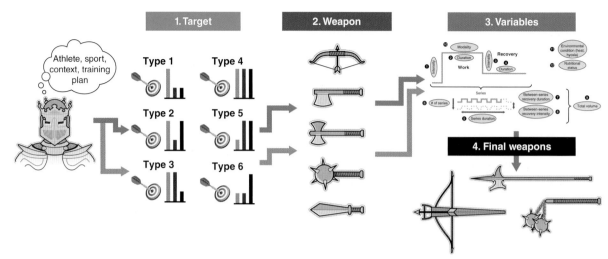

Figure 5.1 The thought patterns that can be used in programming. The more common thought pattern when it comes to HIIT weapon selection is to think format/weapon first. Our challenge to the reader is to think differently: what do you want (HIIT type/target), how do you do it (format/weapon), what variables do you adjust to hit your targets before final creation of your weapon.

As highlighted in the decision tree outlined in figure 1.5, all these factors merge toward establishing the desired physiological objectives of the HIIT session. Are we after aerobic, anaerobic, or neuromuscular responses (proxy adaptation) that we outlined in chapter 3 to develop our athletes appropriately, depending on where things sit in the calendar year relative to our sport performance aims? Again with respect to context, are we clear on the needs related to periodization (e.g., training blocks, within-cycle programming to avoid interference and maximize stimulus; chapter 6)?

Finally, once we're clear on the aim, we can go forward like a four-star practitioner in selecting the appropriate weapon to hit our target (figure 5.1).

We've mentioned the analogy before, but it might be good to review. If we think like a full general given a military assignment by his president, he must consider the targets based on the objectives. He has an arsenal of options at his disposal. He can use a weapon of mass destruction, hitting his target of course, but also everything else in its wake, including civilian casualties or collateral damage. Or, he can use military intelligence, call on his Navy Seal team, bring in Rambo, and be more specific with his approach. While occasionally mass destruction weapons must be used in the context of real-world training application, our preference is to keep collateral damage to a minimum and select a specifically targeted approach (recall toothpaste analogy, chapter 4). Thus, the aim of this chapter

is to enhance our military intelligence by outlining the target types available for each HIIT weapon. This knowledge means we can make better-informed decisions when we select our weapons and adjust these in accordance with how they function to best hit our three main physiological targets: the oxidative, anaerobic, and neuromuscular systems.

By way of emphasis, note that it is not one weapon that achieves a certain HIIT target type but rather multiple weapons that can be used to hit the specific target depending on how they are manipulated. To recap, we suggest there are six key target combinations to aim for to enhance the related systems (outlined in figure 1.5):

Type 1, metabolic, eliciting essentially large requirements from the cardiopulmonary system and oxidative muscle fibers;

Type 2, metabolic as per type 1, but with a certain degree of neuromuscular strain;

Type 3, metabolic as per type 1, but with a large degree of anaerobic glycolytic energy contribution;

Type 4, metabolic (oxidative/anaerobic) as per type 3 plus a certain degree of neuromuscular strain;

Type 5, essentially a large anaerobic contribution combined with neuromuscular strain; and

Type 6, essentially a large neuromuscular strain, with limited metabolic contribution (neither oxidative nor anaerobic).

This chapter describes each weapon, and using our combined experience and history in the academic (121) and applied areas (50, 51), we describe the magnitude of the aerobic oxidative, anaerobic glycolytic, and neuromuscular responses to acute HIIT variable manipulations.

Long Intervals

We lead off this chapter with our first weapon, the long-interval format. Recall that long intervals typically consist of intervals performed near $\dot{V}O_2$max speed and power, over durations of 2 to 5 min. Long intervals are the weapons we can use to hit target types 3 and 4.

$\dot{V}O_2$ (Oxidative) Responses to Long Intervals

When we think of long intervals, we typically focus on targeting the top end of the aerobic system. As outlined in chapter 3, the hallmark measure of aerobic system function is $\dot{V}O_2$max, considered a proxy of maximal aerobic locomotor function and highly related to endurance exercise performance. Thus, how long (time) we can perform at $\dot{V}O_2$max, referred to as T at $\dot{V}O_2$max (or Tmax), becomes a generic measure we can use to observe how the manipulation of different HIIT variables affects the acute oxidative response. While not definitively proven, the principle of specificity suggests that if $\dot{V}O_2$max is important, then it makes sense to work on strategies that allow the accumulation of T at $\dot{V}O_2$max. This section focuses on the intricacies of manipulating variables within long intervals to enhance $\dot{V}O_2$max. As long intervals are long, such intervals naturally target type 3 and 4 acute oxidative responses (figure 4.13).

Exercise Intensity During Long Intervals

As shown in both chapters 2 and 4, work intensity close to v/p$\dot{V}O_2$max is needed to elicit a maximal $\dot{V}O_2$ response. When we look to the scientific literature, these responses are typically described during single constant-speed or power exercise, not always applicable to the repeated nature of interval training exercise, but it's a place to start. In an attempt to determine the velocity and exercise intensity associated with the longest T at $\dot{V}O_2$max during a run to exhaustion, six physical education students performed four separate runs at 90, 100, 120, and 140% of their v$\dot{V}O_2$max (17 km/h) (23). Not surprisingly, time to exhaustion (T_{lim}) was inversely related to the

running intensity. T at $\dot{V}O_2$max during 90% and 140% conditions was trivial (i.e., <20 s in average), but reached substantially *larger* values at 100% and 120%: 190 ± 87 (57% of T_{lim}, ES > +2.8) and 73 ± 29 s (59%, ES > +1.7). In another study, middle-distance runners did not manage to reach $\dot{V}O_2$max while running at 92% of v $\dot{V}O_2$max (110). The ability to reach $\dot{V}O_2$max during a single run at vΔ50 (i.e., the velocity between the maximal lactate steady state and v$\dot{V}O_2$max, ≈92%-93% of v$\dot{V}O_2$max (23)) via the development of a $\dot{V}O_2$ slow component (5) might be fitness dependent (20), with more highly trained runners less able to reach $\dot{V}O_2$max, possibly due to their higher fat oxidation rates and greater fatigue resistance (105). In addition, as the determination of vΔ50 is impractical in the field, work intensities of ≥95% v/p$\dot{V}O_2$max are recommended to maximize T at $\dot{V}O_2$max during single isolated runs.

Of course, in practice, athletes do not exercise to exhaustion, but use intervals or sets. Thus, slightly lower intensities (≥ 90% v/p$\dot{V}O_2$max) are often used when considering repeated exercise bouts such as long-interval sessions and game-based HIIT, since interval $\dot{V}O_2$ is likely to increase with successive repetitions due to the development of a $\dot{V}O_2$ slow component (5). As suggested by Astrand in the 1960s (5), exercise intensity does not need to be maximal during an HIIT session to elicit $\dot{V}O_2$max.

Time to Reach $\dot{V}O_2$max and Maximizing Long-Interval Duration

As alluded to in chapter 4, the concept of optimizing long-interval duration with respect to achieving the longest time possible at $\dot{V}O_2$max was of particular interest to Paul in the early 2000s, and this was one of the primary areas of research investigated during his doctoral studies (121). If $\dot{V}O_2$max is to be reached during the first interval of a sequence, its interval duration must be at least equal to the time needed to reach $\dot{V}O_2$max. Thus, with short intervals, as during typical HIIT sessions (work interval duration < time needed to reach $\dot{V}O_2$max), $\dot{V}O_2$max is usually not attained on the first interval. The time needed to reach $\dot{V}O_2$max during constant-speed/power exercise to exhaustion has received considerable debate in the past (17, 102, 108-110, 123). As shown in figure 5.2, the marker shows considerable variability across a number of factors including fitness, gender, and age, with ranges from 97 s (17) to 299 s (110), along with high inter-subject variability (20%-30% (108, 110, 123) to 40% (102)).

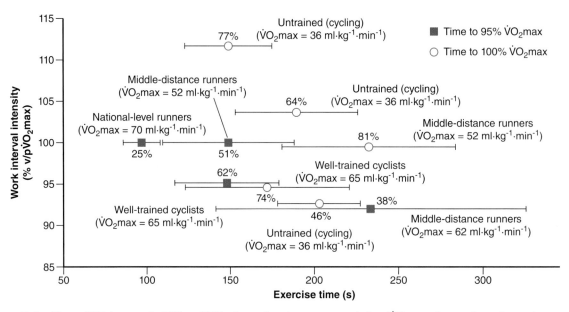

Figure 5.2 Time (SD) to reach 90% or 95% of maximal oxygen uptake ($\dot{V}O_2$max) as a function of exercise intensity in various sports and populations.

While methodological differences likely explain some of these discrepancies (i.e., whether 95% or 100% of $\dot{V}O_2$max is considered, the presence and type of pretrial warm-up), the variability is consistent with those shown in $\dot{V}O_2$ kinetics at exercise onset. $\dot{V}O_2$ kinetics, that is the time it takes for oxygen delivery to respond to the demands of exercise, are generally affected by exercise intensity (114), accelerated during running compared with cycling (107) and faster in trained individuals (143). The relationship between $\dot{V}O_2$ kinetics at exercise onset and $\dot{V}O_2$max, however, is less clear, with some studies reporting relationships (42) and others showing no correlation (11, 53, 153), suggesting that the $\dot{V}O_2$ kinetics at exercise onset is more related to training status (118, 143) than $\dot{V}O_2$max per se. For intervals shorter than the time needed to reach $\dot{V}O_2$max, $\dot{V}O_2$max can still be reached during consecutive intervals, through the priming effect of an adequate warm-up and/or a series of preliminary intervals, which accelerates $\dot{V}O_2$ kinetics (79, 93) and the development of the $\dot{V}O_2$ slow component (5). As illustrated clearly by Burnley et al. (62), a second bout of heavy exercise speeds $\dot{V}O_2$max attainment by about 2 min (figure 5.3).

As an alternative to the use of fixed long-interval durations, using 50% to 70% of the T_{lim} at v/p $\dot{V}O_2$max has been suggested as an alternative to individualizing interval training (15, 21, 122, 123, 167, 168). While the rationale of this approach is

sound (50% to 70% is the average proportion of T_{lim} needed to reach $\dot{V}O_2$max), this method lacks practical application in the field. To our knowledge, prescribing training based on time to exhaustion is very rare compared to how endurance athletes actually train for a number of reasons.

1. In addition to v/p$\dot{V}O_2$max, time to exhaustion at v/p $\dot{V}O_2$max must be determined, which is only a moderately reliable measure (CV = 12% (134) to 25% (22)), is exhaustive by nature and highly depends on the accuracy of the v/p$\dot{V}O_2$max determination (135).

2. The time required to reach 100% of $\dot{V}O_2$max has frequently been reported to be longer than 75% of T_{lim} in some participants (108-110).

3. Intervals lasting 70% of T_{lim} have been reported as very difficult to perform, likely due to the high anaerobic energy contribution required (167).

4. For athletes presenting with exceptionally long T_{lim}, repeating sets of 60% of T_{lim} is typically not attainable (123).

5. There is no link between T to $\dot{V}O_2$max and T_{lim} (108, 123).

In light of these nuances, since a given percentage of the T_{lim} results in vastly different times spent at $\dot{V}O_2$max, the most logical way to use T to $\dot{V}O_2$max to individualize interval length (108) may be to

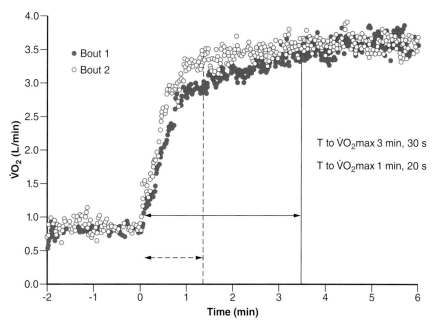

Figure 5.3 The $\dot{V}O_2$ response of a typical subject to a first and second bout of heavy exercise. Note that $\dot{V}O_2$ projects to a higher value after about 2 min in the second bout, indicative of an increased primary $\dot{V}O_2$ amplitude or a faster rate of engagement in the aerobic oxidative energy system.

Adapted by permission from M. Burnley, J.H. Doust, D. Ball, and A.M.Jones, "Effects of Prior Heavy Exercise on VO2 Kinetics During Heavy Exercise Are Related to Changes in Muscle Activity," *Journal of Applied Physiology* 93 no. 1 (2002): 167-174.

take the T to $\dot{V}O_2$max (if known) and add 1 or 2 min. If the T to $\dot{V}O_2$max cannot be determined (as is often the case), we recommend using fixed long-interval durations of 2 to 5 min. These can be adjusted in accordance with the athlete's exercise mode and training status, with less-trained individuals performing at a lower training intensity but with longer intervals. If we consider that the time constant of the primary phase of the $\dot{V}O_2$ kinetics at exercise onset (τ) in the severe intensity domain is generally in the range of 20 to 35 s (107, 110, 153), and that a steady state ($\geq 95\%$ $\dot{V}O_2$max) is reached after exercise onset within $\approx 4\,\tau$, $\dot{V}O_2$max should theoretically be reached from between 1 min, 20 s to 2 min, 20 s when long intervals are repeated, irrespective of training status and exercise mode. This is consistent with the data shown by Vuorimaa et al. (180) in national-level runners (v$\dot{V}O_2$max = 19.1 ± 1 km/h), where $\dot{V}O_2$max values were reached during 2 min intervals but not during 1 min intervals (work:rest ratio 1:1). Similarly, Seiler and Sjursen (163) showed in well-trained runners (v$\dot{V}O_2$max = 19.7 ± 1 km/h) that peak $\dot{V}O_2$ was only 82% ± 5% of $\dot{V}O_2$max during 1 min intervals, while it reached 92% ± 4% during 2 min intervals. Extending the work duration fur-

ther did not modify these peak values (93% ± 5% and 92% ± 3% for 4 and 6 min intervals, respectively) (163). Although performed on an inclined treadmill (5%), these latter sessions were completed at submaximal self-selected velocities (i.e., 91%, 83%, 76%, and 70% v$\dot{V}O_2$max for 1, 2, 4, and 6 min intervals, respectively (163)), which probably explains why $\dot{V}O_2$max was not reached (23).

Volume of HIIT With Long Intervals

Another variable that will contribute to the T at $\dot{V}O_2$max is the number of long-interval repetitions completed. In reality, few studies have actually examined HIIT sessions or programs consistent with the sessions that athletes actually perform in the field, and research describing T at $\dot{V}O_2$max in this regard is limited. Billat (15, 21) has often promoted using $2.5 \times T_{lim}$ for an athlete's individualized target training volume (figure 5.4). Cumulated high-intensity (>90% v/p$\dot{V}O_2$max) exercise time during typical sessions in well-trained athletes has been reported to be 12 min (6 × 2 min or 6 × ≈600 m (136)), 15 min (5 × 3 min or 5 × ≈800-1000 m (48)), 16 min (4 × 4 min or 4 × ≈1000-1250 m (116)), 24 min (6 × 4 min or 6 × ≈1000-1250 m (162); 4 × 6 min or

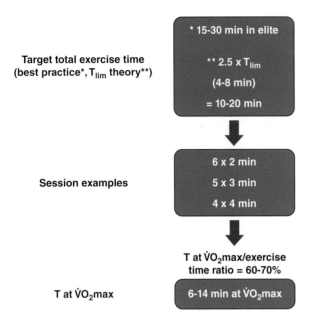

Target total exercise time (best practice*, T_{lim} theory**)

* 15-30 min in elite

** 2.5 x T_{lim}

(4-8 min)

= 10-20 min

Session examples

6 x 2 min

5 x 3 min

4 x 4 min

T at $\dot{V}O_2$max

T at $\dot{V}O_2$max/exercise time ratio = 60-70%

6-14 min at $\dot{V}O_2$max

Figure 5.4 Process used to define target time spent at or near $\dot{V}O_2$max (T at $\dot{V}O_2$max) during HIIT with long intervals. Data from elite athletes (* best practice) or Billat's recommendations (**T_{lim} theory (21)) suggest that overall exercise time should be between 10 and 30 min. Once total volume is broken into sets, and knowing the average portion of exercise time that is actually spent at or near $\dot{V}O_2$max during each interval (T at $\dot{V}O_2$:exercise time ratio), it is possible to estimate the actual T at $\dot{V}O_2$max associated with those prescribed sessions.

$4 \times \approx 1500$ m (163)) and 30 min (6×5 min or $5 \times \approx 1300$-1700 m (76)), enabling athletes to accumulate, depending on the HIIT format, from 10 min >90% (48, 136) to 4-10 min >95% (76, 136) at $\dot{V}O_2$max. In our experience, elite athletes typically tend to accumulate a greater T at $\dot{V}O_2$max for a given HIIT session at some point of the season. Also of note is that such training can be highly stressful, and inappropriate (excessive) prescription can rapidly lead to signs of overtraining (see chapter 7).

Recovery Interval Characteristics During Long-Interval HIIT

Recovery interval characteristics, both the duration and intensity, were highlighted as one of the 12 manipulation factors of importance in chapter 4. As we discussed, these two variables must be considered in light of maximizing work capacity during subsequent intervals (by increasing blood flow to accelerate muscle metabolic recovery, e.g., phosphocreatine

(PCr) resynthesis, H+ ion buffering, regulation of inorganic phosphate (Pi) concentration and K+ transport, muscle lactate oxidation) and maintaining a minimal level of O_2 to speed T to $\dot{V}O_2$max during subsequent intervals (i.e., starting from an elevated baseline) (15, 132). While performing active recovery between interval bouts is appealing to accelerate T to $\dot{V}O_2$max, and in turn, induce a higher fractional contribution of aerobic metabolism to total energy turnover (79), its effects on performance capacity (T_{lim}, and hence, T at $\dot{V}O_2$max) are not straightforward.

As we determined in chapter 4, and in the context of long-interval HIIT, passive recovery is recommended when the relief interval is less than 2 to 3 min. If an active recovery is chosen for the abovementioned reasons (15, 79, 132), relief intervals should last at least 3 to 4 min at a submaximal intensity (12) to allow the maintenance of high-intensity exercise during the following interval. Made even simpler, about 2 min of passive walking seems simple best practice for maximizing T at $\dot{V}O_2$max (refer to figure 4.5 and related text for details).

Uphill Running During HIIT With Long Intervals

Recall that hill running was variable 10 (work modality) of the many means we can manipulate to adjust physiological stress during HIIT (chapter 4). Despite its common practice (19), the cardiorespiratory responses to field-based HIIT sessions involving uphill or staircase running have received relatively little attention. Laboratory studies have shown that for a given running speed, $\dot{V}O_2$ is higher during uphill running compared to level running after a couple of minutes, probably due to the increased forces required to move against gravity, the subsequently larger motor units recruited, the greater reliance on concentric contractions, higher step frequency, increased internal mechanical work, shorter swing/aerial phase duration, and greater duty factor (185), all potential initiators of the $\dot{V}O_2$ slow component (152). However, in practice, athletes generally run slower on hills versus the track (165). Gajer et al. (90) found in elite French middle-distance runners ($v\dot{V}O_2$max = 21.2 ± 0.6 km/h, $\dot{V}O_2$max = 78 ± 4 mL·min⁻¹·kg⁻¹) that T at $\dot{V}O_2$max observed during a hill HIIT session (6×500 m (1:40), 4 to 5% slope [85% $v\dot{V}O_2$max]/1:40 [0%]) was lower compared to a reference track session (6×600 m (1:40) [102% $v\dot{V}O_2$max]/1:40 [0%]). While $\dot{V}O_2$ reached 99% and 105% $\dot{V}O_2$max during the hill and track sessions, respectively, the T at $\dot{V}O_2$max:exercise time ratio was *moderately* lower during the hill HIIT (27% versus 44%, ES ≈ −1.0). The reason for the lower T at $\dot{V}O_2$max during the hill HIIT is unclear. Despite the expected higher muscle force requirement during hill running (165), this is unlikely enough to compensate for the reduction in absolute running speed. If we consider that running uphill at 85% v$\dot{V}O_2$max with a grade of 5% has likely the same (theoretical) energy requirement as level running (or treadmill running with a 1% grade to compensate for wind resistance (154)) at ≈ 105% (138), the differences observed by Gajer et al. could have been even greater if the flat condition were run at a faster (and possibly better matched) speed (105% versus 102% (90)). As well, intervals in these sessions might not have been long enough to observe the additional slow component generally witnessed with uphill running (≈2 min (152)).

More recently, Barnes et al. (10) used the same approach to examine multiple variable manipulations (slopes) as the study by Stepto and colleagues (169) described in chapter 4. Here the authors used five different hill repeat-interval programs (2 times/wk) in small groups (3 to 5 runners) over 6 wk. Intervals were performed using gradients ranging from 4% to 18%, with associated longer or shorter bout durations (faster or slower run speeds) accordingly. Like Stepto et al. (169), no clear winner was observed from the formats in 5 km time trial performance. Interestingly, however, in the two middle groups performing intervals in the long-interval domain (G3 and G4) at 100% and 90% of v$\dot{V}O_2$max, with interval repetitions of ~2.5 and ~5 min, respectively, the trend was toward improving $\dot{V}O_2$max the most after 6 wk. However, these findings likely relate simply to the specificity of the HIIT programs used. (The specific long-interval format improved $\dot{V}O_2$max the most as it often does.) From a practical and applied standpoint, training programs are not ever exclusive to a single format, and an athlete's brain (central governor) will always lower and raise intensity in accordance with what is manageable and appropriate. Nevertheless, with respect to long intervals and hill gradient, research would suggest that a 7% to 10% gradient is an appropriate slope for performing hill-based long intervals in well-trained runners.

Summary of Oxidative Responses to Long Intervals

The long interval is a key weapon in our arsenal that we can use to enhance the oxidative response to HIIT. To achieve the necessary oxidative response (proxy adaptation), we have learned that for long intervals

* intensity should range from 92% to 102% of p/v$\dot{V}O_2$max,
* duration should span 2 to 5 min, at a repetition number that achieves ~10 min of T at $\dot{V}O_2$max,
* recovery intervals should be passive (i.e., walking) for about 2 min, and
* in the case of runners using hills, a 7% to 10% gradient appears appropriate.

However, despite this ideal HIIT profile, practitioners use many format variations in their programs (i.e., longer intervals, different work:rest ratio, etc.). The decision to use a variation of this weapon over another depends on numerous factors, including an athlete's needs, the sport's needs, and context. Figure 5.5 shows how four different HIIT sequences, which all possess a similar oxidative target by allowing an athlete to spend 8 to 10 min at $\dot{V}O_2$max, can vary substantially in terms of training volume, anaerobic contribution, and musculoskeletal and neuromuscular strain (total distance and distance at high speed). There is no right or wrong option, but practitioners may choose between options to either increase training volume (2 sessions in the middle of figure 5.5, >35 min) or limit blood lactate accumulation (session on the left) and high-speed running volume (SSGs, on the right). Note in this example the different responses in populations examined (runners for the three sessions on the left versus handball players for the SSGs). This explains the high lactates after the SSGs for the handball players, who would probably not cope with the running sessions applied to the runners (figure 5.5).

The following sections will extend our reasoning for the manipulation of the different HIIT variables to better control anaerobic contribution and musculoskeletal or neuromuscular strain during long intervals.

Anaerobic Glycolytic Energy Contribution to Long-Bout-Duration HIIT Sessions

Though not typically considered relative to the larger aerobic contribution to long intervals, the anaerobic glycolytic energy contribution to long intervals can be substantial. For example, in endurance-trained athletes performing constant-speed efforts at

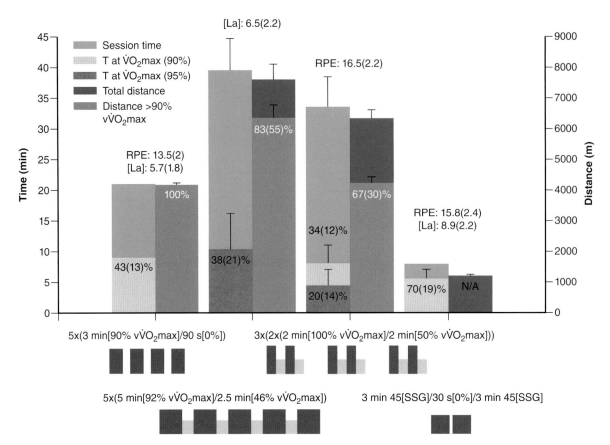

Figure 5.5 $\dot{V}O_2$ responses of four distinct long-interval HIIT sessions, highlighting the impact of different variable manipulations on T at $\dot{V}O_2$max, distance run, and session time (48, 56, 76, 136). Mean ± SD of total session time, T at $\dot{V}O_2$max, total distance, and distance run above 90% of v$\dot{V}O_2$max during four different long-interval HIIT sessions. Percentages (mean ± SD) refer to T at $\dot{V}O_2$max relative to the total session time and distance run above 90% of v$\dot{V}O_2$max relative to the total distance run. RPE and [La] (mmol/L) are provided as mean ± SD when available. HIIT: high-intensity interval training; [La]: blood lactate concentration; N/A: not available; RPE: rating of perceived exertion; SSGs: small-sided games (handball); $\dot{V}O_2$max: maximal oxygen uptake; T at $\dot{V}O_2$max: time spent above 90% or 95% of $\dot{V}O_2$max; v$\dot{V}O_2$max: minimal running speed associated with $\dot{V}O_2$max.

Reprinted by permission of Springer Nature from M. Buchheit and P.B. Laursen, "High-Intensity Interval Training, Solutions to the Programming Puzzle: Part I: Cardiopulmonary Emphasis," *Sports Medicine* 43, no. 5 (2013): 313-338.

v$\dot{V}O_2$max, over interval durations longer than ~90 s, the initial rise in blood lactate ranges from 5 to 7 mmol·L^{-1}·5min^{-1} (figure 5.6) (17, 76, 133, 162, 167, 170). Thus, long intervals can be manipulated to target the anaerobic glycolytic energy component associated with type 3 and 4 acute responses.

Effect of Work Interval Intensity on the Anaerobic Glycolytic Response to Long Intervals

While manipulation of HIIT variables can modulate the anaerobic glycolytic response, it must be appreciated that blood lactate accumulation is additionally related to training status (14) (figure 5.6). For example, in elite French middle-distance runners (v$\dot{V}O_2$max = 21.2 ± 0.6 km/h) performing repeated 600 m bouts (~1:40, work:relief ratio = 1), the initial rate of blood lactate increase was in the lower range of the values reported, i.e., ≈5 mmol·L^{-1}·5min^{-1} (90). The shorter work duration in this example (100 s) also illustrates the important concept that shorter interval repetitions will lower the lactate response (see subsequent section).

Despite the lack of a direct examination, study comparisons suggest that higher work intensities performed during long intervals likely elicit increased rates of blood lactate production (proxy anaerobic glycolytic energy contribution) (162, 167, 170).

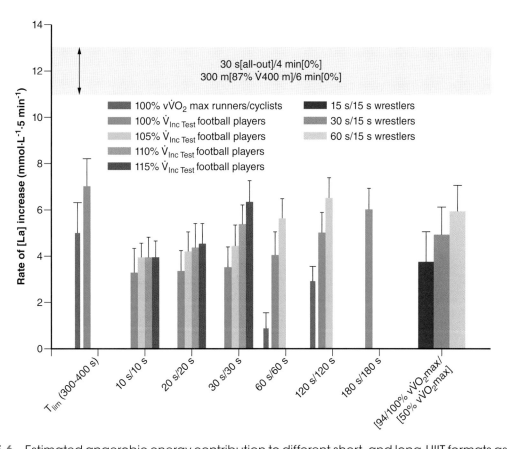

Figure 5.6 Estimated anaerobic energy contribution to different short- and long-HIIT formats as inferred from the initial rate of blood lactate accumulation ([La]). Values are mean±SD. Exercise intensities are % of the peak speed reached in the 30-15 intermittent fitness test (V_{IFT}), speed or power associated with maximal oxygen uptake (v/p$\dot{V}O_2$max), or peak incremental test speed ($V_{Inc,Test}$). Gray rectangular box represents the initial rate of blood lactate accumulation during lactate production training, i.e., all-out sprints or at the speed maintained during a 400 m run (V400m).

Reprinted by permission of Springer Nature from M. Buchheit and P.P. Laursen, "High-Intensity Interval Training, Solutions to the Programming Puzzle: Part II: Anaerobic Energy, Neuromuscular Load and Practical Applications," *Sports Medicine* 43 no. 10 (2013): 927-954.

Effect of Work Interval Duration on the Anaerobic Glycolytic Response to Long Intervals

Extending the interval duration of a long-interval HIIT session without altering the relief interval duration clearly increases the anaerobic glycolytic energy contribution, as more work must be completed in a given time period. In practice, however, coaches generally maintain the work:relief ratio when they manipulate their HIIT variables. In these latter conditions, an increase in work interval duration additionally is likely to increase anaerobic glycolytic energy contribution. For instance, doubling interval duration (2 min versus 1 min run at v$\dot{V}O_2$max, work:relief ratio = 1) leads to substantial

increases in anaerobic glycolytic energy contribution (figure 5.6) (180). Accumulated O_2 deficit ($\approx$25±2 versus 21±2 mL/kg, ES = +2.3) and end-session blood lactate measurements (8.8±3.6 versus 4.8±1.1 mmol/L, ES = +1.7) were *very largely* and *largely* higher, respectively. Likewise, in distance runners (v$\dot{V}O_2$max = 19.5±0.7 km/h), increasing the interval duration run at v$\dot{V}O_2$max from 2:10 to 2:30 (+15%) with a work:relief ratio of 1:2 resulted in an almost twofold increase in the initial rate of blood lactate accumulation (from $\approx$6 to $\approx$10 mmol·L^{-1}·5min^{-1}) (167). Of note, however, is that a decrease in work intensity (i.e., from 93% to 84% of v$\dot{V}O_2$max on a treadmill) can compensate for the effect of work interval extension from 1 to

6 min (work:relief ratio = 1) and maintains blood lactate at manageable levels (i.e., 4-5 mmol/L post exercise) (163).

Effect of Recovery Interval Characteristics on the Anaerobic Glycolytic Response to Long Intervals

As we stated with this factor in chapter 4, the influence of HIIT recovery interval duration on the subsequent bout's anaerobic glycolytic energy contribution is not straightforward. Maintaining a work:relief ratio of 1, accumulated O_2 deficit in the first min of a 2 min/2 min sequence run at $v\dot{V}O_2$max has been shown to be markedly greater than a 1 min/1 min set (23.8 ± 1.6 versus 20.5 ± 1.9 mLO₂/kg, ES = 1.9) (180). This is likely related to the lower total $\dot{V}O_2$ attained in the longer 2 min rest period condition, which increases the O_2 deficit for subsequent intervals (160). When the duration of the exercise interval is fixed, things are a bit different, and a shortening of the recovery interval would be typically associated with higher anaerobic glycolytic energy contribution due to the increased exercise load (greater total work done in less time). However, following self-selected 4 min work interval intensities ranging from 83% to 85% $v\dot{V}O_2$max (with a 5% grade), reducing the relief interval from 4 to 1 min did not affect end-session blood lactate levels (6-7 mmol/L) in moderately trained runners ($v\dot{V}O_2$max = 17.6 ± 1 km/h) (162). It is worth noting, however, that despite the inclined treadmill, the exercise intensity was submaximal in these studies (162, 163). It is expected that for sessions run at $v\dot{V}O_2$max, blood lactate responses would be higher and more responsive to relief interval manipulation (167). It is also worth noting that blood lactate concentration, as a systemic measure with a certain inertia, is likely a less sensitive measure of anaerobic glycolytic energy contribution than accumulated O_2 deficit, which may explain the differences between the studies by Vuorimaa et al. (180) and Seiler and Hetlelid (162).

When the relief interval duration is >3 to 4 min, active recovery (60%-70% $v\dot{V}O_2$max) can be used to accelerate blood lactate clearance compared to passive conditions (3, 12), leading to a lower accumulation throughout the session. While the effect of short (≤2 min) passive versus long (>3-4 min) active recovery on the anaerobic energy contribution to exercise has not been studied, it is worth noting that reductions in blood lactate may be indicative of effective lactate shuttling and high

lactate consumption in working skeletal muscles (31). As we touched on in chapter 4, blood lactate gets a bad name in the press, when at the end of the day it's simply a metabolite in flux. Its so-called removal, or lack thereof, in most contexts, is typically irrelevant.

Work Interval Modality Effect on the Anaerobic Glycolytic Response to Long Intervals

While field-based HIIT sessions involving hill repeats, sand running, stair climbing, and plyometric work are very common in the applied setting, there is surprisingly limited data showing the anaerobic energy contribution of such exercise. In elite French middle-distance runners ($v\dot{V}O_2$max = 21.2 ± 0.6 km/h, $\dot{V}O_2$max = 78 ± 4 mL·min⁻¹·kg⁻¹), blood lactate accumulation during a self-paced HIIT hill session on the road (6 × 500 m [~1 min, 40 s, work:relief ratio = 1], slope: 4%-5%) was *largely* lower compared with a reference self-paced track session (6 × 600 m) ([La] post-series: 8.5 ± 2.2 vs. 13.2 ± 4 mmol/L, ES = −1.5) (90). Nevertheless, this could have been due to the lower absolute running speed attained during the inclined condition used in this study that did not compensate for an eventual higher mechanical muscle demand and/or change in muscle pattern activation (165). Further studies are needed to compare the effect of different exercise modes (e.g., running versus cycling versus rowing) on anaerobic glycolytic energy contribution during actual HIIT sessions in athletes. In general, however, for coaches and athletes in the applied setting, exercise mode has a much lower impact on anaerobic glycolytic impact relative to key aspects such as intensity and duration of the work bout.

In summary, while HIIT with long intervals is likely the best format for adapting cardiopulmonary oxidative function, blood lactate accumulation (and likely anaerobic glycolytic energy contribution) can still reach high levels (rate of accumulation >5 mmol·L·5min⁻¹ and end-session values >10 mmol/L) (167) (figure 5.6), type 3 and 4. Therefore, for coaches striving to limit the anaerobic glycolytic contribution, the use of different forms of HIIT, such as short intervals, may be warranted (15).

Neuromuscular Responses to Long Intervals

The importance of quantifying the effect that an HIIT bout has on the neuromuscular system was highlighted in chapter 3. Long intervals can be used to hit type 4 targets, which represent an important musculoskeletal and neuromuscular strain. With respect to long intervals, manipulating interval duration on changes in CMJ height were examined in national level runners ($v\dot{V}O_2$max = 19.1 ± 1 km/h) by Vuorimaa et al. (179), who showed no within- or between-HIIT differences in CMJ height with 1 versus 2 min interval sessions (1:1 work:rest ratios) ran at $v\dot{V}O_2$max (179). Similarly, there was no effect on stride length throughout successive intervals (179). These findings may relate to the endurance-trained athlete's particular neuromuscular profile, the fact that running speed was similar between the 2 HIIT sessions, and that blood lactate levels remained moderate, even during the 2 min intervals (8.8 ± 3.6 mmol/L). Typically, neuromuscular impairment of muscle function during high-intensity exercise is accompanied by high blood lactate levels, i.e., >10-12 mmol/L (99, 144).

The effect of running speed or intensity on neuromuscular load can be indirectly inferred from results reported in highly trained young runners ($v\dot{V}O_2$max = 18.6 ± 0.9 km/h) (48). Here, Buchheit et al. (48) examined CMJ height and 5 m sprint times before and after long intervals (5 × 3 min) in normoxia (90% $v\dot{V}O_2$max) and normobaric hypoxia (inspired O_2 fraction = 15.4%, simulated altitude of 2400 m, 84% $v\dot{V}O_2$max). For both HIIT protocols, no changes in CMJ height were found, either immediately or 20 min after. Interestingly, while there was no change in sprint times following the runs completed at 84% $v\dot{V}O_2$max, sprint times were improved after the runs completed at 90% $v\dot{V}O_2$max immediately after the session (ES for difference in changes = 0.2-0.5), suggestive of a postactivation potentiation effect (figure 5.7) (113). However, this response was no longer evident 4 h later.

Last, compared to a reference track session (6 × 600 m), stride frequency (2.98 versus 3.1 strides/s) and amplitude (185 versus 203 cm) tended to be lower during a road-based HIIT hill session (6 × 500, 4%-5% incline) (90), suggesting that hill training can be effective at lowering hamstring muscle loading. In alignment with this, inclined (5%) 250 m sprints were associated with reduced stride length (−14%) and rate (−7%) and a +27% increase in push-off time, compared with 300 m sprints on the track (165). Importantly, despite no adjustment in quadriceps muscle activation, hamstring muscles were also less activated. Finally, in middle-distance runners ($v\dot{V}O_2$max = 21.8 ± 1.8 km/h), performance measures reflecting muscle power have also been

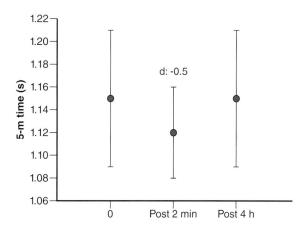

Figure 5.7 Changes in 5 m split time (SD) after long interval HIIT run at 90% $v\dot{V}O_2$max. Changes in 5 m split time were improved immediately (post 2 min) after the HIIT session run at 90% $v\dot{V}O_2$max, however, there was no substantial change in sprint time following the HIIT session run at 84% in hypoxia (i.e., consistently 1.15 ± 0.06 s).

shown to be lower for uphill versus horizontal incremental running performance (149). Taken together, these data (90, 149, 165) and others (100) suggest that incline running lowers hamstring strain in runners, which could be beneficial to prevent injuries during maximal and/or high-volume sessions (178). However, since athletes might be required to run downhill to prepare for the next interval, care should be taken with respect to potential acute muscle damage arising from the downhill phase (63).

Thus, HIIT hill sessions represent a useful alternative for reducing overall acute hamstring strain and appear well suited for high-volume training cycles, but strategies to avoid the downhill running phase should be considered by coaches. It is also worth noting that over longer time frames (once acute muscle damage is recovered), downhill running can be considered advantageous as it has a prophylactic effect (63) (i.e., repeated-bout effect) and can additionally be effective training for preventing future musculoskeletal injuries (see chapter 14; road running).

The level of neuromuscular strain during long intervals for cyclists can be manipulated by varying cadence or pedaling rate and associated resistance per pedal stroke. For example, Nimmerichter et al. (142) compared the effects of a low- (60 rpm uphill) or high-cadence (100 rpm level ground) long-HIIT (6 × 5 min) in well-trained cyclists over 4 wk. The 60 rpm group increased power output during both up (4.4% ± 5.3%) and flat (1.5% ± 4.5%) time trials, while changes in the level-ground HIIT group were less impressive (−1.3% ± 3.6% and 2.6% ± 6.0%, for uphill and level ground, respectively). Thus, increased neuromuscular demands (higher forces per pedal stroke) during long-interval HIIT in cyclists may also be beneficial to cycling performance, as alluded to further in our specific application chapter on this sport (see chapter 15, Road Cycling).

Short Intervals

The next weapon we'll describe in detail is the short interval. This is probably the most useful and versatile format for practitioners due to the fact that we can hit almost all HIIT target types and explains why the weapon has received so much attention in the research literature. As alluded to in chapter 4, Martin is particularly passionate about this weapon based on his history, beginning in his youth and continuing through to his coaching and research work. In this section, we will show how short intervals, with bout durations ranging from 10 to 60 s, can be used to target type 1, 2, 3, and 4 acute responses.

O₂ (Oxidative) Responses to Short Intervals

The marker of acute aerobic response, T at $\dot{V}O_2$max, during short-interval runs to exhaustion has largely been shown to be related to the total exercise time (i.e., T_{lim}) (132). This intuitively implies that the first approach you can make toward maximizing T at $\dot{V}O_2$max during such sessions should be to focus on how you can adjust aspects of the interval format (intensity and duration of work and relief bouts) to increase the T_{lim}. In practice, of course, coaches will almost never prescribe HIIT sessions to exhaustion; they prescribe a series or set of short intervals (56, 136, 137, 173). In this context, it's important to consider the strategies needed to maximize T at $\dot{V}O_2$max within a given time period or to define time-efficient HIIT formats with respect to the T at $\dot{V}O_2$max/ exercise time ratio. That is, we need to determine the greatest T at $\dot{V}O_2$max that can be achieved within the total duration of the HIIT session we have available, not including the warm-up. In team sports especially, conditioning coaches often have only 10 to 20 min per session to develop the aerobic qualities of their players (see team sport chapters), so they need to ensure this time is used wisely.

Let's explore the variables we can manipulate to achieve this objective.

Exercise Intensity During Short Intervals

Billat et al. (18) were the first to show the effect of exercise intensity on T at $\dot{V}O_2$ during HIIT using 15 s/15 s short intervals in a group of senior (average age 52 yr) distance runners (v$\dot{V}O_2$max = 15.9 ± 1.8 km/h). While the concurrent manipulation of the relief interval intensity (60%-80% of v$\dot{V}O_2$max, which maintained an average HIIT intensity of 85%) might have partially influenced the $\dot{V}O_2$ responses, the authors showed that increasing work interval intensity from 90% to 100% of v$\dot{V}O_2$max was associated with a *small* improvement in the T at $\dot{V}O_2$/ exercise time ratio (81% versus 68%, ES = +0.5). However, the T at $\dot{V}O_2$/exercise time ratio (85%) was not substantially greater when the work interval was increased to 110% compared to 100% of v$\dot{V}O_2$max (ES = +0.2). The differences may be related to the fact that the lower amplitude (difference between exercise and recovery intensities) likely accelerates the T to $\dot{V}O_2$max (see figure 5.8).

Using a fixed relief interval intensity (figure 5.9) (83, 137, 175), increasing work intensity from 100% to 110% of v$\dot{V}O_2$max during a 30 s/30 s format in trained young runners (v$\dot{V}O_2$max = 17.7 ± 0.9 km/h) induced a *moderate* increase in the T at $\dot{V}O_2$/exercise time ratio (ES = +0.6), despite *very large* and *moderate* reductions in T_{lim} (ES = −4.4) and T at $\dot{V}O_2$max (ES = −0.7), respectively (175). A slight increase in work intensity from 100% to 105% of v$\dot{V}O_2$max during a 30 s/30 s short-interval format in well-trained triathletes (v$\dot{V}O_2$max = 19.8 ± 0.93 km/h) was associated with a *large* improvement in the T at $\dot{V}O_2$/ exercise time ratio (ES = +1.2) (137). The twofold magnitude difference in the Millet et al. (137) study compared to Thevenet et al. (175) (ES: +1.2 versus +0.6) is likely due to the fact that Millet's runs were not performed to exhaustion but implemented with predetermined sets. It is therefore possible that if the runs at 100% had been performed to exhaustion (137), this would have compensated for the lower efficiency of the protocol and decreased the difference in T at $\dot{V}O_2$max observed. Similarly, increasing the work intensity from 110% to 120% of v$\dot{V}O_2$max during a 15 s/15 s format in physical education students (v$\dot{V}O_2$max = 16.7 ± 1.3 km/h) led to a *large* improvement in the T at $\dot{V}O_2$/exercise time ratio (ES = +1.8) (83). Interestingly, in the study by Millet et al. (137), individual improvements in T at $\dot{V}O_2$ with the increase in work intensity were inversely correlated with the athletes' time constant for $\dot{V}O_2$ kinetics at exercise onset (r = 0.91, 90% CL (0.61; 0.98)), sug-

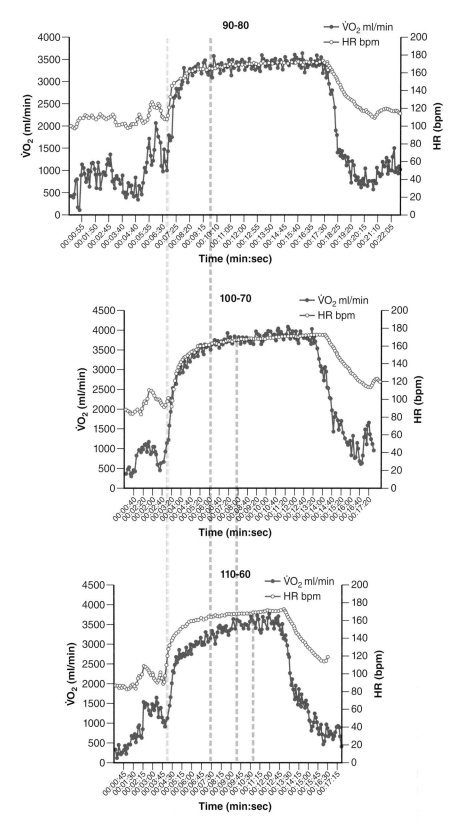

Figure 5.8 Lower amplitude (difference between exercise and recovery intensities) accelerates the T to V̇O₂max (red vertical dotted lines), as shown in the study by Billat et al. (18) using 15 s/15 s short intervals with work:relief intensities of 90%:80%, 100%:70%, and 110%:60% of vV̇O₂max.

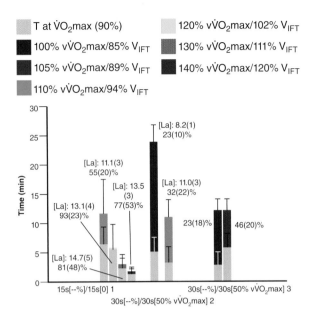

Figure 5.9 Mean ± SD total time and T at V̇O₂max during different short-interval HIIT as a function of changes in work interval intensity. Percentages refer to the mean ± SD T at V̇O₂max relative to total session time (83, 137, 175). [La]: post-exercise blood lactate.

Reprinted by permission of Springer Nature from M. Buchheit and P.B. Laursen, "High-Intensity Interval Training, Solutions to the Programming Puzzle: Part I: Cardiopulmonary Emphasis," *Sports Medicine* 43, no. 5 (2013): 313-338.

gesting that the time constant could be an important variable to consider when selecting HIIT variables (35, 137). Practically speaking, this data could imply that coaches should program short intervals at slightly higher intensities for athletes presenting with slow V̇O₂ kinetics (i.e., older/less trained (143)), or for athletes exercising on a bike (107). However, since increasing exercise intensity has other implications (e.g., greater anaerobic energy contribution, higher neuromuscular strain), such programming manipulations need to take a cost/benefit approach.

With respect to the use of very high exercise intensities (>102%/120% V_{IFT}/vV̇O₂max) for HIIT, while the T at V̇O₂/exercise time ratio is high (81 and 77% at 130 and 140% of vV̇O₂max, respectively), exercise capacity is typically impaired and hence, total T at V̇O₂ for a given HIIT session is usually relatively low (83) (i.e., 5 min, 47 s at 120% vV̇O₂max (83)). Nevertheless, the use of repeated series of such training can allow the accumulation of a sufficient T at V̇O₂max. Additionally, well-trained athletes are generally able to perform HIIT at this intensity for longer periods (i.e., >8 min (54, 56,

60, 80)), especially when V_{IFT}, instead of vV̇O₂max, is used (34).

Effect of Work Interval Duration on T at vV̇O₂max

The effect of work interval duration on systemic V̇O₂ responses during short-interval HIIT was one of the first parameters examined in the HIIT literature (6, 68). Surprisingly, however, there is little data available on repeated efforts lasting less than 15 s (figure 5.10), despite the common approach used by coaches (e.g., 10 s/10 s, 10 s/20 s) (26, 74). During very short runs (<10 s), energy requirements in working muscle are met predominantly by oxidative phosphorylation, with more than 50% of the V̇O₂ used derived from oxymyoglobin stores (6). During the recovery periods, oxymyoglobin stores are rapidly restored and then available for the following interval (6). As a result, the cardiopulmonary responses of such efforts are relatively low (13), unless exercise intensity is set at a very high level and/or relief intervals are short and intense enough so that they limit complete myoglobin resaturation. Therefore, in the context of HIIT involving short intervals (100%-120% vV̇O₂max or 89/105% V_{IFT}), work intervals ≥10 s may be required to elicit high

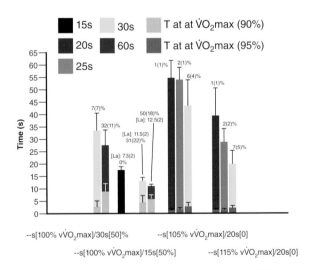

Figure 5.10 Mean ± SD total time and T at V̇O₂max during different short-interval HIIT as a function of changes in work interval duration. Percentages refer to the mean ± SD T at V̇O₂max relative to total session time. [La]: post-exercise blood lactate.

Reprinted by permission of Springer Nature from M. Buchheit and P.B. Laursen, "High-Intensity Interval Training, Solutions to the Programming Puzzle: Part I: Cardiopulmonary Emphasis," *Sports Medicine* 43, no. 5 (2013): 313-338.

$\dot{V}O_2$ responses. Indeed, prolonging exercise duration increases the relative aerobic energy requirements (91) and increasing work interval duration, while keeping work relief intervals constant, also increases T at $\dot{V}O_2$max (136, 159, 181). For example, extending work interval duration from 30 to 60 s using a fixed-relief duration of 30 s in well-trained triathletes (v$\dot{V}O_2$max = 19.9 ± 0.9 km/h) induced *very large* increases in T at v$\dot{V}O_2$max (9 versus 1.5 min, ES = +2.4), despite a shorter total session time (28 versus 34 min, ES = −0.9; change in the T at v$\dot{V}O_2$max/exercise ratio, ES = +2.8) (136). Similarly, in wrestlers (v$\dot{V}O_2$max = 16.3 ± 1.1 km/h), Rozenek et al. (159) showed that increasing running work interval duration from 15 to 30 s led to *very large* increases in T at $\dot{V}O_2$max (4 versus 0 min, ES = 2.9); a further increase in the interval duration to 60 s extended T at $\dot{V}O_2$max to 5.5 min (ES = 0.5 versus the 30 s condition). Considering the importance of $\dot{V}O_2$ kinetics for extending T at $\dot{V}O_2$max (137), these data suggest that longer work intervals (e.g., 30 s/30 s versus 15 s/15 s) are preferred for individuals with slow $\dot{V}O_2$ kinetics (i.e., older/less trained (143)) or for exercising on a bike (107).

Characteristics of the Recovery Interval Intensity and Its Impact on T at $\dot{V}O_2$max During Short Intervals

In concert with the HIIT recovery bout discussion started in chapter 4, recovery bout intensity also plays a major role in the $\dot{V}O_2$ response during HIIT involving short intervals since it affects both the actual $\dot{V}O_2$ during the sets and exercise capacity (and hence, indirectly T_{lim} and T at $\dot{V}O_2$max; figure 5.11 (85, 174, 176)). Compared to passive recovery, runs to exhaustion involving active recovery are consistently reported to be 40% to 80% shorter (81, 82, 85, 174, 176). Therefore, when considering runs to exhaustion during 15 s/15 s exercises, the absolute T at $\dot{V}O_2$max might not differ between active and passive recovery conditions (81) (ES = −0.3), but the T at $\dot{V}O_2$max/exercise time ratio is substantially greater when active recovery is implemented (ES = +0.9), a factor of clear importance when implementing predetermined sets of HIIT (56, 136, 173). During a 30 s/30 s exercise model, compared with passive recovery, recovery intensities of 50% and 67% of v$\dot{V}O_2$max were associated with *small* and *very large* increases in T at $\dot{V}O_2$max (ES = +0.4 and +0.1 compared to passive recovery, respectively) and the T at $\dot{V}O_2$max/exercise time ratio (ES = +2.3 and +4.1), respectively (174, 176). Increasing the recovery

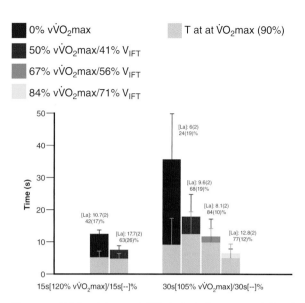

Figure 5.11 Mean ± SD total time and T at $\dot{V}O_2$max during different short-interval HIIT as a function of changes in relief interval intensity. Percentages refer to the mean ± SD T at $\dot{V}O_2$max relative to total session time. Mean ± SD [La] mmol/L is provided when available.

Reprinted by permission of Springer Nature from M. Buchheit and P.B. Laursen, "High-Intensity Interval Training, Solutions to the Programming Puzzle: Part I: Cardiopulmonary Emphasis," *Sports Medicine* 43, no. 5 (2013): 313-338.

intensity to 84% (the speed associated with the lactate threshold) *moderately* lowered T at $\dot{V}O_2$max (ES = −0.6) but *very largely* increased the T at $\dot{V}O_2$max/exercise time ratio (ES = +3.4).

In addition to limiting the drop in $\dot{V}O_2$ during the relief interval, which allows a greater $\dot{V}O_2$ to be reached during the subsequent exercise interval, active recovery also accelerates T to $\dot{V}O_2$max (figure 5.12). T to $\dot{V}O_2$max during different work and relief interval intensities involving short HIIT (30 s/30 s) was examined in young endurance-trained athletes (174-176). Not surprisingly, these studies showed shorter T to $\dot{V}O_2$max values for work intensities ≥105% v$\dot{V}O_2$max and relief intensities ≥60% v$\dot{V}O_2$max. Conversely, using slightly lower work and/or relief interval intensities (i.e., work 100% and relief 50% v$\dot{V}O_2$max) caused the runners to take more than 7 min to reach $\dot{V}O_2$max. Despite no statistical differences (174-176), all ES between the different work/relief ratios examined were *small* to *very large* (figure 5.12).

In the field then, T to $\dot{V}O_2$max might be accelerated by manipulating HIIT variables during the first interval of the session, i.e., using more intense

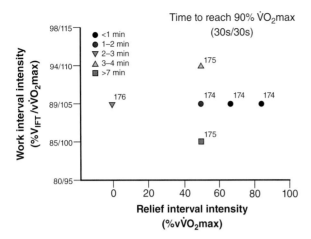

Figure 5.12 Time to reach $\dot{V}O_2$max during HIIT with short intervals as a function of both work and relief interval intensities. Generally higher intensities of work and relief interval combinations speed the T to $\dot{V}O_2$max. (175); (176); (174). Numbers refer to references.

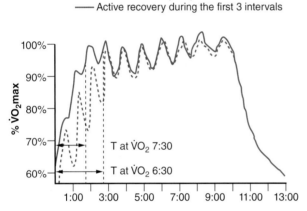

Figure 5.13 Effect of active recovery during the three first intervals only (the rest being passive) on $\dot{V}O_2$ during HIIT with short intervals.

work and/or relief interval intensities during the first 2 to 3 intervals or using longer work intervals and/or shorter relief intervals. This effect is illustrated in figure 5.13, where T to $\dot{V}O_2$max was shown to be faster when active versus passive recovery was used during the first three intervals of a short-interval sequence. The fact that active recovery had a likely greater impact on T at $\dot{V}O_2$max during the 30 s/30 s (174, 176) compared with the 15 s/15 s (81) exercise model is related to the fact that $\dot{V}O_2$ reaches lower values during 30 s of passive rest, which directly affects $\dot{V}O_2$ levels during the following effort.

In general, the characteristic of the recovery interval intensity can be aligned with the work intensity, with higher relief interval intensities used for lower work interval intensities (18) and lower relief exercise intensities used for higher work interval intensities and durations (83, 137, 175).

Series Duration, Sets, and T at $\dot{V}O_2$max for Short Intervals

Dividing HIIT sessions into sets has been consistently shown to lower the total T at $\dot{V}O_2$max (56, 136, 173). For example, in endurance-trained young runners ($v\dot{V}O_2$max = 17.7 ± 0.3 km/h), performing 4-min recoveries (30 s rest, 3 min at 50% $v\dot{V}O_2$max, 30 s rest) every 6 repetitions (30 s/30 s) was associated with a *moderately* lower T at $\dot{V}O_2$max (ES = −0.8) despite *very large* increases in T_{lim} (ES = +4.3). The T at $\dot{V}O_2$max/exercise time ratio was therefore *very largely* reduced (ES = −2.3) (173). This is likely related to the time these athletes needed to return to high $\dot{V}O_2$ levels after each relief interval, irrespective of the active recovery used. While reviewing such studies could infer we advise athletes to consistently run short intervals to exhaustion to optimize T at $\dot{V}O_2$max, this would likely be challenging, psychologically speaking, for both coaches and athletes alike. This is likely why HIIT sessions to exhaustion are rarely practiced. In the field, the number of intervals programmed should be related to the goals of the session (total load or total T at $\dot{V}O_2$max expected), as well as to T to $\dot{V}O_2$max and the estimated T at $\dot{V}O_2$max/exercise time ratio of the session.

If we consider that a goal T at $\dot{V}O_2$max of ≈10 min per session is appropriate to elicit important cardiopulmonary adaptations, athletes should expect to exercise for a total of 30 min using a 30 s [110% $v\dot{V}O_2$max]/30 s [50% $v\dot{V}O_2$max] format, since the T at $\dot{V}O_2$max/total exercise time ratio is approximately 30%. While it's unrealistic to perform a single 30 min session, we can break such a session into 3 sets of 10 to 12 min (adding 1-2 min per set or series to compensate for the time needed to regain $\dot{V}O_2$max during the second and third sets). This is a typical session used regularly by elite distance runners in the field. A lower volume (shorter series or less sets) is also used in other sports (i.e., in team sports, a T at $\dot{V}O_2$max of 5-7 min is likely sufficient (35)) and/or for maintenance during unloading or recovery periods in an endurance athlete's program. In elite handball for example, 2 × (20 × 10 s [110% V_{IFT}]/20 s [0] for a series duration of 10 min) is common practice, and might enable players to spend ≈7 min at

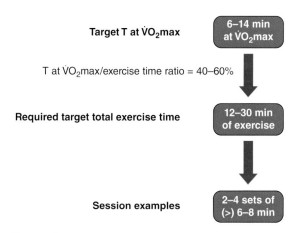

Figure 5.14 In the absence of best practice or scientific guidelines (15, 16, 21), the target total exercise time of short-interval HIIT can be defined using both T at $\dot{V}O_2$max and the T at $\dot{V}O_2$/exercise time ratio. A good target T at $\dot{V}O_2$max will range from 6 to 14 min at $\dot{V}O_2$max with a T at $\dot{V}O_2$/exercise time ratio of 40% to 60%. Total target exercise time will correspondingly range from 12 to 30 min.

$\dot{V}O_2$max (considering a T at $\dot{V}O_2$max/exercise ratio of 35%, see chapter 27, Handball). In soccer, HIIT sessions such as $2 \times (12\text{-}15 \times 15$ s $[120\%$ $V_{Inc.Test}]/15$ s [0]) are often implemented (80), which corresponds to ≈ 6 min at $\dot{V}O_2$max (14 min with a T at $\dot{V}O_2$max/ exercise time ratio of $\approx 45\%$ (81)). See for example chapter 30, Soccer. It is however worth noting that throughout the years, Martin and some of his colleagues involved in elite team sports have had the tendency to decrease the volume of HIIT work with their athletes (e.g., $2 \times$ series of 4-5 min rather than 2-3 $\times$ 6-10 min as during their early careers), without any clear indication of a detrimental effect on physiological adaptations and performance. While only anecdotal, the minimum volume of HIIT required to elicit adaptations and improve performance in this population may be less than previously thought, and this should be a topic for future research.

A summary of the oxidative response recommendations for short intervals is shown in figure 5.14.

Short Versus Long Intervals and T at $\dot{V}O_2$max

A direct comparison between long- and short-HIIT sessions, with respect to T at $\dot{V}O_2$max, has to our knowledge only been reported twice in highly trained athletes. Gajer et al. (90) compared T at $\dot{V}O_2$max between 6 × 600 m (track session, 102%

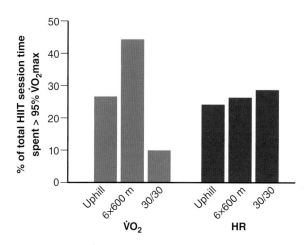

Figure 5.15 $\dot{V}O_2$ and HR responses during uphill and track HIIT with long intervals and HIIT with short intervals. Note: SD not provided by the authors. Note once more the dissociation between $\dot{V}O_2$ and HR.

Data from B. Gajer, C. Hanon, D. Lehenaff, and J.C. Vollmer, "Analyse comparée de différentes séances de développement de VO2max," in *Expertise et Sport de Haut Niveau: Actes des Entretiens de l'INSEP*, Novembre 2002, edited by D. Lehénhaff and C. Mathieu (Paris: INSEP, 2003).

v$\dot{V}O_2$max, run in ≈ 1 min, 40 s) and 10 repetitions of a 30 s/30 s HIIT session (work/relief intensity: 105/50% v$\dot{V}O_2$max) in elite middle-distance runners (v$\dot{V}O_2$max = 21.2 ± 0.6 km/h). While $\dot{V}O_2$ reached 105% v$\dot{V}O_2$max during the track session, $\dot{V}O_2$max was not actually attained during the 30 s/30 s session (figure 5.15). If the track session is considered as the reference session (T at $\dot{V}O_2$max/exercise time ratio: 44%), T at $\dot{V}O_2$max was *very largely* lower during the 30 s/30 s intervals (10%, ES ≈ -2.6). Similarly, Millet et al. (136) showed that performing 2 min/2 min intervals enabled triathletes to attain a *very largely* longer T at $\dot{V}O_2$max compared to a 30 s/30 s session (ES = +2.2, T at $\dot{V}O_2$max/exercise time ratio = +2.2). Long intervals were, however, *moderately* less efficient than the 60 s/30 s effort model (T at $\dot{V}O_2$max/exercise time ratio, ES = −0.8) (136). Taken together, these data suggest that long intervals and/or short intervals with a work/relief ratio >1 should be preferred due to the greater T at $\dot{V}O_2$max/exercise time ratio, when focus on aerobic development is important.

Anaerobic Glycolytic Energy Contribution to Short Intervals

As with long intervals, in which the aerobic oxidative system is the primary physiological response apparent, there is still substantial involvement from the anaerobic glycolytic energy contribution for short intervals. Thus, short intervals can be manipulated to target the anaerobic glycolytic energy component associated with type 3 and 4 acute responses, while lowered contributions enable the type 1 and 2 responses.

Work Interval Intensity and Duration

When we consider short-interval HIIT sessions (i.e., 15 s/15 s) of a similar mean intensity (i.e., 85% of $v\dot{V}O_2$max), perhaps not surprisingly, we find that higher work interval intensities elicit greater blood lactate responses and also shorten time to exhaustion (18). For example, blood lactate at exhaustion was 9.2 ± 1.3 mmol/L for work/relief intensities of 90/80% of $v\dot{V}O_2$max, 9.8 ± 1.4 mmol/L for work/relief intensities of 100/70% (ES=0.4 vs. 90/80%), and 11.3 ± 1.3 mmol/L for work/relief intensities of 110/60% (ES=1.6 and 1.1 vs. 90/80% and 100/70%, respectively) (18). The effect of work duration on anaerobic contribution is also straightforward, with the longer high-intensity exercise periods eliciting larger draws on the glycolytic system. Interestingly however, as shown in figure 5.16, the repetition of very short efforts (i.e., 10 s) will in fact achieve a very limited engagement of anaerobic energy contribution, thanks predominantly to the use of the muscle's myoglobin stores. These myoglobin stores enable more reliance on the aerobic energy system during such very short duration intervals, and as a result, limit the anaerobic contribution.

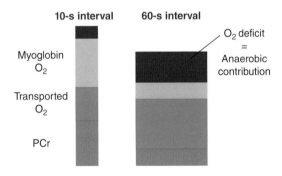

Figure 5.16 Theoretical illustration of the role that the stored oxygen in myoglobin plays during HIIT with short intervals of different durations, relative to the energy provided by transported oxygen (O_2) and phosphocreatine (PCr). The O_2 deficit (and resulting anaerobic energy contribution) is highly limited for very short intervals, during which the O_2 linked with myoglobin supplies most of the energy demands.

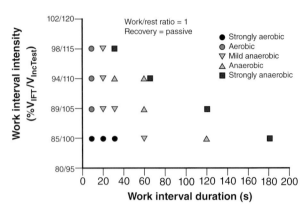

Figure 5.17 Schematic illustration of the energy system requirements for different forms of HIIT, with respect to blood lactate accumulation. Clearly, anaerobic involvement relates to higher work interval intensities and longer work interval durations. Strongly aerobic: <3 mmol·L⁻¹·5 min⁻¹; aerobic: 3 mmol·L⁻¹·5 min⁻¹; mildly anaerobic: 4 mmol·L⁻¹·5 min⁻¹; anaerobic: 5 mmol·L⁻¹·5 min⁻¹; strongly anaerobic: 6 mmol·L⁻¹·5 min⁻¹. T_{lim} time to exhaustion, $v\dot{V}O_2$max, minimal velocity associated with maximal oxygen uptake.

Reprinted by permission of Springer Nature from M. Buchheit and P.B. Laursen, "High-Intensity Interval Training, Solutions to the Programming Puzzle: Part II: Anaerobic Energy, Neuromuscular Load and Practical Applications," *Sports Medicine* 43 no. 10 (2013): 927-954.

The respective effects of work interval intensity and duration on blood lactate accumulation have also been examined in semiprofessional soccer players (peak incremental test running speed, $V_{Inc.Test}$ (figure 5.6) = 16.5 ± 2.3 km/h), during HIIT that included intervals lasting 10 to 30 s (17, 26, 76, 83, 133, 159, 162, 167, 180). Combined with data collected in other studies (e.g., see (55, 180)), this latter experimentation (26) shows how the selection of the appropriate combinations of different HIIT variables may be needed to reach specific blood lactate accumulation targets (figure 5.6). For exercise at 100% of $V_{Inc.Test}$, only work intervals longer than 1 min tend to be associated with high blood lactate levels. With work intensities of 110% $V_{Inc.Test}$, however, anaerobic glycolytic energy contribution is already likely increased when exercise is longer than 30 s. At a fixed work interval intensity, increasing the work/relief ratio is associated, not surprisingly, with substantial increases in the initial rate of blood lactate accumulation (figure 5.17) (159). Overall, however, with all data pooled from both long- and short-interval weapons (figure 5.6), it is clear that many short-interval formats will allow lactate to remain well below long-interval HIIT levels, which may be the key advantage of using the short-HIIT weapon in certain cases (type 1 and 2 versus type 3 and 4).

Finally, it is worth noting that for extremely high exercise intensities (i.e., 20 s at 170% of pVO$_2$max interspersed with 10 s rest periods for 2 min), the accumulated O$_2$ deficit may reach maximum levels (172) (i.e., similar to the anaerobic capacity of the subjects, defined as the maximal accumulated O$_2$ deficit during an exhaustive 2-3 min of continuous exercise) (129) (chapter 3).

Glycogen Use With Short Intervals

As discussed in chapters 1 and 3, high-intensity exercise specifically draws on greater rates of carbohydrate oxidation, predominantly from a limited stored glycogen reserve. Its high use with HIIT is important to appreciate so as to appropriately manage (see factor 12 discussion in chapter 4). Figure 5.18 shows the glycogen degradation following different short-interval formats that all display the same intensity and work:rest ratio, differing only in their durations (7). Note from the figure how the longer exercise durations elicit higher blood lactate levels and larger decrements in muscle glycogen. Thus, longer short-interval formats will have a marked effect on both lactate production and the muscle glycogen use, and such training

needs to be managed and programmed appropriately (183, 184).

Recovery Period Intensity and Duration

As most authors examining the impact of the recovery period intensity during HIIT on blood lactate accumulation have used runs to exhaustion, which are not typically done in practice, the specific impact of the recovery interval intensity on blood lactate accumulation during actual field-based HIIT sessions performed by athletes is not clear (81, 174, 176). With increasing recovery intensity during a supramaximal 30 s (105% vVO$_2$max)/30 s effort model, a progressive increase in blood lactate has been shown at exhaustion, despite a progressive decrease in exercise time (estimated from pH values: ≈6±2, 10±2, and 12.5±2 mmol/L for recovery period intensities of 50%, 67%, and 84% of vVO$_2$max, respectively) (174, 176). In contrast, compared to passive recovery, active recovery (40%-50% vVO$_2$max) during a repeated submaximal 15 s (102% vVO$_2$max)/15 s HIIT model has consistently been associated with *slightly* lower blood lactate values at exhaustion (10.7 ± 2.0 versus 11.7±2.1 mmol/L, ES=−0.5 (81) and 12.6±1.7 versus 13.1±2.7 mmol/L, ES=−0.2 (85)). In the only study in which HIIT (15s [102% vVO$_2$max]/15 s) was examined over comparable durations, active recovery

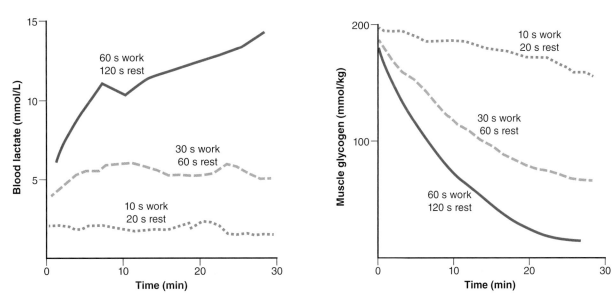

Figure 5.18 Lactate and glycogen levels during HIIT with constant work intensity, equivalent work:rest ratio, but varying bout durations.

Reprinted by permission from B.S. Rushall, "Interval Training, High-Intensity Interval-Training, and USRPT, Version 1.1," *Swimming Science Bulletin* 55 (2015), https://coachsci.sdsu.edu/swim/bullets/55%20ITHIITUSRPT.pdf. Adapted from P.O. Åstrand and K. Rodahl, *Textbook of Work Physiology: Physiological Bases of Exercise*, 2nd ed. (New York: McGraw-Hill, 1977).

was shown to be associated with *moderately* higher post-HIIT blood lactate values (10.7 ± 2.0 versus 9.2 ± 1.4 mmol/L, ES = +0.9 (82)). If we consider that the lower muscle oxygenation level apparent with active recovery (85) (chapter 4) generally triggers anaerobic glycolytic system contribution during HIIT (69, 70), then an active recovery during short-interval HIIT is more likely to be associated with a *higher* anaerobic contribution (85). If we also consider that active recovery may be the preferred method for increasing T at $\dot{V}O_2$max during HIIT with short intervals, programming active-recovery HIIT sessions and achieving low blood lactate levels may be difficult. In practice, reducing the work/relief ratio and using passive recovery, as during a supramaximal HIIT format (e.g., 10 s [>100%V_{IFT}]/20 s [0], holding V_{IFT} for the final speed reached at the end of the 30-15 intermittent fitness test, figure 5.6), provides an interesting alternative with respect to achieving both a high T at $\dot{V}O_2$max with moderate lactate production (i.e., type 3). In the latter case, the work interval duration prevents excessive anaerobic energy release yet is still great enough to achieve a high O_2 and the passive recovery duration allows for partial phosphocreatine (PCr) resynthesis (103), while limiting the drop in O_2 (figure 5.16). An alternative approach is to use a submaximal work interval intensity ($\leq$100% v$\dot{V}O_2$max, which is less likely to trigger anaerobic glycolytic energy contribution) with active recovery periods ($\geq$50% v$\dot{V}O_2$max) (24) (i.e., type 1). It is also worth noting that all field-based HIIT formats with short intervals are associated with low initial rates of blood lactate accumulation compared with long intervals (5, 68). As a result, the short-interval format may be a more sustainable, regular training weapon to use in the programs of some athletes, and less likely to elicit excessive sympathetic nervous system engagement that could lead to overtraining (chapter 7).

Work Interval Modality

The introduction of changes of direction (COD) into HIIT has been shown to moderately increase blood lactate accumulation, irrespective of the work intensity and duration (ES $\approx$ +1, for all short-HIIT models tested, i.e., 10 s/10 s, 15 s/15 s, and 30 s/30 s) (74). This is not surprising given the increased mechanical demands of the repeated accelerations inherent with consecutive COD (148) and the fact that on average, the actual running speed is higher with COD (to compensate for the time lost while changing direction). In fact, COD running is likely to increase peripheral (particularly biarticular locomotor muscles) and, in turn, systemic O_2 demands (with a possibly greater upper-body muscle participation). Therefore, while absolute anaerobic energy contribution is likely higher with COD (2, 104), the percentage contribution to total energy expenditure may be lower during high-intensity runs (47). When the intensity of the work intervals during HIIT was adjusted for the time lost with COD (figure 5.19), blood lactate values were surprisingly similar or even lower compared to HIIT without COD (37). The acute blood lactate responses to different short-interval HIIT formats with 10 s/20 s, including either running, sprinting, hopping, or squatting efforts every second work interval, were also compared in 8 highly trained adolescent handball players ($V_{Inc.Test}$ 16-17 km/h; figure 5.20) (72). Compared to the running-only condition, there were *very large* lower blood lactate concentrations following the sprinting (ES = −3.5) and squatting (ES = −2.9) conditions, but there was no clear difference with hopping (ES = 0.0). While the cardiorespiratory responses to these specific sessions should also be considered, these latter results provide relevant information for coaches wanting to manipulate the anaerobic glycolytic contribution to HIIT sessions within their periodized training plans.

Finally, running surface is another variable that likely affects anaerobic glycolytic energy release during HIIT. When team sport athletes (3 km running time = 12 min, 34 s) performed 3 sets of 7 × 25 to 45 s intervals performed at the highest sustainable intensity (W/R ratio 1/2 to 3) in the sand, their end-session blood lactate was largely greater (ES = +1.0) than when they did the same session on grass (25).

Neuromuscular Responses to Short-Interval HIIT Sessions

Short-interval HIIT can be manipulated to adjust for the degree of neuromuscular response. The neuromuscular response is emphasized in type 2 and 4 short intervals, while the response is attenuated in type 1 and 3 short intervals.

The acute neuromuscular responses to 5 × 300 m runs (77% of maximal sprinting speed [MSS], $\approx$120%-130% v$\dot{V}O_2$max) interspersed by 1 min recovery periods (100 m walk-jog) was examined in well-trained middle- and long-distance runners (164). Despite nonsignificant changes in maximal torque during a knee extensor MVC (−5%, with ES $\approx$ −1.2, which still shows a large effect), the HIIT session caused severe acute peripheral fatigue, as

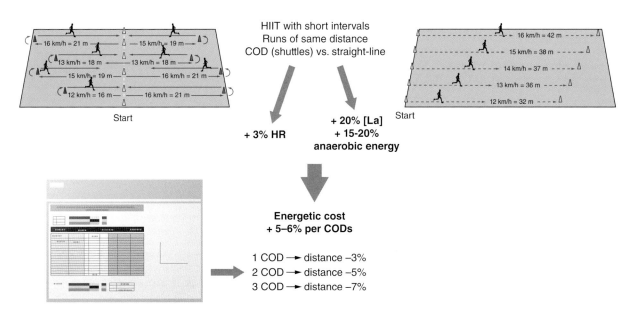

Figure 5.19 Empirical method used to account for the extra energetic cost of 180° changes of direction (COD). The additional energy requirements from oxidative and anaerobic systems when comparing COD versus straight-line runs is estimated to be around 5% to 6% during typical short-interval HIIT. This is based on the 3% higher heart rates (HR, upper left panel) (74), 20% higher blood lactates [La] (lower left panel) (74), and greater anaerobic contribution at maximal intensity (upper right panel) (47) during runs including COD compared to straight-line efforts. To compensate for this additional energy cost, practitioners are advised to remove 2% to 3% from the target running distance per COD (47). The free spreadsheet that allows such calculations is available via the 30-15$_{IFT}$ app at https://30-15ift.com.

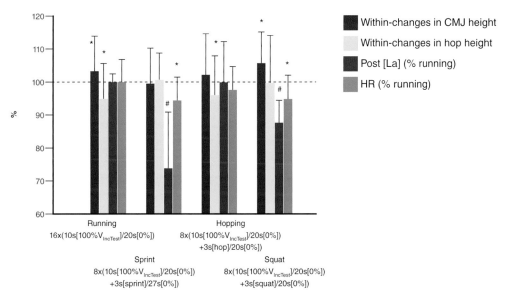

Figure 5.20 Changes in physiological responses and neuromuscular performance following different high-intensity interval training formats. Values are mean±SD. Changes in countermovement jump (CMJ) and hopping (Hop) height following four different high-intensity interval training sessions (short intervals [10 s/20 s] including running and, every second work interval, either running again or sprinting, hopping, or squatting efforts) and differences in mean heart rate (HR) and post-exercise blood lactate ([La]) compared to the running-only condition (*: moderate standardized difference; #: large standardized difference).

Reprinted by permission of Springer Nature from M. Buchheit and P.B. Laursen, "High-Intensity Interval Training, Solutions to the Programming Puzzle: Part II: Anaerobic Energy, Neuromuscular Load and Practical Applications," *Sports Medicine* 43 no. 10 (2013): 927-954.

evidenced by reduced efficiency of excitation-contraction coupling (e.g., –28% for twitch torque, ES >–5). Muscle contractile function was recovered and even improved within 10 min following the session (e.g., +11% for twitch torque, ES >1), while maximal torque during the MVC remained depressed for at least 120 min (≈–5%-6%, ES < –1.2). Due to the task dependency of acute muscular fatigue (86), the potential carryover effects of HIIT-related fatigue on subsequent training sessions involving sport-specific movement patterns (e.g., sprints, squats) is not straightforward and requires further research. In one study that assessed neuromuscular performance after an HIIT session (3 sets of 7 × 25 to 45 s intervals performed at the highest sustainable intensity, W/R ratio 1/2 to 3), most measures showed a return to baseline within 24 h (25). As well, the recovery of some measures was slightly better when the session was performed on sand versus grass. It is possible, therefore, that longer recovery periods may be required when sessions are performed on a harder surface (e.g., track, road). As well, consideration for the run surface and its influence on the neuromuscular load should be considered when programming run training.

While direct comparisons between long- and short-bout HIIT have yet to be documented, the acute neuromuscular load may be greater with short intervals for the following reasons.

1. Work intensity is generally higher with shorter intervals. While the majority of muscle fibers might already be recruited during long intervals (considering a minimal recruitment threshold at >75%-85% v$\dot{V}O_2$max for both type I and II fibers (4, 98)), the firing rate and relative force development per fiber is likely greater during short intervals (106).

2. Short intervals require frequent accelerations, decelerations, and reaccelerations (the occurrences of which are increased if the intervals are performed over shuttles). In addition to the increased metabolic and muscle force demands during acceleration phases of high-intensity exercise (78, 148), the completion of short intervals requires achievement of a greater absolute speed. For example, for a shuttle run completed at 120% of v$\dot{V}O_2$max in the field, a small portion (i.e., 1-3 s) of such a run may in fact need to be run at 135% to compensate for the time lost during both the acceleration and deceleration phases (figure 5.21) (82). When this high-speed

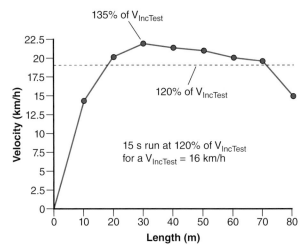

Figure 5.21 Example of the velocity versus distance relationship for a subject running 80 m in 15 s during a shuttle run (120% of V$_{IncTest}$, equal to 16 km/h). Portions of such a shuttle run actually need to be run at 135% of V$_{IncTest}$ to account for the required changes of direction, which has direct effects on neuromuscular load.

Reprinted by permission of Springer Customer Service Centre GmbH from G. Dupont, N. Blondel, and S. Berthoin, "Performance for Short Intermittent Runs: Active Recovery vs. Passive Recovery," *European Journal of Sport Physiology* 89 no. 6 (2003): 548-554.

portion of HIIT is considered in relation to the percentage of MSS and anaerobic speed reserve achieved (>80% and >50%, respectively), the level of neuromuscular engagement is high (106) and should be considered within the context of training load and injury management (especially hamstring muscles (178) and traumatic-type injuries (88, 147, 166)).

3. For unique athletes, such as extremely tall or heavy basketball or rugby players, the musculoskeletal load of long intervals might actually be higher than during short intervals, due potentially to poor running technique and economy. Therefore, for these particular athletes, long run-based intervals should be avoided, or implemented on soft surfaces (e.g., sand, grass (25)), bikes, or rowing ergometers to prevent injuries.

While the specific impact of COD on the neuromuscular system during field-based HIIT sessions has yet to be examined in detail, it may exacerbate lower-limb muscular fatigue compared to straight-line running due to the additional accelerations and decelerations required (32). The impact of a strength-oriented HIIT session on the neuromuscular system was also examined in 8 high-level endurance runners ($V_{IncTest} = 20.7 \pm 1.7$ km/h) (72, 77). Interestingly, when repeating six 200 m runs at 90%-95% of $v\dot{V}O_2$max (36-38 s) with alternate 30 s dynamic or explosive strength exercises, the runners avoided impairment in leg stiffness during running (8.08 ± 1.49 versus 7.87 ± 1.31 kN/m, ES < -0.2). While this might be related to the specific population of athletes (distance runners), this finding suggests that such training is well tolerated by distance runners and might have limited carryover effects on subsequent sessions. Whether injury risk is increased from such training is not known, but the increased load on the musculoskeletal system should be considered (77). Finally, the impact of different running patterns and exercise modes on acute neuromuscular responses during HIIT with short intervals was also examined in adolescent handball players (see chapter 27, Handball) (72). The acute neuromuscular responses to the four different HIIT sessions were protocol specific, with improvements in CMJ height shown following the running and squatting formats (possible postactivation potentiation (113)), and reductions in hopping height shown following the running and hopping conditions (possible neuromuscular fatigue related to localized overload on these muscle groups; figure 5.20). While the effect of these sessions on neuromuscular fatigue over longer durations (i.e., 24-48 h) is unknown, these data suggest that in team sport players, running patterns and exercise modes have important implications for programming, which should be considered with respect to other training sessions to avoid overload or injury (see chapter 7) and maximize adaptation.

Finally, in direct alignment with the anaerobic contribution, running surface has likely an acute effect on neuromuscular function. For example, it's reasonable to assume that softer surfaces (e.g., sand) will reduce impact force on the lower limbs compared to harder surfaces (e.g., grass or track (92)), which is likely to be of help for athletes returning from injuries or during periods of high training volume. Whether these acute loading differences substantially influence neuromuscular recovery in the following hours or days requires further research. Nevertheless, 24 h following intense short HIIT on the grass, these team sport athletes (25) moderately increased their CMJ and maintained repeated sprint performance, while after the same session performed in the sand, their CMJ was unaffected and their

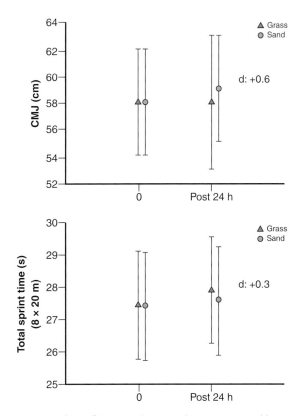

Figure 5.22 Change in countermovement jump (CMJ) and total repeated sprint time following HIIT with short intervals performed either on the sand or on grass (25).

repeated-sprint performance was slightly impaired (figure 5.22) (25).

Repeated-Sprint Training

Repeated-sprint training (figure 4.15), or a repeated-sprint sequence (RSS), is generally defined as the repetition of more than two short ($\leq$10 s) all-out sprints interspersed with a short recovery period ($<$60 s) (95). Recall that RSSs are used for type 4 and 5 targets, involving varying blends of acute oxidative, anaerobic glycolytic, and neuromuscular responses.

O₂ (Oxidative) Responses to Repeated-Sprint Sequences

To bring this section on RSS into proper context for the reader, it may be helpful to review figure 4.6, which shows the mean $\dot{V}O_2$ during six all-out 4 s running sprints in team sport athletes (44). Indeed, compared to the extensive data available on cardiorespiratory responses to long and short HIIT, relatively little has been presented on the acute responses

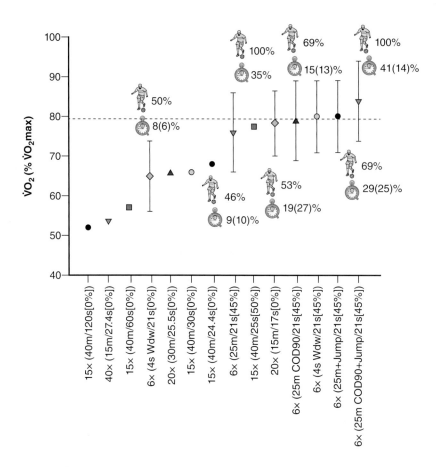

Figure 5.23 Mean±SD $\dot{V}O_2$ responses during selected repeated-sprint sequences. The intensity of the relief interval (i.e., [percentage]) is expressed as a fraction of the $\dot{V}O_2$max. When available, both the percentage of participants that reached $\dot{V}O_2$max (runner) and the mean±SD time spent above 90% of $\dot{V}O_2$max (clock) are provided.

Reprinted by permission of Springer Nature from M. Buchheit and P.B. Laursen, "High-Intensity Interval Training, Solutions to the Programming Puzzle: Part I: Cardiopulmonary Emphasis," *Sports Medicine* 43 no. 5 (2013): 313-338.

to RSS. Early in the 1990s, Balsom et al. (8, 9) demonstrated that RSSs were aerobically demanding and showed that this form of training can induce an aerobic response in excess of 65% $\dot{V}O_2$max. Dupont et al. (84) have also shown that soccer players can reach $\dot{V}O_2$max with repeated sprinting. As shown in our two-part review, shown here in figure 5.23, we reanalyzed data from previous studies (36, 43, 44, 52) to provide T at $\dot{V}O_2$max values for several forms of RSS (8, 9, 36, 43, 44, 52, 84). This analysis showed that when manipulating key variables already described (figure 2 in (33)), $\dot{V}O_2$max is often reached and sustained for 10% to 40% of the entire RSS duration. If RSSs are repeated 2 or 3 times a session, as is often done (29, 57, 60), the majority of athletes will spend up to 2 to 3 min at $\dot{V}O_2$max during the sprints.

As illustrated in figure 5.24, to increase T at v$\dot{V}O_2$max during an RSS, sprints or efforts should

last at least 4 s and recovery should be active and less than 20 s (8, 9, 36, 43, 44, 52, 84). The introduction of jumps following the sprints (36) and/or changes in direction (43) are also useful since these may increase systemic O_2 demand without the need for increasing sprint distance, which could lead to inappropriate muscular strain and/or greater injury risk. Nevertheless, with very short passive recovery periods (i.e., 17 s), some athletes can reach $\dot{V}O_2$max by repeating only 3 s sprints (15 m). Nevertheless, with RSS, players do not always reach $\dot{V}O_2$max and T at $\dot{V}O_2$max shows high inter-individual variations (CV = 30%-100%) (84). For example, when considering the four different forms of RSS performed in the same group of 13 athletes (36, 43), it was observed that 6 athletes (45%) reached $\dot{V}O_2$max on four occasions, 1 (8%) on three, 4 (31%) on two, and 2 (15%) never reached $\dot{V}O_2$max during any of the RSSs. When

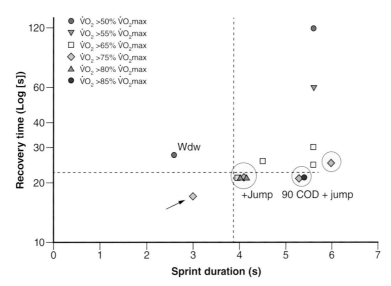

Figure 5.24 The mean $\dot{V}O_2$ responses during the repeated-sprint sequences presented are categorized into six color-coded families (based on the % of $\dot{V}O_2$max elicited) and then plotted as a function of sprint and recovery duration. The dashed lines represent the shorter sprint and recovery durations likely needed to achieve at least 80% of $\dot{V}O_2$max. Circles indicate active recovery. Note (see arrow) that 75% of $\dot{V}O_2$max can be achieved with very short sprints (i.e., 15 m) with passive recovery when sprints are interspersed with very short pauses (i.e., 17 s). COD: changes of direction; $\dot{V}O_2$: oxygen uptake; $\dot{V}O_2$max: maximal $\dot{V}O_2$; v$\dot{V}O_2$max: minimal running speed required to elicit $\dot{V}O_2$max. Wdw refers to sprints performed on a nonmotorized treadmill.

Reprinted by permission of Springer Nature from M. Buchheit and P.B. Laursen, "High-Intensity Interval Training, Solutions to the Programming Puzzle: Part I: Cardiopulmonary Emphasis," *Sports Medicine* 43 no. 5 (2013): 313-338.

the data from the four RSSs were pooled, the number of times that $\dot{V}O_2$max was reached was inversely related to $\dot{V}O_2$max (r = −0.61, 90% confidence limits, CL (−0.84;−0.19)). Similarly, the total T at $\dot{V}O_2$max over the four different RSSs was inversely correlated with $\dot{V}O_2$max (r = −0.55, 90%; CL (−0.85;0.00)). These data indicate that, with respect to T at $\dot{V}O_2$max, the use in athletes of high fitness for targeting an acute oxidative response is questionable.

Anaerobic Glycolytic Energy Contribution During RSS

The all-out sprint nature of RSS naturally elicits a large anaerobic glycolytic contribution component in its acute response, and hits both type 4 and 5 targets. As shown in figure 5.25, end-exercise blood lactate values reported for RSS can range from 6 to 18 mmol/L (1, 8, 9, 36, 44, 46, 52, 64, 84, 125, 140) and can reach very high levels, i.e., similar to those reached with lactate production training (all-out 30 s efforts (115) or 300 m run at the speed maintained during a 400 m run (v400m) (99)). While methodological inconsistencies can partly explain the differences between studies, these data show that

manipulating the sprint distance or duration, the recovery intensity or duration, and work modality substantially impacts the anaerobic glycolytic contribution to an RSS.

Work:Relief Ratio

When sprints are longer than 4 s (i.e., >25 m) and when the recovery interval is less than 20 s and generally active, the initial rate of blood lactate accumulation is consistently high (i.e., >10 mmol·L^{-1}·5min^{-1}; figure 5.26). In contrast, shorter sprints and/or longer recovery durations can be less taxing on the anaerobic energy system. The initial rate of blood lactate accumulation during an RSS is also largely related to the work/relief interval, irrespective of the sprinting distance (figure 5.26). Interestingly, extremely high initial rates of blood lactate accumulation, that is, greater than those observed for all-out 30 s efforts (115) or 300 m run at 400 m sprinting speed (99)), can be reached when repeating 4 s sprints on a nonmotorized treadmill (44) or when long sprints (>6 s) are separated by short recovery durations (≈17 s) (140). These observations are of particular interest for team sport coaches wanting to implement lactate production

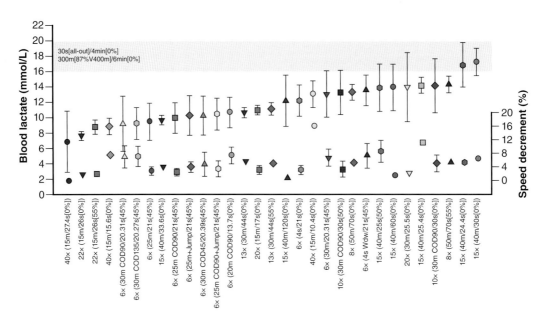

Figure 5.25 Estimated anaerobic energy contribution to different repeated-sprint sequence formats. Blood lactate measured following the different repeated-sprint sequences and their associated speed decrement (values are mean±SD when available). The gray rectangular box represents the initial rate of blood lactate ([La]) increase during lactate production training, i.e., all-out sprints or at the speed maintained during a 400 m run (v400m).

Reprinted by permission of Springer Nature from M. Buchheit and P.B. Laursen, "High-Intensity Interval Training, Solutions to the Programming Puzzle: Part II: Anaerobic Energy, Neuromuscular Load and Practical Applications," *Sports Medicine* 43 no. 10 (2013): 927-954.

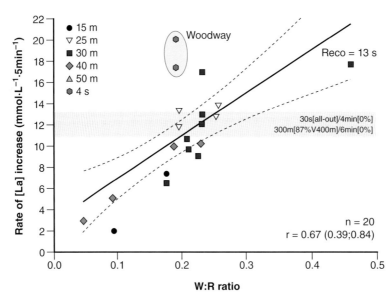

Figure 5.26 Relationships (r [90% confidence limits]) between the initial rate of blood lactate ([La]) increase during select repeated-sprint sequences and work:rest (W:R) ratios. Correlation coefficients are provided with 90% confidence intervals. The gray rectangular box represents the initial rate of blood lactate increase during lactate production training, i.e., all-out sprints or at the speed maintained during a 400 m run (v400m). The black oval highlights the two sprints performed on a nonmotorized treadmill (i.e., Woodway).

Reprinted by permission of Springer Nature from M. Buchheit and P.B. Laursen, "High-Intensity Interval Training, Solutions to the Programming Puzzle: Part II: Anaerobic Energy, Neuromuscular Load and Practical Applications," *Sports Medicine* 43 no. 10 (2013): 927-954.

training since RSSs are more team sport specific and might improve motivation in players reluctant to train on a track and/or perform longer sprints.

Work Modality

In addition to the work:recovery ratio, incorporating COD and/or jumps into RSS has the potential to influence the blood lactate response. When 25 m sprints (departing every 25 s, relief intensity = 7 km/h) are repeated over a shuttle run (180° COD), blood lactate can be increased (9.3 ± 2.4 versus 10.0 ± 10.7 mmol/L, ES = +0.3) (43). However, when RSSs are matched for initial sprint time (requiring a reduction in sprinting distance as COD angles increase), RSS with or without 90° COD angles are recommended to either minimize or maximize blood lactate accumulation, respectively (46). For RSSs that involve 0°, 45°, 90°, or 135° COD angles, Δ[La] (post-resting values) of 10.1 ± 2.2, 8.0 ± 2.3, 6.1 ± 2.5, and 7.4 ± 2.3 mmol/L have been reported, with *moderate-to-large* differences between those COD angles shown (except 45° and 135°). While it's intuitive to think that muscle recruitment (and blood lactate) increase with larger COD angles, associated absolute sprinting speed would be lower in this particular setting (due to the shorter distances) (46) (figure 5.27). Finally, jumping after each sprint is also associated with *small* increases in blood lactate accumulation (ES = +0.2-0.3) (36),

probably as a consequence of the increased total muscular work (figure 5.28).

Neuromuscular Responses to RSS

As with the anaerobic glycolytic component, the all-out nature of RSS naturally elicits large demands on the acute neuromuscular response, enabling us the ability to reach both type 4 and 5 targets. During RSS, the reduction in running speed observed reflects the progressive increase in overall locomotor stress, as evidenced by an impaired force production, changes in stride patterns (lower stride frequency and stride length), decreased musculoskeletal stiffness (96), and both neuromuscular adjustments and metabolic disturbances at the muscle level (95). Despite its poor reliability (145), the percentage of speed decrement (%Dec) is still the more commonly reported index used to assess acute fatigue during RSS, a marker that varies from 1% to 12%, depending on the RSS format (figure 5.29).

With respect to neuromuscular load, %Dec values should be interpreted with caution. While a high %Dec is likely associated with an increased (muscle) fatigue in the acute setting, the actual musculoskeletal strain of the sequence (with respect to possible muscle damage and/or injury risk) is more likely related to running patterns and the running speed maintained during each repetition (i.e., individuals with higher running speeds and low %Dec may have

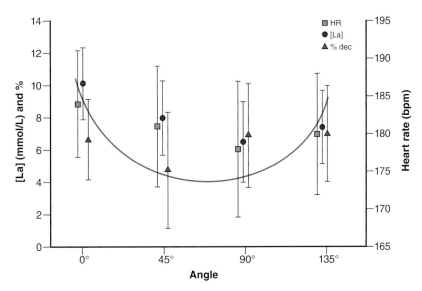

Figure 5.27 Heart rate (HR), blood lactate ([La]), and speed decrement (%Dec) responses to repeated-sprint sequences including straight-line (0°), 45°, 90°, or 135° change-of-direction sprints.

Data from M. Buchheit, B. Haydar, and S. Ahmaidi, "Repeated Sprints With Directional Changes: Do Angles Matter?" *Journal of Sports Sciences* 30 no. 6 (2012): 555-562.

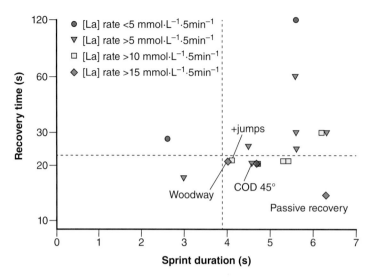

Figure 5.28 Rate of blood lactate increase during different repeated-sprint sequences as a function of recovery and sprint duration. The dashed lines represent the shortest sprint and recovery duration likely needed to achieve a rate of blood lactate increase (10 mmol·L·5 min⁻¹) with the exception of one repeated-sprint sequence performed with 45° changes of direction (COD) (5 mmol·L·5 min⁻¹). All repeated-sprint sequences leading to a rate of blood lactate increase (10 mmol·L·5 min⁻¹) included an active recovery, except for one with passive recovery. COD: changes of direction, with associated angle; Woodway refers to sprints performed on a nonmotorized treadmill.

Reprinted by permission of Springer Nature from M. Buchheit and P.B. Laursen, "High-Intensity Interval Training, Solutions to the Programming Puzzle: Part II: Anaerobic Energy, Neuromuscular Load and Practical Applications," *Sports Medicine* 43 no. 10 (2013): 927-954.

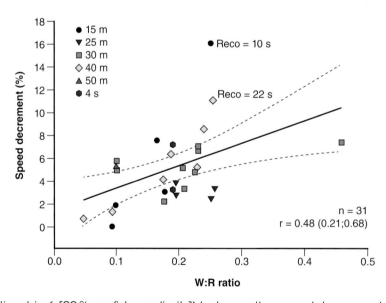

Figure 5.29 Relationship (r [90 % confidence limits]) between the speed decrement of various repeated-sprint sequences and work:relief (W:R) ratios. Correlation coefficients are provided with 90% confidence intervals.

Reprinted by permission of Springer Nature from M. Buchheit and P.B. Laursen, "High-Intensity Interval Training, Solutions to the Programming Puzzle: Part II: Anaerobic Energy, Neuromuscular Load and Practical Applications," *Sports Medicine* 43 no. 10 (2013): 927-954.

a high musculoskeletal strain). When data from these studies were pooled, %Dec was moderately and positively correlated with the work:relief ratio ($r = 0.48$, 90% confidence limits (0.21; 0.68), figure 5.29). A higher work:relief ratio is generally associated with reduced PCr resynthesis and an accumulation of blood lactate (figure 5.26) and metabolites in the muscle, which may partially explain the greater impairment of repeated-sprinting capacity (95). It is, however, worth noting that for extremely short recovery periods (i.e., 10 s (125)), the percentage of speed decrement is dramatically increased (see outlier data point, figure 5.29). Since this latter format might impose a substantial load on the musculoskeletal system, it should be implemented only with consideration for the timing of the other neuromuscular-oriented training sessions to avoid overload.

In addition to variations in sprint duration and work:relief ratio, the introduction of COD to RSS can also affect the fatigue profile and hence acute neuromuscular load. Compared to straight-line sprinting, for example, RSS with 180° COD were associated with a *slightly* lower %Dec (ES = −0.4) (43). When comparing the effect of COD angles *per se* (on sprints adjusted for initial sprint duration), the fatigue response to the RSS has been shown to be angle dependent (46). Values for %Dec were 6.7 ± 2.5, 4.8 ± 3.6, 7.0 ± 3.2, and $7.1 \pm 3.0\%$ for straight line, 45°, 90°, and 135°, respectively (with %Dec for 45° being substantially lower than for the three other conditions) (46) (figure 5.29). Running with 45° COD required variation in muscle activation compared to straight-line running (slowing down slightly to turn), without the need to apply large lateral forces, such as with the greater angles (135°) (32). This finding suggests that repeated sprints involving 45° COD may be an effective alternative to reducing acute neuromuscular load during RSS. Another important point to consider when it comes to introducing COD into RSS is the likely modification in lower-limb neuromuscular control. In fact, compared to repeated straight-line high-intensity 16.5 m runs, runs with 90° COD (performed within 4 s, departing every 20 s) were associated with both an increased stabilization time after a single-leg drop jump and a selective reduction of electromyography activity in hamstring muscles (101). Therefore, due to potential transient loss of ankle and knee stability, RSS including sharp COD might expose athletes to higher risk of ankle sprain and knee injuries, especially for athletes not used to performing such movement patterns at high speed (e.g., combat sport athletes,

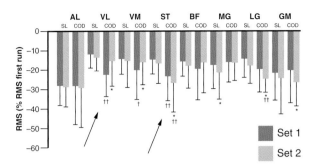

Figure 5.30 Changes in electromyography amplitude (RMS) for eight muscles during and after high-intensity intermittent efforts, with (COD) or without (i.e., straight line, SL) changes of direction. *: possible within-condition difference versus first set; †: possible difference versus SL; ††: likely different. AL: adductor longus; VL: vastus lateralis; VM: vastus medialis; ST: musculus semitendinosus; BF: biceps femoris; MG: medial gastrocnemius; LG: lateral gastrocnemius; GM: gluteus medius. SL: straight line; COD: change of direction; n = 11.

gymnasts). In practice, in addition to modulating the metabolic aspects reviewed above, changing direction during RSS might be an effective training practice to promote long-term COD-specific neuromuscular adaptations aimed at improving performance and knee joint stability (figure 5.30).

The specific impact of deceleration during RSS has the potential to increase acute muscle fatigue (i.e., impaired repeated sprinting performance), but only when a large number of sprints are performed, i.e., >11 sprints (119). Finally, adding jumps after each sprint during RSS is also likely to increase neuromuscular load. This was shown by a *moderately* greater %Dec for sprints, with (ES = +0.7) and without (ES = +0.8) shuttles (180°) (36). Finally, when jumps were added to RSS that involved shuttles, the %Dec for jump performance was highest (12 ± 4 versus $8 \pm 4\%$ for shuttle versus straight sprints, ES = +0.8), which suggests that this latter RSS format is likely more demanding on lower limbs. With respect to traumatic injuries, the introduction of COD during RSS has the advantage of restricting sprinting distance and stride length, which might help prevent hamstring overload and acute injuries. In contrast, as for HIIT with short intervals, RSS including COD might expose athletes to a higher risk of ankle sprain.

Finally, the time needed to recover from acute neuromuscular fatigue following RSS is important for RSS programming (158). In cycling studies, it has been shown that when a second RSS was performed 6 min after the first, fatigue was accelerated (i.e., %Dec of 17 versus 13% for the second versus the first set) (131), suggesting that a certain level of neuromuscular fatigue remained. When interspersing run-based RSS with 5 min rest, followed by 6 min active recovery and then a short specific warm-up (total time ≈15 min), repeated-sprint performance was not impaired during the second set (36). Explosive strength, however, had not fully recovered, since CMJ height was 5% lower (ES = −0.4) than before the first set (36). Compared to cycling, however, changes in neuromuscular coordination and stride adjustments appear to compensate for the acute fatigue during sprints to maintain running performance (160). This data suggests that when RSSs are repeated within a short time period (i.e., within 2 to 5 min (29, 57, 60)), neuromuscular fatigue, as evaluated from post-exercise jump tests, is heightened. To implement quality RSS sessions (if this is indeed possible (38)), a prolonged and likely active recovery period should be implemented between sets (possibly >15-20 min) to maximize muscle recovery.

Sprint Interval Training

Sprint interval training (SIT, figure 4.16), also termed speed endurance training, is another form of HIIT that involves near to maximal (all-out) efforts (115). Compared to the RSS format, efforts and recovery periods are typically longer (e.g., repeated 30 s sprints interspersed with 2-4 min of passive recovery (115)). SIT is similar to RST or RSS in that both are performed all out, so they can be prescribed without the need to pretest the individual (i.e., v/p$\dot{V}O_2$max is not specifically needed to calibrate the intensity). SIT differs from RST/RSS only in terms of the time range. RST/RSS could be described as short sprints, and tend to range from 3 to 10 s, while SIT is sometimes called long sprints, and usually last from 20 to 30 s in duration (94, 115). SIT is exclusive to type 5 targets in terms of their acute responses, requiring predominantly anaerobic glycolytic and neuromuscular responses.

$\dot{V}O_2$ Responses to Sprint Interval Sessions

As with our understanding of the RSS in the previous section, it may be prudent to review the all-out sprint training background in chapter 2, and specifically

with reference to figure 2.10, which shows the power output, $\dot{V}O_2$, and muscle tissue oxygenation index response during a SIT session. Notwithstanding the important research that demonstrates its benefits (94), only a small number of studies show the acute physiological responses to typical SIT sessions that might be implemented in practice. Tabata et al. (172) showed that $\dot{V}O_2$max was not reached (peak of 87% O₂max) during repeated 30 s cycling efforts (at 200% p$\dot{V}O_2$max, and therefore not actually all-out) interspersed by 2 min passive recovery. In contrast, we have shown (41) during a fully all-out SIT session that most athletes reached values close to (or above) 90% of their $\dot{V}O_2$max and HRmax (figure 2.10). In this study, T at $\dot{V}O_2$max was only 22 s on average (range 0 to 60 s, with two athletes not reaching >90% $\dot{V}O_2$max) (41), and $\dot{V}O_2$max was reached by only five subjects (50%). These important individual $\dot{V}O_2$ responses to SIT sessions were partly explained by variations in cardiorespiratory fitness (i.e., there was a negative correlation between T at $\dot{V}O_2$max and both $\dot{V}O_2$max (r = −0.68; 90% CL (−0.90;−0.20)) and $\dot{V}O_2$ kinetics at (submaximal) exercise cessation (r = 0.68; 90% CL (0.20; 0.90)). As with RSS, there was no link between T at $\dot{V}O_2$max and $\dot{V}O_2$ kinetics at exercise onset. Finally, it is worth noting that although pulmonary $\dot{V}O_2$ is not high during SIT, muscle O₂ demand is, especially as the number of sprint repetitions increase (figure 2.10). It has been shown that there is a progressive shift in energy metabolism during a SIT session, with a greater reliance on oxidative metabolism when sprints are repeated (27, 150). Along these same lines, muscle deoxygenation levels and post-sprint reoxygenation rates have been shown to become lower and slower, respectively, with increasing sprint repetition number. This response implies a greater O₂ demand in the muscle with increasing sprint repetition, since O₂ delivery is likely improved with exercise-induced hyperemia (blood excess in muscle bed supplying vessels) (41).

Anaerobic Glycolytic Energy Contribution During SIT

As with RSS, the all-out nature of SIT naturally engages a high anaerobic-glycolytic response. When physical education students repeated 4 × 30 s sprints at 200% of p$\dot{V}O_2$max interspersed with 2 min rest periods, the accumulated O₂ deficit reached 67% of their anaerobic capacity (172), defined as the maximal accumulated O₂ deficit during an exhaustive

2 to 3 min continuous exercise (129). Total accumulated O_2 deficit over the four sprints, however, was three times higher than the anaerobic capacity. Blood lactate levels generally reach 16 to 22 mmol/L (28, 42, 115, 128), which corresponds to blood lactate accumulation rates >10 to 15 mmol·L^{-1}·5min^{-1} (figure 5.26). While few researchers have manipulated SIT variables to examine their effect on the anaerobic glycolytic energy contribution, it is expected that slightly shorter sprints and/or lower intensities would reduce its input. As well, sprints >45 s are more likely associated with a greater contribution from the aerobic system (i.e., >40% (91)), which lowers anaerobic glycolytic energy demand in ensuing sprints. Thus, a general rule is that recovery periods should be long enough (i.e., >1.5-2 min) to allow for the aerobic system to return to resting levels, and thus enable an O_2 deficit to occur at the onset of the following exercise (160). Since an increased intramuscular H^+ concentration may inhibit glycolysis (89, 155), extending the recovery period might also allow for subsequent sprints to be achieved with a higher acid/base status, allowing, in turn, a greater anaerobic glycolytic energy contribution. For instance, post-exercise blood lactate levels were shown to *moderately* increase from 13.3 ± 2.2 to 15.1 ± 1.7 mmol/L (ES = +0.9) in well-trained team sport athletes (V_{IFT} = 18.9 ± 1.5 km/h) when the recovery between 30 s all-out shuttle sprints was increased from 30 to 80 s (45). Maximal blood lactate values were also reported to be greater when 30 s sprints were interspersed with 4 min of recovery (≈ 17 (28) and 22 (127) mmol/L) compared to 2 min (15.3 ± 0.7 mmol/L) (41). Finally, in elite Spanish 400 m runners (92% of the world record times) performing 300 m sprint repetitions (run in 40-45 s with varying inter-sprint recoveries), blood lactate after the sixth sprint was higher for sessions run at 87% of v400m (≈75%-80% of MSS) with 6 min recovery (17-19 mmol/L) compared to sessions involving sprints at 91% of v400m (>80% MSS) but separated by only 3 min of recovery (≈10 mmol/L) (99). Again, these results show how SIT variable manipulation can lead to different blood lactate levels, which has direct implications for HIIT programming.

Neuromuscular Responses to SIT

As with the anaerobic glycolytic system, the all-out nature of SIT additionally will engage a large response from the neuromuscular system. The large speed or power decrement score generally observed (20% for repeated 30 s cycling sprints (41, 127), 5%-20% for track sessions involving repeated 300 m runs (99)) suggests that neuromuscular function is largely impaired following a SIT session. Studies suggest that in contrast to other forms of HIIT (e.g., short duration and/or nonmaximal efforts (120, 151)), central mechanisms may be the primary origin of the impairment to MVC performance following long sprint repetition (87). There is, however, little data available examining the neuromuscular response to SIT variable manipulation. Neuromuscular fatigue (as assessed by jump height) following an HIIT session in elite 400 m runners (personal best = 92% of world record) is likely protocol dependent (99). The magnitude of the SIT-induced reduction in CMJ height was shown to be positively correlated with initial CMJ height and is affected by between-run recovery duration, with longer recovery durations (and hence the greater the anaerobic glycolytic energy contribution) showing greater impairments in jump height (99). When examining the neuromuscular responses in team sport athletes to single maximal sprints lasting 15 s (100 m), 31 s (200 m), and 72 s (400 m), Tomazin et al. (177) showed that knee extensor MVC reduction was apparent immediately and 5 min after the 72 s sprint and was fully recovered 30 min post-sprint.

In run-based sports, SIT is often implemented in a straight-line fashion or over an arcing shape of >200 m (running over half of a soccer pitch, for example). While this setting can allow players to reach very high running speeds (close to their MSS for the first intervals), it can dramatically increase hamstring injury risk (178). SIT sessions should therefore be considered using a cost-benefit approach. It is clear that SIT is unlikely to develop MSS (38, 58). However, when an appropriate warm-up is used and when distance is built up over the sessions, such SIT formats can, in addition to triggering the well-known metabolic adaptations in muscle (94), serve as a prophylactic intervention (i.e., preparing lower-limb muscle and tendons to tolerate the extreme tensions associated with maximal sprinting). For a safer option (or for the initial sessions of a SIT program), coaches can implement SIT sessions using 40 m shuttles (58).

Game-Based High-Intensity Interval Training

Recall from chapter 4 that game-based HIIT (GBHIIT) involves an aspect of play and decision-making when the format is being conducted. While much research has been published in the area of GBHIIT, and specifically team sport–based SSGs (with the great majority published in soccer) (112), it is beyond the scope of our book to exhaustively summarize all findings, since the effects of SSG-related variable manipulation are sport-, population-, and context-specific. We have therefore opted to present the main trends observed (but not the magnitude of the effects, as we have done for run-based HIIT) so as to illustrate examples of how this specific puzzle piece can be shaped, mainly with data arising from the soccer context. It is also worth noting that because of the inherent tactical and technical components of SSGs, many team sport practitioners program these using more tactical rather than physiological considerations (e.g., chapter 23, Basketball). There is obviously no right or wrong way to do this. For example, Martin still programs GBHIIT using physiology-based objectives (see soccer and handball chapters) and for consistency with the other chapters, we have kept the structure of this weapon similar to the others so as to be consistent in describing its acute physiological responses. Indeed, GBHIIT can be used to hit type 2 through 4 acute target responses.

GBHIIT is an HIIT format that differs substantially from the other four weapons for several reasons:

1. With the other weapons already presented (figures 4.13 to 4.16), exercise mode is typically an option. With GBHIIT, however, work modal-

ity must be sport specific by default, i.e., athletes practice their own sport under specific rules and contexts (e.g., number of players, specific areas).

2. Work intensity can't be prescribed as a function of given physiological entities such as $V/P_{IncTest}$, V_{IFT}, or CP/CV. Therefore, in contrast to the four other formats, exercise intensity is more affected by the manipulation of GBHIIT-specific variables (e.g., player number, field size, rules), which indirectly affects a player's effort and subsequent intensity (figure 5.31).

3. The important skill or tactical component is a two-edged sword. While it creates a fantastic opportunity to reinforce and even develop key aspects of team sport, together with a metabolic stimulus (table 5.1, figure 5.32), the highly variable quality and density of player interactions lead to a more variable and less predictable metabolic response, which can be limiting when a specific biological adaptation is being targeted.

Table 5.1 provides a thorough description of the advantages and disadvantages of using SSGs over traditional run-based HIIT in team sports.

Stratton et al. (171) have developed a simple model to characterize sport activities, with the view of enhancing skill acquisition and motor learning. The model is based on the respective levels of variability and randomness of game situations, and assumes that the variability within a practice environment

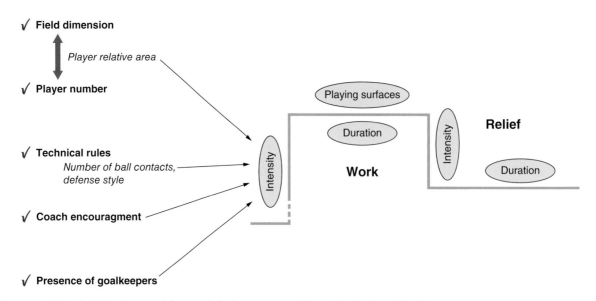

Figure 5.31 Methods used to modulate exercise intensity during GBHIIT.

Table 5.1 Advantages and Disadvantages Associated With Physical Training Using Soccer Drills and Generic Running

Soccer drills	Traditional running
A small-sided game with specific constraints (scoring, targets, balls, players, rules, and area)	A controlled running session with players exercising for a specific time or distance
Advantages	
Improved motivation	Exact work intensity can be easily controlled
Enhanced training of movement efficiency	Improvements can be monitored objectively
Improvements in tactical awareness	Comparisons can be made between players
Improvements in technical skill	Gain insight into player character or motivation
Optimizes training time and physical load	
Potential decrease in injuries	
Disadvantages	
Exact work intensity is difficult to control	Less movement associated with match play
Often difficult to organize optimal training structure	Players do not practice technical skills
Increased risk of contact injuries and overuse injuries (repeating over and over the same movement patterns)	No game-based tactical elements
Need numbers to make up session	Players do not like running
Certain degree of technical ability required	May increase risk of some injuries (tendonitis, lumbopelvic problems) due to unaccustomed running
Possible ceiling effect for very fit players	

Reprinted by permission from T. Little, "Optimizing the Use of Soccer Drills for Physiological Development," *Strength and Conditioning Journal* 31 no. 3 (2009): 67-74.

elicits a more flexible generalized motor program, allowing the natural variety of similar (but different) situations encountered in competition. The effects of such variable practice may also enhance an athlete's performance potential outcome due to the random versus blocked (predictable) practice conditions enabled. In a blocked practice condition, players are required to practice a single skill such as passing, shooting, or hitting during the session. In contrast, under random (game-based) practice conditions, skills are performed randomly, in an ad hoc manner, as they must be in the competition environment. While blocked practice may be better for short-term performance, random practice conditions might enhance skill-based learning. Figure 5.32 illustrates where traditional HIIT and SGG formats reside within this classification, and illustrates the importance of GBHIIT for team sport and racket-based athletes, irrespective of their metabolic responses.

V̇O₂ Responses to GBHIIT

Despite its important use in the field, only a few investigations have actually measured V̇O₂ during GBHIIT. This is mainly due to both logistics (e.g.,

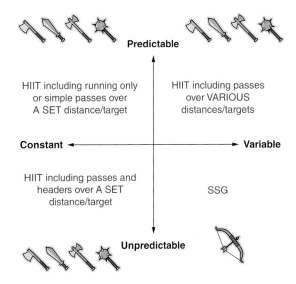

Figure 5.32 The Stratton model and its use for characterizing sport activities with respect to skill acquisition and motor learning, based on the respective levels of variability and randomness of training situations. The five weapons are positioned with respect to the two axes. SSG examples in red.

Adapted from G. Stratton, T. Reilly, A.M. Williams, and D. Richardson, *Youth Soccer: From Science to Performance* (Abingdon, Oxon: Routledge, 2004).

number of both gas analyzers and player availability) and complexity (e.g., disruption of technical skills, potential harm caused by analyzer in case of contact, etc.) of such measures during game play. The $\dot{V}O_2$ demands of run or cycling-based HIIT discussed in the first sections of the chapter are generally examined by testing one athlete after the next consecutively, using a single gas analyzer (one athlete per testing session, 12 athletes tested = 12 experimental sessions, a task that is feasible for any research team). In contrast, when it comes to monitoring the $\dot{V}O_2$ responses of SSGs, 3 to 5 gas analyzers are needed to characterize the $\dot{V}O_2$ demands of multiple players at the same time—a costly endeavor for any organization. In fact, due to the respective interactions between the 6 to 8 players typically involved during GBHIIT, every experimental GBHIIT must involve almost the entire participant pool (with a portion of players using a gas analyzer). This means that if we were to use only one gas analyzer, and considering the intense demands of GBHIIT that preclude repeating a high number of sets on the same day (i.e., player fatigue), and considering that at least two trials per athlete are required to compensate for the well-known SSG-to-SSG variability in locomotor patterns (see chapter 2; in turn, leading to more variability of energetic demands), participants would in effect be required to visit the lab a ridiculous number of times to allow each individual player to be tested. If you add to this the manipulation of some of the programming variables (e.g., exercise intensity, exercise length, and tactical rules, figure 5.31), it becomes almost impossible to monitor the $\dot{V}O_2$ responses of different variations in GBHIIT formats. In the real world, this simply wouldn't happen. For this reason, the majority of researchers to date have used HR responses to SSGs to characterize the metabolic responses and effects of various programming manipulations, since HR can easily and effectively be collected simultaneously in all players. The aforementioned intermittent exercise HR/$\dot{V}O_2$ dissociation that naturally arises during the phases that characterize GBHIIT (especially at exercise onset and in recovery, see figures 2.3 and 5.33) adds a degree of uncertainty when using HR as a proxy marker of the oxidative response. As with using blood lactate measures to infer anaerobic energy demands, we must accept the HR/$\dot{V}O_2$ limitations so as to begin to understand how SSGs can be manipulated to solve the puzzle. While the $\dot{V}O_2$/HR relationship issue limits direct interpolation of actual $\dot{V}O_2$ demands per se, this issue plays less of a role when assessing the relative effect of GBHIIT variable manipulation.

The limited literature available describing actual $\dot{V}O_2$ responses shows that some forms of SSGs can be used to achieve high levels of $\dot{V}O_2$ (4v4 handball SSGs: >90% $\dot{V}O_2$max (56) or 2v2 in basketball: 80% $\dot{V}O_2$max (67)), but not others involving more players (5v5 indoor soccer: peak values reached = 75% $\dot{V}O_2$max (65)). When it comes to assessing the effects of SSG manipulation on $\dot{V}O_2$ responses in the same population, there is even less data available. The study from Castagna et al. (67) in junior basketball players ($\dot{V}O_2$max 55 mL·min^{-1}·kg^{-1}) showed that mean $\dot{V}O_2$ responses increased linearly by 5% when player number was reduced from 5v5 (average response 69% of $\dot{V}O_2$max) to 3v3 (74%) and 2v2 (79%). Further considerations regarding the effects of SSG manipulation that follow are based on HR measures only.

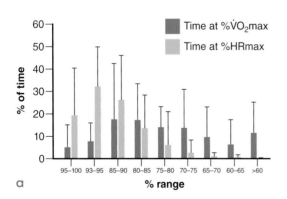
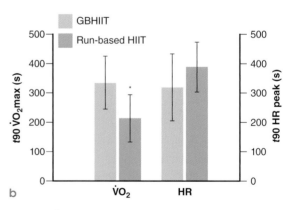

Figure 5.33 (a) Percentage of game time spent in selected $\dot{V}O_2$ and HR intensity zones (mean and 95% CI) during futsal game play (66). (b) Mean (95% CI) time spent above 90% of maximal oxygen uptake (t90 $\dot{V}O_2$max) and above 90% of maximal heart rate (t90 HRpeak) during handball SSGs (game-based HIIT, GBHIIT), and HIIT with short intervals (run-based HIIT) (56). *Significant difference between GBHIIT and run-based HIIT.

Work Intensity

The different options available for practitioners to modulate exercise intensity during GBHIIT are summarized in figure 5.31. Varying a player's relative area via changes in either player number and/or field size are the two most adjusted variables used in the field. Since comparable player areas can be achieved using different variations of either player number or field size, HR responses to player area variations have presented mixed findings in the literature. When player number is constant, an increase in field size is generally associated with increased HR responses (since greater space allows for more running, figure 5.34), while in some circumstances findings are not as clear (figure 27.8). The lack of consistency in this regard is likely related to the fact that over very small playing areas, changes in velocity, direction, and contacts tend to increase compared to the larger pitch size (73), and in turn compensate for the reduced running demands (56, 73).

Similarly, lower player numbers in SSGs tend to increase the HR response, due in part to increased ball involvement associated with the reduced teammate number (figure 5.34). The third most-used component when it comes to modulating the exercise intensity of SSGs is adjustment of the technical rules, such as varying the number of ball contacts allowed (the lower the number, the greater the HR demands (75)), the defensive style (e.g., man marking, which also increases HR (141)), and adding extra rules (e.g., the need for the attacking team to have all players in a specific area of the pitch—half or third side of the opponent's goal—which tends to increase HR (111)). The inclusion of goalkeepers (GK) into SSGs has shown varying effects on HR (increases without GK when players run more to score on smaller goals, but additionally when GK increase player motivation (112)). Coach encouragement can also motivate player exertion and HR (figure 5.34) (112).

Work Duration

As with long-interval HIIT, the optimal work duration for SSGs of low player number (i.e., 3v3 or 4v4) is between 2 and 4 min (112, 124). The duration should be long enough for $\dot{V}O_2$ to reach high levels (T to $\dot{V}O_2$max) but not so long as to cause excessive fatigue that could impair technical efficiency and the ability to maintain a high T at $\dot{V}O_2$max. In fact,

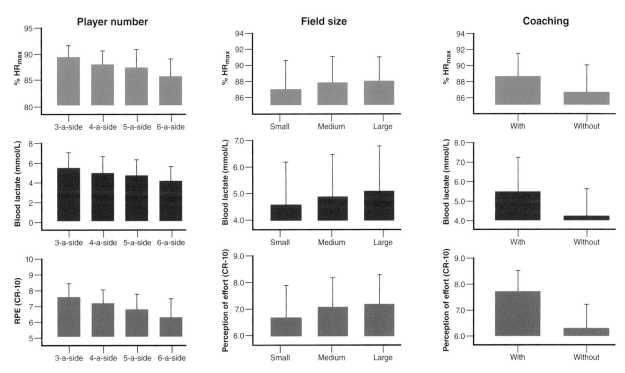

Figure 5.34 Effect of variations in player number, field size, and coach encouragement on heart rate (HR), blood lactate, and rating of perceived exertion (RPE) responses during typical small-sided games (SSGs) in soccer players.

Data from E. Rampinini, F.M. Impellizzeri, C. Castagna, G. Abt, K. Chamari, A. Sassi, and S.M. Marcora, "Factors Influencing Physiological Responses to Small-Sided Soccer Games," *Journal of Sports Sciences* 25 no. 6 (2007): 659-666.

fatigued players will more frequently lose the ball, which inappropriately breaks the activity and lowers overall exercise intensity. Exercise intensity needs also to be balanced with the exercise duration, i.e., longer durations for lower intensities and higher intensities for shorter durations. For example, SSG durations that involve more players (e.g., 8v8) are generally programmed over longer durations (8-10 min) (see chapter 30, Soccer (126)). These longer intervals likely target more threshold-like responses (>80%-90% HRmax (124)) rather than V̇O₂max (>90%-95% HRmax) (112).

Playing Surface

In the only study to date (30) investigating the effect of playing surface on metabolic responses to SSGs, active young male adults performed 2×5v5 SSGs for 10 min (separated by 5 min passive recovery) on either sand, artificial turf, or asphalt. Total distance and sprint number were 2585±208 m and 7±2; 3726±121 m and 13±2; and 3895±39 m and 21±2, respectively. The results, summarized in figure 5.35, showed that, in opposition to locomotor demands (asphalt > artificial turf > sand), artificial turf tended to elicit the highest HR, blood lactate, and rating of perceived exertion responses, followed next by asphalt and then sand, respectively (small to moderate differences between all conditions). In practice, however, while it might be feasible to program in recreational beach soccer at some stages of the preseason, it would be difficult to rationalize playing on asphalt given the overall increased injury risk that such a session would expose.

Between-GBHIIT Recovery Periods

As detailed in chapter 4, decreasing duration or increasing intensity of the between-set recovery period impairs the restoration of W′, which can be detrimental to technical performance during the following work period (figure 5.36). Since GBHIITs are first about a player's technical interaction, care should be taken to ensure a minimum level of skill proficiency (limiting fatigue), but also the maintenance of exercise intensity and, in turn, metabolic responses and T at V̇O₂max. Rest periods ideally should be 2 to 4 min and completely passive (112).

Anaerobic Glycolytic Energy Contribution During GBHIIT

In contrast to run-based HIIT, research indicates that the oxidative and anaerobic contributions tend to follow the same pattern of response to HIIT variable manipulation during GBHIIT (71). This implies that the general effects of SSG manipulation on anaerobic energy contribution may be similar to those discussed earlier for HR (and hopefully V̇O₂) responses. Increases in field dimension, decreases in player number, lowered number of ball contacts, man-to-man marking, goalkeeper integration, and coach encouragement all tend to increase anaerobic contribution to exercise (figures 5.34 and 5.36). In contrast, shorter SSG duration and longer between-SSG breaks tend to lower anaerobic contribution.

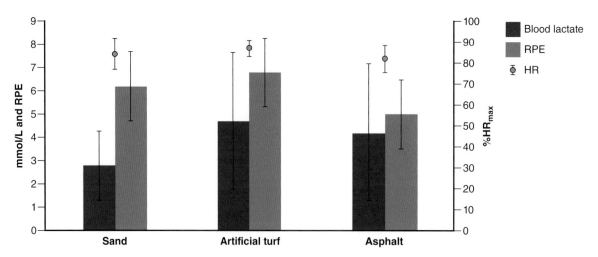

Figure 5.35 Heart rate (HR), blood lactate, and rating of perceived exertion (RPE) response to 5v5 SSGs performed on different surfaces.

Data from J. Brito, P. Krustrup, and A. Rebelo, "The Influence of the Playing Surface on the Exercise Intensity of Small-Sided Recreational Soccer Games," *Human Movement Science* 31 no. 4 (2012): 946-956.

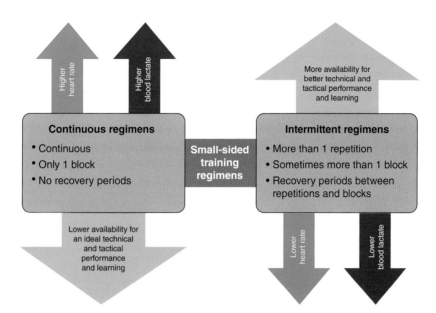

Figure 5.36 Schematic representation of the effect of continuous versus intermittent regimens (and by extension the impact of the between-set recovery characteristics) when using SSGs (182).

Neuromuscular Responses to GBHIIT

The neuromuscular impact of GBHIIT has probably received the least attention in the literature. The work intensity, duration, between-set recovery, and playing surface should all be considered for this aspect of the weapon's target (type 2 and 4 responses).

Work Intensity, Duration, and Between-Set Recovery

Since the actual neuromuscular load is likely to be exercise intensity dependent (the greater the exercise intensity, the more associated mechanical load), the same relationship as described for the oxidative and anaerobic contribution should apply. It is, however, worth noting that the type of neuromuscular fatigue is likely different for large- and small-size SSGs, since it involves different types of locomotion. In fact, while small fields tend to increase mechanical work (i.e., the number and magnitude of acceleration/ deceleration and changes of direction, which stress lower-limb extensors such as quads and glutes), larger fields likely create more total distance run (figure 27.8) at higher speeds, which stresses hamstring muscles (157) (see also chapter 30, Soccer, for discussion on the relative contribution of the lower-limb muscle as a function of the type of locomotor actions). In support of the greater neuromuscular load associated with smaller player number SSGs, sprint ability over

5 and 15 m tests (acceleration phases, involving the extensors more) decreased moderately after a 4v4 + GK, but not after an 8v8 + GK (157).

Playing Surface

Playing surface also impacts the development of acute neuromuscular fatigue with GBHIIT independent of other physiological responses. For example, when active young male adults performed two 5v5 SSGs for 10 min (5 min passive recovery between) on either sand, artificial turf, or asphalt, sprint performance wasn't substantially affected. In contrast, there were small reductions in CMJ for artificial turf and asphalt (figure 5.37) (30). As discussed earlier, however, there may be only a limited number of practitioners who would actually program SSGs on asphalt for the reasons mentioned earlier (greater injury risk, etc.). Therefore further research should focus on artificial turf versus natural grass.

The main effects of GBHIIT variable manipulations are summarized in figure 5.38.

Analysis and Comparison of HIIT Weapons

We finish chapter 5 with a short section comparing all formats against one another, in terms of their oxidative, anaerobic glycolytic, and neuromuscular acute responses.

Comparison of V̇O₂ Responses Among HIIT Weapons

Throughout chapter 5, we have highlighted the V̇O₂ responses to various forms of HIIT. It appears that most HIIT formats, when properly manipulated, can enable athletes to reach V̇O₂max. However, important between-athlete and between-HIIT format dif-

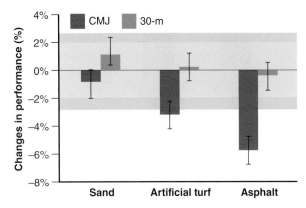

Figure 5.37 Changes in countermovement jump (CMJ) and sprint times following 5v5 SSGs performed on sand, artificial turf, or asphalt. Gray and orange zones represent trivial changes for sprint and CMJ performance, respectively.

Data from J. Brito, P. Krustrup, and A. Rebelo, "The Influence of the Playing Surface on the Exercise Intensity of Small-Sided Recreational Soccer Games," *Human Movement Science* 31 no. 4 (2012): 946-956.

ferences exist with respect to T at V̇O₂max. RSS and SIT sessions allow for a limited T at V̇O₂max compared to HIIT that involve long and short intervals (figure 5.39). Combined, data from high-level athletes (90, 136) suggests that long intervals and/or short intervals with a work:relief ratio >1 should enable a greater T at V̇O₂max/exercise time ratio during HIIT sessions. Table 5.2 also provides overview comparisons of the impact of the various HIIT weapons in terms of their physiological response types.

Comparison of the Anaerobic Glycolytic Responses Between HIIT Weapons

The anaerobic glycolytic energy contribution during an HIIT session is HIIT parameter dependent. SIT- and RSS-type HIIT weapons are typically associated with elevated rates of blood lactate accumulation (figure 5.40). During RSS sessions, sprint durations greater than 4 s with work relief intervals less than 20 s lead to the highest blood lactate accumulation. In contrast, SIT sessions require relief interval durations equal to or longer than 4 min to maximize the anaerobic glycolytic energy response. As shown, the manipulation of HIIT variables with short intervals may allow practitioners to vary the level of anaerobic glycolytic energy contribution to a given session. In general, longer interval durations and higher interval intensities (when > vV̇O₂max) will elicit

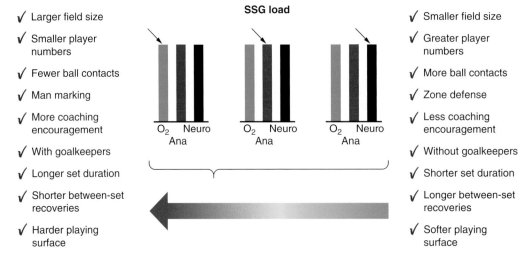

Figure 5.38 Main physiological responses in relation to variations in some of the programming aspects of GBHIIT and small-sided games (SSGs). Note that compared with run-based HIIT, and with the exception of the impact of playing surface, there is a tendency for all physiological responses (oxidative, anaerobic, and neuromuscular systems) to respond in a similar fashion.

Table 5.2 Recommendations for the Design of Run-Based HIIT Protocols for Optimizing Time at Maximal Oxygen Uptake (T at $v\dot{V}O_2max$), Ordered From Lowest to Highest in Terms of Expected Oxidative Response

Format	W duration	W intensity	Modality	R duration	R intensity	Reps and series[c]	Between-set recovery Duration	Between-set recovery Intensity	Expected T at $v\dot{V}O_2max$	Acute demands
SIT	> 20 s	All-out	Sport specific	≥ 2 min	Passive	6-10			0-1 min	Peripheral ++++
RST	> 4 s (> 30 m or 2×15 m)	All-out	COD Jumps Explosive efforts	< 20 s	≈ 55% $v\dot{V}O_2max$ /40% V_{IFT}	2-3 RSS (each > 6 sprints)	≥ 6 min	≤ 60-70% $v\dot{V}O_2max$ [b]	0-3 min	Central + Peripheral +++
Game-based training	> 2-3 min	Self-selected RPE > 7	Sport specific[d]	≤ 2 min	Passive	6-10×2 min 5-8×3 min 4-6×4 min			> 8 min	Central ++ Peripheral +++
HIIT with long intervals	2-3 min[a]	≥ 95% $v\dot{V}O_2max$	Sport specific	≤ 2 min ≥ 4-5 min	Passive ≤ 60-70% $v\dot{V}O_2max$[b]	6-10×2 min 5-8×3 min 4-6×4 min			> 10 min	Central ++++ Peripheral ++
HIIT with short intervals	≥ 15 s[a,c]	100-120% $v\dot{V}O_2max$ (85-105% V_{IFT})	Sport specific	< 15 s ≥ 15 s	Passive ≤ 60-70% $v\dot{V}O_2max$ (45-55% V_{IFT})	2-3 × ≥ 8-min series	≥ 4-5 min	≤ 60-70% $v\dot{V}O_2max$[b]	> 10 min	Central ++ Peripheral ++

Specific recommendation for manipulating various forms of high-intensity interval training (HIIT), including long or short intervals, repeated-sprint training (RST), and sprint interval training (SIT). Intensities are provided as percentages of the speed associated with maximal oxygen uptake ($v\dot{V}O_2max$) and the speed reached during the 30-15 intermittent fitness test (V_{IFT}).
(a) To be modulated with respect to exercise mode (longer for cycling vs. running, for example), age, and fitness status (shorter for younger and/or more-trained athletes).
(b) These can also be game-based (moderate intensity) in team sports.
(c) To be modulated with respect to the sport, i.e., longer for endurance and highly trained athletes than team-sport and less-trained athletes.
(d) To be modulated with respect to physiological training objectives (manipulating playing number, pitch area, etc.) and so specific rules are added for the fittest players to compensate for the fitness-related responses, which will parallel the HIIT sessions.

W: work; R: relief; reps: repetitions; RPE: rating of perceived exertion; COD: changes of direction; SSG: small-sided games; T at $v\dot{V}O_2max$: time at $v\dot{V}O_2max$.
The number of symbols (+) indicate the magnitude of the expected adaptations.

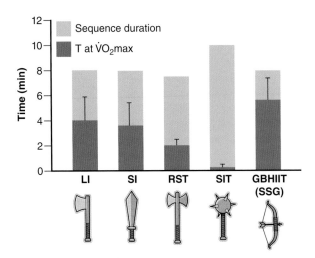

Figure 5.39 Total exercise time and time spent at or near maximal oxygen uptake (T at V̇O₂max) for typical HIIT formats: 2×2 min/1 min long intervals (LI), 1×8 min series of short intervals (15 s/15 s, SI), a repeated sprint sequence (RST, 2 sets of 6 sprints), a sprint interval session (SIT, 4 sprint repetitions), and an 8 min small-sided game (SSG, one of the most common forms of game-based HIIT, GBHIIT).

Data from M. Buchheit and P.B. Laursen, "High-Intensity Interval Training, Solutions to the Programming Puzzle: Part I: Cardiopulmonary Emphasis," *Sports Medicine* 43, no. 5 (2013): 313-338.

higher blood lactate levels. While the evidence is limited, increasing the intensity of exercise during the recovery interval in short HIIT bouts may also increase blood lactate accumulation. Interestingly, anaerobic glycolytic energy release can also be manipulated during GBHIIT (i.e., SSG) via changes in rules and/or player number and pitch dimension (112) so that blood lactate accumulation can be maintained at low levels despite a prolonged T at V̇O₂max (56). A comparison of the anaerobic glycolytic energy contribution and response type to different HIIT weapons is shown in table 5.3 and figure 5.40.

Comparison of the Neuromuscular Responses Among HIIT Weapons

While the magnitude of neuromuscular loading during HIIT can be modulated through the manipulation of HIIT variables (e.g., work intensity or duration, exercise mode or pattern; figure 5.41), the responses are highly athlete profile dependent, with endurance-type athletes showing low levels of acute fatigue and speed decrement, and team sport athletes typically showing high levels of neuromuscular fatigue following HIIT (figure 5.42). There is likely a

Table 5.3 Recommendations for the Design of Run-Based HIIT Protocols With Respect to Blood Lactate Accumulation, Ordered From Lowest to Highest in Terms of Expected Lactate Response

Format	W duration	W intensity	Modality	R duration	R intensity	Expected initial rate of blood lactate accumulation
HIIT with short intervals	≥20 s <30s	<100% vV̇O₂max (<89% V_IFT)	Straight line	≥20 s <30s	≈55% vV̇O₂max (40% V_IFT)	<5 mmol·L⁻¹·5 min⁻¹
	<15 s	<120% vV̇O₂max (<100% V_IFT)	Straight line	≥20 s	Passive	<5 mmol·L⁻¹·5 min⁻¹
Game-based training	3-4 min	Self-selected RPE >7	Sport specific	≤2 min ≥ 4-5 min	Passive 55% vV̇O₂max (40% V_IFT)	≤5 mmol·L⁻¹·5 min⁻¹
HIIT with long intervals	<2 min	<100% vV̇O₂max	Straight line	2 min	Passive	≈5 mmol·L⁻¹·5 min⁻¹
HIIT with short intervals	>25 s	>110% vV̇O₂max (>90% V_IFT)	COD	>15 s <30 s	60%-70% vV̇O₂max (45%-55% V_IFT)	≈6-7 mmol·L⁻¹·5 min⁻¹
HIIT with long intervals	>3 min	≥95% vV̇O₂max	Straight line, sand, hills	>3 min	Passive	≈6-7 mmol·L⁻¹·5 min⁻¹
RST	<3 s	All-out	45°-90° COD	>20 s	Passive	≤10 mmol·L⁻¹·5 min⁻¹
RST	>4 s	All-out	Straight line + jump	<20 s	≈55% vV̇O₂max (40% V_IFT)	>10 mmol·L⁻¹·5 min⁻¹
SIT	>20 s	All-out	Straight line	>120 s	Passive	>10 mmol·L⁻¹·5 min⁻¹

Specific recommendation for manipulating various forms of high-intensity interval training (HIIT), including long or short intervals, repeated-sprint training (RST), and sprint interval training (SIT). Intensities are provided as percentages of the speed associated with maximal oxygen uptake (vV̇O₂max) and the speed reached in the 30-15 intermittent fitness test (V_IFT). W: work; R: relief; RPE: rating of perceived exertion; COD: changes of direction.

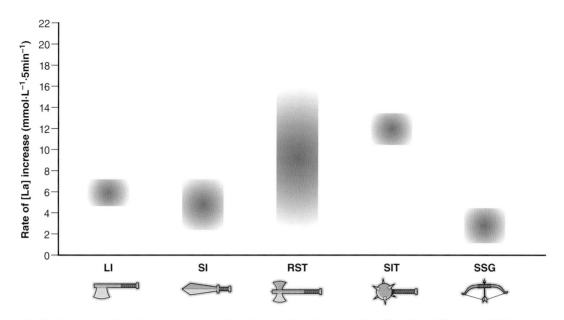

Figure 5.40 Range of lactate accumulation typically observed for the five different HIIT formats.

Data from M. Buchheit and P.B. Laursen, "High-Intensity Interval Training, Solutions to the Programming Puzzle: Part II: Anaerobic Energy, Neuromuscular Load and Practical Applications," *Sports Medicine* 43 no. 10 (2013): 927-954.

bell-shaped relationship between exercise intensity and acute neuromuscular performance responses, with too low (≤85% v$\dot{V}O_2$max) and too high (all-out) an intensity having not enough and acute detrimental effects, respectively (figure 5.43). Work intensities >80%-85% v$\dot{V}O_2$max require recruitment of fast-twitch fibers (97), induce post-activation potentiation, and possibly lead to long-term structural adaptations that allow fatigue resistance to high-speed running (161). In contrast, supramaximal-to-maximal (≥120% v$\dot{V}O_2$max, ≥100% V_{IFT}) intensity exercises are likely associated with acute impairments in muscular performance. The residual fatigue from HIIT sessions that persists over time may have large implications for subsequent training (carry-over effect), but there is limited data documenting the recovery course of neuromuscular function following HIIT. Finally, in addition to mechanical work intensity, the associated metabolic responses and potentially accumulated metabolites within muscle should also be taken into account when examining the acute neuromuscular load of a given ses-sion. Coaches can choose to balance the level of neuromuscular engagement associated with a given HIIT format, based on both the expected training-induced adaptations (either through the HIIT session itself or the associated sessions and possible additive effects) and the acute changes in neuromuscular performance (table 5.4). Running pattern (e.g., COD, introduction of jumps during the recovery periods), exercise mode (e.g., cycling, running, bouncing), or ground surfaces (e.g., pavement, synthetic track, grass, sand, treadmill) and terrain (uphill, downhill) also may have direct implications on traumatic and overuse injury risk, and should be chosen for programming based on a risk-benefit approach (figure 5.43). Similarly, before programming an HIIT training cycle, coaches should also consider that in team sports, physical fitness is unlikely to have the same impact on match running perfor-mance for all players, as playing position, systems of play, and individual playing styles directly affect the relationship between physical fitness and match running performance (59, 61, 130, 139).

Table 5.4 Recommendations for the Design of Run-Based HIIT Protocols in Reference to Acute Neuromuscular Performance and Potential Injury Risk

Format	W duration	W intensity	Modality	Ground surface	R duration	R intensity	Acute change in muscular performance[a]	Injury risk level
Game-based training	> 2-3 min	Self-selected RPE > 7	Sport specific	Sport specific	≤ 2 min	Passive 55% $v\dot{V}O_2$max (40% V_{IFT})	SSG format-dependent	Traumatic ++ (contacts, joint sprain) Overuse +
HIIT with long intervals	> 2-3 min[b]	≥ 95% $v\dot{V}O_2$max	Straight line	Grass or treadmill	2 min	Passive	From improved ++ to impaired ++	Traumatic - Overuse +
	> 2-3 min[b]	≥ 95% $v\dot{V}O_2$max	Straight line	Track	4-5 min	60-70% $v\dot{V}O_2$max (45-55% V_{IFT})	From improved + to impaired +	Traumatic ++ (tendons) Overuse +++
	> 2-3 min[b]	≥ 85% $v\dot{V}O_2$max	Hill	Road	2 min	Passive	From improved + to impaired +	Traumatic - Overuse ++ (downhill = shocks)
HIIT with short intervals	< 15 s	< 120% $v\dot{V}O_2$max (< 100% V_{IFT})	Straight line	Track, indoor	> 15 s but < 30 s	60-70% $v\dot{V}O_2$max (45-55% V_{IFT})	From improved + to impaired +	Traumatic - Overuse - (since short series)
	≤ 20 s	< 110% $v\dot{V}O_2$max (> 90% V_{IFT})	Straight line	Track, indoor	≤ 20 s	Passive	From improved + to impaired ++	Traumatic - Overuse ++ (since long series)

	Work duration	Intensity	Exercise mode	Surface	Recovery duration	Recovery type	Effect on fitness	Injury
	≤ 20 s	< 110% v$\dot{V}O_2$max (> 90% V_{IFT})	COD	Track, indoor	≤ 20 s	Passive	From improved + to impaired ++	Traumatic ++ (ankle sprain) Overuse ++
	≤ 20 s	< 110% v$\dot{V}O_2$max (> 90% V_{IFT})	COD	Grass	≤ 20 s	Passive	From improved - to impaired +++	Traumatic ++ (ankle sprain and adductors) Overuse +
RST	≤ 5 s	All-out	Distance < 20 m 45-90 degree COD	Sport specific	≤ 25 s	passive	Impaired - to ++	Traumatic ++ (ankle sprain)
	> 3 s	All-out	Straight line > 20 m	Sport specific	≤ 30 s	≈ 55% v$\dot{V}O_2$max /40% V_{IFT}	Impaired + to +++	Traumatic ++ (hamstring)
	≤ 3 s	All-out	Straight line < 20 m, COD, and jump	Sport specific	≤ 30 s	≈ 55% v$\dot{V}O_2$max /40% V_{IFT}	Impaired ++ to ++++	Traumatic -
SIT	> 20 s	All-out	Straight line	Sport specific	> 120 s	Passive	Impaired ++ to ++++	Traumatic +++ (hamstring)

Specific recommendations for manipulating various forms of high-intensity interval training (HIIT) sessions including long or short intervals, repeated-sprint training (RST), and sprint interval training (SIT). Comparisons between muscular fatigue following runs over different surfaces are adapted from the work of Sassi et al. (A. Sassi, A. Stefanescu, P. Menaspa, A. Bosio, M. Riggio, and E. Rampinini, "The Cost of Running on Natural Grass and Artificial Turf Surfaces," *J Strength Cond Res* 25, no. 3 (2011): 606-611.) (with an energy cost of running lower for hard surface < sand < grass < treadmill) and Gains et al. (G.L. Gains, A.N. Swedenhjelm, J.L. Mayhew, H.M. Bird, and J.J. Houser, "Comparison of Speed and Agility Performance of College Football Players on Field Turf and Natural Grass," *J Strength Cond Res.* 24, no. 10 (2010): 2613-2617.). While additional combinations between the different surfaces and exercise modes can be implemented (e.g., uphill running on a treadmill), these examples illustrate the main logic behind the selection of HIIT variables. The level of injury rate is estimated as a function of the number of (+) symbols.

(a) Fatigue responses are likely athlete-dependent.
(b) To be modulated with respect to exercise mode (longer for cycling vs. running for example), age, and fitness status (shorter for younger and/or more trained athletes).
SSG: small-sided game; W: work; R: relief; RPE: rating of perceived exertion.

Intensities are provided as percentages of the speed associated with maximal oxygen uptake (v$\dot{V}O_2$max) and the final speed reached in the 30-15 intermittent fitness test (V_{IFT}).

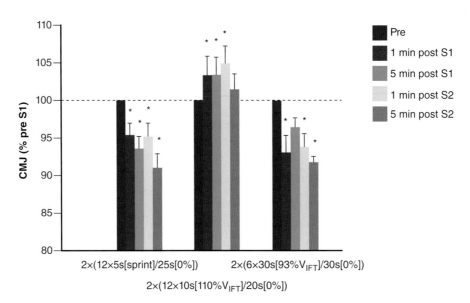

Figure 5.41 Changes in countermovement jump (CMJ) height following three different high-intensity interval training sessions (repeated-sprint sequence and high-intensity interval training of either 10 s/20 s or 30 s/30 s format) performed over two series (146). S1: first series; S2: second series; V_{IFT}: peak speed reached in the 30-15 intermittent fitness test; * indicates moderate standardized difference; # indicates large standardized difference.

Reprinted by permission of Springer Nature from M. Buchheit and P.B. Laursen, "High-Intensity Interval Training, Solutions to the Programming Puzzle: Part II: Anaerobic Energy, Neuromuscular Load and Practical Applications," *Sports Medicine* 43 no. 10 (2013): 927-954.

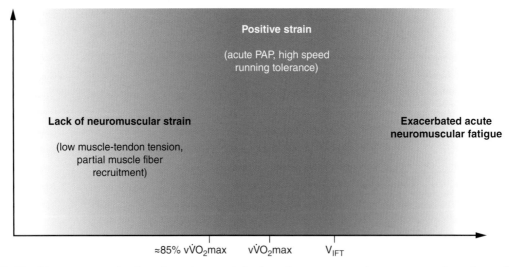

Figure 5.42 Neuromuscular load and associated performance outcomes as a function of running speed during typical high-intensity interval training sessions. PAP: post-activation potentiation; V_{IFT}: peak speed reached at the end of the 30-15 intermittent fitness test; $v\dot{V}O_2max$: lowest running speed required to elicit maximal oxygen uptake.

Reprinted by permission of Springer Nature from M. Buchheit and P.B. Laursen, "High-Intensity Interval Training, Solutions to the Programming Puzzle: Part II: Anaerobic Energy, Neuromuscular Load and Practical Applications," *Sports Medicine* 43 no. 10 (2013): 927-954.

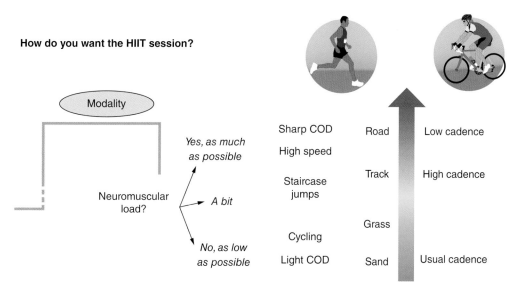

Figure 5.43 The effect of work modality during HIIT sessions on the expected neuromuscular and musculoskeletal demands.

Summary

To summarize chapter 5, we have gone deep into the science to review how the key moving parts of HIIT variable manipulation (chapter 4) can be used to adjust the physiological responses in the five key HIIT weapons to hit our desired targets. As illustrated originally in figure 1.5, long intervals (figure 4.13) can effectively be manipulated to hit type 3 and 4 targets; short intervals (figure 4.14) are versatile formats that can be used to hit the majority of HIIT targets (types 1-4); RST (figure 4.15) is useful for hitting type 4 and 5 targets; while SIT (figure 4.16) is a specialist weapon used to hit type 5 targets. The master team and racket sport weapon is the GBHIIT (figure 4.17), which is a highly flexible tool for hitting type 2 through 4 targets. The decision tree model originally offered in figure 1.5 provides a roadmap solution to the programming puzzle, which can be used alongside the fine-tuning details offered in this chapter to help more precisely guide the manipulation of HIIT sessions in line with target-type goals. The complexities and the science encompassing the integration of concurrent type 6 speed and strength targets, shown in figure 1.5, are described in chapter 6.

6

Incorporating HIIT Into a Concurrent Training Program

• • • • • •

Jackson Fyfe, Martin Buchheit, and Paul Laursen

To maximize performance across a number of sports, most athletes require not only high levels of cardiorespiratory fitness but also aspects of enhanced maximal strength, power/rate of force development, and speed (50), with varying degrees of these traits needed across different sports (see figure 1.6). For example, enhanced maximal strength and power/rate of force development is associated with improved performance in sport-specific skills, including sprinting, jumping, and change of direction (see reviews by 23, 95). Resistance training can also enhance both short- and long-duration performance (often termed *endurance*), due largely to neuromuscular adaptations that improve exercise efficiency (87), as outlined already in chapters 3, 4, and 5. It is therefore common practice for athletes to engage in some form of resistance (i.e., strength) training in combination with training aimed at enhancing cardiorespiratory and metabolic fitness (e.g., high-intensity interval training, HIIT). From this perspective, concurrent training represents an additional piece of the programming puzzle that practitioners must consider when prescribing endurance training modalities, including HIIT, with athletes.

The simultaneous integration of both strength and endurance training into a periodized training regime is termed *concurrent training*, a topic that has received considerable scientific interest since the first concurrent training studies appeared in the literature (47, 48). While concurrent training provides clear benefits for athletic performance by satisfying both ends of the strength-endurance continuum (77), this approach also presents additional logistical challenges to the practitioner. In particular, a primary concern with concurrent training is the potential for endurance training to interfere with adaptations primarily associated with strength training (i.e., enhanced maximal strength, power or rate of force development, and muscle hypertrophy) (for reviews see 6, 36)). A number of studies have indeed shown that, relative to performing strength training alone, concurrent training compromises gains in maximal strength (e.g., 9, 30, 34, 38, 41, 46, 47, 53, 57), aspects of power and rate of force development (38, 41, 46, 53, 57, 61), and muscle hypertrophy (9, 57, 82). While it is clear that endurance training may compromise aspects of strength training adaptation, the majority of evidence suggests that concurrent training does not attenuate improvements in $\dot{V}O_2max$ compared to endurance training performed alone (100). Taken together with the aforementioned evidence that strength training positively influences both cycling and running performance (87), these observations demonstrate the predominantly unidirectional nature of the interference effect. Put simply, endurance training may limit strength and power development during concurrent training, but strength training should not compromise endurance capacity and instead will likely enhance it (figure 6.1). This does not mean that inclusion of strength training in any weekly training plan does not pose challenges for the programming of HIIT and other forms of metabolic conditioning; as will be discussed later in this chapter, there is also the potential for strength training to influence performance in the opposing mode (as well as vice versa).

It is important to note that the concurrent training field is rife with conflicting evidence regarding the existence and nature of the interference effect to strength training adaptations. For example, not all studies suggest endurance training (referred to hereafter as *metabolic conditioning*) causes any interference to strength training adaptations during concurrent training (e.g., 7, 26, 70, 78). When an interference effect with concurrent training is observed, there is evidence for certain aspects of strength training adaptation to be compromised more than others. For example, attenuated training-induced improvements

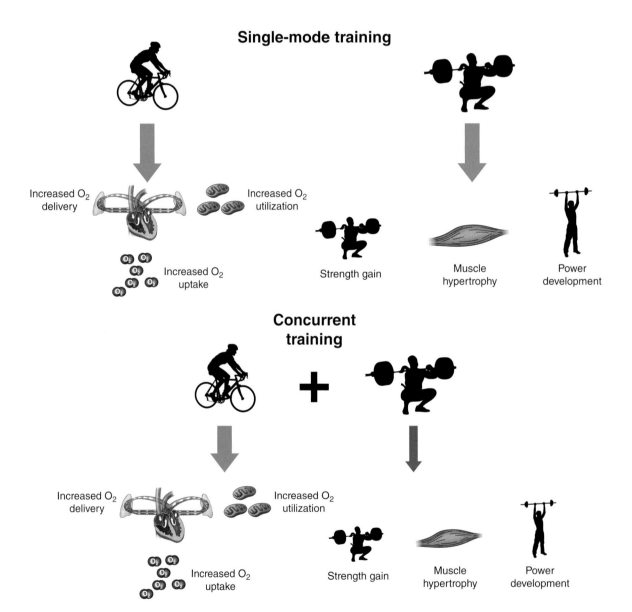

Figure 6.1 The interference effect illustrated. When performed separately, endurance and strength training lead to quite specific long-term adaptations. When performed concurrently, metabolic conditioning may limit strength and power development; however, strength training is unlikely to reduce (and instead will likely enhance) endurance performance (i.e., average power or speed maintained over prolonged durations or the ability to repeat high-intensity actions over time).

in power or rate of force development may occur without any measurable interference to strength gain or muscle hypertrophy (41). Interestingly, there is evidence that short-term concurrent training may even potentiate improvements in muscle hypertrophy (but importantly, not strength gain) (56, 66) versus strength training performed alone. The conflicting evidence base on the existence and magnitude of any so-called interference effect or concurrent training effect illustrates the complexity of the concurrent training field. These observations also suggest the interference effect is likely influenced by the specific manipulation of both training and nontraining (e.g., training status, nutrient availability) variables within the concurrent training program (36). As concurrent training involves the prescription and integration of both metabolic conditioning and strength training into the overall program, key training variables naturally include those related to the metabolic conditioning component (e.g., intensity, volume, type, modality), the strength training component (e.g., intensity, volume, type), and additional between-mode considerations (e.g., order in which endurance and strength training are performed in succession, length of between-mode recovery, nutritional intake around training sessions). When prescribing concurrent training, the programming puzzle challenge for the practitioner is to manipulate these variables to minimize any interference effect to strength training adaptations, while simultaneously maximizing improvements in cardiorespiratory fitness via metabolic conditioning. This then begs the question: how exactly do we minimize the interference effect when prescribing concurrent training? To answer this important question, and for practitioners to employ an evidence-based approach to limiting the interference effect during concurrent training, an understanding of the key factors responsible for the interference effect is required.

Potential Mechanisms for the Interference Effect and Ways to Minimize Possible Interference During Concurrent Training

Despite published evidence for the interference effect with concurrent training first appearing in the early 1980s (47), the mechanisms responsible are still incompletely understood. Although the exact factors are unclear, the interference effect likely is caused by:

- a compromised quality of strength training sessions, and/or
- a blunting of post-exercise processes that underpin aspects of strength training adaptation (e.g., attenuated post-exercise increases in rates of muscle protein synthesis and/or exacerbated rates of protein breakdown).

A compromise of either of these factors will likely result in suboptimal strength training adaptation. Variations of these two theories have been termed the *acute* and *chronic* hypotheses for the interference effect, respectively (24, 63).

The acute (or neuromuscular) hypothesis for the interference effect is based on the premise that metabolic conditioning simply limits the ability of the athlete to successfully perform strength training at the desired intensity and/or volume, consequently limiting strength training adaptation. In other words, metabolic conditioning simply ruins the quality of strength training sessions, leading to suboptimal development of strength, power or rate of force development, and/or muscle hypertrophy. In practice, it is easy to imagine how heavy strength training (e.g., squats and deadlifts performed at ≥85% 1RM) is considerably more challenging to perform both at the required intensity (i.e., load) and for the desired number of repetitions or sets at a given load when the lower-body musculature is prefatigued from metabolic conditioning performed in the hours or days prior. If this situation is repeated over time, training-induced gains in strength, power, and/or muscle mass may be less than if strength training were performed in isolation. It is important to consider, however, that while strength training does not appear to inhibit long-term improvements in endurance performance, there is the potential for the residual effects of strength sessions to negatively influence metabolic conditioning sessions performed subsequently, for example, by influencing running kinematics and reducing economy (32). The practitioner must therefore be mindful of the potential for both strength training and metabolic conditioning to influence session performance in the opposing exercise mode, and that in some circumstances, performance during key HIIT or strength sessions may need to be prioritized over the other.

An alternate (but not necessarily mutually exclusive) theory for the interference effect has been termed the chronic (or molecular) hypothesis. This theory is based largely on the specificity of training adaptation and the apparent incompatibility between large muscle fiber sizes and high levels of oxidative (endurance) capacity (98). Clearly, strength training and metabolic conditioning lead to quite specific long-term adaptations, although initially these adaptations may be less mode-specific compared to that seen following long-term training (22). In previously untrained individuals, for example, strength training can also improve $\dot{V}O_2$peak (48), while aerobic exercise (specifically cycling, but not running) can promote type I muscle fiber hypertrophy (43, 44). This concept also brings us back to the toothpaste theory (initially described in chapter 4) when we discussed aspects of exercise prescription for elite athletes. While most forms of exercise do a decent job of squeezing from the middle of the tube (i.e., gaining some level of physiological adaptation and training outcome), after some time, it becomes an ineffective strategy to get the toothpaste out. Squeezing strongly and consistently on just one side before the other (i.e., a proper strength workout for strength development before appropriate HIIT for metabolic conditioning) and not squeezing just from the middle allows a more efficient means of dispensing toothpaste on our brush. Indeed, the higher the training status of an individual (and the less toothpaste in the tube), the more important it is that we squeeze our tube properly. At the extremes of the strength-endurance continuum, the specificity of training adaptation may be best illustrated by comparing the vastly divergent body types (i.e., phenotypes) of marathon runners to powerlifters, but similar differences can even be seen clearly within the same sport (i.e., sprint versus hill climbing cyclists and heavy versus lightweight rowers; chapters 15 and 16, respectively).

At the cellular level, the molecular factors responsible for this specificity of training adaptation in skeletal muscle are becoming increasingly clear (although these factors are certainly not yet completely understood). Adaptation to strength training (specifically, muscle fiber hypertrophy) has been primarily associated with the molecular factors governing muscle protein synthesis (i.e., the mechanistic target of rapamycin complex 1 (mTORC1) signaling pathway) (68), whereas endurance training adaptations in skeletal muscle have been linked to signaling pathways that regulate mitochondrial biogenesis (via activation of the transcriptional coactivator PGC-1α, including the AMPK, CaMK, SIRT1, and p38 pathways) (51). It has been suggested that strength and endurance training stimulate a distinct

activation of these molecular signaling pathways within skeletal muscle, and that when repeated over time, these pathways largely underpin the divergent phenotypes induced by chronic training in either mode (consider marathon runners versus powerlifters as an example) (5).

Research investigating the molecular basis for the specificity of training adaptation has also provided clues to a potential mechanism for the interference effect with concurrent training. A classic study by Atherton and colleagues (5) aimed to replicate the stimuli associated with strength training and metabolic conditioning by electrically stimulating isolated rat muscles in either a strength training-like (repeated, high-intensity stimulation) or metabolic conditioning-like (prolonged, low-intensity stimulation) manner to investigate the molecular underpinnings of mode-specific training adaptations in muscle. The results suggested strength training-like electrical stimulation selectively activated the mTORC1 signaling pathway and increased the synthesis rates of contractile (i.e., myofibrillar) muscle proteins, whereas the metabolic conditioning-like electrical stimulation tended to activate only the AMPK/PGC-1α signaling pathway, without any increase in the synthesis rates of contractile muscle proteins. These researchers also noted that the metabolic conditioning-like stimulation seemed to block the activation of the mTORC1 pathway, which may explain why myofibrillar protein synthesis was not increased by this type of stimulation. Based on these observations, it was suggested this so-called master-switch mechanism could potentially explain the specific adaptations caused in muscle by strength training and metabolic conditioning (5). This blunting of anabolic responses may also be explained by the ability of AMPK, which functions as a cellular energy sensor, to switch off the mTORC1 pathway in conditions of cellular energy stress such as those muscle cells experience during metabolic conditioning (54). In other words, when AMPK is activated by energy stress caused by endurance training (or at least endurance-like electrical stimulation), AMPK might act as a molecular brake on the mTORC1 pathway, which may blunt muscle protein synthesis rates and, in turn, potentially long-term muscle hypertrophy.

The next question, then, is can this master switch hypothesis explain why strength training adaptations (i.e., improvements in maximal strength, power, and muscle hypertrophy) may be blunted with concurrent training? Since the Atherton and colleagues (5) study was published, many studies have investigated whether this molecular interference phenomenon actually occurs in human skeletal muscle following concurrent training. Despite the observations of the AMPK/mTORC1 master-switch mechanism occurring in rat muscle, at present there is virtually no evidence of a similar mechanistic function in human muscle during exercise. For example, in moderately trained individuals ($p\dot{V}O_2max = 361$ W), post-exercise anabolic responses in skeletal muscle after strength training were not impeded by prior HIIT cycling (5×4 min at 85% $\dot{V}O_2$peak/3 min at 100 W), despite prior HIIT increasing skeletal muscle AMPK activity (~90%) (3). There is also even evidence that anabolic responses (i.e., mTORC1 signaling) in skeletal muscle are increased to an even greater extent with concurrent training versus strength training alone (37, 65). Put simply, the ability of strength training to activate anabolic processes that regulate skeletal muscle growth appears not to be impeded in humans when preceded by a bout of strenuous metabolic conditioning, such as HIIT. It is also important to consider that metabolic conditioning itself is sufficient to activate anabolic processes (both mTORC1 signaling and increased rates of muscle protein synthesis) in human muscle (69), an effect that appears greater with higher-intensity metabolic conditioning (29). Additionally, training status is a key influencer of early post-exercise molecular responses in skeletal muscle (99), so further work is needed to investigate whether there is a molecular basis for the interference effect in more highly trained individuals.

When discussing the potential mechanisms underpinning the interference effect with concurrent training, it is perhaps important to consider that any molecular basis to the interference effect can likely only explain interference to muscle hypertrophy, as opposed to strength and/or power development. While muscle hypertrophy has traditionally been considered an important contributor to strength development (74), this notion is now being challenged (15), while it is also clear that increases in strength can occur with strength training in the absence of measurable changes in muscle size (101). The implications of any potential interference to muscle hypertrophy versus interference to strength development with concurrent training for the development of sport-specific physical capacities should also be considered by the practitioner. For example, while there is evidence that higher levels of strength

and power are associated with improved performance in sport-specific skills such as jumping, sprinting, and changes of direction (23, 95), evidence for the importance of muscle hypertrophy per se in developing these qualities is lacking. Because of the clearer links between strength and power development and sport-specific skill development, the implications of interference to strength and power development (as opposed to hypertrophy) with concurrent training are perhaps a more relevant consideration for the practitioner.

Nevertheless, while there is limited evidence of a molecular basis for the interference effect, it is acknowledged that training adaptation in skeletal muscle is largely mediated by the cumulative effects of early post-exercise responses to repeated training bouts (81). These include the molecular signaling events that underpin key adaptations to strength and metabolic conditioning, such as muscle hypertrophy and mitochondrial biogenesis (35). An understanding of the influence of concurrent training organization on early post-exercise responses, summarized for the reader in figure 6.2, may be potentially important for understanding the implications for long-term adaptations to concurrent training.

Linking the Metabolic and Neuromuscular Demands of HIIT With Their Potential Influence on Concurrent Strength Training

As discussed in chapter 4, prescribing HIIT requires the manipulation of at least 12 different variables, any of which may affect the short-term physiological responses to an HIIT session. Also described in chapter 5 was the concept that any given HIIT session will challenge, at differing respective levels, both the metabolic and neuromuscular physiological systems (chapter 3). In the context of prescribing HIIT in concurrent training programs, particularly important considerations include the neuromuscular demands of individual HIIT sessions (type 6 targets; figure 1.5) and how these demands may then influence performance during subsequent strength training sessions.

As discussed earlier in the chapter, an ideal scenario is whereby strength training sessions are undertaken when the neuromuscular system is less fatigued, so that strength training performance may

KEY POINTS

To summarize, prescribing concurrent training (as shown in most sports you'll find in the application chapters) presents unique challenges for the practitioner, given the potential for endurance training to interfere with the development of strength, power, and/or muscle hypertrophy induced by strength training. Although concurrent training likely benefits endurance performance over the long term, the potential for strength training to also compromise performance during key HIIT sessions should also be considered. Possible mechanisms for attenuated strength training adaptations with concurrent training include compromised strength training quality (i.e., the acute or neuromuscular hypothesis) and/or a compromised activation of anabolic processes after strength training sessions that underpin muscle hypertrophy (i.e., the chronic or molecular hypothesis; figure 6.2). While there is limited evidence for any molecular interference effect occurring in human muscle with concurrent training, there is certainly evidence that prior metabolic conditioning training can compromise subsequent strength training performance, as will be shown in the following section, lending support to the neural hypothesis for the interference effect. Because of the lack of evidence for any molecular basis for the interference effect, it is difficult to provide practical recommendations for minimizing

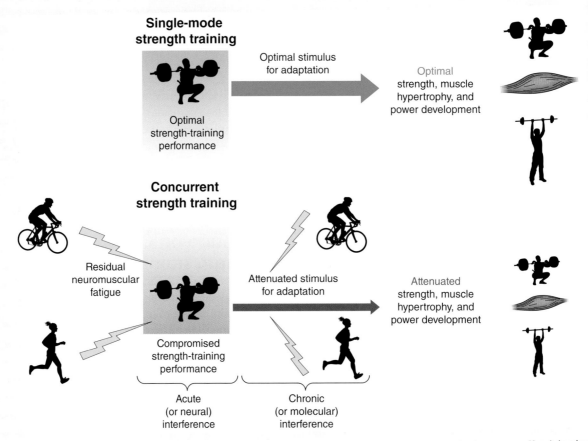

Figure 6.2 Conceptual framework outlining the potential mechanisms for the interference effect, including compromised resistance training quality and/or recovery from resistance training sessions. When strength training is performed alone (i.e., single-mode strength training), performance is maximized as minimal residual fatigue is present. This allows for an optimal stimulus for adaptation and, subsequently, optimal development of classic strength training adaptations (strength, muscle hypertrophy, power development). With concurrent training, the metabolic conditioning component likely causes residual neuromuscular fatigue that may compromise both strength training performance and potentially the adaptive response to strength training sessions. Both of these factors will likely limit the stimulus for adaptation, resulting in attenuated development of classic strength training adaptations.

interference with concurrent training based solely on the molecular responses to single concurrent exercise bouts. Rather, practical recommendations may be derived by considering factors related to metabolic conditioning sessions that are likely to compromise subsequent strength training performance, therefore likely leading to an interference effect. Practitioners integrating HIIT within concurrent training programs must therefore have a sound understanding of the physiological (anaerobic and neuromuscular in particular) demands of different HIIT formats (chapters 3 and 5) and how the residual effects of individual HIIT sessions may influence subsequent strength training performance, thereby influencing adaptation to concurrent training programs.

be maximized. This is because a less-fatigued athlete can likely:

- lift heavier absolute loads (at a higher percentage of his or her 1RM) for a given number of repetitions,
- perform more repetitions at a given percentage of the 1RM load, and/or
- perform repetitions at faster intended and/or actual concentric velocities (as a percentage of the maximum velocity possible with a given load).

These factors likely ensure the strength training stimulus (type 6, figure 1.5) is maximized, and therefore, the potential for adaptation to that strength training session likewise is optimized. As such, the challenge for the practitioner is to schedule concurrent HIIT and strength training sessions so that the residual effects of the HIIT sessions do not have a substantial negative influence on strength training performance.

The practitioner must consider that two HIIT sessions may similarly challenge the cardiopulmonary and oxidative systems, while at the same time involve distinctly different anaerobic energy contributions and/or neuromuscular strain (chapter 5). Any HIIT session that evokes a large neuromuscular strain component (i.e., types 2, 4, or 5) will likely result in more substantial residual fatigue of the exercised musculature, compared to HIIT sessions with smaller neuromuscular strain components (i.e., types 1 or 3). For this reason, HIIT sessions characterized by larger neuromuscular demands will likely further compromise subsequent strength training performance for a period of time after HIIT cessation, compared to HIIT sessions of lower neuromuscular demands. Similarly,

it is likely that strength sessions (type 6) may also compromise performance during subsequent HIIT sessions with high neuromuscular demands (i.e., types 2, 4, or 5). As you will see in later sections of this chapter, the practitioner must consider the relative priority of key HIIT or strength sessions within any given training week and manipulate the organization of these sessions to minimize the potential for negative interactions between training modes.

There is strong evidence that the force-generating capacity of exercised musculature is compromised in the subsequent hours following metabolic conditioning performed at various intensities (2, 10, 11, 60, 61). As discussed, residual fatigue from endurance training may compromise performance during a strength training session conducted within this period, primarily by limiting the number of repetitions possible at a given absolute or relative intensity, thereby limiting total session volume (28, 59, 83, 92, 96). This attenuation of within-session strength training performance is likely to, at least partially, mediate the interference effect during periods of concurrent training (24, 63).

From a practical perspective, it is useful then to consider the effects of HIIT variable manipulation on the neuromuscular demands of HIIT and, subsequently, the potential implications for subsequent strength training performance. Currently, however, there are considerable gaps in our knowledge surrounding the influence of HIIT variable manipulation on neuromuscular demands, and particularly the implications of these demands for performance during subsequent training sessions (e.g., strength training). Current understanding of the factors modulating the neuromuscular demands of HIIT are well described in chapters 3, 4, and 5; however, these factors are summarized for the reader in figure 6.3.

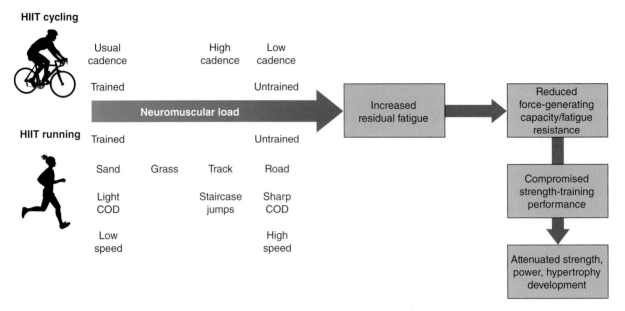

Figure 6.3 Conceptual framework summarizing the practical factors that might influence residual fatigue following HIIT, and therefore may further negatively influence subsequent strength training performance.

The factors outlined in figure 6.3 should be considered when integrating HIIT with strength training, given that residual effects of such metabolic conditioning examples may negatively influence strength training performance. Indeed, a number of studies (e.g., 28, 59, 83, 92, 96) have investigated the consequences of prior metabolic conditioning (of various relative intensities) on subsequent strength training performance. While most studies show a negative effect of prior metabolic conditioning on subsequent neuromuscular and/or strength training performance (28, 59, 83, 92, 96), others instead show no effect (62). These equivocal findings suggest that, like the interference effect itself, this phenomenon likely depends on the intricacies of the prescription of both training- and nontraining-related variables within a concurrent training program. The reality of these complexities is highlighted in the application chapters in part II, written by coaches and sport scientists charged with the daily delivery of evidence-based practice in elite sport. Although much further work is needed to identify optimal strategies for integrating HIIT into concurrent training programs, existing evidence has begun to shed light on the potential effects of training (e.g., HIIT work intensity, volume, and modality) and nontraining (e.g., within-session training order, length of between-mode recovery, and the potential influence of training status or age) variables on subsequent strength training performance.

Effect of HIIT Work Intensity

Given the focus on HIIT, the potential effects of HIIT work intensity in modulating the interference effect with concurrent training is a highly relevant practical consideration. There is evidence that the compromising effect of metabolic conditioning on subsequent force-generating capacity and strength training performance may be somewhat intensity dependent (11, 28, 62). For example, neuromuscular fatigue (indexed by reduced isometric MVC force and quadriceps muscle activation assessed via EMG) of the exercised musculature is evident for at least 6 h after combined continuous/HIIT cycling (30 min at 80% $\dot{V}O_2$max followed by 4×60 s efforts at 120% $\dot{V}O_2$max) in moderately trained triathletes ($\dot{V}O_2$max $= \sim59$ mL·kg^{-1}·min^{-1}) (11), whereas less residual fatigue is often noted following lower-intensity continuous endurance training (28, 62). It follows that the negative impact of metabolic conditioning-induced fatigue on strength training performance is worsened with higher-intensity metabolic conditioning (28, 59, 83). This finding is not universal, however, with detriments to strength training performance in recreationally active athletes

($\dot{V}O_2$max = ~57 mL·kg^{-1}·min^{-1}) shown to be similar when preceded by either submaximal continuous (36 min at 40% p$\dot{V}O_2$max) or HIIT (6 × 3 min at 95%-100% p$\dot{V}O_2$max/3 min at 40% p$\dot{V}O_2$max) cycling (92). Additional work has also shown no difference between moderate-intensity continuous (30 min at 80% of the lactate threshold [LT]) and HIIT (10 sets of 1 min at 120% LT, 1 min passive recovery) cycling on either anabolic responses in muscle to subsequent strength training (37) or 1RM leg press strength gain after 8 wk of training (38). It is important to consider, however, that although these studies highlight the influence of relative endurance training intensity for eliciting residual neuromuscular fatigue and compromising strength training performance or adaptation, virtually nothing is known about the effect of different HIIT work interval intensities on these parameters. For example, whether HIIT work intervals performed at 120% versus 100% v$\dot{V}O_2$max elicit greater neuromuscular fatigue, and how this influences the quality of subsequent strength training sessions, is currently unclear. Regardless of this lack of empirical evidence for the role of HIIT intensity in modulating neuromuscular fatigue, the more conservative option for the practitioner may nevertheless be to reduce HIIT intensity prior to strength training sessions and consequently favor HIIT types 1 and 3 as opposed to HIIT types 2, 4, and 5 (figure 1.5).

Effect of HIIT Volume

Although not specific to HIIT volume per se, there is some evidence that the total volume of endurance training is an important modulating factor for the interference effect during concurrent training (55, 88, 100). A meta-analysis of the concurrent training literature (100) suggested increased weekly frequencies and/or durations of endurance training sessions are associated with greater interference to strength training adaptations. Additional indirect evidence for a volume-dependent interference effect is provided by the absence of interference with lower endurance training frequencies (≤2 sessions/wk) (39, 41, 70), whereas attenuated strength development is observed with higher weekly endurance training frequencies (≥3 sessions/wk) (9, 46, 47, 55, 57). These observations suggest that strategies that limit the frequency and/or session volume of HIIT may be worthwhile for minimizing interference during periods of concurrent training, particularly during training peri-

ods during which the development of maximal strength, power, and/or hypertrophy may be prioritized. Despite this, much further work is required to better define the role of overall HIIT volume in mediating the interference effect.

Effect of HIIT Modality

As discussed in chapters 4 and 5, HIIT may be programmed using multiple metabolic conditioning modalities (e.g., running, cycling, swimming, rowing). It is important to recognize that different training modalities are characterized by unique patterns of muscle recruitment, as well as differences in the magnitude of neuromuscular strain imparted on the active musculature. For example, running and cycling primarily recruit the lower-body musculature, whereas both swimming and rowing involve a considerable element of upper-body muscular work. Despite these obvious between-mode differences in muscle group involvement, comparisons between the neuromuscular demands of different endurance training modalities, i.e., running, cycling, swimming, rowing (particularly in reference to HIIT) are currently lacking. Nevertheless, due to an increased eccentric loading component (71), running likely imparts greater neuromuscular strain on the lower-body musculature compared to cycling, whereas both swimming and rowing will clearly induce greater neuromuscular strain on the upper-body musculature versus either cycling or running. These factors have implications for the integration of HIIT within concurrent training programs because differences in muscle recruitment and neuromuscular strain profiles associated with different HIIT modalities, specific to the exercise mode, are likely to differentially influence performance in particular strength-training exercises performed subsequently. For example, running-based HIIT will likely further compromise subsequent lower-body strength training performance versus cycling-based HIIT, whereas upper-body strength training performance may be limited by both swimming- and rowing-based HIIT. It is also important to note that similar considerations can also be held for the potential influences of strength training on performance during subsequent key HIIT sessions, as discussed previously. While these observations likely provide some insight into the potential effects of different metabolic conditioning modalities on subsequent strength training performance, there is very little published literature available to verify these insights. One study (79) compared the effects of HIIT cycling or treadmill running (15×1 min at v/p$\dot{V}O_2$max/1 min passive recovery) on subsequent strength training performance (4 sets of maximum repetitions of half squats at 80% 1RM) in recreationally active males ($\dot{V}O_2$peak = ~45 mL·kg^{-1}·min^{-1} and ~38 mL·kg^{-1}·min^{-1} measured during running and cycling, respectively) (79). Both HIIT cycling and treadmill running limited the number of repetitions performed and total volume load lifted (in kg) during subsequent sets of half squats, although cycling actually resulted in more prolonged negative effects (79). As the prior cycling- or running-based HIIT did not influence muscle activation (quantified via vastus lateralis EMG activity) during strength training, the authors speculated their findings were mediated by a higher reliance on anaerobic metabolism with cycling (i.e., HIIT types 3 and 5), although markers of this were not measured. It is possible these findings may have also been influenced by the training status of the participants with reference to running versus cycling. Based on the higher reported $\dot{V}O_2$peak values during running (79), it is possible these participants were more accustomed to running versus cycling, which may have led to increased residual fatigue following cycling and, in turn, further compromised strength training performance. Clearly, more work is needed to confirm the effects of different HIIT modalities on residual neuromuscular fatigue and the associated implications for strength training performance.

Effect of Within-Session Order and Recovery Duration Between HIIT and Strength Training Sessions

As neuromuscular fatigue induced by metabolic conditioning is a transient phenomenon (10, 11, 92), the recovery duration allowed between endurance and strength training sessions likely influences the effects of prior metabolic conditioning on strength training performance (and vice versa). Most evidence suggests that neuromuscular fatigue persists for at least 6 h after strenuous endurance exercise (including HIIT), which may be fully resolved after 24 h (10, 11, 92). It should be kept in mind, however, that although often implemented by practitioners, the 6 h window may not always be the magic number for optimal between-mode recovery length, since the recovery rate is likely affected by a number of modulating factors, including the type of exercise performed and an athlete's training status (i.e., figure 6.3). Nevertheless, extended recovery periods after HIIT sessions are likely optimal for resolving any residual fatigue (particularly following HIIT sessions involving large neuromuscular demands) and hence are likewise optimal for maximizing subsequent strength training performance. For this reason, it is also advisable that when strength training and metabolic conditioning are performed within a single training session, strength training should precede the metabolic conditioning component (rather than vice versa) (76). There is indeed some evidence that increasing the recovery periods between endurance and subsequent strength training can limit any negative effects on strength training performance. For example, completing either submaximal continuous (36 min at 40% p$\dot{V}O_2$max) or HIIT (6×3 min at 95%-100% p$\dot{V}O_2$max/3 min at 40% p$\dot{V}O_2$max) cycling compromises strength training (leg press) performance at both 4 and 8 h post-exercise, although these negative effects were resolved after 24 h (92). There is also some indirect evidence for the benefits of increasing between-mode recovery lengths when comparing strength gains to concurrent training when strength and metabolic conditioning sessions are performed on separate days, compared to being performed on the same day. For example, one study (89) showed that performing low-intensity strength training (15-20-RM loads) on different days than HIIT sessions (6-8×3 min cycling bouts at 90%-100% $\dot{V}O_2$max) led to superior 1RM leg press strength gains (but not markers of muscle hypertrophy), compared to undertaking both training modes on the same day. Additional evidence (20) in recreationally trained subjects ($\dot{V}O_2$max = ~40 mL·kg^{-1}·min^{-1}) suggests even supramaximal-intensity cycling (SIT involving 4-6×20 s all-out modified Wingate-style sprints) does not cause interference to maximal strength or hypertrophy responses when performed on alternating days to high-intensity (~85% 1RM) strength training. Increasing the recovery duration between HIIT (3×6 min sets of 15 s 120% MAV/15 s passive recovery) and strength training (from 0 to 24 h recovery) seems to optimize strength and power development in amateur rugby players, even when HIIT sessions were always performed after strength training (86). Since HIIT was not performed prior to strength training in that study (86), it is therefore unlikely these results could be explained by compromised strength training performance. Interestingly however, increasing the between-mode recovery duration also led to larger improvements in $\dot{V}O_2$peak (86), which may reflect compromised HIIT performance when preceded closely by strength training (although this was not directly assessed). Indeed, the potential for residual fatigue from prior strength training sessions to negatively influence performance during subsequent HIIT sessions (as well as vice versa, as previously discussed), including altering factors such as running kinematics and economy (32), is worth considering. For example, single bouts of strength training can compromise subsequent cycling time trial (15 min) performance (17), and both running (31) and arm cranking (33) time to exhaustion. Performing strength training before endurance training can also compromise training-induced improvements in running time trial (4 km) performance, compared to the reverse exercise order (21). While these observations highlight the potential bidirectional interactions between strength and endurance training acutely influencing performance in the opposing mode, the weight of evidence nevertheless suggests strength training can, in the long term, improve various aspects of endurance performance without compromising $\dot{V}O_2$max (1).

Aside from performance enhancement alone, considerations for the order of concurrent training sessions also extends to modulating injury risk during HIIT (64). This is because strength training (e.g., Nordic hamstring lowers) may transiently reduce levels of muscle strength and/or activation, which in turn may expose the musculature to increased loading during high-speed running sessions performed subsequently and potentially increase injury (e.g., hamstring strain) risk (64). In these cases, the practitioner should be mindful of programming high-speed running for a period after strength training sessions and manipulate HIIT formats accordingly to constrain absolute running speeds when performed subsequent to strength training.

Altogether, the available evidence suggests that where possible, strength training should be performed prior to HIIT if performed within the same session or at least 6 h after HIIT sessions if performed within the same day. The ability for strength training sessions to also induce neuromuscular fatigue and then influence performance (and also injury risk) during subsequent HIIT sessions performed must also be considered. Ultimately, the practitioner will need to decide on the relative priority of any given HIIT or strength training session and adjust the weekly training plan accordingly to ensure performance is maximized within priority training session(s).

Role of Athlete Training Status or Age

As discussed in chapter 3, individual training status (that is, the athlete's fitness level or ability to perform a given exercise task) will largely influence the degree of neuromuscular fatigue induced by a given HIIT session, and therefore the likelihood of that session compromising subsequent strength training sessions. Interestingly, there is evidence that for some athletes, neuromuscular performance may be transiently enhanced, rather than compromised, following strenuous HIIT sessions (e.g., 14). This observation has been attributed to a possible postactivation potentiation effect (13), whereby prior high-intensity muscular contractions can acutely enhance performance during subsequent activities (49). The practitioner should therefore consider the possibility that prior HIIT sessions (likely those performed in close proximity to strength training and with a low-anaerobic contribution and/or associated muscle contractile perturbation, i.e., types 1 or 2) may actually enhance, rather than inhibit, subsequent strength training performance in highly trained athletes. It is also possible that in some circumstances, prior strength training sessions may also likewise enhance performance (e.g., power output) during subsequent HIIT sessions (18). However, the factors that modulate this potentiating effect are complex and likely related to the intricacies of both the type of HIIT session performed, the type of subsequent activity or strength training performed, as well as the training status of the athlete. Much further research is required to determine the role of these factors in modulating the influence of prior HIIT sessions on the capacity to acutely enhance or compromise performance during subsequent strength training sessions (as well as vice versa).

Overall it is clear that neuromuscular fatigue from metabolic conditioning can negatively influence performance during subsequent strength training sessions, and this may at least partially explain attenuated strength training adaptation with concurrent training. Understanding of the neuromuscular demands of different HIIT formats allows the practitioner to manipulate HIIT prescription in consideration of the potential consequences of these sessions for other training modalities performed within a weekly microcycle (e.g., strength training). While current evidence has begun to shed light on the neuromuscular demands of different HIIT formats and the impact of metabolic conditioning (including HIIT) on subsequent strength training performance, this evidence is not without limitations, and our understanding of these factors is by no means complete. Although there is no doubt much further work is needed to identify optimal strategies to integrate HIIT into concurrent training programs, existing evidence has nevertheless begun to shape practical recommendations for minimizing the interference effect.

It should also be recognized that in some circumstances, the weekly periodization of strength training and HIIT may be dictated not by what is necessarily optimal but by other practical factors (e.g., coach preference with weekly schedule and/or within-session order of training content, priority of HIIT versus strength training quality, etc.). In some cases (particularly in endurance sports), the quality of key HIIT sessions may often need to be prioritized ahead of strength training sessions (18). In these situations, the practitioner may need to accept compromised strength training quality to allow for this emphasis on HIIT sessions.

Piecing It Together: Practical Strategies for Programming HIIT During Concurrent Training

As discussed throughout the chapter, programming HIIT during concurrent training requires consideration of how individual HIIT sessions may influence performance during subsequent strength training sessions and, in turn, modulate any potential interference effect to strength training adaptations. Although more research is required to evaluate optimal strategies for integrating HIIT within concurrent training programs, a number of practical recommendations for maximizing concurrent training adaptation may be devised based on our current understanding. It should be made clear, however, that these recommendations depend on multiple logistical factors (see part II), including the particular sport itself, the training phase, athlete training status, etc. Nevertheless, here are general recommendations for limiting interference to strength training adaptations with concurrent training.

- Limit neuromuscular fatigue prior to strength training sessions by performing strength train-

ing either before or at least (approximately) 6 h after HIIT sessions.

- HIIT sessions performed in the 24 h prior to strength training sessions should ideally be characterized by lower neuromuscular demands by incorporating lower absolute or relative work intensities associated with lower neuromuscular load (i.e., types 1 and 3). However it is worth noting that using lower HIIT intensities may often need to be associated with longer effort durations (e.g., 3 min at 85% V_{IFT} versus 10 s/20 s at 120% V_{IFT}), and consequently these longer durations may also cause neuromuscular fatigue. There is, in fact, a likely optimum combination between exercise intensity and duration when it comes to neuromuscular responses and fatigue (figure 5.42).

- Limit prescription of all-out HIIT modalities (i.e., RSS, SIT formats, or in general, neuromuscular-demanding HIIT formats, i.e., types 2, 4, and 5).

- Performing running-based HIIT on softer surfaces (e.g., grass or sand instead of road) is likely to impart less neuromuscular strain (figure 5.43).

- Limit the change-of-direction (COD) component (particularly sharp COD) of running-based HIIT or employ cycling-based, rather than running-based, HIIT (depending on the athlete's training specificity).

- Where possible and when individual strength or power development (type 6) may be favored over the metabolic conditioning component, total weekly metabolic conditioning volume should be limited by reducing the weekly frequency of HIIT sessions and/or performing fewer repetitions and/or series during HIIT sessions or by reducing training volume associated with other cardiorespiratory modalities (e.g., prolonged endurance training sessions).

Based on these recommendations, a number of practical scenarios in which HIIT is integrated into concurrent training programs are shown in figures 6.4 and 6.5, with examples of optimal organization of HIIT and strength training within a weekly microcycle of team and individual sport programs, respectively. Excellent team and endurance sport examples of weekly microcycle periodization of concurrent training can additionally be viewed in nearly every chapter in part II.

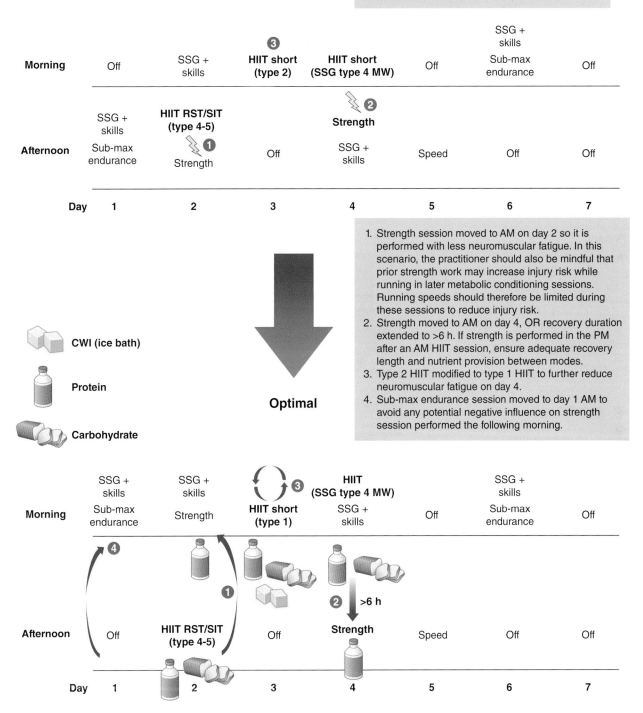

Team sport weekly periodization
example: preseason

Sub-optimal

1. High neuromuscular strain from type 4-5 HIIT will likely compromise subsequent strength session.
2. Type 4 SSG HIIT session will likely cause neuromuscular fatigue for at least 6 h afterward. Strength session likely compromised if performed within this time window.
3. Residual fatigue on day 4 might be worsened by type 2 session performed on previous day.

Morning	Off	SSG + skills	**③ HIIT short (type 2)**	**HIIT short (SSG type 4 MW)**	Off	SSG + skills / Sub-max endurance	Off
Afternoon	SSG + skills / Sub-max endurance	**HIIT RST/SIT (type 4-5)** ⚡① Strength	Off	⚡② **Strength** / SSG + skills	Speed	Off	Off
Day	1	2	3	4	5	6	7

1. Strength session moved to AM on day 2 so it is performed with less neuromuscular fatigue. In this scenario, the practitioner should also be mindful that prior strength work may increase injury risk while running in later metabolic conditioning sessions. Running speeds should therefore be limited during these sessions to reduce injury risk.
2. Strength moved to AM on day 4, OR recovery duration extended to >6 h. If strength is performed in the PM after an AM HIIT session, ensure adequate recovery length and nutrient provision between modes.
3. Type 2 HIIT modified to type 1 HIIT to further reduce neuromuscular fatigue on day 4.
4. Sub-max endurance session moved to day 1 AM to avoid any potential negative influence on strength session performed the following morning.

CWI (ice bath)

Protein

Carbohydrate

Optimal

Morning	SSG + skills / Sub-max endurance	SSG + skills / Strength	**③ HIIT short (type 1)**	**HIIT (SSG type 4 MW)** / SSG + skills	Off	SSG + skills / Sub-max endurance	Off
Afternoon	④ Off	**HIIT RST/SIT (type 4-5)** ①	Off	② >6 h **Strength**	Speed	Off	Off
Day	1	2	3	4	5	6	7

Figure 6.4   Team sport concurrent training program puzzle example.

131

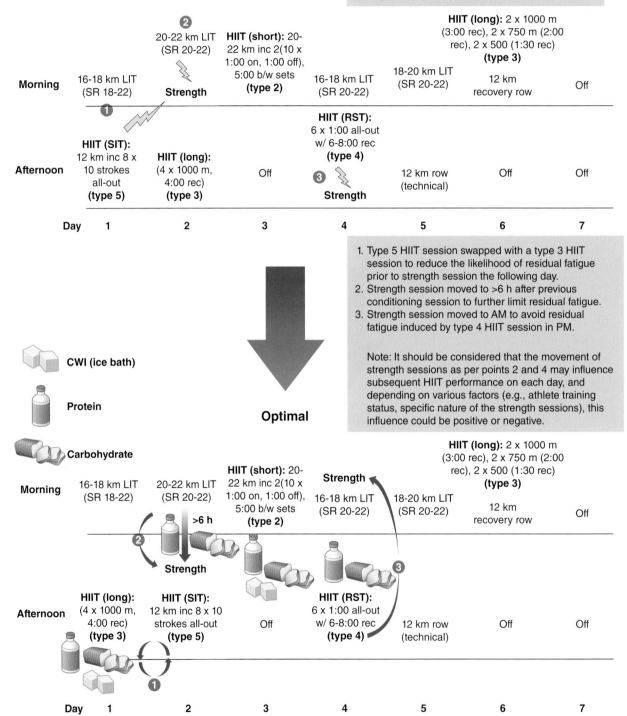

Figure 6.5 Endurance sport concurrent training program puzzle example.

Additional Nontraining-Related Strategies to Mitigate the Interference Effect

As discussed initially in this chapter, the interference effect is likely a result of compromised performance and/or adaptive responses to individual strength training sessions, culminating in attenuated strength training adaptations. Aside from the manipulation of training variables and weekly session organization, there is potential for other nontraining-related strategies to somewhat mitigate any potential negative influence of HIIT on strength training performance and/or post-exercise adaptive responses during concurrent training.

Strategies to Minimize (Acute) Residual Fatigue Prior to Strength Training

The links between HIIT-induced neuromuscular fatigue and the resulting potential for subsequent reductions in strength training performance suggest interventions aimed at attenuating post-exercise neuromuscular fatigue may be beneficial to limit any potential compromise to strength training performance during concurrent training. There is indeed evidence that certain post-exercise recovery modalities, including cold water immersion (CWI) (94) and dynamic pneumatic compression devices (90), can enhance recovery of the declines in muscle strength or increases in muscle soreness after strenuous exercise. However, whether the implementation of recovery modalities following metabolic conditioning can minimize detrimental effects on subsequent strength training performance has not been investigated. While strategies such as cryotherapy have shown promise for accelerating post-exercise recovery (94), one potential downside of cold therapies applied in the hours prior to strength training sessions are potential short-term reductions in force production or rate of force development due to cold-induced decreases in nerve conduction velocity. As such, there is potential for the application of cryotherapy modalities in close proximity to a subsequent strength training session to actually compromise, rather than enhance, performance. It is therefore possible a certain recovery window after application of post-exercise recovery techniques is necessary to allow for an attenuation of neuromuscular fatigue, coupled with a restoration of neuro-

muscular properties (such as nerve conduction velocities), before subsequent strength training is performed. Another potential concern is that the application of CWI may itself interfere with strength training adaptations, as performing CWI immediately (i.e., within 5 min) after strength training sessions has been shown to blunt maximal strength and muscle size improvements after 12 wk of training (85). Whether this negative effect of CWI on strength training adaptations is apparent only when applied immediately following strength training sessions, as opposed to following metabolic conditioning sessions performed at least 6 h prior to strength training, is currently unclear. More work is needed to better understand how the implementation of post-exercise recovery strategies can influence exercise performance and adaptation to concurrent training, and this is indeed a promising area for future research.

Nutritional strategies also have the potential to influence exercise performance, and therefore may be useful for countering residual fatigue during periods of concurrent training. Apart from maximizing post-exercise adaptive responses (particularly anabolism following strength training), nutrient availability between training sessions (e.g., between a morning metabolic conditioning session and an afternoon strength training session) also likely impacts exercise performance during the second session and, likely, the resulting long-term adaptations. Given the links between muscle glycogen content and endurance performance (12), post-exercise glycogen replenishment between concurrent training sessions performed within the same day (or even on alternate days) may play a role in maximizing exercise performance during the second session. It is important to note that glycogen repletion may be further accelerated when carbohydrate is coingested with protein (16), providing another rationale for consuming protein after completion of metabolic conditioning sessions. As such, the ingestion of protein after both metabolic conditioning and strength training sessions is recommended, with carbohydrate (CHO) potentially provided between sessions to assist with muscle glycogen restoration that may influence performance during subsequent training sessions (irrespective of the focus of the second session, i.e., strength training or HIIT).

As well as macronutrient intake, other ergogenic aids, including caffeine (25) and creatine monohydrate (58), can enhance high-intensity exercise performance and may be useful to counter any residual fatigue induced by prior metabolic conditioning during concurrent training (see also related section on caffeine in chapter 4). In one study (27), creatine supplementation prevented the impairment to lower-body strength training performance seen following a bout of HIIT (5 km run performed intermittently at 1 min at $v\dot{V}O_2max$/1 min passive recovery). While these findings are promising, further studies are needed to confirm whether the short-term benefits of creatine supplementation translate into improved adaptation (and less interference to strength training adaptations) following longer-term concurrent training. It also remains to be determined whether caffeine supplementation might be effective for countering residual fatigue induced by a morning (e.g., metabolic conditioning) session and subsequently improving performance in an afternoon (e.g., strength training) session (see chapter 4).

Strategies to Enhance Adaptive (Chronic) Responses to Concurrent Training

Since training adaptations are largely underpinned by the accumulation of adaptive responses to single exercise bouts performed during a training program (45, 81), strategies to maximize these responses are paramount for maximizing training adaptation. Although direct evidence is currently lacking, the notion that metabolic conditioning may interfere with adaptive responses to strength training (45) also highlights the relevance of optimizing post-exercise adaptive responses during concurrent training.

Nutrient availability is a key nontraining-related factor for optimizing adaptation to both endurance and resistance training, and concurrent training is naturally no different (73, 80). Nutritional status can influence both exercise performance (as with CHO availability or caffeine ingestion, for example, which can influence exercise capacity and therefore the quality of the training stimulus itself; see chapter 4), as well as the adaptive responses to exercise (such as when training with low CHO availability or with post-exercise protein intake, both of which influence adaptive responses to exercise in muscle).

Nutrient and energy availability clearly have a profound effect on adaptive responses to both strength training and metabolic conditioning, and in some respects, in a divergent manner. In general, adaptive responses to metabolic conditioning seem to be amplified in an energy-restricted environment, whereas an energy-rich environment may be required

to support anabolism following strength training (42). For example, post-exercise adaptive responses related to mitochondrial biogenesis and substrate metabolism are further enhanced when metabolic conditioning is performed under conditions of low energy (in particular, carbohydrate) availability (8). Interestingly, however, anabolic responses to strength training are no different when performed in a glycogen-depleted state (19), whereas the role of protein (in particular, essential amino acid) ingestion in maximizing post-exercise rates of muscle protein synthesis (97) and subsequently lean mass accretion (75) is well established. It should also be mentioned that post-exercise carbohydrate ingestion does not influence muscle anabolism above protein intake alone (40, 93), suggesting there may be limited need to ingest large amounts of CHO following strength training sessions (at least when not followed by HIIT).

Given that nutrient availability plays a key role in adaptation to both metabolic conditioning and strength training, it likely also influences the interference effect with concurrent training. The fact that HIIT can impart significant energy stress on the active musculature, including glycogen depletion and increased AMPK activity (3), potentially provides a suboptimal environment for anabolic responses to strength training (45). Although there is a lack of evidence for glycogen depletion (19) or increased AMPK activity (3) inhibiting anabolic responses to strength training, post-exercise protein ingestion is nonetheless important for promoting protein turnover and remodeling following both metabolic conditioning (73) and strength training (75). Prolonged metabolic conditioning also promotes increased oxidation rates of amino acids (72) derived from the catabolism of muscle proteins, which can result in a negative muscle and whole body protein balance during exercise (52). Protein ingestion following metabolic conditioning sessions is therefore likely to assist in restoring any disruption caused to net protein balance that may limit chronic lean mass accretion during concurrent training.

Clearly, optimizing nutritional strategies (and protein intake in particular) is an important consideration when undertaking concurrent training. Both the amount (i.e., ~1.2-1.7g/kg body mass per day, or 20 g in a single dose) and pattern (i.e., 4-5 separate intakes of an optimal protein dose over a 12 h period (4)) of protein intake seem important for maximizing the beneficial effects on muscle protein synthesis and/or muscle growth. While 20 g of protein is often considered an optimal dose, higher protein amounts (e.g., 40 g) might be necessary to maximally stimulate muscle protein synthesis following whole-body exercise (67). Higher protein doses (e.g., ~27.5-40 g) may also be necessary to ingest prior to sleep to maximize overnight levels of muscle protein synthesis (84) and subsequently muscle growth (91). Adoption of these protein intake strategies during periods of concurrent training may potentially minimize any interference effect to strength training adaptations, although empirical evidence for this is currently lacking.

Since the interference effect with concurrent training is likely mediated by either a compromised training quality and/or adaptive response to training, the role of nontraining-related strategies in modulating both of these parameters highlights their potential importance in supporting concurrent training adaptation.

The potential role of these nontraining-related strategies for mitigating the interference effect can be summarized as follows:

- Nutritional strategies (such as creatine and caffeine supplementation), as well as the replenishment of muscle glycogen stores between training sessions, may be useful for attenuating residual (acute) neuromuscular fatigue during concurrent training.

- Other nonnutritional recovery strategies (e.g., cryotherapy) may somewhat attenuate residual (acute) neuromuscular fatigue following metabolic conditioning sessions, which may restore performance during subsequent strength training sessions.

- Protein intake following both metabolic conditioning and strength training sessions is essential for maximizing muscle protein synthesis rates to support necessary muscle remodeling and subsequently (chronic) training adaptation.

- Additional post-exercise carbohydrate intake, while useful for muscle glycogen repletion, does not influence anabolic responses to strength training and may even dampen (chronic) adaptive responses to endurance training in some circumstances.

Summary

Integrating both metabolic conditioning (including HIIT) and strength training into the overall training program presents unique challenges for the practitioner. That the residual effects of each training modality likely influence performance in any subsequent modalities highlights the importance of weekly session sequencing when integrating multiple training modes into the program. Although our understanding of how prescription-related factors may exacerbate any interference effect is improving, more work is required to further characterize these factors, so that practical strategies to mitigate any negative interactions between metabolic conditioning and strength training may be informed.

In the context of the HIIT programming puzzle (figure 1.5), the practitioner requires an understanding of factors that modulate the demands of HIIT sessions, particularly neuromuscular strain, as HIIT formats characterized by large neuromuscular demands are more likely to compromise subsequent strength-training performance. The practitioner should also be mindful of the influence of strength training-induced fatigue influencing the quality of key HIIT sessions, of which sessions with larger neuromuscular demands may likewise suffer most. In either case, the practitioner may need to prioritize performance in key HIIT sessions over strength-training sessions (and vice versa) during different stages of the overall program. Although empirical evidence is lacking, such a periodized approach may help to minimize negative interactions between sessions within the weekly program, which may transfer to better long-term adaptations. Aside from the manipulation of training-related variables, the potential benefits of nutritional interventions and post-exercise recovery strategies for maintaining between-session performance may also aid in mitigating the interference effect; however, evidence for their efficacy in concurrent training scenarios is limited. Together, the integration of metabolic conditioning with strength training clearly forms another complex piece of the programming puzzle, which practitioners must solve within their limitations in an attempt maximize the simultaneous development of strength and endurance capacity in their athletes.

HIIT and Its Influence on Stress, Fatigue, and Athlete Health

• • • • • •

Philip Maffetone, Paul Laursen, and Martin Buchheit

Up to this point in the book, we've primarily been focused on the intricate methods involved in skinning the cat when it comes to high-intensity interval training (HIIT) programming for athletic performance. With any approach, however, it implies a linear relationship between the chosen training format and the performance outcome. That is, keep progressing the HIIT stimulus more and more, and performance capacity should follow. This is typically how we think, and we're as guilty as the next person in doing so at various times throughout our careers. Experience in the high-performance setting with coaches and athletes, however, has shown us that this relationship is not as simple as we may have wished. In this chapter, we welcome Philip Maffetone, a colleague with a vast amount of experience as a physician and coach, with involvement in virtually all athlete types ranging from endurance to motor sport, amounting to a 40 yr career as a clinician working with patients and athletes. Together, our aim in this chapter is to take a more holistic view of HIIT in outlining both the benefits and common pitfalls to such training within the context of its effect on stress, fatigue, and athlete health. HIIT has many benefits to performance as we've already outlined. Less discussed in the literature, however, are the potential negative consequences of the practice when things go wrong. As the old coaching saying goes, *speed kills*. This chapter deals with aspects we don't always think about from the fitness standpoint, but need to if we want to prevent illness and injury, help athletes reach their human potential, and extend their performance lives. We must consider their health.

Health and Fitness Defined

The human body is generally quite resilient, as indicated by an athlete's ongoing and improving training and competitive cycles (74). However, injuries, poor health, reduced performance, and occasionally, and most unfortunately, even death, are realities. While we think of athletes and their amazing feats, we often automatically assume they have healthy bodies. However, that is not always the case. This apparent paradox is addressed by defining health and fitness separately (124):

- Health: a state of physical, biochemical, and mental-emotional well-being, in which all bodily systems (neuromuscular, hormonal, immune, digestive, etc.) function in harmony (figure 7.1).
- Fitness: the quality of human performance, the ability to compete at one's athletic potential.

Injuries, illness, and other mostly preventable but common conditions may be the best examples of

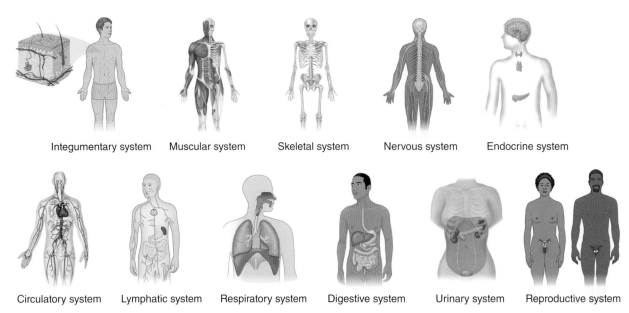

Integumentary system   Muscular system   Skeletal system   Nervous system   Endocrine system

Circulatory system   Lymphatic system   Respiratory system   Digestive system   Urinary system   Reproductive system

Figure 7.1 The 11 major physiological systems of the body that must be considered in the context of athlete health.

athletes who are fit but unhealthy. These conditions can also affect immediate and long-term training and competitive performance, the longevity of an athletic career, and current and future quality of life. By personalizing training and competition, and other lifestyle factors that impact the brain and body, athletes can be both healthy and fit (162).

Balanced Training

The many benefits of HIIT can be significant in helping athletes achieve optimal performances. The main physiological benefits, outlined in chapter 3, include improved aerobic oxidative, anaerobic glycolytic, and neuromuscular function. Additional benefits include enhanced bone remodeling, important for bone strength; support and function of muscles to enable human movement; and hormonal balance that includes the regulation of stress, sex, digestion, and other factors of importance for training, competition, and recovery.

Although the concept of balancing health and fitness in the name of preventing injury and illness to optimally progress performance ability is sometimes a difficult one to implement, a simple training equation may illustrate an important basic concept:

$$Training = workout + recovery$$

Training can be observed as the balance of an athlete's workouts plus recovery from them. Too much of the former, too little of the latter, or both,

can lead to excess training stress commonly called overtraining (104, 144).

In the previous equation, we can assume that training is the lifestyle an athlete chooses to live, which entails not only physical training but also the food consumed, stress management, a social life, and other daily routines including sleep. As such, overtraining refers to an imbalance of an athlete's lifestyle or a lifestyle the athlete is not adapted to (figure 7.2).

While HIIT provides adequate training stress to develop various health and fitness benefits, too much HIIT, either through volume, intensity, or lack of recovery, can add undue stress to the body. The topic of stress is an important one in relation to HIIT.

Stress

It is widely known that exercise offers many health and fitness benefits, the stimulus being a variety of catabolic and other physical and biochemical changes generally referred to as stress. More precisely, the anabolic adaptation mechanisms stimulated by sufficient training stress allow the body to benefit from HIIT. As described in chapter 3, proper adaptation to HIIT improves endurance, power output, or speed for a given metabolic cost, and ultimately performance.

Stress comes in many forms and can be categorized as physical, biochemical, and mental-emotional (153, 196). The molecular and physiological mechanisms of the various types of stress are well known and

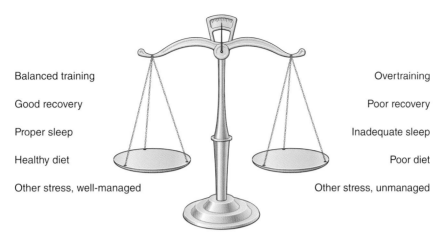

Figure 7.2 Athletes must balance stress in life.

applicable to all sports, and specifically to HIIT. Whether stress involves too much workout volume or intensity (the product of which is referred to as *training load*, see chapter 8), inadequate nutrition, or poor sleep or recovery, excess stress can impair health and ultimately fitness. Stress can be considered as the mechanism used by the body to adapt to the wear and tear of lifestyle. For the athlete, this means the accumulation of training and competition stress, with high-intensity activities typically producing the highest training loads (see chapter 8) and stress responses (195) (see chapter 9).

Defining Stress

Endocrinologist Hans Selye was the first to research biological stress and began demonstrating the existence of the brain-body adaptation mechanism and the hypothalamic-pituitary-adrenal (HPA) axis in the 1920s (197). He categorized the body's progressive response to all stress as the general adaptation syndrome, beginning with an acute stage, progressing to a second excess stress stage if recovery is not implemented, which can lead to a chronic and serious stage of stress. This general triad is outlined here because it is appropriate when describing athletic training, especially in relation to workloads such as HIIT, which can lead to fitness benefits with the potential for excess stress, e.g., overtraining.

In a sporting context, various terms are often thrown around to define the influence of stress associated with training and competition. These include burnout, staleness, failure adaptation, underrecovery, training stress syndrome, and unexplained underperformance syndrome, with the overtraining syndrome (OTS) the most commonly used term today

(103, 144). In addition, the general term *overreaching* is used in reference to increased training stress, with two specific components referred to as *functional overreaching* and *nonfunctional overreaching* (25). All these terms and conditions have an important common denominator—stress. To simplify these and other descriptions of stress, it may be best to consider the process as a spectrum (66, 123), one that also parallels Selye's three stress stages (described below).

HIIT Stress Benefits

An important feature of HIIT is the initiation of the first stage of acute stress. This allows the brain and body to adapt to an increased workload, and in conjunction with the process of recovery, various physical and biochemical adaptations are made that lead to improved competitive performance (see chapter 3). An individual's capacity to respond to this stress can vary, sometimes considerably (95), and occurs through the brain's hypothalamus and pituitary gland and the body's adrenal glands—the HPA axis.

Hypothalamic-Pituitary-Adrenal Axis

The HPA axis (figure 7.3) is a complex stress response mechanism important in the adaptation process to HIIT. A variety of neural and hormonal (neuroendocrine) changes take place as a response to a high-intensity workout, such as increased heart and respiration rates, increased muscle activity and associated energetic processes, electrolyte and hydration adjustments, alongside discomfort and other processes. This response can even begin before the

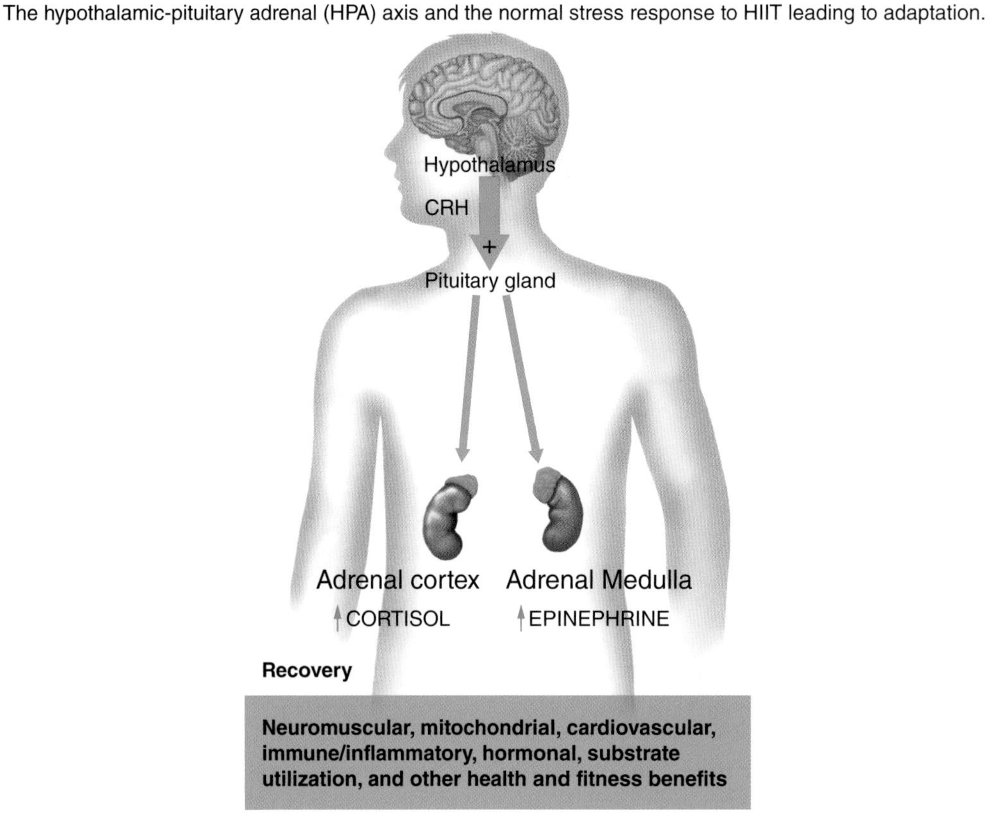

The hypothalamic-pituitary adrenal (HPA) axis and the normal stress response to HIIT leading to adaptation.

Hypothalamus

CRH

+

Pituitary gland

Adrenal cortex   Adrenal Medulla

↑CORTISOL   ↑EPINEPHRINE

Recovery

Neuromuscular, mitochondrial, cardiovascular, immune/inflammatory, hormonal, substrate utilization, and other health and fitness benefits

Figure 7.3 General overview of neuroendocrine and autonomic responses associated with healthy HIIT. HPA: hypothalamic-pituitary-adrenal; ANS: autonomic nervous system.

workout through pretraining anticipation (not unlike that of precompetition) sensed by the brain (40, 228). In addition to the hypothalamus, an area that influences autonomic function, the brain stem (helps control messages between brain and body) and limbic system (emotions) play important roles, too, along with body-wide hormone regulation via the pituitary. The hypothalamus also releases hormones (including corticotrophin-releasing hormone and arginine vasopressin) that act on the anterior pituitary to release adrenocorticotropic hormone (ACTH), which in turn stimulates the adrenal gland's outer cortex to release various hormones that regulate glucose, electrolytes, and blood pressure, and primarily the stress hormone cortisol (which stimulates gluconeogenesis). Increased sympathetic activity releases another stress hormone, epinephrine, from the adrenal medulla. The resulting HPA actions impact the athlete's process of adaptation (with other axes also involved in this process, including hypothalamic-pituitary-gonadal and hypothalamic-pituitary-thyroid), with the inflammatory and immune mechanisms playing key roles.

Exercise is associated with a range of beneficial inflammatory and immune responses (135). HIIT, for example, can induce healthy levels of muscle and bone stress that trigger the process of repair, regeneration, and growth, moderated by inflammation (36). The process includes the release of a variety of proinflammatory cytokines, along with monocytes, neutrophils, and macrophages, along with antiinflammatory chemicals (135). The increased exercise intensity in particular also increases the release of oxygen free radicals (oxidative stress) by muscles (137). In addition to skeletal muscle, some of these actions, most notably the production of cytokine interleukin-6, infer benefits to cardiac muscle as well (138).

As outlined in chapter 3, adaptation to HIIT involves improving the function of mitochondria, the energy (ATP)-generating component of muscle cells, helping to manage oxygen free radicals (251). For example, healthy training adaptation upregulates antioxidant enzymes to cope with oxidative stress, especially in cardiac muscle (94). This process of recovery can last up to 48 h or more and possibly for days (224).

In summary, a healthy response to HIIT activates the neuroendocrine stress mechanisms originating in the HPA axis, resulting in the release of the adrenal cortex stress hormone cortisol and increased sympathetic activity releasing another stress hormone, epinephrine, from the adrenal medulla, with inflammatory and immune activity playing key roles in healthy adaptation. The physiological outcomes include various health and fitness benefits provided proper recovery takes place. Figure 7.3 overviews this mechanism.

While the acute benefits of HIIT can lead to adaptations that lead to improved performance (chapter 3), *excessive* stress from training and/or poor recovery can overwhelm the body's stress adaptation mechanisms leading to health impairments, including injury, illness, and reduced performance.

Athletes: Fit but Unhealthy?

In the pursuit to improve performance through higher training intensities or volumes beyond that which from the body can recover, athletes may inadvertently exceed their stress limits. This can result in various signs and symptoms—stress-related "injuries" that

may be physical, biochemical, or mental-emotional. Some of these are listed in table 7.1. In addition to training, the accumulation of stress from an athlete's lifestyle, such as diet and social factors, can further lead to reduced fitness, as indicated by poor training and competitive performance. While traditional overtraining may be diagnosed *following* reduced performance lasting several months or performance *after* completion of a resting period of several days or weeks (77, 114), this does not allow for the potential of prevention, which is most valuable and preferred.

Assessing Training Stress

The recognition of excess training stress is an important step in preventing continued impairment, and is based on an athlete's current and past health and fitness history. *When* the transition from optimal HIIT to harmful stress occurs, if at all, varies considerably among athletes. Sometimes this appears as a physical injury or sudden onset of illness or extreme fatigue, often preceding diminished performance. Various subjective and objective physiological indications can help coaches and clinicians

Table 7.1 Potential Physical, Biochemical, and Mental-Emotional Signs and Symptoms Associated With Excess Stress in Athletes (103, 144)

Category	Signs and symptoms
Physical	Max and submax performance decrements
	Muscle soreness, stiffness; or fatigue
	General persistent fatigue
	Bradycardia
	Autonomic imbalance (including cardiac)
	Disease conditions such as asthma, thyroid disease, adrenal disease, diabetes mellitus or insipidus, iron deficiency with or without anemia, celiac sprue, hypertension
Biochemical	Excessive oxidative stress or damage
	Increased susceptibility to viral, bacterial, and other infections
	Inflammation
	Malnutrition
	Hormone imbalance
	Reduced muscle glycogen levels
Mental-emotional	Disordered eating
	Depression
	Insomnia
	Disrupted mood or behavior
	Loss of motivation
	Reduced mental concentration
	Anxiety

THE ATHLETE'S HEART AND SUDDEN DEATH

Physiologic adaptations that improve cardiac function are among the benefits of athletic training. They include increased stroke volume and cardiac output, longer diastolic filling time, and decreased oxygen demand, while maintaining normal systolic and diastolic function, with blood pressure and heart rate (HR) trending lower (see chapter 3). Training benefits, which include normal hypertrophic changes to the heart muscle walls, extend far beyond the cardiovascular system and are well known, with exercise far outweighing any health risks in most adults (68). Even extreme exercise training is well tolerated by healthy individuals, with increasing exercise volume and intensity further reducing cardiovascular risk (45). HIIT is recommended as a treatment strategy for patients with cardiovascular disease because it can provide benefits more rapidly than standard cardiac rehabilitation exercise (96).

Unfortunately, in the process of building fitness, athletes can also become unhealthy as discussed above, especially during high-intensity—high-stress—training (124). Combined with reduced health, high-intensity training and its associated increased HR and blood pressure and elevated stress hormones can contribute to sudden death in athletes with known or occult cardiovascular disease (45, 133).

Among the signs evident in unhealthy athletes is sudden death due to various cardiac injuries such as an acute myocardial infarction (heart attack) or arrhythmia (irregular electrical heart beat) (33). These individuals are often asymptomatic until during or within an hour of a cardiac event, and may be seven times more likely to die during activity than at rest (222).

The incidence of sudden cardiac death, the leading cause of death in athletes during exercise, has been estimated in young athletes <35 years of age at 1:917,000 athlete-years, however rates four to five times higher have recently been estimated, with men, African Americans, and male basketball players being at greatest risk (12).

A vital point about this important topic is that sport training in itself is not the cause of most sudden death in athletes, but acts as a trigger for cardiac arrest in the presence of underlying cardiovascular diseases predisposing to a cardiac event (45). In addition, sudden cardiac arrest does not always result in death, with many individuals surviving such an event, which may or may not occur during exercise.

In younger athletes (<35 years), the most common cause of sudden death is hypertrophic cardiomyopathy, accounting for approximately one-third or more of sudden deaths, with congenital coronary anomalies occurring in 15% to 20% of the cases and myocarditis (infection) much less common (45). In those >35 years of age, the most common cause of sudden death is atherosclerotic cardiovascular disease. As such, it is vital for clinicians to differentiate between normal hypertrophy developed from chronic training and its pathological state. Normal changes to an athlete's heart, which can imitate pathology, must be distinguished from serious cardiac disorders. Elite athletes are also not immune to cardiovascular disease (223), nor is it limited to athletes >35 years, and may account for 56% of the sudden deaths in young competitive athletes (132).

Cardiovascular causes for sudden cardiac death in athletes may be mostly preventative. For example, both genetic and lifestyle factors can contribute to pathologic hypertrophic cardiomyopathy, the latter being associated with cardiometabolic impairment including abnormal blood lipids and glucose, prediabetes and diabetes, and chronic inflammation. In athletes, hypertension is the most common risk factor for cardiovascular disease.

In athletes >35 years, the risk of sudden death due to ischemic heart disease increases progressively with age, where coronary artery disease accounts for more than half of the cases of sudden death (45), with atherosclerosis (a buildup of plaque in an artery) being a contributing factor. Coronary artery calcification is specifically associated with chronic high-intensity training (194), with vitamin D important in helping prevent calcification (21).

The prevalence of sudden death in athletes increased by 6% annually between study years 1980 to 1993 and 1994 to 2006, with 31% of the sudden death population occurring between 1980 and 1993 and 69% between 1994 and 2006 (132). As the data were largely limited to sudden deaths that became part of the public domain and records, the increasing number of fatal events observed over the study period may reflect enhanced public recognition caused by increased media attention. Corrado et al. (44) raised a reasonable concern about the reliability of the estimation of athletes' sudden cardiac death that could lead to an incorrectly low number of cardiac events and underestimation of mortality rates. Performance-enhancing drugs could also adversely affect heart health through cardiac toxicity, including anabolic-androgenic steroids, growth hormone, testosterone, erythropoietin (EPO), and others (33).

It is also possible that athletes experiencing fatal events previously had cardiac clinical screening that failed to detect a cardiac condition (180), with Maron et al. (132) estimating 30% of athletes cannot be identified reliably by preparticipation screening, even with ECG. Despite this, early identification of cardiovascular disease risks or cardiac abnormalities through a screening program could prevent sudden cardiac death, as recommended by the European Society of Cardiology, the American Heart Association, the International Olympic Committee, the American Society for Sports Medicine (64), and the American College of Cardiology (131).

Table 7.2 Important Assessment Tools Described in This Chapter

Assessment	Performed by
History and dialogue	Coach, clinician (athlete providing details)
Submaximal performance	Athlete (assessed by coach, clinician, see chapter 9)
Gait analysis	Coach, clinician, gait lab experts
Laboratory analyses (e.g., blood, urine, saliva)	Ordered by athlete, coach, clinician*
Complete clinical evaluation	Clinician
Heart rate variability (see chapter 9)	Athlete, coach, clinician
Dietary analysis	Athlete, coach, clinician
Urine color (hydration)	Athlete
Weight	Athlete, coach, clinician
Waist-to-height ratio	Athlete, coach, clinician

*Based on local regulations or laws.

monitor athletes before, during, and after HIIT, with a number of important assessment tools discussed in this chapter and listed in table 7.2. Chapter 8 focuses on the quantification of training stress for practitioners (termed training load), while chapter 9 examines methods of monitoring the athlete's response to training stress.

History and Dialogue

Sir William Osler, described as the father of modern medicine, said, "Never treat a stranger." Applied here, the quote refers to the importance of knowing each athlete to help assess his or her readiness to start HIIT and whether the positive effects of HIIT stress turn negative. This may be most evident through a dialogue that uncovers various subjective symptoms. However, in our high-tech world (see chapters 8 and 9), reliance on digital devices often replaces some of the basics such as asking athletes about new or worsening symptoms. These subjective evaluations of wellness (see chapter 9) can be more important than high-tech measures (191, 218). These simple, cost-effective, subjective symptomatic evaluations

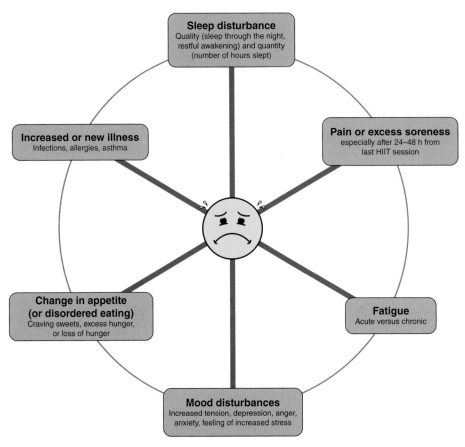

Figure 7.4 Signs and symptoms associated with the excess stress discussed in this chapter. Athletes can compare their current condition with that of "normal," including worse or better than normal. This assessment can be performed weekly or monthly.

can be performed regularly, allowing a rapid adjustment to training schedules or other stress as indicated. The process can also help athletes better understand their own symptomatology and training progress. Examples of early symptoms include acute fatigue, increased illness such as infections, asthma or allergies, mood changes (associated with tension, depression, anger, vigor, fatigue, or confusion), and sleep disturbances (13, 191). Figure 7.4 lists some of these common early symptoms.

Assessing Responses to Submaximal Exercise

As expanded on in chapter 9, noninvasive heart rate assessment of submaximal exercise activity can accurately inform athletes, coaches, and clinicians about training status (25), with improvements in submaximal training HR occurring relatively quickly, sometimes within a week after the start of an endurance

training program (27). Submaximal testing can also reflect a state of overreaching (52, 202), and changes in the response to submaximal exercise may be one of the first objective indications of excess stress (114). In contrast with maximal tests, which are more fatiguing, submaximal intensity-based evaluations are more easily implemented during easy training periods, between HIIT days, and during the competitive season. For example, Buchheit et al. (26) showed that changes in submaximal exercise heart rate running at 9 km/h (5.6 mph) in a 5 min test were inversely related to changes in peak aerobic running speed (i.e., $V_{IncTest}$). Moreover, Le Meur et al. (113) have shown that heart rate recovery following submaximal exercise may be more discriminant than measures taken following maximal exercise for monitoring endurance athletes' responses to training stress.

Normally, periods of high-intensity training and/ or increases in training volume, followed by adequate recovery, result in decreased resting, submaximal, and maximal HR and improved competitive performance (114, 115). This can be evaluated by comparing a constant submaximal HR against run speed, cycling power, or other metrics. Expected training improvements are reflected in faster paces or speed (or increased power) at the same submaximal HR.

While reduced resting and submaximal HR can be considered a sign of improved fitness, measured by increased submaximal run speed, reductions in maximal HR can be reflective of improved competitive performance. However, without adequate recovery and/or excess training intensity or volume, athlete performance responses can be impaired, evidenced through either increased submaximal HR responses, reduced exercise run speed or power output, or both. Surveillance, in terms of the heart rate–exercise intensity response, can be used to monitor athlete progress and health, and is covered extensively in chapters 8 and 9.

Gait Analysis

The ongoing observation of gait can be a useful tool for evaluating excess stress. While even minor physical injuries are known to influence neuromuscular output during running, for example, and can influence gait (141), the accumulation of other physical, biochemical, or mental-emotional stress, possibly related to the intensity or volume of an HIIT session, can also adversely affect gait (67, 241). Fatigue can adversely affect gait through proprioceptive afferent feedback from muscles involved in motor control (146, 169). Specifically, fatigued muscles surrounding a joint can adversely affect the proprioception of that joint leading to potential abnormal movement (169, 207). Fatigue can also influence gait by slowing muscle reaction time (243). Gait analysis is a relatively simple process during on-field workouts and competition, with more in-depth details obtained in a gait analysis facility.

Clinical Assessment

When necessary, additional and more extensive assessments can be obtained by a health practitioner through a complete clinical evaluation based on the athlete's need. The justification for physical examinations, laboratory analysis, and other assessments are made by the clinician and therefore not detailed here. Clinical assessments may include a comprehensive health and fitness history and physical examination. In addition, basic laboratory evaluations

can include blood, urine, and hormone tests for immune, inflammatory, cardiometabolic, and other functions. More specifically, these may include:

- Blood tests such as a complete blood count and blood chemistry, including hematocrit and hemoglobin, liver function, glucose, and tests for electrolytes (Na, K, Ca, Mg), vitamin D, folate, iron and ferritin, along with C-reactive protein (a sign of excess inflammation).
- Urinalysis to help rule out infection, dehydration, and hematuria. It can also test for pregnancy.
- Salivary tests for cortisol or other hormones (98).

While there is no single test or group of tests specific for excess training stress, and most have limitations, a holistic approach that considers all aspects of an athlete's physical, biochemical, and mental-emotional condition is important because individual response to excess stress, and therefore signs, symptoms, and abnormal laboratory findings, can vary considerably (98).

Stages of Training Stress

A number of general stages of stress are outlined in this section with the heightened stage summarized in figure 7.5. The athlete response to stress, along with associated signs and symptoms, are based on the physiological progression of excess stress. Importantly, this is merely a broad-spectrum overview as athlete response to excess stress will vary considerably. For example, it is common for athletes to present with signs and symptoms in more than one stage of categories. Therefore, the following categories are provided only in the interest of offering general benchmarks within the stress severity continuum.

Acute Stress

The first stage of *acute stress*, sometimes referred to as overreaching, plays an important role in HIIT benefits, as discussed earlier (figure 7.3). However, excess stress can begin to affect the athlete's health and fitness in this stage via increased cortisol and sympathetic tone (87), producing abnormal signs and symptoms that may include:

- Reductions in sleep quality that can interfere with recovery, commonly observed as middle-of-the-night awakening, unable to quickly get back to sleep (187).

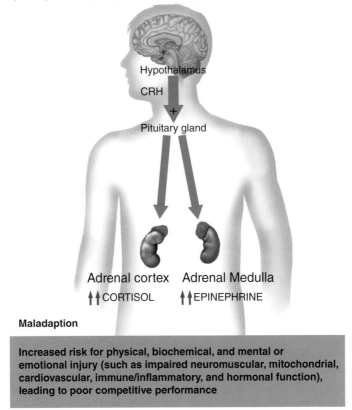

The hypothalamic-pituitary adrenal (HPA) axis and the heightened stress response leading to maladaptation.

Figure 7.5 General overview of heightened neuroendocrine response to excess stress and maladaptation leading to impaired health and fitness. ACTH: adrenocorticotropic hormone; HPA: hypothalamic-pituitary-adrenal; ANS: autonomic nervous system.

• Feelings of depression or anxiety, fatigue, excess soreness, or pain, as the brain's executive functions are sensitive to excess stress. Other symptoms may be difficult for the athlete to precisely verbalize but could still be important (191, 218).

• While increased physical fitness is associated with cardiac vagal modulation that reduces resting and submax HR (26) and improves global heart rate variability (HRV) (176, 213), sympathetic overactivity can lead to *increased* resting HR and lowered global HRV (114). The regular use of a heart rate monitor can be an accurate way to help track HR changes throughout the year (25), the topic of which is expanded on in chapter 9.

With the acute nature of excess stress, the condition is often reversible within several days to weeks (106). Most important is to consider reducing training volume and/or intensity, such as using type 1 HIIT, with increased recovery during and/or between HIIT sessions. This is also an important time for coaches and athletes to consider other lifestyle stress factors, especially diet as discussed below, to prevent progression of stress.

Advanced Stress Responses

The continuation of excess stress is sometimes called sympathetic overtraining, or nonfunctional overreaching, and is associated with increased ACTH from the pituitary with downstream increases in cortisol and epinephrine from the adrenal glands (196). This increased stress may be associated with sleep disturbances, daytime sleepiness, pain, and reduced desire to train. Even an acute bout of HIIT can elicit these neuroendocrine changes (120). The onset of immune (increased illness such as colds, flu and other infections, asthma) and GI dysfunction (from minor indigestion, excess gas or heartburn to vomiting or diarrhea during HIIT or competition) is also possible (51, 196).

Secondary to the now chronic cortisol elevations (figure 7.5), additional problems may include:

• Reductions in testosterone in men and women (102), potentially reducing muscle and bone strength and sex drive, and further increasing fatigue.

- Reduced thyroid function may be the result of inhibition of the peripheral conversion of T4 (thyroxine) to T3 (triiodothyronine) (75). T3 may require up to 72 h following HIIT before returning to normal, with signs and symptoms of excess training stress similar to those of hypothyroidism.

- In female athletes, low energy, menstrual dysfunction, and reduced bone density, separately or in combination, make up the female triad, with the prevalence of at least one of these problems estimated at 60% (219). Disruption of the HPA axis can impair various other hormones including estradiol, testosterone, luteinizing hormone, and others, and cause menstrual dysfunction, such as amenorrhea and oligomenorrhea.

- Sleep disturbances may become more severe (117, 208) and are discussed separately.

- Neurological performance may become impaired, including reduced sensory skills such as keen awareness and fine hand-to-eye coordination required in sports such as soccer, baseball, basketball, racket sports, golf, and others (38, 139, 229). This may also include increased response or reaction time and increased number of mistakes in measures of attention, skills, and processing speed ability (54, 86).

Addressing these and other problems must involve attending to the primary cause(s). For example, prescribing hormone therapy or a sleeping aid may not address primary factors such as excess training stress, diet, or poor recovery.

Athletes with these increased levels of stress may be at risk for exercise-associated hyponatremia (EAH), usually defined by blood levels of sodium less than 135 mmol/L (160). EAH may develop in athletes during or within 24 h of longer and/or harder training or racing. However, low sodium may develop at any time during heightened levels of stress due to reduced aldosterone (secondary to high cortisol) and its influence on sodium retention, especially if combined with excess water intake (hyperhydration). In some athletes, water retention can result, leading to an increase in water weight after training or competition compared to weight before these events. EAH can produce symptoms of fatigue, mental disorientation, gait alterations, or breathing difficulty, or no symptoms at all, making it difficult to diagnose and differentiate from dehydration. To differentiate, blood sodium levels can additionally be monitored during periods of high stress.

Recovery from these increased stress levels can take weeks to months depending on the severity of the athlete's condition. Temporary cessation of HIIT, reductions in training volume, and addressing other lifestyle stresses are important. Figure 7.5 is a general overview of the abnormal neuroendocrine response to excess stress.

Chronic Overtraining

The highest levels of chronic excess stress observed in clinical practice, referred to here as chronic overtraining, is a serious condition dominated by a significant autonomic dysfunction. It is associated with decreased hypothalamic and/or pituitary responsiveness to stress, with reduced growth hormone from the pituitary gland and low adrenal response to ACTH, sometimes called adrenal insufficiency (7, 24). The related adrenal insufficiency leads to abnormally low cortisol and other adrenal hormones, along with impaired hypothalamic-pituitary-gonadal axis function (24, 65).

A relative lack of sympathetic activity can result in an abnormally *decreased* resting heart rate, with continued worsening of both submaximal and competitive performance that can be a serious threat to the athlete's health (114). With their careers in jeopardy, these athletes usually require ongoing help from health practitioner(s) knowledgeable in sports medicine who can properly evaluate all physical, biochemical, and mental-emotional aspects of the patient. Returning an athlete to his or her former high-performance state may be difficult and could take months to years.

Remedies for the excess stress vary considerably with the athlete's particular needs. Some important factors to consider:

- A modification of the training schedule in stage 1 might include relying on lower-stress HIIT sessions (i.e., toward type 1), including shorter intervals and/or more rest between them, more rest or recovery days between HIIT workouts, or combinations of both.

- A *training taper* that includes up to a 50% reduction in training volume and intensity, for example, may further help speed recovery while increasing muscular strength, reducing the risk of injury and illness (119, 152, 155, 225).

- Excess stress associated with lifestyle must be addressed, including the diet.

- A complete clinical evaluation by a health practitioner may be necessary to help uncover physical, biochemical, or mental-emotional impairments associated with poor adaptation to HIIT.

Stress Recovery: Sleep

Good sleep quantity and quality can help athletes improve recovery from HIIT, increasing the opportunity for better training and competitive performance (76, 116, 204) with vital metabolic, immune, muscular, and other recovery processes occurring during specific stages of sleep (187). For example, Mah et al. (129) demonstrated that basketball players who obtained as much extra sleep as possible following 2 wk of normal sleep habits had faster sprint times and increased free-throw accuracy, along with increased vigor and decreased fatigue. Additionally, swimmers who increased their sleep time over their usual amount improved 15 m sprint, reaction time, turn time, and mood (128).

While adults may require a minimum of 7 h of quality sleep, with adolescents needing 8 to 10 h, these general guidelines could increase with the added stress of HIIT (187). As such, those who extend their normal sleep hours and "sleep in" may recover and perform better (116, 128, 129, 204). Unfortunately, the prevalence of poor sleep quality and/or quantity is common in athletes (187), who may be more sleep deprived than the general population (116, 184), with this problem being important feedback for coaches and clinicians (143).

Sleep *quantity* refers to total sleep time, while sleep *quality* refers more to factors such as time required for sleep onset, quality of rapid eye movement (REM) and non-REM sleep attained, waking or not during the night, and restfulness on awakening (161). Poor sleep quantity or quality can lead to:

- Symptoms of depression, tension, confusion, anger, decreased vigor, fatigue, and other mood states associated with neuroendocrine system disturbances (76).
- Both immune and inflammatory dysfunction (58, 61, 151).
- Enhanced daytime pain (which can interfere with nighttime sleep) (111).
- Impaired cardiometabolic factors (99, 210, 230), including poor glucose regulation, insulin resistance, and impaired appetite regulation, which may also increase hunger or cravings for sweets (209).
- Reduced estrogen and testosterone in men and women (50).

In addition to improving sleep quality and quantity, short (e.g. 30 min) naps can also help improve recovery (76). Longer daytime naps, however, may disturb nighttime sleep patterns.

Food, Stress, and Repair

The process of stress adaptation and proper recovery from training requires complex biochemical actions that continuously repair the body through processes

STRESS-RELATED FATIGUE

The normal process of recovery from HIIT is associated with mild to moderate fatigue and is considered a body-wide phenomenon that begins in the brain and affects the working muscles (159). Features of this neuromuscular fatigue include a temporary reduction in power output and submaximal performance of muscles, while increasing the perception of effort necessary to exert a specific force (57, 170). It can affect young healthy men and women who have no other signs or symptoms of dysfunction (243), affecting athletes from a wide variety of sports (4, 136, 207, 245).

Excess training stress can lead to excess fatigue, which can increase injury risk as muscles normally help disperse and share impact loads on joints and bones, with excess muscle fatigue reducing this protective action (182). Excess fatigue may be an acute response during or immediately after an HIIT session, with symptoms sometimes continuing up to the next HIIT session (238). This is an important issue to appreciate and relates to the programming aspects described throughout chapter 5, and the monitoring aspects discussed in chapters 8 and 9.

fueled by the consumption of food. Even a single HIIT session employs untold numbers of nutrients from food, including:

- Macronutrients: carbohydrate, fat, and protein; water; fiber.
- Micronutrients: all vitamins and minerals.
- Phytonutrients: thousands of plant-based compounds such as alpha- and beta-carotene, tocotrienols, and non-vitamin E tocopherols.

The American College of Sports Medicine and the International Society of Sports Nutrition recommend a "well-balanced diet" to meet all macro- and micronutrient requirements (30). However, nutritional deficiencies are not uncommon in athletes, even in those taking dietary supplements (6, 80, 105, 236). These nutritional problems can affect the HIIT response. For example, the very nature of the heightened metabolic requirement of HIIT increases oxygen free radicals that require various antioxidant nutrients from food to avoid unhealthy oxidative stress and poor recovery (216).

The term *diet* can be defined as the sum of energy (calories) and nutrients obtained from foods and beverages consumed regularly by individuals (8). A low-quality *poor* diet would include more processed, packaged, and preprepared foods that have lower nutrient density (such as micronutrients and fiber) versus natural, whole, unprocessed foods higher in nutrient density (43, 147). In addition, processed (refined) carbohydrates, including flour and sugar, foods containing added sugars, and sugar-sweetened beverages, substantially increase the glycemic index of meals and snacks and can contribute to chronic inflammation and other cardiometabolic impairments (206, 212). The name that encompasses these processed, low-quality items is *junk food*, sometimes called fast food, foods that are high in calories and low in nutrients (79).

The availability and affordability of junk food, including convenient or packaged items and those offered in restaurants, vending machines, cafeterias, and elsewhere, has led to an increased prevalence of poor diets, with sugar-sweetened beverages the single largest source of added sugar and the top source of energy intake in the U.S. diet (85). These products can increase hunger and cravings for more sweets (17). High-glycemic foods can also quickly impair fat oxidation rates (234, 240), contribute to the production of inflammation and pain (41, 92), and increase reactive oxygen species production (186).

Refined-carbohydrate foods are also associated with increased levels of insulin, a potent activator of the sympathetic nervous system (108).

Food intake and reward behavior is regulated by the hypothalamus and other areas of the brain (22, 181), especially in relation to the consumption of junk food (91). The combined HPA-axis stress (e.g., neuroendocrine imbalance) alongside the consumption of a high-sugar diet can promote inflammation, metabolic substrate imbalance (reduced fat oxidation), and maladaptation, and contribute to overtraining (figure 7.5) (124).

A major concern about the consumption of junk food, especially when regularly consumed, is that it replaces healthy food that could be providing many valuable nutrients to help recovery and adaptation from HIIT. Reading food labels, which list processed flour and sugar and carbohydrate content, helps make avoiding junk food easier. Natural whole foods are now sold by more stores and in some restaurants. Be aware of packaged products in natural food stores, which also contain many junk food ingredients. Table 7.3 provides examples of both junk food and alternative healthy food sources.

An important first step in assessing an athlete's food habits is performing a dietary analysis to evaluate diet quality. Some dietary analysis programs are available online and are free, such as the Cronometer (https://cronometer.com) and Senza (https://senza.us), and can provide reasonably accurate nutrient assessments, their primary purpose. However, some commercial programs also offer generic guidelines that may or may not be appropriate for a given athlete's individual needs.

Macronutrients

Once athletes eliminate junk food, balancing carbohydrates, fats, and proteins is easier. All three macronutrients are important in a healthy diet for athletes, in particular for those performing HIIT, as fatty acids (from fats) and amino acids (from proteins) are necessary for muscle recovery and repair through the regulation of inflammation and immune function. Balancing macronutrients involves individualizing food choices based on current needs, including eating ad libitum—when hungry rather than following a menu—a process humans have always done until relatively recently. Human research on self-selection of macronutrients associated with sports activity is limited, although it is known that the hypothalamus is associated with

Table 7.3 Common Junk Foods With Healthy Food Alternatives for Daily Meals and Snacks (43, 62, 147, 198)

Junk foods	Healthy alternatives
Prepared breakfast foods (cold cereal, instant oatmeal, pancakes, waffles, etc.)	Whole eggs (i.e., veggie omelet), unprocessed long-cooking whole grain cereals (i.e., oatmeal), fresh fruit and berries
Most bread (bagels, rice cakes, muffins, etc.), including most labeled "whole wheat"	100% whole grain bread products
Fast food (burgers, fishcakes, fries)	Vegetable salad, avocado, meat, fish, dairy
Processed lunch meat and fish (many brands have added sugar)	Whole pieces of meat, fish, or cheese
White rice, most pasta and noodles	Brown rice, lentils, beans
Most energy bars (high in sugar), soda, sports drinks,ᵃ sweetened protein shakes	Water, vegetable juice, coffee, and tea including herbal tea (without sugar)
Sweet snacks and desserts (cake, cookies, pie, sweetened yogurt, ice cream, candy, chocolate or sweetened milk, etc.)	Fresh fruit and vegetables,ᵇ unsweetened yogurt, raw nuts (almonds, cashews, macadamias)
Vegetable oils, trans fats (margarine and shortening)	Butter, olive oil, coconut oil

ᵃ The use of sports drinks around HIIT sessions and during competition could be considered a healthy choice relative to the goals of the session, as discussed in chapter 4.
ᵇ High-glycemic vegetables include white potatoes and corn. High-glycemic fruits include bananas, grapes, watermelon, pineapple, and dried fruits (including raisins), and fruit juice.

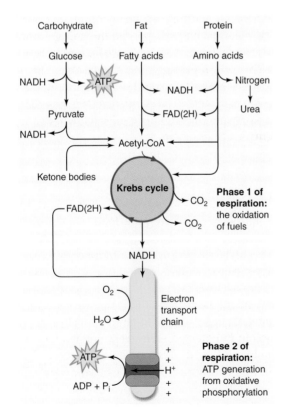

Figure 7.6 The role of food in the production of ATP.

the ability to choose foods based on the body's requirements (19).

Carbohydrate, fat, and protein are important contributors to the production of energy as ATP (chapter 3) and require the actions of micronutrients (see figure 7.6).

Traditional macronutrients for total daily energy in adults, set by the Food and Nutrition Board of the Institute of Medicine (130) is as follows:

- Carbohydrate at 45% to 65%
- Fat at 20% to 35%
- Protein at 10% to 35%.

However, these recommendations are a general guideline and inherently subjective as they don't take individual needs into account. For example, some athletes may perform best with significantly different macronutrient percentages, as discussed below.

Dietary Carbohydrate

Some traditional carbohydrate recommendations for athletes performing high levels of training are 8-12 g/kg per day (29). However, this estimation does not necessarily apply to everyone, nor is it followed. In a study of elite athletes (327 men and 226 women) across a wide range of sports including endurance, team, and strength-focused, normal macronutrient intake was evaluated, with more than half of the individuals consuming <5.0 g/kg of carbohydrate per day (236). As dietary carbohydrate is technically not an essential nutrient, with glycerol (from fats) and a variety of amino acids (from protein) capable of converting to glucose (242), there is a continued interest in lower carbohydrate and higher fat and protein in sports, which challenges traditional recommendations (16, 156, 166, 249). Examples of good sources of carbohydrate are lentil stew with vegetables and fresh fruit and berries.

While there is no official definition of low- or very low-carbohydrate diets, three commonly used terms associated with reduced carbohydrate diets are as follows (59, 158).

Moderate-carb: 26% to 40% of daily meals, with 140 to 210 g of natural carbohydrate per day; fat content is 100 to 130 g or 43% to 57%.

Low-carb: 11% to 25% of daily meals, with 51 to 139 g of natural carbohydrate per day; fat content is 135 to 165 g or 58% to 71%. Low-carbohydrate intake may begin producing measurable amounts of ketone bodies (assessed through blood, urine, and breath) that are used for energy, and may be important health-promoting signaling molecules (233).

Very low-carb: 5% to 10% of daily meals, with 25 to 50 g of natural carbohydrate; fat content is 168 to 182 g or 72% to 78%. Very low-carbohydrate intake leads to higher levels of ketone bodies (beta-hydroxybutyrate concentration >0.5 mmol/L), referred to as *ketogenic*, with individuals in a state of nutritional ketosis.

Various other traditional definitions are sometimes used (8).

Extending further from the information outlined initially for us in chapter 4 (carbohydrate training low), some benefits of reducing carbohydrate foods from traditionally recommended levels include:

- **HIIT and competitive activities.** Increased fat oxidation and glycogen-sparing effects that can help maintain and/or improve power output during repeated sprints for athletes in team sports such as soccer, rugby, and basketball (35), gymnastics (167), and endurance athletes (109, 234, 240).

- **Weight and body fat.** Long-term low-carbohydrate, high-fat eating has been more or less as effective as high-carbohydrate, low-fat eating in reducing body weight and fat mass (28). This is a healthy alternative for athletes in weight-sensitive sports, who, through unhealthy strategies of energy restriction, dehydration, and other dangerous methods to reduce weight, can impair both performance and health (97).

- **Health.** As reviewed by Chang et al. (35), many studies have shown that long-term lower-carbohydrate intake is not harmful provided there is sufficient energy and protein intake and can actually reduce the risk of increased body fat, metabolic imbalances, cardiovascular disease, diabetes, and other conditions.

These changes can occur following metabolic adaptation to a lower-carbohydrate, higher-fat eating routine, which may require at least 2 to 4 wk. Acute withdrawal from a high-carbohydrate diet, however, can temporarily reduce muscle glycogen and blood glucose, increase fatigue, and impair performance (35, 109).

A case study of a professional female triathlete of 13 years demonstrated how the process of individualizing macronutrient intake, resulting in very low-carbohydrate eating, can be accomplished (125). Based on signs and symptoms, including extreme hunger and fatigue, increased need for nutrients (food and drink) during training, menstrual stress (painful and irregular periods), and severe GI distress, especially during races, alongside laboratory evaluations such as elevated fasting glucose, the following dietary recommendations were made:

- eliminate refined carbohydrates,
- reduce natural carbohydrate, and
- make up the caloric difference by increasing dietary fat.

Reducing carbohydrate foods and monitoring symptoms over a period of about 2 to 4 wk resulted in reductions in hunger, fatigue, food needs during training, and GI distress, with the ultimate carbohydrate content decreasing from 73% (475 g) to 12% (78 g) of total calories, whereas fat content increased from 14% (40 g) to 75% (217 g) and protein levels remained constant at 13% (85 g) (see figure 7.7). Within 2 mo, the athlete also reported increased perception of daily energy during and between training sessions, normal menstruation, and reduced need for daytime naps, with normalization of fasting

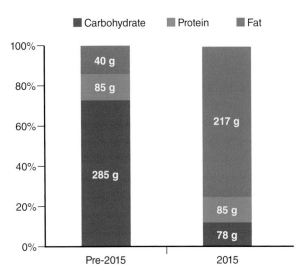

Figure 7.7 Daily macronutrient intake before and after dietary shift and intervention.

Reprinted by permission from P.B. Maffetone and P.B. Laursen, "Reductions in Training Load and Dietary Carbohydrates Help Restore Health and Improve Performance in an Ironman Triathlete," *International Journal of Sports Science & Coaching* 12 no. 4 (2017): 514-519.

glucose. In addition, cycling power output increased by 20 W and run pace increased (12-15 s/km) at the same training heart rate (141 beat/min), and, with the exception of water, nutrition was no longer required during long rides (~4 h). Race calories consumed (based on energy needs) were reduced from ~400 kcal/h in previous years to ~175, 145, and 130 kcal/h over the course of the next three Ironman events. Signs and symptoms of GI stress during competition ceased to occur, and 2 of 3 races were personal best times, with the final event completed in 8 h, 52 min. The levels of carbohydrate were well below typical recommendations (29), with fat intake higher than the ~30% considered appropriate, and ~85 g of protein for this 60 kg (132 lb) athlete, which is within some common recommendations ranging from 1.2 to 2.0 g/kg (174), although Paoli et al. (167) have recommended 1.3 to 2.5 g/kg of protein to ensure the maintenance of muscle mass, gluconeogenesis, and fat oxidation when consuming low-carbohydrate, high-fat diets. While maintaining very low-carbohydrate, high-fat intake, all markers of health and fitness improved, both short and long term.

Dietary Fat

Natural, healthy fats (also called oils) in the diet are necessary to help athletes recover from HIIT and improve overall health. Examples of healthy fats include olive and coconut oils, butter, the fats in

meats, eggs, and dairy, and other foods high in healthy fats such as avocados and raw nuts such as macadamias, almonds, and cashews. These fats can be used by the body for beta-oxidation to provide energy and regulation of inflammation (discussed below). Unhealthy fats include margarine and shortening that contain trans fats, and vegetable oils high in omega-6 fats (corn, peanut, safflower, soy, canola) (93), which can promote inflammation under certain conditions.

After consumption, dietary fat is usually deposited in fat stores. Even the leanest athletes when healthy can use this fat to supply a substantial portion of their total 24 h energy needs and training energy, including for HIIT (48, 81, 183, 233, 249). Generally, the combined amounts of fat and glucose used for energy during training vary with intensity, with increased fat oxidation occurring at lower intensities and lower levels as intensity increases. In addition to movement, fat oxidation provides energy for slow-twitch aerobic muscle fiber function, important to help support bones and joints, vascularization, and antioxidant activity (175).

Fats also help regulate inflammation through the actions of essential fatty acids: omega-6 (containing linoleic and arachidonic acids) and omega-3 (containing linolenic and eicosapentaenoic acids) (20, 93, 247).

Omega-6 oil contains the essential fat linoleic acid (LA), which normally converts to anti-inflammatory chemicals (collectively called eicosanoids). However, poor eating can divert LA to inflammatory chemicals instead through two key mechanisms. Excess intake of LA-containing omega-6 vegetable oils (corn, peanut, safflower, soy, canola), which has doubled in the past 100 years in Western countries (93), especially in junk foods, can convert LA to inflammatory chemicals. Carbohydrate-stimulated insulin (especially high-glycemic foods) further promotes the conversion of LA to inflammatory chemicals. In addition, a poor diet—one low in micronutrients and/or protein and high in trans fats—along with excess stress, can reduce production of anti-inflammatory chemicals from LA. Arachidonic acid (AA) is also an essential fatty acid that normally produces appropriate amounts of inflammatory chemicals (important in recovery from HIIT). The most common dietary source of AA is chicken, with other meat, egg yolk, and dairy containing lesser amounts. However, excess intake of omega-6 fats, which convert to inflammatory chemicals, do so by increasing AA. Beware of the dietary supplements containing primrose, borage, or black currant seed oils (concentrated omega-6 oils containing high levels

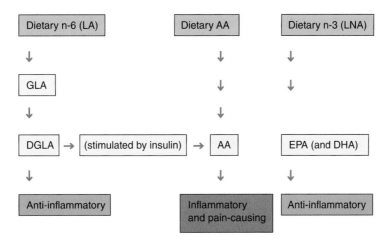

Figure 7.8 The relationship between dietary fats, refined carbohydrates, and inflammation. Excess omega-6 fats (corn, canola, soy, peanut, and safflower oils) and excess sugar or refined carbohydrate-stimulated insulin can drive omega-6 fats away from their potential anti-inflammatory pathways to inflammation through conversion to arachidonic acid. Some foods, especially chicken, also contain arachidonic acid. A different pathway containing omega-3 fats, primarily EPA-containing fish and fish oil supplements, can increase anti-inflammatory chemicals (23, 93). n-6: omega-6 fats; LA: linoleic acid; GLA: gamma linolenic acid; DGLA: dihomo-gamma linolenic acid; AA: arachidonic acid; n-3: omega-3 fats; LNA: alpha linolenic acid; EPA: eicosapentaenoic acid; DHA: docosahexaenoic acid.

of gamma linolenic acid), which can convert to AA in the inflammatory pathway.

Omega-3 fats, common in coldwater fish and seafood, with smaller amounts in beans and flaxseeds, contain the essential fat alpha linolenic acid (LNA) and also play an important role in producing anti-inflammatory chemicals. LNA must first be converted to eicosapentaenoic acid (EPA) (along with docosahexaenoic acid) for anti-inflammatory actions (23), a process requiring micronutrients and protein, but is impaired by trans fat and excess stress. However, in humans, plant-based omega-3 oils (such as from flaxseeds and beans) are poorly converted to EPA. Animal foods, primarily fish, already contain EPA. Coldwater fish such as salmon, anchovies, herring, and sardines have the highest food sources of EPA.

Figure 7.8 shows the relationship between dietary fats, their respective fatty acids, and the production of inflammatory and anti-inflammatory chemicals. Inflammation is also associated with pain.

In summary, the combination of a junk food diet and excess training stress can increase the risk of chronic inflammation (41, 92), which can trigger physical, biochemical, and mental-emotional injuries, including pain. Associated suppression of the immune system also increases the risk of infections, allergies, and asthma (215). These inflammatory and immune responses are comparable to those created by serious trauma and infections, and involve complex mecha-

nisms described elsewhere (100). Figure 7.9 is an overview of this diet and training paradigm.

Dietary Protein

High-quality healthy protein foods include *unprocessed* meat such as beef, pork, lamb, and fish (62), along with eggs and dairy (221). During periods of reduced protein foods (such as during travel), dietary supplements, including healthy protein drinks, may be useful to help avoid lower protein intakes. Reading nutritional labels helps avoid added sugars, common in these foods.

The intake of adequate dietary protein can help ensure athletes recover by enhancing skeletal muscle, bone and tendon adaptation, along with various metabolic benefits (72, 221). Protein may also supply up to 15% of an athlete's energy needs (63).

Protein needs may be more individualized than by that predicated by sport, with general requirements similar between athletes engaged in aerobic and sprint activities and most other sports, although higher intakes are indicated during periods of high-intensity training (221). For example, while the recommended daily allowance (RDA) of protein is 0.8 g/kg, consumption at double this level (1.6 g/kg) or higher can help preserve lean muscle and reduce excess body fat (8, 15, 112). Longland et al. (118) recently showed that during periods of high-intensity interval sprints and resistance training,

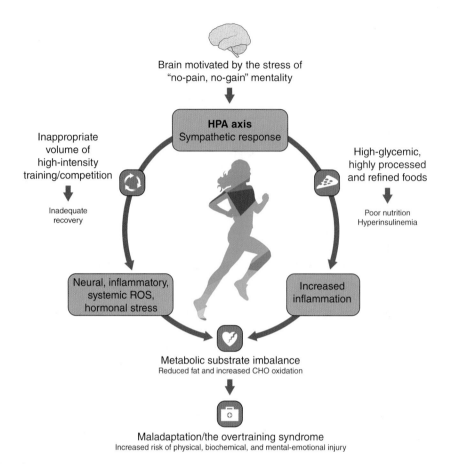

Figure 7.9 The fit but unhealthy eating and training paradigm.

protein intake at 2.4 g/kg caused lean muscle gains (1.2 kg) and fat loss (4.8 kg), while 1.2 g/kg preserved lean mass and fat loss. Instead of daily recommendations, muscle adaptation to training may be maximized by ingesting ~3.0 g/kg body weight following high-intensity training (221). In addition to post-training intake, spreading protein intake relatively evenly throughout the day, such as in 3 or 4 meals or every 3 to 5 h, may help improve digestion, absorption, and utilization (174).

Water

As a macronutrient, water is obviously important for proper hydration in all aspects of health and performance. We are made up of more than 50% water. Daily water needs are satisfied by drinking plain water plus the water content in foods and other beverages. Science is without a consensus on drinking strategies for athletes, as there is likely a range of successful approaches that reflect individual needs (10, 56, 70) and include:

- A fluid plan that follows a certain volume per hour based on the sport, exercise duration, and outside temperature.
- Ad libitum drinking, e.g., whenever and in whatever volume an athlete chooses.
- Drinking to thirst, very similar to ad libitum, and equally effective (47).

As we touched on in chapter 4, increased muscle activity during HIIT increases heat production that is compensated for through sweating, which requires adequate water intake to prevent excess body temperatures (192). Elevations in core body temperature for prolonged periods of time that exceed 40°C (104°F) can increase the risk of exertional heat illness (heat stroke), which is life-threatening. Excess water loss through sweating (and the lungs, kidneys, and intestines) can reduce blood (plasma) levels (hypovolemia), and long periods under this condition can impair the brain and nervous system, cardiovascular function, and other factors that can

INFLAMMATION, PAIN, AND MEDICATION

Exercise-induced muscle damage from HIIT can lead to muscle soreness and pain, and many athletes use over-the-counter or prescription medications when symptomatic (193). While valid indications exist for nonsteroidal anti-inflammatory drug (NSAID) use in sports medicine, these drugs are not regulated (168). A recent review supports the potential for short-term NSAID use after an acute muscle injury (149), however, athletes may also have limited awareness of their effects and side effects (73). All pain medications have the potential for immediate and long-term side effects, including:

- The worsening of existing physical injuries (134).
- Delayed bone healing and muscle weakness (227).
- GI bleeding (even if not noticeable) and dysfunction (3, 231).
- Impaired tendon repair (232).
- Stroke (34).
- Low blood sodium (hyponatremia) (165).

Despite these risks, the high use of NSAIDs and other analgesics is widespread in all sports (46, 84, 226, 237). NSAID use in triathletes, for example, may be as high as 60% (73), with similar prevalence of NSAIDs and other analgesics in marathoners (107), and higher rates in both futsal and association football (172). Despite the lack of evidence on any added benefits of injected versus oral NSAID administration, Pedrinelli et al. (172) found that 15% of futsal (football) players injected NSAIDs. In addition to NSAIDs, other analgesics and muscle relaxants are also commonly used by athletes.

significantly reduce performance and health (221). As outlined in chapter 4, however, short-term periods of mild dehydration in the heat may offer an adaptive response in terms of plasma volume expansion and enhanced adaptation to heat (69).

A normal hydration status can be achieved with a range of total water intake (173). However, individual differences in sweat rates can lead to an array of conditions from dehydration to overhydration (47). In a study examining 2,135 endurance athletes who completed 42 km (26 mi) marathons, 109 km (67.8 mi) cycling events, and 226 km (140.4 mi) Ironman triathlons, about 60% of the athletes were dehydrated whereas 11% were overhydrated, 6% had mild hyponatremia (abnormally low blood sodium, <135 mEq/L), and 1% had severe hyponatremia (160). Excess water intake is even possible in team sport athletes (200). While reduced performance has been reported to occur with dehydration levels in excess of 3% to 5% or more of body weight, performance in the heat is maintained at controlled

and blinded dehydration levels up to 3% of body mass (37, 235), so despite its large exposure in the press, hydration status, at least in terms of dehydration, is typically overblown as an issue in the world of elite sport (47). Indeed, Sharwood et al. (199) showed no increased risk of heat illness associated with high levels of dehydration during the 2000 and 2001 South African Ironman triathlon, and high levels of weight loss did not significantly impair performance.

To help guide athletes performing HIIT in maintaining hydration balance—avoiding excess dehydration and overhydration—consider these suggestions:

- Have fluid available and encourage athletes to drink to thirst and not beyond (47).
- Those with a history of or suspected hydration problem can seek help from a clinician to test urine osmolality, specific gravity, and plasma sodium concentrations.

- Monitor body weight before and after training and competition. In general, a loss of body weight of 1 kg represents approximately 1 L of sweat loss (221), but remember that this is a natural occurrence and the body tolerates this well (47). Hypothetically, this could be countered by drinking 0.4 to 0.8 L/h of fluid (192).

- Body weight gain after training or competition may indicate excess fluid intake or overhydration, with the potential risk of hyponatremia (47).

- For daily self-assessment of hydration status, athletes can observe urine color, with pale (versus darker) yellow urine a general indicator of normal hydration (173). Achieving a pale urine color 2 to 4 h before training may be accomplished by consuming 5 to 10 mL/kg body weight (2 to 4 mL/lb), allowing time to void excess urine (192).

- The addition of sodium (salt) to food and water—to taste—can help fluid retention and improve hydration balance (189, 192).

- Rehydration following HIIT sessions or competition is important. The coingestion of food and water may work as well as sports drinks or milk-based beverages (14, 31).

Popular sports hydration recommendations are frequently influenced by commercial interests, including sports drink companies, sponsoring research (157).

Micronutrients

All vitamins and minerals make up the category of micronutrients and are essential for training, recovery and adaptation, competitive performance, and overall health. For example, various micronutrients are required in most aspects of body functions, playing vital roles in the conversion of macronutrients to energy (ATP), inflammatory regulation, immune function, muscle contraction and relaxation, brain function, hydration, and more.

The most important source of micronutrients is a healthy diet. However, athletes who eat a poor-quality diet or restrict calories from macronutrients may have suboptimal levels of micronutrients (221). Many athletes take dietary supplements, believing that they can improve athletic performance, but with some exceptions this idea is not supported in the scientific literature, and, in fact, some supplements can impair health (148, 171, 220). Like other nutri-

ents, an athlete's individual needs best dictate the use of a dietary supplement, and supplements should not replace a healthy diet. Blood tests for vitamins and minerals are commonly employed; however, many micronutrients don't necessarily reflect levels in muscles and other tissues (145) or reflect low acute dietary intake as indicated by dietary analysis (122).

Four key vitamins are highlighted here because they are commonly low in athletes (221).

Vitamin D

Technically a secosteroid hormone, vitamin D plays a key role in muscle function and recovery from training (164), can increase type 2 fast-twitch muscle fiber size, and may improve athletic performance (32). Related to its effect on bone health through improved calcium absorption and metabolism, vitamin D can help reduce the risk of stress fractures (188) and is important for immune, hormone, and inflammatory regulation (101). Vitamin D *insufficiency* is defined as blood levels of 20 to 30 ng/mL (50 to 75 nmol/L) with *deficiency* <20 ng/mL (<50 nmol/L) (221). However, peak athletic performance may be associated with levels of 50 ng/mL and above (32). Blood levels of vitamin D >100 ng/mL are considered an excess, with levels >150 ng/mL considered toxic (5).

Unfortunately, low levels of vitamin D are common in athletes and are associated with poor recovery, muscle pain and weakness, muscle atrophy, impaired power output, reduced coordination, increased risk for physical injury, and overall reduced exercise performance (32, 110, 201). Up to 94% of athletes in indoor sports and up to 80% in outdoor sports may have abnormally low vitamin D (201). As such, it is important for clinicians to routinely assess blood levels, especially in those with a history of poor vitamin D status. Athletes with darker skin (natural or tanned) and those who use sunscreen, wear protective clothing, have excess body fat, avoid the sun, or live at latitudes >35th parallel or who primarily train and compete indoors may be at higher risk for inadequate vitamin D (201).

The most common cause of poor vitamin D status is reduced sun exposure (110). A healthy range for adults and children of 50 to 80 ng/mL (125 to 200 nM/L) year-round appears adequate, with lower levels in this range found in late winter and early spring and higher levels in late summer (in the northern hemisphere). Measuring the 25(OH)D form of vitamin D versus the 1,25(OH)$_2$D form is a better indicator of vitamin D status and is the standard blood measurement used in clinical trials (90).

Vitamin D is produced by the conversion of 7-dehydrocholesterol in the skin following exposure to ultraviolet B radiation from the sun, the most readily available source of vitamin D for human metabolism (163). Peak skin production following a ~10 min exposure of summertime sun between 10 a.m. and 3 p.m., for example, can produce about 10,000 IU of vitamin D (201).

The most naturally occurring active form of this vitamin produced in the body from sun exposure is D3, or cholecalciferol, and is also found in fish liver oil, while the plant source D2, or ergocalciferol, is the form usually found in the diet (9). Foods provide only small amounts of vitamin D2, mostly through the fortification of junk foods. The use of vitamin D3 fish oil supplements may be necessary to restore and maintain normal vitamin D levels in athletes, with 10,000 IU per day defined as the tolerable upper-intake level without toxicity (reviewed by Jerome et al. (90)). However, deficiencies may require 50,000 IU of vitamin D3 per week for 8 wk under the guidance of a clinician (82).

Iron

A deficiency of iron, which may or may not cause anemia, can impair muscle function and athletic performance and produce symptoms of weakness and fatigue (121). Low iron levels can result from low intake of heme food sources, especially meat (18), with increased iron loss associated with high-altitude training, blood loss (such as gastric or menstrual), rapid growth (such as in adolescence), and, for some athletes, intense training due to iron loss in sweat, urine, feces, and from intravascular hemolysis (221). Low levels of riboflavin (vitamin B2) can also impair iron utilization (178).

Athletes who suspect low iron should visit a clinician who can perform a history, physical exam, and appropriate blood tests, which usually includes serum iron, ferritin (the stored form of iron), and total iron-binding capacity (transferrin) (154).

The use of lower-dose iron-containing dietary supplements as low as 10 mg can be useful to treat a diagnosis of iron deficiency. However, high doses of iron, such as 50 or 100 mg, can increase the risk of iron overload, observed as elevated ferritin that can increase oxidative stress and impair mitochondrial function (211).

Antioxidants

As noted earlier, dietary antioxidants play a key role in regulating inflammatory and immune responses and recovery of high-intensity training, in great part due to their control of oxygen free radicals (177, 239). A healthy diet of fresh fruits and vegetables with meat, fish, and eggs can provide many natural antioxidants, not just vitamins and minerals but various phytonutrients, along with the amino acids cysteine and taurine (140, 177, 239).

However, dietary supplements containing antioxidants, in particular vitamins C and E and the phytonutrient beta-carotene, can become unwanted *prooxidants* and impair mitochondrial function and worsen oxidative stress (39, 140, 203, 248). These dietary supplements can also prevent training increases in $\dot{V}O_2max$ (205).

Folate

As one of the B vitamins found in food, folate plays a key role in the synthesis of DNA, the metabolism of amino acids, red blood cell function (carrying oxygen to muscles), inflammation and oxidative stress regulation, and the prevention of megaloblastic anemia and insulin resistance (1, 179, 250). While blood tests for *folic acid*, an inactive form of folate, may appear normal, high numbers of people have a genetic mutation (called the C677T polymorphism of 5,10-methylenetetrahydrofolate reductase [MTHFR] gene) that impairs the conversion of folic acid (found in most dietary supplements and fortified processed foods) to the active form, folate (83). The MTHFR C677T and similar polymorphisms can be evaluated in a blood test, with folate levels measured in serum and as RBC folate (250). Athletes with a low folate status or the mutation should consider consuming more folate-rich foods (see table 7.4; (49)), avoiding inactive folic acid from dietary supplements (labeled as "folic acid") and processed or fortified foods, including many energy bars and sports drinks, and, under the direction of a clinician, taking the active form (5-methyltetrahydrofolate, or 5-MTHF) as a dietary supplement to maintain normal blood levels. Adequate folate status could be achieved by eating a greater amount of natural folate-rich foods.

Body Composition

Food is sometimes used by athletes in an attempt to manipulate body composition: body fat and lean muscle mass. Many athletes focus on losing weight by reducing total calories. Deficient energy intake of one, two, or all three macronutrients, which can also reduce micronutrient intake, can impair

Table 7.4 Single-Serving Folate-Rich Foods

While there is no scientific definition of serving size, it is generally considered the amount of food customarily or reasonably consumed at one meal or a typical portion. Examples include 1/2 cup cooked vegetables, 1 cup raw vegetables or cooked whole grains, or 3 ounces of meat or fish.

Food	Naturally occurring folate (in mcg)
Turkey	486
Lentils	358
Spinach	263
Asparagus	243
Beef	221
Broccoli	168
Brussels sprouts	157
Beets	136
Leaf lettuce	119
Avocado	118
Papaya	112
Green peas	94
Orange	54

neuroendocrine and cardiometabolic health and lead to poor hormone, bone, immune, protein synthesis, and cardiovascular function (217). This problem, termed *relative energy deficiency in sport*, is a serious health risk in male and female athletes of all sports and ages, and one that can reduce performance (150).

Reducing calories is based on the idea of "calories in, calories out" and interpreted as eat less food and train longer or harder. However, this oversimplified concept is often not successful in long-term weight loss because the metabolism and endocrine response to food is not considered (8). For example, just reducing food calories can lower energy expenditure, increasing fat storage. A more sensible approach is to reduce the unwanted calories of junk food, such as cola or a candy bar, with its metabolic stress response. However, avoid reducing calories of nutrient-dense foods such as vegetables, healthy fats, or proteins. In addition, macronutrient composition influences metabolism and energy expenditure, as protein intake has a much greater thermic effect than carbohydrates or fat (78). Dietary fat is commonly restricted, due to its high caloric content, which can reduce the intake of the fat-soluble vitamins A, E, and K and essential fatty acids (88).

Over the course of a season, especially building up to HIIT with related higher energy expenditure, balanced body composition is important. Whether specifically pursued or naturally occurring, healthy

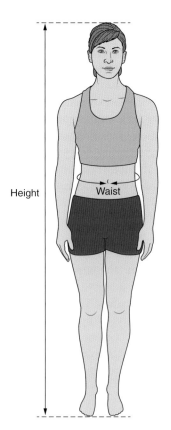

Figure 7.10 The waist-to-height ratio (WHtR) should be <0.5, meaning that the waist should be less than half the height.

changes in lean muscle mass and body fat, with potential weight adjustments, based on the specific needs of each athlete, are possible. Increased lean mass from added muscle can be valuable in sports such as American football (chapter 20), rugby (chapters 28 and 29), and ice hockey (chapter 25), while soccer players (chapter 30), runners (chapters 13 and 14), cyclists (chapter 15), and triathletes (chapter 19), as well as those in weight categories (i.e., combat sports and rowing, chapters 11 and 16, respectively) and aesthetic sports may require reduced weight, especially the loss of excess body fat, for better economy and/or meeting event requirements.

The term *overfat* refers to increased body fat that can impair health (126, 127). While the prevalence of excess body fat in athletes appears to be increasing (55, 244, 246), reducing it can also improve fitness, such as run performance (42, 185).

Measuring fat through body composition evaluation is commonly done with the body mass index (BMI), defined as weight in kg divided by height in m². However, this is not an accurate method that distinguishes lean muscle mass from body fat, with BMI misdiagnosing high numbers of people (127). The use of dual x-ray absorptiometry (DXA) may be the most effective method to accurately monitor body composition in athletes, including percent body fat (214). However, DXA can be costly for regular monitoring and not always accessible.

While there is no universally applicable criterion for body composition assessment (2), skinfolds and DXA are commonly used methods to monitor changes in body compositions (214). The use of skinfold thickness is commonly used to estimate percent body fat, with the American College of Sports Medicine recommending the use of Jackson and Pollock body density equations (142). There are limitations in this approach as fat distribution, subcutaneously and internally, is not similar for all individuals, varying across gender, ethnicity, body type, and age (71, 89).

A practical, simple, and inexpensive indirect measure of body fat that can be performed monthly by athletes, coaches, and clinicians is the waist-to-height ratio (WHtR). This highly accurate risk assessment for being overfat is useful for all ethnicities and ages in adults and children (11, 190). WHtR won't provide body fat percentage, which is without a consensus of normal cutoffs, but comes with a simple recommendation: the waist (measured at the level of the umbilicus) should be less than half one's height, with a healthy ratio below 0.5 (127). This is particularly important for excess abdominal fat, which promotes body-wide low-grade chronic inflammation (60). Assessment of the WHtR is illustrated in figure 7.10.

Disordered Eating

In their extreme desire to change body composition, some athletes may develop unhealthy eating behaviors. Unhealthy eating behavior in male and female athletes, triggered by the desire to change body composition, can adversely affect HIIT due to deficits of energy, antioxidants, fatty acids, protein, and other nutrients. Disordered eating may be common in sports, appearing as a spectrum (53). The *Diagnostic and Statistical Manual of Mental Disorders* characterizes one extreme of the disorder as a gross disturbance in eating behavior that includes anorexia nervosa and bulimia nervosa, with higher numbers exhibiting less-severe but still unhealthy pathogenic eating behaviors (53). Features of the condition may include calorie restriction, fasting, and the use of laxatives, diuretics, diet pills, and vomiting. The problem appears more prevalent in sports requiring a minimum weight, although endurance athletes may mistakenly believe just weighing less will improve performance. Disordered eating may be more prevalent during competitive seasons or exist year-round, with athletes focusing on all foods or only part of the diet such as avoiding fat or protein. Addressing the problem starts with its recognition on the part of athlete, coach, and clinician, and sometimes a mental health practitioner.

Summary

HIIT offers many health and fitness benefits to athletes and can lead to improved performance. However, the combination of excess training stress causing neuroendocrine imbalance and the consumption of a poor diet, one high in sugar, can promote inflammation, metabolic substrate imbalance (reduced fat oxidation), and maladaptation, and contribute to physical, biochemical, and mental-emotional injuries. Athletes, coaches, and clinicians are encouraged to carefully monitor training progress (see chapters 8 and 9) and rely on healthy eating to maximize HIIT.

8

Quantifying Training Load

• • • • • •

Martin Buchheit and Paul Laursen

To this point in our book, we've described the main physiological targets of high-intensity interval training (HIIT), the parameters that form and fine-tune our HIIT weapons, principles to consider when integrating strength training concurrently in the training program, along with important strategies for maintaining health in the context of HIIT. While our key puzzle pieces are nicely taking shape, one key aspect we haven't yet covered is the process of trying to understand the impact of a given HIIT session on the athlete and the contribution that the HIIT session is making toward solving the overall puzzle.

For anything we might try to understand, like training and performance, we ideally need to quantify its moving parts. Sticking with our military context, the term *surveillance* is used. The main purpose of surveillance for military operations is largely management. As the old adage goes, you can't manage what you can't monitor. Ultimately in training for sport, we often talk about the training load, and that we need to manage it. But before we go too deep into the monitoring of training load, we'd better first try to define it.

Training Load: What Is It?

Rarely have we seen training load clearly defined within the literature. If we were to break the concept of training load down into a first principle compo-

nent, it's difficult. While training load is often discussed in the world of training for sport, it is really more or less an abstract concept that we use to describe theoretically how the physical task involved with training creates stress and fatigue (chapter 7) as well as adaptation and fitness (chapter 3). But here's where it gets tricky. Because it's an estimated abstract concept, where we can never truly reach any precise level of assessment, we can only make approximations of it. That's not to say it's not useful to do, but it's important to acknowledge these limitations from the start. We have to do a bit of calculated guesswork in the area. That means we always need to take our calculations with a grain of salt.

The stress of any theoretical training load can be considered from two different but complementary concepts. Training load can be described from either the external standpoint, based on how much physical work (J) is actually completed in training, or from the internal standpoint, referring to the body's acute physiological response to the external work being completed. The latter aspect, the internal training load (i.e., $\dot{V}O_2$, lactate, RPE) is a display of the body's acute reaction, or stress, to the applied external training load performed (figure 8.1). Whichever way we look at it, this training load stress evokes an input to the physiological system.

In this chapter, we'll set our focus on aspects of the training load itself, while we'll devote chapter 9

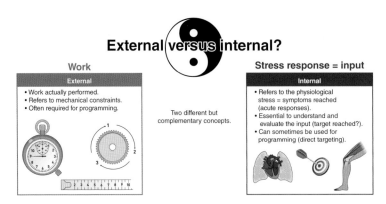

Figure 8.1 Comparing internal (red) versus external (blue) training load concepts. The external training load applied evokes an internal training load stress that provides an input to the athlete's training stress-adaptation system.

to the carryover effects of these training load arsenals, in terms of the damage they inflict or the *response* that the training load stress imparts on the athlete. Beyond these immediate chapters on surveillance, we'll have our expert practitioners show us how they attempt to manage their surveillance systems in the heat of battle. As they'll tell us, this is often easier said than done within the real world of elite sport. Nevertheless, the purpose of these next two chapters is to lay down some groundwork in the area, look to see what might be optimal, consider what is actually practical, and combine science with common sense to give us some surveillance principles we can take to the battlefield of elite sport.

An Aerial View of the Battlefield

If we're just starting out with the process, it might be a good idea to review figure 1.5 to remind ourselves of the importance of context around the sport and individual athlete. What's our individual athlete's characteristics or physiological profile? What is the sport we are talking about? Is it individual or team-based, and what are the associated demands we need to be preparing for?

For the majority of situations, the manipulated variables of an HIIT session outlined in figure 4.5 (i.e., intensity, duration, recovery, etc.) need to be considered first and foremost. Was the completed training in line with what was prescribed? The military would describe such factors as *targeted interceptions*. In military context, it means that these aspects are *marked*—the variables matter—so we need to measure them.

But context is vital. What is the main sport modality we're referring to, and from it can we

easily, noninvasively, reliably, and accurately measure how the parameter evolved over time in an HIIT session, such as the power output or movement speed? How do the internal training load markers evolve during the HIIT session relative to the external training load? From this surveillance, can we gain insight into the likely oxidative, anaerobic glycolytic, and/or neuromuscular responses (i.e., input) to the stress we imparted on our athlete during the HIIT session?

Perhaps one of the most important reasons for surveillance relates simply to the fact that we are all individuals, a factor highlighted throughout nearly every chapter to this point of our book. We all have varying phenotypes, diverse daily psychosocial stresses, different diets, unusual lifestyles, etc. These other stresses, highlighted in chapter 7, can all cause us to respond just a bit differently during the same HIIT workout (i.e., similar external loads but different internal loads). Surveillance and athlete monitoring is an enormous area of research in sports science, with the holy grail thought to be found within the factors that make up the dose-response relationship between training and performance (26).

Once we've collected the data that matters, and we have it in front of us, then what? At first glance, the data collected is more or less just interesting. How do we move from interesting to meaningful and useful, where it becomes a tool that helps us make appropriate decisions toward solving our programming puzzles? For this we require some method of analysis, a method that is as simple and logical to perform as we can make it. We need a system and a process, and it must be relatively easy and practical.

Another important reason for monitoring an athlete's training load relates to the improved probability of lowering an athlete's injury risk. Given the high cost of injuries, especially in team sports (i.e., ~12.5 million dollars per team in the top-four soccer leagues as just one example (2)) and the strong association between injury incidence and a team's performance in the standings (39), it makes sense to invest time and resources into the initiative. Indeed, the last 15 years have witnessed incredibly rapid development of (micro)technology in the field, which is unlikely to slow any time soon (46).

Figure 8.2 provides a schematic representation of the important factors at play in the training prescription and surveillance process. Beginning with the known target of the session (figure 1.5), we can prescribe training from either the external or internal training load perspective in alignment with our target. Take for example the case of a cyclist who requires a type 3 target for the session. We might prescribe an external training load as 5×3 min at 350 W, 2 min passive recovery, while additionally measuring the associated internal training load attained through heart rate and rating of perceived exertion (RPE). Alternatively, if the cyclist lacks a

power meter, we might aim to hit the same target using an internal training load prescription as 5×3 min intervals at 95% HRmax, 2 min passive recovery. While it is difficult to say that one method of prescription is better than the other, we believe that to efficiently shape the puzzle piece, the more information that we can gather (i.e., both internal and external load measures, and possibly different types of each), the greater the precision.

Thus, in the context of training load programming and our surveillance battlefield, practitioners likely need tools to help them:

Program the INPUT: Define a target reference exercise intensity based on the external load demands (power, speed, movement) or directly target certain levels of internal load ($\dot{V}O_2$, HR, lactate, neuromuscular activity, RPE).

Understand the INPUT: Was the prescribed external training load (i.e., HIIT running as bouts of 4 min at 18 km/h) in line with what was intended in terms of the likely physiological response (internal load response, e.g., 95% HRmax)? This information is required to:

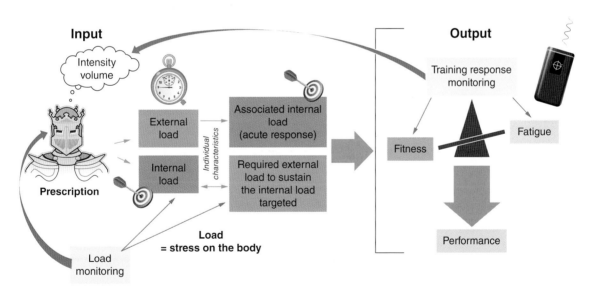

Figure 8.2 An overview of the training load programming and surveillance battlefield. Training, which can be prescribed and monitored as an external training load (blue box) can be seen to impart stress or an input on the athlete, measured additionally as an internal training load (subsequent red box; i.e., HR response to a given power output). Likewise, an internal training load stress can be prescribed and monitored (i.e., 3 min bouts at 95% HRmax) while measuring the related external training load parameters (subsequent blue box, power or speed). The response to the internal training load stress creates the signal for physiological adaptation in the athlete, viewed jointly as both fatigue and resulting fitness. The gain of fitness in the absence of fatigue theoretically enables an athlete to maximize his or her physical performance potential. Blue arrows indicate the retrospective feedback loop that can be used to learn from the surveillance process to adjust subsequent training load prescription.

- Adjust immediate and future external load prescriptions when physiological targets are not reached;
- Adjust immediate and future external load prescription to better fit the puzzle (e.g., cardiorespiratory responses were as expected but anaerobic participation and neuromuscular demands were too high relative to a game scheduled to occur in 48 h); and
- Improve return to full training process with progressive loading in the case of a previous injury.

Understand the OUTPUT: Once integrated into a larger model, the responses or changes to the load can then be used to optimize the process, as will be our focus in chapter 9. This helps us to learn from the past (retrospective analysis showing links with positive versus negative adaptations and outcomes), including physiological adaptations, fitness, and performance; fatigue; and injury.

Targeted Interception Markers for HIIT

Our first priority targeted interception markers within the context of HIIT surveillance need to be those outlined in chapter 4 that describe an HIIT session, and ultimately form the prescribed external training load puzzle piece. As a reminder, these include the:

1. work bout intensity
2. duration of the work bout
3. recovery period intensity
4. recovery period duration
5. number of intervals or series duration
6. number of interval bout series
7. between-series recovery duration
8. between-series recovery intensity
9. total work performed

These all can be measured as either direct or indirect markers of work rate, such as external power output or movement speed, and used to describe the activity in question, to enable us to classify our HIIT weapon (chapter 4) and target type (chapter 5) accordingly. Ideally, a relevant internal training load marker, such as heart rate, used as a proxy measure of $\dot{V}O_2$ (with limitations discussed in chapters 2, 3, and 9), is also captured alongside the external load marker to assess the success of our targeting (or lack thereof).

External load	Internal load
Work done	*Physiological and perceptual responses*
• Video tracking • Accelerometers • GPS tracking • Encoders • Power meters • Feet sensors	• $\dot{V}O_2$ • HR • Blood lactate • RPE • Intelligent shirts • Temperature • Sweat measures • Saliva content • Muscle oxygenation • Core temperature • Foot contact

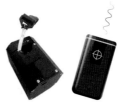

Figure 8.3 The variety of internal and external sensors currently at our disposal to estimate training intensity, and in turn, training load in athletes.

The following section outlines the primary tools currently used to describe markers of internal and external training load in the context of HIIT. As shown in figure 8.3, there are a number of different ways we can measure both the external and internal training loads, and with (micro)sensor technology on an exponential rise, becoming smaller and smaller, the numbers of integrated and embedded devices are expected to rise substantially over the next decade.

As shown in figure 8.3, there are already a number of sensors today at our disposal. While an important role of the sport scientist is to drive innovation in an attempt to gain a fair advantage over competition, it's vital not to lose sight of important day-to-day operations. As first told to us in 2007 by good friend and road cycling chapter contributor Marc Quod, this push for innovation and integration of the most recent technologies into daily training quantification and monitoring practices should not take us away from effective industry practices, simplicity, validity, reliability, and integrity. In Marc's own words, "Occam's razor always applies." Simply put, no more assessment should be used than is really necessary, as overmonitoring will add distracting noise to your daily smooth operation. Experiment with new emerging technologies with staff and colleagues, but on the battlefield, use only what is needed (29).

Training Load Variables

Training load can be quantified as the product of both the intensity and duration of the exercise bout. What follows first in this section is a description of the different ways we can monitor the intensity of exercise. More details on the load calculations (intensity × volume) will be described in the last part of the chapter.

As a first port of call, and in the context of a book on HIIT, we need an objective way to be able to describe how an athlete's HIIT session is actually completed. In chapter 2, we outlined the traditional methods that coaches have used to prescribe HIIT, including the RPE-based method, the maximal aerobic speed and power-based approach, the 30-15 intermittent fitness test, anaerobic speed reserve measures, all-out sprint training, the track-and-field approach, the team sport style, and additionally heart rate and power meter–based methods. In the upcoming 20 sport application chapters, you will read examples of how sport practitioners prescribe and monitor HIIT in the context of their sports. As shown in figure 8.2, the chosen method of surveillance will depend on the sport and available technologies, but in any of these cases, we ideally need to get a handle on relevant markers of both internal and external training loads. Take the case of a cyclist for whom we may have a direct measurement of external load via his cycling power output, but we can additionally measure his internal load using heart rate. In the context of sports that are running based (most), we can usually revert to the track-and-field approach using a simple stopwatch, recording the time it takes the athlete to cover a set distance for any given HIIT session to measure external training load, and typically use a heart rate monitor to measure internal load (if relevant). More advanced technological methods now include global positioning–based systems (GPS), semiautomatic cameras, and radio-frequency systems to measure movement speed. As we will discover shortly, in the context of many sports, the movements and associated stresses are complex, and we need to rely on other methods to gain practical insight into an athlete's experienced internal and external training loads.

External Training Load Variables

This section describes the main external training load marker variables of concern in sport and the technology tools currently available to monitor them. Relevant external training load markers ultimately refer to the mechanical aspect of movement, and the rate at which external work is produced. To be clear, with all of these methods, our aim is to gain insight into the exercise intensity. Variables we can currently measure include an athlete's power output, movement speed, and/or the number or rates of accelerations. The associated external tracking system tools that can be used to monitor these variables include power meters, GPS, local positional systems, semiautomatic video, and linear position transducer technology (4).

Power Output as a Marker of Mechanical Intensity   In the context of HIIT, we really need to get a handle on arguably the most important variable of all, the exercise intensity. Nowadays, power output, or the rate at which work is done, can be measured in watts (J/s), across a number of exercise modes using stationary ergometers, to give us a direct measurement of the exercise intensity. But measurement of power output is no longer exclusive to laboratory-based stationary ergometry. The last two decades have witnessed an explosion in the number of portable measurement devices that can remotely measure, either directly or via estimation, the power produced during exercise completed in the field. Thus, within the context of assessing a target kill for a given weapon (chapter 5), power output or HIIT work rate completed is highly relevant.

Nowhere has the measurement of field-based power output been more successful than in the sport of cycling. In the 1980s, German medical engineer Ulrich Schoberer invented the world's first cycling power meter, consisting of a strain gauge embedded into a bicycle's pedal crank arm. Using the force recorded in the strain gauge, alongside the angular velocity inferred from the cyclist's pedal rate, meant that power output (W) could be accurately measured in the field, just as it was done in the laboratory. Like a GPS can measure speed and total distance across a workout, a cycling power meter provides even better resolution, giving us a direct measure of intensity across any given moment in a ride, in addition to the total work (kJ) applied across any select time period.

Although not without some level of error, Abbiss et al. (1), Quod et al. (55), and others have established the accuracy, reliability, and validity of these devices in the field, and an explosion of related tools and analysis software programs has since followed, capitalizing on improvements in unit size, battery life, and automated wireless data transfer and analysis. Today, systems such as TrainingPeaks, Golden Cheetah, Garmin Connect, and others can automatically receive and analyze the training performed by a cyclist as soon as the session is completed, and in emerging cases, even in real time. Chapter 15 on road cycling expands on this area and describes how these devices and their software systems are used in the field of professional cycling.

Power output can additionally be measured on stationary ergometers that are specific to an athlete's exercise mode, such as for rowing (62), kayaking (51), and cross-country skiing (48, 49). While power output during these exercise modes can be measured in the field (i.e., via strain gauge and accelerometry), the lack of a constant moment arm length (relative to the cycling crank example) makes accuracy currently challenging, with commercial solutions slow to progress relative to the cycling market. Thus, individual sports outside of cycling today mostly rely on accurate GPS, using reference to world best time or pace (see rowing and cross-country skiing chapters as examples). Additionally, estimations of external power output associated with these alternate forms of locomotion are technically possible via combined GPS and accelerometry systems, but are not without limitations (described below).

Locomotor-Based Rates of Movement With the continued development of the (micro)technology industry, athlete movement tracking is today consid-

ered one of the most important components of load monitoring for both individual and team sports (4). In fact, it is difficult today to find an elite individual sport athlete or team without minimally using one or multiple forms of GPS, semiautomatic cameras, or radio-frequency system tracking during both training and competition (4). While coaches and practitioners may monitor a number of different aspects of training load throughout the week, the monitoring of various aspects of HIIT sequences (see chapters on soccer and Rugby Sevens) is of primary importance for optimizing the overall training impact.

The first aspect to consider when it comes to external tracking systems is that despite the vast array of technologies available today (figure 8.4), at varying costs, the overall reliability (how consistent or repeatable is the measure?) and validity (is it measuring what it's supposed to be measuring?) of most systems tend to be about the same (23). While advances in technology in coming years will undeniably improve these features, our view today is that it may not be the technology per se that matters most but rather the selection of the variables that can seamlessly be collected and how practitioners use them to understand load.

When it comes to selecting the best tracking variables available on the market today, the classification of Gray (21) may be useful. Gray uses three distinct

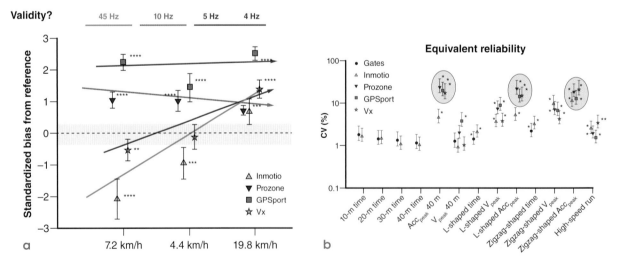

Figure 8.4 (a) Standardized difference in distance covered at various speeds using the different technologies (GPS, semiautomatic video and local positional system). No current technology provides a perfect estimation of actual distance. (b) Reliability of external load tracking variables using current technologies across various drills. The level of reliability is likely similar across the four systems shown. Note the reduced reliability across some of the most important load variables.

Adapted by permission from M. Buchheit, A. Allen, T.K. Poon, M. Modonutti, V. Gregson, and V. Di Salvo, "Integrating Different Tracking Systems in Football: Multiple Camera Semi-Automatic System, Local Position Measurement and GPS Technologies," *Journal of Sports Sciences* 32 no. 20 (2014): 1844-1857, https://www.tandfonline.com/doi/full/10.1080/02640414.2014.942687.

levels to describe the capabilities of current tracking technologies (21):

Level 1 reports the typical distances covered in different velocity zones; old-school-type analysis, provided by all technologies; e.g., 345 m of running above 19.8 km/h.

Level 2 reports events related to changes in velocity, including accelerations, decelerations, and changes of directions; provided by most technologies; e.g., 45 accelerations over 3 m/s across a total distance of 233 m.

Level 3 reports events derived from inertial sensors or accelerometers; microtechnology only, so not available with camera-derived systems; e.g., 17 impacts above 6 G, player load of 456 AU, stride variables (ground force load, contact times), stride imbalances (4% reduced impulse force on right leg).

More specifically, to assess HIIT load for run-based work, the key aspects we need to consider are both the intensity of exercise and the overall volume of the session (total distance or TD). Calculating the TD/min may be the best capture of exercise intensity (level 1 type variable). However, specific neuromuscular constraints must also be considered, including high-speed (HS, level 1) stride work involving large hamstring muscle activation, total HS distance in zones (see below), and the total amount of HS work in a given time period (HS/min), as well as time accelerating, decelerating, or changing direction (level 2, summarized as mechanical work, MW, involving thigh muscles (quads and hamstrings), total and MW/min) (20). Level 3 type variables are used more from a training status surveillance perspective, detailed in chapter 9. Finally, metabolic power has also received growing attention (54). This hybrid measure, based on both level 1 and 2 type variables, aims to provide a good estimate of the overall cost of high-intensity actions by combining the actual cost of HS (level 1) and accelerated (level 2) running (54). Unfortunately, however, practitioners are left with a difficult dilemma when it comes to selecting their variables, since the validity and reliability of each is likely to be inversely related to their load monitoring importance, i.e., high-speed running, acceleration/deceleration work, and metabolic power being the least valid and reliable variables (4, 41). Put another way, the variables believed to be best wind up likely being the least useful (18). This does not mean that such variables should not

be monitored, but rather suggests that greater care must be taken when interpreting their differences or changes (i.e., defining a larger, more conservative smallest worthwhile difference or change; see chapter 9) (19).

In addition to the validity and reliability issues outlined, other important limitations of tracking variables must be appreciated as follows (20):

- Acceleration values attained should be directly related to the time window of recording (in general between 0.2 and 0.8 s) and the signal filtering technique used (20, 41). Consensus regarding the time window and filter optimums has yet to be established, however, a simple solution might be to report such values over a single meter of length (i.e., base International System of Units) (38).

- Commercial systems producing this technology often update their data processing techniques (software or unit chipset updates), creating large differences in data output (24). This makes it difficult to maintain historical databases, except in the unlikely case in which a system is not updated.

- The number of available GPS satellites and their random spread (geometric dilution of precision) with respect to time-of-day location variation, or interfering infrastructures (stadium roofs causing partial blockage), result in unclear readings. Unfortunately, few activity reports readily provide this important detail.

- Large discrepancies in GPS distance are known to occur between Doppler and local coordinate techniques. While Doppler tends to be the preferred method, interbrand inconsistencies remain.

- Speed zone acceleration and distance validity are acceleration (5)- and speed (23)- dependent; i.e., validity is lowered with increases in acceleration and speed. Again, variables of most importance are likely the least useful.

- Increased sampling frequency does not always result in better precision or validity (23).

- Large between-unit variations (up to 50%) have been reported, even between units of the same brand (24). To partially counter this limitation, players should always use the same unit, and we have to remain cautious about our interpretations when comparing player data (using larger magnitude thresholds for meaningful differences) (19).

While we were originally excited about the potential of quantifying metabolic power (MP) from GPS readings (22), we have since reconsidered our stance and today question its usefulness in the field as a tool for monitoring elite-level team sport athletes (i.e., Ferraris). This is essentially related to recent research questioning the validity of the MP construct in the context of team sport–specific movements, combined with the fact that the MP calculation represents an incomplete metabolic assumption of internal load due to its broad external load capture.

At least four (16, 22, 42, 63) distinct and independent research groups have now shown locomotor-related MP assessed via either GPS or local positioning system (P_{GPS}) as being largely different from true metabolic demands as assessed using gold standard indirect calorimetry ($\dot{V}O_2$ measures, $P_{\dot{V}O2}$). P_{GPS} was reported as very largely greater than $P_{\dot{V}O2}$ during walking (16), yet very largely lower during low-speed shuttle runs (63) and soccer (22)-, rugby (42)-, and team sport (16)–specific circuits.

Despite its great potential, at this point in time the questionable accuracy, validity, and reliability of P_{GPS} prevent us from recommending its use as a surveillance tool for team sport–specific efforts with currently available commercial technology (23).

Considering that the agreement between P_{GPS} and $P_{\dot{V}O2}$ appears acceptable only during continuous linear running (but not during walking and intermittent changes of direction) (16), the metabolic underestimation consistently reported (16, 22, 42, 63) appears to be arising from the application of a nonspecific linear sprint acceleration formula to calculate P_{GPS} (34), which is clearly not suited for team sport–specific running patterns (e.g., rest, irregular step frequency and stride length, turns, upper-body muscle activity, static movements) (22). Additionally, if P_{GPS} were to reflect only locomotor-related metabolic activity (as opposed to a systemic measure such as $P_{\dot{V}O2}$), what is the real value of knowing this number anyway? Presently, these identified limitations (figure 8.5) highlight the questionable value of monitoring P_{GPS} in team sports. The usefulness of P_{GPS} is also limited with respect to what practitioners should actually be aiming to monitor in the field. Surveillance should include:

1. Overall estimates of internal training load, which in our view is satisfactorily assessed using HR and RPE measures (4); currently, metabolic load measured exclusively using locomotor-related actions such as P_{GPS} is not comprehensive enough.

2. Precise measures of external load, related directly to specific mechanical muscle group constraints, which have direct implications for training, recovery, and injury risk. However, P_{GPS} is clearly dissociated from actual muscle activation, as shown by the large variations in the P_{GPS}/ electromyography (EMG) ratio with running that involves accelerations and decelerations (38). If P_{GPS} is used as a global marker of mechanical work (combining high-speed running and mechanical work), it does not decipher the underlying specifics of the load (figure 8.5). The more logical approach is to use the accelerating, decelerating, and high-speed running distance since these are more representative of the specific muscle group load. As injuries tend to be more related to inappropriate volumes of accelerations (14) or high-speed running (35), there is little evidence to suggest that spikes in overall energy consumption per se play any role in injury etiology.

In conclusion, while there are many ways we can skin the cat when it comes to team sport surveillance, we believe that current best practice for characterizing the external load of a training session is to monitor a session's total distance, high-speed running distance, and mechanical work (and not metabolic power). Table 8.2 (at the end of the chapter) provides individual session examples in two different athletes performing the same run-based HIIT sequence, alongside the internal and external load markers. Further examples can be found in the chapters on soccer, Rugby Sevens, and field hockey.

Linear Position Transducer

Linear position transducer (LPT) technology allows for measurement of the velocity of many types of gym-based movement. These devices typically take the form of a central processing unit attached to the resistance training equipment (such as a barbell) via a retractable, measuring cable (e.g., Gymaware, Tendo) linked to optical readers that measure cable velocity via its linked wheel rotation (40). LPT devices convert physical attributes (the length of the measuring cable or speed of wheel rotation) into electrical signals that record the displacement of the barbell in this case, other resistance training equipment, or even the athletes themselves. LPT devices

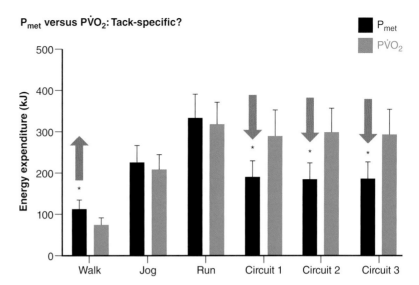

Figure 8.5 Four independent studies (16, 22, 42, 63) that have as of today clearly shown the lack of agreement between metabolic power (P_{met}) assessed via either GPS or local positioning system as being largely different from true metabolic demands as assessed using gold standard indirect calorimetry ($P_{\dot{V}O2}$). P_{GPS} was reported as very largely greater than $P_{\dot{V}O2}$ during walking (16), very largely lower during low-speed shuttle runs (63) and soccer (22), rugby (42), and team sport (16)-specific circuits.

Reprinted from https://martin-buchheit.net/2016/12/01/metabolic-power-powerful-enough-to-drive-ferraris/.

display live, velocity-based feedback via a display screen or secondary device (such as personal computer or tablet device). The measurement error of such devices has been shown to be very low, and both relative and absolute reliability have been shown to be acceptable. Harris et al. (40) provide a comprehensive review of the technology underpinning this equipment for further reading.

With respect to HIIT programming, encoders can help to monitor the velocity and calculated power output of movements during gym-based circuits (see chapter 6), which can be used as a measure of exercise intensity for type 6 targeting in the same way as cycling power and running speed. There is to date however very little, if anything, published regarding how to best use LPT for prescribing an HIIT session with respect to its neuromuscular component (i.e., type 2, 4, and 5 target responses). This is likely related to the fact that HIIT prescription in the past has generally been based on whole-body movements and/or locomotor modes that involve a large number of muscle groups, and in turn, involve high metabolic demands (e.g., v$\dot{V}O_2$max with running or p$\dot{V}O_2$max with cycling). Using gym-based movements is less likely (although not impossible) to trigger high systemic metabolic demands. However, the ability to record movement intensity during HIIT is never-

theless important for better understanding HIIT demands, monitoring changes in external load over time, and examining external to internal ratios (see chapter 9).

Internal Training Load Variables

Markers of training load considered internal refer to those that assess how the body has responded acutely during training, as measured by the external training load (figure 8.2). To be clear here, the internal training load markers we will cover in this section are attempts at understanding the intensity of the exercise from an internal measurement. Calculation of the load (intensity × volume) from our selected internal load marker is covered shortly. Measurement of internal training load is important, as it can offer us solutions to the programming puzzle related to the basic principle of individuality. That is, we all respond differently to any given HIIT session prescription, even one that might be normalized to the individual (i.e., W/kg, % PPO, % v$\dot{V}O_2$max, etc.). When we measure markers of internal relative to external training loads (expanded on in chapter 9), it gives us direct insight into how the internal machinery of the individual is working to produce his or her external movement speed or power output. Thus, internal measurements that can be easily monitored become useful adjuncts to record alongside the external training load markers we identified earlier when it comes to putting good surveillance systems around HIIT sessions. While many means of monitoring internal training load (exercise intensity) potentially exist (figure 8.3), the most relevant and practical field-based markers for practitioners are those that align with the key physiologically relevant HIIT parameters we introduced originally in chapter 3. These markers, with known limitations already identified, can be considered proxy readings of the oxidative, glycolytic, and neuromuscular responses during training. In line with these physiological systems, they include heart rate (aerobic demand and cardiovascular work), blood lactate (anaerobic contribution), and markers of neuromuscular function (neuromuscular demands and musculoskeletal strain), respectively. Notwithstanding these direct physiologically aligned variables, we describe further the gold standard holistic marker of internal training load, the session rating of perceived exertions (s-RPE).

Heart Rate

In chapter 2, we described how heart rate is probably the most commonly measured internal training load marker used to measure exercise intensity in the field (17), being well suited to prolonged and submaximal exercise bouts. Its challenge of course is the loss of relevance for monitoring the intensity of most HIIT sessions. Indeed, HR alone cannot inform on the intensity of physical work performed above $v/p\dot{V}O_2max$ (figure 2.3), representing the large proportion of HIIT prescription (9, 10, 45). Additionally, while HR can reach maximal values (>90%-95% HRmax) during exercise at or below $v/p\dot{V}O_2max$, this is not always the case, especially for short intervals (<30 s) (52) and medium-long intervals (i.e., 1-2 min) (61), due to the previously described exercise onset HR-lag phenomenon, with HR lagging well behind the $\dot{V}O_2$ response (figure 2.3) (27). Additionally, HR inertia continues at exercise cessation (i.e., HR recovery), which can lead to overestimation of training load when measured across recovery periods (61).

Notwithstanding its limitations, heart rate is a valuable internal training load marker to monitor in athletes, and while acknowledging that $\dot{V}O_2$ cannot be directly inferred from heart rate, it is the best we have, and at least it tells us about the actual work intensity of the heart. It is simple to take, relatively nonrestrictive for athletes in most sports, with a number of seamless commercial systems now using automatic uploading via Wi-Fi, Bluetooth, or smartphone direct to software for analysis and communication to external parties.

Use of such a system is shown in figure 8.6, where the simultaneous monitoring of external and internal markers of training load was collected in an elite triathlete during cycling and running short interval sessions (type 4 targets). Note the lag and inertial response of heart rate relative to power and speed, respectively. Nevertheless, the collection of heart rate during such sessions provides good insight into the athlete's health status and function, which will be expanded on further in chapter 9.

Blood Lactate

As we alluded to originally in chapter 3, lactate, or lactic acid when it is dissociated from the H^+ ion, is produced both at rest and during all intensities of exercise from the oxidation of glucose during glycolysis and is an important source of chemical energy (i.e., fuel substrate) during both exercise and in recovery. During steady-state exercise below the lactate threshold, the rate of blood lactate production from glycolysis is matched by the rate of its removal (conversion of lactate to pyruvate via the Cori cycle and lactate shuttle). Lactate produced in working muscle fibers is transported and can flow to adjacent less-recruited muscle fibers to be converted to pyruvate in a process known as the lactate shuttle (15). Here, pyruvate is converted to acetyl-CoA and oxidized through the central energy pathway (figure 3.7). This balanced process is referred to as lactate turnover (11).

Blood levels of lactic acid are increased at exercise intensities above the anaerobic threshold due to the greater ATP demand, and therefore the greater reliance on glycolysis to match the ATP energy requirements. Lactic acid levels begin to accumulate when lactate production rate exceeds its removal rate, and this denotes a high use of the anaerobic glycolytic energy system (type 3, 4, and 5 targets). Changes in pH and bicarbonate accompany these higher lactic acid levels (57). When blood lactate accumulates at a rate in excess of its removal, this causes increases in intracellular acidity, which may cause enzyme disruptions and muscle contraction impairment and ultimately fatigue (11). However, alternative data suggests that higher levels of acidity in the muscle actually assist in the optimization of force production during muscular contraction, making the production of lactic acid during HIIT actually beneficial to muscular contraction (53).

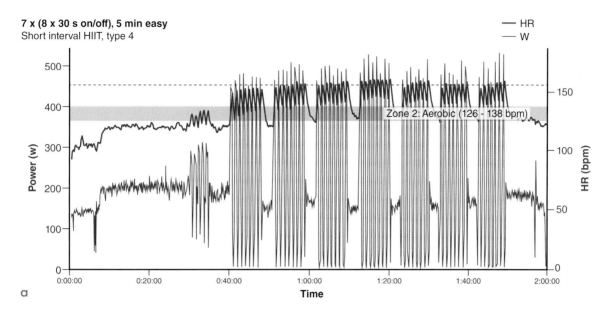

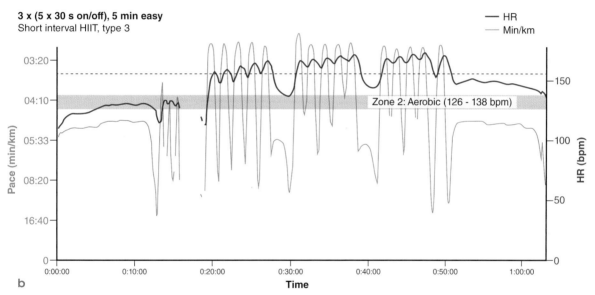

Figure 8.6 Simultaneous monitoring of external and internal markers of training load in an elite triathlete during (a) bike and (b) run short-interval training sessions. Zone 2 (5-zone model) heart rate is highlighted for reference. Note the lag and inertial response of heart rate relative to cycling power (a) and running speed (b).

Regardless of the possible benefits or encumbrances, lactic acid rises during exercise of increasing intensities associated with HIIT, and is a useful variable to monitor when the opportunity is convenient and practical, as it provides insight into the level of anaerobic system participation. In particular, blood lactate is often monitored during progressive exercise testing for endurance athletes during testing phases (see the chapters on rowing, swimming, and cross-country skiing, for example). Coyle et al.

(31) define the lactate threshold as a 1 mmol/L increase in blood lactic acid levels above steady-state levels (figure 3.8). Importantly, however, an individual's lactate threshold will be specific to the exercise intensity (power output or running speed) where the imbalance between the muscle cell's lactate formation and clearance occurs, which depends on training status, diet, and individual characteristics, among other factors. The measurement of lactate can, however, provide a means of

highlighting an athlete's metabolic (aerobic oxidative and glycolytic) responses, and may provide a benchmark for exercise training intensity prescription when incorporated with the associated heart rate, running speed, or power output response. It is important to note that just like the heart rate measurement, the blood lactate measurement will be specific to the mode of exercise due to the neuromuscular blueprint utilized. That is, recruitment of less-trained muscle fibers during unfamiliar exercise modes will alter the lactate response. Thus, the lactate needs to be determined using the mode of exercise specific to the athlete's mode of familiarity.

In the clinical setting, lactate levels are commonly measured using benchtop or portable lactate analyzers. A common benchtop analyzer includes the YSI Lactate Analyzer (12), with the gold standard for lactate analysis thought to be the Radiometer (28). In the field setting, the measurement of blood lactate accumulation (and its rate of accumulation) is the least practical and most annoying internal load measurement for athletes due to its invasive nature. For that reason, in contrast to heart rate, for example, it is currently impossible to measure blood lactate accumulation during every HIIT session. Nevertheless, in some specific circumstances, it can be of great value to confirm or verify the expected anaerobic contribution to a particular HIIT format (see chapter 5), especially when coaches and athletes are seeking to find the best available weapon for hitting their targets within their specific context (e.g., finding no available literature or HIIT data for their given sport or exercise modality). Some of the more common handheld portable lactate analyzers include the Accutrend (36), Lactate Pro (64), and i-STAT (33).

Neuromuscular Function

Assessing neuromuscular engagement (contraction intensity) and musculoskeletal strain during training is now possible via the use of new technology that includes portable EMG systems that measure muscle activity using embedded sensors in clothing, as well as contact time insoles that provide insight into foot work and leg stiffness regulation. While it is difficult to prescribe actual HIIT sessions using this new information, the monitoring of such responses is helpful for understanding whether actual physiological targets have been attained (i.e., type 2, 4, and 5 targets). When such technology is not available, indirect ways we can gain insight into the neuromuscular load of a session is twofold. The first approach is to use typical external load measures

as a proxy of the actual neuromuscular load, since it can be assumed that the greater the high-speed running, mechanical work, or mean cycling or rowing power of the HIIT session, the greater the neuromuscular engagement (i.e., figure 8.6). The second option is to examine pre- versus post-session changes in neuromuscular-oriented performances and/or adjustments during standardized tasks (refer to neuromuscular sections, chapters 3, 4, and 5). While possible post-activation potentiation mechanisms can sometimes occur, it is logical to think that the greater the impairment of neuromuscular performance post-HIIT, the greater the neuromuscular load attained in the session.

Session Rating of Perceived Exertion

The session-RPE method for quantifying exercise intensity was developed originally by Foster et al. (37) using a modification of the Borg scale (13). Instead of asking athletes how they are feeling at any specific point during exercise, about 30 min after they finish their workout athletes are asked the simple question, "How hard was your workout?" and typically use a 1 to 10 scale. This session RPE (sRPE) can then be interpreted as a global proxy of exercise intensity during the session. The reliability of sRPE is only moderate, but its practicality largely outweighs this limitation (43, 58). It is also worth noting that from our experience, accuracy and reliability improve with an athlete's use of the method over time.

Summary of Targeted Interception Markers for HIIT

In summary, markers of internal training load are those that can be used to assess how the various systems of the body respond acutely during training. While we have referred to markers of internal training load, we need to remind ourselves that in actuality we have been referring to markers used to assess the degree of exercise intensity, with direct calculations of load to follow. In line with our three key physiological targets discussed throughout the book, we can gain understanding of the likely internal oxidative load response through measurement of heart rate (notwithstanding limitations), insight into the anaerobic glycolytic response through measurement of blood lactate, and in emerging cases, various means of understanding the neuromuscular and musculoskeletal involvement that were described. Table 8.1 shows that the main internal training load markers of intensity, including heart rate, lactate, and sRPE,

Table 8.1 Typical Five-Zone Training Intensity Model, Including Percentage of Heart Rate Maximum, Blood Lactate Concentration, Rating of Perceived Exertion (RPE), and the Typical Effective Work Time in Zone for Endurance Athletes Performing a Polarized Training Model

These various markers of intensity are more or less correlated, with some exceptions.

Intensity zone	Heart rate (% max)	Lactate (mmol/L)	RPE	Typical effective work time within zone
1	60-72	0.8-1.5	1-2	1-6 h
2	72-82	1.5-2.5	2-3	1-3 h
3	82-87	2.5-4.0	3-4	50-90 min
4	88-93	4.0-6.0	4-6	30-60 min
5	94-100	6.0-10.0	7≥8	15-30 min

Monitoring internal load intensity during daily practice

Lactates and $\dot{V}O_2$
High cost and not practical

HR
Limited for supramax and intermittent exercise

RPE
- Simple
- Can be used with any sort of load → to aggregate different types of load
- Capture something more than HR and [LA] (likely neuro and cognitive load)
- Integrates fatigue status in the responses
- Reflects environmental strain (e.g., heat) that can affect load independently of external load
→ *Best global indicator by far*

Figure 8.7 Pros and cons of the various intensity markers practitioners can monitor to calculate internal training load.

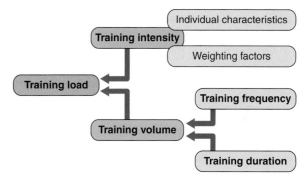

Figure 8.8 Training load is the product of the training intensity and the training volume.

are more or less correlated. While all markers of internal load surveillance have their place, depending on sport context, the global marker of internal training load (intensity) described was that of the session RPE, which can inform on multiple measures of global internal training load. Certain markers of intensity are better choices than others to measure, with specific reference to the practical element, and a summary of the pros and cons of each are shown in figure 8.7.

From Exercise Intensity to Exercise Load

Irrespective of the load marker considered, we acknowledge that quantification of training intensity

in terms of both external and internal load can be confusing, but let's move on. To this point in the chapter, we have outlined the primary means of assessing markers of exercise intensity from both external and internal standpoints. It's now time for us to make some load calculations. To do this, we need to appreciate that exercise stress (load) is not solely due to the exercise intensity but will additionally relate to the duration of the exercise intensity. The training amount (including the duration and frequency) of an exercise is also referred to as the training volume. Combined, training load can generally be considered the product of the training intensity and the training volume (figure 8.8).

Speed/Power-Based Intensity Zones and External Load

To compute an external training load measure, practitioners will generally combine markers of intensity (i.e., speed or power data) with the actual time spent exercising or distance covered across various (3 to 7) preestablished intensity zones. While it is difficult to find a sound rationale for all available training zones, practitioners tend to use both absolute (arbitrary) and relative (individual) key intensity benchmarks that correspond with meaningful training intensity bandwidths of relevance, in accordance with the specificities of the sport. For example, a five-zone power output model of training might be used in an Ironman distance triathlete (see triathlon chapter) as the model can generally capture the time in relevant training zones appropriately. However, this model is unlikely to have the resolution of interest for a cyclist with a sprinting role or focus (see cycling chapter), where the model used might be more likely to involve seven zones. While it makes sense to believe that the use of individual zones would better capture an understanding of exercise intensity at the individual level, it requires testing the athlete, which is not always feasible. The more common procedure used by most coaches across sport is the arbitrary method. The following speed zones are used in both the literature and in the field:

ABSOLUTE AND ARBITRARY SPEED (MAINLY TRACKING DATA IN TEAM SPORTS)

- 14.4 km/h
- 18 km/h
- 19.8 km/h
- 25.2 km/h

INDIVIDUAL (BOTH INDIVIDUAL AND TEAM SPORT ATHLETES)

- Maximal power output (55) or sprinting speed (50)
- Maximal aerobic power (55) and speed (50)
- V_{IFT} (59)
- Speed reached at the end of the Yo-Yo IR1 test (25)
- Speed/power associated with LT_2/VT_2 (3, 32)
- 80% of maximal aerobic power or speed (50)
- Speed/power associated with LT_1/VT_1 (60)

Internal Load-Related Intensity Zones, the Training Impulse, and Internal Load

For the range of endurance-related sports, most national sport governing organizations typically use a guiding intensity scale based on ranges of maximum heart rate and blood lactate concentrations at

associated work rates for given durations. Typically, aerobic endurance training in the intensity range of ~50% to 100% of $\dot{V}O_2$max is divided into five intensity zones shown in table 8.1 (60). Unfortunately, this traditional approach, using a standardized intensity scale, fails to account for individual variation in the relationship between heart rate and blood lactate concentration; activity-specific variation, such as the tendency for maximal steady-state concentrations of blood lactate to be higher in activities that engage less muscle mass (7, 8); or level of neuromuscular engagement as previously mentioned. However, for the practitioner, these potential sources of error seem to be outweighed by the improved communication that a common scale facilitates between coach and athlete, as well as across sport disciplines. Speaking the same training intensity language may be particularly important for improving the link between training intensity prescription from a coach's and an athlete's perspective (60).

In chapter 3, we defined three physiologically based demarcation points based on ventilatory or lactate thresholds (figure 3.8). While not directly comparable with the five-zone model, what is typically identified as lactate threshold intensity, or 2 to 4 mM blood lactate concentration, corresponds well in practice with the intensity zone demarcated by the first and second ventilatory turn points (VT_1, VT_2). So, for practical purposes, the three-zone model and five-zone model (numbered 1-5, table 8.1) are superimposable, with the lowest and highest intensity zones in the three-zone model further divided into two zones. Which intensity zone approach is best? For the young or inexperienced endurance athlete, using a three-training intensity zone model has the advantage of simplicity and makes communicating training intensity goals more straightforward. For the experienced athlete, the five-zone model provides a more precise description of training intensity distribution that may be important for communicating subtle changes in training prescription (60).

Figure 8.8 shows simply that training load can be considered as the product of training intensity and training volume. However, those of us familiar with HIIT know all too well that when intensity reaches the highest levels, the fatigue it generates is considerable. It doesn't take very long for an HIIT session to make a large impact on training load. Thus, the problem with the simple calculation (figure 8.8) is that it does not differentiate between intensity levels of training. Banister (6) was the first to recognize this and noted that blood lactate levels rise exponentially during intense exercise. Using the fractional elevation in heart rate or heart rate recovery plotted against the blood lactate, Banister (6) was able to gauge a weighting factor (y) to reward the hard work.

Training impulse (TRIMP) was the term Banister used to refer to the integration between time, intensity, and his relative weighting (y) of the exercise intensity to describe the exercise dose into a single number as follows:

$$TRIMP = time \times \Delta HR \times y$$

The TRIMP has been used in many research studies as a means of quantifying training load, and it is used extensively throughout endurance and team sports. For example, when the mean heart rate accrues time in a higher heart rate zone, the TRIMP produces a larger number due to the higher weighting factor of the exercise intensity. While these weighting factors attained from the study have been generalized to the whole population, it must be acknowledged that they are really only reflective of the sample population used in the study, given the blood lactate response is individual. As well, average heart rate does not represent the large fluctuation of activity seen in intermittent activities such as team sports.

During low- to moderate-intensity exercise, the heart rate and blood lactate response is linear. However, when intensity increases, blood lactate rises exponentially. Thus, for a more accurate TRIMP, we can use knowledge of the individual blood lactate and heart rate response to calculate an individualized TRIMP (iTRIMP) for every heart beat during an exercise session before summing up all values. Figure 8.9 shows the relationship between iTRIMP and performance in distance runners (47).

Anaerobic Glycolytic and Neuromuscular Load

As just described, and in the lactate section earlier (internal training load variables), blood lactate has a number of moving parts to it (Cori cycle, lactate shuttle, etc.), as well as rising exponentially with intensities above the lactate threshold, making assessment of an anaerobic glycolytic load variable difficult, especially from a practical standpoint. While we are aware of companies developing continuous

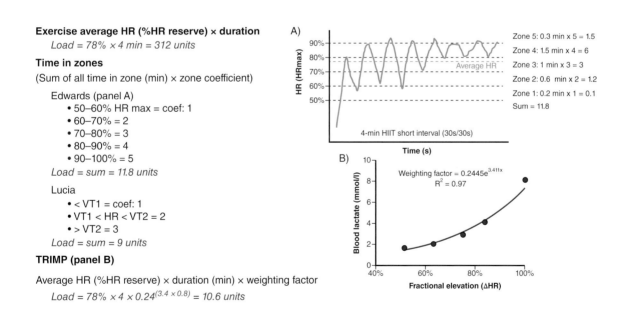

Exercise average HR (%HR reserve) × duration
Load = 78% × 4 min = 312 units

Time in zones
(Sum of all time in zone (min) × zone coefficient)

Edwards (panel A)
- 50–60% HR max = coef: 1
- 60–70% = 2
- 70–80% = 3
- 80–90% = 4
- 90–100% = 5
Load = sum = 11.8 units

Lucia
- < VT1 = coef: 1
- VT1 < HR < VT2 = 2
- > VT2 = 3
Load = sum = 9 units

TRIMP (panel B)

Average HR (%HR reserve) × duration (min) × weighting factor
Load = 78% × 4 × 0.24$^{(3.4 \times 0.8)}$ = 10.6 units

Figure 8.9 Example of the different approaches to measuring cardiovascular load based on heart rate responses. The training impulse approach, originally proposed by Banister (6) was later adapted by Manzi et al. (47), using the individual relationship between blood lactate and heart rate responses to incremental exercise to define the weighting factor.

Graph B: Reprinted by permission from V. Manzi, C. Castagna, E. Padua, M. Lombardo, S. D'Ottavio, M. Massaro, M. Volterrani, and F. Iellamo, "Dose-Response Relationship of Autonomic Nervous System Responses to Individualized Training Impulse in Marathon Runners," *American Journal of Physiology - Heart and Circulatory Physiology* 296 no. 6 (2009): H1733-H1740.

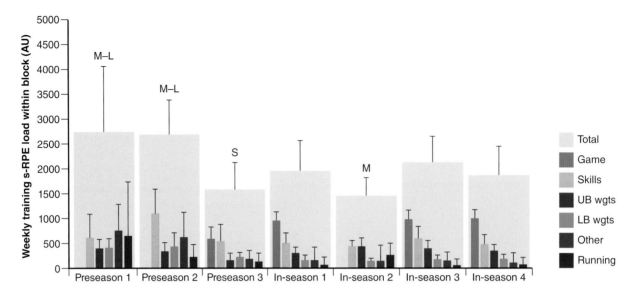

Figure 8.10 Training distribution expressed by RPE per week within block for weekly total load (large bar) and all modes (small bars), mean ± SD. UB: upper-body; LB: lower-body; AU: arbitrary units; M: moderate standardized difference versus in-season 1, 3, and 4; L: large standardized difference versus preseason 3 and in-season 2; S: small standardized difference versus in-season 1, 3, and 4.

Adapted by permission from D. Ritchie, W.G. Hopkins, M. Buchheit, J. Cordy, and J.D. Bartlett, "Quantification of Training Load During Return to Play After Upper- and Lower-Body Injury in Australian Rules Football," *International Journal of Sports Physiology and Performance* 12 no. 5 (2017): 634-641.

blood lactate monitors that work using a subdural microsensor, until such technology is realized, calculation of an internal anaerobic glycolytic load variable (intensity × volume) remains out of the picture. Likewise, with neuromuscular load, while the technologies described earlier in the related section provide promise for the future, as of today we are not able to be confident using their inputs to calculate a neuromuscular-related load variable. Until more progress in the area occurs, the main means of assessing anaerobic/neuromuscular contribution to HIIT remains in blood lactate concentration and accumulation (e.g., 9 mmol/L) and rate of accumulation (e.g., 5 $mmol \cdot L^{-1} \cdot 5min^{-1}$; see chapter 5).

RPE Load

As described previously, the session rating of perceived exertion (sRPE) developed by Foster et al. (37) is among the most commonly used measures for quantifying internal workloads in elite sports. This simple approach involves multiplying the athlete's RPE for a given session by the duration (volume) of the session (in min), to derive a training load in arbitrary units. As such, a session rated as hard (sRPE = 5) over 90 min would be attributed with a

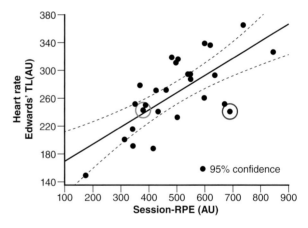

Figure 8.11 Correlation between mean team session-RPE-based training load and HR-based training load (Edwards TL) from 27 training sessions in young soccer players (r = 0.71, P <0.001). Note that while there is a large correlation in overall, there are some large individual variations too. For example, a session with an Edward load of 230 A.U. can be associated with sRPE values from 400 to 700 A.U. (likely reflecting different levels of neuromusclar load for a similar cardiovascular load).

Reprinted by permission from F.M. Impellizzeri, E. Rampinini, A.J. Coutts, A. Sassi, and S.M. Marcora, "Use of RPE-Based Training Load in Soccer," *Medicine & Science in Sports & Exercise* 36 no. 6 (2004): 1042-1047.

KEY POINTS: LOAD

These dissociations highlight the fact that each load marker may be specific to a biological system, which makes load monitoring easier and more precise in practice. As conducted by most practitioners in the field (see sport application chapters), by using a combination of simple field-based measurements, such as HR, sRPE, and locomotor data (power meters and GPS), we can characterize the related acute cardiovascular load (HR), neuromuscular and musculoskeletal load (indirectly from power meters, accelerometers, or GPS readings), and overall training load (sRPE). Doing so allows us to see which system is receiving the greatest strain, and to better understand and program the different types of stress, which is needed for training different systems simultaneously for enhancing adaptations and limiting interferences (see chapter 6 and the chapter on soccer). Table 8.2 shows how the load of an HIIT session can be estimated using both internal (HR, lactate, and RPE) and external (locomotor demands via GPS) measures of training load.

Table 8.2 Load Reports Showing External and Internal Load Using Relative and Absolute Thresholds for Two Athletes Performing the Same Run-Based HIIT Sequence

Both athletes performed the same run-based HIIT sequence (8 min, 15 s straight-line running at 20 km/h (83 m)/15 s passive recovery + 2 min passive + 6 min same sequence), HIIT type 4. Note that in absolute terms both athletes performed the same external load (which in fact was prescribed). However, the internal load responses (average HR, rate of blood lactate accumulation, sRPE, TRIMP, Edwards HR load, RPE load) tend to be greater for athlete B. Note that the greater internal load could be somewhat predicted when looking at external load based on a relative speed threshold (i.e., D>V$_{IFT}$). Note also the small difference in estimated cardiovascular load between TRIMP and Edwards methods, likely related to differences in individual HR profiles.

High-speed running D >19.8 km/h, m)	D > vV$_{IFT}$	Mechanical Work (A.U)	Heart rate (% HRmax)	HR-TRIMP	Edwards HR load	Rate of lactate accumulation (mmol.L.5 min)	sRPE	RPE lOAD
1257	1257	6	90	19.5	52	4	7	112
1262	1698	8	91	20.1	48	4.5	8	128

V$_{IFT}$: maximal speed reached at the end of the 30-15 intermittent fitness test; see chapter 2. D > V$_{IFT}$: distance covered above V$_{IFT}$. V$_{IFT}$: 20 km/h for athlete A, 19 km/h for athlete B. Mechanical work: overall measure of acceleration, deceleration, and change of direction work (18).

Adapted from M. Buchheit, "Player Tracking Technology: What If We Were All Wrong?" presented at 2nd Aspire Sport Science Conference on "Monitoring Athlete Training Loads: The Hows and Whys," Doha, Qatar (February 2016).

load of $5 \times 90 = 450$ units, while a recovery session rated as easy (sRPE = 2) over the same duration would receive 180 units. One benefit of this approach is that it can be used to aggregate and quantify the various training modalities undertaken by team sport athletes and other mixed-training groups (see the chapter on combat sports, for example). An example of how different training loads arising from resistance training or other sport-specific conditioning and skill sessions can be compiled together with the sRPE method is shown in figure 8.10 from Ritchie et al. (56). In addition, the sRPE method has been shown to relate favorably with objective load measures including heart rate, blood lactate (30), and other factors, such as collisions. Thus, the sRPE method represents an inexpensive and highly practical tool for the monitoring of training loads in diverse sport settings (see combat sport chapter, figure 11.7, for example).

Assessing Training Load in Practice

While there is typically the tendency for all load types (internal versus external) or methods (absolute versus relative thresholds) to be correlated, those correlations are never perfect. For example, there is a tendency for RPE to reflect cardiovascular strain (13), but on an individual session basis, there is often dissociation between RPE and heart rate responses (i.e., when the session involves substantial neuromuscular loading coupled with low cardiovascular strain; e.g., type 5 target). This indicates that the RPE measure is telling us something more than just heart rate. For example, Impellizzerri et al. (44) applied the session-RPE method proposed by Foster et al. (37) in young soccer players across 27 different training sessions to compare internal training load calculations. Relationships with heart-rate-based training load calculations were assessed. As shown in figure 8.11, the heart-rate-based Edwards training load calculation was well correlated with the session-RPE method. However, there were distinct outliers across the comparison, reflective likely of these individual dissociations mentioned, reflecting the fact that different stressors outside of cardiovascular load were impacting the athlete (i.e., neuromuscular, cognitive-mental-emotional, thermal; figure 8.7). Thus, heart rate and sRPE markers collectively provide complementary surveillance as they together give insight into the effect a training session likely had on more than just a single physiological target.

Summary

In summary, we have shown the importance of putting surveillance systems in place across HIIT sessions through monitoring the stress of training. The stress of training is theoretically calculated as the training load, which can be assessed using markers of external (outside the person) or internal (inside the person) exercise intensity, which is subsequently used to estimate exercise load when integrating exercise volume. Our main methods of monitoring external training load included measures of power output and locomotor activity (power meter and GPS), while internal monitoring loads can be assessed using markers of oxidative metabolic and cardiovascular strain (through HR), blood lactate, and various indices of neuromuscular and musculoskeletal strain. The global marker of exercise training load, and the one that takes advantage of the athlete's own inbuilt sensor of stress, the brain, was termed the sRPE. In the name of application and practicality, and to apply Occam's razor (29), the simple variables in the field are usually enough, with our top three including power or GPS, heart rate, and sRPE. The monitoring of all three provides comprehensive surveillance over the ACTUAL demands, which in addition to providing important programming clues, permits the important assessment of internal-to-external load ratios to be used in the context of training status surveillance, discussed next in chapter 9.

Response to Load

• • • • • •

Martin Buchheit, Paul Laursen, Jamie Stanley, Daniel Plews,
Hani Al Haddad, Mathieu Lacome, Ben Simpson, and Anna Saw

In our last chapter, we explored the concept of training load as it relates to HIIT. However, many coaches and practitioners often get confused with a related, but independent, concept: the response to training load. As these are exclusively different concepts, we need a unique set of tools and understanding to have impact. Importantly, our athlete's load *response*, commonly termed *training status*, is not uniform across all athletes and clearly depends on the training and individual characteristics. Recall from figure 8.2 that the training load (internal and external) can be considered the INPUT, whereas the response to the load can be considered the system's OUTPUT. Providing meaningful surveillance over an athlete's unique response to training, and especially HIIT, has been considered the holy grail of coaching and applied sport science. Just as with internal and external markers of training load (chapter 8), development of microsensor technology has equipped scientists and practitioners with a vast array of tools for describing this response to training load. We have many at our disposal, and a secondary purpose of this chapter is to describe those we find useful for the practitioner.

As we just learned in chapter 8, training load, the theoretical input marker of training stress (chapter 7), can be considered from both an external (mechanical work) and internal (metabolic, cardiovascular, neu-romuscular) standpoint (figure 8.2). While we can use these load concepts to program training intelligently, they tell us little with respect to how exactly athletes have reacted or responded to HIIT, the output, and where an athlete actually lies from a readiness-to-train perspective. Without somehow gaining insight into the output response, we're really just guessing as to what's going on in the athlete. It's precisely via the monitoring response to the training load that we can assess fitness and readiness to perform. We need tools therefore to gain insight into the output response.

In simple terms, insight into fitness and readiness to train will be gained by examining:

- Markers of fitness, fatigue, and health, which taken together may inform on performance capacity, as well as
- Efficiency or cost/output models, such as the ratios between the internal and external responses to training, in which the lower the ratios, the greater the performance capacity.

As highlighted in chapter 7, for any type of stress, the body's survival response is the process of adaptation or putting defense systems in place so that it may better remain in homeostasis should the stressor be encountered again. As we've emphasized from the beginning, we all respond uniquely to any form of stress. This unique response provides the opportunity to modify the training content through programming to keep athletes on track and progressing toward their performance goals. Therefore, this unique response to training forms the final step in the process to help us solve our programming puzzle. Understanding an athlete's unique response to training can help us to:

- understand the athlete's individual response to training, i.e., training status;
- estimate fitness, fatigue, and performance potential;
- determine whether athletes are adapting to their training programs, i.e., gaining fitness or assessing fatigue and associated need for recovery; and
- minimize risk of nonfunctional overreaching, injury, and illness (chapter 7).

The aims of this chapter then are to:

1. highlight current training response markers that appear useful to monitor for both individual and team sports,
2. describe the current and ever-evolving challenges that practitioners face when monitoring an athlete's response to training and health status,
3. offer a framework, including simple statistics, that may be used in an applied setting to assess meaningful changes in training status, and
4. provide guidance on how to improve data visualization and increase coaching staff buy-in for sport scientists embedded in larger high-performance programs.

Combined through the diverse team of authors assembled, our aim is to provide readers with the opportunity to improve their ability to make informed decisions that assist them when solving their training program puzzles, with particular reference to HIIT, and positively impact an athlete's future performance. The overarching concepts that gain us insight into fitness, fatigue, and readiness to train and perform are illustrated in figure 9.1. As the figure shows, potential performance capacity, or training status, can be inferred using direct or indirect measures. Direct markers include races and competitions, fitness and strength tests, as well as maximal efforts in training (including HIIT, such

as key sets), whereas indirect markers of performance capacity include fitness and fatigue responses, and internal-to-external load ratios. We will begin by outlining the main indirect training response category tools that we will discuss in the chapter.

Training Response Markers

As discussed throughout chapter 8, athlete tracking is considered one of the most important initiatives for both individual and team sports. For the weapons we implemented in training (chapters 4, 5, and 6), how lethal were they in terms of the damage they inflicted in our athletes? We need to understand this damage response to the applied training load weapons, or the carryover effect of the load. These incidences occur after the load has been applied, providing insight into the body's response to training in the period following (hours to days after). These responses provide insight into an athlete's performance level without directly measuring it.

Training responses in athletes are generally related to the training stimuli (e.g., relative or internal training load; chapter 8) (16). While both too much or not enough training load can contribute to fatigue (nonfunctional overreaching or overtraining; chapter 7), the appropriate training dose at the individual level may allow for optimal improvements in fitness and performance (16, 20, 55, 76, 78, 115, 116). It is therefore vital that an athlete's fatigue, fitness, and/or performance responses during the various training phases of an athlete's periodized calendar are under surveillance, so training load and its contents can be adjusted and individualized, both during and between training cycles (16, 97, 142, 159).

When it comes to monitoring athlete fatigue and/or performance responses to training load, various tools and methods can be used, such as the monitoring of saliva and specific blood variables (82, 121), the use of psychometric questionnaires (16, 47, 83, 153), and of course, generally knowing the athlete on a personal level and regularly communicating with him (remember to never treat a stranger; chapter 7). Changes in blood lactate can be used to track changes in fitness (chapter 8) (11), but its usefulness to inform on fatigue is, in our opinion, unlikely (109, 121). Moreover, in addition to being painful and inconvenient for frequent monitoring, the actual value of blood sampling is also questionable (81, 123).

We believe there are primarily three distinct families of key importance, each related to specific aspects of training status, that may all be useful in

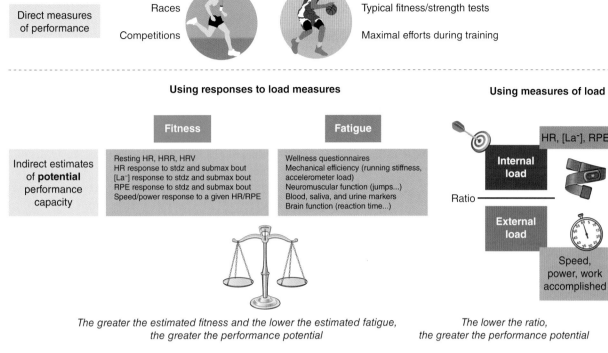

Figure 9.1 Best practice determinants of potential performance capacity. Performance capacity, or training status, can be inferred using direct or indirect measures. Direct markers include races and competitions, fitness and strength tests, and maximal efforts in training. Indirect markers of performance capacity include fitness and fatigue responses and internal-to-external load ratios.

assessing performance potential or readiness to train. Alongside experts in these respective areas, we herein describe each of these three categories with the tools we believe best represent them. Globally, and very simply for the practitioner, these include:

1. Internal metabolic, cardiopulmonary, and autonomic status, with heart rate the tool chosen to infer on the status of that system;

2. Neuromuscular and external force production and locomotor efficiency using a global positioning system (GPS) and accelerometers;

3. Overall health, fatigue, and mood (psychology); wellness questionnaires are a simple means of gaining insight into this important (and global) aspect.

Tool 1: Heart Rate Measures

With Jamie Stanley, Daniel Plews, and Hani Al Haddad

Today, there is high interest in the ability of noninvasive surveillance tools to monitor divisions of biology and physiology. Arguably the key player in the physiological domain is the autonomic nervous system (ANS), the body's central controller of, and responder to, all physiological systems, whose main role is homeostasis and balance maintenance. Conveniently for the practitioner, the ANS has a direct influence on the heart rate (HR), which can be observed through the level and variability of HR at rest (142, 159), following exercise (43, 45-47), during exercise (43, 46, 70, 147), and during recovery after exercise (59). The measurement of heart rate is noninvasive, inexpensive, time efficient, and can be applied routinely and simultaneously in large numbers of athletes. While the collection of beat-to-beat heart rate was initially only possible with expensive laboratory-based electrocardiograph recorders, the recent availability of valid and portable recorders, such as heart rate monitors (68, 167, 168), specifically designed systems (54, 135), and smartphone applications (66, 145) has substantially boosted the use of heart rate variability (HRV) monitoring in the field.

In this section, we specifically describe how heart rate measurements can be used successfully to monitor acute fatigue and recovery responses to isolated periods of endurance-based training, which allow us to adjust training load daily, and both positive and negative adaptations to blocks of endurance-based training. The application of each measure, together with statistical guidelines to assist interpretation, is outlined along with a simple decision process to assist practitioners in selecting the heart rate variables most suited to their needs.

One Simple Variable, Multiple Complex Indices

The measurement of a person's heart rate is simple and straightforward. It can be measured during sleep, upon waking, during exercise, or in the period following exercise. Analysis of heart rate can be as simple as reporting a 20 s value or as complex as delving into the beat-by-beat variance, more commonly known as the HRV. All methods and conditions have their advantages and disadvantages, with different determining factors (36), adaptation time courses (46), and sensitivities to fitness (43, 46, 47). For example, heart rate–derived indices such as exercise heart rate (HRex) and post-exercise heart rate recovery (HRR) can occur relatively rapidly (<1 wk after the start of an endurance training program), yet changes in resting HRV can take much longer to manifest (i.e., 4 wk of training (46)). While all measures of heart rate relate to ANS activity, the findings suggest that different indices provide insight into diverse physiological aspects of adaptation to training load and HIIT (30, 36, 46). Their use in combination therefore might improve surveillance of individual athletes. Although the appropriate combination, timing, and data collection methods need determining, it has become clear that the regular monitoring of a few simple markers can substantially improve the training process (46, 142). In the following section we present the physiological determinants and practical usefulness of each heart rate measurement.

Resting Measures

The physiological determinants, reliability, and sensitivity of the different heart rate measures are shown in table 9.1. The basic principle behind monitoring such indices repeatedly over time relates to our attempts to understand the cardiac ANS status in response to training. Since ANS activity is highly sensitive to environmental conditions (e.g., noise, light, temperature (1)), it is important to standardize recording conditions to isolate the training-induced

effects on the ANS. While evening (nocturnal) recordings theoretically represent the best (more standardized) recording condition for HR(V) monitoring (21, 138), the effects that differences in sleep patterns (132) and quality (51) have on HRV, independent of training-related changes in ANS status, can unfortunately result in misinterpretation (figure 9.2). To overcome such limitations, HRV data measured during select slow wave sleep (SWS) episodes, which offers the best signal stability, might be preferred (21, 40). However, a typical day's activity level tends to affect the night HRV during the early hours of sleep, when the higher proportion of SWS occurs (127). As will be detailed, consideration of the day's training load that precedes the measure is crucial to correctly interpret the changes in ANS status interpreted from HRV recordings.

Currently, the best practice for athletes tends to be short-term (1-5 min) measurements of HR(V) after waking in the morning (figure 9.3) (64, 128, 142, 159). While both supine and standing recordings are often used in the literature (156), the supine condition is better tolerated by athletes and is simple to do in the morning after waking, especially using smartphone applications that use the camera lens (photoplethysmography) to measure heart rate through the fingertips, a method that has been validated against chest strap and echocardiogram (145). These morning resting measures overcome the limitations of overnight recordings while still offering a level of standardization (e.g., same bed and same time most days, quiet environment, without the immediate effect of daily activities). Measurement using such systems is simple, convenient, and therefore highly practical for athlete and team practitioner.

Surprisingly, while morning resting heart rate has been used for decades by coaches, scientists have essentially focused their research on morning resting HRV, considering it to be a more powerful tool than heart rate. However, the possibly greater sensitivity of HRV is unlikely as large as previously thought. Indeed, we recently showed only a slightly stronger trend toward nonfunctional overreaching detection from vagal-related HRV indices over morning resting HR (r = 0.88 vs. 0.81) (139). Similarly, the relationship between changes in resting HRV and 10 km running performance (r = 0.76) were only slightly greater compared to changes in HR (r = 0.73) (141).

There is no shortage of methods for assessing HRV (161). The most common methods include time domain and spectral analyses, while nonlinear methods such as entropy and symbolic analyses have also

Table 9.1 Determinants, Reliability, and Sensitivity of Different Heart Rate Measures

	Determinants	Monitoring variable(s)	Typical error, expressed as coefficient of variation	Signal-to-noise ratio*	Smallest worthwhile change*
Resting HR	Cardiac morphology, plasma volume, ANS, and baroreflex	Wellness, fitness, readiness to perform	~10%	0.7	~−2%
Resting vagal-related HRV indices	Genetics, plasma volume, ANS, and baroreflex	Wellness, fitness, readiness to perform	Index-dependent, e.g., ~12 (Ln rMSSD) to ~80 (LF/HF) %	0.8	~+3%
Exercise HR	Fitness, plasma volume	Aerobic fitness	~3%	1.6	~−1%
Exercise HRV	Intensity-dependent: ANS< VT1, respiration >VT2	In theory, aerobic fitness	Index-dependent, e.g., ~60 (Ln rMSSD) to ~150 (LF/HF) %	N/A	N/A
Post-exercise HRR	Theoretically ANS and genetics but essentially metaboreflex	In theory, wellness, fitness, and readiness to perform. In practice, more fitness because of its link with relative exercise intensity.	Index-dependent, e.g., ~25 (HRR$_{60s}$) to ~35 (HRRτ) %	1.3	~+7%
Post-exercise vagal-related HRV indices	ANS and baroreflex, but the metaboreflex has the greater effect	In theory, wellness, fitness, and readiness to perform. In practice, more fitness because of its link with relative exercise intensity.	Index-dependent, e.g., ~16 (Ln rMSSD) to ~65 (LF/HF) %	1.1	~+4%

HR: heart rate; HRR$_{60s}$: HR recovery within 60 s following exercise; HRRτ: time constant of HR recovery derived from monoexponential modeling; HRV: HR variability; N/A: not available. Typical error: see text for related references. Signal-to-noise ratio refers to the magnitude of the change observed in (31) divided by the typical error reported in (4). See text for the methods used to calculate the smallest worthwhile change. *: for positive training adaptations.

gained some interest (161). Each index captures a different feature of the ANS, with some indices more likely to reflect cardiac sympathetic activity and others cardiac parasympathetic activity (161). In practice, however, when it comes to selecting the more appropriate HRV indices to monitor athletes in the field, time domain indices (e.g., rMSSD (square root of the mean of the sum of the squares of differences between adjacent normal R-R intervals) or SD1 (standard deviation of instantaneous beat-to-beat R-R interval variability measured from Poincaré plots), both reflecting parasympathetic modulation, appear to be the best. These measures can be captured reliably over a very limited time (e.g., 10 s to 1 min (74, 130, 131)) and are compatible with the short duration of recordings usually performed by athletes. As well, the sensitivity of rMSSD and SD1 to breathing patterns is very low compared to spectral indices (136), which is useful for day-to-day monitoring under spontaneous breathing conditions in athletes (148). Importantly, the day-to-day variations of time domain indices during short

(5-10 min) recordings in the field are likely lower than those of spectral indices (table 9.1). While the absolute magnitude of a CV is not an issue per se (see below), large CVs may lower the signal-to-noise ratio, which could compromise the sensitivity of the measures.

To conclude, the priority should be to collect resting HR and time domain HRV indices such as rMSSD. Despite large discrepancies in the literature (probably related to methodological issues), these indices, when interpreted correctly, are two promising tools for monitoring changes in general fatigue, fitness, and performance both over short- (159) and longer-term training periods (142).

Exercise Measures

Cardiovascular-related measures that can be measured practically during exercise to gather insight into training readiness and/or fitness or fatigue include heart rate during exercise and the variability of heart rate (HRV) during exercise.

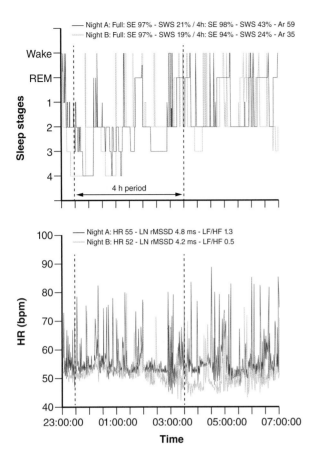

Exercise HR

With resting heart rate, heart rate measured during exercise (HRex; figure 9.3) is probably the simplest measure to collect in individual athletes and does not require anything specialized such as beat-to-beat sampling. Depending on the intensity, exercising for about 3 to 4 min will generally allow heart rate to reach a steady state during submaximal exercise (56), and the last 30-60 s of data is generally used for analysis (e.g., (45, 46)). Since heart rate is closely related to O_2 uptake during continuous exercise, HRex (when expressed as a percentage of maximum) provides a good marker of an athlete's exercise intensity (chapter 8), where lower relative heart rates at a given exercise intensity are generally indicative of a fitter athlete (114). Monitoring submaximal HR is common today in elite team sports clubs (35, 164). Many clubs use a 4 to 5 min steady state (~12-14 km/h) run-based monitoring on a weekly or monthly basis as an index of cardiovascular fitness. Generally speaking, an increase in heart rate should not be used as a marker of either fatigue and/or fitness impairment (43), although in the particular context of high-altitude camps, large increases (i.e., >4%) in HRex accompanying increased training loads could be predictive of illness (48). In summary, HRex is a highly recommended surveillance tool for monitoring positive aerobic-oriented training adaptations (43, 155).

Notwithstanding the ideal controlled scenario just mentioned, it unfortunately isn't what happens in

Figure 9.2 Overnight hypnogram and heart rate (HR) patterns during two nights subjectively rated as very good (i.e., 5/5 on a 5-point scale) by a 25-year-old team sport athlete. Physical activity (no intense exercise) preceding each night was similar (resting day, i.e., 2809 versus 2826 Kcal, as measured by triaxial accelerometers) (21, 40). Note that while both sleep efficiency (SE) and total slow wave sleep (SWS) time are similar over the two complete nights (which is consistent with the subjective rating of the night), the actual sleep stage distribution and fragmentation between the first 4 h of the two nights differ markedly (i.e., greater proportion of SWS during the first part of night A, 43% versus 24%, and more arousals (Ar, changes in sleep stages), 59 versus 35). The greater sleep fragmentation during night A is associated with more HR arousals, which directly increases the number of rapid (beat-by-beat) changes in HR (reflected by both the power density in the high frequencies (HF) or the square root of the mean of the sum of the squares of differences between adjacent normal R-R intervals, Ln rMSSD) and, more importantly, the power spectral density in the low frequencies (LF), which, in turn, increases dramatically the LF/HF ratio. Compared to night B, this results in a paradoxical autonomic response, in which a greater vagal activity (Ln rMSSD) is superimposed to a greater sympathetic background (greater HR and LF/HF ratio). Autonomic coactivation may explain these observations (165), however, more likely it is a limitation of the HRV analysis methods to capture the actual ANS state during nonstationary periods such as sleep. Additionally, the greater Ln rMSSD and LF/HF values are inconsistent with the greater proportion of SWS during the first part of night A, since SWS is generally associated with both reduced Ln rMSSD and LF/HF (21, 132). Therefore, the calculation and interpretation of HRV indices over a large period of sleep, with no consideration of the actual sleep stage patterns, is particularly challenging and remains questionable for monitoring purposes. REM: rapid eye movements.

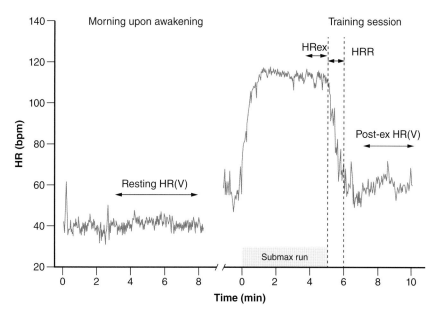

Figure 9.3 Example of the different HR recording conditions during the day. HR: heart rate; HRex: exercise HR; HRR: HR recovery over 60 s; HRV: HR variability.

Reprinted by permission from M. Buchheit, "Monitoring Training Status With HR Measures: Do All Roads Lead to Rome?" *Frontiers in Physiology* 27 (2014): 73 under the terms of the Creative Commons Attribution 4.0 International License (http://creativecommons.org/licenses/by/4.0/).

the life of most high-performance athletes and teams. Athletes and teams travel to different locations in the world at different times of the year, and environmental conditions change frequently. Because of the likely effect of heat on HR responses (especially during exercise performed outside), assessment of an athlete's fitness status must be made with consideration of the confounding influence that heat has on HR to avoid a false-positive assessment (result that indicates HR is elevated and fatigue is present). One way to avoid this is to perform the monitoring inside, where the environment can be controlled (47). However, in the likelihood of limited indoor space available for run-based monitoring, testing athletes on cycle ergometers is a good alternative (164), but perhaps less engaging for run-based team sport players. With most team sports, run-based monitoring on the pitch is the preferred option, so the temperature effect on HR must be known.

We showed that a 10°C drift in temperature leads roughly to a 1% shift in the fractional utilization of HRmax during a 4 min HRex monitoring run (figure 9.3) (102). From July and the summer training camp in hot conditions (temperature >35°C) to the cold winter of France (temperature <0°C), large variations in temperature can occur. Such variations independent of fitness changes can lead to changes of up to ±2% in HR%, which are higher than the SWC and thus meaningful. To avoid misinterpretation

(i.e., players are assessed as unfit while the shift in HR% is due to hot temperature), it is necessary to adjust the HR values recorded based on outside temperature (figure 9.4b).

HRV During Exercise

With respect to the measurement of HRV during exercise (figure 9.3), while attempts have been made to gain further insight into training-induced changes in fatigue and/or fitness (13, 101), there are still too many limitations with the method (24). Until new evidence is presented, the monitoring of HRV during exercise remains an interesting scientific toy but not a useful training monitoring tool.

Post-Exercise Measures

With respect to gaining insight into training readiness and/or fitness or fatigue from cardiovascular-related measures that can be assessed practically after exercise, the main variables we should consider include the post-exercise heart rate recovery and the post-exercise heart rate variability (figure 9.3).

Post-Exercise Heart Rate Recovery

Post-exercise heart rate recovery is reflective of a general hemodynamic adjustment in relation to body position, blood pressure regulation, and metabore-flex activity, which partly drive sympathetic withdrawal and parasympathetic reactivation (36, 59).

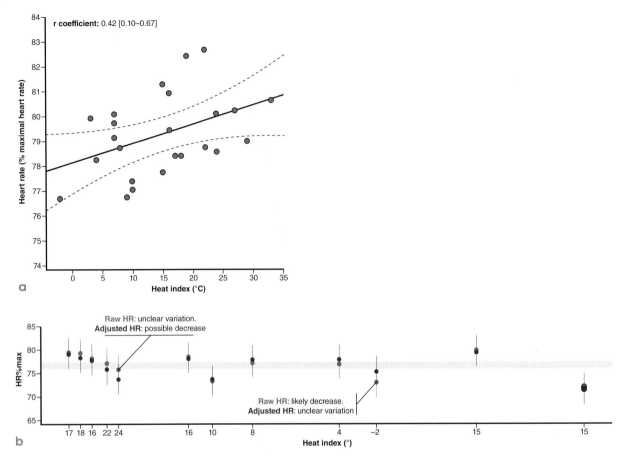

Figure 9.4 (a) Relationship between heat index (index that combines air temperature and relative humidity to determine the human-perceived equivalent temperature, °C) and HR response during a 4 min submaximal monitoring run. Regression coefficients (r) are presented as mean (±90% CL). (b) Intra-player changes in HR response (unadjusted (blue) and adjusted (red) based on heat index) to the 4 min submaximal monitoring run. During the fifth run, the unadjusted HR value suggests an unclear variation in fitness, however, the adjusted heat index (+24°C)-related HR suggests a possible improvement (decreased HR). During the tenth run, the temperature was –2°C; unadjusted data suggest a likely increased fitness, while the variation appears in fact unclear when considering adjusted HR. Created with Tableau 10.2.

Reprinted by permission from M. Lacome, B.M. Simpson, and M. Buchheit, "Monitoring Training Status With Player-Tracking Technology. Still on the Way to Rome," *Aspetar Sports Medicine Journal* 7, Targeted Topic: Football Science Evolution (June 2018): 54-66.

We can measure HRR a number of ways, from the number of beats recovered within a given time (e.g., 60 s, HRR_{60s}) to signal modeling via linear or (mono) exponential models (36). In practice, however, as good relationships between changes in simple HRR variables (i.e., HRR_{60s}) and changes in endurance performance and fatigue are reported (with the greater the increase in HRR, the better the performance) (59), HRR emerges as a relevant training surveillance tool for tracking positive changes in high-intensity exercise performance with individual athletes. However, increases in HRR have also been reported following functional overreaching (108),

which suggests that care should be taken when interpreting HRR changes and that other monitoring measures should be considered in parallel assessment (see limitations section). Nevertheless, changes in HRR have not always correlated with performance changes, in team sport athletes especially (43, 47), with correlations of lower magnitude than HRex.

Post-Exercise Heart Rate Variability

Post-exercise HRV (figure 9.3) has received some interest in sport science research, with the idea that it might offer deeper insight into training adaptations over and above that provided by resting HRV or HRR (171). The determinants of post-exercise HRV are multiple and include blood pressure regulation, baroreflex activity, and especially metaboreflex stimulation following exercise, which drives sympathetic withdrawal and parasympathetic reactivation (36, 159). High exercise intensities that drive blood acidosis and metaboreflex stimulation slow the HRR and lower the vagal-related HRV indices. Thus, to assess the true autonomic influences on HRV, independent of the metaboreflex stimulation, the use of submaximal exercise only ($\leq VT_1$) has been suggested (36). Indeed, if exercise intensity is not low enough, post-exercise HRV is related to the exercise intensity only and additionally becomes less reliable (table 9.1). Thus, as post-exercise HRV offers no further insight over HRex, and is no more practical to implement in the field, being influenced by too many factors outside of even the exercise itself, its measurement is currently not considered of any use to monitor in athletes.

Acute Responses

The natural day-to-day training load variations associated with the programs of most successful athletes are coupled by large daily variations of cardiac ANS activity (i.e., CV = 10%-20% for Ln rMSSD (38, 47)). In general, intense exercise acutely lowers vagal-related HRV indices for 24 to 48 h (figure 9.5), likely a sign of the body's homeostasis restoration, and generally runs parallel to improvements in perceived levels of whole body recovery (159).

In line with such observations, HRV has been used experimentally to guide daily training content, in which subjects performed high-intensity training only when vagal-related HRV indices were at normal levels (98, 100, 159). While these HRV-guided training approaches have been shown to result in greater improvements in endurance performance compared to traditional programming (98, 100, 159), such an approach is not as simple as it sounds. For example, in association with heavy training loads in the heat, increased, not decreased, vagal-related HRV indices are observed in the following 24 h period, despite acute decreases in perceived wellness (47). Additionally, in the 2005 Marathon des Sables, an intense multiday desert race (running 253 km over 7 d in extremely hot conditions), after an expected initial drop in vagal-related indices during the first 3 d (22), we observed a clear increase in cardiac parasympathetic activity, which was opposite the increased fatigue and lowered running performance (figure 9.6). These inverse associations between vagal-related HRV indices and acute fatigue suggest that in addition to the load of the preceding session(s) (chapter 8), environmental conditions and hydration status

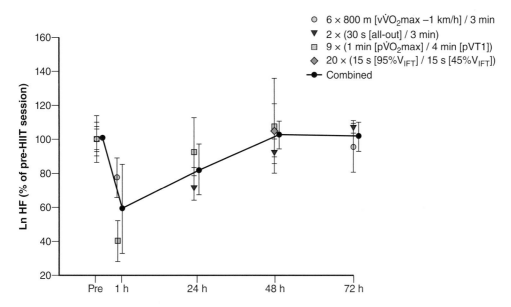

Figure 9.5 Changes in the logarithm of the high-frequency component of heart rate variability (Ln HF) before (Pre) and following different HIIT sessions. pVT1: power associated with the first ventilatory threshold.

Adapted from James et al. (2002); Niewiadomski et al. (2007); Mourot et al. (2004); Buchheit et al. (2009).

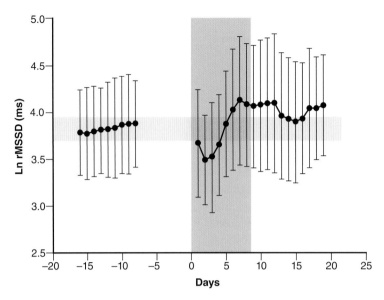

Figure 9.6 Average changes (90% CI) in the logarithm of the square root of the mean of the sum of the squares of differences between adjacent normal R-R intervals (Ln rMSSD) measured at rest after awakening in six runners (4 M, 2 F, 38.2±1.8 yr, 170.7±7.9 cm, 65.0±11.6 kg, 6.8±2.1 h of training per week) before, during, and after the 20th Marathon des Sables (2005, 253 km in 7 d in a hot environment, with temperature sometimes exceeding 50°C). The increase in Ln rMSSD after the fourth day of the race is unlikely reflective of general fatigue and fitness (which were reported to be deteriorated by the runners) but rather reflects changes in plasma volume due to the combination of exercise-induced hypervolemia (37) and heat acclimatization responses (47, 103).

Unpublished data (Buchheit, Leprêtre, and Billat).

must also be considered for correct interpretation of the ANS response to exercise (47, 159). This is due to the fact that plasma volume increases occur in response to both intense aerobic-oriented exercise (71) and heat acclimatization (103), which tends to increase beat-to-beat HRV independently of clear changes in fatigue and/or fitness (37, 47, 158). Additionally, other factors that influence cardiac autonomic activity recovery time include hydrotherapy and sleep, which should also be considered when interpreting daily HRV changes (4, 160).

Chronic Responses

HRV and HRR are known to fluctuate in accordance with training load periodization features, including volume, intensity, and overall load (46, 69, 93, 95, 117, 137, 138, 146). Moderate training loads are generally associated with increased vagal-related HRV indices, while high training loads are associated more with lowered vagal-related HRV indices (137, 138) and slower HRR (14). However, several studies in elite endurance athletes and/or athletes with a long training history do not always follow these trends,

with relationships in fact described more as bell shaped (93, 95, 110, 117, 142) (figure 9.7). In these particular endurance athlete subtypes, cardiac autonomic regulation is typically shown to improve during the first part of the training phase (e.g., building-up or extensive endurance phase, likely leading to functional overreaching), but decrease over the weeks preceding competition (i.e., tapering (91)). Since this particular pattern has been observed both in highly successful athletes (World and Olympic champions (93, 142)) and recreational athletes with long training histories successfully completing their first marathons (91, 95, 117), it may reflect an optimal training response. Importantly, performance has been reported to continually improve despite a lowered cardiac parasympathetic activity (figure 9.7), such that the relationship between these two variables appears reversed during the final stages of preparation. In support of this, while there are generally positive correlations between vagal-related HRV indices and markers of aerobic performance across large groups of athletes of varying training status (30, 46, 137), negative and large correlations are reported in homogeneous groups of well-trained athletes (17, 42). Reasons to explain these training phase- or load-specific relationships are not fully understood, but might be related to the training intensity distribution during the different training phases (140, 142, 159), independent of fatigue. Indeed, low-intensity exercise, representing the greater proportion of training during high-volume training, is likely to acutely increase vagal-related HRV indices the day after exercise, while intense exercise, representing the greater proportion of training during tapering, lowers those indices for 24 to 48 h (159). This highlights the importance of considering training context (phases, training load and its distribution) when interpreting changes in HR-derived indices. Making inferences on the training status of an athlete based on HR measures without consideration of the training context is likely to be misleading. While assessing training load and training intensity distribution is straightforward in endurance sports (chapter 8), this is more difficult in team sports since the load arises from stress applied to countless biological systems simultaneously (see below). Therefore, whether the impact of training load (and intensity distribution) on

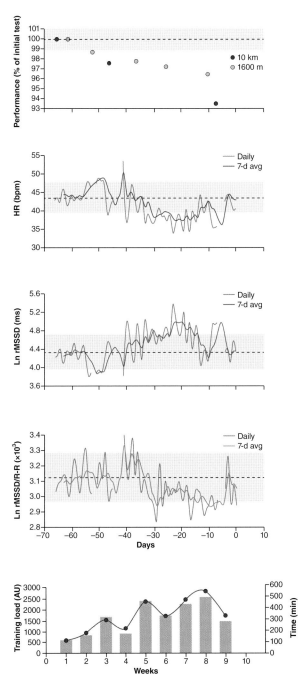

Figure 9.7 Changes in running performance (best time over a self-paced 5×1600 m interval training session and an all-out 10 km run), resting heart rate (HR), logarithm of the square root of the mean of the sum of the squares of differences between adjacent normal R-R intervals measured at rest after awakening (Ln rMSSD), the Ln rMSSD to mean R-R interval (Ln rMSSD/R-R), and training load (perceived exertion, CR-10 Borg scale×training duration (94)) and volume in a distance runner (32-yr-old, $\dot{V}O_2$max = 59 mL·min^{-1}·kg^{-1}, v$\dot{V}O_2$max = 18 km/h) over the 9 wk training program leading to his first

marathon (3 h, 15 min). The shaded areas represent trivial changes. Ln rMSSD and running performance change as a function of the training progression. While running performance improves continuously throughout, Ln rMSSD changes follow a bell-shaped relationship, with an initial increase followed by two consecutive reductions during the last phase of training. Interestingly, while the decrease in Ln rMSSD during week 7 to 8 is concomitant with a plateau of the Ln rMSSD/R-R ratio, the decrease observed during week 9 occurs with an increase of the Ln rMSSD/R-R ratio. This suggests that the decrease during week 7 to 8 is likely related to the saturation phenomenon (further increase in vagal activity), while that seen at week 9 is more likely related to decreased vagal activity and increased sympathetic activity (which might be required to reach greater exercise intensities during competition). This interpretation has important implications for using HRV to help guide the training process, which is only possible when using the combination of both indices.

Reprinted by permission from M. Buchheit, "Monitoring Training Status With HR Measures: Do All Roads Lead to Rome?" *Frontiers in Physiology* 27 (2014): 73 under the terms of the Creative Commons Attribution 4.0 International License (http://creativecommons.org/licenses/by/4.0/).

HR-derived indices described in endurance sport (140) is the same in team sports is not clear.

Saturated HRV Profile

At first glance, athletes who show a low vagal-related HRV index are thought to be fatigued, under a heavy training load, or on the receiving end of some unexplained stress in their lives. But as we just alluded to, this is not actually the case in a number of athletes, even when such athletes are without fatigue, not training hard, and rested. Typically, the observation occurs in athletes with long training histories and is likely due to two different mechanisms. The first reason is a lowered global level of parasympathetic activity due typically to the polarized training load distribution (see chapters 3 and 8), reinforced by possible pre-competition stress (118, 124). This increased sympathetic activity is likely beneficial for HIIT performance, as it allows the attainment of greater levels of exercise intensity, often referred to as *maximal sympathetic mobilization* (79, 107, 133, 134). The second is what is known as the *saturation phenomenon* (99), which occurs independently of fatigue and/or sympathetic overactivity (40, 44, 99). This reduction in vagal-related HRV indices occurs with low HR levels and is actually the consequence of an increase, not a decrease, in vagal activity. The underlying mechanism can be understood if one understands any physiological saturation phenomenon. The one that is best understood today is that of insulin resistance, which happens when a person's cells become resistant to the hormone insulin. Ultimately the insulin has little effect on its main job of glucose disposal in cells at its setpoint concentration, thereby requiring more and more insulin to have any effect on lowering glucose concentration. Likewise with HRV, it is the saturation of the vagal-influenced acetylcholine in its receptors at the myocyte level, where this heightened level of vagal tone gives rise to a sustained parasympathetic control of the sinus node, thereby eliminating respiratory heart modulation, resulting in reduced vagal-related HRV indices (112). As the vagal-related HRV indices are more reflective of the magnitude of modulation in parasympathetic outflow as opposed to an overall parasympathetic tone per se (80), we observe a decrease in the HRV, despite increased vagal activity (i.e., typically shown as a high HRV response). Figure 9.8 shows an example in an athlete displaying the HRV saturated profile at low heart rates (higher R-R intervals).

The next point is critical for practitioners who want to interpret meaning from HRV measured in their athletes. Since the saturation phenomenon (figures 9.7 and 9.8) can confound the interpretation of training-induced adaptations, a number of approaches have been developed. These include using sitting (98), standing (46, 156), or post-exercise (45, 46) measures, which induce a minimal level of sustained sympathetic activity, constraining vagal activity below the tipping point of saturation (i.e., R-R interval >1000 ms (99, 139, 142)). When using the convenient resting supine or seated method, the only way of knowing whether a lowered vagal-related HRV index is related more to sympathetic overactivity versus saturation is to compare changes against resting heart rate. In practice with athletes, we recommend using the Ln rMSSD/R-R ratio (139, 142) (figure 9.8 and table 9.2). In the case of a sympathetic-driven lowering of Ln rMSSD, the R-R intervals should also be shortened (heart rate is higher), which means you see maintenance or an increase in the ratio. While moderate increases can sometimes be optimal (increased maximal sympathetic mobilization mentioned above), extreme increases in the ratio might reflect maladaptation to training, and in turn, lowered performance (142). In the case of saturation, the R-R is increased (heart rate is lower) and the ratio is substantially reduced (142). Whether saturation is beneficial for performance is unknown, as each athlete likely displays his or her own unique Ln rMSSD/R-R ratio profile (141), which may also be training cycle-dependent, suggesting that longitudinal monitoring over months or years is needed to maximize surveillance across each athlete (141). For an athlete showing a saturated profile during extensive training periods, a sudden loss of saturation suggests either increased readiness to perform (positive adaptation (142)) or fatigue/negative adaptation (15, 19)). To decipher between these two scenarios, practitioners need to consider the magnitude of the increase in the Ln rMSSD/R-R ratio (see above), alongside psychometric measures and/or face-to-face conversations with the athlete (47, 119).

Interpreting Changes in Measures

In sports, so-called significant changes (i.e., changes determined based on null-hypothesis testing) in both performance tests and physiological variables, including HR-derived indices, GPS and accelerometry data, and wellness markers, are typically con-

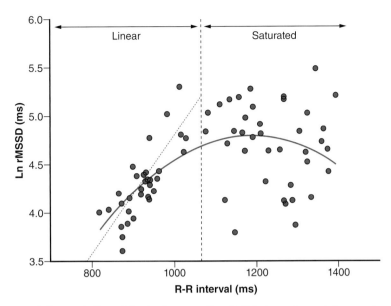

Figure 9.8 Example of the relationship between the R-R interval and the natural logarithm of the square root of the mean sum of the squared differences between R-R intervals (Ln rMSSD) in a subject with increasing bradycardia. Here, a saturation of heart rate variability is seen with long R-R intervals. Note how at shorter R-R intervals there is a linear relationship between Ln rMSSD (dotted line), which becomes disassociated as the duration of the R-R interval increases, indicating heart rate variability saturation.

Reprinted by permission of Springer Nature from D.J. Plews, P.B. Laursen, J. Stanley, A.E. Kilding, and M. Buchheit, "Training Adaptation and Heart Rate Variability in Elite Endurance Athletes: Opening the Door to Effective Monitoring," *Sports Medicine* 43 no. 9 (2013): 773-781.

sidered as having almost no practical relevance. Conversely, nonsignificant changes using null-hypothesis testing (P-value statistics) often have meaningful effects (87).

In order to avoid the embarrassing situation detailed in the sidebar Appropriately Appreciating Signal with Respect to Noise: Avoiding Russian Roulette Programming, we need a robust procedure. What actually matters to practitioners is whether the training-related change in a measure of relevance (such as HR) is actually important. Put another way, we want to know whether the magnitude of change

is essentially greater than the smallest practical or meaningful change or effect. Nowadays, we typically refer to this as the smallest worthwhile change (SWC) (10, 90). Additionally, when we compare the *average* changes in a performance or physiological variable of interest in a number of team sport athletes, across different metrics, and/or with heterogeneous between-athlete variances, the findings are often misleading (32).

For groups of athletes, an attractive option for assessing meaningful changes in any given variable we feel that matters and/or comparing changes in

STATISTICS ARE OUR WEAPONS

"Statistics are our weapons" was first told to us by Dr. Nick Broad, 1974-2013. Dr. Broad was an English soccer nutritionist who worked for some of Britain's largest soccer clubs, including the Blackburn Rovers, Birmingham City, and Chelsea Football Club, and in Paris, for Paris Saint-Germain. Broad was a close friend of former Chelsea manager Carlo Ancelotti and graduated from Aberdeen University. He died on January 19, 2013, age 38, in an accidental traffic collision (169). We remember him also for his important message.

Table 9.2 Guidelines for Interpreting Chronic Training Status Based on Different Scenarios in the Changes of Heart Rate–Based Measurements

Changes in rMSSD	Changes in HR	Changes in rMSSD/RR ratio	Occurrence	Likely mechanisms	Practical interpretation
Resting HRV and HR					
↑	↓	Maintained or moderate ↓	Very frequent following a short-term training program in moderately trained athletes and/or during the building-up phase of elite athletes (high-volume and low-intensity training)	Increase in overall parasympathetic activity	Coping well with training
↑	↑	Large ↑	May occur at the beginning of a training block, likely observed in previously saturated athletes	Increase in sympathetic activity that reverses the saturation phenomenon	1. If occurring during tapering, increased readiness to perform 2. If not, accumulated fatigue
↓	↑	Maintained or moderate ↑	Frequent during tapering	Increase in sympathetic activity	1. If occurring during tapering, increased readiness to perform 2. If not, accumulated fatigue
↓	↓	Large ↓	Frequent in elite athletes or others with a long training history	Increase in overall parasympathetic activity that causes saturation	1. Elite athlete or athlete with long training history coping well with training, likely high-volume and low-intensity training 2. If prolonged and not reversed with tapering, can inform on an overtraining state
Exercise HR					
↓			Frequent, in relation to changes in training load	Decrease in relative exercise intensity, plasma volume expansion	Cardiorespiratory fitness improvements
↑			Frequent, in relation to changes in training load	Likely increase in relative exercise intensity or only reduction in plasma volume	Unclear; doesn't indicate decreased performance capacity
Post-exercise HRR					
↑			Very frequent following a short-term training program in moderately trained athletes and/or during the building-up phase of elite athletes (high-volume and low-intensity training)	Increase in overall parasympathetic activity	1. If occurring during tapering, increased readiness to perform 2. If prolonged and not reversed with tapering, can inform on an overtraining state
↓			Frequent during tapering	Increase in sympathetic activity	1. If occurring during tapering, increased readiness to perform 2. If not, accumulated fatigue

Note that all changes need to be considered in relation to training context for appropriate interpretation. HR: heart rate; HRV: HR variability; rMSSD : square root of the mean of the sum of the squares of differences between adjacent normal R-R intervals, reflecting cardiac parasympathetic activity; HRR: HR recovery.

APPROPRIATELY APPRECIATING SIGNAL WITH RESPECT TO NOISE: AVOIDING RUSSIAN ROULETTE PROGRAMMING

Martin Buchheit

One of the best examples of naïve data interpretation in the field that I can recall, which was unfortunately followed up with inappropriate decisions related to training, relates to a strength coach I used to work with long ago. The coach was fond of using technology to monitor workouts, though at the time we were in the infancy of understanding linear transducer technology and these types of innovative tools (see chapter 8). His main presumption (not a bad one actually) was that fatigued athletes needed to rest (or cycle easily on a stationary bike) and should avoid lifting weights at all. Conversely, fresh and fit athletes should double up their session efforts and go harder. While his idea had merit, his monitoring approach, being solely reliant on this technology, was excessive and, more importantly, lacked any sort of an established basis for making decisions. Sadly this cost him his job in the end. In fact, the transducer data were so unreliable at the time (notwithstanding the overall split-squat movement technique used to assess readiness) that athletes often had power data two times greater, or smaller, than those recorded in prior gym sessions. Immediate increases or reductions in power shown by the linear transducer machine, irrespective of magnitude, formed nonnegotiable indicators of training adaptation in his mind, with the resulting instructions to either do nothing or go hard. As the numbers were so detached from an athlete's perception of fatigue and readiness to train, his start-of-the-session split squat assessment became viewed a bit like Russian roulette or a random number generator. What my mate had forgotten in his monitoring approach was that what mattered most in any measured variable was the magnitude of change *relative* to the noise of the measurement. Without appreciating both means we'll often make the wrong decision.

variables of different metrics is using the concept of standardization (90). We can standardize any observed change by following Cohen's effect size principle, which is simply the change in the mean divided by the between-athlete SD of baseline test data. From this, the magnitude (standardized unit) can then be compared with magnitude-based thresholds that can be considered as small (>0.2-0.6), moderate (>0.6-1.2), large (>1.2-2), or very large (>2) (90). Because the SWC is generally ~0.2 standardized units, the assessment of substantial changes becomes relatively straightforward. However, because of individual responses in a team for example (evidenced by confidence intervals [CI] that will be large), meaningful inferences about the observed magnitude must be made to assess whether the effect is substantially beneficial or detrimental (clearly

greater than the SWC), trivial (clearly within the SWC), or eventually unclear (CI overlaps zero and/or the SWC). These inferences can be achieved using a specifically designed spreadsheet (i.e., post-only crossover for within-team changes (84)), where both the individual response (CI around the average change) and SWC are taken into account to make our final assessment (90).

In practice, however, practitioners need to monitor each athlete in isolation to individualize his or her training process, which requires a specific approach (88). As detailed in the following sections, the observed individual change in any given variable (such as heart rate) needs to be assessed in relation to its SWC (whether it is greater than the SWC, and if yes, by how much), while considering the possible error of measurement (see figure 9.9). The following

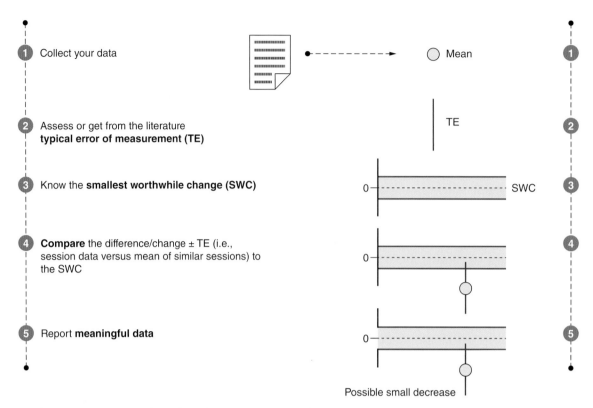

1. Collect your data
2. Assess or get from the literature **typical error of measurement (TE)**
3. Know the **smallest worthwhile change (SWC)**
4. **Compare** the difference/change ± TE (i.e., session data versus mean of similar sessions) to the SWC
5. Report **meaningful data**

Mean

TE

0 — SWC

0 —

0 —

Possible small decrease

Figure 9.9 Best-practice five-step statistical process for assessing changes in surveillance variables in an individual athlete.

Reprinted by permission from M. Lacome, B.M. Simpson, and M. Buchheit, "Monitoring Training Status With Player-Tracking Technology. Still on the Way to Rome," *Aspetar Sports Medicine Journal* 7, Targeted Topic: Football Science Evolution (June 2018): 54-66.

sections will detail how these two key elements can be determined.

Acknowledging Uncertainty Within the Measure

When it comes to monitoring an individual athlete's normal variation of measurement, or her within-athlete day-to-day variability, we use the typical error of measurement (TE), expressed as a coefficient of variation (CV) (85) (figure 9.9). The variability in each measure can be obtained either from the research literature or by using repeated measures of the variable collected in your athletes (88). The magnitude of these variations depends on both the variable itself (such as HR) and the recording conditions (i.e., HR measure CVs range from 3% to 190%, table 9.1) (149). For example, the CVs for time-domain HRV indices at rest are generally lower than those of spectral indices (especially for ratios, table 9.1) (5). Supine HR measures will show lower CVs than standing and exercise measures (149), while the CV for HRV during exercise is large, with values ranging from 120% to 190% (111, 120, 170). The

CVs for our recommended HRex or HRR measures (3%-35%, table 9.1) are much lower than those of exercise HRV (5, 18, 62), and CVs decrease slightly with exercise intensity increases (104, 106). As only submaximal exercise can be used as a warm-up for most sports, using HIIT to derive less variable HRex and HRR data is not practical. Moreover, while HR monitoring is often used as a diagnostic measure, it is unlikely that any coach would implement an intense exercise bout in an athlete already suspected to be overreached (chapter 7).

Importantly, it is not the absolute TE (or CV) of any measure that matters but the magnitude of its noise compared to the usual observed changes (signal) and the change that matters, or the one that has a practical effect (i.e., >SWC) (88) (figure 9.9). A measure showing a large TE but one that responds largely to training can actually be more sensitive and useful than one with a low TE but with a poor response to training. The greater the signal-to-noise ratio, the greater the sensitivity of the measurement. To understand the possible sensitivity of the different HR measures to positive adaptations to training,

training-induced changes in all HR variables (46) can be put in relation to the TE reported in the literature using a similar population (5). The comparison of the signal-to-noise ratio, calculated for each variable (range 0.7-1.6, table 9.1) suggests that HRex might be the most sensitive measure for tracking positive aerobic-oriented training adaptations. Importantly, however, these results often only apply within the context of the selected study (46) (e.g., short training period aimed at improving aerobic-related performance). The sensitivity of HRex to performance improvements can decrease over longer training periods (155), and whether it can be used to track other types of performance improvements (i.e., nonaerobically related) needs to be determined. Limited data exists on the sensitivity of HR measures for monitoring negative responses to training, and importantly, we know of no study in which all HR variables have been simultaneously reported, which would be required to compare the sensitivity of each HR index. In the study by Schmitt et al. (156), the signal (difference between fatigued and nonfatigued state)-to-noise ratio was shown as being greater for HRV indices (i.e., 3 for a vagal-related index) compared to resting HR (1.3) in the supine position. This difference in apparent sensitivity is consistent with the stronger trend shown toward nonfunctional overreaching for resting vagal-related HRV indices compared to resting HR (r = 0.88 versus 0.81) reported by Plews et al. (139). Considering that HRex does not always track impairments in physical performance (43), these data collectively suggest that HRV might be the more sensitive HR measure related to fatigue, but further studies are needed to confirm this.

The magnitude of the TE can also be reduced when repeating measurements, since noise will decrease by a factor of $1/\sqrt{n}$ (i.e., 4 tests half the noise) (88). Interest in repeated measures has been shown in endurance athletes, where correlations with running performance in healthy (141) and overreached (110) athletes were observed using the average of at least 3 to 4 d of HR and HRV data, as opposed to isolated measures taken on single days (141, 144). However, we want a test with a TE that is lower or at least equal to the SWC; the ideal scenario is one with a TE less than half the SWC. Any change in the measure that is greater than the SWC will be almost certainly substantial (88). For other scenarios, practitioners are advised to use common sense and consider (visually) the degree of noise relative to the SWC band and whether it overlaps

(figure 9.9). When extreme precision in the interpretation is required, a specifically designed spreadsheet (assessing an individual (86)) can provide the practitioner with assessment of the chances (%) that the observed change is substantially greater or lower than the SWC.

Determining the Smallest Worthwhile Change While defining the SWC of any variable is a key aspect of the monitoring process (88) (figure 9.9), it is often overlooked in the literature (15, 59, 156, 166). A change that is clearly greater than the TE isn't necessarily practically meaningful. Indeed, it must be clearly greater than the SWC to arrive at this conclusion. Defining the appropriate magnitude of the SWC is complex, however, and will depend on training context, the adaptation type being monitored, and the variable itself.

For individual sports performance, expressing changes as a fraction of the within-athlete variation in performance is probably the best way of standardization, where we retain the ability to compare the obtained scores with magnitude thresholds. One-third of within-athlete variation in performance between competitions is generally considered as the SWC, while 0.9, 1.6, and 2.5 refer to moderate, large, and very large changes (88, 90). Simulations have shown that as much as $0.3 \times CV$ performance improvements may result in a top athlete gaining one extra medal for every 10 races (89). However, when it comes to defining the SWC for individual changes in physiological markers, such as HR variables (that are not actually performance measures), the appropriate magnitude for the SWC is less straightforward (7). For HR(V) data, for example, in which day-to-day variability varies largely between individuals, using the within-athlete CV is likely the best option (25, 28, 29) (i.e., SWC = from 0.5 (110) to 1 (139, 142) × individual CV). For performance variables in team sports (e.g., vertical jump, bench press), the magnitude of the between-athlete SD is related to group heterogeneity, which can be seen as a limitation; however, fractions (i.e., 0.2) of the between-athlete SD are still recommended (25, 28, 29, 46, 47). Since the magnitude of the between-athlete SD is related to group heterogeneity and it doesn't consider the variations inherent to repeated measures, using the (individual) CV (139, 142) as the reference for the SWC is intuitively a better choice. It is also worth noting that because of the training context dependency of HRV changes (143), the actual magnitude of the SWC may need to vary throughout the training phases. HRV responses to either isolated sessions (159) or prolonged training phases (142) are also highly individual, so that the magnitude of the SWC for HR variables should also be individualized. However, there is no evidence that changes greater than any fraction/multiple of the CV are actually meaningful in practice with respect to actual changes in training status and/or performance. Therefore, to provide a starting point for understanding the magnitude of the SWC for each HR variable, group-average changes in HR variables following a successful endurance training period were extracted from the literature and related to the associated changes in performance variables for running (41, 43, 45-47) and cycling events (105, 114). The SWC for performance was considered as 1% for peak incremental test speed (43, 46) and 10 km running (46) and 40 km cycling (105, 114) time, and 0.2× the between-athlete SD for the Yo-Yo intermittent recovery (41, 47) and repeated-sprint ability (45) tests. The HR-variable change corresponding to the performance-related SWC was then linearly extrapolated from the group-average Δperformance/ΔHR relationship in each study and considered as the SWC for the HR variable of interest (table 9.1). The SWCs obtained from each study were then averaged to produce a single SWC estimate for each HR measure. This group-average approach was preferred over within-individual modeling for two main reasons:

1. individual data points were not available for all studies, and

2. the noise inherent within HR measures can compromise the performance/HR relationships at the individual level.

Since the time course of HR can be bell-shaped when training is prolonged over several months, as with elite rowers (93, 141), triathletes (110, 139), or runners preparing for a marathon (95, 117) (figures 9.7 and 9.8), the use of the SWC provided in table 9.1 should be limited to moderately long training periods (build phases) and/or performance improvements within the range of those observed in Buchheit's study (46). While this bell-shaped time course likely reflects an optimal scenario (rowers were gold medalists at the Olympics and all runners ran their personal bests), the fact that HR variables returned to baseline levels by the end of the tapering phase and the lack of information on performance changes throughout the training programs means

that a clear estimation of the SWC in such cases isn't really possible. However, we can suggest that a 4% to 9% increase in vagal-related HRV indices during the build phase may be needed for athletes to compete optimally following the taper (93, 110, 139, 141) (figure 9.7). Because of the limited literature available on negative HRV responses to training and the lack of consensus on the expected relationships between HR variables and poor training status, the SWC magnitude for assessing negative adaptation remains. Until new evidence is provided, we suggest using, for convenience, the same threshold used for positive adaptations (4%-9%).

To close, we highlight what we feel is current best practice based on our previous work (25, 28, 29), and this framework is detailed in figure 9.9 for the practitioner.

Making Decisions Guidelines for interpreting changes in the different HR measures are shown in table 9.2. As emphasized throughout the book, training context is always crucial for interpreting changes correctly. When we monitor an athlete, there is always risk of finding either a false negative (no decision made when you should have) or a false positive (decision taken when you shouldn't have) error. In elite sport, such errors can be considered drastic in the context of performance optimization. Therefore, we recommend taking a conservative approach in our attempt at reducing the incidence of false negatives (48). It is better that we overcall and reduce training load (chapter 8) in athletes suspected of becoming tired or sick (chapter 7) even if they are not, versus the opposite. In this regard, using a lower SWC for our negative adaptation might be an option. Once a substantial impairment threshold in an HR index is identified, practitioners need to decide whether to make their decision immediately (i.e., alter training content in line with the diagnostic) or wait and see if the changes persist over 2 or 3 consecutive days (23). These rules of engagement can be either gradual or index dependent. For example, after observing a substantial decrease in resting rMSSD with the maintenance of training load, the training intensity distribution across a number of sessions can be shifted from intense to low, which should increase rMSSD without reducing overall load. If this marker was to further decrease after initial training adjustments, enforced rest could be applied (depending on associated fatigue; see neuromuscular and wellness sections below) and/or specific reconditioning could be completed (in the case of detraining, in conjunction with other markers, see below). Finally, further analyses over larger numbers of athletes showing clear changes in training status are needed to determine the precision of sensitivity (proportion of true cases) and specificity (proportion of true noncases diagnosed as noncases) of each HR measure.

If a practitioner has the goal of using HR-derived measurements to help guide the daily training prescription, the only appropriate option really is the use of the morning resting HRV (98, 100, 159). Commercial smartphone technologies have made this very convenient for athletes, coaches, and scientists alike. The first advantage of the method is that there is often time for the data to be analyzed, typically before the training commences, so training can be modified accordingly, although this is not always the case for athletes who start training at the crack of dawn. Second, resting HRV measures can be repeated at any time (77) to assess the detailed recovery time course of the cardiac ANS following training (159). In contrast with exercise and post-exercise measures, which are generally performed during the session warm-up, there is no analysis time needed prior to training. Additionally, the data collection frequency to track ANS recovery time course can be limited to the times when the athletes exercise (e.g., no measure until later in the day (77)) (159).

When it comes to selecting the most appropriate measure of moderate- to long-term training monitoring in athletes throughout the season, practitioners need to consider the balance between the power of a given measure (e.g., its relevance in relation to changes in fitness, fatigue, or both (32)) and common sense (e.g., ability to implement daily versus weekly). This directly determines the overall usefulness of the monitoring system. Consideration of the needs and the time constraints of each athlete, a measure that can be collected with high resolution (i.e., more frequently) is likely more useful than a possibly more powerful measure that can be collected only occasionally. Increasing measurement frequency allows us to define more accurately the normal ranges of individual variation and decreases the noise of measurement by a factor of $1/\sqrt{n}$, which in turn, improves our ability to adjust training content. The perfect scenario is to collect a combination of the most powerful measures daily.

Figure 9.10 shows a simple decision chart for helping practitioners select the most appropriate HR mea-

sure(s) to use in their monitoring system, based on their sport and measurement timing. The minimum number of daily recordings per week required to assess meaningful changes in training status from HRV is an important consideration with respect to an athlete's compliance. Endurance athletes might be advised to collect HRV on awakening 3 or 4 times a week (144) for the data to be averaged (110, 141, 142) and to supplement these measures once a week with HRex and HRR. Endurance athletes typically are at a greater risk of overtraining than team sport players, therefore requiring a more complete assessment. This population is also typically familiar with frequent monitoring and cope well with (almost) daily HR recordings. In contrast, implementing HR measures more frequently than once a week is unrealistic in the team sport setting, as home-based measurement in this population is outside of cultural acceptance and difficult for such athletes to implement. The only viable option in such groups is to collect HRex and eventually HRR each week on a standardized training day. Furthermore, the practitioner can implement the measurement of HRex into the team warm-up, which tends to be acceptable by coaches and fits well into the time available in elite team sports.

Limitations of HR Measures

It is important to highlight here that HR measures cannot inform on all aspects of wellness, fatigue, and performance, especially as it relates to the response to HIIT, and especially the response to neuromuscular-related type 2, 4, 5, and 6 targets (31, 159). For example, while cardiac ANS recovery may align with muscular performance potential (57), there tends to be no association between this marker and blood creatine kinase or perceived muscle soreness following both a soccer game (41) and a 53 km mountain trail run (figure 9.7). Similarly, one has to wonder how cardiac ANS could possibly track metabolic recovery aspects such as glycogen resynthesis (31, 159). Finally, the time course of HRex and HRV adaptation during a training camp at 3600 m in highly trained young soccer players has been shown to be dissociated from both the changes in the RPE response to a submaximal run and psychometric measures of altitude tolerance (49). While mechanisms remain to be elucidated, the lack of sensitivity of HR measures to most neuromuscular, metabolic, or psychometric perturbations likely relate to the fact that HRV is only a marker of the *cardiac*

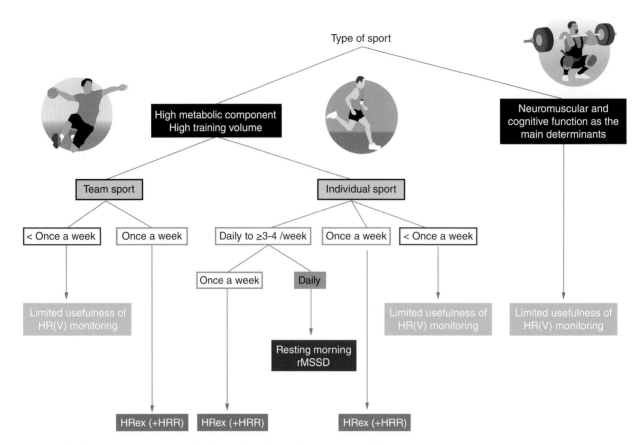

Figure 9.10 Decision chart for the selection of heart rate (HR) measures based on sport participation and implementation possibilities. HRV: heart rate variability; Ln rMSSD: logarithm of the square root of the mean of the sum of the squares of differences between adjacent normal R-R intervals measured after exercise; HRex: submaximal exercise heart rate; HRR: heart rate recovery.

ANS and nothing more (161) (see also figures 9.11 and 9.12). Therefore, the use of HR measures in combination with noninvasive neuromuscular-related markers found in GPS systems alongside countermovement jump scores (38, 58, 73) as well as general wellness and fatigue markers (83) may provide the complete solution for monitoring training status and response to HIIT load across most athletes and teams (47, 119). Therefore, assessment of changes in all relevant markers is needed to make the critical decision when it's required. The sport scientist needs to decide on the variable and physiological system that needs attention. As shown in figure 8.11, during congested periods of play in young soccer players, different time courses of adaptation may occur for individual players; fatigue can occur at the neuromuscular level without impaired cardiorespiratory fitness, and the converse. A last limitation of HR measurements is that athletes are generally required to use a chest belt, which is not

always convenient. There is however no doubt that future technological developments, where heart rate is collected via other sensor types (e.g., wrist-only monitors, clothes, sheets), will further increase the interest of HR monitoring in athletes.

Summary of Tool 1

In summary, from a measure as simple as HR, a large number of indices related to internal metabolic, cardiopulmonary, and autonomic status can be gathered. In as little as 1 to 5 min, morning resting HR(V) can capture a snapshot of an athlete's cardiac parasympathetic activity on that day (142, 159), whereas a period of submaximal exercise HR (last min of a 4-5 min cycling/running) is additionally a useful monitoring variable. Resting HRV measures can be collected frequently to examine acute (daily recordings (159)) and chronic (at least 3-4 d per week (144))

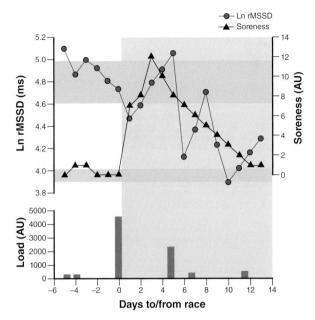

Figure 9.11 Time course of the logarithm of the square root of the mean of the sum of the squares of differences between adjacent normal R-R intervals measured supine at rest in the morning (Ln rMSSD) and perceived muscle soreness (Soreness, 0-10 scale) in a distance runner (32-yr-old, $\dot{V}O_2$max = 59 mL·min^{-1}·kg^{-1}, v$\dot{V}O_2$max = 18 km/h) before and after his first mountain trail (53 km, 4400 of positive ascent in 8 h, 22 min). Training/competitive load was provided as perceived exertion (CR-10 Borg scale) × training/race duration (94). All sessions were run-based except the one at post-race +5, which was a bike session. The green area represents the post-race recovery period. Gray areas represent trivial changes for both Ln RMSSD and soreness. Note that post-race Ln rMSSD recovers within 2 d and rebounds above pre-race levels within 5 d. The recovery time course of Ln rMSSD unexpectedly mirrors the dramatic increase in post-race soreness. The impressive increase in soreness (12/10 scale!) is likely related to the fact that the runner was used to running on flat courses only (i.e., marathon training, figure 9.6) and not specially prepared for mountain running at that time.

responses to training, and are likely sensitive to both positive and negative adaptations. Exercise HR may inform more on chronic and positive adaptations.

Correct interpretation requires each variable to be considered (1) in relation to the actual training phase and/or load the athlete is under (Chapter 8), while (2) considering both the individual TE and the SWC. Finally, since HR measures cannot inform on all aspects of wellness, neuromuscular-related fatigue, and performance (31, 159), their use in combination with other markers, including GPS/accelerometers and psychometric/wellness markers (see Tool 2 and 3, respectively, below) may provide a complete solution to monitoring responses to training load in athletes (47, 119).

Tool 2: GPS and Accelerometers

With Mathieu Lacome and Ben Simpson

Traditional methods used to quantify recovery and fatigue in athletes, such as maximal physical-performance assessments (figure 9.1), are typically not feasible for assessing fatigue status throughout competitive periods in team sport athletes, nor are they practical. Faster, simpler, and nonexhaustive tests, such as athlete self-reported measures (below), autonomic nervous system response via heart-rate-derived indices (above), and to a lesser extent, various protocols assessing neuromuscular function, may serve as promising tools to quantify and establish the big picture of an athlete's fatigue status in elite team sport athletes. While this section will focus on the needs within the team sport-specific context, there are nevertheless many concepts that are applicable to the individual athlete. Irrespective of the team versus individual athlete context, the implementation of appropriate, reliable, and sensitive measures of fatigue can provide important information to key stakeholders in any high-performance sport environment.

Current Practices and Associated Challenges in the High-Performance Sport Setting

Since the early 2000s, there has been an exponential rise in research concerning training status monitoring in high-performance sports (6, 60, 61, 72), providing the foundation on which sport scientists may base their analyses. Extending from the aforementioned section on the key metabolic, cardiovascular, and autonomic monitoring aspects, the aim of the second section of this chapter is to attempt to look into the crystal ball of monitoring and outline the most relevant means of assessing neuromuscular performance aspects, including external

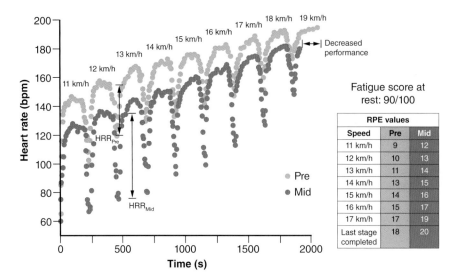

Figure 9.12 Typical example of HR and RPE responses before and after the overload training period in a participant developing functional overreaching (i.e., decreased performance and high perceived fatigue). Note that the HR and HRR responses at the beginning of the test (i.e., low-intensity running) could suggest good adaptation to training when considered in isolation. However, the combination of these markers with RPE value analysis indicates the development of the functional overreaching state.

Reprinted by permission from Y. Le Meur, M. Buchheit, A. Aubry, A.J. Coutts, and C. Hausswirth, "Assessing Overreaching With Heart-Rate Recovery: What Is the Minimal Exercise Intensity Required?" *International Journal of Sports Physiology and Performance* 12 no. 4 (2017): 569-573.

force production and locomotor efficiency. While there is today evidence that neuromuscular-oriented performances, such as jump or groin squeeze tests or maximal sprints, can directly inform on the status of athletes' neuromuscular function (157), there remain important limitations to their implementation in the elite setting, at least in some sports. For example, in elite soccer (chapter 30) or basketball (chapter 23), players are required to play every 2 to 4 d; it is simply not possible to perform such tests maximally between games. Therefore practitioners need to find other means of assessing the neuromuscular-related training status of athletes. Being personally involved in such a particular setting, we (102) have developed a specific monitoring approach based on various measurements that can be collected daily during normal training without the need for formal testing sessions and without requiring players to perform maximally. This section is a summary of our experience using GPS and accelerometry-based technology (102).

GPS Tracking With Basic Metrics

In high-level soccer clubs, it was shown that 40 of 41 surveyed teams collected heart rate and GPS data in every player during all field-based training sessions (2). Among the top-10 ranked variables used to quantify training load and response to load in

practice, distance covered in speed zones, accelerations, heart rate–related variables, and accelerometry metrics (e.g., PlayerLoad (8)) were the most frequently used markers. Referring to the classification of Gray in chapter 8, level 1 and 2 type data tends to be the most used in elite team sports. Since activity patterns of players are more influenced by contextual variables (e.g., rules, coach interventions, score lines, drills used) over player fitness status (53), locomotor-related variables (level 1 and 2) may not be the most vital markers used to directly monitor player training status (33). Additionally, given the diversity of team sport playing positions and/or player profiles that induce large between-player differences in locomotor activity, comparing locomotor performance between players is not very useful. It makes more sense to look at an individual player's change in such variables. One potential option, although limited, is the use of standardized drills (such as D-1 game simulations, see chapter 30, Soccer, i.e., 9v9 + GKs (33)) to assess changes in an individual player's movement strategy (relative to himself) to gain insight into his training status. However, drill standardization is not always feasible in practice. For example, key players are often not available to train for various reasons, while congested fixtures (playing very often) means minimizing the team's ability to perform a drill of interest.

To compensate for the limitations of level 1 or 2 variables in the absence of standardized drills, sport scientists generally examine a player's activity using two types of normalization:

1. Within-player analyses (102): A player compared with himself over multiple days, using historical data, i.e., intra-player trends.

2. Between-player normalization (102): A player compared with the team, with player locomotor activity systematically examined relative to the team or group of athletes.

These main two normalization aspects will be described in the following sections.

Within-Player Analyses

Within-player analysis can include the daily readiness approach, as well as the acute–chronic workload ratio.

Daily Readiness With the daily readiness approach (table 9.3), practitioners can monitor changes and track trends in an individual player's activity using historical data to track eventual signs of acute fatigue or rebound in freshness and readiness to perform (33). In fact we can estimate a player's readiness to perform by comparing any activity on a given day across the range of an expected activity's intensity or volume (e.g., mean drill response ± SD for a particular player for a D+3 and D-2 session; see soccer chapter). However, as differences in a session's content (e.g., an added finishing drill compared to a usual D-1 session) or context (i.e., playing a Champions League game versus the bottom league team the next day in soccer) can create more of an effect on a player's locomotor activity versus changes in her fitness status per se. As a result, definitive conclusions become difficult to call.

Acute–Chronic Ratio Recently, the acute–chronic (A/C) workload ratio has received growing interest for monitoring injury risk (113, 126). The model does not aim to compare a specific session's varying locomotor response but rather tracks respective changes in a predefined acute (5-7 d) and chronic (21-28 d) load, using either internal and/or external load measures. Put simply, the A/C ratio gives us insight into the simple concept of "Am I doing too much work recently, relative to what my body is trained for?"

While the concept is promising, several limitations prevent a number of team sport clubs from fully utilizing the model (26). First, team sport scientists need to achieve the following:

1. Collect enough data (at least one full year of training load and injury data) to build an in-house specific model for the team.

2. Find the most meaningful A/C ratio time windows (e.g., 7/28 versus 6/21) that fit their sport's context (52).

3. Calculate the optimal A/C ratios for each measurement that matters (i.e., sRPE, high-speed

Table 9.3 Reliability and Smallest Worthwhile Change for the Different GPS and Accelerometer Measures

Variable	Technology	Monitoring variable(s)	Typical error, expressed as coefficient of variation	Smallest worthwhile change
Daily readiness	GPS	Readiness to perform	Total distance: ~6% Dist >14.4 km/h: ~18% MechW: ~14%	Total distance: ~6% Dist >14.4 km/h: ~18% MechW: ~14%
Between-player Comparison	GPS	Readiness to perform		Total distance: ~2% Dist >14.4 km/h: ~5% MechW: ~5%
HRΔ	GPS and HR	Energetic cost of locomotion	3%	~1%
vL/fL	GPS and accelerometer	Locomotor efficiency	7.2±4.1%	2%
Leg stiffness (K)	Accelerometer	Locomotor efficiency	11±3.5%	4%

HRΔ is calculated as the difference between the HR responses to standardized drills such as small-sided games and the predicted HR for such drills based on individual multiples regression using GPS data as the independent variables. MechW: mechanical work; vL/fL: velocity load/force load.

running, mechanical work) since there are likely to be variable-specific sweet spots for decreased injury risk.

One important limitation that many elite team sports have to deal with are the periods when teams switch from club to international team and vice versa, which can sometimes be frequent. As one example, top soccer clubs in Europe have 60% to 75% of their players selected to perform on their national teams (A or U23-U19) at various times for international competitions. Because of little data-sharing between club and international team staff and the need for 21 to 28 d off to compute a chronic ratio, calculation of the A/C ratios is difficult (figure 9.13). With one international break every month from September 1 to mid-November, the use of A/C ratios will be

compromised during the first part of the season. While data can be estimated (26), this requires extensive work and adds uncertainty to the calculation. Figure 9.13 shows an example of an international soccer player. During the first part of his season, three international breaks required practitioners to estimate a substantial portion of the data (gray bars), lowering the confidence in the ratio calculated during the 3 mo period with the club. Additionally, the A/C window used (7:28 versus 4:18) means that we can have different interpretations of the same data (i.e., sweet spot versus increased injury risk).

Another limitation in our experience is the increasingly high number of false-positive outcomes that can be observed nearly every day (65), especially when using exponentially weighted moving averages (26) (e.g., ratio can be very high but players

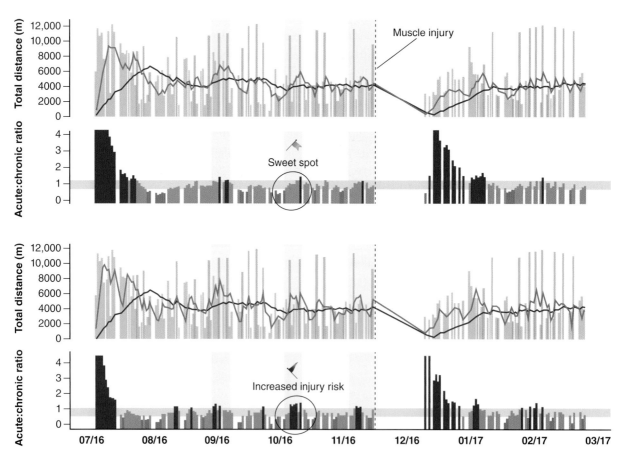

Figure 9.13 Measurement of total distance (m) in an elite soccer player over a 7 mo period. Acute (blue line) and chronic (red line) loads are calculated using 7 and 28 d periods (upper panel) and 4 and 18 d periods (lower panel), respectively. Dark gray zones represent international breaks when workloads were estimated based on the data obtained from the player's national team sports scientist. Total distance panels: gray bar, training session; yellow bar, match. Acute–chronic ratio panels: blue bars represent unloading (acute < chronic load) and red bars represent loading periods (acute > chronic load). Created in PowerBI (v2017-2.45).

remain injury free). As a result, players can directly discredit sports scientists who alarm coaches and medical staff on potential injury risk that doesn't manifest. Additionally, the fact that injuries can still occur in the 1 to 3 wk period (92) following a spike in load helps the defenders of the method to justify its interest to predict injury. Indeed, recurrent spikes in load are frequent in team sports, making it easy and convenient to find such occurrences to apply causation to the data set once a player is injured retrospectively (102).

Based on these highlighted limitations, we would encourage sport scientists willing to track (neuromuscular) fatigue and injury risk to consider other methods of data analysis, such as the normalization of individual player locomotor activity.

Between-Player Normalization

Player activity normalization (table 9.3) relative to the mean or median of the team or a group of specific players (same profile, same position) is another way to view data (equation 1). The main interest of this approach is that it is less likely affected by possible changes in session content for a given day (e.g., D+3, D-2 load), since all players can be considered. Additionally, the method can be used immediately on return from a national break, for example, since the metric doesn't rely on the previous week's load. Once historical data are available (e.g., previous season), insight into a player's fitness and/or early sign of fatigue can be gained while following the trends of these normalized data over several consecutive training days. In fact, sport scientists can use any variable (total distance, high-speed distance, accelerations, mechanical work-related variables/min) to construct similar models. Another possibility is the creation of a standardized value for each player based on the mean or median value of a typical drill used on a given day alongside the known standard deviation of the drill (equation 1). For example, following examination of the variability of most soccer drills we know, we have chosen to use only game simulations including goalkeepers (GS), possession-based games (PO), and some tactical and technical drills (102). Warm-ups have been removed due to the large between-player variability and overall low activity volumes. For our model, as the mean number of players is highly variable and generally less than 20 for the majority of the drills, the normalization is completed using the median value rather than the mean because it better represents the central tendency of small populations.

$$\text{Individual player readiness} = \frac{\text{drill locomotor value (TD)} - \text{drill group median (TDmed)}}{\text{standard deviation of the drill}}$$

Despite its promise, there are still limitations to this methodology, especially when training a small group of players (top-up sessions, position-specific sessions), since the variability of the metrics likely increases with the lower number of players, or in player return to play (since the player trains by himself, no comparison can be made).

Optimizing the Model

The quest of every practitioner working in elite sport is to continually search for an area of improvement in the collection, analysis, and reporting of data to the coaching staff (figure 9.13). To move forward, sport scientists can consider a simple yet effective framework for continual improvement by using:

1. adjustment of previously used variables based on contextual factors to reduce noise/TE,
2. relationships between existing variables, and
3. integration of new and useful variables to strive for insight into a player's fitness, readiness to perform, and/or fatigue (figure 9.14).

For outdoor sports, weather and environmental conditions, as previously discussed (figure 9.4), contribute noise or variation to the measurements that ultimately become confounding factors in the model and need to be accounted for when interpreting data. Understanding the influence (or lack thereof) of the various contextual variables that can affect training load metrics is of great importance. With the recent use of advanced metrics (level 3 metrics (33)), sport scientists can record contact time, flight time, and/or leg stiffness (K) (34, 39), which means that understanding the player-pitch interaction is of interest. Yet little is known currently regarding how pitch surface (hardness, shear strength) can influence such metrics. While preliminary internal studies have shown that slight variation in pitch stiffness, as measured with Clegg Hammer (~70 to 85 kN), has no clear influence on metrics related to neuromuscular efficiency during running (K) (figure 9.15) (102), investigation into potential factors that could influence accelerometry data should be of interest in coming years. It is our responsibility as sport scientists to seek out every contextual variable that could increase the noise of the model, and in turn, lower our ability to detect meaningful changes in an athlete's

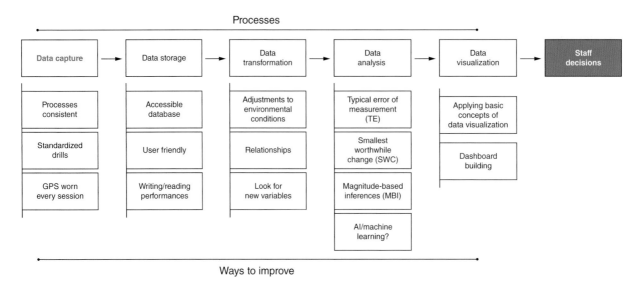

Figure 9.14 Framework for continual optimization of training load response monitoring models.

Reprinted by permission from M. Lacome, B.M. Simpson, and M. Buchheit, "Monitoring Training Status With Player-Tracking Technology. Still on the Way to Rome," *Aspetar Sports Medicine Journal* 7, Targeted Topic: Football Science Evolution (June 2018): 54-66.

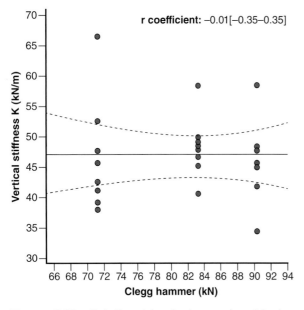

Figure 9.15 Relationships between heat index (index that combines air temperature and relative humidity as an attempt to determine the human-perceived equivalent temperature, °C) and pitch hardness measured with Clegg Hammer (kN) and leg stiffness (K). Regression coefficients (r) are presented as mean (± 90% CL).

Reprinted by permission from M. Lacome, B.M. Simpson, and M. Buchheit, "Monitoring Training Status With Player-Tracking Technology. Still on the Way to Rome," *Aspetar Sports Medicine Journal* 7, Targeted Topic: Football Science Evolution (June 2018): 54-66.

fitness or fatigue state and/or a factor that would cause us to make the wrong interpretation.

Building Relationships Between Existing Variables

In various team sports clubs around the world, compound metrics created by the combination of two or more variables are often used, requiring appropriate internal validation. For example, the ratio between velocity load (or m/min) and force load (or Player-Load) can provide a representation of the amount of force or ground impulses required per unit of displacement. Such a metric can be used to assess neuromuscular and running efficiency (the greater the ratio, the better the efficiency) and in turn neuromuscular freshness during standardized drills such as box-to-box runs or small-sided games (35, 39). While this metric requires proper validation, the concept in itself and preliminary results are promising.

To assess locomotor or work efficiency, and in turn infer potential fatigue and readiness to perform outside of the laboratory, sport scientists should assess the internal-to-external load ratios as a key marker of athlete readiness (figures 8.1, 8.2, and 9.1; table 9.3). In other words, simple internal-to-external load ratios can provide insight into an athlete's training status and may be helpful in making decisions concerning training load adjustments. Using existing metrics to build relationships between internal- and external-related training load variables can be a simple way to assess internal load relative to the external load as a cost/output relationship (50). For example, an increase in internal load relative to a standardized external load (e.g., monitoring run) can infer athlete fatigue or reduced fitness, while a decrease in internal load (e.g., a lower heart rate or perception of effort during a standardized external load) likely indicates that an athlete is gaining fitness and coping well with training. We used a ratio between RPE and relative total distance (RPE:m/min) to assess the overall acclimatization and fatigue trends during a training camp in a hot environment preceded by a long-haul flight (35). Akubat et al. (3) observed that the ratio between total distance (TD) and iTRIMP (chapter 8, compound measure based on HR) (TD:iTRIMP) during a standardized soccer-specific exercise was related to measures of fitness (vOBLA, vLT; chapter 3), suggesting that such a ratio might be used as a measure of readiness to perform.

As recently shown in Australian football (see chapter 21), measures of internal load (here RPE) are related to various external load metrics, while being highly individual (9). As such, individual relationships between internal load- and external load-related metrics could be assessed during a predetermined period to be used later as a prediction model. Subsequently, external load metrics (e.g., GPS metrics) can be used as independent variables to predict the dependent variable internal load (e.g., HR) after sessions. Therefore predicted HR responses could be compared to the real HR responses and a HR_{real}: $HR_{predicted}$ ratio could in theory inform on whether the athlete was gaining fitness and coping well with training or alternatively gaining fatigue (see figure 9.16, panel Predicted vs Real (%)). Figure 9.16 summarizes these considerations and shows total distance covered in a player over 2 mo, across the start of his rehabilitation post-injury period to his full return to play. The different panels present (from top to bottom) total distance covered and the different ways to monitor injury risk or potential signs of fatigue: acute–chronic ratios, readiness index, and internal–external load relationships with $HR_{predicted}$ versus HR_{real} comparisons.

Potential for New Variables

With the ever-evolving advances in technology, a new array of GPS technology will soon be available (GPSport Evo, Statsport APEX, and Catapult G5, to cite a few), which incorporate improved GPS chips (≥15Hz) and accelerometers (≥400 Hz). Sport scientists will encounter new challenges and opportunities in their athlete monitoring. Whereas Occam's razor (chapter 8) must still apply, level 3 (accelerometers, inertial measurement units)-type data will be easily available and likely more accurate than in the past. Thus, innovative and promising variables will be available for every session, and in turn, fatigue monitoring could become easier and more precise. With that in mind, practitioners should today consider the following opportunities related to force load and stride characteristic assessments in team sports.

Force Load (fL)

With the Athletic Data Innovation (ADI) analyzer, force load (table 9.3; (33)) refers to the sum of estimated ground reaction forces during all foot impacts, assessed via an accelerometry-derived magnitude vector. fL reflects only locomotor-related impacts and provides better estimates of overall footwork and impulses than total distance or PlayerLoad (8), especially when the session includes static movements and little displacements (i.e., rondos, free kicks).

During a given standardized drill, in relation to the average velocity (vL), vL/fL can be used to assess neuromuscular and running efficiency (the greater the ratio, the better the efficiency). Recently, the vL/fL ratio during box-to-box runs was shown to increase following soccer-specific endurance and speed sessions, suggesting a loss of efficiency in horizontal force application capability, likely due to the fatiguing effect of large amounts of high-speed running or training volume on posterior chain function (39). Also, moderate-to-large increases in vL/fL were observed 2 d after the end of an intense training camp in the heat, suggesting an increase in neuromuscular efficiency, which likely related to a rebound in the players' neuromuscular freshness (35).

fL can be compared between right and left legs during any locomotor actions (e.g., accelerating versus running at high speed, which is likely related to the use and potential weaknesses of different muscle groups (34).

Stride Characteristics

Stride characteristics refer to contact and flight time calculated from accelerometry data. From these two variables, it is possible to calculate vertical stiffness (K, table 9.3), which has been shown to decrease substantially with neuromuscular fatigue (125). While the typical error for K is slightly greater when calculated in the field (i.e., box-to-box monitoring) compared to standardized runs on an indoor treadmill

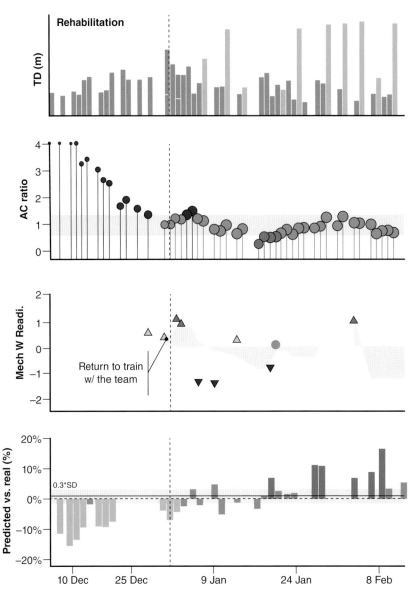

Figure 9.16 Training load (TD, m), acute–chronic ratio (AC ratio), readiness index (based on mechanical work, MechW Readi.), and HR response expressed as a percentage of predicted HR (Predicted vs Real (%)) in a typical player returning to training following injury. Vertical dashed line stands for the date of return to training with the whole group. TD (m): gray bar, training sessions; yellow bar, games. AC ratio: size of the circle related to chronic load (m); red circle, A:C >1.5; blue circle, A:C< 0.8; gray area represents the theoretical sweet spot (0.8-1.5); A:C ratio >1.5 during the rehabilitation phase due to preceding prolonged period without training. MechW Readiness: each form stands for one session standardized mechanical readiness (equation); blue form, MechW readiness >0.2; red form, MechW readiness <0.2; gray zone, rolling average over the last three sessions. Predicted vs Real (%): differences between GPS-based predicted HR and real session mean HR; orange bar, predicted < real, which means poorer than usual fitness; blue bar, predicted > real, which means better than usual fitness; in the absence of a clear value to define the smallest worthwhile change, the gray area was defined as 0.2* between-player standard deviation. Following a prolonged period without training, A:C ratio progressively returns into a zone of reduced risk. At the same time, the difference between predicted and observed HR increases, which likely means that the player is gaining fitness. Created with Tableau 10.2.

Reprinted by permission from M. Lacome, B.M. Simpson, and M. Buchheit, "Monitoring Training Status With Player-Tracking Technology. Still on the Way to Rome," *Aspetar Sports Medicine Journal* 7, Targeted Topic: Football Science Evolution (June 2018): 54-66.

(11%±4.5% (34) versus 6%±1.5% (39)), the error remains small. The constant monitoring of stride characteristics during standardized running bouts in the field provides new perspectives for the monitoring of neuromuscular status under ecologically valid conditions.

Figure 9.17 shows how such variables can be used in practice. Panel A shows the symmetry calculated from the fL of all foot impacts when either running above 14.4 km/h, changing direction (COD), or accelerating (>2 m/s) for all sessions of a player suffering from a tibiofibular inferior ligament sprain (right ankle). Following his injury, there was a clear force deficit on the left side, which progressively returned to baseline as long as the return-to-play program advanced. With these new metrics now available, especially due to the fact that the force load imbalances can be locomotor-phase specific (i.e., COD versus accelerations versus high-speed running), detailed injury-related patterns can be revealed. For example, in panel C, a player with a medial collateral ligament (MCL) sprain in the right knee presented with much greater strength imbalances during COD phases than during high-speed running and/or accelerations, likely due to the specificity of the strain associated with this injury. (The MCL is mainly

involved in protecting the knee against lateral force and is less affected by anteroposterior movements.) The diagnosis of strength imbalances is thus locomotion dependent, allowing sport scientists to complement and confirm the physician's or physiotherapist's manual testing protocols. This allows the provision of a fully functional diagnosis of the sprain or imbalance.

Summary of Tool 2

When it comes to using technology to gain insight into an athlete's fitness, readiness to perform, and fatigue, we believe that a clear vision of the framework needed to develop, optimize, and improve the models over time is required. In fact, the measures themselves are unlikely to provide much information directly (in contrast to HR responses to a submaximal run, for example). It's more the way that data are analyzed and presented that make such measurements useful and relevant (27). In this regard, applying the right methods of analyses (stats, understanding the noise and SWC of each variable, table 9.3) and combining this information with those derived from other monitoring variables is what becomes useful (i.e., internal physiology with HR

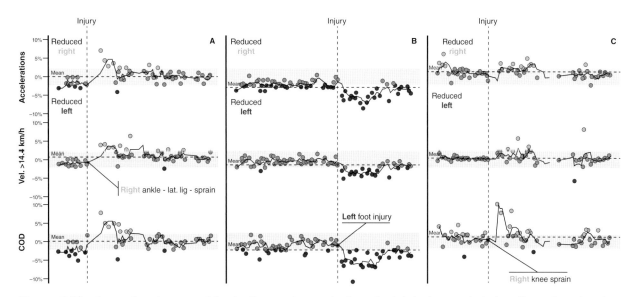

Figure 9.17 Force load symmetries in three players before their injuries and during the return-to-play period following tibiofibular inferior ligament sprain of the right ankle, left foot sprain, and medial collateral sprain of the right knee. The symmetry is calculated from the force load of all foot impacts during (from top to bottom) accelerations, running phase above 14.4 km/h, and changes of directions. Orange circle: right-leg force deficit >2%; red circle: left-leg force deficit >2%; red-dashed lines: injury date. Created in Tableau Software 10.2.

Reprinted by permission from M. Lacome, B.M. Simpson, and M. Buchheit, "Monitoring Training Status With Player-Tracking Technology. Still on the Way to Rome," *Aspetar Sports Medicine Journal* 7, Targeted Topic: Football Science Evolution (June 2018): 54-66.

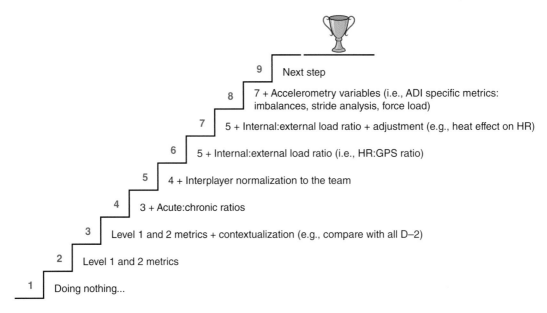

Figure 9.18 The way to Rome: A summary of training load monitoring practices.

Reprinted by permission from M. Lacome, B.M. Simpson, and M. Buchheit, "Monitoring Training Status With Player-Tracking Technology. Still on the Way to Rome," *Aspetar Sports Medicine Journal* 7, Targeted Topic: Football Science Evolution (June 2018): 54-66.

measures, tool 1, and global health with wellness measures, tool 3).

A summary of the different training load monitoring options for practitioners, with specific reference to team sports, is shown in figure 9.18.

To this point in the chapter, we've assessed two of our three key families of importance for assessing performance potential or readiness to train, namely, our internal metabolic, cardiovascular, and autonomic marker of heart rate as well as our neuromuscular and external force efficiency markers through GPS and accelerometry systems. The final family of importance that we must acknowledge and respect in the context of HIIT and training load is the measurements that can offer insight into health and fatigue and what's inside an athlete's mind: the athlete's psychology and wellness.

Tool 3: Wellness

With Anna Saw

Wellness is used in this book as an all-encompassing term to refer to an athlete's physical, psychological, and/or social well-being. While some insight into physical wellness may be gathered from the biological markers already described, simply asking an athlete to report her perceived wellness may be the most holistic and meaningful approach (153). Wellness

measures typically take the form of a series of items with associated rating scales that can be either paper based or electronic, and which are completed on a regular, often daily, basis. The relative simplicity, accessibility, and universal nature of wellness measures make them a popular monitoring tool across all sports and participation levels. Even in well-resourced high-performance sport settings, wellness measures tend to be the most commonly adopted monitoring tool, used in approximately 80% of programs (162).

The use of wellness measures in practice was recently addressed in a systematic literature review, which provided strong empirical support for subjective wellness to reflect an athlete's response to training (2, 153). Specifically, subjective wellness was shown to decrease in response to an acute increase in training load (chapter 8) and improve in response to an acute decrease in training load. The sensitivity and consistency by which wellness measures reflect the response to training load makes them ideal as surveillance tools.

Consider the following scenario in which a team of athletes attend a 2 wk training camp in the lead-up to a major competition. The first week is a solid training block, with more HIIT than the athletes had been completing in their home training environment. An acute increase in training load coupled with the additional stresses associated with the training camp environment is expected to elicit a decrease in subjective wellness. Indeed, this pattern is seen across the team and the practitioner can be reassured that the desired training effect is being achieved. However, two individual athletes are flagged for deviating from this expected and typical team response. One athlete's wellness remains high, requiring the practitioner to investigate whether the athlete is not being sufficiently stressed by the training load. The other athlete has a disproportional decrease in wellness, requiring the practitioner to investigate whether the training load is excessively stressing the athlete or perhaps other nontraining factors are negatively affecting the athlete. The second week of the training camp is a taper week leading into competition. As such, subjective wellness is anticipated to improve. Similarly, the practitioner flags any athlete whose wellness does not improve as anticipated or deviates from the team's response.

This scenario illustrates how wellness measures can be used as an effective monitoring tool. However, achieving this textbook scenario in practice is no simple feat and requires both preliminary and ongoing efforts. Initially, careful consideration must be given to selecting a measure that has acceptable validity and reliability to enable the collection of meaningful data (figure 9.9). Data quality is then dictated by athlete compliance and honesty, which is influenced by how the measure is set up, supported, and used. Each of these factors is addressed in the following sections.

Selecting a Wellness Measure

We have noted that wellness measures are both widely adopted in high-performance sport and well supported in the literature. However, we must acknowledge the divergence between research and practice when it comes to the particular measures employed. Experimental support for wellness measures is limited to established measures in the literature (153), yet practice tends to favor brief, custom measures (162). Recently, applied research using custom measures has noted similar responses to training as empirical measures (67, 163, 164), however, this is yet to be systematically evaluated. In order to avert the risk of less valid and reliable measures becoming repeatedly adopted and published (63), the following recommendations pertain to selecting an existing research-based measure.

Research-supported wellness measures assess one or more of the dimensions (overarching constructs) of mood, stress, recovery, symptoms, and emotions (table 9.4). Scales and items may relate to general wellness (e.g., I was fed up with everything (96)) or be sport specific (e.g., I felt frustrated by my sport (96)). It may be argued that sport-specific items are more applicable to, and better received by, athletes. Alternatively, the argument that the training response also manifests as general wellness signs and symptoms suggests general items or a composite measure may be more appropriate for athlete monitoring.

Measures of subjective mood disturbance, perceived stress and recovery, and symptoms of stress have additionally been shown as being responsive to acute changes in training load (153). Therefore, there is no one dimension that may be recommended as the best option for athlete monitoring. Selecting multiple dimensions allows for variable athlete responses and avoids emphasizing one aspect of the training response over others.

The assessment of symptoms provides useful clinical insight into physical (e.g., headache, sore throat, digestive complaints) or behavioral (e.g., ability to work, eating habits) manifestations of the training response. However, in practice, it may be more advantageous to monitor mood disturbance and perceived stress and recovery in order to detect maladaptation prior to the appearance of symptoms (122).

The decision of which empirical wellness measure to implement will ultimately be dictated by the intended purpose and practicalities of the sport context (154). There should be a clear intention for how the data obtained will be used (i.e., to inform practices on a daily basis and/or with a longer-term perspective of improving understanding of athletic preparation for the future). Commitment of the coaching team to the process is of utmost importance, while efforts should also be invested in developing the buy-in of athletes, support staff, and the sports organization (152).

The selected measure must also be feasible in regards to the time and effort required of athletes and practitioners, in addition to the associated financial costs. It is important for sports to consider both the initial investment needed to set up the measure and monitoring process, ongoing costs of maintaining the measure (e.g., software updates), and interpreting and applying the data (e.g., practitioner time) as described below.

Setting Up the Measure

Beyond the measure itself, the instruction given to athletes and the time and location of completion can affect the validity and reliability of responses. Athletes must understand the items and scales, however, it is

Table 9.4 Empirically Supported Wellness Measures

Measure	Primary dimension(s)	General or sport-specific	Scales (n)	Items (n)	Time frame*
Profile of Mood States (POMS)(186)	Mood	G	6	65	1 week
POMS-Short Form (POMS-SF)(192)	Mood	G	6	37	1 week
POMS-Abbreviated (POMS-A)(175)	Mood	G	7	40	1 week
POMS-Adolescents/Brunel Mood Scale (BRUMS) (193, 194)	Mood	G	6	24	1 week
Brief Assessment of Mood (BAM)(173)	Mood	G	6	6	1 week
POMS energy index(182)	Mood	G	2	15	Now
POMS training distress scale (190)	Mood	G	2	7	1 week
Multi-component Training Distress Scale (MTDS) (185)	Mood, stress, symptoms	G,S	6	22	1 day
Daily Analyses of Life Demands for Athletes (DALDA)(191)	Stress, symptoms	G,S	2	34	Now
Training Distress Scale (TDS)(174)	Symptoms	G,S	1	19	2 days
Perceived Stress Scale (PSS)(172)	Stress	G	1	14/10	1 month
Recovery-Stress Questionnaire for Athletes (RESTQ-Sport)(96, 179)	Stress, recovery	G,S	19/19/12	76/52/36	3 days/ nights
Acute Recovery and Stress Scale (ARSS)(176, 180)	Stress, recovery	S	8	32	Now
Short Recovery and Stress Scale (SRSS)(177, 180)	Stress, recovery	S	8	8	Now
Recovery-Cue (181)	Stress, recovery	G,S	7	7	1 week
Perceived Recovery Status Scale (PRS)(183)	Recovery	S	1	1	Now
Emotional Recovery Questionnaire (EmRecQ)(184)	Emotions	G	5	22	Now
Rating of Fatigue Scale (ROF)(187)	Fatigue	G	1	1	Now

*Time frame reflects response set of originally developed measure, however, this may be modified to meet requirements of context if permitted by the manual. G: general wellness; S: sport-specific wellness.

Adapted by permission from A.E. Saw, M. Kellmann, L.C. Main, and P.B. Gastin, "Athlete Self-Report Measures in Research and Practice: Considerations for the Discerning Reader and Fastidious Practitioner," *International Journal of Sports Physiology and Performance* 12 Suppl 2 (2017): S127-S135.

not necessary for this understanding to be universal among athletes. Athletes should complete the measure on their own and never discuss their responses with other athletes. As well, a standardized time and frequency for completion should be established (152), which will be related to the selected measure. However, some measures may need to be modified to suit the specific sport context.

A wellness measure can be set up as paper-based or electronic form or may be incorporated into one of the many commercial monitoring software platforms now available. Each mode has advantages and limitations, which should be weighed by the sport. Consideration should be given to the athlete completing the data, the practitioner overseeing compliance, and the individual- and group-level responses, with more in-depth insight completed as required. In

recent years, the accessibility of smartphones and the Internet has negated many of the previous limitations associated with electronic measures (152). Software applications now provide a simple and appealing solution for both athletes and practitioners.

It is important for software applications to be user friendly. Software that seems cumbersome, has glitches, or is not optimized for viewing on different devices will quickly deter use (152). As such, it is important that resources are invested in developing or purchasing a system that is simple, intuitive, and visually appealing. Ongoing investment is also necessary to ensure the software remains current and compatible with technological advances. Compatibility with other data sources, including training load, heart rate, and GPS measures (chapter 8 and above), is also desirable to facilitate integrated monitoring.

Creating a Positive Environment to Support Use

The sporting environment will either serve to support or hinder the use of a wellness measure. In order to avoid the common pitfalls of poor compliance or dishonesty, it is important to invest in creating an environment in which athletes and practitioners buy in to the process, and athletes feel comfortable to disclose poorer states of wellness (152).

Prior to implementing the measure, practitioners should establish a clear purpose for the data, specify who will have access to the data, and how the data will and will not be used (including selection) (154). This process must be communicated to the athletes and reaffirmed through ongoing transparency and feedback. In sports programs in which several practitioners are involved in athlete monitoring, it is recommended that there is one key practitioner who coordinates input to ensure a consistent message is being fed back to the coaching team and athlete (129).

Introducing a wellness measure early in an athlete's career may serve to develop the habit of completion and also allow time for appreciation of the value of the measure to develop (12). Use of coercion or punishment to enforce compliance will undermine the long-term success of the measure and should be avoided (152).

Interpreting and Acting on the Data

The interpretation of data requires the assessment of whether or not a change is meaningful. Interpretation of a meaningful change in wellness scores needs to take into account the individual's reporting habits. Some athletes habitually report within a very narrow range of values while others fluctuate considerably. Furthermore, the value an athlete considers as his normal may be the midpoint on the scale or at the lower end or upper end of the scale. To account for this, it is recommended that practitioners establish the CV for each individual from repeated measures between which no change in state is anticipated to have occurred (see previous section in this chapter). Once the individual CV is known, responses that exceed 1.5 to 2.0 times the CV may be flagged (85), however, this threshold has yet to be empirically established.

While attention typically is focused on detecting a meaningful change in an individual's data, it may be equally telling to detect a *lack* of change when one is expected. For instance, an athlete whose subjective wellness remains stable rather than improving with a decrease in training load should be flagged, compared to their peers all being flagged for improving as expected.

Flagged wellness responses simply alert the practitioner to a potential issue and provide direction for further investigation (151). The practitioner must first consider the context of the wellness response (e.g., the training phase and expected wellness response, information from other monitoring tools, and knowledge of the athlete and her current situation) (151). If justified, follow-up actions include talking to the athlete and modifying training and recovery variables as appropriate. This process is illustrated in figure 9.19, which operates simultaneously with the self-monitoring (conscious or subconscious) of the athlete.

Additional Benefits Beyond Monitoring the Training Response

When implemented effectively, wellness measures become a vehicle for improved communication between athletes and practitioners and also among practitioners. The measure provides an additional communication channel that enables athletes to disclose information they otherwise might not have. Athlete responses also serve as both a prompt and an invitation to discuss any concerns, whether it is the athlete approaching a practitioner or a practitioner approaching the athlete or other practitioners. Additionally, practitioners not working with the athlete daily can be kept informed on what the athlete is doing and how she is responding.

Strengthening relationships and collaboration among athletes and practitioners may serve to enhance the belief and confidence in a training program and that performance-related factors are accounted for and managed appropriately (72, 75, 151). Improved communication between practitioners facilitates the collaboration of different areas of expertise and perspectives to develop a more coordinated approach to athletic preparation. Furthermore, attention is directed to the importance of wellness for both performance and life. Indeed, use of a wellness measure may promote athletes to become more active and educated participants in their athletic preparation, both independently and by drawing on the support of practitioners (150). Furthermore, use of a wellness measure, independent of any practitioner involvement, is associated with improved athlete sporting self-confidence (150).

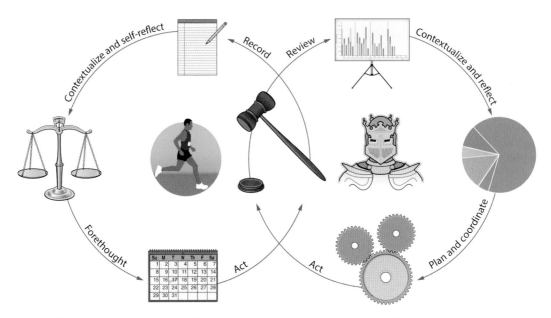

Figure 9.19 Conceptual model of the process of incorporating a wellness measure into practice for both the athlete (left) and practitioner (right).

Adapted by permission from A.E. Saw, "Self-Report Measures in Athletic Preparation." PhD dissertation in School of Exercise and Nutrition Sciences. Deakin University, 2015.

Summary of Tool 3

The relative simplicity and efficacy of wellness measures makes them a staple for every practitioner's surveillance toolkit. However, it is important for practitioners to appreciate that this efficacy depends on establishing strong foundations for data quality and continuing to invest in the process. As discussed in previous sections, incorporated wellness measures can aid in the interpretation of HR and GPS measures. Similarly, these objective measures can provide additional context to wellness measures to guide action for the coach and practitioner.

Summary

In summary, the stress of training (chapter 7), quantified as training load (chapter 8), elicits a response to training that is highly individual. As this response to training is unique across athletes, understanding it is critical when assessing fitness, fatigue, and performance potential, determining adaptation, or assessing maladaptation or overreaching and injury risk. In this chapter, we have detailed the three distinct families of key training load response variables, each related to specific aspects of training status, which may all be useful in assessing performance potential or readiness to train. The categories, alongside the tools we believe best rep-

resent them, include the internal metabolic, cardiopulmonary, and autonomic status via heart rate; the neuromuscular or external force production and locomotor efficiency via GPS and accelerometry; and finally overall health and psychology from wellness questionnaires, describing the perceived global fatigue aspect of HIIT and the training load response.

Before finishing this chapter, there's one final point we'd like to highlight for tomorrow's sport scientist. In most elite sports (see chapters 11-30), the sport science department supports the coaching staff or performance manager, but the coach or coaches dictate the training program and, in turn, often the majority of the HIIT and training load (2). Effective communication to increase coach buy-in is now one of the more important, if not the most vital, of all soft skills needed for sport scientists working in the high-performance setting (27).

Today, coaches and performance managers need to delegate time to player demands, media requests, and sponsors, which highlights the importance of time-efficient practices for preparation, debriefing sessions, and/or the training plan. That said, it is unreasonable to think that most decision makers would spend more than 3 to 5 min reading any report; they simply don't have the time. Therefore, feedback must be accurate, straight to the point, and delivered in a timely manner.

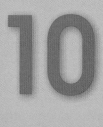

Putting It All Together

• • • • • •

Paul Laursen and Martin Buchheit

We've reached our final chapter describing the science behind high-intensity interval training (HIIT). Understanding the science is important for a practitioner because it instills us with the power to be able to manipulate the contents of training to form and fine-tune our HIIT weapons. If we have the right intelligence behind our weapons, we can operate more like Rambo, moving through the battlefield more astutely, hitting our desired physiological response targets, as opposed to having nothing but shock-and-awe-type operations in our repertoire, which leave nothing but collateral damage in their wake. Taking the targeted approach to HIIT application we have outlined provides our solutions to the programming puzzle.

In this chapter, we take the opportunity to briefly review each chapter (figure 10.1), simplify the key points, and bring them all together before delving into their specific application in the 20 most popular individual and team sports in the world that use prescribed HIIT as a key preparation tool. Here, you will read about how practitioners immersed in your favorite sport, or even those outside of your current interest perhaps, apply the science of HIIT within the confines of their specific world—elite or high-performance sport.

Chapter 1: Genesis and Evolution of High-Intensity Interval Training

In chapter 1, we started with some background in the area, describing the origin, history, and evolution of HIIT, before arriving at our current state of understanding its best practice application today. HIIT is simply defined as repeated bouts of high-intensity exercise performed above the lactate threshold (a perceived effort of hard), interspersed with either low-intensity exercise or complete rest. Ultimately, this broken exercise format of HIIT can allow either a more manageable training session with an equal training stress, or alternatively, the accumulation of a greater total volume of high-intensity exercise when the sequence is repeated. By performing a portion of our training in the HIIT format, as opposed to continuous exercise at an equivalent average work rate only, we can apply a better global training stimulus, alongside adaptations that can be made specific to a given biological system and/or sport demands.

From its beginnings in the early 1900s, long-distance runners were documented performing high-intensity repetitions on the track prior to winning Olympic medals, but as described in the

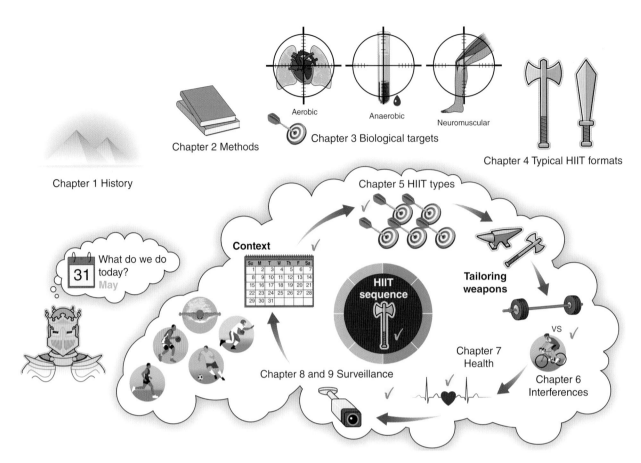

Figure 10.1 Putting it all together. A synopsis of the science and application of the high-intensity interval training journey we have taken in our book.

middle-distance running chapter by J. C. Vollmer (chapter 13), it wasn't until the 1950s when physiologists began describing the response in scientific journals. Team sports took hold of the method in the 1970s, where successful soccer coaches were witnessed using various forms of HIIT to prepare players. The computer, Internet, television, and other technological advances in media helped facilitate the global rise in sport interest over the last five decades into the multibillion-dollar industry it is today. As appropriately applied HIIT is considered a key preparatory tool in reaching individual athlete and team goals, its scientific interest has grown in parallel, where today it now ranks as the highest interest topic by leading organizations in sports science and sports medicine (15).

One of the primary aims of the book was to show the reader how HIIT can be used as a tool or weapon to solve a practitioner's programming puzzle. Indeed, by manipulating the different features of HIIT, we can create various types of weapons through their associated metabolic and neuromuscular responses,

alongside the resulting adaptations that ensue. But before we dive into the intricacies of making weapons, if we are to actually have an impact in our sport of interest, we need to be very clear about certain aspects of our sport—that is, sport context, and specifically just how appropriate, or not, it might be to launch such military weapon engagements (figure 1.4). While we are fortunate to have the research available to understand and describe our tools (5, 6), such information can be used effectively only when we clearly understand the real-world operations of our athletes inside the sport of interest (3). HIIT needs to be applied at the right place and the right time. To this effect, the primary figure used throughout the text, figure 1.5, provides a global synopsis of the situation and highlights how we must understand the individual athlete and his or her physiological profile, the phase of training the athlete is in (micro-, meso-, macrocycle), and the athlete's needs relative to the sport demands (figure 1.6), prior to selecting the appropriate HIIT session to use. Once we clearly see the features of the battlefield before us, only then can we send in our Navy Seal team to hit the precise physiological target responses needed to generate the adaptations we are after. What we are trying to get away from, and where we feel some may be doing their sport a disservice, is when we enthusiastically take the shock-and-awe approach with its associated collateral damage and uncertain outcomes for athletes. Indeed, it would be best if the term "no pain, no gain" were removed from our vernacular.

Chapter 2: Traditional Methods of HIIT Programming

We used chapter 2 to step back and understand the lay of the land, so to speak, in the world of HIIT science and application, looking at traditional methods of HIIT programming. Certainly there are many useful concepts in the area we need to appreciate, which have been developed over time from leading coaches and practitioners across the years, methods we still use today. Techniques included the rating of perceived exertion technique, the maximal aerobic speed and/or maximal aerobic power-based methods, the 30-15 intermittent fitness test (30-15 IFT), the use of proportions of the anaerobic speed reserve, all-out sprint training, the track-and-field or team sport approaches, and also heart rate- and power meter–based approaches. All approaches are considered useful in the right context; all have their pros and cons, and none are perfect. However, it is important to have different tools in the toolbox to apply what's best at the right place, at the right time. We will not elaborate further on these methods here, but please return to review chapter 2 as necessary for details related to any of these traditional methods (6).

Chapter 3: Physiological Targets of HIIT

In chapter 3, we began the process of describing how different forms of HIIT can be used to alter physiological responses. Notwithstanding the multitude of biochemical and physiological aspects that are impacted during various forms of HIIT (11), we tried to follow Einstein's advice, when he said famously, "things should be made as simple as possible, but no simpler." Here, we expanded on the detail we started in our two-part review (5, 6), by describing the key physiological aspects that are affected with HIIT. These included:

- Aerobic oxidative metabolic response targets, including cardiac output, aerobic enzymes, mitochondrial function as well as respiratory work;
- Anaerobic glycolytic metabolic response targets that may cause changes primarily in energetic flux, lactate kinetics, and glycogen depletion; and
- Neuromuscular and musculoskeletal strain targets seen through various aspects including soreness, muscle function and muscle strength or power, and changes in movement characteristics.

The manipulation of the different HIIT parameters, outlined in chapter 4, can form our HIIT target types (figure 1.5) that we can fine-tune further from knowledge gained in chapter 5.

Chapter 4: Manipulating HIIT Variables

In chapter 4, we used a strange English saying that "there's more than one way to skin a cat" when it comes to HIIT, before introducing the 12 different factors that can be manipulated to form our primary HIIT weapons. While the main factors were the intensity and duration of the work bouts, other variables included the intensity and duration of the recovery interval, the number of interval bouts or series duration, the number of interval bout series, their between-series recovery duration and intensity, the total work performed, the exercise mode and/or ground surface used for run-based HIIT, the environment (heat and altitude), and nutritional elements manipulated around the HIIT session.

The chapter highlighted that, depending on how you skin the cat, in general, there were five main classifications of HIIT weapons we can form, including:

1. Long intervals, that include repeated bouts of exercise around v/p$\dot{V}O_2$max (95%-105%) or 80% to 90% of V_{IFT}, involving durations longer than a minute, separated by short durations (1-3 min) of passive recovery, or longer durations (2-4 min) of active recovery up to 45% of V_{IFT} or 60% of $V/P_{IncTest}$.

2. Short intervals, consisting of interval bouts performed at between 90% and 105% of V_{IFT} (100%-120% $V/P_{incTest}$) for less than 60 s, and

repeated in comparable short-time-duration recovery periods that range in intensity from passive to 45% V_{IFT}/60% V/$P_{IncTest}$.

3. Repeated-sprint training (RST), which involves 3-10 s all-out efforts with variable recovery durations (majority <30-45 s) ranging from short and passive to 45% V_{IFT}/60% V/$P_{IncTest}$.

4. Sprint interval training (SIT), consisting of all-out maximal sprinting efforts, ranging from 20 to 30 s. Recovery for such intervals is passive and generally long (typically 1-4 min).

5. Last but not least, we have game-based HIIT (GBHIIT), which includes small-sided games that ultimately wind up forming game-based forms of long intervals that are sport specific. Importantly, GBHIIT involves decision-making and interactions with opponents (at least one in the case of racket sports) and teammates, which make these unique and different from typical sport-specific intervals (often in the form of HIIT with short intervals with athletes reproducing sport-specific movements). GBHIIT usually involves intervals that last 2 to 4 min at a sport-specific intensity of effort, with recovery durations of 90 s to 4 min that are typically passive.

Figure 10.2 offers a summary of the intricacies pertaining to the five key HIIT weapons and their associated targets.

Chapter 5: Using HIIT Weapons

After we established our five primary weapons from chapter 4, we shifted focus in chapter 5 and began to consider how these weapons could be manipulated to hit the primary physiological targets of importance discussed in chapter 3. Depending on how we skinned the cat, HIIT manipulations could allow us to form five different target types, depending on the degree of oxidative, glycolytic, and neuromuscular emphasis the manipulation evoked (figure 10.2). Remember here that the HIIT formats or weapons (long intervals, short intervals, RST, SIT, GBHIIT; figure 10.2) are different than the physiological targets (chapter 3) that we're aiming to hit. The HIIT target types relate to the combination of physiological responses they elicit (degree of oxidative, glycolytic, or neuromuscular response; figure 10.2). Importantly, format does not obligatorily imply target type and different weapons can be

used to hit the same, or alternate, targets. The informed decision is up to you, the four-star practitioner (figure 10.1).

To recap, we suggested that there were primarily six key targets we can aim for to enhance the related systems using our five basic weapons (figure 5.1). These were outlined for us originally in figure 1.5 and included:

- Type 1, metabolic, but eliciting essentially large requirements from the cardiopulmonary system and oxidative muscle fibers;
- Type 2, metabolic as per type 1, but with a certain degree of neuromuscular strain;
- Type 3, metabolic as per type 1, but with a large degree of anaerobic glycolytic energy contribution;
- Type 4, metabolic as per type 3, plus a certain degree of neuromuscular strain;
- Type 5, metabolic, with essentially an important anaerobic glycolytic energy contribution and a large neuromuscular strain;
- Type 6, not considered HIIT, but exercise involving a high neuromuscular strain only, referring typically to speed and strength training.

To manipulate the acute responses to HIIT in terms of cardiopulmonary, anaerobic, and neuromuscular strain, and specifically so as to reach the different targets, the following programming aspects should be considered.

Manipulate the Cardiopulmonary Responses

Most HIIT formats, if properly manipulated, can enable athletes to reach $\dot{V}O_2max$ while achieving a prolonged T at $\dot{V}O_2max$. However, RSS and SIT sessions allow limited T at $\dot{V}O_2max$ compared to HIIT sessions involving long and short intervals. The $\dot{V}O_2$ responses during RSS and SIT appear to be fitness dependent, with fitter athletes less able to reach $\dot{V}O_2max$ during such training. Overall, the following general recommendations can be made:

- To individualize exercise intensity and target specific acute physiological responses, v/p$\dot{V}O_2max$ and ASR/APR or V_{IFT} are likely the more accurate references needed to design HIIT with long (>1-2 min) and short (<45 s) intervals, respectively. For run-based HIIT sessions, compared to the ASR, V_{IFT} integrates

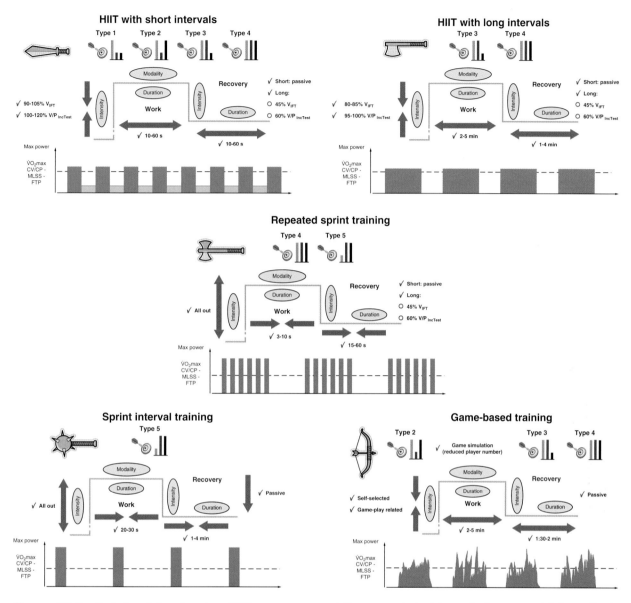

Figure 10.2 Details of the five key HIIT weapons and the associated targets they can hit from their manipulations. See text for details, and additionally chapter 4.

between-effort recovery abilities and COD capacities, which make V_{IFT} especially relevant for programming short, supramaximal intermittent runs performed with COD, as implemented in the majority of team and racket sports (see chapter 2).

- Especially in well-trained athletes who perform exercises involving large muscle groups, and assuming the accumulation of T at $\dot{V}O_2max$ may maximize the training stimulus to improve performance potential, we recommend long- and short-bout HIIT with a work:relief ratio >1.

Additionally there should be little delay between the warm-up and the start of the HIIT session so that T to $\dot{V}O_2max$ is accelerated. Warm-up intensity can be ≤60% to 70% v/p$\dot{V}O_2max$ or game-based (moderate intensity) for team and racket sport athletes. Combined data from high-level athletes suggest that long intervals and/or short intervals with a work:relief ratio >1 should enable a greater T at $\dot{V}O_2max$/exercise time ratio during HIIT sessions. Total session volume should enable athletes to spend between ≈5 min (team and racket sports) and ≈10 min (endurance sports) at $\dot{V}O_2max$.

Manipulate the Anaerobic Contribution

In practice, some HIIT formats are associated with a large anaerobic glycolytic energy contribution. It is possible to minimize the anaerobic system participation by using certain forms of HIIT, including short intervals, and possibly some types of GBHIIT. When appropriately manipulated, HIIT sessions (especially RSS or SIT) can, in contrast, be a powerful stimulus for producing high levels of blood lactate, a marker of the anaerobic glycolytic response.

Manipulate the Neuromuscular Load and Musculoskeletal Strain

In practice, while the magnitude of neuromuscular load during HIIT can be modulated through the manipulation of HIIT variables (e.g., work intensity or duration, exercise mode or pattern), the responses are highly athlete profile dependent, with endurance-type athletes showing low levels of acute fatigue and speed decrement, and team sport athletes typically showing high levels of neuromuscular fatigue following HIIT. There is likely a bell-shaped relationship between exercise intensity and acute neuromuscular performance responses, with too low ($\leq 85\%$ v$\dot{V}O_2$max) and too high (all-out) an intensity having not enough and acute detrimental effects, respectively. Practitioners can choose and balance the level of neuromuscular engagement associated with a given HIIT format, based on both the expected training-induced adaptations (either through the HIIT session itself or the associated sessions and possible additive effects) and the acute changes in neuromuscular performance. Running pattern (e.g., COD, introduction of jumps during the recovery periods), exercise mode (e.g., cycling, running, bouncing), or ground surfaces (e.g., pavement, synthetic track, grass, sand, treadmill) and terrain (uphill, downhill) also may have direct implications on traumatic and overuse injury risk, and should be chosen for programming based on a risk/benefit approach.

Chapter 6: Incorporating HIIT Into a Concurrent Training Program

In chapter 6, Jackson Fyfe took us through the topic of concurrent training, defined as the simultaneous integration of both strength and metabolic training within a periodized training regime, which represents a clear challenge for the practitioner's programming puzzle, with particular appreciation for the type 6 target and response (figure 1.5). While concurrent training has the potential to compromise aspects of strength training adaptation, current evidence suggests it does not attenuate improvements in factors such as $\dot{V}O_2$max and endurance performance, and in general appears to mostly benefit running and cycling performance. Thus, the main programming puzzle challenge for the practitioner is to manipulate HIIT variables (chapter 4 and 5) so that any interference effect to strength training adaptations is minimized, while simultaneously maximizing improvements in cardiorespiratory fitness via metabolic conditioning. When strength training is performed alone (i.e., single-mode strength training; type 6 target), performance is maximized, as residual neuromuscular fatigue should be minimal, thereby allowing for an optimal adaptation stimulus for strength, muscle hypertrophy, and power development. The practitioner should consider that a less-fatigued athlete can likely:

- lift heavier absolute loads (at a higher percentage of 1RM) for a given number of repetitions,
- perform more repetitions at a given percentage of the 1RM load, and/or
- perform repetitions at faster intended and/or actual concentric velocities (as a percentage of the maximum velocity possible with a given load).

The metabolic conditioning (i.e., endurance and HIIT sessions) component of concurrent training however, likely causes residual neuromuscular fatigue that may compromise both strength training performance and potentially the adaptive response to strength training sessions. Both of these factors may limit the stimulus for adaptation, resulting in attenuated development of classic strength training adaptations.

In the context of prescribing HIIT in concurrent training programs, particularly important considerations include the neuromuscular demands of individual HIIT sessions, and how these demands may then influence performance during subsequent strength training sessions (figure 1.5). Any HIIT session that evokes a large neuromuscular strain component (i.e., type 2, 4, 5) will likely result in more substantial residual fatigue of the exercised musculature, compared to HIIT sessions with smaller neuromuscular strain components (i.e., type 1, 3). Similarly, it is likely that strength sessions (type 6) may also compromise performance during subsequent HIIT sessions with high neuromuscular demands (i.e., type 2, 4, 5). Thus, practitioners should consider the relative priority of key HIIT or strength sessions within any given training week and manipulate the organization of these sessions to minimize the potential for negative interactions between training modes.

Here are our general recommendations for limiting interference to strength training adaptations with concurrent training.

Limit neuromuscular fatigue prior to strength training sessions by performing strength training either before, or at least (approximately) 6 h after, HIIT sessions.

HIIT sessions performed in the 24 h prior to strength training sessions ideally should be characterized by lower neuromuscular demands. This can be achieved by several tactics:

- Incorporate lower absolute/relative work intensities that are associated with lower neuromuscular load (i.e., type 1 and 3). It is however worth noting that using lower HIIT intensities may often need to be associated with longer effort durations (e.g., 3 min at 85% V_{IFT} versus 10 s/20 s at 120% V_{IFT}), and consequently these longer durations may also cause neuromuscular fatigue.

- Limit prescription of all-out HIIT modalities (i.e., RSS, SIT formats, or in general, neuromuscular-demanding HIIT formats, i.e., type 2, 4, and 5).

- Perform running-based HIIT on softer surfaces (e.g., grass or sand instead of road) likely to impart less neuromuscular strain.

- Limit the change-of-direction (COD) component (particularly sharp COD) of running-based HIIT.

- Employ cycling-based, rather than running-based, HIIT (depending on the athlete's training specificity).

Where possible, and where individual strength/power development is favored over the metabolic conditioning component, total weekly metabolic conditioning volume should be limited by:

- reducing the weekly frequency of HIIT sessions and/or performing fewer repetitions and/or series during HIIT sessions, and

- reducing training volume associated with other cardiorespiratory modalities (e.g., lowering volume of long duration aerobic conditioning sessions).

Chapter 7: HIIT and Its Influence on Stress, Fatigue, and Athlete Health

In chapter 7, Philip Maffetone showed us a new perspective on HIIT that needs to be contemplated when we're considering our athletes. Exercise is a type of stress, and HIIT can represent one of its most potent forms. In this chapter, our aim was to present more of a holistic understanding of stress before more objectively attempting to specifically quantify the stress associated with exercise training (load; chapter 8) as well as the individual response to that training load that arises in the athlete (chapter 9). Thus, chapter 7 was devoted to understanding not only the stress of HIIT but the stress of other confounding variables, including food, that can impact an athlete's physiology, attenuate or compound overall stress, and subsequently improve or derail progress.

In this regard, it was important first to define health and fitness separately. *Fitness* was defined as the quality of human performance and the physical ability to compete at one's athletic potential. *Health* was defined separately more as a state of physical, biochemical, and mental-emotional well-being in which all bodily systems (metabolic, neuromuscular, hormonal, immune, digestive, etc.) function in harmony. Stress does not necessarily need to be considered in a negative light, as it is important, creating the stimulus that enables the body to adapt to the wear and tear of lifestyle, including sport and exercise. However, whether training involves too much workout volume or intensity (load; chapter 8), inadequate nutrition, or poor sleep or recovery, excess stress can impair health and ultimately fitness. Too much stress without adequate recovery quickly manifests in a lack of health, seen as illness, injury, or both. A holistic perspective on HIIT can be appreciated when we consider it across other physiological systems that are affected by it. The hypothalamic-pituitary-adrenal (HPA) axis, which serves as a primary-link between the nervous and endocrine systems, was described as a key regulator of the stress response, and one that is important to appreciate when stress reaches chronic levels that may manifest in what is more commonly known as the overtraining syndrome.

Sleep and adequate nutrition were singled out as the critical factors of importance for eliciting repair and adaptation to stress. A person's diet is considered the sum of energy (calories) and nutrients obtained from foods and beverages consumed regularly, and requires adequate levels of macronutrients, micronutrients, and phytonutrients. A low-quality, poor diet is one that includes more processed, packaged, and preprepared foods that have lower nutrient density (such as micronutrients and fiber) versus natural, whole, unprocessed foods higher in nutrient density. In addition, processed (refined) carbohydrates, often termed junk food, including flour- and sugar-containing foods, substantially increase the glycemic index of meals and snacks, and can contribute to chronic inflammation and stress through the HPA axis. Indeed, the combination of excess training stress, including HIIT, can create a neuroendocrine imbalance, which will be manifested by the consumption of a poor diet. A diet high in sugar can promote inflammation, metabolic substrate imbalance (reduced fat oxidation), maladaptation, and contribute to physical, biochemical, and mental-emotional injuries. Athletes, coaches, and clinicians need to carefully monitor training progress with sound surveillance methods (chapters 8 and 9) and rely on healthy eating to maximize outcomes from HIIT.

Chapter 8: Quantifying Training Load

In chapter 8 we learned how to put surveillance systems over the markers that matter and monitor them. The primary variable of interest when it comes to HIIT stress and trying to quantify it is the theoretical concept of training load, where training load is defined as the product of training intensity and training volume. These training load parameters can be considered from either an external (occurring outside of the person, e.g., power output or movement) or internal (measured as something going on inside the person, e.g., heart rate during exercise) standpoint. External training load parameters are often used for programming HIIT (i.e., perform 4×3 min at 350 W cycling, 3 min rest; or 4×3 min at 3:15/km running, 2 min rest), while the internal training load refers to the internal training stress of the measured system (heart rate, lactate, etc.) generated during the exercise. Understanding both is important, as either parameter can be useful to appreciate in light of the other. However we want to skin it (using internal or external loads), we appreciate that these loads represent the likely input marker of stress on the body. This load is required both for programming as well as for understanding what has actually occurred in training (prescribed versus actual training).

Nowadays, we have a surplus of potential technology and its associated data available to consider as being useful. External training load markers should be specific to the athlete's sport and could include power meters, GPS, local positional systems, and semiautomatic video. Relevant internal training load parameters involve those that offer surveillance over the oxidative, glycolytic, and neuromuscular parameters, and might include heart rate, lactate, and rating of perceived exertion.

Finally, in the spirit of Occam's razor, where the simplest explanation tends to be the right one, it can be useful to break down training and HIIT into its relevant intensity brackets by describing training in terms of time accumulated in certain training-intensity bandwidths or zones. Thus, speed, power, and heart rate zone descriptions of athlete training have become useful methods of providing surveillance over athlete training. In the case of the field-based practitioner, the simple and most relevant markers to monitor for load surveillance include power output and/or locomotor movement (GPS), heart rate, and rating of perceived exertion. While the important glycolytic (lactate) load may be absent from our model, this measurement today is currently too impractical for most field-based scenarios, and we await with interest as to whether technology helps create this missing puzzle piece.

Chapter 9: Response to Load

In chapter 9, we explored aspects of the right side of figure 8.2, with particular attention on the output of our training system, or our *response* to training. As load versus response to load are exclusively different concepts, we need a unique set of tools and understanding. Importantly, our athlete's training load response, commonly termed training status, is not uniform across all athletes, and clearly depends on the training and individual characteristics.

We identified three key families of training load response markers that we need to monitor. First is internal metabolic, cardiopulmonary, and autonomic status with heart rate (HR) the tool chosen to infer on the status of that system. From a measure as simple as HR, we identified a large number of indices that could inform us globally concerning metabolic, cardiopulmonary, and autonomic fitness. In as little as 1 to 5 min, morning resting HR(V) can capture a snapshot of an athlete's cardiac parasympathetic activity on that day, while a period of submaximal exercise HR (last min during 4-5 min cycling or running) is additionally a useful monitoring variable. Resting HRV measures can be collected frequently to examine acute (daily recordings) and chronic (at least 3-4 d per week) responses to training and are likely sensitive to both positive and negative adaptations. Exercise HR may inform more on chronic and positive adaptations.

Next is neuromuscular status and locomotor efficiency using GPS and accelerometry. While insights into an athlete's neuromuscular status in response to training can be gained via different approaches, we focused exclusively on the methods available to practitioners in the field. The most relevant methods include regular vertical jump testing and more importantly microtechnology-derived indices relating to locomotor efficiency and stride characteristics. The use of those latter variables is still in its infancy, but there is no doubt that the development of these technologies in the future will increase our ability to collect better data at a greater frequency, allowing for an improved monitoring sensitivity.

Finally we turn to overall health, fatigue, and mood (psychology) using wellness questionnaires as a simple means of gaining insight into this important (and global) aspect. The relative simplicity of using wellness measures makes them an easy go-to tool for every practitioner's surveillance toolkit. However, it is important for practitioners to appreciate that this effectiveness depends on establishing strong foundations in data quality and continuing to invest in the process. Incorporating wellness measures can aid in the interpretation of HR and GPS measures. Likewise, these former markers give enhanced context to wellness measures to guide action for the practitioner.

Note here that we don't tend to monitor anaerobic-related responses in parallel with the lack of surveillance around this system in load monitoring (chapter 8).

In summary, we've come full circle now and our feedback loop is complete. You, the four-star coach or practitioner in the operation (figure 10.1), understand your battlefield, are aware of the athlete or team in front of you, know the sport and factors of importance, and as a result, clearly see the context by which you can now appropriately apply your HIIT. With this knowledge at the forefront, alongside the physiological responses you're after (i.e., the three main physiological targets we have been discussing throughout the book—oxidative, glycolytic, neuromuscular), it's time to start planning. You know the types of weapons you can formulate and the factors you can manipulate to fine-tune them to hit your HIIT target types. You put the plan in place, as well as appreciating concurrent training aspects if relevant. With a holistic appreciation of stress, it's time to appropriately monitor both the load and the response to load using simple surveillance techniques. This response helps you to adjust and repeat the process to continuously improve the probability of enhanced outcomes for your individual athletes or teams. In the following application chapters, written by experienced practitioners embedded in some of the world's most popular sports, we'll learn exactly how they go about doing this, and we hope you'll be able to use this information to help refine your own practice.

Application of HIIT in Sport: Thinking Outside the Box

In the forthcoming chapters, expert practitioners will begin by describing their sports and the factors involved with successful campaigns. They will tell us where and when HIIT is important and additionally where and when its relevance takes a back seat to preparation for performance. The targets of physical performance (oxidative, glycolytic, neuromuscular) will be highlighted, and in the case of team sports, how these targets are often different across the various playing positions. Then it's about taking aim at those targets. Here is where the formation and manipulation of the most relevant HIIT weapons, within the context of each sport, is described. Some practitioners even show how their HIIT programs progress and develop from a longitudinal standpoint, as well as offering strategies for structuring the HIIT program within the confines of the sport's controllable and uncontrollable factors. The load and response to load monitoring tools used within each sport are also shown. Finally, example training programs, some with very fine detail pertaining to HIIT and other aspects, are provided throughout most sport chapters. You'll discover that the depth of information gifted by each practitioner is immense, and we know of little else currently available providing as rich a content as you'll find offered by our team. While traditionally such information is considered top secret by professional teams throughout the world, this group of practitioners holds a different philosophy on the matter, are selfless, open-minded, and are driven more to share with others. These individuals think outside the box (4), and we would describe them as being archetype 3 individuals (figure 10.3).

We believe that the concept of *thinking outside the box* is extremely important both for practitioners working in applied sport and for academics in universities who are passionate about contributing to sport science. Indeed, we often witness the *sport* aspect of sport science as somewhat lost these days in some organizations. Whether you're an academic or a practitioner embedded in sport, or those who strive to do both, we believe that those who embrace the concept described herein and strive to be individuals that fall into personality archetype 3 will have the most impact in both sport science application and research. These individuals are prepared to break from the pack and do what the others are not prepared to do. It is these developed character traits associated with the archetype 3 personality that allow them to do this.

The three personality archetypes in relation to people's ability and willingness to grow, share knowl-

edge, collaborate, and adopt an open-minded attitude are highlighted in figure 10.3, and are based on the idea that people's mindset travels continually back and forth through an infinity-shaped loop, between more (left) and less (right) comfortable zones. It is where people tend to reside for most of the time that defines their profile and that will allow them to make a substantial difference (or not) (4).

Archetype 1

Archetype 1s may be considered to have a balanced profile, reflective of the mindset of most people. They spend most of their time in their comfort zone, but can, when required and/or when pushed by others, step out briefly to grow and make progress. Most won't stay long in the danger zone, however, either through laziness and/or naively believing that "it will be okay." A strong drive for improvement and/or self-confidence to make archetype 3 is missing. Their chance to have impact in both applied sport and/or research is limited.

Archetype 2

Archetype 2s are not our favorite. These individuals we come across often have been working in high-level positions for a long time, both at the academic (e.g., head of faculty or departments, journal editors)

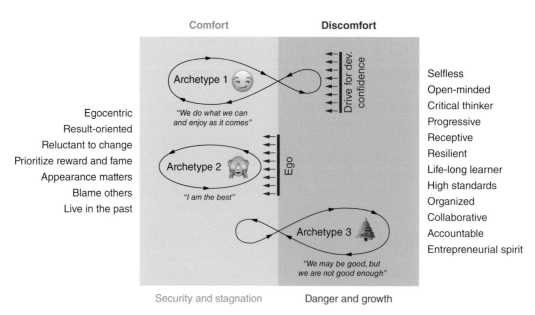

Figure 10.3 Schematic representation of the three personality archetypes. The archetypes are based on the idea that people's mindset travels continually back and forth through an infinity-shaped loop between more (left) and less (right) uncomfortable zones. Drive for dev: drive for development.

Adapted by permission from M. Buchheit, "Outside the Box," *International Journal of Sports Physiology and Performance* 12 no. 8 (2017): 1001-1002.

and practitioner (e.g., head coaches, head physios, and strength coaches) levels. They have chosen to be rather than to do, even though this has meant compromising their own integrity at certain stages of their career. Unfortunately this has little consequence for them, as long as their titles, salaries, and public roles are secured, which satisfies their egos and allows them to feel important. Centered on themselves, they tick the boxes and continue in their same looping comfort zone. They purposely avoid challenge and can't be bothered listening to others. They are more satisfied with old problems than committed to finding new solutions (12). When it comes to giving lectures, they teach what they know and not what the students need. They want their names on papers as last authors, but would be unable to collect the data or discuss the stats and study findings. Their blindness keeps them away from the recent literature and the reality of journal requirements (i.e., topics, quality, designs), which inevitably leads to inappropriate and irrelevant submissions, likely to be rejected by editors. In some extreme scenarios, people keep digging deeper against the evidence. For example, while the need to move away from the null hypothesis testing approach is in the process of being accepted (2, 14), those running in their own circle (or staying in orbit (3)) still ignore effect magnitudes (8) and choose to further decrease the P value threshold to make decisions (<0.005) (1) (see also chapter 9).

In high-performance sports, archetype 2s don't read research papers and never update their skills and methods. They avoid using new technologies and continue delivering outdated programs. They purposely don't share what they do to protect themselves. Their focus on their own personal comfort is so prevalent that it often derails the optimal training or recovery process of the athletes they oversee. "They want to wear the tracksuit but not run the laps" (7). Providing advice to help those individuals is a waste of time unfortunately, as their ego prevents them from seeing outside the box (figure 10.3). Their future depends on their political and survival strategies.

Archetype 3

Our archetype 3 individuals are featured in the subsequent chapters. These individuals have taken the ultimate progression from the archetype 1 personality toward the right side of the shape (figure 10.3). They are selfless, open-minded, curious, ambitious, and accountable for their actions and show a critical mind. They know well that getting "out of the box" is necessary to learn, grow, innovate, create, and, eventually, succeed. They have understood that life is continuously brought into question and are always willing to do better. They have embraced the uncomfortable truth that natural assets and talent can be outmatched through consistent efforts, deliberate practice (10), and in turn, the development of skills. They are open to constructive criticism (9) and listen more than they talk. They are not afraid to ask for help. They accept and acknowledge their errors to learn from them. They set very high standards for themselves, apply strict self-discipline, and tend to be life-long learners (13). They read daily, listen to podcasts from various fields, travel, seek information in different disciplines, and always say yes when it comes to sharing their experience and knowledge (chapters 11-30). They are more concerned by the process than by the results. They are interested in doing and act to keep their integrity. They treat everyone the same, regardless of their status (13).

For the future sport scientists reading this volume, both in research and as applied practitioners, we feel that getting out of the box is likely a compulsory trait needed to advance our field in the long term. Embrace the challenge, and please continue to advance our field forward!

PART II

Sport-Specific Application of High-Intensity Interval Training

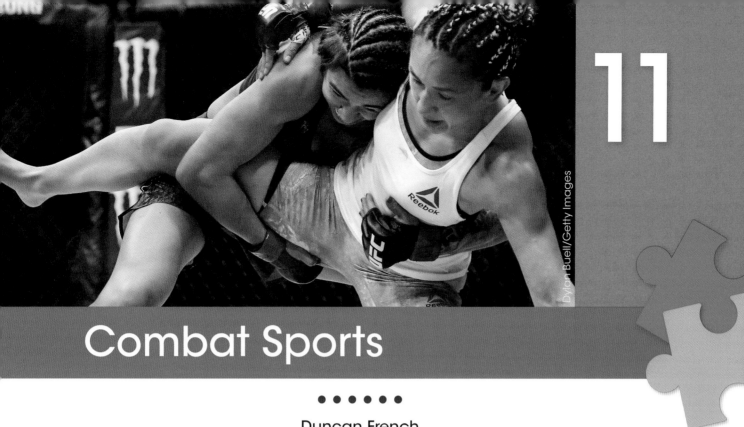

Dylan Buell/Getty Images

Combat Sports

• • • • • •

Duncan French

Performance Demands of Combat Sports

Combat sports encompass a wide variety of full-contact martial arts and fighting disciplines, many of which have indigenous regional and national forms. Depending on each discipline and the discrete rules of competition, competitors employ strikes with their fists, elbows, knees, shins, or feet (e.g., boxing, karate, taekwondo, and Muay Thai), engage in wrestling and grappling techniques (e.g., judo, sambo, freestyle or Greco-Roman wrestling, and Brazilian jiu-jitsu), or utilize a mixture of fighting styles in a hybrid fashion (e.g., mixed martial arts (MMA), wushu, and hapkido).

Sport Description and Factors of Winning

Combat sports have grown in popularity over the past decade, with MMA now recognized as the fastest growing sport in the world. The global popularity of combat sports is reflected by the Ultimate Fighting Championship (UFC) holding more than 400 events in 133 cities within 22 countries around the world. MMA now exceeds all other combat disciplines in popularity, consistently achieving more pay-per-view viewers than boxing. In 2016, UFC 202 exceeded previous records by attracting 1.65 million pay-per-view buys.

Combat sports have amateur and professional tiers of competition in which men and women compete. The majority involve one-on-one full-contact fighting, however, some combat sports such as Karate and Taekwondo have team competitions that can also be contested. Owing to the different technical, physical, and physiological characteristics found between combat disciplines, competition structures vary greatly. Bouts can comprise anywhere from 3 to 12 rounds, with individual rounds lasting between 2 to 5 min, or be contested during continuous matches ranging from 5 to 30 min. Winning is achieved by a variety of methods, including disabling an opponent at any point during the fight via knockout or submission or by rendering the opponent unable to continue; by an official's intervention to stop the fight; or by outscoring an opponent based on electronic scoring or a judge's decisions (11). The complexities of combat sports mean a fight can be over in an instant or see competitors completing the required number of rounds in their entirety.

Relative Contribution of Physical Performance

The physical demands of combat sports make them among the most complex of all sports, with athletes requiring high levels of metabolic conditioning concurrently with the ability to generate explosive knockout strength and power. While the characteristics of individual fighting disciplines vary, combat sports are collectively defined as high-intensity intermittent exercise in which force must be repeatedly exerted against an external resistance in the form of an opponent. High-force-generating qualities are required to manipulate the mass of an opponent, withstand collisions, or underpin high-velocity techniques such as strikes, throws, and takedowns (30). These actions must be expressed concurrently with levels of metabolic conditioning that meet the energetic requirements of each particular discipline. Attempts have been made to quantify workload in combat sports, but it remains difficult to clearly define the physiological requirements of competition. Instead, effort:pause ratios during each round of a fight have been used as a proxy of physiological load, with judo, wrestling, and karate reported to have typical effort:pause ratios of 2:1 (5, 43), boxing is approximately 3:1 (34), taekwondo ranges from 1:3 to 1:6 (25, 40), Brazilian jiu-jitsu matches are near to 10:1 (51), and MMA ranges from 1:2 in regional events, and up to 1:4 in the UFC (18, 41) (see figure 11.1).

Targets of Physical Performance in Combat Sports

Effort:pause characteristics can be used to define workload distribution, and from these insights appropriate training strategies can be developed. This can be particularly challenging for hybrid combat sports, however, as the large combination of techniques necessary to succeed places great demand on divergent physiology (e.g., explosive striking versus sustained grappling). Figure 11.2 shows the relative importance of the three main physical qualities of speed, strength, and endurance for elite participation in combat sports and the general relative importance of skills, tactical awareness, and physical capacities.

Combat athletes must also consider the importance of body composition and weight management, as most competitions have weight classifications in which athletes are matched by body weight. The majority of combat athletes therefore attempt to maximize lean tissue and minimize body fat, all while minimizing total body weight and maintaining optimal performance standards (53). When pooling all weight classes together, unpublished data in professional UFC

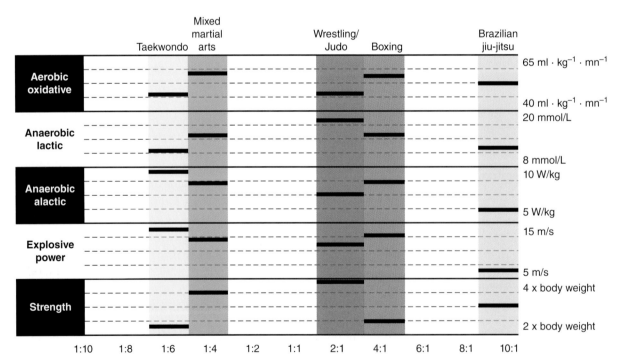

Figure 11.1 Schematic representation of the physiological attributes associated with combat sport disciplines, N.B. data not to scale.

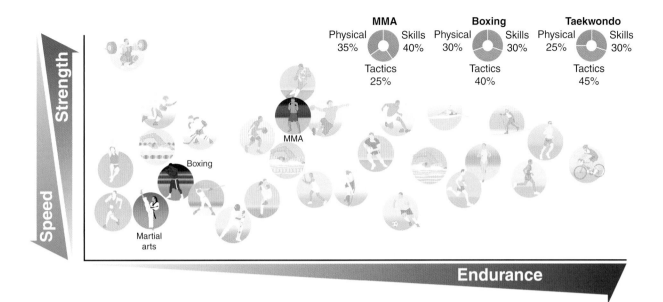

Figure 11.2 The position of the combat sport athlete on the three axes illustrates the relative importance of the three main physical qualities of speed, strength, and endurance for elite participation, acknowledging this varies between categories. Outside of critical psychological components, which are difficult to quantify, the pie charts show the general relative importance of skills, tactical awareness, and physical capacities for combat sport athlete success.

Adapted from G.A. Nader, "Concurrent Strength and Endurance Training: From Molecules to Man," *Medicine & Science in Sports & Exercise* 38, no. 11 (2006): 1965-1970.

fighters indicates athletes vary between an average of 19.1% body fat when off camp, to 17.3% early in camp, 14.0% midway through a fight camp, and are approximately 13.3% at the latter stages of a fight camp when measured by duel-energy X-ray absorptiometry. The following section describes the physiological demands of each combat sport category in greater detail.

Striking

Striking sports, such as boxing, karate, taekwondo, and Muay Thai, involve highly complex motions of the arms or legs to inflict physical damage on an opponent. Striking techniques including punches, elbows, knees, and kicks are extremely dynamic in nature and occur in a fraction of a second. Primarily a function of the high-energy phosphate system, mean impact velocities range from 8.9 to 9.14 m/s for a boxing punch (4, 39, 52) to 7.3 to 14.4 m/s for karate, taekwondo, and kung-fu kicks (19, 45). Anaerobic energy production is critical for striking disciplines, with the high-energy phosphate (i.e., ATP-PCr) and glycolytic systems providing the primary sources of energy for high-impulse movements. Peak (~9.3 W/kg) and mean (~6.7 W/kg) anaerobic power is similar among the striking sports

of boxing (14), taekwondo (7), and karate (13), but somewhat lower than standards found in wrestlers (53). Oxidative energy production is also an important consideration in striking sports (17, 48), as aerobic metabolism supports the athlete's ability to maintain repetitive high-intensity actions during a bout, accelerate the recovery processes between discrete high-intensity efforts, and fulfill chronic work rates throughout the duration of a fight. Interestingly, mean aerobic power is comparable between all striking disciplines, with the value of 44 to 65 ml·kg^{-1}·min^{-1} reported for boxers similar to that found in karate (47 to 61 ml·kg^{-1}·min^{-1}) (13) and taekwondo (44 to 63 ml·kg^{-1}·min^{-1}) fighters (7).

Wrestling

Wrestling techniques are used in judo, sambo, freestyle or Greco-Roman wrestling, wushu, and MMA. To win in wrestling you must attempt to pin your opponent by forcing both shoulder blades to touch the mat using maneuvers such as takedowns, reversals, and escapes. Like all combat sports, the physiological requirements of wrestling are challenging, as matches can last a matter of seconds or as long as 9 min, possibly stressing explosiveness of the lower body or muscular endurance of the upper body. Having greater absolute strength than an opponent, or by achieving greater relative strength based on weight class, can give wrestlers a competitive advantage in a sport in which manipulating the body weight and resistance of an opponent is critical. In comparisons of successful versus less successful wrestlers, absolute strength levels are greater in more successful athletes, particularly in the upper body (49).

Energy expenditure during a wrestling match has been estimated to be 13 to 14 kcal/min, giving wrestling one of the highest rates of expenditure among all sports (26). Anaerobic peak power and mean power (i.e., anaerobic capacity) are critical physical attributes associated with the explosive high-impulse maneuvers that lead to control of an opponent. The maintenance of anaerobic power for the duration of a bout is essential in wrestling and is likely due to an athlete's ability to utilize and replenish anaerobic glycolytic capacity and buffer metabolic acids. In junior wrestlers, anaerobic power and capacity are as much as 13% higher in elite performers compared to recreational age- and bodyweight-matched opponents (27). Elite Korean wrestlers have been shown to have venous lactate concentrations of 10 to 13 mmol/L following 5 min of wrestling competition (54), while Kraemer et al. (35) reported concentrations as high as 20 mmol/L in NCAA collegiate wrestlers. When comparing aerobic power (i.e., $\dot{V}O_{2peak}$) in wrestlers, both successful and less successful wrestlers from Olympic, collegiate, and scholastic populations have similar values of 53 to 56 ml·kg^{-1}·min^{-1} (27, 53). Owing to the complex energetic demands of wrestling, effective high-intensity interval training (HIIT) modalities are an essential way to augment both the aerobic and anaerobic systems that regulate a wrestler's ability to sustain high-intensity workloads.

Grappling

Grappling techniques can be used in judo, sambo, freestyle or Greco-Roman wrestling, Brazilian jiu-jitsu, and MMA. Instead of trying to pin an opponent, grappling uses submission holds (e.g., chokes, arm bars, and leg locks) to place opponents in positions that cause extreme pain, fear of injury, or loss of consciousness, thereby forcing them to submit out of a match. In comparison to wrestling, in some forms of grappling, lying on your back underneath your opponent can actually be advantageous, as it gives fighters the opportunity to hold their opponent with their legs and perform submission holds. A typical jiu-jitsu grappling match comprises intervals of ~170 s of activity, of which 25 ± 7 s is standing combat and 146 ± 119 s is groundwork, interspersed with 13 ± 6 s intervals of active rest (51).

Elite-level jiu-jitsu fighters have excellent levels of abdominal and upper-body strength endurance (3). These same athletes have moderate to low levels of maximal leg strength, perhaps indicative that grappling relies more on ground-based chokes and submission holds rather than the explosive throwing movements normally seen in judo and wrestling. Brazilian jiu-jitsu fighters have limited maximal isometric strength levels in comparison to judo and wrestling athletes, but they are able to maintain sustained levels of strength throughout a fight, with upper-body strength endurance a critical attribute for grappling disciplines (44). Metabolically, grappling elevates several biochemical markers relating to the high physiological stress induced by intense exercise, as well as severe microtrauma to muscle tissue (6). Aerobic power (i.e., $\dot{V}O_{2max}$) in elite Brazilian jiu-jitsu fighters is approximately 50 ml·kg^{-1}·min^{-1}, somewhat lower than the values seen in both judo athletes (12, 20) and wrestlers (26, 53). These findings most likely reflect that the metabolic cost is diminished somewhat by athletes lying semipassively on their backs for sustained periods of activity. The specific characteristics of grappling influence the need to select appropriate training modalities, with HIIT focusing less on explosive force expression and more on the need for sustained work output for longer durations.

Hybrid

Combining all combat modalities, hybrid combat sports such as MMA, wushu, and hapkido utilize a mixture of striking, wrestling, and grappling techniques. Hybrid disciplines distinguish themselves by the highly complex skillsets athletes must possess. Victory is not only influenced by a fighter's ability to land strikes (e.g., Muay Thai) but also by his proficiency in defending against or successfully achieving takedowns (e.g., wrestling) and then executing ground fighting techniques (e.g., grappling). These complex requirements place significant demand on divergent physiology, making training for hybrid sports very complex and multifactorial (figure 11.1). In professional MMA, high-intensity epochs of activity occur for approximately 8 to 10 s, interspersed with periods of lower-intensity activity (e.g., clinch work, grappling) lasting 2 to 3 times as long (41). Notably, 77% of all MMA contests are ended during high-intensity phases of activity (18). The challenging performance dynamics of hybrid combat sports lend themselves to intermittent HIIT strategies, as the need to develop the physiological attributes that support both explosive force production (i.e., striking) and prolonged work output (i.e., wrestling/grappling) can be effectively distributed throughout a training phase using this approach.

High-level MMA fighters possess greater upper- and lower-body strength levels than lower-level fighters (31). When comparing hybrid athletes from MMA with other combat disciplines, MMA fighters are most physiologically similar to judo players and least like kung fu athletes (47). Del Vecchio et al. (18) report that approximately twice as many MMA fights end during high-intensity groundwork sequences (50%) than intense striking exchanges (26.9%), further reinforcing the need for high levels of muscular strength to support grappling techniques. However, striking is an essential part of MMA, particularly when an athlete has achieved an advantageous top position (e.g., full mount). Indeed, 80.4% of fighters who record four or more significant strikes per bout while in a dominant position on the ground ultimately go on to win the fight (32). Significant ground strikes landed per minute, total strikes landed per minute, and striking accuracy all contribute to success in MMA (32).

Hybrid combat sports place demand on both anaerobic and aerobic energy pathways (figure 11.1). With greater than three-quarters (i.e., 77%) of MMA fights ending during high-intensity episodes lasting only a few seconds (18), there is a need for athletes to have a well-developed neuromuscular system that support strikes, throws, and takedowns. Anaerobic supply of ATP accounts for 90% of energy contribution for maximal efforts lasting ~10 to 15 s (21). However, repeatedly executing high-intensity episodes also challenges glycolytic capacity and the ability to tolerate extremely high metabolic acidosis. Lactate levels up to 20 mmol/L are reported following both MMA training and competition (2). Because of repeated high-intensity effort, it is likely that even greater lengths of time are spent operating near maximal aerobic power (i.e., >90% $\dot{V}O_{2peak}$). Hybrid combat sports recruit type II muscle fibers in combination with high levels of cardiac output, which is ultimately driven by increased stroke volume and associated myocardium enlarge-

ment (36). Superior aerobic power is therefore a critical physiological parameter, with MMA fighters at a regional level reported to have $\dot{V}O_{2peak}$ values of 55.5 ± 7.3 ml·kg^{-1}·min^{-1} (47) and professional fighters in the UFC as high as 62.75 ± 4.8 ml·kg^{-1}·min^{-1} (1). The variety of ways in which HIIT can be manipulated to target specific physiological (i.e., high-energy phosphates, anaerobic glycolysis, or oxidative phosphorylation) and neuromuscular systems means it represents a valuable approach to the physical preparation of hybrid fighters.

Key Weapons, Manipulations, and Surveillance Tools

The complexity of combat sport physiology means a variety of HIIT methods are required to adequately target both the metabolic and neuromuscular characteristics that determine success. This section discusses some of the HIIT approaches used in combat sports, the distribution of which is outlined in figure 11.3.

HIIT Weapons

Aerobic, anaerobic lactic, and anaerobic alactic contributions depend on the changing intensities and duration of each combat discipline. To develop the physiological attributes required for performance in combat sport, metabolic conditioning must address

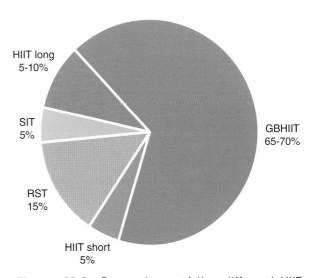

Figure 11.3 Percentage of the different HIIT weapons (formats) used throughout the annual season in combat sports. HIIT: high-intensity interval training; RST: repeated-sprint training; SIT: sprint interval training; GBHIIT: game-based HIIT in the form of fight-based HIIT (FBHIIT).

the five key bioenergetic and neuromuscular load targets (figure 1.5):

1. Aerobic oxidative (HIIT type 1)
2. Aerobic oxidative + neuromuscular (HIIT type 2)
3. Aerobic oxidative + anaerobic glycolytic (HIIT type 3)
4. Aerobic oxidative + anaerobic glycolytic + neuromuscular (HIIT type 4)
5. Anaerobic glycolytic + neuromuscular (HIIT type 5)

The most effective training programs coordinate all aspects of fight preparation and skill training with supplementary strength and conditioning activities (type 6 response; chapter 6). The distribution of each load target (i.e., HIIT types 1 to 5) within a training plan is critical to achieving the desired adaptations, with combat sports placing great demand on all respective metabolic and neuromuscular systems. It is important to realize that HIIT induces distinct effects on all systems of the body, and therefore the way HIIT is distributed between training phases is fundamental in determining the adaptations that can be achieved.

Manipulations of Interval Training Variables

Manipulating HIIT variables must first be observed at the most fundamental level of training variation (i.e., periodization). Based on the specific combat discipline and the level of participants, athletes will either have a defined competition structure (e.g., scheduled open tournaments, national or world championships, Olympics; see figure 11.4) or be randomly assigned to fight bouts (e.g., contractually signed to professional fight cards) throughout the year. Generally, fighters can be considered either in out-of-competition or off-camp (≥8 to 12 wk from their next bout) phase or in a fight preparation phase or fight camp (normally ≤8 to 6 wk prior to the next fight or tournament). In simple terms, the primary goal of out-of-competition conditioning is to augment *maximal energy production* capabilities (i.e., metabolic power), while fight camps should focus on developing the *efficiency to utilize energy* (i.e., metabolic efficiency) (33).

HIIT With Long Intervals

Organized into multiple rounds with intermittent rest periods, many combat sports are ideally suited to long training intervals. Long-interval HIIT develops both aerobic and anaerobic energy pathways (9, 10) and impacts bioenergetic target types 3 and 4. In combat sports, long intervals are typically performed between 90 s to 5 min at 80 to 95% HR_{peak}, and are often used to replicate specific competition structures (e.g., 2 min rounds for taekwondo, 3 min rounds for boxing, 5 min rounds in MMA). Heart rate zones used in conjunction with ratings of perceived exertion (RPE) are a valuable tool to gain insight to training intensity for combat sports, as reference speeds like maximal aerobic speed (MAS) for running is rarely used. As most combat training strategies do not involve running, they therefore must be interpreted with caution, as certain modalities may challenge physiological responses in different ways (e.g., the effort required to achieve 80% to 95% HR_{peak} via grappling versus striking bags). Some combat categories (e.g., wrestling, grappling) do, however, adopt extremely long work intervals of up to 15 min continuous activity during out-of-competition training phases to overload both muscular strength and endurance. Long-interval strategies are easily applied to a variety of sport-specific drills, as well as more generic strength and conditioning activities such as metabolic circuits and machine-based intervals (see table 11.1).

The crossover between anaerobic and oxidative pathways occurs at ~2 min of the first interval, meaning that during 2 min intervals approximately 50% of the total ATP during the first interval may be derived from anaerobic pathways and 50% from aerobic pathways (figure 11.5). Over a 4 min effort, approximately 60% would be derived aerobically and 40% anaerobically; in 6 mins, 75% would be aerobic and 25% anaerobic, and so on (38). Metabolic limitations to long-interval HIIT are therefore mechanisms that limit anaerobic power (e.g., glycolytic enzyme kinetics) and capacity (e.g., H^+ tolerance and buffering capacity), as well as those that limit maximal aerobic power (e.g., oxidative enzyme kinetics, stroke volume, myocardial enlargement; chapter 3). Using long-interval HIIT to develop anaerobic capacity as well as the oxidative system not only improves energy supply but also aids in processing the removal of metabolic by-products and the replenishment of muscle glycolytic capacity. Without a well-developed aerobic system, a fighter's anaerobic capabilities are essentially limited, as it will ultimately take longer before he or she is able to produce alactic and lactic energy again to enable the critical combat

Olympic Games Plan

Year	Month	Week commencing	Weeks to major	Phase	Period	Competitions	Other events and info
2011	June	5/30/2011	63	Out-of-competition	R1 – General		Austrian Open
		6/6/2011	62				
		6/13/2011	61				
		6/20/2011	60				
		6/27/2011	59				
	July	7/4/2011	58		Specific	Korean Open	
		7/11/2011	57				
		7/18/2011	56				
		7/25/2011	55				
	August	8/1/2011	54	Fight camp	R1 Specific		
		8/8/2011	53				
		8/15/2011	52				
		8/22/2011	51				
		8/29/2011	50				
	September	9/5/2011	49		R2 Competition		Russian Open
		9/12/2011	48				Polish Open
		9/19/2011	47				Israel Open
		9/26/2011	46			British Open	
	October	10/3/2011	45		R2 Specific		
		10/10/2011	44				
		10/17/2011	43				Serbian Open
		10/24/2011	42				
		10/31/2011	41				Croatian Open
	November	11/7/2011	40	Fight camp	Competition		
		11/14/2011	39				
		11/21/2011	38				
		11/28/2011	37			French Open	
	December	12/5/2011	36	Out-of-competition	R3		
		12/12/2011	35				
		12/19/2011	34				
		12/26/2011	33				
2012	January	1/2/2012	32		General		
		1/9/2012	31				
		1/16/2012	30				
		1/23/2012	29				
		1/30/2012	28				Swedish Open
	February	2/6/2012	27		R4		
		2/13/2012	26	Fight camp	Specific		
		2/20/2012	25				
		2/27/2012	24		Competition	German Open	
	March	3/5/2012	23				
		3/12/2012	22		R5	Dutch Open	
		3/19/2012	21				
		3/26/2012	20	Fight camp	Specific		Belgian Open
	April	4/2/2012	19			Junior Worlds	Spanish Open
		4/9/2012	18				
		4/16/2012	17		Competition		
		4/23/2012	16				
		4/30/2012	15			European Champs	
	May	5/7/2012	14		R6		
		5/14/2012	13	O-of-c	General		
		5/21/2012	12				
		5/28/2012	11				
	June	6/4/2012	10				
		6/11/2012	9		Specific		Overseas training camp
		6/18/2012	8				
		6/25/2012	7	Fight camp			Preparation camp
	July	7/2/2012	6		Competition		
		7/9/2012	5				
		7/16/2012	4				
		7/23/2012	3				
		7/30/2012	2				
	August	8/6/2012	1		R7	Olympic Games	
		8/13/2012	44				
		8/20/2012	43				
		8/27/2012	42				

Figure 11.4 Sample combat sport (taekwondo) macrocycle for Olympic Games preparation. The distribution of phases (i.e., out of competition and fight camp) throughout the year is based on a set competition schedule. Phases are further divided into general, specific, and competition periods to further define the focus of preparatory activities throughout the year and peak performance standards for competition. Note, competitions are identified as primary (black) or secondary (white) based on the amount of ranking points available, with the major focus of the year (i.e., Olympic Games) shown in gold.

Table 11.1 Combat Sport-Specific High-Intensity Interval Training (HIIT) Workouts With Long Intervals

These long-interval (approximately 90 s to 5 min at 80% to 100% HR_{peak}) HIIT workouts focus on the development of physiological attributes associated with bioenergetic target types 3 and 4.

	Striking (boxing)	Wrestling (freestyle)	Grappling (BJJ)	Hybrid (MMA)
Target	↑ oxidative capabilities of ST and FT fibers	↑ cardiac output, ↑ mitochondrial proliferation, and ↑ oxygen utilization	↑ maximum rate of oxygen delivery and the ability of FT fibers to utilize oxidative metabolism	↑ maximum rate of oxygen delivery and oxidative capabilities of ST and FT fibers
HIIT type	4	3	3	4
Modality	Boxing the heavy bag	Shadow wrestling	Technical drilling	Metabolic circuit (auxiliary strength and conditioning)
Format	Simulated boxing rounds using various punching techniques to hit the heavy bag	Shadow wrestle by moving in all directions, intermittently simulating double-leg or high crotch takedowns or sprawl defense. Focus on stance and movement.	Semicompetitive drilling with sustained defensive pressure from partner.	Circuit of five auxiliary exercises that challenge force expression and max work rates (e.g., VersaClimber, battle ropes, Airdyne, strongman variants, throws)
Intensity	Moderately high (80% to 90% HR_{max})	Moderate (70% to 85% HR_{max})	Moderately high (80% to 95% HR_{max})	High (85% to 100% HR_{max})
Volume	12 × 3 min	10 × 2 min	3 × 8 min	2 × (3 × 5 min), 3 min between sets
Work:Rest	3:1	3:1	2:1	5:1

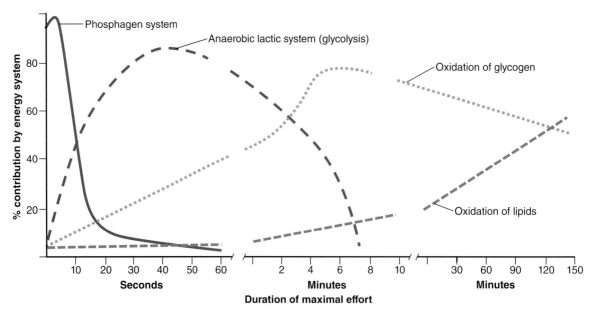

Figure 11.5 Relative contribution of the four energy-delivery systems according to the duration of the event or working interval (time of maximal effort).

maneuvers (33). Long-interval HIIT is primarily used to develop oxidative power during out-of-competition training and during the early stages of a fight camp where *metabolic efficiency* is the priority.

HIIT With Short Intervals

Short intervals in combat sport training are primarily used to develop the high-energy phosphate (i.e., alactic) and lactic systems, which impact bioenergetic target types 2, 3, and 4. In combat sports, short-interval HIIT ranges from repeated single near-maximal-intensity efforts (i.e., type 2) that stress alactic neuromuscular power (e.g., kickboxing strikes or medicine ball throws) to intervals of 10 sec-on/10 sec-off up to 40 sec-on/180 sec-off (i.e., types 3 and 4), which develop lactic power (e.g., takedown drills or clinch defense). High-energy phosphates are critical to the high-impulse movements required in combat sport. Short intervals increase enzymatic activities that facilitate alactic energy production as well as increase the stores of readily available phosphocreatine within the working muscles (38). Primarily used during fight camps, short intervals

develop metabolic efficiency to support the high-velocity movements essential to striking and takedown maneuvers.

The maximal rate of lactic ATP production can also be increased by short-interval HIIT. Lactic power intervals and explosive repeats can be performed with fight-specific drills (e.g., takedowns, throws, striking, and passing) or generic cardio exercises (33), and are often performed out of competition to augment maximal anaerobic lactic power. As with any training method focusing on increasing power, short-interval HIIT should be performed at ≥ 100% intensity with very high work rates. The majority of combat sports adopt 10 to 40 s bursts of maximal intensity effort, including wrestling takedowns, combination punches, or repeatedly kicking bags (see table 11.2). These drills place great demand on fast-twitch power output during sustained high-velocity movements, and therefore promote energy production via alactic and lactate metabolism (i.e., lactate power). They do, however, induce high levels of metabolic fatigue, and for this reason should be prioritized away from competition.

Table 11.2 Combat Sport-Specific High-Intensity Interval Training (HIIT) Workouts With Short Intervals

These short-interval (approximately 10 to 60 s at 90 to 100% HR_{peak}) HIIT workouts focus on the development of physiological attributes associated with bioenergetic target types 1, 2, 3, and 4.

	Striking (taekwondo)	Wrestling (judo)	Grappling (BJJ)	Hybrid (MMA)
Target	↑ alactic energy production and power output of FT fibers ↑ enzymatic activity and stores of readily available PCr	↑ alactic power ↑ neuromuscular strength and power characteristics	↑ alactic power and power output of FT and ST fibers ↑ oxidative process of recovery	↑ alactic power output of FT fibers ↑ enzymatic activity and stores of readily available PCr
HIIT type	3	2	1	4
Modality	Leg kick combinations against partner's body armor, heavy bag, or double kick pads	Repeat hip throws (O-Goshi technique)	Technical drilling of transitions	Striking to takedown transition drills
Format	Fighters throw high velocity leg kick combinations for a set high-intensity interval, focusing on executing the maximal number of repetitions in the set time.	Athletes complete the maximal amount of hip throws against partners offering passive resistance in the set time	Simulated technique transitions from top position to submission hold (full speed) with semipassive resistance	Work with partner striking Muay-Thai kick/knee combinations then immediately transitioning into takedowns to a dominant top position
Intensity	Near maximal (85% to 100% HR_{max})	Near maximal (85% to 100% HR_{max})	Near maximal (85% to 100% HR_{max})	Near maximal (85% to 100% HR_{max})
Volume	4 × (4 × 15 s), 45 s rest between sets	8 × 30 s	2 × (8 × 20 s), 30 s rest between sets	3 × (30 s striking + ≤ 30 s to achieve takedown × 5), 90 s rest between sets
Work:Rest	1:3	1:4	1:3	1:3

Repeated-Sprint Training

Maximal effort repeat-sprint intervals provide the most effective stimulus to upregulate glycolytic enzymes and increase anaerobic lactic capacity (38). Repeat-sprint training is a valuable HIIT weapon for combat sports and primarily used to hit target type 4. It is widely accepted that repeat sprints promote the ability to tolerate high levels of metabolic acidosis (i.e., H$^+$). A variety of methods from sport-specific bag or pad work, wrestling takedowns, or grappling transitions can be used, to more generic sprint intervals on a track or nonmotorized treadmill (e.g., 12 × ≥ 30 sec-on/30 sec-off). It is important to note that primary adaptations occur in the muscles that actually perform the work, so when planning the use of repeat sprints exercise selection should be taken into consideration.

Anaerobic lactic capacity is essential for fighting styles that require repetitive high-power output for short to moderate durations (e.g., boxing, wrestling). As such, repeat-sprint HIIT is an important strategy for combat sports with repeated explosive epochs of activity or a high effort:pause ratio. Common work intervals include 15 to 40 s of maximal intensity exercise, with no more than 10 to 30 s of rest. Negative work:rest ratios of 20 sec-on/10 sec-off, as popularized by Tabata et al. (50), are also popular among combat athletes. The ability to maintain repetitive explosive efforts under fatigue is a key factor in the later rounds of combat bouts, along with recoverability between rounds. For these reasons repeat-sprint HIIT is used to increase lactic ATP production (i.e., lactate power) and promote better buffering mechanisms to improve *lactic tolerance*.

Sprint Interval Training

Sprint intervals are associated with energy contributions via alactic metabolism (target 5) with large amounts of neuromuscular fatigue (e.g., maximal intensity striking combinations or bike sprints). All combat disciplines require explosive anaerobic power to be expressed at critical points during a fight, be it to throw punches and kicks, go for a takedown, improve a ground position, or finish a fight with a submission. Alactic power can improve up to 30% by increasing the enzymes of alactic energy production, elevating phosphocreatine storage capacity, and increasing the strength of fast-twitch muscle fibers (33, 38). Surprisingly, using sprint intervals to train the alactic system to produce ATP at

extremely fast rates is also closely associated with oxidative metabolism as aerobic pathways support the replenishment of phosphocreatine reserves (e.g., 4 × 3 × ≤ 30 sec-on with 60 to 90 s rest between repetitions and ~180 s rest between sets). Sprint intervals elevate the magnitude of anaerobic power and are therefore commonly performed out of competition when athletes can be exposed to high levels of neuromuscular fatigue. This modality of HIIT can also be used sparingly in the later stages of fight camps as a mechanism to stimulate higher-order motor units, but it is important that volume load is reduced significantly.

Fight-Based Training

Fight-based HIIT drills, combat sport's version of GBHIIT, are a well-established approach to metabolic conditioning in all combat sports, with simulated rounds, technique drills, or situational fighting used to develop both aerobic and anaerobic metabolism (see table 11.3). Fight-based training adds an additional layer of complexity to the physical demands of long-interval HIIT, in that situational and scenario-based fighting drills concurrently challenge decision-making, the need to reactively execute a variety of offensive and/or defensive techniques, as well as the potential to change intensity level during any given repetition (i.e., moving from controlled clinch work to rapid flurries of striking). Fight-based training is largely specific to each respective combat discipline, as it often involves the technical skills discrete to that sport. For example, MMA fighters often train against multiple sparing partners and rotate 1 min epochs of takedown defense, grappling techniques, and striking for 5 min rounds (i.e., shark tank drill). Fight-based training strategies can be used to isolate specific techniques and see athletes placed under duress for the duration of an interval. A good example of this can be found in judo and wrestling, where specific throwing techniques (e.g., leg sweeps, hip throws) are executed repeatedly at high speed, with athletes looking to perform the maximal number of throws possible in a given time period. An important consideration when adopting fight-specific HIIT is that mechanical and metabolic fatigue impacts the quality of fighting techniques, and executing technical skills while fatigued can have detrimental effects on skill development. Consequently, when considering fight-based training methods, athletes should consider the effect that HIIT will have on technical as well as physiological responses.

Table 11.3   Fight-Based High-Intensity Interval Training (HIIT) Workouts Using Fight-Specific Training Methods

These short-interval HIIT workouts focus on the development of physiological attributes associated with target types 1, 2, 3, and 4.

	Striking (Muay-Thai)	Wrestling (wrestling)	Grappling (BJJ)	Hybrid (MMA)
Target	↑ alactic energy production and power output of FT fibers ↑ peak blood lactate accumulation ↑ oxidative process of recovery	↑ oxidative capabilities of ST and FT fibers ↑ cardiac output, ↑ mitochondrial proliferation, and ↑ oxygen utilization	↑ oxidative capabilities of ST and FT fibers ↑ alactic power and power output of FT and ST fibers ↑ lactic ATP energy production	↑ peak blood lactate accumulation ↑ lactic power and capacity, and ↑ maximal rate of ATP production ↑ oxidative process of recovery
HIIT type	4	1	2	3
Modality	Counter sparring drill	Endurance work	Fight gone bad drill	Shark tank conditioning drill
Format	Fighter is positioned on the ropes or in a corner. Working with a partner, the fighter must throw counter combinations against pressure.	Working with a partner, fighter drills technical work in a continuous semisparring fashion for extended work periods.	Fighter deliberately starts the drill in a compromised tactical position, then works to escape from poor defensive positions. Reset start position following each escape	One fighter competes against five other fighters, rotating between 1 min of boxing, bottom-position BJJ, Muay-Thai, takedown defense, and clinch work for the period of a 5 min interval
Intensity	High (80% to 90% HR_{max})	Moderately high (80% to 95% HR_{max})	Moderately high (80% to 95% HR_{max})	Near maximal (90% to 100% HR_{max})
Volume	4 to 8 × (3 × 60 s), 30 s recovery between sets	15 to 30 min	5 to 10 min	3 to 5 × 5 min (1 min epochs of different MMA techniques)
Work:Rest	3:1 to 1.5	Continuous work	Continuous work	5:1

Metabolic Responses to Changes in Ring Dimensions   Competition areas in combat sports vary, and can range between 5.5 m (18 ft) boxing rings to 9.1 m (30 ft) octagons. Whereas the shape and dimension of the competitive areas differ, there is little evidence to suggest metabolic demands are impacted significantly based on the size of the competition area. Indeed, it is not uncommon for boxing rings, wrestling mats, and MMA octagons to be found in a host of different regulation dimensions for competition. However, as combat sports are largely contested between two athletes in close proximity, there is little requirement to move over significantly large distances. Consequently, unlike expansive court- and field-based sports such as handball and soccer, where changing the pitch dimensions can drastically affect the physiological demand, such responses are equivocal in combat sports. Interestingly, finishing rates are found to differ in MMA based on octagon dimensions, with a 48% finishing rate in 9.1 m (30 ft) octagons and 60% in 7.6 m (25 ft) octagons. However, there is little supporting evidence to indicate that these differences are consequent to altered metabolic demand.

Locomotor Responses to Changes in Ring Dimensions   Locomotor responses to changes in ring dimension are observed. In particular, the shape of the competition area, be it a circle, square, or octagon, can ultimately impact fight tactics, which in turn influences locomotion. For example, octagons and circles don't have corners, whereas boxing rings do. From a tactical perspective, boxers and Muay Thai fighters can use specific movement patterns to trap an opponent in a corner in order to gain a more dominant attacking position. In an octagon there is greater opportunity to circle and move around the competition area without becoming trapped. Changes in movement patterns then support these tactical considerations be it more sideways movement or aggressive forward pressure, etc. Furthermore, an important consideration in most hybrid sports is that locomotor patterns are constantly changing as athletes transition between different fighting styles. The energetic requirements of boxing and striking movements, clinch work in wrestling, or the various postures achieved during ground fighting all present different energetic demands. Boxing and striking largely hit type 2 targets; wrestling challenges targets types 3, 4, and 5; while grappling targets HIIT types 1 and 3.

Longitudinal Training Effects of HIIT

While cross-sectional data detailing the performance standards of various combat sports, includ-

ing karate, taekwondo, boxing, and MMA, has been presented (7, 12-14, 31), understanding of the longitudinal effects of HIIT in combat disciplines is very limited. Indeed, there is no published data detailing the influence of specific HIIT interventions in combat sports. This is largely due to the fact that HIIT is rarely employed in isolation in combat sports but instead is combined with traditional fight-training modalities (e.g., sparring). Furthermore, combat sports differ greatly from field and invasion games, where HIIT modalities have traditionally been utilized. This makes it hard to fully determine the impact of HIIT on overall fighting performance, as it can be unclear as to which stimuli is causing any training adaptations (i.e., HIIT or fight training). Figure 11.6 indicates longitudinal changes in metabolic performance of world-level Olympic taekwondo fighters.

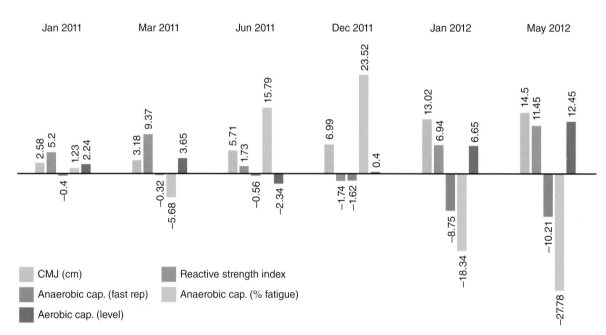

Figure 11.6 Percent change in performance standards for selected physiological measures in elite international taekwondo players preparing for the 2012 Olympic Games. These data are consequent to the distribution of HIIT represented in figure 11.3. Note, the London Olympic Games were in August 2012. Countermovement jump (CMJ) height (cm) was used as an assessment of lower-body power, while reactive strength index was measured as a proxy of explosive strength (calculated as flight time [ms]/ contact time [ms] during a 40 cm drop jump). A 300 m shuttle test (12 × 25 m) was performed twice with a 3 min rest between efforts and used to estimate anaerobic capacity. During the 300 m shuttle, the fastest repetition was measured and the percent of fatigue between the fastest and slowest repetitions was determined. Aerobic capacity was monitored using the YoYo Endurance test (level 2).

Load Surveillance and Monitoring Tools

The relationship between *intrinsic* physiological stress and the *extrinsic* time-motion characteristics (see chapter 8) is a representation of *training load.* Presently there is a dearth of information reporting chronic training load characteristics in combat sports, and load surveillance is a relatively new concept to the fight community. As described in chapter 8, calculating session-RPE (rating of perceived exertion [RPE] × session duration) is a cost-effective way to monitor intrinsic training load (15). Importantly, session-RPE can be aggregated from multiple training modalities, be they combat-specific drills or strength and conditioning activities, to give a holistic overview of total load (see figure 11.7). This can be particularly valuable when monitoring the collective contributions of training techniques in hybrid sports. Elsewhere, heart rate monitoring represents a common method to quantify internal load. By reporting heart rate variables (e.g., max or mean beats/min) against training duration, it is possible to establish a training impulse (TRIMP) as a proxy of training load (24).

Current advances in technology (e.g., GPS) have revolutionized extrinsic load monitoring in sports such as soccer, rugby, and Australian rules football. Interestingly, the use of wearables, inertial sensors, and tracking technologies remains in its infancy in combat sport. Stand-up fight disciplines such as boxing, karate, and taekwondo lend themselves to potentially using wearable technologies to provide crude biomechanical assessment of strike count, velocities, and power. Indeed, monitoring like this can give awareness of how training stimuli impact performance standards. However, for ground-fighting disciplines (e.g., judo, wrestling, jiu-jitsu, MMA) the monitoring of extrinsic load using inertial sensors placed on the body remains a challenge. This is largely due to the fact that reliability can be affected by opponents pulling on monitors, the sensors becoming dislodged during grappling and wrestling, or the potential for injury if athletes land on a sensor during a throw or takedown.

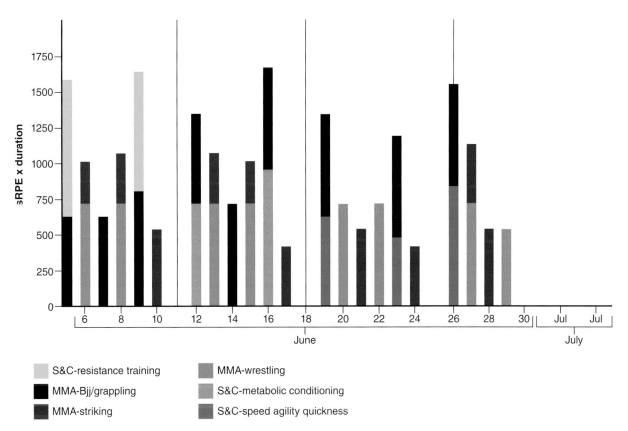

Figure 11.7 One-month training load surveillance in a professional MMA athlete using session-RPE (sRPE). Note, sRPE can be used to aggregate different types of training sessions on a single day, in order to give a holistic overview of total training load exposure.

Training Status Surveillance and Monitoring Tools

Tools to monitor training status in combat sports are often limited to noninvasive cost-effective solutions. For example, wellness monitoring using simple questionnaires, such as those described in chapter 9, gives valuable insight into an athlete's perception of health, well-being, and his ability to tolerate the training load (46). Wherever possible, wellness monitoring should be associated with an objective assessment of readiness to train (RtT). The concept of RtT is adopted by performance specialists as a reflection of intrinsic physiological status. For example, monitoring heart rate variability (HRV; see chapter 9) using technologies such as Omegawave and Morpheus provides insight into sympathetic and parasympathetic activity, with the understanding that training overload can suppress aspects of neurological activity (chapter 7). HRV has been shown to be an effective tool to detect physiological sensitivity to training stimuli and to understand if athletes are able to accommodate a specific training load or if there is suppression of physiological systems (8, 37). Other methods used as a proxy of RtT can include simple jump testing diagnostics (e.g., countermovement and/or drop jumping). High-impulse activities like jumping require rapid neuromuscular drive, and changes in peak jump height or a reactive strength index (RSI; [flight time/contact time] during a drop jump) can be indicative of suppressed neuromuscular capabilities consequent to heavy training (16, 22). Some combat sports also have punch meters that can be used as a crude assessment of training status. Monitoring sport-specific parameters such as striking force, power, and/or velocity can give valuable insights as to how performance standards are impacted by longitudinal training strategies.

Efforts to undertake longitudinal surveillance of training load are important, as understanding acute:chronic workload variation over time can be useful (28). Acute workload is defined as the absolute workload performed in 1 wk, whereas chronic workload is the 4 wk average or exponentially weighted moving average. Murray et al. (42) have indicated that accentuated spikes in acute:chronic load should be avoided, as they are associated with heightened injury incidence. Longitudinal monitoring of the acute:chronic ratio, in association with session-RPE and other intrinsic and extrinsic monitoring tools, provides invaluable surveillance insights that can be used to regulate HIIT prescription.

Strategies for Structuring the Training Program Using HIIT

Optimal physiological adaptations do not just come from the use of effective training methods but more importantly the application of the right methods at the right time and in the right way (33). Organizing the distribution of HIIT effectively between out-of-competition and fight camp training is important. Indeed, the correct sequencing of HIIT stimuli throughout the competition year is critical in order to ensure optimal development of both metabolic and neuromuscular systems. Furthermore, consideration must be given to the residual effects of training, be they acute, accumulated, or delayed (33), as poorly managed fatigue and excessive overload can present diminishing returns in response to poorly managed training.

Controllable and Uncontrollable Factors

The greatest challenge to the use of HIIT in combat sports is often the need to navigate around injuries and biomechanical accommodations (e.g., limited shoulder range of motion) that impact an athlete's capacity to execute drills in a desired fashion. Owing to the daily rigors of fight preparation, combat athletes are susceptible to injuries that require either minor adjustments in exercise selection and duration or whole-scale changes due to more severe contraindications (e.g., concussion). In addition to unforeseen injury, without a clearly defined competition structure, as found in some combat sports, it can be challenging to gain awareness for longitudinal periodization of training. Indeed, for many professional combat athletes who rarely have set annual structures but negotiate their addition to fight cards in a random fashion, it can be challenging to consistently plan the distribution of HIIT training blocks throughout the year.

Program Structure and Progression

For periodization purposes, combat athletes can be considered either out of competition or in fight camp. In those sports with set competition schedules, out-of-competition training can potentially be further periodized into a *general preparation* or *accumulation* phase, during which general fitness and strength are built, and a *specific preparation* or *transmutation* phase, in which general abilities are transferred to

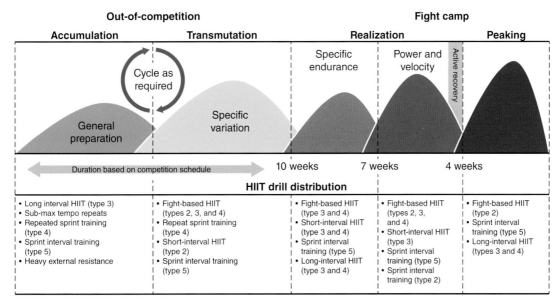

Figure 11.8 An example of the correct sequencing of training blocks and associated distribution of high-intensity training stimuli during out-of-competition and fight camp training phases for combat sport athletes.

special abilities (29). Fight camps represent the *peaking* or *realization* phase when athletes become acutely prepared for competition (see figure 11.8). Sadly, for the majority of combat athletes, the fight camp mesocycle is traditionally the only phase given specific attention regarding clear structure and progression, as athletes focus on an 8 to 12 wk process of reducing body weight for the official weigh-in and optimizing performance for the fight or tournament. However, performance standards within a fight are limited by the training athletes complete between fights, not just the training done in the weeks leading up to it. Working around the limitations of knowing a competition structure or not, a comprehensive training plan for combat sports needs to include out-of-competition phases that systematically improve the level of physical preparedness throughout the year. Distribution of training stimuli should be managed annually rather than just within an 8 to 12 wk fight camp, thereby giving adequate time for specific systemic adaptations to occur. This reduces the desire to use fight camps as the *only* phase to address all aspects of conditioning. Indeed, by utilizing longitudinal periodization and the concept of *phase potentiation* (23), combat athletes can elevate their performance standards beyond those achieved during 8 to 12 wk fight camps alone.

Out-of-competition phases (off-camp) should cycle between *accumulation* and *transmutation*, during which fighters need to prioritize the progression of structural and functional adaptations that enhance aerobic, lactic, and alactic metabolic power. These complex physiological adaptions (e.g., mitochondrial biogenesis, H^+ buffering capacity, oxidative enzyme kinetics, myocardial enlargement) are the foundations on which fight-specific fitness is optimized, and in many cases the realization of these adaptations requires months to become apparent. Philosophically, out-of-competition training is about "putting money in the physiological bank" so that the value of these savings can be returned during fight camp.

When an athlete finally enters a fight camp phase, the focus is *realization* of metabolic efficiency specific to the characteristics of the fight (figure 11.8). This differs relative to each combat discipline (i.e., effort:pause ratio), and for hybrid sports such as MMA it can also be affected by the style of opponent (e.g., "predominantly a striker," "strong ground game") or the way an athlete feels he can dominate a fight. Fight camps themselves should cycle training blocks that emphasize the progression of physiological characteristics such as local neuromuscular endurance, cardiovascular capacity, and high-intensity speed (33), so that at the end of the 8 to 12 wk camp athletes can express very high-intensity epochs of neuromuscular power with the metabolic capacity to replicate these efforts continuously over time.

Incorporation of HIIT

In a combat athlete's out-of-competition training, accumulation and transmutation phases should be cycled for 3 to 8 wk. A week of de-loading would preferably separate the phases, and as soon as clarity around a fight schedule becomes apparent, appropriate planning to cease out-of-competition cycles should be planned for 8 to 12 wk prior to a fight. The priority of an accumulation phase is to develop maximal power capabilities and a general level of conditioning in all neuromuscular and metabolic systems (figure 11.8). This includes maximizing the contractile properties of fast- and slow-twitch fibers, developing glycolytic capacity and H^+ tolerance, and elevating the rate at which the body can process energy via oxidative metabolism, i.e., $\dot{V}O_{2peak}$ (29, 33, 38). The most appropriate HIIT modalities for the accumulation block include:

- High-intensity long intervals (cardiac output)—types 3 and 4
- Submaximal tempo repeats (oxidative capacity)—types 1 and 3
- Repeat-sprint intervals (lactate tolerance)—types 4 and 5
- Sprint intervals (neuromuscular power)—type 5
- And, outside of HIIT, heavy resistance work (developing contractile properties; type 6)

A transmutation or transition phase includes more sport-specific training factors and a reduction in general preparatory activities. Essentially, the general physical abilities developed in the accumulation phase are *transmutated*, or transitioned, into event-specific readiness. In some nomenclature the transmutation phase is also referred to as a *special preparation phase*. The focus of the transmutation phase is to emphasize the neuromuscular capabilities of specific muscle groups, challenge the metabolic demands of competition, and promote recoverability through enhanced regenerative qualities of the oxidative system. The selection of appropriate HIIT modalities is critical in a transmutation phase, so as to realize the potential of the general

training that has been completed before, but not to overload specific attributes that could potentially lead to detrimental fatigue (see figure 11.8). HIIT strategies would include:

- Fight-based training (cardiac output)—types 1, 2, 3, and 4
- Repeat-sprint intervals (lactate capacity)—types 4 and 5
- Short intervals (alactic power)—type 2
- Sprint intervals (neuromuscular power)—type 5

Finally, when an athlete moves from out-of-competition conditioning to fight camp, the focus shifts to specific conditioning that allows an athlete to make an 8 to 12 wk progression to competition standards. Much of the training done during this block is focused on fight-based HIIT, including sparing, simulated rounds, and high-intensity technique work. Within fight camp, athletes should cycle through shorter training blocks of 2 to 3 wk, moving progressively from high-volume capacity work to high-intensity explosive efforts and active recovery. The fight camp (e.g., effort:pause ratio) should build on out-of-competition adaptations and maximize their influence on fight-specific skills. HIIT modalities should include:

- Fight-based training (lactic capacity)—types 3, 4, and 5
- Short intervals (lactic power)—types 3 and 4
- Short intervals (alactic power)—type 2
- And, outside of HIIT, speed-strength resistance work (developing neural activation)
- Active recovery

Sample Training Programs

Tables 11.4 and 11.5 provide sample HIIT programs used in various combat sports during different phases of training, including both out of competition and fight camp. Each of these programs has very specific physiological objectives, and they demonstrate how HIIT is a central aspect of the programming strategy in combat sports.

Table 11.4 Weekly Plan for an Out-of-Competition Accumulation Phase in Elite Olympic Taekwondo Players

	Monday	Tuesday	Wednesday	Thursday	Friday	Saturday	Sunday
0700							
0800		0800-0930 **S&C** (Type 3) Long-interval HIIT	0800-0930 **TKD** (Type 4) High volume striking			0800-0930 **S&C** (Type 5) Repeat sprint intervals and lactate tolerance work	
0900	0900-1030 **TKD** (Type 1) Technical drilling and technique volume				0930-1100 **TKD** (Type 1) Technical drilling and technique volume		
1000							
1100		1130-1330 **TKD** Technique work in the clinch	1130-1300 **S&C** Heavy resistance training (Type 6)	1130-1330 **TKD** (Type 3) Movement and agility to scoring chances			
1200							
1300							OFF
1400	1400-1530 **TKD** (Type 2) Speed/high tempo striking				1400-1530 **TKD** (Type 2) Speed/high tempo striking		
1500							
1600				1630-1800 **TKD** (Type 4) Sparring			
1700		1730-1830 **TKD** Individual technique work					
1800	1800-1900 **S&C** Power emphasis resistance training (Type 6)				1800-1900 **S&C** Heavy resistance training (Type 6)		
1900							

TKD = taekwondo-specific workout; S&C = supplementary strength and conditioning workout

Table 11.5 Weekly Plan for the Fight Camp Phase of a Professional MMA Fighter

	Monday	Tuesday	Wednesday	Thursday	Friday	Saturday	Sunday
0700							
0800							
0900							
1000							
1100	1100-1300 **Grappling/ BJJ** (Type 3) Long-interval HIIT	1100-1300 **Wrestling** (Type 3) Technical drilling and long-interval HIIT		1100-1300 **Muay-Thai/ Striking** (Type 2) Speed/high-tempo striking and short-interval HIIT	1100-1300 **Grappling/BJJ** (Type 1) Technical drilling and long-interval HIIT	1600-1800 **MMA Sparing** (Type 5) Repeat intervals and lactate tolerance work	
1200							
1300							OFF
1400							
1500							
1600	1600-1800 **S&C** (Type 6) Heavy resistance training	1600-1800 **Muay-Thai/ Striking** (Type 2) Explosive speed and max power short interval HIIT	1600-1800 **MMA Sparing** (Type 4) Explosive speed and max power short-interval HIIT	1600-1800 **Wrestling** (Type 3) Anaerobic capacity and lactate tolerance work	1600-1800 **S&C** (Type 6) Power-emphasis resistance training		
1700							
1800							
1900							

BJJ = Brazilian jiu-jitsu; MMA = mixed martial arts; S&C = supplementary strength and conditioning workout

CASE STUDY

Shortly following the 2012 London Olympics, I became the head strength and conditioning coach for the Great Britain Olympic Taekwondo team, with the remit of directing the team's physical preparations for the Rio Olympics in 2016. Expectations were high with the team having achieved its most successful Olympic Games ever in London, winning gold and bronze medals. Sadly, however, London 2012 was a frustrating experience for Bianca Walkden, who was the team's up-and-coming +67 kg heavyweight. Two years prior to the London Games, Bianca agonizingly ruptured the ACL in her left knee, an injury that effectively ended her chances of securing a place to compete at London 2012.

Fast-forward 2 yr, and fueled by her desire not to miss out on another Olympic Games, Bianca was committing all her energies to becoming the best fighter she could be. An absolute coach's dream, Bianca gave everything to her physical preparation. Things were coming together, her physical standards were increasing exponentially, and in 2014 Bianca secured her maiden European crown at the European Championships in Baku, Azerbaijan. Two months later, tragedy struck again! At the world Grand Prix in Turkey, Bianca was dominating her opponent with powerful leg kicks, but after landing awkwardly she fell to the ground clutching her left knee. Heartbroken, she knew straightaway what it was, and she couldn't believe it was happening with the next Olympics less than 2 yr away. The ACL in her left knee had ruptured again.

After surgery Bianca regrouped and targeted the 2015 World Championships in Chelyabinsk, Russia, as her comeback in a major championship. This was only 8 mo away! As a support team we felt this was ambitious given that knee injuries in a kicking sport like taekwondo can significantly affect performance. However, we set about her rehabilitation and I dedicated my efforts to progressively increasing her physical capabilities to compete again at the most elite level. We built out the physical development plan alongside her rehabilitation needs and the coaches' integration of taekwondo-specific drills. With 8 mo, we periodized the steady reconditioning of her bioenergetics through a variety of continuous and HIIT modalities. Progress didn't happen as planned, and we were at a loss to understand why. Local muscular endurance was improving, and metabolic conditioning was getting better, but her repaired knee was still an issue and things weren't right. After much consultation, the decision was made by the medical team to go back into her knee 2 mo after the initial ACL surgery, make minor surgical repairs, and hope that healing would be accelerated as a consequence. Eight months of preparation time for the Worlds crazily became 6 mo, the first two of which she would be very limited in any sport-specific capabilities. We all felt like this was an impossible task to get her to the Worlds, but with crucial Olympic ranking points for Rio on the line it was almost nonnegotiable that she had to fight, otherwise her dreams of competing at the Olympics would once again be ruined.

Immediately the periodization of metabolic conditioning changed significantly. We moved to four HIIT sessions a week, two of which were focused on neuromuscular and metabolic power, and two that truly challenged her glycolytic system and the ability to tolerate high levels of metabolic acidosis. Many of the early sessions had to be performed in nontraditional fashions as we attempted to accelerate the metabolic conditioning, all the time working around the injured knee. Adopting a reverse-periodization strategy, the overarching focus became the development of the highest levels of anaerobic and aerobic power possible, and then use of HIIT strategies to build capacity/endurance against newly found levels of performance.

Only 6 mo following the second surgery on her torn ACL, Bianca was walking out to compete at the World Championships in Russia. It was truly remarkable, and knowing the dedication she had given to the rigorous HIIT schedule we prescribed, it was truly one of the most rewarding moments of my career. I never thought we would get her there, but with a clearly defined HIIT plan and unwavering commitment, Bianca made it to the Worlds! She

(continued)

was operating with about 80% neuromuscular power in her left leg, but her glycolytic and oxidative conditioning levels were the highest they had ever been. It was a punt, but she was willing to take the chance against the world's best.

At great surprise to everyone who knew what Bianca had been through, she began to progress through the tournament, winning through the early rounds and ultimately making it to the final round. In the final, she was going up against a French athlete who was recognized as one of the most powerful and dominant female fighters of recent times. Following a crazy fight, much to everyone's surprise, Bianca won!! Eight months after an ACL rupture, 6 mo after a secondary knee surgery, and essentially following 4 months of high-intensity training, Bianca had become world champion!! It was a remarkable turnaround, and for me it reiterated how valuable it is to have a clearly defined training plan that is aligned to the specific needs and demands of competition.

The story didn't end there! Bianca immediately got back to work, continuing to work on her physical conditioning. Amazingly, 12 mo after becoming world champion she retained her European title and was the number one ranked fighter in the world. She had amassed enough ranking points in half the amount of time to other competitors to confirm her place at the Rio Olympic Games. She took home a Bronze medal at the Olympic Games and was somewhat disappointed. But this was an amazing achievement for an athlete who had won two European championships, a world championship, and a Bronze medal at the Olympic Games just over 2 yr after a potential career-ending knee surgery.

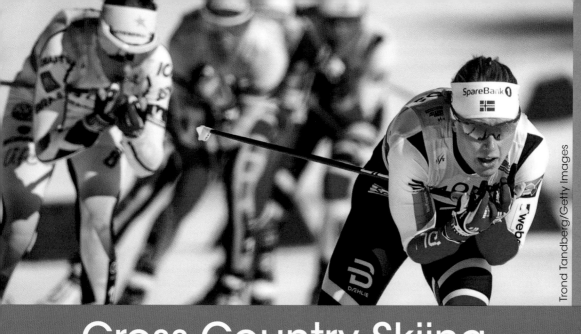

Trond Tandberg/Getty Images

12

Cross-Country Skiing

● ● ● ● ● ●

Øyvind Sandbakk

Performance Demands of Cross-Country Skiing

Cross-country (XC) skiing involves long-duration competitions across varying terrain, where whole-body exercise involves the gearing between different subtechniques of the classical and/or skating styles (8, 18). A XC skiing competition itself demands interval-based, high-intensity efforts, and many of the competitions, involving mass-start races with fields of 6 to 100 athletes, are often decided in a final sprint. Accordingly, XC skiers design their training to concurrently improve their aerobic endurance capacity, high-speed ability, as well as technical and tactical expertise.

Sport Description and Factors of Winning

XC skiing has been an Olympic event since the first Winter Games of 1924 in Chamonix, France. The sport is especially popular in the northern part of the European and American continents, although athletes from more than 60 countries compete in international championships. Since XC skiing is also employed in the biathlon and Nordic-combined events, 27 gold medals in the 2018 Winter Olympics were won utilizing XC skiing techniques. This sport then comprises more than a quarter of the overall number of medals available across the modern Winter Olympic Games.

International XC skiing competitions extend throughout a variety of different endurance formats. On the shorter high-intensity side, these include multiple ~3 min races in sprint skiing (i.e., a qualification time trial and 3 knockout heats), while the more prolonged endurance distances involve races of 30 km (women) and 50 km (men) lasting 1.5 to 2 h. In terms of terrain, most race courses tend to be approximately one-third uphill, one-third flat, and one-third downhill, with ~50% of the total time spent racing uphill due to the slower invoked speed working against gravity (5, 6, 26). Elite performance then requires a skier to master many different techniques and to efficiently transition between these, at speeds ranging from 5 to 70 km/h on inclines ranging from -20% to +20% gradients. In addition, 10 of the 12 competitions in international championships involve mass starts, where tactics and sprint ability are crucial determinants of the final result.

Speed during XC skiing events must be adapted to the track profile, snow conditions, and the competition altitude (0 to 1800 m above sea level). Skiers tend to use a positive-pacing strategy (1), whereby speed is slightly reduced throughout races, although the best performing skiers are able to maintain speed better than their lower performing counterparts (6, 13, 26). However, throughout a given race, skiers must perform more metabolic work during uphill sections (20), followed by reduced intensity and recovery on downhill sections (3, 6, 24). Thus, the race format of XC skiing is interval based itself, with the highest work rates (and largest performance separations between competitors) arising on the uphill sections. In mass-start events, the importance of drafting behind other skiers and the ability to maneuver into a position that allows for the utilization of an athlete's individual strengths is also important. Indeed, races are often decided by attacks in uphill sections at the end of races or in a final sprint to the finish line.

Relative Contribution of Physical Performance

Physical performance is of crucial importance in XC skiing (figure 12.1), with various indices of endurance capacity, including $\dot{V}O_2$max, speed at anaerobic thresholds and gross efficiency being the strongest correlates of performance (17, 21, 22, 25, 26). On average, the aerobic proportion of the total energy expended during XC skiing competitions (i.e., 70% to 75% in sprints and 85% to 95% across longer distances) is comparable to the corresponding values for other sports over similar racing times. However,

the requirements for higher intensity on uphill terrain push metabolic demands considerably above those required to elicit $\dot{V}O_2$max, resulting in energy requirements as high as 40% and 15% to 20% above that of aerobic energy capacity in sprint and distance races, respectively (15, 24). Hence, XC skiers additionally require high levels of anaerobic capacity (24). Further, upper-body strength is important in order to achieve a high maximal movement speed using propulsive force production during XC skiing (28). Accordingly, a combination of physical and technical skills is required to produce sufficiently long cycle lengths combined with rapid cycles (4, 10, 19). This is exemplified in explosive male skiers who produce peak double-poling forces as high as 430 N within 0.05 s, as well as forces greater than 1600 N during leg push off when skating (27, 29).

Targets of Physical Performance in Cross-Country Skiing

World-class XC skiers have shown some of the highest $\dot{V}O_2$max values ever reported among all athletes, with values of >6.5 and >4.5 L/min and 80 to 90 and 70 to 80 mL·kg⁻¹·min⁻¹ for men and women,

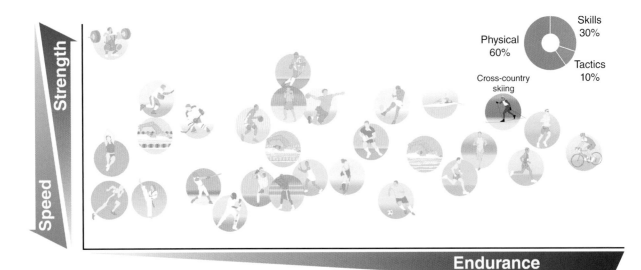

Figure 12.1 The position of the cross-country skier on the three axes illustrates the relative importance of the three main physical capacities of importance for elite participation in this sport, acknowledging this varies slightly between the different competition disciplines. Outside of critical psychological and team chemistry components, which are difficult to quantify, the pie chart shows the general relative importance of skills, tactical awareness, and physical capacities for cross-country skiing success.

Adapted from G.A. Nader, "Concurrent Strength and Endurance Training: From Molecules to Man," *Medicine & Science in Sports & Exercise* 38, no. 11 (2006): 1965-1970.

respectively (9, 25, 32). The absolute $\dot{V}O_2$max values measured by elite sprint and distance skiers are similar, although sprint skiers are often heavier and their $\dot{V}O_2$max may be slightly lower when normalized to body mass (11). In addition, XC skiers need to elevate their $\dot{V}O_2$peak to $\geq 95\%$ of $\dot{V}O_2$max when using all of the subtechniques in classic and skating technique, even when employing subtechniques that involve relatively little muscle mass (8). Overall, the fractional utilization of $\dot{V}O_2$max during races, which reflects the aerobic energy utilized (i.e., performance $\dot{V}O_2$), is a main determinant of performance. In this context, the so-called anaerobic threshold (or critical power, chapter 4) is of importance, although the constraints of XC skiing lead to utilization of different techniques where this threshold may differ. These technique changes at constantly varying workloads also emphasize the importance of being able to alter O_2 kinetics rapidly from one technique to the next.

Anaerobic power in XC skiing is correlated to sprint performance (12) and anaerobic capacity appears to become higher when training is intensified during the competitive period (14). However, since the relative contribution from anaerobic energy decreases as the competition period proceeds, it becomes less important at longer distances. While the muscles of well-trained athletes contain higher levels of both glycogen and intramyocellular triglyceride stores, energy availability may still limit XC skiing performance over the longer competition duration (16). In the case of both sprint and distance XC skiing, the ability to transform metabolic energy efficiently into speed is a key determinant of performance (2, 20, 21). This likely reflects the technical complexity of XC skiing, with the numerous degrees of freedom and constraints for timing force generation by both arms and legs. Speed over a short distance and maximal strength/power in movement-specific exercises naturally tend to correlate with sprint performance (5, 29). In this context, upper-body strength and power generation have become of particular interest for both researchers and XC skiers, due to its large potential for enhancement, especially in female athletes (28, 33).

Key Weapons, Manipulations, and Surveillance Tools

Low-intensity endurance training ($<VT_1$, aerobic threshold) makes up the major proportion of an elite XC skier's training time. The 800 to 950 h of annual training (including 700 to 850 h of endurance) by the best skiers comprise approximately 80% of the training time at low-intensity ($<VT_1$), 4% to 5% moderate (VT_1-VT_2), and 5% to 8% high-intensity interval training (HIIT; $>VT_2$), and the remaining 10% as strength and speed work (17, 18). Endurance training time is calculated using the modified session goal approach (30), and although HIIT might seem to be only a small component of the overall training, these HIIT sessions are believed to be the key sessions involved in solving a skier's programming puzzle, and make up ~20% of the overall session number (races + HIIT).

Most XC skiing competitions involve considerable racing time at intensities above 90% of $\dot{V}O_2$max, and therefore have similar metabolic and neuromuscular responses as typical HIIT sessions programmed in training (i.e., type 2 and 3 targets). For this reason, races can be considered as additional high-intensity components of a XC skier's programming puzzle, and local or national competitions may be used instead of a specific HIIT session. Therefore, while the topic of this book is to present the different HIIT weapons used in the field and how practitioners can best implement and program such training components, these high-intensity races have been mentioned where necessary to allow a better understanding of the context required for optimal HIIT programming (see figure 12.2).

Approximately 60% of the training time tends to be performed between May and October (preparation phase), while the remaining 40% of training time occurs during the competition period from November to April. The preparation period includes extensive volumes of low-intensity training interspersed with regular HIIT sessions, and is followed by the competition period, which uses a more polarized training pattern, with less volume and more high-intensity training (including competitions). Tables 12.1 and 12.2 illustrate typical training programs of all-around XC skiers during the preparation and competition periods, respectively. In comparison to these programs, skiers specializing in the sprint distances appear to train slightly less, but use more speed and strength training. In all elite athletes, roller skiing using special tracks with competition-specific terrain and techniques, running on varying terrain, and cycling form the predominant modes of endurance exercise from May to October, with only 5 to 10 d of snow-based training per month. From November until the end of the competition period, most training involves skiing on snow.

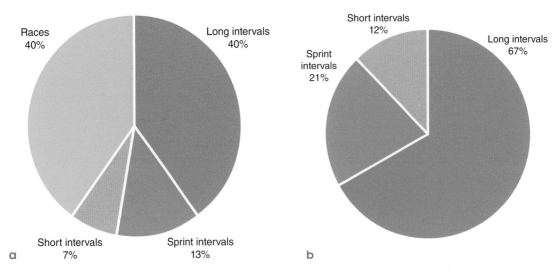

Figure 12.2 Percentage of the different HIIT components seen throughout the annual season in an elite cross-country skier: (a) races + HIIT; (b) HIIT only.

Table 12.1 Typical Training Week for a World-Class XC Skier at Low Altitude (<800 m Above Sea Level) During the Preparation Period

Day	Hard training week	Easy training week
Monday	a.m.: 6×5-min HIIT, uphill running with poles (type 1)	a.m.: 2 hrs LIT, running on easy/moderate terrain
	p.m.: 1.5 h LIT, classical roller skiing with double poling on easy terrain	p.m.: Rest
Tuesday	a.m.: 1.5 h, LIT roller ski skating on easy/moderate terrain	a.m.: 5×4 min HIIT, uphill running/walking with poles (type 1)
	p.m.: Strength training# including 5×30 s sprint interval double poling (type 5)	p.m.: 30 min LIT, easy cycling
Wednesday	a.m.: 2.5 h LIT, classical roller skiing on varied terrain	p.m.: 1.5 h LIT, roller ski skating on varied terrain, including 10×12 s sprints
	p.m.: 1.5 h LIT, running on hilly terrain with a soft surface	p.m.: Rest
Thursday	a.m.: 50 min continuous MIT/HIIT,* roller ski skating on a roller ski track (type 2)	a.m.: 2.5 h LIT, classical roller skiing on varied terrain
	p.m.: 10×10 maximal jumps+strength training#	p.m.: Rest
Friday	a.m.: 1.5 h LIT, roller ski skating on varied terrain, including 10×12 s sprints	a.m.: 6×5 min HIIT,* roller ski double poling (type 2)
	p.m.: Rest	p.m.: 1.5 h LIT, running on hilly terrain with a soft surface
Saturday	a.m.: 5×8 min HIIT* with 15 s final sprints, roller ski classic on a roller ski track (types 2 and 3)	p.m.: 1.5 h LIT, classical roller skiing on easy/moderate terrain, including 6×15 s double-poling sprints
	p.m.: 60 min LIT, easy cycling	p.m.: Rest
Sunday	a.m.: 3.5 h LIT, running on terrain of moderate incline with a soft surface	a.m.: 3 h LIT, running on terrain of moderate incline with a soft surface
	p.m.: Rest	p.m.: Rest

LIT=low-intensity training; blood lactate concentration <2.5 mmol/L, heart rate <80% HRmax.

MIT=moderate-intensity training; blood lactate concentration 2.5 to 4.0 mmol/L, heart rate 80% to 90% HRmax.

HIIT=high-intensity interval training; blood lactate concentration >4.0 mmol/L, heart rate >90% HRmax.

* Competitions and HIIT sessions routinely included approximately 30 to 45 min of LIT, followed by 10 to 15 min of MIT/HIIT. Cooldown involves 15 min of LIT.

\# Strength sessions typically consist of a 30 min warm-up (running/cycling at LIT) followed by 15 to 30 min maximal movement-specific strength exercises for the upper body and thereafter 30 to 45 min of more general core/stabilization exercises.

Table 12.2 Typical Training Week for a World-Class XC Skier During the Competition Period

Day	Hard training week	Competition week
Monday	a.m.: 2.5 h, LIT ski skating on moderate terrain	a.m.: 2 h LIT, classical skiing on easy terrain
	p.m.: 1.5 h LIT, classical skiing with special focus on double poling on easy terrain	p.m.: Warm-up+30 min strength training
Tuesday	a.m.: 8×4 min HIIT, skating on uphill terrain (type 2)	a.m.: 5×4 min HIIT,* skating on varied terrain with included 10 s attacks or sprints (types 2 and 3)
	p.m.: 1.5 h LIT, classic on easy terrain	p.m.: 30 min LIT, running on treadmill
Wednesday	a.m.: Strength training#	a.m.: 1.5 h LIT, ski skating on relatively flat terrain
	p.m.: 1.5 h LIT, ski skating on varied terrain, including 10×12 s sprints	p.m.: Rest
Thursday	a.m.: 2.5 h LIT, classical skiing on varied terrain	a.m.: Travel
	p.m.: Rest	p.m.: 1 h LIT, skating on moderate terrain including 5×10 s sprints
Friday	a.m.: 5×8 min MIT/HIIT,* ski classic on a competition track (type 2)	a.m.: 45 min LIT on the competition track followed by 3×5 min MIT/HIIT.* Classical skiing (type 2)
	p.m.: 30 min LIT, running on a treadmill	p.m.: Rest
Saturday	a.m.: 1 h LIT, ski skating on varied terrain + strength training#	MO: Morning jog 30 min, strides and jumps a.m.: 15-km classic competition* (type 2)
	p.m.: 1.5 h LIT, classical skiing on easy/moderate terrain, including 8×20 s double poling sprints (type 5)	p.m.: Easy skiing 45 min, stretching/massage
Sunday	a.m.: 3.5 h LIT, skating on relatively easy terrain	a.m.: 30 km skiathlon competition* (type 2)
	p.m.: Rest	p.m.: Travel

LIT = low-intensity training; blood lactate concentration < 2.5 mmol/L, heart rate < 80% HRmax.

MIT = moderate-intensity training; blood lactate concentration 2.5 to 4.0 mmol/L, heart rate 80%-90% HRmax.

HIIT = high-intensity interval training; blood lactate concentration >4.0 mmol/L, heart rate >90% HRmax.

* Competitions and HIIT sessions routinely included approximately 30 to 45 min of LIT, followed by 10 to 15 min of MIT/HIIT. Cooldown involves 15 min of LIT.

Strength sessions typically consist of a 30 min warm-up (running/cycling at LIT) followed by 15 to 30 min maximal movement-specific strength exercises for the upper body and thereafter 30 to 45 min of more general core/stabilization exercises.

HIIT Weapons

For XC skiing, the majority of high-intensity sessions are competitions (40% of all high-intensity sessions, occurring mainly in the competition period), while long intervals above 2 min work duration make up another 40% of all high-intensity sessions (figures 12.2 and 12.3). The remaining 20% of all high-intensity sessions include a combination of short intervals and sprint intervals. While the latter category might seem small, many of the competitions and long intervals also include shorter bouts of increased and reduced intensity along the varying terrain described above. The fact that some short intervals and sprint intervals are included in these sessions is discussed below and described in the training programs presented in tables 12.1 and 12.2.

When the competitions are excluded from the overall high-intensity training components in the program, 60% to 70% are long intervals, whereas 10% to 15% are short intervals, and 15% to 25% are sprint intervals. For full context, figure 12.2 shows how the high-intensity component of training is broken down either in light of overall high-intensity work or with respect to HIIT specific sessions, while figure 12.3 shows the placement of both high-intensity components throughout the annual season in an example for a world-class XC skier.

Manipulations of Interval Training Variables

As described in chapters 4, 5, and 6, not only are the type and number of HIIT sessions of importance

Period	1. Preparation period			2. Preparation period			Competition period					Recovery	
Testing	T	T		T	T	T	T		T		T	T	
Training camps	L	L	L	L	H H H	L H H H	L	H H		H H			
	May	June	July	August	Sept.	Oct.	Nov.	Dec.	Jan.	Feb.	March	April	SUM
Training hours	70	80	85	90	90	85	75	60	60	50	45	35	825
Number of HIIT/month													
Sprint races							2	2	2	2	2		10
Time-trial races							2	2	2	2	1	1	10
Mass-start races							1	2	4	3	3		13
Relays								1	1	1			3
Other competitions	1	2	1	2	1	0						1	8
Long intervals	3	3	4	4	5	5	4#	4#	4#	4#	4#		44
Short intervals	1	1	1	1	1	1	1					1	8
Sprint intervals	1	2	2	2	2	2	1	1		1			14
SUM intervals	5	6	7	7	7	8	6	5	4	5	4	1	66
SUM all HIIT	6	8	8	9	9	8	11	12	13	13	10	3	110

Figure 12.3 Annual training plan of a world-class XC skier competing in sprint and distance races. Example shows weeks of testing and training camps, as well as monthly training hours, number of competitions, and other HIIT sessions. T = laboratory testing; L = training camp at low-land altitude; H = training camp at high altitude; # Half of these are performed with 50% to 60% of the work duration.

but equally crucial are the manipulation of the work interval and session quality. Uniquely for XC skiing, a particular emphasis is on the choice of exercise mode (see chapter 4), since HIIT models should develop a XC skier's performance in his specific subtechniques. Skiers mainly use skiing, roller skiing, and running with poles on different terrains. These techniques load the upper and lower body to different extents across the constantly changing competition terrain. Accordingly, skiers must purposefully choose the HIIT terrain and thereby determine the extent to which they train their different subtechniques. For example, since ~50% of racing time is spent uphill, HIIT training of uphill techniques is especially important. The constantly changing terrain also leads to interactions between the different factors involved in manipulating training that coaches need to consider. For example, when doing an 8 min interval of varying terrain, the 8 min could include external work rates varying from 400 Watts uphill to 0 Watts downhill, although the fluctuations of the metabolic demands are slightly less. This is illustrated in figures 12.4 and 12.5.

Races

A relatively large part of the high-intensity training component of a XC skier involves competitions. Throughout a year, elite XC skiers perform around 45 competitions, with approximately 30 to 40 of these performed skiing on snow in the competitive season and 5 to 10 performed as roller ski competitions, running races, and/or cycling races during the dryland period. For an elite XC skier, the different races tend to be distributed as follows:

- On a single day, ~10 sprint competitions that involve 1.3 to 1.8 km (i.e., 2 to 4 min) time trials, including a qualifying time trial race and three subsequent knockout heats. Recovery periods become progressively shorter between heats, i.e., from 60 to 20 min, and the overall event takes 3 to 4 h to complete, including warm-up with preparation sprints and some high-intensity skiing of 30 s.

- 10 individual time trials, mainly over 10 km (women) or 15 km (men).

- 15 mass-start races, as 10 to 30 km (women) or 20 to 50 km (men) pursuit (i.e., changing from classic to skating technique midway) or mass-start races.

- A few relay competitions, of differing types, such as relays with four skiers from each team performing a 5 or 10 km section or a sprint relay that involves a qualifying race and a final heat where two skiers on each team perform three 1.3 to 1.8 km sections each.

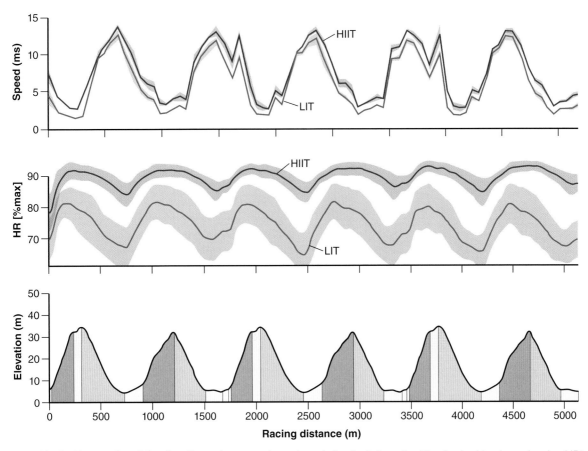

Figure 12.4 Example of fluctuations in speed and metabolic intensity (illustrated by heart rate; HR) in a 5 km bout of a continuous high-intensity interval training (HIIT, red) session performed on varying terrain while skiing using the skating technique (n = 8 elite XC skiers). This is contrasted to low-intensity (LIT, blue) exercise in the same track under the same external conditions.

• Of the 5 to 10 competitions during the dry-land period, approximately 50% to 60% are roller ski competitions (either sprint, time trials or mass starts, evenly distributed) whereas 40% to 50% are running or cycling competitions.

These competitions are the most specific high-intensity sessions that relate to XC skiing performance, and target all required systems to varying degrees, with sprint races mainly hitting type 3 and type 4 HIIT targets (see descriptions in chapter 5), whereas the long-distance competitions mainly hit a type 2 HIIT target (with cycling/running races type 1). It is worth noting that women compete over shorter distances (and durations) than men and that both sexes ski in the same tracks. This slightly influences the energetic demands of the race, with male and female skiers using somewhat different subtechnique proportions (e.g., loading of upper and lower extremities).

HIIT With Long Intervals

The most common long-interval type HIIT sessions performed in the preparation period involve total work interval durations that range from 20 to 40 min, with recovery periods of approximately 25% to 50% of the work duration. These HIIT weapons use leg or whole-body exercise modes, where large muscle mass engagement can fully task cardiovascular system capacity. Still, in order to perform these extensive sessions at an intensity at or above 90% of $\dot{V}O_2$max, athletes must be extremely well trained. My impression is that elite athletes do not get sufficient stimulus to further enhance their aerobic power when performing shorter total work duration of intervals, which contradicts what has repeatedly been shown as being effective among populations with lower endurance capacity (7). This is also supported by our previous studies where long-interval HIIT completed at slightly lower intensity was more

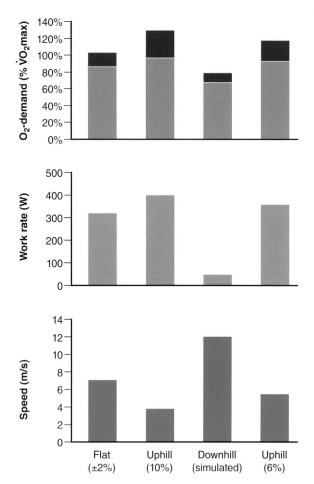

Figure 12.5 Example of speed, work rate, and O_2 demand (aerobic metabolic rate, green; anaerobic metabolic rate, red) during four 3 min HIIT intervals, with 2 min recovery at different inclines while roller ski skating on a large treadmill. The athlete was allowed to self-select the speeds.

effective at enhancing most endurance performance indices compared with short-interval HIIT done at higher intensity (23, 31).

Examples of long-interval HIIT sessions performed as either roller skiing, skiing, or running (with poles) are described below (type 1 or 2 targets):

- 4 or 5 × 8 min intervals with 2 to 3 min recovery periods (90% to 92% of HR_{max})
- 6 to 8 × 4 min intervals with 1 to 2 min recovery periods (92% to 95% of HR_{max})
- 5 or 6 × 5 min intervals with 2 min recovery periods (90% to 94% of HR_{max})
- Continuous natural interval sessions of 20 to 40 min (i.e., Fartlek training, chapter 1) where

effort is increased uphill, maintained on the flat, and reduced downhill (90% to 95% of HR_{max})

- Various types of pyramid intervals (e.g., 5/6/7/8/7/6/5 min) with similar work durations as those above (90% to 95% of HR_{max})

Note that women compete at shorter distances than men do and could in some cases prefer interval models with slightly shorter work duration than men (more sessions with total work duration of 20 to 30 min versus more commonly 30 to 40 min in men). The same applies to younger athletes, in an earlier stage of their career, and for male and female elite skiers in periods with less training load or in the competition period when the aim is to trigger the cardiovascular system and competition speed without creating excessive fatigue. The latter sessions might have a 30% to 50% reduced work duration of each interval compared to those described above, but with similar recovery periods as the full sessions. Typical examples are (type 1 or 2 targets):

- 5 × 4 min intervals with 2 min recovery periods (90% to 94% of HR_{max})
- 8 × 2 min intervals with 2 to 3 min recovery periods (92% to 95% of HR_{max})
- 2 or 3 × 5 min intervals with 2 min recovery periods (90% to 92% of HR_{max})
- 15 min of continuous work in the competition track (90% to 95% of HR_{max})

In all recovery periods described above, XC skiers use active recovery by moving with a pace corresponding to low-intensity training.

The long-interval HIIT sessions are mainly performed on skis or roller skis using either the classical or skating techniques, or as running with poles. Some sessions might include pure double poling to create an extra stimulus on the upper body and reduce the effort on the legs. These sessions mainly target the metabolic O_2 system (type 1), although technique is essential in the ski-specific sessions (type 2). In addition, there is an anaerobic component that might develop that system concurrently in some athletes (type 3). Note that many of these sessions are performed in relatively steady terrain in the first preparation period (table 12.1), whereas more competition-specific terrain is chosen when the competitive season approaches (table 12.2). The latter includes more variations in workload within the intervals, with the recovery periods in the downhill phases slightly lowering overall O_2 demand (i.e., figures 12.4 and 12.5). However, the local muscle's metabolic demand varies considerably, with inconsistent demands placed on arm and leg musculature over undulating and varying technique (mode). Both coaches and athletes need to be aware of this when designing sessions. A potential means of addressing this might be to include uphill attack simulations and a final sprint during some of the intervals as the competitive season approaches, in order to develop these key components for success in international cross-country ski races.

HIIT With Short Intervals

The variations of intensity when skiing in varying terrain, both during competitions and with longer intervals, facilitates work that can almost be characterized as short-interval HIIT, with the greatest work completed over uphill periods normally lasting from 15 to 60 s. Thus, some defined short-interval sessions are used in many programs. For example, typical intervals of 45 s work durations, with 15 s active recovery at an easy pace, performed over 10 to 30 min are used by some athletes. Such sessions are often done while running or roller skiing on constant terrain, and more commonly performed by XC skiers who need to work with high speed to optimize their technique close to competition speed, and specifically target types 2 and 3 responses. Other short-interval sessions that target type 3 (and type 4) responses could include 10×1 min efforts with 30 s to 1 min active recovery, with work intervals done at very high intensity where both aerobic and anaerobic metabolic systems are targeted. Such sessions need to be done using specific technique, and personally, I like to use modes and terrains that are of particular importance at the end of races, such as attacks in uphill terrain or the final sprint. It is also important that good technique and high speed are maintained throughout the session.

Sprint Interval Training

Some of the additional HIIT sessions used by XC skiers can be categorized as sprint interval training. These weapons are included in other sessions (attacks, final sprints) as described previously. However, some sessions are also specifically designed as 5 or 6×20 to 30 s maximal sprints with 2 to 3 min recovery as part of a speed session, 10×30 s double

poling or ergometer poling in the gym to load the upper body, as well as gym sessions (circuits) with 20 to 45 s maximal work periods followed by 30 to 60 s recovery phases. Such sessions are often developed specifically for individual athletes or teams in order to develop specific areas or weaknesses. These sessions target type 5 responses for elite athletes (although in less-trained skiers these might also stimulate the O_2 system), with sessions done technique specific with good form maintained throughout the entire session.

Load Surveillance and Monitoring Tools

Due to the uncontrollable environmental conditions during much of the training of a XC skier, speed is often not a good measure of training load, and external work rate is difficult to measure and interpret. Thus, various measures of perceived exertion and internal intensity, such as those addressed in chapter 8, are used to monitor training. Most commonly, XC skiers use some kind of rating of perceived exertion (RPE) measures, as well as heart rate in combination with GPS to track distance, altitude climbed, and speed during sessions. These data are uploaded to an online training diary, which separates sessions into different intensities and exercise modalities, together with athlete/coach comments on execution, design, manipulation aspects, and other lifestyle factors such as health-and-fitness status (chapter 9). Together, these objective measurements alongside the training diary become important tools used to understand the load of the various sessions, as well as the response to load, and are especially useful for facilitating good dialogue between athlete and coach. A coach's observations and playback of video recordings of sessions are equally important, but there are limitations to how much coaches are able to observe since athletes cover long distances in outdoor terrain. Today, large treadmills can be used for roller ski sessions where coaches can observe their athletes over long durations, athletes can be tracked in more detail with GPS during training and competitions (6), and also new sensors and drone camera technology combine to provide the coach with more insight into training and performance than ever before. While we have only started to use such technology, these tools have promising future potential in sports such as XC skiing, where a coach cannot always follow the athletes.

Training Status Surveillance and Monitoring Tools

As mentioned before, the online training diary (www.olt-dagbok.net) used by our skiers is also an important tool for monitoring training status. In this context, resting heart rate has been one of the measures used for decades by XC skiers, although today, many use HRV to track their recovery status (see chapter 9). In addition, we use regular treadmill testing, with both maximal (e.g., $\dot{V}O_2$max and time to exhaustion tests) and submaximal tests (e.g., physiological responses to standardized bouts) to control and understand the progression (compared to the expected development) during the preparation period, so that capacities may be maintained at a high level during the competition period. Such tests are mostly done roller skiing on a large treadmill using standardized protocols (21, 22, 25), but some athletes also prefer having regular treadmill running tests used, which has been the traditional standard test regimen in most countries for decades. In between these formal tests, skiers also have standard training sessions where performance is monitored, while roller skiing at standardized conditions on the treadmill can also indicate training status (e.g., HR, RPE at a given workload). Many athletes also have their own 15 to 30 min running tests (most often over uphill terrain) or double-poling tests that have been used throughout their whole career without using any fancy equipment other than a stopwatch (23). Hematological status is taken regularly in elites, both in cases where the athlete is not responding well to training as well as before and after altitude camps, with the primary markers of interest being blood volume and total hemoglobin mass. Additionally, lung function is regularly measured, especially in athletes with asthma.

Strategies for Structuring the Training Program Using HIIT

Strategies for structuring the training program used by XC skiers are described and discussed next, with a special emphasis on how HIIT sessions are planned and incorporated.

Controllable and Uncontrollable Factors

As XC skiing is an individual sport, many of the factors influencing the training program and overall load can be individualized. However, external factors will influence the load of sessions and the subsequent recovery extensively, e.g., due to changes in weather conditions, training environment, training group situations, and various other lifestyle factors. For example, sudden changes in snow conditions might change static friction (grip) during the push off in classical skiing, gliding friction in both styles can be affected for various reasons, as well as a variable softness of surface where forces from poles and skis are applied. These factors change the speed and subtechniques employed, thereby altering the overall load of the session. In some cases, there is lack of snow and/or sudden changes in snow conditions that makes on-snow training impossible, even during the wintertime. Sometimes it is not possible to use roller skis in training as compensation for skiing on snow, which leads skiers to use various other training modes in their HIIT sessions or adjust the programming puzzle with the session performed on another day. Very cold temperatures sometimes force skiers to keep training intensity lower than originally planned (due to cold-inflicted muscle/respiratory temperatures and its physiological effects) or even skip an HIIT session due to the increased risk of bronchospasm. Another important factor altering the training program or execution of sessions is the behavior of competitors in competitions and how teammates pace during interval sessions. These aspects influence the training stimuli gained from the session, which might have consequences for the recovery and subsequent sessions. Another factor influencing the programming is the fact that most skiers need to qualify for the important competitions, and whether or not they are qualified and/or need to qualify might change throughout the season and subsequently dictate how training is structured. Finally, elite athletes are humans with emotions and health issues just like the rest of us, and all these factors can be difficult to control or predict, but need to be taken into consideration in the training process.

Program Structure and Progression

The yearly plan (figure 12.3) for an elite XC skier typically involves a 6 mo preparation period (table 12.1), followed by a 5 mo competition period (table 12.2) and 1 mo of recovery. Most elite skiers periodize their training volume relatively constantly from week to week during the 6 mo preparation period from May to October, training mostly around 20 to 25 h per wk, with some weeks involving <15 h following extensive periods of training (25). In this case, the frequency of HIIT sessions tends to be on average twice per week. However, a greater emphasis on high-intensity training, often periodized more in HIIT blocks due to periods with an extensive number of competitions, are placed on the period of competition. However, also within the preparation period, there is a gradual progression with an initial increase in training volume from May to July, before the load of the HIIT sessions is increased by either longer intervals and/or more repetitions at the same intensity or by increasing intensity of the sessions. In addition, the specificity of HIIT sessions is altered toward the competition period, including more HIIT sessions on competition-specific terrain, on snow and at competition intensity. Within the preparation period, there tends to be a natural periodization of training that involves a cycle of:

1. 5 to 10 d training camps at low altitude with stable volume/load but increased focus on HIIT (1 or 2 more sessions than normal),
2. 2 to 3 wk altitude camps with reduced HIIT components (normally only 1 per wk), but higher volume of low-intensity training, and
3. individualized training with a slightly easier load between camps.

In the competition period, the competition blocks are interspersed with a couple of 2 or 3 wk periods with higher training volumes and less HIIT, often done at altitude.

While the yearly plan is set at the beginning of the year (i.e., figure 12.3), each month starts with an analysis of what was done in the previous month and how the progression is appearing. Test/competition results and the quality of HIIT sessions are key factors for the decision-making and possible modification of the training program. Furthermore, daily and weekly adjustments are done using close dialogue between athlete and coach, with modifications made for example if the athlete experiences sudden changes in how he responds to training. Especially in the competition period, continuous dialogue between athlete and coach is vital.

Incorporation of HIIT

HIIT sessions are always the first sessions included in the training program. After the HIIT sessions are planned, the other components of the program are included. In the preparation phase, moderate-intensity sessions and the longest low-intensity sessions are programmed secondary to the HIIT sessions, as these provide an important stimulus during this phase. Thereafter, strength and speed training are puzzled in before overall load/volume is regulated by other low-intensity sessions. In the competition period, speed sessions might also be included after the HIIT sessions and used to ensure freshness for the HIIT sessions.

An elite athlete who had previously shown good performance progression contacted me after experiencing stagnation in training/performance and lack of advancement over the last season. He was close to reaching the absolute world-class level, and although he and his coach believed that he trained harder and better, his performance over the last year was not as expected, which was also in line with lower values of performance physiology attained in testing. The athlete and coach were obviously both frustrated with the situation and the condition was not for a lack of trying. The conclusions from an extensive analysis of the athlete's training and lifestyle were as following:

- Training content, overall training load, and recovery balance seemed appropriate, with progression in training load being approximately +5% during each of the two years, and all indices of recovery appearing normal.
- Both low-intensity and HIIT sessions looked to be performed at an appropriate intensity, with most of the sessions performed close to the target heart rate and blood lactate concentration.
- The choice of HIIT models and training terrain/techniques seemed relevant for the demands of the key event they were preparing for.
- There had been no major occurrence of illness, changes in lifestyle, or other changes in cognitive or emotional stressors over the last years.

However, by observing a few of their key HIIT sessions, I had a feeling that something was lacking. The athlete seemed to be too instrumental in his approach. Things were done "by the book," but he and his coach lacked a level of playfulness and passion in their training, and they did not strive to continuously develop their key sessions or incorporate new elements that could create further progression. Although intensity was always correct (heart rate, lactate, etc.), the speed was not as high as I would have expected, the technique lacked "punch," and the minor aspects that might decide a race were not present in the key sessions. For example, the athlete did not accelerate out of each turn, he changed his subtechniques at just a moment too late, he did not work extra hard over each hilltop, and stopped sprinting 3 m before the finish line. While each aspect individually might seem minor, together they were causing a major impact on his performance, and were additionally indicative of a lack of freshness. My impressions were that the athlete was not 100% "in the moment" and in full contact with the situational demands during his key sessions. I also had the feeling that the athlete and coach focus was too much on exercising with the correct internal intensity instead of focusing on the most important aspect of skiing—moving faster!

So what did we do? After a discussion with the coach and the athlete about these aspects, we decided not to change the overall training plan but rather to focus on developing each session and making minor adjustments to optimize the training quality and adaptations. The two following areas were specified as those to work on:

HUNT THE OPTIMAL HIIT SESSIONS

- Planning: Sessions need to be continuously developed and improved. Each session needs to be prepared with a clear aim of the session, where the HIIT design, choice of terrain, intensity, training partners, etc., match the specific development focus of each session.
- Performing: Be 100% present during the HIIT session, "in one" with the terrain, playing with the constraints and letting the body search for its optimal technical solutions that accelerate the body; placing the main focus on optimizing technique and speed, with internal intensity being secondary; having only a few checkpoints to reinforce the specific focus areas that are clarified with the coach (e.g., using video, feedback, etc.).
- Debriefing: Reflect on what went well as soon as possible after the session, and discuss what could be done better next time. Get frustrations out directly with open communication, agree with the coach on areas of needed learning.
- Relax and recover.

AIM FOR OPTIMAL HIIT ADAPTATIONS

- Key HIIT sessions should be completed with the highest possible quality and prepared first in the programming puzzle. Other sessions are secondary.
- Measure time/speed on key sessions to continuously measure performance indices and ensure expected progress.
- Evaluate training by output (i.e., progress, adaptation), in order to regulate future input.

These changes in focus for the pair gave an immediately positive response. They changed many of the HIIT sessions slightly in order to make them more specific and/or of higher quality. This ensured a positive process, which was also reflected in better test results (higher $\dot{V}O_2$max and lower physiological stress on standardized submaximal load), positive emotions, and passion for the training process. Thanks to the subsequent adaptations, performance progress was improved, and in the following season the athlete performed really well and took the final step into the world of the elite. For me, this was an important lesson on the various factors involved in the development process of athletes the programming puzzle is much more than just a training program on a piece of paper.

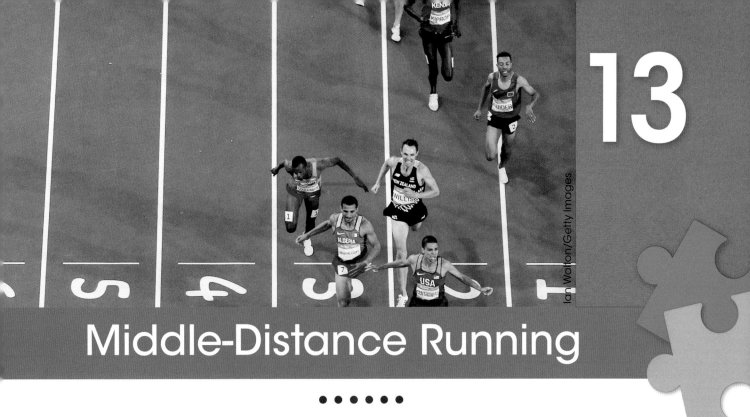

13

Middle-Distance Running

• • • • • •

Jean Claude Vollmer and Martin Buchheit

Performance Demands of Middle-Distance Running

In this section, we introduce track and field's 1500 m event and discuss the various factors of importance and the relative contribution that physical performance, running technique, and tactics make toward winning races. Note that the data presented and analyzed throughout the chapter was mostly available from male athletes, and slight differences may be apparent when comparing across genders. The chapter is written predominantly from the point of view and experience of coach Jean Claude Vollmer, with the scientific interpretation of Martin Buchheit.

Sport Description and Factors of Winning

In the sport of track and field, or athletics, the middle-distance (MD) events refer to distances run over 800 to 2000 m on an athletic track, including the 1500 m and 1 mile races, which are run at relatively high speeds (table 13.1). Middle-distance events differ from long-distance races (3000 m, 5000 m, 10,000 m), which must be run at slower speeds (i.e., 24.5 to 22.82 km/h for 3000 to 10,000 m WR speeds, respectively). It is important to note however that the average speed of the 1500 m is only 2.3 km/h slower than that of the 800 m, despite being almost twice as long, while it is 1.9 and 2.4 km/h faster than the 3000 m and 5000 m races, respectively. In terms of running demands, the 1500 m event is a race that sits right in the middle between short, very high speed races (800 and 1000 m), which require high muscle power and strength, and longer endurance events (3000 and 5000 m), which require more muscular endurance. This explains the related observation, whereby, in addition to runners with a specific 1500 m profile, the 1500 m event features both 800 m and 3000/5000 m profile athletes, who can all be successful. Thus, determining a runner's locomotor profile is a compulsory practice for MD coaches to

Table 13.1 Middle-Distance Events, World Record Times, and Associated Running Speeds

Event	World record time (min:sec)	Speed (km/h)
800 m	1:40:91	28.54
1000 m	2:11:96	27.28
1500 m	3:26:00	26.21
Mile	3:43:13	25.28
2000 m	4:44:79	25.28

be able to highlight strengths and weaknesses and consequently determine training priorities.

My analysis (personal observation, J.C. Vollmer) of 800 m to 5000 m race performances of the top 51 all-time 1500 m performers (as of July 21, 2017, range: 3:26.00 world record to 3:30.77) is rich in lessons. These athletes' performances over distances in the ballpark of the 1500 m event are revealing with respect to each athlete's likely phenotypic makeup. For example, we can take performances achieved by these 51 athletes over specific distances ranging from 800 to 5000 m, so long as an athlete is within 98% of the mean fastest distance-specific run time. Doing so provides us with the following results:

- 800 m (n = 44): mean 1:45:18, range 1:41:73 to 1:49:86
- 1000 m (n = 40): mean 2:16:07, range 2:12:18 to 2:20:33
- Mile (n = 49): mean 3:48:81, range 3:43:31 to 3:55:62
- 2000 m (n = 24): mean 4:55:1, range 4:44:79 to 5:06:34
- 3000 m (n = 41): mean 7:39:0, range 7:23:09 to 8:08:08
- 5000 m (n = 32): mean 13:18:95, range 12:50:24 to 14:19:19

From this data, we can divide these short-, middle-, and long-distance specialists into three respective groups:

- Group 1: 17 runners, best performers over 800 m, 1000 m, and 1500 m
- Group 2: 18 runners, best performers exclusively over 1500 m
- Group 3: 16 runners, best performers over 1500 m, 2000 m, 3000 m, and 5000 m

Note that the distances of 1000 m, 2000 m, and 3000 m are not official competition distances in championships, although the 3000 m is an official indoor distance. The merging of the runners into these three groups shows how the 1500 m event is a race distance of energetic convergence, bringing together runners with very different locomotor profiles.

The first profile group (800, 1000, and 1500 m, n = 17) (figure 13.1) had an average 1500 m time of 3:29:57. Athletes show the following performances: 800 m (n = 17) 1:43:5, 1000 m (n = 17) 2:14:3, mile (n = 17) 3:48:5, 2000 m (n = 8) 4:54:3, 3000 (n = 13) 7:47:7, 5000 (n = 7) 13:31:9. These runners display excellent anaerobic capabilities and speed qualities (all runners able to run at around 46.5 over 400 m), which allows them to be in the finals and on podiums in big event championships over 800 m. If they can still perform well over 2000 m, these runners rarely venture beyond their favorite shorter distances. The upper limits of the longer distances include Cram in 4:51:3 over 2000 m, Ngeny in 7:35:5 over 3000 m, and Ramzi with 13:10:7 in the 5000 m. The only one to present a notable performance over 10,000 m is Webb at 27:34:7. Extremely powerful over 1000 m, their performance is typically limited over 3000 m.

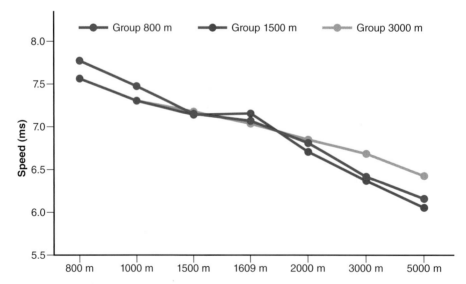

Figure 13.1 Running speed over the different race distances. Error bars omitted for clarity.

Table 13.2 Winners of Major Championships Since 1980 Appearing in the World Top 50 as a Function of Their Locomotor Group Profile

Group 800 m (n=8 athletes for 12 titles)	Group 1500 m (n=3 athletes for 3 titles)	Group 3000 to 5000 m (n=3 athletes for 10 titles)
Coe (Olympics 1980 and 1984)	Rono (Olympics 1988)	Morceli (Worlds 1991, 1993, 1995, Olympics 1996)
Cram (Worlds 1983)	Cacho (Olympics 1992)	El Guerrouj (Worlds 1997, 1999, 2001, 2003, Olympics 2004)
Bile (Worlds 1987)	Centrowitz (Olympics 2016)	Lagat (Worlds 2007)
Ngeny (Olympics 2000)		
Ramzi (Worlds 2005)		
Kiprop (Olympics 2008, Worlds 2011, 2013, 2015)		
Kamel (Worlds 2009)		
Makloufi (Olympics 2012)		

Previous championships (Olympics only) won by Walker (group 1, 1976), Vasala (group 1, 1972), Keino (group 3, 1968), Snell (group 1, 1964), Elliott (group 1, 1960), Delany (group 1, 1956), Barthel (group 1, 1952), and Eriksson (group 2, 1948).

The second profile group (1500 m, n = 18) (figure 13.1) had an average 1500 m time of 3:29:9. Athletes show the following performances: 800 m (n = 16) 1:45:6, 1000 m (n = 14) 2:17:3, mile (n = 17) 3:44:7, 5000 m (n = 9) 13:46:0. This group represents athletes who can perform really well in only the 1500 m. While they are capable of adequate performances over 800 m, they cannot reach podiums. For the most part, they also do not perform well in the upper distances (apart from Cacho, who ran 7:32:9 over 3000 m). They are true 1500 m distance specialists who have developed the relevant physiological capacities and motor skills.

The third profile group (1500, 2000, 3000, 5000 m, n = 16) (figure 13.1) had an average 1500 m time of 3:28:9. Athletes show the following performances: 1000 m (n = 10) 2:17:1, mile (n = 17) 3:48:8, 2000 m (n = 11) 4:51:7, 3000 m (n = 14) 7:29:0, 5000 m (n = 17) 12:58:5. Equipped with exceptional aerobic capacity, this group can also challenge on the world stage over 5000 m. They reach a limit at the 10,000 meters (except for Farah, who developed into a 5000 m to 10,000 m runner). Their great aerobic potential allows them to finish quickly on the last lap.

It should be noted that only one runner, Saïd Aouita (5000 m Olympic champion in Los Angeles), who is a 1500 m (3:29:5), 2000 m (4:50:8), 3000 m (7:29:5), 2 mile (8:13:5), and 5000 m (12:58:0) world record holder, could also claim a group 1 position, with a 1:43:3 over 800 m. Unique in history, he won the bronze in 800 m in Seoul, but got injured and withdrew from the 1500 meters.

Interestingly, the short- and long-distance group profiles tended to have better results in the 1500 m

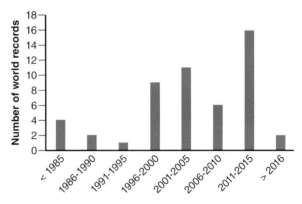

Figure 13.2 Time course of the 51 world best performances in the 1500 m, as of July 21, 2017. Note that this data set included 51 races, where the 50th and 51st performances elicited the exact same time.

event than the 1500 m specialist group profiles in terms of personal bests and podiums at major competitions (table 13.2). As well, there were five runners in group 3, three in group 2, and two in group 1 in the world top 10, as well as ten in group 3, six in group 1, and four in group 3 in the world top 20 for 1500 m.

Note that runners were already running pretty fast over 1500 m more than 30 years ago. The 50 best performances (n=51) ranging from 3:26:0 (world record) to 3:30:77 were achieved at different times (figure 13.2). Comparing the periods of achievement of the top 50 best performances in the various disciplines, it can be seen that while for the 800 m event, seven performances were achieved before 1989, there were no top 50 performances prior to 1996 in the

5000 and 10,000 m events. This shows that disciplines with a strong aerobic dominance continued to progress more than the races relying on more mixed energetic profiles. Among the 51 best performances ever in the 1500 m, 23 were performed in Monaco; 7 in Brussels; 4 in Zürich; 3 in Berlin, Rome, and Paris; 2 in Rieti and Nice; and 1 in Cologne, Doha, Lausanne, and Seville. The Monaco meeting has become the fastest meeting in history, and even more in recent years. Among the 18 best performances of the top 51 that were performed since 2012, 17 were achieved in Monaco on the Louis II Stadium track.

Relative Contribution of Physical Performance

As outlined, the metabolic and neuromuscular underpinnings of a 1500 m runner are essential, and even the phenotype engine makeup of the individual may be a performance determinant (i.e., groups 1 to 3). However, tactics also play a major role in performance outcome, as this impacts how the engine may actually be used during a race.

Championship Race: Twelve competitors will qualify to start during a final of a world championship or Olympic Games. Historically, this number decreased from 12 to 9 at the Melbourne Olympics (10 at the Munich Olympics) before returning to 12 since the Helsinki World Championships in 1983. The number of runners on the starting line influences a key aspect of this event: the tactics, which are an important determinant of success (figure 13.3). If the race objective was essentially to run as fast as possible, as it is for a record race, we might see hares launch during a race to help achieve this objective. During a championship race, it's a completely different story. The 12 runners on the starting line of a major finals all have the will to win, bringing 12 different strategies or racing tactics to the fore, which evolve during the race according to the circumstances. Occurrences might include starting quickly in the first 100 m; running at a constant pace "on the train" (i.e., one after the other) at a sustained high speed; using intermittent accelerations, a progressive acceleration, a sudden surge, or sometimes even teamwork tactics as each country can have three runners start if they manage to qualify during the preliminary rounds. Thus, the position of a runner in the peloton at key moments during the race is essential, especially toward the end of the race. These aspects all need to be addressed and simulated in situational training sessions to prepare the athlete.

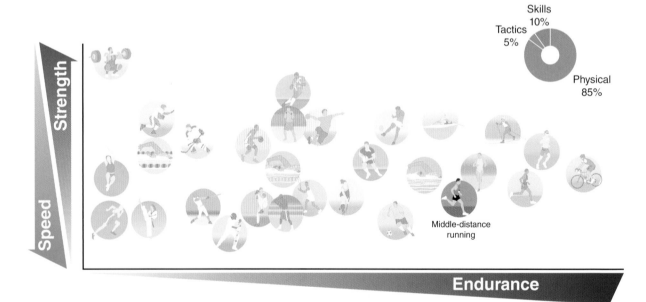

Figure 13.3 The position of the runner on the three axes illustrates the relative importance of the three main physical capacities for elite middle-distance 1500 m competition. Outside of critical psychological aspects, which are difficult to quantify, the pie chart shows the general relative importance of physical competence (85%), skills (10%), and tactical awareness (5%) for success.

Adapted from G.A. Nader, "Concurrent Strength and Endurance Training: From Molecules to Man," *Medicine & Science in Sports & Exercise* 38, no. 11 (2006): 1965-1970.

Another aspect that can't be neglected comes from the impact of successive races occurring before the final in qualifying rounds (series, semifinals, finals, interspersed by a rest day). Like a Tour de France road cyclist who must perform day after day, the MD runner must have an aerobic system that is highly engaged to facilitate recovery between rounds. Since the end of the 1980s, few runners double across the 800 m and 1500 m male competitions. Exceptions include Coe in Los Angeles (winner in 1500 m and second in the 800 m) and P. Elliott in Seoul in 1988 (fourth in the 800 m and second in the 1500 m). While runners more often double across 5000 m and 10,000 m (they have one week of recovery between events), few have ever doubled across 1500 m and 5000 m, with the exception of El Guerrouj in Athens. Most recently, however, Makloufi completed the 800 m and 1500 m double successfully (2 × 2nd) in 2016, which is remarkable considering the difficulty of the sequencing of the races, inducing a high density of work in a very short period of time at the highest level.

To gain further insight into the role that pacing and tactics play in 1500 m performance outcomes, we analyzed performance results of the major championships of the modern era (28 Olympic finals and World Championships since the Munich Olympics in 1972). Here, we found the average time of the winner was 3:35:55 (± 4.10), with performance times ranging from 3:27:66 (Hicham El Guerrouj) at the 1999 World Championships in Seville to Matthew Centrowitz's victory at the Rio Olympics in 3:50:01 (the worst winning time in an Olympics final since 1932!). This extremely large (22.45 s) time difference between winners demonstrates the large role that tactics play in 1500 m race outcomes (figure 13.3). For example, in a study of world mile records, Noakes et al. (12) showed that the slowest lap occurred in 90% of the races in either the second (34%) or third (56%) laps. The last lap was only ever slowest in two races (6%), while in 24 races (76%) it was either the fastest (38%) or second fastest (38%). Record races are special events generally organized for a single runner, in which the only goal is to break the record time. These types of races do not have the richness of a championship, with its wavering pacing strategies and twists and turns. As shown by Thiel (16) in his study of MD events at the Beijing Olympic Games, the profile of a championship race is completely different, including random occurrences and a pace marked by microvariations throughout, even when pace might appear regular to the casual

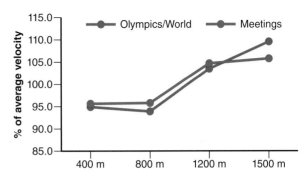

Figure 13.4 Comparison of the pacing profiles during Olympics and World Championships (in which runners chase medals) versus meetings or record races (in which runners try to break records).

observer. The only consistent occurrence is that the gold medal always is won at the end by a sprint over the last 400 m. Our analysis of the 28 finals of the 1500 m at Olympics and World Championships since 1972 shows the pacing pattern illustrated in figure 13.4, alongside the comparison profile of a typical meeting or record race.

Only at the World Championships in Seville (1999) and the Sydney Olympics (2000) did these typical patterns (figure 13.4) not occur. At those races, the first 400 m was markedly faster than the second and third laps due to team tactics; the pace was pushed to the benefit of Hicham El Guerrouj.

Typically, the faster the first 800 m, the slower the last 400 m due to energetic aspects. Thus, fatigue resistance is a particularly important element to train for in the 1500 m event to meet two important requirements:

1. being able to respond to a rapid first 800 m start without burning out metabolically speaking, and

2. being able to finish quickly over the last lap of the race whatever the race situation (table 13.3).

In general, the race is decided across the last 100 m of the 1500 m race, irrespective of the preceding antics.

Nevertheless, over 1500 m, runners can lose a race because of too fast a start or inappropriate accelerations applied at certain moments of the race to gain positions, but what is clear is that 1500 m races are won predominantly in the second part of the race. To win, exceptional fatigue resistance and a high top speed are essential characteristics of all podium athletes.

It should be noted also that the last 200 m of a 1500 m event are often run faster than the last 200 m

Table 13.3 Average, Slowest, and Fastest Running Times (With Average Speed) Measured Over Select Running Portions of the World Top 50, 1500 m Event Performances

Lap	Average time (s)	Slowest time (s)	Fastest time (s)	Average speed (m/s)
Last 800 m	1:50:15 ± 1:33	1:54:07 (Sydney Olympics 2000)	1:46:78 (Athens Olympics 2004)	7:27
Last 500 m	1:06:42 ± 1:24	1:08:93 (Edmonton 2001)	1:04:24 (Stuttgart 1993)	7:58
Last 400 m	52:30 ± 1:24	54:6 (Edmonton 2001)	50:46 (Barcelona 1992)	7:69
Last 300 m	39:30 ± 1:18	41:18 (Edmonton 2001)	37:57 (Barcelona 1992)	7:69
Last 200 m	26:50 ± 0:70	28:03 (Edmonton 2001)	25:18 (Montreal 1976)	7:69

of the 800 m event. Thus, the aerobic aspect is vital in the 1500 m to preserve the important anaerobic resources and neuromuscular freshness. Put another way, an athlete's aerobic foundation spares his speed reserve so it can be released on command.

Conversely, when racing starts too fast (over the first 400 m), which is often the case in record races, achieving a good result also requires high levels of fatigue resistance toward the end of the race. Clearly, the 1500 m event is a complex race requiring both exceptional aerobic capabilities and also top anaerobic abilities (basic speed and fatigue resistance). The 1500 m runner is therefore a particularly complete runner, which is why the 1500 m may be the most interesting middle-distance running race and is often termed a blue-ribbon event in athletics.

Targets of Physical Performance in Middle-Distance Running

Studies have shown that the contribution of aerobic energy supply to a 1500 m simulated race ranges from 77% (5) to 84% ± 1% for well-trained male runners (14) and about 86% for women (5). Note that even from these comparisons across genders, where it's expected that males would have a greater degree of muscularity due to the influence of higher basal testosterone levels, that an individual's degree of muscularity appears related to his or her anaerobic capabilities (18). $\dot{V}O_2$max values of 1500 m runners have been reported as 72 ± 2 ml·kg^{-1}·min^{-1} for well-trained males (5), 75.1 ± 6.1 ml·kg^{-1}·min^{-1} for national-level runners (1) and 78.1 ± 3.7 ml·kg^{-1}·min^{-1} (v$\dot{V}O_2$max: 20.44 ± 1 km/h) for elite French runners (6). Two of the best French runners ever, Baala (3:28:98, 12th fastest performance of all time;

1:43:15 for 800 m; two gold medals at European Championships; 2003 silver medalist; Beijing Olympic bronze medalist) and Bob Tahri (3000 m steeplechase specialist; 3:32:79 for 1500 m; World bronze medalist in 2009; two-time medal winner at the European Championships; two-time Olympic finalist; six-time finalist in the world from 2003 to 2011; retained European record in the 3000 m steeplechase in 8:06:91 and then 8:01:18) displayed $\dot{V}O_2$max values of 79.11 ml·kg^{-1}·min^{-1} and 81.49 ml·kg^{-1}·min^{-1}, respectively.

Interestingly, Boileau et al. (2) showed $\dot{V}O_2$max to be more correlated with performance for middle distance (68.9 ml·kg^{-1}·min^{-1}, r = 0.70) versus long-distance runners (76.9 ml·kg^{-1}·min^{-1}, r = 0.32), suggesting the importance of this physiological variable for predicting 1500 m event success. This may be related to the fact that $\dot{V}O_2$max would be reached during the event approximately 78 ± 17 s after the start, corresponding to a distance of 464 ± 67 m in runners finishing a 1500 m race in 4:08 ± 9 (7, 8). Once $\dot{V}O_2$max is achieved, $\dot{V}O_2$ generally drops correspondingly with the reduction in running speed before stabilizing during the middle portion of the race and then clearly dropping during the last 300 m; in fact, the final acceleration relies strongly on the anaerobic metabolic contribution.

Despite Tahri's very high $\dot{V}O_2$max (81.49 ml·kg^{-1}·min^{-1}) and exceptional performances from 3000 m to 10,000 meters, he only ever presented very good, but not top, performance over 1500 m (3:32:79). Tahri's profile confirms that to be a world top performer over 1500 m, qualities other than $\dot{V}O_2$max are required. In fact, Ingham et al. (10) showed, using an allometric model, that the maximal speed associated with $\dot{V}O_2$, in direct relation to running economy, can explain 95.9% of the performance variance. Anaerobic capacity is also a determinant, as evidenced by the relatively high blood lactate values measured post race (18.4 mmol/L^{-1}) following a 1500 m event (11). Other measures of anaerobic work capacity and neuromuscular power, such as the Margaria stair climbing test and vertical jump power, respectively, have also been shown as being related to 1500 m event outcome (9).

As a consequence, 1500 m runners have a very complete physiological and locomotor profile, as described by top coaches including Peter Coe (4), the father and coach of S. Coe (former 800 m and 1500 m world record holder) and H. Wilson (19), coach of S. Ovett (former world record holder of the 1500 m) as well as from academic studies (3, 13, 15, 17). A nonexhaustive list of the required qualities for successful 1500 m participation are provided in detail in table 13.4 and illustrated simply in figure 13.5.

Table 13.4 Typical Characteristics of Successful 1500 m Runners

Height	The longer the event, the shorter the runners (18) • 800 m: 182.5±6.2 cm • 1500 m: 179.8±5.2 cm • 3000 m steeplechase: 178.2±4.2 cm • 5000 m: 175.5±2.6 cm • 10,000 m: 174.8±3.2 cm
Body mass	The longer the distance, the lighter the runners (18) • 800 m: 67.6±4.8 kg • 1500 m: 64.8±4.9 kg • 3000 m: 65.0±4.8 kg • 5000 m: 61.5±4.7 kg • 10,000 m: 60.3±4.6 kg
Metabolic aspects	• A high $\dot{V}O_2$max and, most importantly, a high v$\dot{V}O_2$max (linked to running economy) • A high anaerobic threshold (the endurance factor, 1500 m runners are also capable of performances over 5000 m and 10,000 m). The aerobic factor is essential because it allows the runner to release his speed.
Neuromuscular aspects	• A good race economy, which influences v$\dot{V}O_2$max • A high anaerobic capacity and power • High lower-limb neuromuscular power (leg strength and power, foot quality) • A good level of basic speed with the ability to accelerate • Good running technique and lower-limb efficiency
Tactical intelligence	1500 m runners must have good awareness of their capacities in relation to the race situation, and be able to adapt their plan accordingly to maximize their outcome.
Strong ability to tolerate pain	Every race inevitably elicits very high blood lactate levels (and associated acidosis) (11).
Age	1500 m runners are relatively young when compared to runners in other events. The average age of the top 50 all-time 1500 m runners is 24.8±3.0 years. Excluding those runners still active who are likely to beat their best performances in the future, the average becomes 25.2±3.2 yr. This average age has decreased slightly compared to a study conducted in 1995 (average age=25.5 yr). This difference can be explained by the arrival of Kenyan runners at earlier maturity but likely similar training ages. In general, Caucasian runners tend to mature later, between 2 to 3 yr later on average. The breakdown by age group is as follows for the world top 50: • <20 yr: 3 • 20 to 23 yr: 12 • 23 to 26 yr: 14 • 26 to 29 yr: 15 • 29 to 32 yr: 5 • >32 yr: 2 The oldest top performer was William Tanui (33 years old). This average age is slightly higher than that of 800 m runners (24.2±3.2 yr) but less than that of 3000 m steeplechase runners (25.9±2.8 yr), 5000 m runners (26.2±3.7 yr), and 10,000 m runners (26.4±3.9 yr).

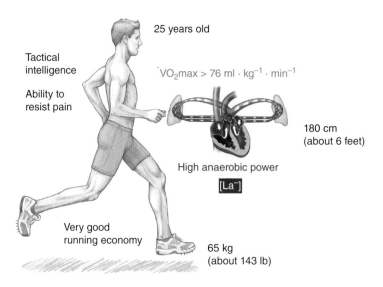

Figure 13.5 Ideal profile of a top 1500 m performer.

Key Weapons, Manipulations, and Surveillance Tools

Recall that weapons refer to the high-intensity interval training (HIIT) formats we can use to target the physiological responses of importance. In this section, we present the different HIIT weapons used within a 1500 m runner's training program, their manipulations, and ways to monitor their effectiveness (surveillance).

HIIT Weapons

The distribution of training content (% of total weekly volume) for an elite 1500 m runner is as follows:

- Aerobic work carried out as both continuous (submaximal) and in intermittent (HIIT) forms represents 80% (winter period) to 70% of the training content depending on the season,

- Race and speed technique work represents 5% to 10%,

- General physical preparation and strength work represents 5% to 10%,

- Work around the specific race pace represents 0% (winter period) to 15%, and

- Miscellaneous work (e.g., other sporting activities such as cycling, swimming, cross-country skiing, mountain biking, etc., to add variety) represents 0% to 5%.

With a greater volume of metabolic conditioning completed as continuous submaximal running (80%

to 90%) and with the intensity determined, depending on the time of year and athletes, using percentages of $v\dot{V}O_2max$, HR_{max}, lactate threshold, race-specific speed or even RPE, HIIT sessions become the key and nonnegotiable components of training used to improve race performance, despite making up only 10% to 20% of all training sessions combined. As detailed throughout the book, the majority of practitioners, if not all, use different forms of HIIT, which vary in terms of the intensity or format. To prepare for the 1500 m, as with other distances, HIIT is used for three main reasons (or targets) when it comes to:

1. Improving oxidative function, namely ($\dot{V}O_2max$ (type 1, 2, 3, 4 targets),

2. Improving anaerobic function, namely anaerobic power and capacity (type 3 and 4 targets), and

3. Targeting and developing responses and adaptive comfort at race-specific speed (type 4 targets), with specific emphasis on achieving adaptations at the neuromuscular level.

At different times of the preparation, and depending on the athlete's profile, I (JCV) will use many forms of HIIT as either short (50%) or long intervals (50%; figure 13.6), with the respective proportion between the two varying according to the training phases. Runs last from 10 s to 8 min (i.e., time to exhaustion at $v\dot{V}O_2max$), using repetitions from 80 to 3000 m at an intensity ranging from 90% of $v\dot{V}O_2max$ (3000 m) to almost maximal (10 s).

Number of repetitions (3 to 20) and series become a direct function of the work interval duration and session objectives.

Manipulations of Interval Training Variables

The attainment of specific HIIT responses, or hitting select target types, for each individual runner, at key moments in preparation, is achieved via the manipulation of at least one of the 12 variables presented in chapter 4 (figure 4.2). Figure 13.7 illustrates this in a 1500 m runner, using a 300 m repetition example, in which adjustment of the recovery characteristics (and only this) allows us to reach three distinct targets.

Continuing with the 300 m repetition example using sessions designed for a top 1500 m runner (PB: 3:36 s, vV̇O₂max 22.5 to 22.8 km/h), HIIT target types (figure 1.5) can additionally be manipulated using several variables at a time, such as the intensity of the work interval and recovery characteristics (table 13.5). Given the importance of running at the right intensity, and in turn, targeting the right acute biological responses, controlling running speed is paramount. It is important not to start too fast in these HIIT sessions, as doing so creates excessive fatigue that can compromise both the quality of the training and the ability of the athlete to complete session repetitions. Several strategies can be used to ensure that runners run at the desired intensity, including:

- Run one or two straight lines (100 m) at the end of the warm-up at the target pace,
- Give split times (using whistle or voice) during rehearsals,

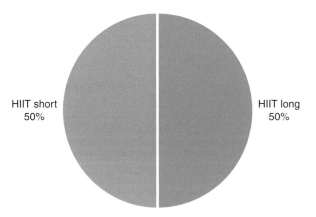

Figure 13.6 Percentage of the different HIIT formats (weapons) used throughout the annual season for elite 1500 m runners. Note here that medium-length intervals (1-2 min) are used often for middle-distance runners, referred to as long intervals consistently throughout the rest of the book.

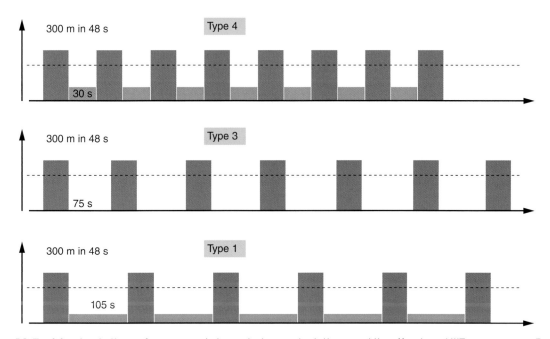

Figure 13.7 Manipulation of recovery interval characteristics and its effect on HIIT responses. Recovery = 30 s at 50% vV̇O₂max (type 4); recovery = 75 s passive (type 3); recovery = 105 s easy jog (type 1).

- Use an external pacing beeper to give the athlete the right rhythm, or have the athlete set the splits on his watch (although this may require reprogramming or readjustment if the coach changes the session during training),
- Coach uses bike to pace runner appropriately, and
- Use of other experienced runners as pacers.

Additionally, specific HIIT target-type example sessions I've (JCV) used with my athletes are shown in tables 13.6 to 13.10.

HIIT with long intervals typically run 94% to 96% of vVO$_2$max across durations ranging from 2:30 to 8:00 (and possibly up to 10:00) or distances from 800 m to 3000 m. This work can be done both outdoors (forest, soccer pitch, the preferred option) or on a track. HIIT with moderate-duration intervals typically run 98% to 104% of vVO$_2$max over 1 to 2 min duration. This work is mostly done on the track. HIIT with short intervals can be run 105% to 108% of vVO$_2$max over durations of less than 1 min, and are systematically executed on the track.

Table 13.5 HIIT Variable Manipulation Effects on Target Types Using 300 m Intervals

HIIT target	Session	Work intensity	Recovery duration	Recovery modality	Between series
Type 1	15 × 300 m	95% vVO$_2$max (49 to 50 s)	45 s	Jog	
Type 2	2 × (6 × 300 m)	105% vVO$_2$max (45.5 to 46 s)	1 min, 30 s	Jog	6 min walk or jog
Type 3	8 × 300 m	115% vVO$_2$max (41 to 41.5 s)	3 min	Walk and jog	
Type 4	6 × 300 m	120% vVO$_2$max (38.5 to 39 s)	8 min	Walk	
Type 5	4 × 300 m	Near max speed (36 s)	12 min	Sitting or walking	

Table 13.6 Example of Type 1 HIIT Sessions Used to Prepare for a 1500 m Race

Session	Work intensity	Recovery duration	Recovery modality	Between series
2 × (3 × 1000 m)	95% vVO$_2$max	2 min	Jog	4 min jog
4 × 1500 m	92% vVO$_2$max	2 min, 30 s	Jog	
12 × 400 m	98% vVO$_2$max	1 min	Jog	

Table 13.7 Example of Type 2 HIIT Sessions Used to Prepare for a 1500 m Race

Session	Work intensity	Recovery duration	Recovery modality	Between series
Fartlek (30 to 45 min)	Near vVO$_2$max (RPE) for 45 s to 3 min, outdoors for a total of 15 to 20 min	30 s to 1 min, 45 s	Jog	
2 × (300/400/500/600/500/400/300 m)	100% vVO$_2$max for 45 s to 1 min, 30 s	45 s to 1 min, 15 s	Jog	6 min walk or jog

Table 13.8 Example of Type 3 HIIT Sessions Used to Prepare for a 1500 m Race

Session	Work intensity	Recovery duration	Recovery modality	Between series
2 (6 × 300 m)	110% vVO$_2$max	2 min, 30 s	Walk, jog	6 min walk
3 (3 × 500 m)	105% vVO$_2$max	1 min, 30 s	Jog	4 min walk

Table 13.9 Example of Type 4 HIIT Sessions Used to Prepare for a 1500 m Race

Session	Work Intensity	Recovery duration	Recovery modality	Between series
3×(800 m+400 m)	800 m at 1500 m speed 400 m at 800 m speed	3 min	Jog	8 min walk
5×(400 m+200 m)	400 m at 1500 m speed 200 m at increasing speed	None		6 min walk
2 (4×300 m)	>1500 m speed	3 min	Walk	8 min walk

Table 13.10 Example of Type 5 HIIT Sessions Used to Prepare for a 1500 m Race

Session	Work intensity	Recovery duration	Recovery modality
500 m+400 m+300 m	800 m speed	10 to 12 min	Walk
3×500 m	>1500 m speed	6 min	Walk
4×400 m	>1500 m speed	3 min, then 2 min, then 1 min	Walk

Load Surveillance and Monitoring Tools

To quantify training load in my runners, I tend to count repetitions at different specific speeds (e.g., race pace, v$\dot{V}O_2$max) and look at cumulated training time and distance run across each macrocycle. I also often ask my runners for their post-session RPE as a way of judging session intensity, although I don't use RPE as part of a global load measure.

Training Status Surveillance and Monitoring Tools

While nothing will ever replace the coach's eye, the main training status monitoring tool I use is the stopwatch. The monitoring of laps or split times during repetitions (average times but also progression of these split times throughout the session) is very useful for gauging progress and detecting a fatigued state. I also measure lactate and HR responses in certain HIIT sessions (i.e., tables 13.8 to 13.10) and especially HR drift between HIIT repetitions, as well as post-session HR recovery as indices of both fitness and freshness. Along these same lines, but for longer run types only, I observe the GPS-speed/HR relationship as a proxy of running economy.

The standardized HIIT sessions, generally performed indoors to avoid environmental fluctuations and associated reduced reliability, might include:

- Post aerobic cycle training assessment (every 8 weeks): 4 × 1000 m at v$\dot{V}O_2$max (interspersed with 1 min, 45 s of passive rest with lactate measured after 1 min) + 5 min passive recovery + all-out 400 m (lactate sample after 3, 10, and 15 min).

- Race pace target session: 4 × 1000 m at 1500 m speed (interspersed with 5 min passive rest with lactate measured after 3 min) + all-out 500 m (lactate sample after 3, 10, and 15 min).

- Anaerobic capacity on a treadmill: 40 s at v$\dot{V}O_2$max on a 10% grade + 15 min passive rest with lactate measured after 3, 10, and 15 min + run to exhaustion at v$\dot{V}O_2$max on a 10% gradient. I use the difference between the post-40 s lactate and post-run-to-exhaustion lactate as a measure of anaerobic capacity.

Strategies for Structuring the Training Program Using HIIT

The implementation of HIIT within the overall program is as much a science as it is an art. Here, I use a blend of experience, combined with an understanding of physiology, biology, and an athlete's history and profile to come up with what I believe is the ideal HIIT option that will best develop the athlete appropriately at any particular time in the program.

Controllable and Uncontrollable Factors

I have mostly always worked with professional athletes, whose lives and daily duties have been mostly planned around their training times. For this reason, we rarely need to compromise training for work or other commitments. This factor makes training the priority and shapes the athlete's life around the most important training sessions to permit optimal recovery. Following these guidelines and, in particular, having these programmed an especially long time ahead of the main competitions provides good control over the training cycles and daily content. While you can always be caught off guard by last-minute details (e.g., family, traffic, media obligations) that can derail the process, the programming for MD runners can typically be well implemented.

Program Structure and Progression

I generally organize my yearly plan using five typical macrocycles:

1. Preparatory phase/development phase 1 (October to March)
2. Preparatory phase/development phase 2 (March to mid-May)
3. Precompetition (mid-May to end of June)
4. Competition (July to August)
5. Taper (before main competition)

Each of these cycles has different aims in terms of their physiological adaptation goals and performance development, with the quantity and type of HIIT sequences varying accordingly (table 13.11).

Incorporation of HIIT

HIIT sequences are generally part of a complete training session, which also include warm-up drills (running technique, often before HIIT) and sometimes strength and coordination exercise (before or after). The form of these sessions often influences the training contents and sequences, e.g., running drills before an HIIT sequence are more likely to be performed on a track or the grass part of the track than in a forest.

Sample Training Programs

In this section, I present several examples of the typical HIIT weapons that I program within each macrocycle (table 13.11) to target each specific HIIT type for two 1500 m runners who display the contrasting locomotor profiles described in the first part of the chapter, namely a group 1 versus group 3 individual (figure 13.1).

Preparatory Period (October to Mid-May)

The preparatory period is the longest overall period of the year and lasts from October to mid-May for most runners without indoor competition.

The 20% of HIIT training time in phase 1 sees a distribution as follows: type 1, 15% (table 13.12); type 2, 3% (table 13.13); type 3, 2% (table 13.14); type 4, 0%; type 5, 0%. This breakdown is detailed in tables 13.12 through 13.14. Note: There are no

Table 13.11 Typical HIIT Target Type Emphases Throughout the Season for Elite 1500 m Runners

Macrocycle	% of HIIT HIIT sessions/total weekly sessions	Type 1	Type 2	Type 3	Type 4	Type 5
Preparatory phase\development phase 1 October to March	20% (2 or 3 HIIT/12 sessions)	15%	3%	2%		
Preparatory phase\development phase 2 March to mid-May	25% (3 HIIT/12 sessions)	10%	5%	5%	5%	
Precompetition mid-May to end of June	20% (2 or 3 HIIT/12 sessions)			5%	10%	5%
Competition June to August	15% (2 HIIT/12 sessions)		5%		5%	5%
Taper (before main competition)	10% (2 HIIT/12 sessions)				5%	5%

Table 13.12 HIIT Type 1 (15%) in Developmental Phase 1 of the Preparatory Period in Elite 1500 m Runners With Group 1 Versus Group 3 Profiles

HIIT with long intervals at 92% to 96% of v$\dot{V}O_2$max for effort times from 2 min 30 s to 8 min (and possibly up to 10 min) or distances from 800 m to 3000 m. This work can be done both outdoors (forest, soccer pitch) or on a track.	
800 m/1500 m profile (Group 1)	**1500 m/5000 m profile (Group 3)**
• 4 × 1200 m in steps of 400 m to 92%/94%/96% of v$\dot{V}O_2$max with a jog recovery of 3 min • Fartlek as 3 min, 4 min, 2 min, 2 min, 4 min, 3 min (pace between 92% to 94% of v$\dot{V}O_2$max) with jogged recoveries of 1 to 2 min (duration and pace of sensations) • Fartlek as 2 min, 3 min, 2 min, 4 min, 3 min, 2 min, 3 min, 2 min (pace between 94% and 96% v$\dot{V}O_2$max) with recoveries of 1 min to 1 min, 30 s of active jog (duration and pace by feel)	• 3 × 6 min or 3 × 2000 m at 95% v$\dot{V}O_2$max with active recovery of 1:30 between sets and 3 min active recovery between series • 2 (3 × 3 min) or 2 (3 × 1000 m) to 95 or 96% of v$\dot{V}O_2$max with active recovery of 1:15 and 4 min between series • 3000 m/2000 m/1000 m at 92%/94%/96% of v$\dot{V}O_2$max with active recovery of 3 min and then 2 min • 1000 m/2000 m/2000 m/1000 m at 96%/95% of v$\dot{V}O_2$max with 2 min, 3 min, 2 min jog recovery
HIIT with moderate-duration intervals (duration of 1 to 2 min effort) from 98% to 102% of v$\dot{V}O_2$max.	
800 m/1500 m profile (Group 1)	**1500 m/5000 m profile (Group 3)**
• 3 (400/600/400 m) at 100%/102%/102% v$\dot{V}O_2$max with passive recovery of 90 s between reps and 4 min passive between series • 2 (5 × 400 m) at 102% of the v$\dot{V}O_2$max with passive recovery of 1:30 between reps and 4 min passive recovery between series • 3 (600 + 500 + 400 m) at 100%/102% of v$\dot{V}O_2$max with 1:30 and then 1:15 of passive recovery between reps and 4 min passive between series	• 3 (2 × 800 m) to 98%/102% of v$\dot{V}O_2$max with active recovery of 1:45 and 4 min between series • 4 (2 × 600 m) of 100% to 102% of v$\dot{V}O_2$max with recovery of 1:30 jog and 3 min between series • 2 (4 × 500 m) from 100% to 102% v$\dot{V}O_2$max with recovery of 1:15 jog and 5 min between series
HIIT with short intervals (duration of effort less than 1 min) from 104% to 106 % of v$\dot{V}O_2$max	
Both profiles	
• 2 (6 × 300 m) at 104% v$\dot{V}O_2$max with light jog recovery and 3 min passive between series • 3 (6 × 200 m) at 106% v$\dot{V}O_2$max with 1:00 to 1:15 jog recovery and 6 min passive between series • 4 (200/300/200 m) at 106%/104%/106% v$\dot{V}O_2$max with 1:45 jog recovery and 6 min passive between series	

Table 13.13 HIIT Type 2 (3%), Metabolic (O_2 Plus Neuromuscular), in Developmental Phase 1 of the Preparatory Period in Elite 1500 m Runners With Group 1 Versus Group 3 Profiles

HIIT with long intervals: none HIIT with moderate-duration intervals: none HIIT with short intervals: 106% to 108% of the v$\dot{V}O_2$max	
800 m/1500 m profile (Group 1)	**1500 m/5000 m profile (Group 3)**
• 3 (4 × 250 m) at 106% v$\dot{V}O_2$max with recovery (alternating walking and jogging) of 2:15 passive between reps and 6 min passive between series • 4 (300 + 200 + 200 m) to 108% v$\dot{V}O_2$max with recovery (alternating walking and jogging) of 2 min between 300 and 200 and then 1:30 between the 200s, and 5 passive min between series	• 3 (4 × 300 m) at 106% of the v$\dot{V}O_2$max with recovery (alternating walking and jogging) of 1:45 passive and 6 min active between series • 3 (6 × 200 m) to 108% of the v$\dot{V}O_2$max with a recovery (alternating stepping and jogging) of 1:30 between reps and 5 min active between series

This work can be carried out uphill (5%-7% slope) by decreasing the quantity by a smaller number of series (two instead of three) or by reducing the number of repetitions per series and by adjusting the pace (about 10% less than the v$\dot{V}O_2$max pace). Examples: 2 × (4 × 300 m) or 3 × (4 × 200 m) uphill. Light jog recovery on descent. More than twice the effort time between repetitions and 6 min walk between runs.

Table 13.14 HIIT Type 3 (2%), Metabolic (O_2 Plus Anaerobic), in Developmental Phase 1 of the Preparatory Period in Elite 1500 m Runners With Group 1 Versus Group 3 Profiles

HIIT with long intervals: paces greater than 102%/104% v$\dot{V}O_2$max	
800 m/1500 m profile (Group 1)	**1500 m/5000 m profile (Group 3)**
• 4×800 m in form (600 m to 102% v$\dot{V}O_2$max + last 200 m with maximum acceleration), passive recovery of 8 min between repetitions • 5×600 m in form (400 m to 104% v$\dot{V}O_2$max then acceleration over 200 m), recovery of 6 min (walking and jogging) between repetitions	• 3×1200 m in form (400 m to 104% v$\dot{V}O_2$max + 400 m average pace 102% v$\dot{V}O_2$max + 400 m to 104% v$\dot{V}O_2$max), passive recovery 12 min between repetitions • 3×(1000 m + 400 m) at 100% v$\dot{V}O_2$max for 1000 m and 102%/104% v$\dot{V}O_2$max for 400 m with recovery of 2 min jog between 1000 m and 400 m and 8 min between repetitions
HIIT with moderate-duration intervals. Average intervals: paces greater than 110% v$\dot{V}O_2$max	
800 m/1500 m profile (Group 1)	**1500 m/5000 m profile (Group 3)**
2×(3×400 m) • First series: first 400 m at 106% v$\dot{V}O_2$max, second 400 m faster at 108% v$\dot{V}O_2$max, third 400 m at 110% v$\dot{V}O_2$max, recovery of 3 min between repetitions and 10 min before the second series • Second series: first 400 m at 110% v$\dot{V}O_2$max, second 400 m at 108% v$\dot{V}O_2$max, third 400 m pace at 110% v$\dot{V}O_2$max, recovery 3 min between 400 m	2×(2×600 m) in form (500 m at 108% v$\dot{V}O_2$max + last 100 m faster), recovery of 6 min between repetitions and 10 min between series
HIIT with short intervals: from 110% to 114% v$\dot{V}O_2$max	
800 m/1500 m profile (Group 1)	**1500 m/5000 m profile (Group 3)**
2×(5×200 m) at 112% v$\dot{V}O_2$max for the first three 200 m repetitions and 114% v$\dot{V}O_2$max for the fourth and fifth 200 m repetitions, recovery of 2 min (marching) between repetitions and 8 min between series	6×300 m at 110% v$\dot{V}O_2$max for 200 m then finish faster in the last 100 m, 2 min recovery (stepping) between repetitions

objectives touching type 4 metabolic (anaerobic plus muscle neuro) and type 5 metabolic (peripheral O_2 plus anaerobic and muscle neuro).

For phase 2 (March to mid-May), HIIT distribution moves to 25% with the following breakdown of target types: type 1, 10% (table 13.15); type 2, 5% (table 13.16); type 3, 5% (table 13.17); type 4, 5% (table 13.18); type 5, 0%. The objective of this phase is to maintain the quality developed during the previous months. The breakdown of this phase is detailed in tables 13.15 through 13.18. Note: There are no objectives touching target 5 metabolic (peripheral O_2 plus anaerobic and muscle neuro).

Precompetitive Period (Mid-May to End of June)

The precompetitive period runs from mid-May to the end of June, with the 20% of HIIT work broken into the following distribution of target types: type 1, 0%; type 2, 0%; type 3, 5% (table 13.19); type 4, 10% (table 13.20); type 5, 5% (table 13.21). This breakdown is detailed in tables 13.19 to 13.21. Note:

There are no objectives touching type 1, metabolic O_2, or type 2, metabolic (O_2 plus neuromuscular).

Competitive Period (June to August)

The competitive period is primarily comprised of races. These races are separated by aerobic-type work, aimed at aiding recovery. The forms of HIIT reappear as part of a new work cycle preparatory to the main objective and sometimes as a small reminder between races if races are separated by sufficient time. The distribution of HIIT work shifts to 15%, with a target distribution as type 1, 0%; type 2, 5% (table 13.22); type 3, 0%; type 4, 5% (table 13.23); type 5, 5% (table 13.24). The breakdown is detailed in tables 13.22 to 13.24. Note: There are no objectives touching type 1 or type 3.

Tapering Period Before Main Competition

The tapering period occurs in the week before major competitions. The aim is to gain freshness. The distribution of HIIT work shifts to 10% with

Table 13.15　HIIT Type 1 (10%), Metabolic O_2, in Developmental Phase 2 of the Preparatory Period in Elite 1500 m Runners With Group 1 Versus Group 3 Profiles

HIIT with long intervals: from 94% to 98% of the $v\dot{V}O_2$max on times from 3 to 6 min. This work can be done both on track and in nature (fields or forest).	
800 m/1500 m profile (Group 1)	**1500 m/5000 m profile (Group 3)**
• 2× (1500 m+400 m) at 94% $v\dot{V}O_2$max (1500 m) and 100% $v\dot{V}O_2$max (400 m), recovery of 1:30 (jogging) between 1500 m and 400 m and 1:30 active between series • 3×1200 m (400+400+400 m progressive pace at 94%/95%/96% $v\dot{V}O_2$max), 4 min active between series • Fartlek as 2 min, 3 min, 4, min, 4 min, 3 min between 92% and 95% $v\dot{V}O_2$max, active recovery of 1 min to 1:30 • 2× (3×800 m) at 98% $v\dot{V}O_2$max, recovery of 1:45 (jogging) and 6 min between series by feel	• 2× (6 min+3 min) or 2× (2000 m+1000 m) to 95% $v\dot{V}O_2$max, passive recovery of 1:45 and 4 min (jogging) • 4×3 min or 4×1000 m to 98% $v\dot{V}O_2$max, passive recovery of 1:15 to 1:30 (jogging) • 2000 m+1000 m+1000 m at 95% and 96% $v\dot{V}O_2$max, recovery of 1:30 (jogging) • 1000 m+2000 m+1000 m at 98% and 96% $v\dot{V}O_2$max, recovery of 1:45 (jogging)
HIIT with moderate-duration intervals: from 100% to 104% of $v\dot{V}O_2$max	
800 m/1500 m profile (Group 1)	**1500 m/5000 m profile (Group 3)**
• 2× (5×400 m) to 104% $v\dot{V}O_2$max, recovery of 1 min (jogging) and 6 min between series • 3× (400+500+400 m) at 102%/100%/102% $v\dot{V}O_2$max, 1:15 recovery (jogging) and 4 min between series • 2× (600+500+400 m) at 98%/100%/102% $v\dot{V}O_2$max, passive recovery of 1:15 and 5 min (jogging) between series	• 3× (2×600 m) at 100% $v\dot{V}O_2$max, recovery of 1 min (jogging) and 4 min between series • 2× (4×500 m) at 102% $v\dot{V}O_2$max, recovery of 1:15 (jogging) and 6 min between series • 3× (500 m+600 m+500 m) at 102%/103% $v\dot{V}O_2$max, recovery of 1:30 (jogging) and 3 min between series
HIIT with short intervals: 104% $v\dot{V}O_2$max	
Both profiles	
• 2× (6×300 m) at 104% $v\dot{V}O_2$max, recovery 1:30 (light jogging) and 6 min passive between series • 3× (5×200 m) at 104% $v\dot{V}O_2$max, recovery 45 s (light jogging) and 6 min passive between series	

Table 13.16　HIIT Type 2 (5%), Metabolic (O_2 Plus Neuromuscular), in Developmental Phase 2 of the Preparatory Period in Elite 1500 m Runners With Group 1 Versus Group 3 Profiles

HIIT with long intervals: no objective HIIT with moderate-duration intervals: no objective HIIT with short intervals: 106% to 108% of $v\dot{V}O_2$max	
800 m/1500 m profile (Group 1)	**1500 m/5000 m profile (Group 3)**
• 3× (200+300+200 m) at 108%/106%/108% $v\dot{V}O_2$max, passive recovery of 5 min (after first 200) and 2 min (after 300), alternating walking and jogging, and passive recovery of 6 min between series • 4× (250+200+200 m) at 106%/107%/108% $v\dot{V}O_2$max, recovery of 4 min (alternating walking and jogging) and passive 6 min between series	• 5× (200+300+200 m) at 106%/108% $v\dot{V}O_2$max, passive recovery of 1:45 and 4 min active between series • 4× (300+300+200) to 108% $v\dot{V}O_2$max, passive recovery of 1:30 (after first 300) and 1:15 (after second 300), alternating walking and jogging, and 4 min active recovery between series

This work can be carried out uphill (% of the slope 5% to 7% difference in level) by decreasing the quantity by a smaller number of series (two instead of three) or by reducing the number of repetitions per series and by adjusting the intensity (about 10% less than the $v\dot{V}O_2$max pace). Examples: 2× (4×250 m) or 3× (3×200 m) uphill. Light jog recovery on descent. Greater than twice the effort time between repetitions and 6 min walk between runs.

Table 13.17 HIIT Type 3 (5%), Metabolic (O_2 Plus Anaerobic), in Developmental Phase 2 of the Preparatory Period in Elite 1500 m Runners With Group 1 Versus Group 3 Profiles

HIIT with long intervals: up to 110% v$\dot{V}O_2$max	
800 m/1500 m profile (Group 1)	**1500 m/5000 m profile (Group 3)**
3 × (500 + 400 m) with 500 m to 108% v$\dot{V}O_2$max then after passive recovery of 3 min a 400 m at 110% v$\dot{V}O_2$max and 8 min passive between series	3 × 1000 m in progressive form (500 m + 300 m + 200 m) • 500 m at 106% v$\dot{V}O_2$max • 300 m at 108% v$\dot{V}O_2$max • 200 m at 110% v$\dot{V}O_2$max Recovery passive of 8 min between repetitions
HIIT with moderate-duration intervals: paces greater than 110% v$\dot{V}O_2$max	
800 m/1500 m profile (Group 1)	**1500 m/5000 m profile (Group 3)**
2 × (3 × 300 m) • first series: first 300 m at 112% v$\dot{V}O_2$max, second 300 m faster at 114% v$\dot{V}O_2$max, third 300 m at 112% v$\dot{V}O_2$max, passive recovery of 2:30 between repetitions and 8 min passive before second series • second series: first 300 m at 110% v$\dot{V}O_2$max, second 300 m at 112% v$\dot{V}O_2$max, third 300 m at 114% v$\dot{V}O_2$max, passive recovery 2:30 between repetitions	3 × (2 × 500 m) in the following form: first 300 m at 108% v$\dot{V}O_2$max + the last 200 m faster (110% v$\dot{V}O_2$max), passive recovery of 4 min between repetitions and passive 8 min between series
HIIT with short intervals: paces greater than 114% v$\dot{V}O_2$max	
800 m/1500 m profile (Group 1)	**1500 m/5000 m profile (Group 3)**
3 × (200 + 250 + 200 m) at 114% v$\dot{V}O_2$max for the first 200 m then 112% v$\dot{V}O_2$max for the 250 m then 114% v$\dot{V}O_2$max for the 200 m, passive recovery of 2 min between repetitions and 6 min passive between series	2 × (4 × 250 m) at 114% v$\dot{V}O_2$max for the first two 250 m, with progressive acceleration for the third and fourth repetitions, passive recovery of 3 min and 2:30 and 2 min, passive recovery of 10 min between series

Table 13.18 HIIT Type 4 (5%), Anaerobic Plus Neuromuscular, in Developmental Phase 2 of the Preparatory Period in Elite 1500 m Runners With Group 1 Versus Group 3 Profiles

HIIT with long intervals: no objective HIIT with moderate-duration intervals: from 108% to 112% v$\dot{V}O_2$max	
800 m/1500 m profile (Group 1)	**1500 m/5000 m profile (Group 3)**
• 3 × (300 + 400 + 200 m) to 108%/106%/110% v$\dot{V}O_2$max, passive recovery of 1:45 between reps and 6 min passive between series • 3 × (400 + 200 + 300 m) to 108% v$\dot{V}O_2$max, passive recovery of 2 min between repetitions and 6 min passive between series	• 2 × (2 × 600 m) to 108% v$\dot{V}O_2$max with the last 150 m in acceleration, passive recovery of 2:30 between 600 m and 6 active min between series • 2 × (500 + 400 + 300 m) to 108%/110%/112% v$\dot{V}O_2$max, passive recovery of 2 min between 500 and 400 m and 1:45 between 400 and 300 m and 6 min active recovery between series
HIIT with short intervals from 112% to 115% v$\dot{V}O_2$max	
800 m/1500 m profile (Group 1)	**1500 m/5000 m profile (Group 3)**
• 4 × (250 + 200 + 150 m) at 112/114/115% v$\dot{V}O_2$max, recovery of 3 min (passive) between the 250 m and 200 m and 2 min between the 200 m and 150 m, 6 min walk between the series • 3 × (150/200/150/200 m) at 114/112/114/112% v$\dot{V}O_2$max, recovery of 2:30 passive between repetitions and 6 min passive between series	• 3 × (4 × 250 m) to 112% v$\dot{V}O_2$max accelerating the last 100 m, recovery of 3 min (passive) between repetitions and 8 min (walk) between series • 3 × (5 × 200 m) at 115% v$\dot{V}O_2$max, passive recovery of 2:30 between repetitions and 6 min active between series

Table 13.19 HIIT Type 3 (5%), Metabolic (O_2 Plus Anaerobic), in the Precompetitive Period in Elite 1500 m Runners With Group 1 Versus Group 3 Profiles

HIIT with long intervals: ranges from 108% to 116% vVO_2max and above	
800 m/1500 m profile (Group 1)	**1500 m/5000 m profile (Group 3)**
• 3×800 m in form 600 m to 110% vVO_2max + 200 m with maximum acceleration, recovery of 8 min between series • 2×1000 m in progressive form (600/400) with 600 m to 114% vVO_2max then after 400 m to 110% vVO_2max, passive recovery of 10 min between the 2 repetitions	• 2×1200 m with first 400 m at 108% vVO_2max + 400 m at 106% vVO_2max + 400 m at 108% vVO_2max, passive recovery 12 min between series • 2×1000 m in progressive form (500/300/200), 500 m at 110% vVO_2max then 300 m at 112% vVO_2max then 200 m at 114% vVO_2max, recovery of 3 min (jogging) between the 2 repetitions
HIIT with moderate-duration intervals: paces from 112% to 116% vVO_2max (and above)	
800 m/1500 m profile (Group 1)	**1500 m/5000 m profile (Group 3)**
2×(3×400 m) • first series: first 400 m at 112% vVO_2max, second 400 m faster at 114% vVO_2max, third 400 m at 112% vVO_2max, passive recovery of 3 min between repetitions and passive 10 min before the second series • second series: first 400 m at 114% vVO_2max, second 400 m at 116% vVO_2max, third 400 m at maximum pace, passive recovery 3 min between repetitions	2×(2×600 m) in the following form: 400 m of the 600 m at 116% vVO_2max + 200 m faster, passive recovery of 6 min between repetitions and passive 10 min between series
HIIT with short intervals: paces greater than 116% vVO_2max	
800 m/1500 m profile (Group 1)	**1500 m/5000 m profile (Group 3)**
• 2×(5×200 m) at 118% vVO_2max for the first four 200 m and close to the maximum for the fifth 200 m, passive recovery of 2 min between repetitions and 8 min passive between series • 3×(200/250/200 m) at 114% vVO_2max for the first 200 m then 116% vVO_2max for 250 m then 118% vVO_2max for 200 m, passive recovery of 2 min between repetitions and 6 min passive between series	• 6×300 m at 115% vVO_2max for 200 m then finish the last 100 m faster, passive recovery of 2 min between repetitions • 2×(4×250 m) at 116% vVO_2max for the first two 250 m, in progressive accelerations for the third and fourth repetitions, progressive passive recovery of 3 min and 2:30 and 2 min and 10 min passive between series

the distribution as follows: type 1, 0%; type 2, 0%; type 3, 0%; type 4, 5% (table 13.25); type 5, 5% (table 13.26). The breakdown for types 4 and 5 is detailed in tables 13.25 and 13.26. Note: There are no objectives touching type 1, type 2, or type 3.

If needed and if time is available, a type 1 (metabolic O_2) workout can be used as a reminder between competitions:

Fartlek: 3×(1 min/2 min/1 min) near 98% to 100% vVO_2, recovery of 1 min (jogging) between repetitions, recovery 2 min (active jogging) between series

Table 13.20 HIIT Type 4 (10%), Anaerobic Plus Muscle Neuro, in the Precompetitive Period in Elite 1500 m Runners With Group 1 Versus Group 3 Profiles

HIIT with long intervals at 110% to 114% vVO$_2$max	
800 m/1500 m profile (Group 1)	**1500 m/5000 m profile (Group 3)**
3 × (600 m + 400 m) with the 600 m at 112% vVO$_2$max and the 400 m at 114% vVO$_2$max, passive recovery of 3 min between 600 m and 400 m and 8 min passive between series	• 800 m + 400 m with 800 m at 110% vVO$_2$max followed by a passive recovery of 2 min and then 400 m at 114% vVO$_2$max followed by a passive recovery of 8 min, and then 600 m + 300 m with 600 m at 112% vVO$_2$max followed by a passive recovery of 3 min (jogging) and then 300 m at 116% vVO$_2$max
HIIT with moderate-duration intervals at 112% to 114% vVO$_2$max	
800 m/1500 m profile (Group 1)	**1500 m/5000 m profile (Group 3)**
• 2 × (3 × 400 m) to 112% vVO$_2$max, passive recovery of 2:30 between 400 m and 8 passive min between series • 3 × (3 × 300 m) to 114% vVO$_2$max, passive recovery of 2 min between 300 m and 6 min passive between series	• 4 × (400 + 300 m) at 112% vVO$_2$max for the 400 m and 114% vVO$_2$max for the 300 m, passive recovery of 2 min between the 400 m and 300 m and 6 min active between series • 3 × (500 + 300 + 300 m) to 110% vVO$_2$max for the 500 m and then 112% vVO$_2$max for the first 300 m and 114% vVO$_2$max for the second 300 m, passive recovery of 2 min between the 500 m and the 300 m and 1:45 between the 2 × 300 m and 8 min active between series
HIIT with short intervals at 112% to 116% vVO$_2$max	
800 m/1500 m profile (Group 1)	**1500 m/5000 m profile (Group 3)**
• 3 × (300 + 300 + 200 m) at 114% vVO$_2$max then 115% vVO$_2$max and 116% vVO$_2$max, passive recovery of 2 min between repetitions and 8 min passive between series • 4 × (300 + 200 + 150 m) at 114%/116% vVO$_2$max, passive recovery of 1:45 between repetitions and 6 min passive between series	• 2 × (4 × 300 m) at 114% vVO$_2$max, passive recovery of 2 min between repetitions and 6 min active between series • 2 × (6 × 200 m) at 116% vVO$_2$max, passive recovery of 1:45 between repetitions and 8 min passive between series

Table 13.21 HIIT Type 5 (5%), Anaerobic (Peripheral O$_2$ Plus Anaerobic Plus Muscular), in the Precompetitive Period in Elite 1500 m Runners With Group 1 Versus Group 3 Profiles

HIIT with long intervals: no objective HIIT with moderate-duration intervals: pace 108% to 110% vVO$_2$max	
800 m/1500 m profile (Group 1)	**1500 m/5000 m profile (Group 3)**
• 3 × (300 + 400 + 300 m) at 110%/108%/110% vVO$_2$max, passive recovery of 1:45 between repetitions and 8 min passive between series • 4 × (400 + 300 + 300 m) to 108% vVO$_2$max, passive recovery of 2 min between repetitions and 6 min passive between series	• 3 × (2 × 600 m) at 108% vVO$_2$max with the last 150 m in acceleration, passive recovery of 2:30 between repetitions and 6 min active between series • 3 × (500 + 400 + 300 m) to 108%/109%/110% vVO$_2$max, passive recovery of 2 min between 500 and 400 m and 1:45 between 400 and 300 m and 6 min active between series
HIIT with short intervals from 110% to 115% vVO$_2$max	
800 m/1500 m profile (Group 1)	**1500 m/5000 m profile (Group 3)**
• 4 × (250 + 200 + 150 m) at 110%/112%/115% vVO$_2$max, passive recovery of 3 min between the 250 m and 200 m and 2 min passive between the 200 m and 150 m and 8 min passive between series • 3 × (150/200/150/200 m) at 114%/112%/114%/112% vVO$_2$max, recovery of 2:30 between repetitions and 6 min (passive) between series	• 3 × (4 × 250 m) to 110% vVO$_2$max accelerating the last 100 m, passive recovery of 3 min between repetitions and 8 min passive between series • 3 × (5 × 200 m) at 115% vVO$_2$max, passive recovery of 2:30 between repetitions and 6 min active between series

Table 13.22 HIIT Type 2 (5%), Metabolic (O$_2$ Plus Neuromuscular), in the Competitive Period in Elite 1500 m Runners With Group 1 Versus Group 3 Profiles

HIIT with long intervals: from 108% to 110% of vVO$_2$max	
800 m/1500 m profile (Group 1)	**1500 m/5000 m profile (Group 3)**
800 m + 200 m then 600 m + 300 m then 500 m + 400 m • 800 m + 200 m: 800 m at 108% vVO$_2$max, recovery 3 min (jogging and walking), then 200 m at 116% vVO$_2$max, passive recovery of 8 min • 600 m + 300 m: 600 m at 110% vVO$_2$max, passive recovery 2:30, then 300 m at 116% vVO$_2$max, passive recovery 8 min • 500 m + 400 m: 500 m at 110% vVO$_2$max, passive recovery 3 min, then 400 m at 116% vVO$_2$max passive 8 min	4 × 800 m at 108% vVO$_2$max on the first 600 m with progressive acceleration over the last 200 m (finish quickly), active recovery of 6 min (jogging and walking) between repetitions
HIIT with moderate-duration intervals: from 110% to 112% of vVO$_2$max	
800 m/1500 m profile (Group 1)	**1500 m/5000 m profile (Group 3)**
• 4 × (2 × 400 m) at 110% vVO$_2$max, passive recovery of 2 min between repetitions and 4 min passive between series • 3 × (4 × 250 m) at 112% vVO$_2$max, passive recovery of 1:45 between repetitions and 6 min passive between series	• 2 × (3 × 500 m) at 110% vVO$_2$max, passive recovery of 2:30 between repetitions and 8 min passive between series • 2 × (500 + 400 + 400 m) at 110%/112%/112% vVO$_2$max, recovery of passive 2 min between repetitions and 8 active min between series
HIIT with short intervals: from 112% to 115% of vVO$_2$max	
800 m/1500 m profile (Group 1)	**1500 m/5000 m profile (Group 3)**
• 3 × (4 × 200 m) at 116% vVO$_2$max, passive recovery of 2 min (stepping) between repetitions and 6 min passive between series • 4 × (300 m + 200 m) with 300 m at 116% vVO$_2$max, passive recovery 2 min, then 200 m progressive and fast finish, recovery 8 min passive between series	• 2 × (3 × 300 m) at 112% vVO$_2$max for first and second repetitions, 114% vVO$_2$max for third repetition, passive recovery of 2 min between repetitions and 6 min active between series • 2 × (4 × 250 m) with first two 250 m at 114% vVO$_2$max, 115% vVO$_2$max for third and fourth repetitions, recovery 3 min (jogging and walking) between repetitions and 8 min active between series

Table 13.23 HIIT Type 4 (5%), Metabolic (O$_2$ Plus Anaerobic Plus Neuromuscular), in the Competitive Period in Elite 1500 m Runners With Group 1 Versus Group 3 Profiles

HIIT with long intervals: no objective	
HIIT with moderate-duration intervals: at 112% to 116% vVO$_2$max	
800 m/1500 m profile (Group 1)	**1500 m/5000 m profile (Group 3)**
• 2 × (300 + 400 + 300 m) at 112%/110%/112% vVO$_2$max, passive recovery of 2 min between repetitions and 8 min passive between series • 3 × (400 + 300 + 200 m) at 112% vVO$_2$max, passive recovery of 2 min between repetitions and 6 min passive between series	• 3 × (2 × 600 m) to 112% vVO$_2$max with the last 150 m with acceleration, passive recovery of 2:30 between repetitions and 6 min active between series • 2 × (500 + 400 + 300 m) to 112%/114%/116% vVO$_2$max, passive recovery of 2:15 between the 500 and 400 m and 1:45 between the 400 and 300 m and 6 min active recovery between series
HIIT with short intervals of 114% to 118% vVO$_2$max	
800 m/1500 m profile (Group 1)	**1500 m/5000 m profile (Group 3)**
• 3 × (250 + 200 + 150 m) at 114%/112%/116% vVO$_2$max, recovery of 3 min (passive) between 250 m and 200 m and 2 min (passive) between 200 m and 150 m and 6 min passive recovery between series • 4 × (200 + 150 + 200 m) at 116%/114%/116% vVO$_2$max, passive recovery of 2:30 between repetitions and 6 min passive between series	• 3 × (3 × 250 m) at 114% vVO$_2$max accelerating the last 100 m, passive recovery of 3 min between repetitions and 8 min active between series • 3 × (4 × 200 m) at 118% vVO$_2$max, passive recovery of 2 min between repetitions and 8 min active between series

Table 13.24 HIIT Type 5 (5%), Anaerobic (Peripheral O_2 Plus Anaerobic Plus Neuromuscular), in the Competitive Period in Elite 1500 m Runners With Group 1 Versus Group 3 Profiles

HIIT with long intervals: no objective HIIT with moderate-duration intervals: no objective HIIT with short intervals of 114% to 116% of $v\dot{V}O_2max$	
800 m/1500 m profile (Group 1)	**1500 m/5000 m profile (Group 3)**
• 6×300 m to 114% $v\dot{V}O_2max$, passive recovery of 3 min between repetitions • 2×(4×200 m) to 118% $v\dot{V}O_2max$, passive recovery of 1:45 between repetitions and 8 min passive between series • 3×(300+200+150 m) at 116% $v\dot{V}O_2max$ for the 300 m and 200 m, 150 m at maximum speed, passive recovery of 3 min between the 300 m and the 200 m and 2 min between the 200 m and the 150 m, recovery of 8 min passive between series	• 3×(300+300+200 m) at 114% $v\dot{V}O_2max$ for 300 m and 116% $v\dot{V}O_2max$ for 200 m, passive recovery of 2 min between 300 m and 1:45 between 300 m and 200 m and 8 min active between series • 3×(400+300 m) at 112% $v\dot{V}O_2max$ for the 400 m and 114% for the 300 m, passive recovery of 2 min between repetitions and 10 min passive between series • 2×(3×400 m) at 114% $v\dot{V}O_2max$, passive recovery of 3 min between repetitions and 10 min passive between series

Table 13.25 HIIT Type 4 (5%), Anaerobic Plus Neuromuscular, During the Tapering Period in Elite 1500 m Runners With Group 1 Versus Group 3 Profiles

HIIT with long intervals: no objective HIIT with moderate-duration intervals: paces 116% to 118% $v\dot{V}O_2max$	
800 m/1500 m profile (Group 1)	**1500 m/5000 m profile (Group 3)**
• 3×(2×300 m) with 200 m at 118% $v\dot{V}O_2max$+last 100 m in acceleration, passive recovery of 3 min between repetitions and 8 min passive between series • 3×(300+300+200 m) at 116% $v\dot{V}O_2max$ for the 300 m and 118% $v\dot{V}O_2max$ for the 200 m, passive recovery of 3 min between 300 m and 2 min between the 300 m and the 200 m and 10 min passive between series	• 2×(2×500 m) with 300 m at 114% $v\dot{V}O_2max$+last 200 m with progressive acceleration, passive recovery of 3 min between repetitions and 10 m passive in between series • 2×(3×400 m) at 114% $v\dot{V}O_2max$ for the first 400 m then 116% $v\dot{V}O_2max$ for the second and then 118% $v\dot{V}O_2max$ for the third, passive recovery of 4 min between the first and second then 3 min between the second and third 400 m, 12 min passive between series
HIIT with short intervals: 120% maximum speed	
800 m/1500 m profile (Group 1)	**1500 m/5000 m profile (Group 3)**
• 6×150 m alternately: first 150 m progressive, second 150 m quick release, third 150 m in 50 m increments, fourth 150 m progressive, fifth 150 m in steps, sixth 150 m at maximum pace, passive recovery of 6 min between repetitions • 10×100 m at a speed close to the maximum (95%), passive recovery of 3 to 4 min between repetitions • 3×(150+200+150 m) at a speed close to the maximum (95%), passive recovery of 6 min between repetitions and 10 min passive between series	• 2×(4×200 m) at 120% $v\dot{V}O_2max$ with a finishing acceleration, passive recovery of 4 min between repetitions and 10 m passive in between series • 3×(2×250 m) close to maximum speed over distance (95%), passive recovery of 6 min between repetitions and 12 m passive in between series • 4×(200 m+150 m) at a speed close to maximum for the 200 m (95%) and maximum speed for the 150 m, passive recovery of 6 min between repetitions and 10 min passive between series

Table 13.26 HIIT Type 5 (5%), Metabolic (Peripheral O_2 Plus Anaerobic Plus Neuromuscular), During the Tapering Period in Elite 1500 m Runners With Group 1 Versus Group 3 Profiles

HIIT with long intervals: no objective HIIT with moderate-duration intervals: no objective HIIT with short intervals: from 116% to 118% $v\dot{V}O_2max$	
800 m/1500 m profile (Group 1)	**1500 m/5000 m profile (Group 3)**
• 5×300 m to 118% $v\dot{V}O_2max$, recovery of 3 min between repetitions • 3×(3×200 m) at 120% $v\dot{V}O_2max$, passive recovery of 2 min between repetitions and 8 min active between series • 3×(250+200+150 m) at 116% $v\dot{V}O_2max$ for the 250 and 200 m, recovery of 2 min between the 250 and 200 m, then passive recovery of 1:30 before the 150 m at maximum speed, recovery of 8 min passive between series	• 2×(400+300+200 m) at 116% $v\dot{V}O_2max$ for the 400 m and 118% $v\dot{V}O_2max$ for the 300 and 200 m, passive recovery of 2 min between 400 and 300 m and 1:45 between 300 and 200 m, recovery of 8 min active between series • 3×(400+300 m) at 114% $v\dot{V}O_2max$ for the 400 m and 116% $v\dot{V}O_2max$ for the 300 m, passive recovery of 2 min between repetitions and 10 min passive between series • 2×(3×300 m) at 116% $v\dot{V}O_2max$, passive recovery of 3 min between repetitions and 10 min passive between series

Jean Claude Vollmer

During my career as a club coach, then as a national coach with the French Athletics Federation, I had the chance to coach many runners, work with athletes and their coaches at different moments of my career and I have always learned a lot from them. Competitors I have trained over 1500 m include Christian Grunder (French junior champion), Blandine Bitzner in her debut (selected at the Atlanta Olympics), Guy Nunige (3:36:84 in 1992, France), Frédérique Quentin (selected at the 1996 Olympics, several times French champion), Nadir Bosch (3:32:94 world finalist, selected for 3000 m steeplechase at the Atlanta Olympics, nine French championship titles), Bryan Cantero (3:36:08, two-time champion of France in the 1500 m indoor), Morhad Amdouni (3:34:55, semifinalist at the 2015 World Championships, several times champion of France), and training them from their junior years before their emergence as world-class runners Mehdi Baala (3:28:98 over 1500 m, World silver medalist 2003, bronze medalist at the 2008 Olympic Games) and Bob Tahri (3:32:94 over 1500 m, third at the World Championships in the 3000 m steeplechase and former European repeat-record holder in the 3000 m steeplechase, 8:06:91, 8:02.19, and finally 8:01:18).

My mission as a national MD coach has allowed me to meet many first-class national and international runners and their coaches. Thanks to these meetings, I was able to exchange, observe, and study their approaches to 1500 m training. Performance over 1500 meters is the product of complex parameters, more than any other distance, as described. Each athlete, through his unique profile, will grasp the distance, the confrontation with his opponents, alongside his strengths and weaknesses. Weaknesses in one area may be compensated by a strong point in another, and tactics must be adapted accordingly to expose a competitor's potential weaknesses as well. Each coach has a personal approach to his runner's training, ideas, convictions, and training methods, but to be successful, he must also be able to adapt his training routines to the profile of his athlete. All coaches are familiar with this reality, in that training content applied in one runner may be entirely ineffective for another. The 1500 m race is the aggregation of the highly demanding requirements of the distance together with the unique profile of an individual runner. Forty years of coaching have shaped my beliefs on the determinants of 1500 m performance, which is (to me at least) becoming clearer and clearer: a well-developed aerobic system allows a runner to release the all-important speed component, allowing the runner to access the performance he desires. To reach the highest level, this takes talent, but talent is far from sufficient. It is also necessary to train very hard every day for years to become a world-class runner. Along these lines, I appreciate the quote of Kevin Durant: "Hard work beats talent when talent fails to work hard." For example, unlike Bosch (the runner with the greatest talent I ever worked with), Baala had the chance to start in a club that specialized in middle distance with qualified coaches and many high level partners. This allowed him to be involved in more-structured training, but above all, allowed him to build an extremely solid foundation, a necessary condition needed to be able to gradually increase workload both in terms of the required volume and intensity, elements that remained hidden from Bosch unfortunately.

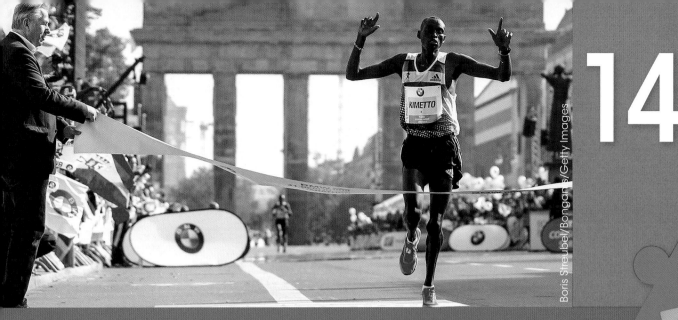

14

Road Running

• • • • • •

Jamie Stanley and Carlos Alberto Cavalheiro

Performance Demands of Road Running

This chapter describes the sport of road running with a particular focus on the marathon. Various factors contributing to elite distance runner success will be discussed, in parallel with the application of high-intensity interval training (HIIT).

Sport Description and Factors of Winning

Road running involves a race run over a measured course on an established road as opposed to an off-road cross-country event or athletics track (i.e., middle distance, chapter 13). The sport's popularity is highlighted in a 2015 statistic, in which there were more than 17 million reported finishers from more than 30,000 events held across all road running distances. Road running events are classified as long-distance in athletics terminology and range from 10 km to 42.195 km (the marathon; 26.2 miles). World-class times to complete such events for men and women range from 26 to 27 min and 30 to 31 min for the 10 km, to 2:03:00 to 2:08:00 and 2:15:00 to 2:20:00 for the marathon, respectively (30). A range of factors, including the topography and layout of the course, environmental conditions, tactics, and strategy, influence success in each of these events (37). However, an athlete's physical capacity is fundamental to successful performance. Figure 14.1 shows the relative importance of road running skills (mechanics), tactics, and physical capacities, alongside other sports covered in the book.

The main physiological factors of importance for distance running success include a high maximal aerobic power (7, 8, 31, 53), the ability to perform at a high fractional utilization of maximal aerobic power throughout the duration of a race (31, 61), and running economically, or possessing a low energetic demand at a given running velocity (3, 31, 61). Key factors that differentiate top- versus high-class elite marathon runners include a high peak oxygen uptake and the capacity to draw on a fast running speed (i.e., > marathon pace) in a prefatigued state (8). Other factors associated with exceptional running performance include the ectomorphic somatotype, consistency of aerobic training from a young age, and a high motivation to succeed in the sport (61). A synopsis of these factors is shown in figure 14.2.

Relative Contribution of Physical Performance

Road running, particularly the marathon, differs from middle- to long-distance track running or

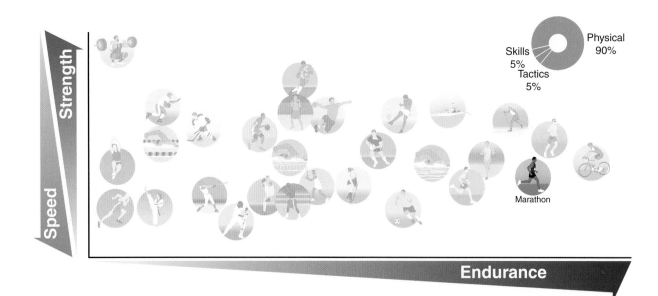

Figure 14.1 The position of the road runner on the three axes illustrates the relative importance of the three main physical capacities of importance for elite participation, acknowledging this varies slightly between race distances. Outside of critical psychological aspects, which are difficult to quantify, the pie chart shows the general relative importance skill, tactics, and physical capacities for road running success.

Adapted from G.A. Nader, "Concurrent Strength and Endurance Training: From Molecules to Man," *Medicine & Science in Sports & Exercise* 38, no. 11 (2006): 1965-1970.

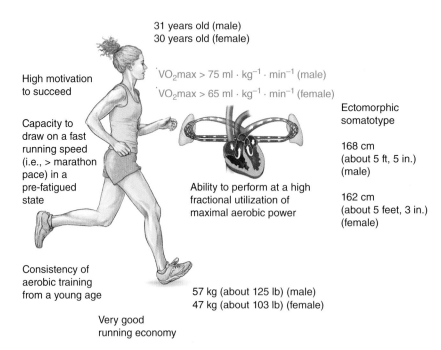

Figure 14.2 Key traits and factors identified as being related to successful marathon performance in elite-level road runners.

cross-country running with respect to the fact that tactical changes in pace are less defining to the overall performance outcome (40, 48). The distance of the marathon, coupled with large incentives for athletes to run the fastest time possible rather than simply being first across the finish line, means that a marathon runner can know the precise physiological requirements of his next race. For example, if an event is likely to be won in a time of ~2:05:00, or if there is monetary incentive (30) to break an existing course record of 2:04:30, then the required pace and associated physiological parameters needed to achieve this time can be reverse engineered. HIIT sessions can then be prescribed and tailored appropriately to meet the athlete's current status alongside the physiological demands associated with the known running performance. There are instances where the race may not be as fast as expected, but this may be due to a lack of direct financial incentive or environmental factors such as hot conditions due to the timing of an event (i.e., World Championships and Olympic Games).

Targets of Physical Performance in Road Running

The key adaptation targets of HIIT for marathon athletes are based on the physiological factors that are critical to marathon performance as described in the previous section (i.e., aerobic power, high fractional utilization of aerobic power, and economy). Therefore, prescription of HIIT for marathon runners should be focused on maximizing adaptations that benefit the physiological factors critical to marathon performance.

Aerobic Power

As described in chapter 3, aerobic power, or the maximal volume of oxygen uptake ($\dot{V}O_2max$), refers to the highest amount of oxygen that can be consumed during maximal exercise. When running at close to maximal velocity over distances >3000 m, oxidative metabolism contributes to >90% of the energy requirements (33). Therefore, the duration of the marathon dictates that aerobic metabolism must be the primary energy source (6). $\dot{V}O_2max$ has been shown to differentiate elite marathon runners (8). Therefore, many believe that the accumulation of training time at $\dot{V}O_2max$, or at velocities associated with $\dot{V}O_2max$ ($v\dot{V}O_2max$), is likely to be the most

effective training stimulus for improving $\dot{V}O_2max$ (11). For training sessions specifically targeting this adaptation, total session time should allow athletes to accumulate ~10 min at $\dot{V}O_2max$ (see chapter 5). In practice, this may be best achieved by minimizing the time between the end of the warm-up and commencement of the HIIT component of the session, and prescribing a work:rest ratio of >1 (e.g., 4 × 5 min with 2 min active recovery). Additionally, the velocity required to accumulate time at $\dot{V}O_2max$ may be manipulated by performing HIIT on an incline or on flat terrain.

High Fractional Utilization of Aerobic Power

Logic dictates that it is impossible to maintain the same $\dot{V}O_2$ for a marathon as running maximally over 3000 m. Therefore, the ability to utilize the highest possible fraction of one's maximal capacity is another key trait required for successful marathon outcomes. Accumulation of time at or just above marathon velocity (75% to 80% $v\dot{V}O_2max$ (6) up to >85% $v\dot{V}O_2max$ in top-class marathon runners (8)) may be the most appropriate stimulus for improving the fractional utilization of aerobic capacity. This is supported by the fact that training at this intensity comprises 10% to 15% of an elite marathon runner's weekly training volume (e.g., 3 × 8 to 9 min at 90% $v\dot{V}O_2max$ with 2 min active recovery, or 2 × 20 min at 85% $v\dot{V}O_2max$ with 3 min active recovery at 70% $v\dot{V}O_2max$) (7, 8). These longer duration intervals are thought to improve buffering capacity and/or metabolic aspects, including blood lactic shuttling and enhanced fat relative to carbohydrate oxidation rates (32).

Economy

Running economy can be improved by influencing metabolic, biomechanical, and/or neuromuscular efficiency (3). HIIT training, targeting $\dot{V}O_2max$ and high fractional utilization of $\dot{V}O_2max$, also has been shown to enhance biomechanical factors influencing running economy. For example, studies have shown improvements in running economy from 1% to 3% using HIIT completed on a 10% incline, such as 9 × 2 min at ~100% $v\dot{V}O_2max$ with 4 min recovery (2), and 4 × 4 min at ~106% $v\dot{V}O_2max$ with 2 min recovery (21). Neuromuscular efficiencies may also be improved by targeting changes in muscle/tendon characteristics through loading patterns that exaggerate relevant mechanical needs of distance runners such as plyometric exercises. Within the specific context of HIIT, prescription of intervals completed downhill or on the decline (e.g., -10% gradient, 2 × 10 min intervals at 85% to 90% vV̇O₂max with 1 min recovery between sets (15)) can be utilized to target such adaptations.

Key Weapons, Manipulations, and Surveillance Tools

In this section, we present the different HIIT weapons, their manipulations, along with ways by which we can monitor their effectiveness (surveillance) for road runners. Like many endurance athlete programs presented throughout the book (i.e., rowers, cyclists, triathletes), the weekly training intensity distribution of an elite marathon runner generally follows the polarized model whereby about 80% of the training volume is completed at submaximal intensities, with the remaining 20% completed at marathon race pace or faster (7, 8, 50). The low- to medium-intensity (50% to 80% HR$_{max}$, 40% to 80% vV̇O₂max i.e., <80% marathon race velocity) component of training provides an important foundation because it builds the resilience (psychological and neuromuscular/ musculoskeletal) (33), body composition, economy (3), aerobic capacity (17, 18, 33), and fat oxidation rates (27) required for the marathon distance.

While HIIT typically forms only ~15% of the total training volume, it provides a stimulus that critically contributes to marathon performance (5-8). Fundamental HIIT targets for road running include types 1 through 4, with type 1 and 3 targets being particularly important for improving maximal aerobic power and fractional utilization of maximal aerobic power, and type 2 and 4 targets important for improving running economy.

HIIT Weapons

The overall breakdown of HIIT weapons used throughout a season in elite marathon runners is shown in figure 14.3. Given the requirements of the marathon, the dominant forms of HIIT tend to be long intervals, using work:rest ratios >1 and terrain (i.e., flat versus incline versus decline) manipulated to emphasize types 1 through 4 targets. Short-interval HIIT is also used to a much lesser extent to target types 2, 3, and 4 during specific phases of preparation (see figure 4.14) (12).

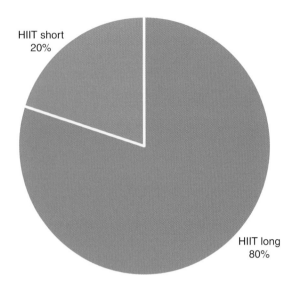

Figure 14.3 General percentage breakdown of HIIT formats (weapons) used in road running across a season at the elite level.

Manipulations of Interval Training Variables

The running intensity and modality of each HIIT session can be modulated such that a specific metabolic, neuromuscular, and locomotor response can be targeted. While manipulation of the work:rest ratio and volume are the primary means by which to modify metabolic HIIT targets, manipulation of the modality (i.e., uphill or downhill running) where HIIT is performed can target specific neuromuscular and locomotor responses.

HIIT With Long Intervals

Long-interval HIIT for road runners typically ranges from 60 s to 15 min work durations at intensities at or faster than marathon race velocity (85% to 100% vV̇O₂max), with work:rest ratios >1 (see examples in figure 14.4). The total duration of time accumulated at these intensities is typically 20 to 40 min, which may be split into 1 to 5 sets of equal or varying duration. A classic long-interval HIIT session is 5 × 5 min at 90% to 95% vV̇O₂max with 2 min active recovery at 40% vV̇O₂max. Two other common long-interval HIIT sessions for a marathon runner would be 25 × 400 m at 95 to 100% vV̇O₂max with 15 to 20 s recovery, or four sets of 5 × 400 m at 100 to 115% vV̇O₂max with 45 s recovery between repetitions and 60 s between sets (figure 14.4). The desired metabolic load for both sessions is similar. However,

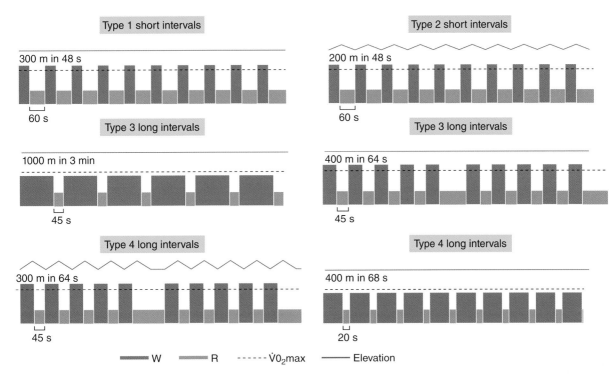

Figure 14.4 Examples of short and long intervals and the various HIIT target types commonly used in marathon training. Note the effect of manipulating work:rest ratios and modality (i.e., elevation, red line) on HIIT target type. W: work; R: recovery; $\dot{V}O_2max$: level associated with maximal oxygen uptake.

the manipulation of the work:rest ratio results in different neuromuscular load. For example, the first session has shorter recovery and therefore a greater neuromuscular load (type 4), whereas the second session, broken into four sets with greater recovery duration and faster pace, has less neuromuscular load (type 3). Further, changing the modality and completing the second session on an incline (i.e., uphill) compared to on the flat, will increase the neuromuscular load, shifting the targets from type 3 to 4 (see figure 14.4).

HIIT With Short Intervals

Short-interval HIIT for road runners typically ranges from 30 s to 45 s work durations at intensities faster than marathon race velocity (>110% $v\dot{V}O_2max$), with work:rest ratios between 1:2 and 1:3. The total duration of time accumulated at these intensities is typically 10 to 20 min and can be done in combination with a long-interval HIIT session. An example session might be 3 × 2000 m at 90% $v\dot{V}O_2max$ with 90 s active recovery (type 3 long interval), 4 min of active recovery at 40% to 50% $v\dot{V}O_2max$, then 12 × 300 m at 115% to 130% $v\dot{V}O_2max$ with 60 s

active recovery (type 1 short interval). If the short-interval HIIT is done as a standalone session with passive recovery, the metabolic targets become type 4. However, combining it with the prior long-interval HIIT session allows all HIIT targets (types 1 to 4) to be met. Similar to long-interval HIIT, different HIIT targets can be achieved by manipulating the work:rest ratio and modality (see figure 14.4).

Load Surveillance and Monitoring Tools

Running is a bodyweight-loaded activity that involves both concentric and eccentric loading, therefore requiring large aerobic oxidative and neuromuscular demands. During high-volume training weeks that many elite road runners perform (~200 km), a runner may accumulate 148,000 to 168,000 steps (i.e., 740 to 840 steps per km, depending on speed). This means that for a typical marathon runner weighing 65 kg, and assuming the impact force of each step is ~3 times that of gravity (i.e., 195 kg per step), the total weekly load becomes 28 to 35 million kg (51). Therefore, load surveillance is of upmost importance for ensuring that training load is progressed appropriately and the risk of lower-limb overuse injury is minimized.

With recent advances in technology, monitoring and/or quantifying individual session/workout and longitudinal training load has become highly data driven. Wrist-based global-positioning systems with built-in accelerometers and integrated heart rate (HR) monitors have made collection of key running metrics (e.g., instantaneous pace, stride frequency, and heart rate) accessible to the masses. This data can be used to provide insight into the physiological response to training and competition intensity and compared alongside laboratory test data to monitor changes in physiological capacities, allowing more specific prescription in training programs (e.g., prescribed pace to run an HIIT session involving type 1 versus 2 or type 3 versus 4 targets when the desire is to increase or decrease neuromuscular load). In addition, such data can be used to calculate training load. Most simply, training load can be defined as the product of exercise intensity and duration. Exercise intensity can be derived from either the external (distance, run pace, power output) or internal (oxygen consumption, heart rate, blood lactate concentration, rating of perceived exertion) loads (chapter 8). There are many models available to derive training load (19), including training stress score from power output (54), training impulse using heart rate (1), and session RPE based on the perceived exertion of the training session (20). Examination of longitudinal trends in training loads such as acute and chronic training load and training stress balance metrics are increasingly being used to model fitness/load progression to minimize injury risk (22, 23), with many commercial software packages now available with the necessary analysis tools to calculate these metrics (see chapter 8).

Training Status Surveillance and Monitoring Tools

There are many tools available to monitor an athlete's training status or readiness to train. The primary tool used by coaches who have regular (i.e., daily) contact with their athletes is to monitor training status or readiness to train using simple visual and audible feedback. This primarily involves a simple conversation with the athlete, asking, "How do you feel?" An experienced coach's intuition based on visual assessment of body language and attitude prior to or during a training session is also important. While

such parameters might be considered qualitative, this daily face-to-face contact is an invaluable surveillance tool used by the most experienced coaches. More quantifiable monitoring tools are generally limited to noninvasive measures such as daily wellness metrics (49), daily resting HR and heart rate variability (HRV) and exercise HR (10), and GPS/accelerometer-derived data. Specifically, analyzing trends in daily wellness, waking HR and HRV in relation to the training context (internal and external loads, i.e., exercise HR and GPS data) provide a powerful tool to confirm an athlete's readiness to perform or assess how an athlete is adapting to the training program (56) (see chapter 9). Although not as accessible to all athletes, blood testing can be used to inform on training status (e.g., overtraining state (34), adaptation to altitude (35), or heat stress (42)) in a similar way to how the biological passport system is used to monitor potential doping practices (44). A benefit of using quantifiable training status tools is that they provide historical information that can be retrospectively analyzed and used to plan future seasons or for understanding how an athlete has adapted to a specific training stimulus.

Strategies for Structuring the Training Program Using HIIT

Strategies for structuring HIIT programming in road running may be confined by various controllable and uncontrollable factors, before proper progression and periodization can be appropriately implemented. This section discusses some of the nuances of training program and HIIT structuring in road running. As discussed, marathon runners generally adopt a polarized training intensity distribution (50) throughout the entire season, with the specific contents of each HIIT session manipulated to suit the desired physiological outcome. Additionally, the timing of HIIT sessions within a weekly microcycle is often manipulated (e.g., from 24 to 72 h) to alter the physiological outcomes based on variable recovery kinetics (55).

Controllable and Uncontrollable Factors

Most elite marathon runners will focus on two or three competitions to peak for each year. Unless there are specific qualification requirements for particular events (e.g., world championships, Olympic Games), athletes have reasonable flexibility in choosing the peak events they prefer to target because there are events all over the world each month of the year. This makes planning a season relatively simple compared to other sports that may have 40 to 90 competitions or race days per year (see chapter 15, Road Cycling).

Program Structure and Progression

Compared to many other sports, periodization for road running, particularly the marathon, is relatively straightforward. Most elite marathon runners typically target only two or three key events per year. The duration between these peak events (i.e., 12 to 25 wk) usually allows for progressive and periodized training blocks that can target key physiological adaptations (28). In general terms, the training phases of a marathon runner's season follow a classic progression (figure 14.5). As outlined in the previous section on load surveillance, it is imperative that training load is progressed appropriately to minimize the risk of overuse injuries and illness.

Macrocycle

For most elite marathon runners, the season is periodized over a 12 month cycle with two or three primary competition objectives or peaks. Within each macrocycle, an athlete might complete 3 to 5 mesocycles progressing from general to specific to competition focus.

Mesocycle

Depending on the time between key events, mesocycles may vary from 3 to 6 wk, with 2 to 5 loading weeks separated by 1 or 2 recovery or de-loading weeks. Due to the weight-bearing nature of running, shock or block mesocycles of high training load

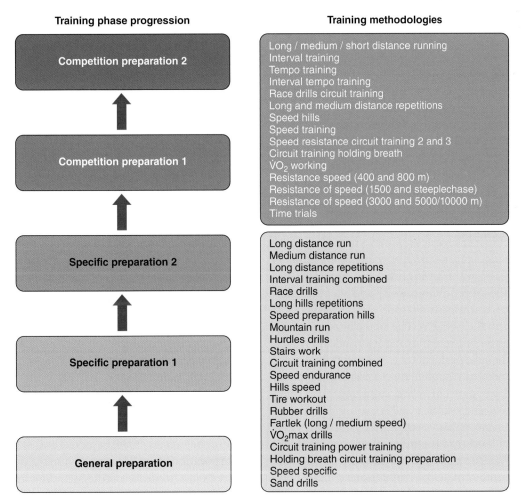

Figure 14.5 Progression of training phases (left panels) with the training methods (right panels) employed.

common in other endurance sports such as cycling (45, 46) or cross-country skiing (47) are typically not as used unless the additional load is composed of cross-training activities such as water running or cycling. This relates to the large neuromuscular demands of weight-bearing running as outlined.

Microcycle

The microcycle of a marathon runner is traditionally, but not always, structured around 7 days. During various phases of mesocycles, a microcycle may comprise up to 11 running-based sessions, 2 or 3 strength and conditioning sessions, 2 or 3 drill sessions, and 1 or 2 water-based sessions. The 11 running-based sessions may include 2 or 3 HIIT sessions (completed on the track, road, hills, or on a treadmill), 1 or 2 long-distance runs (>20 km), which may be steady or increasing in pace, as well as 4 to 6 medium-distance runs (10 to 15 km) at a steady moderate/easy pace. The timing and specific nature of weekly HIIT sessions varies depending on the mesocycle and the desired physiological adaptation objective. For example, during the early general preparation mesocycle, a 7 d microcycle may include 3 HIIT sessions separated by 1 or 2 d. Conversely, during a competitive season mesocycle, only 2 HIIT sessions may be prescribed separated by 2 or 3 d. Modulation of the timing between HIIT sessions may affect recovery kinetics, potentially resulting in differing adaptation responses (55). The detailed periodization examples across the different mesocycles in a world-class marathoner that follow offer real-world examples for the reader to consider.

Hypoxic Stress

While not all successful elite marathon runners undertake altitude training, there is general consensus in the athletic community and scientific literature that training at altitude *may* improve sea level performance (9, 25). The underlying physiological adaptations from training at altitude that may positively benefit performance include an increase in erythropoietin response increasing hemoglobin mass and oxygen-carrying capacity (26) and improved oxygen extraction and economy (25). These adaptations may enhance adaptations during a subsequent sea level training block or upcoming competition (9, 25), although not always (36). The minimal number of peak competitions a marathon runner competes in throughout a year means that periodization of altitude training blocks is relatively straightforward. However, the training content

(including the incorporation of HIIT sessions) in the lead up to and during altitude exposure can greatly influence the adaptation response, and individual athlete fatigue and recovery profiles need to be closely monitored (52). The HIIT response associated with hypoxic training is described in chapter 4.

Heat Stress

Many of the big city marathons are held during cooler times of the year. However, the Olympic Games and World Championship events are often completed in hot environments. Acclimating to the environmental conditions is common practice and generally involves training in a competition-specific (hot/humid) environment for 2 to 3 wk (43). For most athletes, it is not feasible to travel to such locations due to the associated costs involved. Therefore, alternative modalities can be used to provide the appropriate heat stress required to initiate the desired physiological adaptations, including passive sauna exposure (57) or training in an environmental chamber (24). Further, heat stress itself has also emerged as a potential ergogenic aid for enhancing various aspects of training adaptation (14) (see also chapter 4).

Periodized Nutrition

Given the high training volumes completed by marathon runners, nutrition naturally plays an important role in supporting both low-intensity training and HIIT sessions, as well as recovery and altering body composition. Additionally, manipulation of fuel availability (i.e., carbohydrate) before and after each training session can influence the physiological adaptation (see also chapter 4). For example, adopting a train high, sleep low periodization of carbohydrate availability approach, whereby an HIIT session may be performed with high carbohydrate availability but a subsequent low-intensity session the following day is performed with low carbohydrate availability, has been shown to improve submaximal economy, supramaximal capacity, and race pace performance (38). Additionally, the nutritional support required for HIIT or low-intensity training can affect the quality/intensity of the session, as well as the molecular pathways that drive adaptations within the muscle (16) (chapters 3 and 4). Therefore, incorporation of such strategies into the overall periodized plan needs to be considered (4, 29). On race day, the ability to effectively utilize carbohydrate and fat oxidation throughout the entire race will allow for the highest fractional utilization of aerobic power. A recent study suggests that it may be the enhanced ability to use fat metabolism while exercising at high intensities that differentiates well-trained versus recreational endurance athletes (27), highlighting the importance of periodizing nutrition to promote enhanced fat metabolism (38). Nutrition on race day is also fundamental for achieving the full expression of performance capacity. Given the duration and intensity that the marathon is completed in, appropriate individualized nutrition is thought of as being vital for success (58). Adopting a low-residue diet during the days prior to competition may also help minimize potential gastrointestinal disturbances (13). The use of nutritional supplements such as dietary nitrates (e.g., beetroot juice) (39) and caffeine (41) have also been shown to improve economy and delay fatigue, however, athletes should trial any sort of supplement strategy well beforehand so as to be well familiarized prior to race day.

Incorporation of HIIT

As described before, HIIT can be incorporated into the training program during all phases of training. It is important that the overall adaptation response or goal be considered when planning a training program. This is because the timing between HIIT sessions within the week, the modality of HIIT sessions, and the interaction between varying stimuli such as other training, environmental stress, or nutritional strategies will influence the adaptation response.

Sample Training Programs

The following examples are from the specific 25 wk preparation of Brazilian marathon runner Carlos da Costa for the 1998 Berlin marathon, where he broke the world record at that time, crossing the finish line in a time of 02:06:05. This result was the first time in history that a man averaged <3 min per km for the

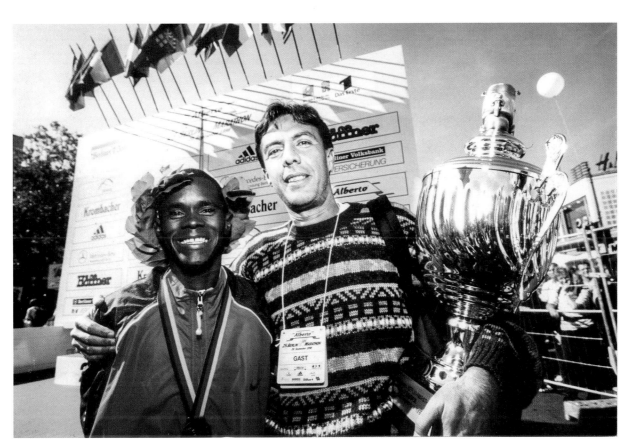

Brazilian marathon runner Carlos da Costa with coach Carlos Alberto Cavalheiro after setting the world record at the 1998 Berlin marathon in a time of 02:06:05.

Victor Sailer/Photorun.

marathon distance. As described in the previous section (figure 14.5), this preparation was broken into one 5 wk general preparation phase (figure 14.6), two 5 wk specific preparation phases (figure 14.7), and finally two 5 wk competition preparation phases (figure 14.8). In each mesocycle, the timing and nature of weekly HIIT throughout each microcycle is shown to change so as to target the desired adaptation response. In the general preparation phase (figure 14.6), there is an emphasis on HIIT target types 2, 3, and 4. Three HIIT sessions are programmed per weekly microcycle, with 48 to 72 h of recovery (low-intensity sessions) to allow more recovery. Neuromuscular load is also relatively high during this phase with the aim of developing resilience, strength, and economy. For example, two HIIT sessions per week include type 2 and 4 targets, supplemented with 2 weekly strength and conditioning (i.e., resistance training in the gym) sessions. During the specific preparation phases, variations of long-interval HIIT type 3 predominate with the introduction of moderate intensity (race pace) training. There is reduced emphasis on neuromuscular loading (no HIIT targets but strength and conditioning sessions remain). Interestingly, the race pace session is programmed within 24 h of the second weekly HIIT session, which means the athlete is likely completing this session in a prefatigued or not completely recovered state. Finally, during the competition preparation phase (figure 14.8), all specific neuromuscular-loading sessions are removed (no HIIT types 2 or 4 or strength and conditioning). However, there is further emphasis on developing race pace ability with the incorporation of race pace work in the long-interval HIIT type 3 sessions. Due to the demanding nature (volume) of each HIIT or race pace session, at least 24 to 72 h separates them to allow for more complete recovery.

General prep 1	Monday	Tuesday	Wednesday	Thursday	Friday	Saturday	Sunday
Morning	S&C + LIT	HIIT (type 3 long)	LIT	S&C + LIT	HIIT (type 3 long + type 4 short)	LIT	HIIT (type 2 short + type 3 long)
Afternoon	LIT	LIT			LIT		

HIIT (type 3 long) 4 × 5 [5 × 400 m at 1:12-1:14 with 45 s active recovery] 60 s active recovery between sets	HIIT (type 3 long + type 4 short) 6 × 1200 m at 3:36-3:42 with 1:15 active recovery + 4:00 active recovery + 12 × 200 m at 32-35 s with 60 s active recovery	HIIT (type 2 short + type 3 long) 25 × 100 m > 75% intensity uphill with 1:30 jogging back recovery + 15 × 2:00 on the flat with 60 s active recovery

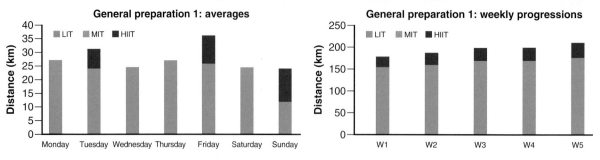

Figure 14.6 A sample general preparation mesocycle consisting of 5 microcycles (weeks). The basic structure and distribution of training sessions within each 7 d microcycle is summarized in terms of the strength and conditioning (S&C) training/resistance training in the gym; low-intensity training (LIT) at <75% $\dot{V}O_2max$, <75% HR_{max}; moderate-intensity training (MIT) at 76% to 85% $\dot{V}O_2max$, 78% to 87% HR_{max}; high-intensity interval training (HIIT) at >85% $\dot{V}O_2max$, >88% HR_{max}. Examples of specific HIIT sessions undertaken by former world record holder Carlos da Costa during the general preparation phase are provided. The average breakdown of intensity distribution throughout a microcycle and the weekly progression of volume and intensity distribution are described.

Specific prep 1	Monday	Tuesday	Wednesday	Thursday	Friday	Saturday	Sunday
Morning	S&C + LIT	HIIT (type 3 long)	LIT	S&C + LIT	HIIT (type 3 long)	LIT/MIT	LIT
Afternoon	LIT	LIT			LIT		

HIIT (type 3 long)
15 x 1000 m at 2:54-2:58 with 35-45 s active recovery

HIIT (type 3 long)
4 x [1600 m at 4:36-4:45 with 50 s active recovery, 800 m at 2:14-2:20 with 90 s active recovery]

LIT/MIT
25 x 100 m > 75% intensity uphill with 1:30 jogging back recovery + 15 x 2:00 on the flat with 60 s active recovery

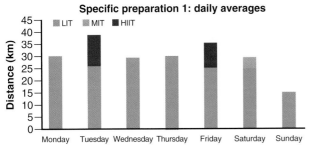

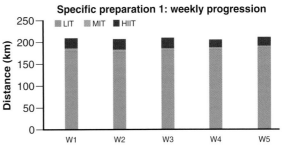

Specific prep 2	Monday	Tuesday	Wednesday	Thursday	Friday	Saturday	Sunday
Morning	LIT	HIIT (type 3 long)	LIT	LIT	HIIT (type 3 long)	LIT/MIT	Rest or LIT
Afternoon	LIT	LIT			LIT		

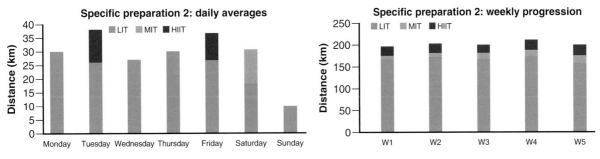

Figure 14.7 A sample of two specific preparation mesocycles consisting of 5 microcycles (weeks). The basic structure and distribution of training sessions within each 7 d microcycle is summarized in terms of the strength and conditioning (S&C) training/resistance training in the gym; low-intensity training (LIT) at <75% $\dot{V}O_2$max, <75% HR_{max}; moderate-intensity training (MIT) at 76 to 85% $\dot{V}O_2$max, 78% to 87% HR_{max}; high-intensity interval training (HIIT) at >85% $\dot{V}O_2$max, >88% HR_{max}. Examples of specific HIIT sessions undertaken by former world record holder Carlos da Costa during the general preparation phase are provided. The average breakdown of intensity distribution throughout a microcycle, and the weekly progression of volume and intensity distribution are described.

Competition prep 1	Monday	Tuesday	Wednesday	Thursday	Friday	Saturday	Sunday
Morning	LIT	MIT/HIIT (type 3 long)	LIT	LIT	HIIT (type 3 long)	LIT	LIT/MIT
Afternoon	LIT	LIT			LIT		

MIT/HIIT (type 3 long)
15 x 1000 m at 3:02-3:06 with 20-25 s active recovery

HIIT (type 3 long)
5 x [3000 m increasing pace for each at 9:30-9:25-9:20-9:10-9:00 with 3:00 active recovery, 800 m at 2:14-2:20 with 90 s active recovery]

LIT/MIT
30 km long run progressing pace every 10/8/5/4/2/1 km as 3:35-3:30-3:25-3:20-3:15-3:10 over flat terrain

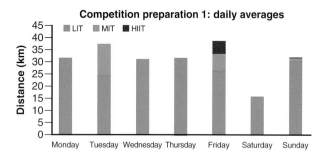

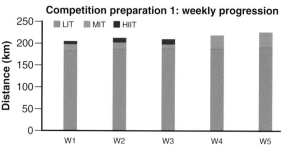

Competition prep 1	Monday	Tuesday	Wednesday	Thursday	Friday	Saturday	Sunday
Morning	LIT	MIT/HIIT (type 3 long)	LIT	LIT	HIIT (type 3 long)	LIT	LIT/MIT
Afternoon	LIT	LIT			LIT		

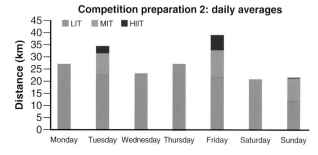

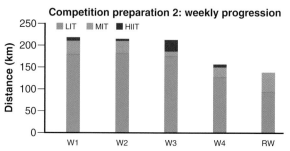

Figure 14.8 A sample of two competitive period mesocycles consisting of 5 microcycles (weeks). The basic structure and distribution of training sessions within each 7 d microcycle is summarized in terms of the S&C, strength and conditioning training/resistance training in the gym; LIT, low-intensity training at <75% $\dot{V}O_2max$, <75% HR_{max}; MIT, moderate-intensity training at 76 to 85% $\dot{V}O_2max$, 78 to 87% HR_{max}; HIIT, high-intensity interval training at >85% $\dot{V}O_2max$, >88% HR_{max}. Examples of specific HIIT sessions undertaken by former world record holder Carlos da Costa during the general preparation phase are provided. The average breakdown of intensity distribution throughout a microcycle, and the weekly progression of volume and intensity distribution are described.

Jamie Stanley

Often in elite sport, the perennial question on a coach's mind may be either "how can we do more?" or "how can we fit more into a program?" to further improve performance. While there is a strong relationship between the volume of training done and the performance outcome, this approach, if poorly implemented can lead to overtraining, maladaptation, injury/illness, and ultimately a compromised preparation and suboptimal performance outcome. As a sport scientist, I like to challenge this approach and ask the alternate question, "What is the minimum stimulus required to achieve the optimal adaptation and performance?" This is commonly termed today as the *minimum effective dose*. As a former elite-level long-distance triathlete accustomed to training 20 to 25 h per wk, I decided to adopt the minimum effective philosophy as a self-experiment during the personal preparation for my first marathon, with the following constraints:

goal time = <2 h 30 min

average training <80 km per wk

6 mo preparation time

About 14 mo separated my final elite half-ironman distance competition (1.9 km swim, 90 km cycle, 21.1 km run) of my career, before commencing my marathon training, during which I exercised only for social and health purposes (running, cycling, and resistance training), including a weekly training volume of 25 km per wk running, 184 km per wk cycling, and 80 min per wk resistance training.

I split my 6 month marathon preparation into three phases. The first phase, lasting 2 mo, was focused on building resilience to the increased running volume. During this phase, weekly run mileage progressed with predominately frequent low-intensity running, before being supplemented with one weekly specific downhill session (to improve neuromuscular and mechanical efficiency as discussed before). The second phase, lasting 3 mo, incorporated the bulk of the "work" and consisted of 6 to 8 runs per week. Each week included one HIIT session on flat terrain (rotation of Mona-fartlek, 90 s to 15 s short intervals at ~95% to 150% v$\dot{V}O_2$max; Yasso 800s, 5 to 10 × 800 m at ~115% to 130% v$\dot{V}O_2$max; and 3 or 4 × 2 km at ~95% v$\dot{V}O_2$max), one HIIT session or fartlek on hills (e.g., 4 × 4 min ~100% $\dot{V}O_2$max) and the occasional 5 or 10 km road race. During these first two phases, weekly bike volume included ~60 km at low intensity to supplement the aerobic training load. Periodized weekly blocks of passive heat exposure (sauna and hot tub) and a 4 wk live-high, train-low hypoxic exposure (altitude tent) was implemented to further enhance cardiovascular and potential molecular adaptations.

The final phase included a 4 wk, three-phase taper whereby training volume and load were initially reduced to 40% to 50% of maximum for 1 wk, returning to 80% to 90% of maximum for the next 2 wk, before finally being reduced for race week. This nontraditional taper was inspired by my father (John Stanley, 02:17:04 marathon best, Australian national team during the 1970s and 1980s) and recent papers detailing preparations of elite Norwegian XC skiers (59) and orienteers (60).

Approximately every 4 wk across the entire preparation I completed a progressively longer long run, commencing with a 20 km steady state (~40% v$\dot{V}O_2$max [4:33 min/km]) progressing to the final run of 36.1 km (the first 15 km was run at ~65% v$\dot{V}O_2$max [3:59 min/km] and the final 21.1 km at marathon pace ~80%v$\dot{V}O_2$max [3:33 min/km], which was actually a personal best half-marathon for me. This final run was a personal psychological and physiological test inspired by the legendary Percy Cerruty (coach of Australian runner Herb Elliot), termed a "will power" session. As Percy himself said, "This session is the one that makes you who

(continued)

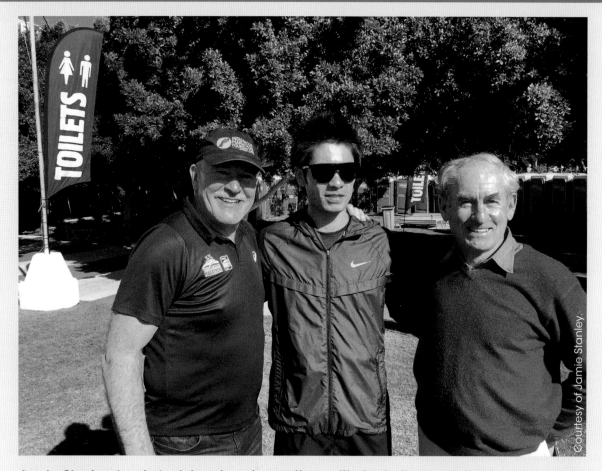

Courtesy of Jamie Stanley.

Jamie Stanley (center) pictured post marathon with Australian marathon record holder Robert de Castella (left) and father John Stanley (right), Australian national team member 1973 to 1985.

you are. Defines what you want to be and gives enlightenment to the individual of oneself. You only ever grow as a human being if you're outside your comfort zone." Percy's infamous "will power" session was done on a sand dune of about 30 to 60 m and the athletes were instructed to run up it as many times as their will allowed.

Throughout the entire preparation, I monitored my adaptation state with heart rate variability, which gives me useful insight, particularly when additional environmental stress loads (heat/hypoxia) were incorporated. In the end, I fell just short of my sub 02:30 debut marathon goal, completing it in 02:32:10 (at the time it was the 21st fastest marathon by an Australian in 2017) off an average weekly running distance of 79.1 km and working full time. To improve, I think that (slightly) more running volume might be required. However, this experiment proved to me that it's not all about "how can we do more?" and that asking "what is the minimum stimulus required for an optimal performance?" is equally an important question we can adopt to produce an optimal performance. In the words of Martin Buchheit, "The process of training is a journey of endless learning, but to learn one must have awareness of how the body adapts to a specific training stimulus."

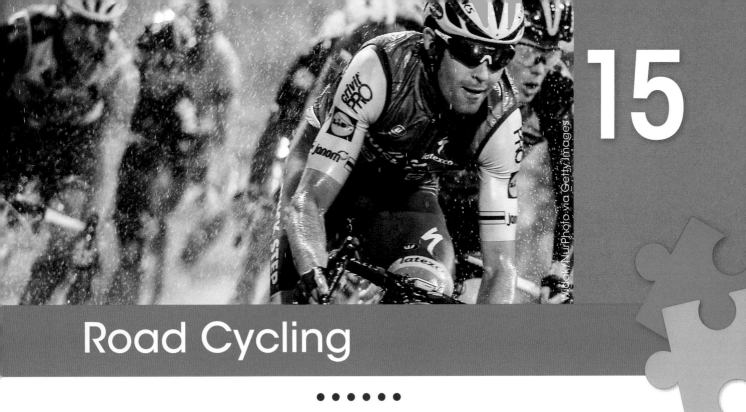

Road Cycling

• • • • • •

Marc Quod

Performance Demands of Road Cycling

This chapter describes the sport of professional road cycling, discussing the various factors of importance for success, and how high-intensity interval training (HIIT) contributes to a cyclist's physical development.

Sport Description and Factors of Winning

One of the most universal sports in the world, road cycling is most popular in Western Europe, centered historically in France, Spain, Italy, and the low countries. Since the mid-1980s, the sport has diversified with professional races now held on all continents of the globe, all governed by the Union Cycliste Internationale (UCI). Road cycling incorporates a large range of competition types, with standalone, single-day races being competed over distances of 3 to 300 km, or a series of races competed over 2 to 21 consecutive days. As well as the UCI's annual World Championships for men and women, the biggest event is the Tour de France, a 3 wk race that can attract more than 500,000 roadside supporters a day. Success in road cycling is influenced by a range of factors including terrain, environmental conditions, tactics, and strategy. However, the primary predictor of performance in a cycling road race is the cyclist's physical capacity. Similar to rowing, swimming, running, and triathlon, success is largely determined by an athlete's physiological capacity over skill or technique. In road cycling, the physiological traits of primary importance are those related to endurance capacity, such as the interrelated qualities of maximum aerobic power, economy, and fatigue resistance.

Due to such large variation in the duration and topography of races, there is equal variation in the type of physiology that is successful in the different events (figure 15.2). As such, many different athlete phenotypes can be competitive in road cycling, as different phenotypes are advantageous in different aspects of the race. Contrasting examples of this are a mesomorphic "sprinter" who relies on an ability to produce a very high peak power output for a very short period of time and an ectomorphic "climber" who needs to maintain a high power output for a much longer duration.

One aspect common to both of these examples, and the reason why power output is expressed in relative terms (W/kg), is the significant impact of mass/gravity on performance. For both the sprinter and the climber alike, their ability to overcome the effect of inertia/gravity is influenced by their body mass, making this a critical part of cycling performance.

297

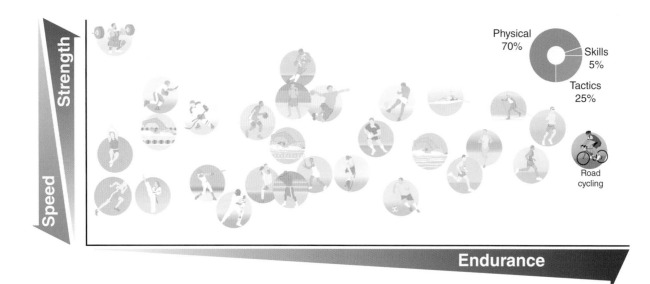

Figure 15.1 The position of the cyclist on the three axes illustrates the relative importance of the three main physical capacities for elite participation, acknowledging this varies slightly between rider type. Outside of critical psychological aspects, which are difficult to quantify, the pie chart shows the general relative importance of skills (5%), tactical awareness (25%), and physical capacities (70%) for cycling success.

Adapted from G.A. Nader, "Concurrent Strength and Endurance Training: From Molecules to Man," *Medicine & Science in Sports & Exercise* 38, no. 11 (2006): 1965-1970.

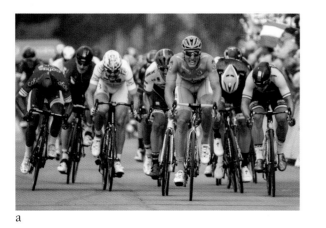
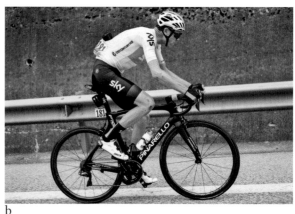

a   b

Figure 15.2 Contrasting examples of (a) Marcel Kittel, a mesomorphic sprinter; and (b) Chris Froome, an ectomorphic climber.

a. Chris Graythen/Getty Images; b. Justin Setterfield/Getty Images.

Road cycling is not without its skill requirements. Descending narrow mountain roads at speeds of up to 100 km/hr requires balance, cornering, and braking skill as well as focus. The ability to ride and navigate "road furniture," dirt and cobbled sections of a course within a fast-moving peloton of up to 200 riders while simultaneously making decisions about the race situation/tactics, requires quick reflexes, fast thinking, and sustained concentration over a long event. These aspects of the sport clearly require practice, skill, and experience, but compared with sports such as American football or tennis, the requirement for skill is comparatively low, making road cycling a sport primarily about the athlete's physiology.

In addition to physiological capacity, there are other important factors that play a role in road cycling success. These include:

1. **An ability to quickly adapt and roll with the punches.** Cycling events take place throughout the year and in different parts of the world. Consequently, environmental factors such as altitude, snow, rain, heat, wind, and cold (sometimes each within a single race) are significant external challenges.

2. **There's a kingpin, but it's a team sport.** A cycle race is competed between teams but has an individual winner, and the winner typically depends on the support of the team to achieve success.

3. **Multiple teams on the pitch make things interesting.** Most team sports are adversarial (team A versus team B), however, in a professional cycle race, 15 to 25 teams of 5 to 9 riders compete at the same time.

4. **Prizes galore add further to complexity.** Within a given cycle race, there are multiple classifications to compete for. In addition to the race winner (first across the line), competitions for points (sprint, mountain, combination) as well as team classifications and total accumulated time (in multiday events) are included, making cycling a game of chess on wheels.

Each of these factors creates an array of incentives and temporary alliances that impact tactics and strategy. As a result, the specific physical requirements that are successful in any given event can vary greatly. The competition requirements for a sprinter in athletics or a rower are clearly established before the competition and do not change. This is not necessarily the case in professional road cycling. As such the specific goal of training depends on an individual rider's strengths and weaknesses, the type of race, and terrain being prepared for, and the likely tactic or strategy to be employed by the team. A benefit of HIIT training is that it can be infinitely varied to tailor the demand of training sessions to replicate the specific physiological requirements that are important in a cyclist's targeted events.

Physical Performance Contributions to Winning

Unlike many other physical capacity–based sports (athletics, rowing, swimming, and running), cycling is competed over much longer durations (up to 300 km for single-day events and ~3500 km across 21 consecutive days of racing in Grand Tours). It is an extreme endurance event (13); consequently, endurance capacity is a key performance indicator.

Figure 15.1 highlights these aspects for cycling in relation to the other sports discussed in this text. In addition, unlike other endurance-based sports, which require athletes to maintain a consistent, maximal-paced effort for a given duration, during a cycling race, the pace is variable. Road cycling is a dynamic event characterized by periods of sustained power output with alternating periods of high and low intensity, the combination of which can be infinitely variable (2).

Figure 15.3 highlights the variable competition demands encountered by a cyclist within and across different stages of a single race. During a flat/sprint stage, the power demands are particularly variable, requiring short maximal accelerations as well as accumulating substantial amounts of time at very low intensity (<100 W). However, during a mountain stage, the power output is less variable but incorporates long periods at sustained moderate intensities. This inherent variability means that every race that a cyclist starts has a unique set of physical demands.

Contrary to popular belief, it is not *necessarily* the cyclist with the highest $\dot{V}O_2max$, or greatest sustainable power output, who wins a road race. The combined impact of tactics, drafting, constantly changing terrain, and associated variable energetic demands means the outcomes of mass start road races are typically determined at one or more critical periods of the races. These distinct periods require the cyclist to produce maximal power output for a race-specific duration. Therefore, depending on the nature of the race (figure 15.3), the winner can potentially be the cyclist who produces the lowest average power output over the duration of the race but produces a maximal effort that is greater than his or her competitors at a critical moment(s) (20). Such acute moments can vary greatly, being as short as 10 s in the final 100 m of the race, to a sustained 5 h effort in a solo breakaway, with every foreseeable combination in between (7, 16).

In summary, to be competitive, a road cyclist requires:

1. A large aerobic capacity, which enables prolonged medium intensity exercise, repeated over sequential days, and

2. An ability to produce a relatively high power output for race-specific periods, the duration of which is variable and may need to be repeated an undefined number of times.

Maximizing the necessary energy systems required to perform this large variation in competition

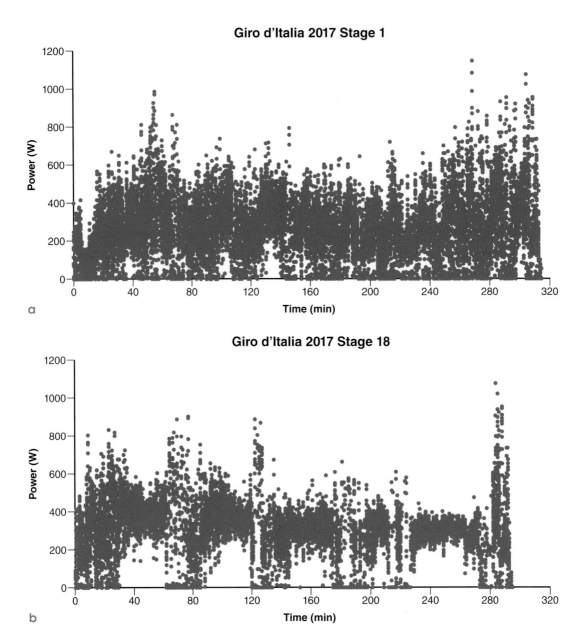

Figure 15.3 Power versus time for the same cyclist during two different stages in the 2017 Giro d'Italia: (a) a flat sprint stage (stage 1); (b) a mountain stage (stage 18). Data are 1 s averages, measured by an SRM power meter.

demands provides an interesting programing challenge for the cycling coach.

Targets of Physical Performance in Road Cycling

As discussed above, road cycling success is built primarily on an aerobic foundation, but anaerobic capacity often dictates the winner. Highlighting the aerobic component of road racing, an analysis of more than 300 flat, semimountainous, and mountainous road races has shown that riders' heart rates average between 50% and 60% of HR_{max}, with average power output during flat and mountainous races reported as 220 W (3.1 W/kg) and 246 W (3.6 W/kg), respectively (18, 19). At first glance, these numbers appear relatively low. However, over the duration of a typical road race, a large number (>100) of very short (<15 s) efforts at power outputs greater than

70% of a rider's peak aerobic power are required (7). Combined with the typical long durations of such road races, these factors create very large energy expenditure and replenishment requirements (~25 MJ/d) (5). The mechanism enabling the expenditure of such large amounts of energy over consecutive days is the cyclist's endurance capacity, which is traditionally measured by maximal oxygen consumption ($\dot{V}O_2max$) and/or maximal aerobic power (MAP). Cyclists tend to have very high values of $\dot{V}O_2max$ and MAP with typical $\dot{V}O_2max$ values ranging between 75 and 85 ml·kg^{-1}·min^{-1} and MAPs of substantially greater than 6.5 W/kg. Chris Froome, the winner of the Tour de France in 2013, 2015, 2016, and 2017, has a reported $\dot{V}O_2peak$ of 5.9 L/min (84 ml·kg^{-1}·min^{-1}), which occurs at a power output of 525 W (7.5 W/kg) (4).

While a large aerobic capacity is a requirement for success, this feature alone is not what separates good cyclists from the best. Comparing submaximal thresholds (see chapters 3 and 4) of elite and professional cyclists, both aerobic (i.e., first ventilatory threshold; VT_1) and maximal lactate steady-state/critical power (i.e., or second ventilatory threshold; VT_2) thresholds occur at significantly higher exercise intensities, with submaximal lactate levels substantially lower in professional compared to elite-level cyclists (14). These physiological adaptations enable cyclists to repeatedly sustain relatively high percentages of their $\dot{V}O_2max$ (>85%) for prolonged periods of time (30 to 60 min) within a road race. In addition, the lowered physiological disturbance at submaximal intensities enabled by high thresholds enhances fatigue resistance and a cyclist's ability to recover both within a race and across multiple days.

It has been highlighted that race-winning moves in road cycling are typically much shorter than the event itself. These moments can vary infinitely in duration, intensity, and pacing pattern, but can be grouped into three general categories:

1. **Sprints:** a maximal sprint in the final meters of a race, which can be as short as 10 s at >17 W/kg (17);

2. **Short attacks:** a repeated series of efforts, designed to distance rivals before reaching the finish line, of between 30 s and 5 min at 7 to 10 W/kg;

3. **Sustained efforts**: a maximally paced effort, typically over the final 10 to 60 min of a race at 5.5 to 7 W/kg (13).

Naturally, these effort types do not occur in isolation. Throughout a race, riders will be required to produce an unknown combination of each of these types of efforts. Cycling is clearly dominated by aerobic and anaerobic capacities, and as the efforts described above occur with relatively slow muscular contractions, the neuromuscular component of training is small compared to many other sports. While this aspect of training should not be overlooked for any athlete, the focus of HIIT training sessions for cyclists tends to be on developing aerobic and anaerobic metabolic capacity.

Cyclists in a professional team are not assigned positions as is the case in most team sports. Rather, their individual physiology (see figure 15.2) and relative ability to perform each of these three types of effort determines the role that is undertaken in each race. Corresponding with the three general categories of effort, there are three general types of rider:

1. **The sprinter:** Sprinters such as Marcel Kittel, Andre Greipel, Mario Cipollini, and Mark Cavendish target the final 200 m of a (normally flat) race. Up to this point they are looked after by their teammates with the goal to expend as little energy as possible throughout the race, saving this for a maximal acceleration in the final meters of the race. The sprint is typically between 10 to 15 s in duration and at power outputs of greater than 17 W/kg (17). Consequently, training tends to focus on short, high-intensity efforts that maximize the athlete's ability to deplete energy stores rapidly. However, while anaerobic adaptations are the focus for these riders, sprints occur at the end of 3 to 7 h of racing and across consecutive days. In addition, the ~10 min prior to the final sprint becomes progressively more difficult and requires a series of near maximal sprints to maintain position in the peloton (17). Therefore, to be fit enough to arrive at the finish line with the competition, aerobic and fatigue resistance aspects of fitness cannot be overlooked.

2. **The all-rounder:** As the name implies, these types of riders may not have a single aspect of performance that they are the best at, but rather, are very capable in many different situations. Riders such as Peter Sagan, Philippe Gilbert, Paolo Bettini, and Eddy Merckx are famous examples of an all-rounder. As these riders are capable across varied terrain, the focus of training will depend on their goal in upcoming races and will span the breadth of aerobic and anaerobic training variables. Due to the versatile strength of these types of riders, they

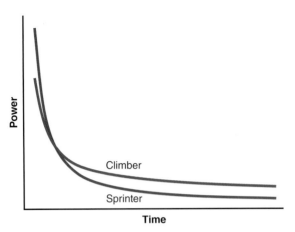

Figure 15.4 A generic power profile that illustrates the relative differences in ability to produce power for two different types of cyclist (climber versus sprinter). For short durations of time, the sprinter can produce very high power outputs, however, as the duration of the effort extends, the relative power produced by the climber exceeds that of the sprinter. The power profile of the all-rounder will often fall between these two extremes.

are often the ones called upon to work during a road race. This can include riding at the front of the peloton for multiple hours at medium intensity to maintain a specific time gap to the breakaway group, returning to a following support vehicle to collect food and drinks for the team leaders, or riding in front of a team leader throughout a race, providing him with an aerodynamic draft and easy ride in the peloton. In these situations, the all-rounder's job is to expend his energy so that the team leader can conserve his own.

3. The climber/general classification (GC): The climber is at the opposite end of the spectrum to the sprinter (as illustrated in figures 15.2 and 15.4). Climbers such as Chris Froome, Alberto Contador, or Nairo Quintana lack the ability to produce very high absolute power outputs required to win a bunch sprint. Rather, they excel by repeatedly sustaining high relative workloads as they ascend mountains. Races typically classified as mountainous include routes that can accumulate up to 5500 m of vertical ascent requiring the climber to accumulate up to 2.5 h at intensities greater than 75% of $\dot{V}O_2$max. Consequently, maximizing aerobic capacity and the sustainable percentage of that capacity are the primary targets of training sessions for the climber.

Key Weapons, Manipulations, and Surveillance Tools

For a professional cyclist, the majority of training hours (10 to 30 h per week) are spent accumulating volume at low intensities (50% to 80% of HR_{max}, 40% to 70% $\dot{V}O_2$max). This relatively unstructured part of the training program is important as it replicates the volume of exercise required in races, as well as positively influencing body composition, economy, and aerobic capacity (10, 12). In addition to the large amount of time spent at low intensities, cyclists also complete a substantial amount of time training at medium, or mid-zone, intensity. Typical aerobic/medium intensity intervals are completed over durations of 15 to 60 min at intensities of 80% to 90% HR_{max} or 70% to 85% $\dot{V}O_2$max. Given the event requirements, this is the aspect of fitness and training that cyclists prioritize.

For most cyclists, HIIT contributes considerably less time to the training schedule (<10%) compared to low- and medium-intensity training. However, even though it contributes only a small percentage of total training time, HIIT remains a critical component of the training program. Road races are won (or lost) in a moment of maximum effort, and HIIT is particularly important for maximizing the adaptations of both oxidative and nonoxidative energy systems that fuel these maximal efforts (see chapter 3). The structure of the various HIIT intervals that are relevant to cycling performance varies greatly, along with the diverse range of competition requirements within road races. The key weapons, or HIIT formats, including their manipulations and surveillance (monitoring) tools, are described next.

HIIT Weapons, Targets, and Manipulations

As shown in figure 15.5, the most common HIIT formats or weapons included in cycling training programs primarily include long interval, short interval, and sprint interval training, aimed at type 1 through 5 targets, with a metabolic emphasis. Repeated sprint training, which incorporates very short duration efforts (3 to 7 s), are used infrequently by road cyclists.

Long Intervals

Long HIIT intervals usually take the form of 1 to 6 min work durations at intensities of 85% to 95%

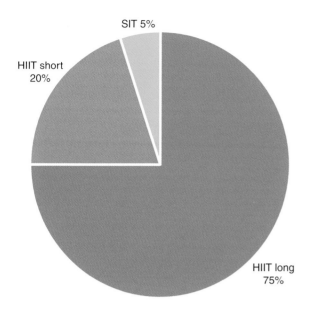

Figure 15.5 Percentage of the different HIIT formats (weapons) used throughout the annual season in professional cycling.

of HR_{max}, 85% to 100% of $\dot{V}O_2max$/MAP, generally with work:rest ratios between 1:0.5 and 1:2. Total accumulated duration at these intensities during such interval sets is typically 20 to 40 min split between 1 to 5 sets. A traditional and common long HIIT interval session for a cyclist is 5×5 min intervals at 80% to 90% MAP with recovery intervals of 5 min at a very low intensity. The desired metabolic load for these HIIT sessions includes type 2, 3, and 4 targets. These different targets can be achieved by manipulating the work:rest ratio. For example, reducing the work period (<90 s) and increasing the rest period (>90 s) will focus the session toward using more anaerobic metabolism. Conversely, increasing the work period (>3 min) while reducing the recovery period (<3 min) will emphasize use of aerobic metabolism.

Short Intervals

Short HIIT intervals for road cyclists usually take the form of 20 to 60 s work durations at intensities of 100% to 140% of MAP, generally with work:rest ratios between 1:0.5 and 1:1. Total accumulated work duration for these interval sets is generally between 10 to 20 min, split between 3 to 10 sets. An example of a short HIIT session for a cyclist would be a series of 6×6 min intervals of alternating 20 s at 110% MAP with 10 s at very low intensity, with recovery between the series of 4 min. The desired metabolic load for these HIIT sessions includes type 1, 2, 3,

and 4 targets. Similar to long HIIT intervals, these different targets can be achieved by manipulating the work:rest ratio. Alternatively, the intensity of both the work or rest period can be adjusted to shift the balance between anaerobic and aerobic metabolism (see chapter 5).

Sprint Interval Training

Sprint intervals for road cyclists tend to be the domain of the "pure" sprinters, although they are relevant to all cyclists who want to improve their sprints. Sprint intervals are composed of maximal efforts between 10 and 30 s, with recovery periods of 2 to 10 min. As the goal of these intervals is to reach maximal values, the number of sprints is typically low (1 to 5), and time between sets relatively long (>30 min). The desired load for these HIIT sessions includes type 5 targets.

Manipulations of Interval Training Variables

A marathon runner is acutely aware of the precise physiological requirements of his next race and HIIT interval sessions can be tailored and periodized appropriately for the specific energy system requirements of a 2 h marathon (see chapter 14). However, the competition demands of a road race vary considerably from race to race (as highlighted in figure 15.3) and are not always predictable. Consequently, each of the 12 different HIIT variables (chapter 4) are important factors in each HIIT session and can be manipulated depending on the type of race a cyclist is targeting.

Physiological parameters such as critical power (CP), onset of blood lactate accumulation (OBLA), MAP, and lactate and ventilatory thresholds are often utilized to guide HIIT interval sessions. In cycling, the use of power meters built into the bicycle, combined with measurement of heart rate, has allowed for very precise prescription and measurement of exercise intensities relative to various physiological markers (see chapter 8). With this technology, the cyclist is able to ride at a specific power output that is associated with the physiological parameter of interest. The advantage of this approach to HIIT interval prescription is that it allows the coach to focus on and isolate the underlying physiology and energy systems that support a given competition demand.

In addition, similar to the track-and-field approach to the prescription of HIIT sessions (chapter 2), the expected competition demands of an upcoming race can also be used to develop specific HIIT training sessions. Using GPS technology and historical records of the speed/power relationship over different sections of terrain, it is possible to make predictions as to the critical sections of upcoming races. For example, a circuit race that includes 15 repetitions of a 1 km climb will require repeating ~2.5 min efforts at >6 W/kg each lap. This critical section of the race can be used to design an HIIT training session. While the components of these sessions are manipulated without reference to the body's energy-delivery systems, the advantage of this method is that the HIIT sessions replicate the specific competition requirements.

The primary factors of any HIIT session include the intensity and duration of the work and rest periods. Typically, as most HIIT work intervals are relatively short in duration, power (W) is best used to prescribe the intensity. There are no required or recommended durations that should be incorporated in a cyclist's HIIT training session, rather the choice of appropriate duration should be anchored by either upcoming competition demands or the limits of the relevant energetic systems. Similarly, the number of intervals in a series, the series duration and time between each series of HIIT intervals will depend on the specific competition demand or the physiologic or metabolic system being targeted by the coach.

Modality is also an important HIIT variable in cycling. Typically, this component of an HIIT session is manipulated by altering terrain (positive, negative, or neutral gradient) and cadence (rpm).

Choice of terrain for HIIT sessions is primarily dictated by the type of terrain that the rider will encounter in upcoming races. However, a secondary benefit of utilizing different gradients in training is the ability to impact the inertial load encountered by the rider. As shown in figure 15.6, due to the disparity in speed while climbing versus riding on the flat, for a given power output, the inertial load during these activities and the associated self-selected cadences are different (9).

Similarly, manipulating the cadence (rpm) during a work interval will impact the balance between muscular strength and coordination as well as the neuromuscular and metabolic demands. For example, a 5 min work interval completed at 80% of MAP and 60 rpm will differ from an interval done at the same intensity but with 120 rpm. This is because power is a product of torque and angular velocity. While the power remains constant across these two work intervals, due to the change in cadence (angular velocity), the torque requirements in the low-cadence condition (60 rpm) are double that of the high-cadence condition (120 rpm). Using cadence to manipulate the torque requirements of a work interval is analogous to focusing on strength versus speed in the gym (see chapter 6).

Because road races are not constantly paced efforts, there is also opportunity to add additional layers (complexity) to HIIT interval sessions to replicate race demands. Specifically, levels of intensity during the work and rest periods can be varied. An example may include a period of moderate-hard intensity work immediately prior to a maximal sprint in a sprint interval training session. This replicates the demands of a sprinter in a race situation, fighting to maintain good position in the peloton in the lead up to her final maximal acceleration. Alternatively, periods of medium-hard intensity may follow a maximal effort prior to the rest period. This type of effort replicates the demand of an all-rounder who needs to accelerate maximally to distance himself from the peloton midway through a race, but then needs to maintain a moderate intensity to maintain this distance to the finish line.

Finally, as training sessions tend to be relatively long in duration (2 to 7 h), the decision of where to place an HIIT interval within a training session is important. Placing HIIT intervals in the beginning, middle, or end of a session changes the initial state of fatigue and energy availability (glycogen stores) that the interval session is commenced with (chapter 4). An athlete who is looking to increase absolute power production in a sprint may choose to complete sprint-specific HIIT intervals in the first hour of a training session to maximize quality and achieve peak power outputs, whereas a rider looking to improve fatigue resistance may complete the intervals in the final hour of training when fatigue is relatively high and glycogen stores are already depleted.

Surveillance and Monitoring Tools

The primary surveillance and monitoring tools used by professional cyclists are the power meter, heart rate monitor, and their associated analysis software. Other useful monitoring tools include a cycling computer that records speed, time, and distance as well as the vertical distance accumulated. Databasing and analyzing trends in these variables over time allows an athlete to precisely track progress,

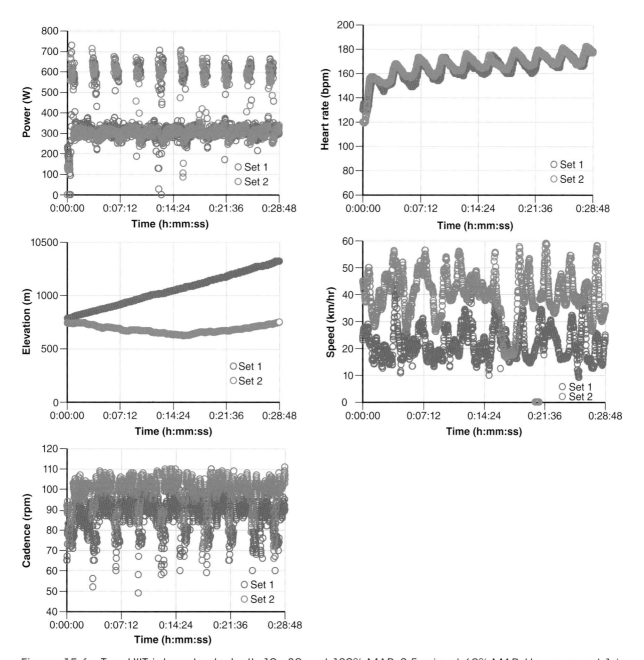

Figure 15.6 Two HIIT interval sets, both 10×30 s at 120% MAP, 2.5 min at 60% MAP. However, set 1 is completed on a climb (average gradient of 5%), whereas set 2 is completed on level ground. Although the power output and heart rate response are almost identical between the two interval sets, the influence of road gradient on speed and subsequently self-selected cadence, torque, and in turn, neuromuscular load, is different.

highlight breakthroughs in performance or aspects of training that have been overlooked.

Load

Intensity prescription based on heart rate is the most commonly used strategy to control and monitor exercise intensity, though it is best suited to prolonged submaximal exercise. The high intensity and

relatively short duration HIIT intervals and the associated lag in HR response (see chapters 2, 8, and 9) preclude the use of HR for prescribing HIIT intervals. The best method for prescribing and monitoring intensity during HIIT sessions is with a power meter attached to the bicycle. These technological innovations allow for accurate and reliable measures of both power output (external work/stress) and heart rate (internal work/strain), which makes cycling a privileged sport in the realm of exercise science and has allowed for numerous laboratory- versus field-based comparisons of performance (1, 8).

Training Status

With the use of power meters, during the course of training or racing, strengths and weaknesses of riders can be identified on any portion of the power-duration continuum where a maximal effort occurs (chapter 4; i.e., W′, CP). For example, markers of sustainable threshold power output are commonly used for road cyclists, and include a 20 or 60 min power output, popularly referred to as functional threshold power (FTP) (3).

The information derived from power meters, heart rate monitors, and their array of associated analysis technologies has proven useful in a number of applications for the cycling scientist and enthusiast. The ability to review a session after training by coach, support team, and athlete allows informed decisions with respect to training and recovery. When the data and analysis (such as the power:heart rate ratio) is compared alongside an athlete's rating of perceived exertion or informal comments, the combined information provides for a sound global indicator of an athlete's state of readiness to perform. Additionally, as much information is freely available today, many athletes research and learn this information and compare their power output numbers to published records. As a result, many athletes in the sport are informed and well versed when it comes to commonly used cycling-specific training lingo, including normalized power, power:heart rate ratio, training stress score, training stress balance (TSB), and chronic training load (CTL) (3).

Given the large training volumes, and the general belief that more training is always better, the risk of developing chronic overreaching is very real (see chapter 7). To help predict or minimize this risk, it is possible to accurately track long-term training load, however the predictive ability of various training load calculations (such as TSB) remains limited and tied to rules of thumb. Advances in other monitoring tools such as heart rate variability are helping (chapter 9), but again, their predictive power is limited.

Despite all this data and technology at our fingertips, there are still many unanswered questions in the world of road cycling. The systematic collection of reliable power and heart rate data has existed for many years, yet we are still some way from understanding the optimal balance of training variables. The varying and diverse rules and goals of the sport, the inherent uncertainty of race demands, and the infinite uniqueness of individual athletes maintains this challenge.

Strategies for Structuring the Training Program Using HIIT

Implementing an HIIT program in the real world of road cycling is a complex task. As with most sports, there are numerous uncontrollable factors that must be considered.

Controllable and Uncontrollable Factors

The World Tour is the top tier of professional cycling and includes 37 races (175 individual race days) spread throughout the world including Australia, China, North America, the Middle East, and Europe. Professional teams consist of 24 to 30 riders and compete in the World Tour as well as other lower-level races each season. Individual riders typically complete 40 to 90 race days each year, spread primarily between January and October. Given the large number of races available, the competition schedule for an individual rider can vary from year to year. As cyclists compete in substantially more races than other endurance athletes, this variable and relatively large race program is the primary factor that impacts an individual's training program.

Due to the extreme nature of road races, the physiological load of a race is typically much higher than can be achieved in training. Therefore, appropriate periods need to be built in to training programs both before (taper) and after (recovery) each race to avoid overreaching and negative training outcomes. Depending on the context, these recovery periods can be 2 d to 2 weeks.

Finally, travel requirements are another challenge that road cycling teams must consider. Races are conducted all over the world, and training camps (typically in hot climates or at altitude; chapter 4) are often in difficult to reach places. Thus, recovery from travel stress as well as time for circadian adaptation to the time zone needs to be considered; otherwise, the health of the athlete may be compromised (chapter 7).

Program Structure and Progression

There are a number of different approaches utilized in cycling, and all have been used successfully at one time or another, from classic to block periodization models, and everything in between. As the competition program is irregular, and to some degree chosen by the athlete, there is vast scope for variation and individualization of the training program and its periodization. Due to high volumes of training in nearly all programs, appropriate progression of training load remains a key to avoiding overuse injuries in road cyclists. Despite this variation, some general observations can be made across the macro-, meso-, and microcycles observed in the majority of the road cycling peloton.

Macrocycle

A road cyclist's season is typically periodized over a 12 month cycle with key racing objectives or peaks lasting 3 to 6 wk. The best cyclists tend to have just one or two primary objectives each season. For these athletes, a classic Matveyev approach (high to low volume, low to high intensity) to periodization is common (15). The duration between season peaks allows for progressive training blocks with targeted physiological overloads. However, many in the peloton are required to be at a high level of fitness for sustained periods, often a series of three to five objectives separated by brief periods of 1 to 3 wk. For these cyclists, periodization can be similar to many team sport athletes who build a high level of fitness in the preseason and then maintain that through a long competitive period. The German athletics coach Peter Tschiene has described this approach to periodization, where all aspects of fitness are trained at a high level at the same time by systematically varying each component of fitness (21, 22). Incorporating the use of frequent, short recovery periods enables the athlete to maintain a readiness to compete throughout a long competitive season.

Mesocycle

A typical basic or preparatory mesocycle in cycling follows the traditional 4 wk approach, with 3 loading weeks and 1 recovery week. However, this will vary depending on the available time between races and can include shock mesocycles (~1 or 2 wk), precompetition or transition mesocycles (~2 to 4 wk), competition mesocycles (~3 to 6 wk), and recovery mesocycles (~1 to 4 wk).

Microcycle

The microcycles of a road cyclist's program tend to be variable. Whereas 2 and 3 day training blocks separated by a single recovery day are the most common and traditional, single day and up to 10 day microcycles are not uncommon. This variation is in line with the competition requirements of the sport. Cyclists who are targeting single-day races are more likely to include single-day training blocks with a focus on maximal expenditure of energy in a single day, whereas a cyclist targeting the overall classification in a 3 wk Grand Tour will incorporate longer microcycles to reflect the recovery and repetition aspects of competition demands.

Periodized Nutrition

As outlined in chapter 4, periodized nutrition also plays an important role in the life of a road cyclist. Not only is nutrition important in controlling a cyclist's weight but manipulating the fuel available for a training session can alter the adaptations to that session (6).

Carbohydrate is the most common macronutrient to be targeted as glycogen stores and availability can be easily influenced by the amount of carbohydrate consumed before, during, or after a training session (11). Performing training sessions with low glycogen stores or minimal exogenous carbohydrate availability (popularly termed *train low*) and consuming carbohydrate at a rate >100 g/h during a training session (popularly termed *train high*) are typical methods of carbohydrate manipulation (11).

Today, carbohydrate quantity is a programmed component of nearly every training session a rider does, and can be incorporated into HIIT sessions, low- and medium-intensity training sessions, as well as being a component of the overall periodization plan.

Sample Training Programs

An example of a cyclist's training program, including planning during the preparation and competition phases alongside HIIT integration and target types, are shown in figure 15.7.

Macro-cycle	10	11	12	13	14	15	16	17	18	19	20
Phase	Preparation 2					Transition 1					Competition 1
Race		Training camp	Training camp			Altitude camp	Altitude camp	Altitude camp			Tirreno-Adriatico
Meso-cycle	1	2	3	4	R	1	2	3	R	1	2
Mon	Medium intervals		Type 1		Volume	Acclimation	Volume	Aerobic intervals			
Tues	Strength	Aerobic intervals	Strength	Type 1		Acclimation					
Wed	Volume	Medium intervals	Volume	Medium intervals		Volume	Strength	Type 2		Medium intervals	
Thu	Aerobic intervals	Strength	Aerobic intervals	Strength		Volume	Medium intervals	Volume			
Fri		Volume		Volume			Volume			Recovery	
Sat	Type 1		Medium intervals			Strength		Type 2	1 day race	Recovery	
Sun	Volume		Type 1	Aerobic intervals		Aerobic intervals	Type 2		1 day race	1 day race	

Macro-cycle	21	22	23	24	25	26	27	28	29	30	31
Phase	Competition 1 (continued)		Transition 2						Competition 2		
Race	Tirreno-Adriatico	Volta Catalunya	Altitude camp	Altitude camp	Altitude camp	Altitude camp	Altitude camp		Giro d'Italia	Giro d'Italia	Giro d'Italia
Meso-cycle	3	4	R	1	2	3	R	R	1	2	3
Mon				Strength + volume		Medium intervals					
Tues				Volume							
Wed				Medium intervals	Type 3 + strength	Type 2	Medium intervals				
Thu					Medium intervals	Medium intervals					
Fri				Strength + volume							
Sat	Medium intervals			Volume	Type 2	Type 3 + strength	Aerobic intervals				
Sun				Medium intervals	Volume	Volume	Volume				

Figure 15.7 Preparation phase of a cyclist's training plan. Details of individual HIIT sessions are: long-interval HIIT type 1 = 5 x 5 min at 85% MAP (5 min easy); short-interval HIIT type 2 = 3 sets of 10 to 16 x (35 sec at 110% MAP, 100+ rpm [25 s at 60% MAP]); long-interval HIIT type 3 = 2 sets of 6 x 3 min at 90+% MAP (3 min easy).

The Team Time Trial World Championship is an event competed over distances of 30 to 60 km (45 to 70 min depending on the terrain) in teams of six riders. Each rider takes a turn at the front of the group while the other riders follow in the lead rider's draft. The goal of the event is to get at least four of the team of six riders from point A to point B in the least amount of time.

Historically, to win this event requires an average speed of 52 to 57 km/h. Depending on the composition of the team and the terrain, riders take turns at the front of the group for 20 to 90 seconds. The power requirement while riding at the front of the group at these speeds is roughly 110% to 120% MAP. After each rider's turn at the front, the rider moves to the back of the line of riders, rotating through to the front sequentially. While following teammates, the power output in the aerodynamic slipstream is reduced significantly. The second rider in line is required to produce ~80% of the power produced by the lead rider, third ~65%, and fourth to sixth ~55%, typically around 60% to 70% MAP. Although dictated primarily by the terrain, the length of time between turns at the front is typically 2 to 5 min. As you can see, the Team Time Trial is essentially an HIIT session, alternating high-intensity work periods with lower-intensity recovery periods.

In an ideal situation, preparation for the Team Time Trial involves the selected six riders training together over a course that replicates the race. However, due to other team objectives and the proximity of other races, it is not always possible to get all six riders together prior to the event. In 2016, our team had riders coming from very different backgrounds: two riders had recently competed in the Olympic Games in the Team Pursuit (an event that lasts <4 min), three had completed the Tour de France (>3300 km across 3 wk, 8 wk prior to the event) and one had completed the Vuelta España (>3100 km across 3 wk, 3 wk prior to the event). The diversity in training and racing in the lead-up to the event meant that each of the six riders had different recovery and training requirements. In addition, different race programs immediately prior to the event precluded any group training sessions.

The two riders coming from the Olympic Games and Team Pursuit training had already completed a lot of work to maximize their ability to produce power over short durations (<4 min), but the 2016 Team Time Trial World Championships were expected to take ~45 min to complete the 40 km course. Conversely, the remaining riders had recently completed Grand Tours and had spent 80+ hr over 3 wk at a medium intensity; they were undoubtedly fit but lacked the exposure to the specific high-intensity work required for the Team Time Trial.

As the riders coming from the Olympic Games lacked the required aerobic adaptations necessary to repeat efforts over a 45 min event, type 1 HIIT sessions, short intervals of 10 to 30 s at 110 to 130% MAP, were targeted in their training. Conversely, the riders coming from the Grand Tours needed to improve their ability to produce a high-power output while at the front of the team. Consequently, type 3 HIIT sessions, long intervals of 60 to 90 s at 90% to 110% MAP, were incorporated in their training.

Unfortunately, the team was not able to win the World Championships in 2016, but with the help of individualized HIIT training sessions, a group with limited opportunity to train together and from vastly different training backgrounds achieved a podium result, finishing within 1.5% of the winner's time.

This experience highlights the value in the inherent variability of HIIT sessions, which provided a distinct advantage in this situation. While the optimal way to prepare for such an event may be to have the whole team training together, by targeting and manipulating each of the 12 HIIT variables (see figure 4.2), it is possible to bring a diverse group of athletes together and be competitive as a team.

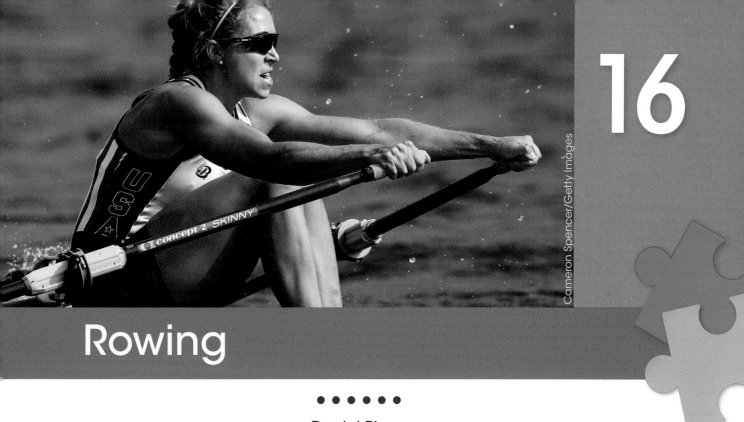

Rowing

Daniel Plews

• • • • • •

Performance Demands of Rowing

This chapter describes the sport of elite rowing, the various factors that are important for success in the standard Olympic distance 2000 m event, and how high-intensity interval training (HIIT) contributes to physiological development.

Sport Description and Factors of Winning

Rowing, often referred to as crew in the United States, is a sport with origins back to ancient Egyptian times, and it is one of the oldest Olympic sports. The sport is based on propelling a boat (racing shell) on water using oars. By pushing against the water with an oar, force is generated to move the boat. Modern rowing as a competitive sport can be traced to the early 10th century when races were held between professional watermen on the river Thames in London, United Kingdom. Amateur competition began toward the end of the 18th century with the arrival of boat clubs at the British public schools of Eton College and Westminster School, progressing to present day's annual Boat Race held between the University of Oxford and the University of Cambridge crews. The International Rowing Federation (in French, the Fédération Internationale des Sociétés d'Aviron, or FISA), responsible for international governance of rowing, was founded in 1892 to provide regulation at a time when the sport was gaining popularity. Across six continents, 150 countries now have rowing federations that participate in the sport.

Each year the World Rowing Championships, staged by FISA, sees 22 boat classes raced. In Olympic years only the non-Olympic boat classes are raced at the World Championships. Rowing competitions take place over 2000 m for both men and women. Races are held for sculling (where the rower holds two oars) and sweep boats (where each rower holds one oar), and include pairs, fours, and eights, as well as sometimes the inclusion of a coxswain, although "coxed" fours and pairs are no longer events in the Olympic schedule. The single scull boat is raced by an individual rower (both genders) using two oars. There are additionally lightweight rowing events for both male and female divisions. The different types of rowing classes result in marginal variation in the time taken to complete the 2000 m event, ranging from 5 min (men's eight rowing) to 7 min (women's single scull). The Olympic boats (as of the last Olympics) are outlined in table 16.1. The table shows the associated abbreviations that will be used throughout the chapter.

Table 16.1 Olympic Rowing Boat Classifications

Boat	Number of athletes in boat	Rowing type	Abbreviation
Men's single scull	1	Scull	M1x
Women's single scull	1	Scull	W1x
Men's pair	2	Sweep	M2-
Women's pair	2	Sweep	W2-
Men's double	2	Scull	M2x
Women's double	2	Scull	W2x
Men's lightweight double	2	Scull	LM2x
Women's lightweight double	2	Scull	LW2x
Men's four	4	Sweep	M4-
Men's lightweight four	4	Sweep	LM4-
Men's quad	4	Scull	M4x
Women's quad	4	Scull	W4x
Men's coxed eight	8 + 1 × cox	Sweep	M8+
Women's coxed eight	8 + 1 × cox	Sweep	W8+

Classifications as of the Rio Olympic Games.

Rowers are typically large in terms of both body mass and stature. This is advantageous for creating a long distance per stroke. Anthropometric values for open-class males and females are 94.3±5.9 kg and 76.6±5.2 kg, respectively. Comparatively, lightweight rowers, who are classified in their division by weight, average 72.5±1.8 kg and 58.5±1.5 kg, respectively, while typical statures average 1.95±0.05 m and 1.81±0.05 m for open-class males/females and 1.82±0.04/1.69±0.05 m for lightweights (7).

The body composition of rowers is varied, but generally athletes have higher levels of fat-free mass versus other endurance-like sports. This is because their weight is supported by the boat. The average sum of 8 skinfolds in elite-level rowers for males and females has been reported to be 65.3±17.3 mm and 89.0±23.6 mm, respectively. Conversely, lightweight rowers generally carry very little fat-free mass (figure 16.1), possessing an average sum of 8 skinfolds of 44.8±8.1 mm and 59.7±12.4 mm for males and females, respectively, levels near those of other endurance-sport athletes (i.e., triathletes, cyclists, runners) (7).

Like many other water-based sports (i.e., swimming, kayak, etc.), rowing has a large technical component that is needed to apply force effectively in the water medium. Rowing is characterized by a complex sequence of movements, which in its simplest terms can be broken down into the *drive phase* and the *recovery phase*. This is what allows the athlete to propel the boat from one point to the next in the fastest possible time. Coaches in their training programs nearly always emphasize rowing technique, with specific drills often used to improve distance per stroke and synchronicity/timing between crewmembers. Often, there can be discrepancies between performance on the indoor Concept 2 rowing machine (which requires only raw power and little technique) and that of on-water performance (which is highly technical), thus showing the importance of on-water rowing technique (13). Raw physical power by itself cannot win in this sport.

Traditionally, the intensity of rowing is set by stroke rate (SR) rather than heart rate or speed. The SR chosen during 2000 m racing depends on the boat, with smaller boats rating at lower SRs (30 to 34 strokes per minute; SPM) and larger boats at higher SRs (38 to 41 SPM). The relationship between SR and speed is generally linear (8), making this an important consideration in training program design. Figure 16.2 shows a typical training intensity prescription for an elite M2-, based on the linear speed-to-SR model (8). Interestingly, despite the differences in the SRs associated with race pace, the typical approach I have observed among rowing coaches is one where SR is set at a fixed rate across multiple crew boats, regardless of the chosen SR during competition. This results in a varied training intensity between boats training at the same time. For example, if an M1x has a racing SR of 31, and an M8+ has a racing SR of 39, both might still be asked to rate at 25 SPM during a training session completed together. As a

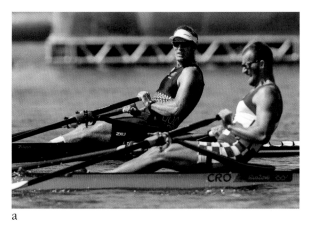 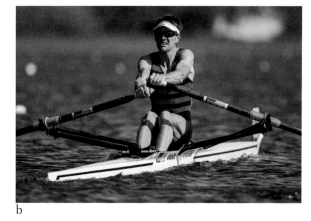

a
b

Figure 16.1 The distinctly different physical and proportional anthropometric characteristics of (a) open-class and (b) lightweight rowers.

a. Christian Petersen/Getty Images; b. Joel Ford/Getty Images.

World record training zones					
Grade elite World (%)	Boat M2- Speed km/hr	Time per 500 m	HIIT format	HIIT targets	Target stroke rate
77	15.0	1:59.6	18		18
78	15.2	1:58.1		Aerobic endurance (LIT)	
79	15.4	1:56.6			
80	15.6	1:55.2	20		20
81	15.8	1:53.7			
82	16.0	1:52.3	20		20
83	16.2	1:51.0		Threshold intensity (MIT)	
84	16.4	1:49.7	23		23
85	16.6	1:48.4	24		24
86	16.8	1:47.1			
87	17.0	1:45.9	26		26
88	17.2	1:44.7	28		28
89	17.4	1:43.5			
90	17.6	1:42.4			
91	17.8	1:41.2			
92	18.0	1:40.1	32		32
93	18.2	1:39.1	34		34
94	18.4	1:38.0			
95	18.6	1:37.0			
96	18.8	1:36.0			
97	19.0	1:35.0	35	Long intervals	Type 3 and 4	35
98	19.1	1:34.0			
99	19.3	1:33.1	37		37
100	19.5	1:32.1	38		38
101	19.7	1:31.2	39	Short intervals	Types 1, 2, 3, 4	39
102	19.9	1:30.3	40		40
103	20.1	1:29.4	41	Repeated sprint training	Type 4 and 5	41
104	20.3	1:28.6			
105	20.5	1:27.7			
106	20.7	1:26.9	Open rate	Repeated sprint training	Type 5	Open rate
107	20.9	1:26.1			
108	21.1	1:25.3			
109	21.3	1:24.5			
110	21.5	1:23.7			

Figure 16.2 Typical training intensity prescription model for an elite M2- based on the general linear speed-to-SR relationship. Recommendations for stroke rate relative to training intensity, HIIT type, and boat speed (percent of world best time) are shown.

result, the intensity will be much higher for the single scull rower compared to the M8+ crew. Figure 16.2 shows how this linear relationship can be extrapolated to training intensity prescription across typically performed training sessions for an M2-.

When comparing across boats, rowing coaches often use a prognostic model, which was developed by British Rowing in the 1980s. This model compares the speed at which a boat travels relative to current world best time (WBT) over 2000 m in that boat class.

Physical Performance Contributions to Winning

As successful rowing performance depends on correct technique mastery combined with physical capacities, rowers typically perform large volumes of training. Training regimes each week classically consist of around 20 h of training, rowing 150 to 200 km on the water. This volume-based training approach means that the training intensity distribution is generally described by a polarized model, with most training taking place at an intensity below the lactate threshold (LT_1; figure 16.3; see chapter 3).

The physiological attributes that determine success in rowing are well documented. The strongest predictor of 2000 m rowing performance is the power output at $\dot{V}O_2max$ and maximal power/force during 5 peak strokes (r = 0.95), highlighting that both aerobic fitness and strength play key roles. Other strong relationships include absolute $\dot{V}O_2max$ (r = 0.88) and the $\dot{V}O_2$ at blood lactate threshold or power associated with a 4 $mmol^{-1}$ blood lactate reading (r = 0.92; i.e., LT_2) (5, 21). As such, it is clear that successful rowing performance is highly dependent on both aerobic and anaerobic energy production, with both the power at $\dot{V}O_2max$ and 5 stroke peak power showing strong correlations with performance (5).

Specific weight training generally constitutes a significant proportion of a rower's typical training week (although not in every case (16)), where rowers generally complete 2 or 3 weight-training sessions per week. Rowers are relatively strong (i.e., high force produced for specific movement tasks) when compared to other endurance athletes (3), with elite male rowers displaying the ability to generate a force of more than 2000 N in an isometrically simulated rowing position. In layman's terms, this means rowers for 1 RM are able to deadlift, back squat, and bench row 1.9, 1.9, and 1.2 times their body weight (10). Accordingly, strength clearly plays an important role in rowing performance, with studies showing the bench pull power and 1 RM power-clean as strongly related to peak stroke power (11).

Targets of Physical Performance of Rowing

As mentioned, there are clear contributions from both the aerobic/anaerobic energy systems and strength in rowing. Estimated requirements of both aerobic and anaerobic systems have been estimated at 70% to 80% and 20% to 30%, respectively, over a 2000 m ergometer performance (12). While the aerobic pathway may be the dominant system used across a 5 to 7 min all-out event, both systems must be addressed appropriately in training so as to ensure event success (figure 16.4). As pacing strategies normally take a "U"-shaped approach during 2000 m races, the anaerobic pathway may be of primary importance during the initial sprint and final phases of the race.

Given that the fastest time over the 2000 m event in the world is 5:18.7 (men's eight rowing), versus 7:07.7 for the women's single scull (slowest Olympic

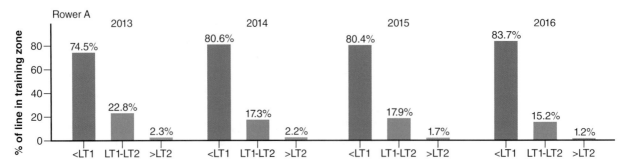

Figure 16.3 The yearly training intensity distribution of an Olympic champion rower each year prior to the Olympic Games or World Championships event. LT_1: first lactate threshold; LT_2: second lactate threshold.

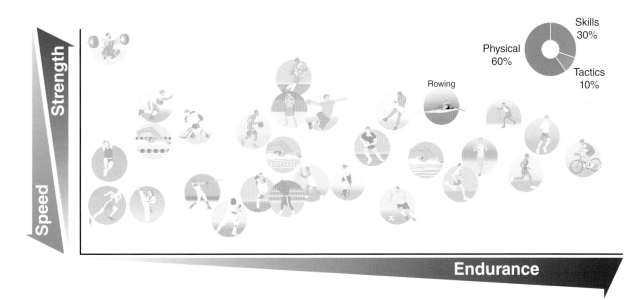

Figure 16.4 The position of the rower on the three axes shows that rowing is a sport requiring high levels of strength and endurance.

Adapted from G.A. Nader, "Concurrent Strength and Endurance Training: From Molecules to Man," *Medicine & Science in Sports & Exercise* 38, no. 11 (2006): 1965-1970.

Table 16.2 Global Physiological Targets for a Rower Based on Event and Its Respective World Best Times

Event	V̇O₂max	Anaerobic capacity	PS	VT₁	VT₂	Male WBT (August 2016)	Female WBT (August 2016)
Single scull (x)	++++++	++	++	+	+++	6:30:7	7:07:7
Rowing pair (–)	++++++	+++	++	+	++	6:08:5	6:49:1
Rowing double (x)	++++++	+++	++	+	++	5:59:7	6:37:3
Rowing four (–)	++++++	++++	++	+	++	5:37:8	6:14:4*
Rowing quad (x)	++++++	++++	++	+	++	5:32:3	6:06:8
Rowing eight (–)	++++++	+++++	+++	+	+	5:18:7	5:54:2
Lightweight double (x)	+++++	+++	++	+	++	6:05:4	6:47:7

–= single oar; x= double oars; PS = peak speed; WBT = world best time; * = non-Olympic

rowing event), these percent energy system contributions change slightly relative to both the boat class (table 16.1) and individual. This indicates that the relative importance of each energy pathway or physical attribute (figure 16.4) should be viewed at a boat-by-boat level. Indeed, successful World and Olympic rowing champions in the single sculls are known to spend considerable time cycling at an aerobic intensity. A boat class that has a greater aerobic contribution than other boat classes may indicate why such a strategy is successful for the single scull. Indeed, the current Olympic champion Mahe Dry-sdale performed ~53% of his total training time cycling in the year 2012 before his gold medal success at the London Olympics. The proposed importance of each physiological requirement is outlined in table 16.2 and figure 16.5.

The energy system contributions and physical requirements not only vary on a boat-to-boat basis, but also may vary equally at an individual level. Indeed, two rowers producing the same power output over 2000 m might do so using different energy system contributions (16). However, as shown using theoretical data (figure 16.5), we should aim to

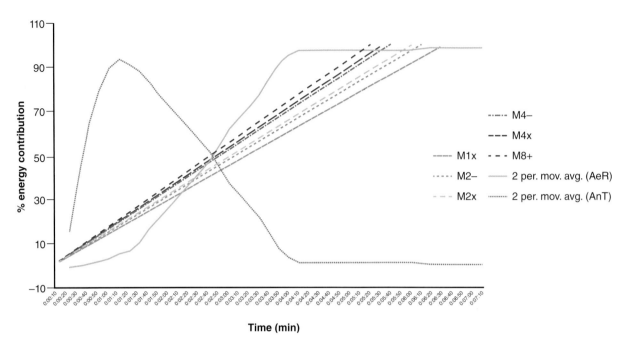

Figure 16.5 Theoretically derived aerobic (AeR) and anaerobic (AnT) energy system contributions to the 2000 m rowing event. The percent contribution from the various energy pathways can vary in accordance with boat class. In this example, differences are apparent when comparing the M8+ (red-dotted line) and M1x (gray line).

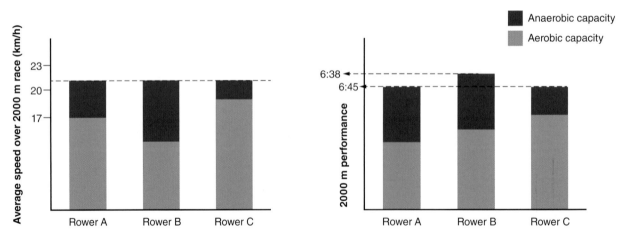

Figure 16.6 Theoretically differing individual energetic contributions over 2000 m (rowers A, B, and C). The aim of the training program should be to develop either (or both) systems to improve overall performance.

increase various aspects of these energy pathways to increase total power over the 2000 m event using an appropriate stimulus of training.

In summary, the physical attributes of successful rowers are predominantly aerobic endurance, with a relatively high strength component. However, as shown (figure 16.6), anaerobic glycolytic metabolism is also important. The key target of training often is to build or maintain a rower's natural area of talent, without compromising any weakness (if any; i.e., figure 16.6). When all systems are maximized, high levels of performance may be achieved. HIIT plays a pivotal role in optimizing the required physical attributes, and when used appropriately, becomes a critical tool in the coach's and support team's toolbox.

Key Weapons, Manipulations, and Surveillance Tools

Like other endurance sports (14, 15, 22), most rowing training hours (15 to 25 h per wk) are spent accumulating large volumes of training at low exercise intensities (<LT_1 or SR of 18 to 22 SPM). Accordingly, given the dominance of the aerobic system within the rowing event (70% to 80%), this part of the training plays an important role, as it develops the aerobic foundation needed to support the development of $\dot{V}O_2$max, economy, and thresholds ($\dot{V}O_2$ at blood lactate thresholds; chapter 3) (9, 19). As well as the large amounts of time training at low intensities, rowers also complete specific pace work at medium, or mid-zone, intensities. This is often known as threshold training, and the relevant intensities are shown in figure 16.2. These pieces are typically longer in duration (i.e., 5 or 6 × 2 k, 2 × 4 k, 2 × 5 k, or 3 × 3 k), with the total distance of work ranging from 8 to 12 km.

As with other endurance sports, HIIT contributes less to the total training time in rowing, but is a very important part of the overall training program design. This is particularly the case in the final build to key events, such as a World Championship or Olympic Games. Rowers generally follow the polarized model of training, with roughly 80% of training performed as low intensity (<LT_1), and about 20% of the total training in the form of HIIT. The HIIT work is generally completed at, or just above, race intensity. HIIT is vital for developing the oxidative, anaerobic, and neuromuscular/musculoskeletal properties needed to enable fatigue resistance over prolonged durations (see chapter 3). The key weapons or HIIT formats used to achieve this, including their manipulations, will be described.

HIIT Weapons, Targets, and Manipulations

The most common HIIT formats or weapons included in rowing training programs primarily involve long-interval, short-interval, and sprint-interval training (above 2000 m race pace). The purpose of these intervals is to aim for type 1 through 5 targets, with a metabolic emphasis. Repeated sprint training, which incorporates very short-duration efforts (3 to 7 s), are generally used for start practices. Although physiological intensity (in terms of $\dot{V}O_2$max and HR) is described below, in practice on water, training is typically prescribed via stroke rate and/or speed (pace per 250/500 m).

Long Intervals

Long-interval HIIT usually takes the form of 2 to 8 min (rowing 500 to 1500 m of distance), with work intensities of 85% to 95% of HRmax (≥ 2000 m race SR), 85% to 100% of $\dot{V}O_2$max, generally using work:rest ratios between 1:0.5 and 1:2 on water. On the rowing ergometer this would mean 95% to 97% of 2000 m ergometer power. Total accumulated duration at these intensities during such interval sets is typically 20 to 40 min split between 3 and 8 repetitions, aiming generally for type 2, 3, and 4 targets. These different targets can be achieved by manipulating the work:rest ratio. For example, reducing the work period (<90 s) and increasing the rest period (>90 s) alters the focus of the session toward anaerobic metabolism (type 3). Conversely, increasing the work period (>3 min) and reducing the recovery period (<3 min) emphasizes the aerobic metabolic response (type 4; table 16.3).

Short Intervals

Short-interval HIIT for rowing usually takes the form of 30 to 60 s work durations at intensities of 100% to 102% of race speed (normally measured in time pace per 250/500 m), generally with work:rest ratios between 1:0.5 and 1:1. For typical rowing prescription, short interval durations are typically between 30 and 60 s, or use a maximal number of strokes from a stationary position or from a rolling start (i.e., 20 to 30 maximal strokes).

Total accumulated work duration for these interval sets is generally between 10 and 20 min, split from 1 to 5 sets. Example sets can be seen in table 16.4. For elite rowers, the aim is to perform short intervals at a target stroke rate above that which they would race at, with a corresponding speed of

Table 16.3 Typical Long-Interval HIIT Parameters for Rowing Training

Mode	Work intensity (% $\dot{V}O_2$max)	Stroke rate (spm)	% of WBT (elites)	Work duration	Rest intensity	Rest duration	Rep number	Series	Target types
Rowing	85%-100%	32-38	97%-100%	3 min	50%	2 min	4	1	3 and 4

Table 16.4 Typical Short-Interval HIIT Parameters for Rowing Training

Mode	Work intensity (% V̇O₂max)	Stroke rate (spm)	% of WBT (elites)	Work duration	Rest intensity	Rest duration	Rep number	Series	Between series recovery	Target types
Rowing	100%-110%	35-42	100%-102%	30 s	50%	30	8	2	4 min	1, 2, 3, 4

~100% of WBT. The desired metabolic load for these HIIT sessions includes type 1, 2, 3, and 4 targets. Similar to long-interval HIIT, these various targets can be achieved by manipulating the work:rest ratio. Alternatively, the intensity of both the work or rest period can be adjusted to shift the balance between anaerobic and aerobic metabolism.

Sprint Interval Training

SIT is used frequently by rowers as competition approaches, often combined as start practice. However, if SIT is performed as maximal speed efforts (from rolling rather than standing, for example), it is important to carry out the interval with correct technique and within the functional stroke rate range. Rather than over a specific duration, SIT in rowing is normally composed of maximal efforts across a number of counted strokes (5 to 15, lasting 10 to 25 s), with recovery periods that range between 2 and 10 min. The goal of these intervals is to produce maximal force and high speed rates as fast as possible. The number of sprints is typically low (1 to 5), with time between sets relatively long (>30 min). SIT aims for type 5 targets.

Manipulations of Interval Training Variables

The beauty of rowing is that athletes and coaches are acutely aware of the precise physiological requirements of their race. Notwithstanding unforeseen changes in weather conditions (i.e., high wind suddenly picking up to impact front, rear, or side trajectory, including wake/wave effects), each race is almost identical, taking place over a 2000 m course and typically in a relatively calm lake. As such, HIIT interval sessions can be tailored and periodized appropriately for the specific energy system requirements of a typical 2000 m race.

As mentioned, the physiological parameters of rowing include an important contribution from both anaerobic and aerobic demands, with a higher emphasis on the aerobic requirements. Accordingly, V̇O₂max, power/speed associated with V̇O₂, and

maximal force over short time frames (10 to 60 s) are important considerations. At the same time, however, the importance of economy, efficiency, and threshold levels cannot be overlooked. V̇O₂ at lactate threshold and power at onset of blood lactate accumulation (OBLA) are also important determinants of rowing success (5). These key requirements should help guide training program design and HIIT implementation in a rowing program.

The primary factors of any HIIT sessions include the intensity and duration of the work and rest periods. Typically, as most HIIT work intervals are relatively short in terms of duration, stroke rate and speed are best used to prescribe the intensity in rowing (figure 16.2). The selection of an HIIT session should be mainly governed by the appropriate physiological adaptations sought after for the individual or crew. Similarly, the number of intervals in a series, the series duration, and time between each series of HIIT intervals will depend on the specific physiologic/metabolic system being targeted (i.e., chapters 3, 4, and 5). The selection of HIIT is not always an easy task in the sport of rowing; as with crew boats, all individuals have differing physiological requirements but must perform the same training when on the water. In such instances, this sometimes means that HIIT is best performed on an indoor rowing machine so as to individualize the important HIIT session.

Manipulating the stroke rate (measure of SPM) during a work interval will impact the balance between muscular strength and coordination, as well as the neuromuscular and metabolic demands (as described in chapters 4 and 5). For example, a 3 min work interval completed at either 25 or 30 SPM will not only be performed at differing intensities but will additionally differ in the applied force and associated neuromuscular characteristics. Lower stroke rates are thought to perhaps promote development of muscular strength and alter neuromuscular demands. For long intervals, lower- and upper-end SR (e.g., 35 versus 39) (figure 16.2) provides succinctly different metabolic outputs and neuromuscular responses.

The typical scheduling of HIIT as competition approaches is also a critical consideration. Early season training generally consists of mostly aerobic training with intermittent threshold work. However, as key races approach, more focus is moved toward long and short intervals, with the final 4 wk preparatory period consisting of all three interval types (long, short, and SIT) (see tables 16.5 and 16.6).

Surveillance and Monitoring Tools

The main surveillance and monitoring tools used in rowing include GPS devices (integrated wrist watches and on-boat devices) and heart rate. In some instances, these integrated systems can stream their data via Bluetooth and Wi-Fi to real-time systems that can be instantaneously viewed by the coach. These data can be used extensively in many applications (i.e., Training Peaks, Golden Cheetah; chapter 8) that advise the coach and practitioner regarding a rower's overall training load and training status.

Load

Intensity prescription for rowing training will vary, but has historically been based on kilometers rowed, HR, and RPE × duration (2). When dealing with large squads of athletes, HR monitoring can be a very attractive tool, as it has superior practical application and little practitioner intervention. However, the high-intensity and relatively short-duration HIIT intervals and the associated lag in HR response (see chapters 2, 8, and 9) prevent the use of HR for prescribing HIIT in any of the event disciplines. A more suitable approach is to monitor HIIT using rowing speed (%WBT) and time spent at targeted stroke rates (speed and SR measured via GPS and accelerometers). Rowing load can be calculated using various software systems that use Banister's classic fitness-fatigue modeling or training impulse calculation (TRIMP) scores in each respective discipline (1) (see also chapter 8).

Table 16.5 Typical Training Week for an Elite Rower During the Preparation Period, Including a Hard and Easy Week

In the early season, typically more time is spent performing moderate-intensity training (MIT), with more HIIT applied as the race season approaches.

	Hard training week	Easy training week
Monday	a.m.: 20-22 km LIT SR 20-22 p.m.: Rowing erg: 5×4′ at HIIT, with 3′ recovery (long intervals, type 4)	a.m.: 16-18 km LIT SR 20-22 p.m.: Rowing erg: 2×(10×30″ at HIIT, 30″easy), 5′ between repetitions (short intervals, type 3)
Tuesday	a.m.: 24-26 km LIT SR 20-22 p.m.: Weight followed by 6-12 km TECH	a.m.: 24-26 km LIT SR 20-22 p.m.: Weights only
Wednesday	a.m.1: 20 km row with 2×5 km MIT (SR 28-32), 5′ recovery threshold a.m.2: 45′ LIT on indoor rowing machine p.m.: REST	a.m.: 18 km row with 1×5 km MIT (SR 28-32), 5′ recovery threshold p.m.: REST
Thursday	a.m.: 20-22 km LIT SR 20-22 p.m.: Weight followed by 6-12 km TECH	a.m.: 16-18 km LIT SR 20-22 p.m.: Weights only
Friday	a.m.: 20-22 km row included 4×8′ MIT with bungee for added resistance p.m.: 12 km row 18-22 SR LIT	a.m.: 20-22 km row included 6×3′ MIT (3′ recovery) with bungee for added resistance (long intervals, type 4) p.m.: 30′ on indoor rowing erg low LIT
Saturday	a.m.: 26-28 km row including 1×8 km MIT threshold p.m.: REST	a.m.: 26-28 km row including 2×4 km MIT threshold p.m.: REST
Sunday	REST	REST

LIT = low-intensity training: blood lactate concentration <2.5 mmol/L, heart rate <80% HRmax.
MIT = moderate-intensity training: blood lactate concentration 2.5 to 4.0 mmol/L, heart rate 80% to 90% HRmax.
HIIT = high-intensity interval training: blood lactate concentration >4.0 mmol/L, heart rate >90% HRmax.
TECH = Easy row, focusing on technical skills and drills.

Table 16.6 Typical Training Week for an Elite Rower During the Competition Period

Presentation of the competition week assumes a normal World Cup regatta, running Friday to Sunday, which is different than the Olympic Games or World Championship events that normally run over a 1 wk period. During the hard training phase, long-interval HIIT, viewed as one of the key sessions for elite rowers, is performed every 5 d.

	Hard training week	Competition week
Monday	a.m.: 16-18 km LIT (18-22 SR) p.m.: 4 × 1000 HIIT with 4' recovery (long intervals, type 4)	a.m.: 18 km row include 8 × 1 km MIT with 1' recovery threshold p.m.: 12 km of TECH
Tuesday	a.m.: 20-22 km LIT SR 20-22 p.m.: Weights followed by 12 km included 8 × 10 strokes all-out from start (SIT, type 5)	a.m.: 24-26 km LIT SR 20-22 p.m.: 12 km row include 6-8 × 8-12 stroke starts all-out (SIT, type 5)
Wednesday	a.m.: 20-22 km include 2 × (10 × 1' on 1' off) 5' between sets (short intervals, type 4) p.m.: REST	a.m.: 12-14 km row included 1 × 1000 and 2 × 250 HIIT (5' recovery) (long and short intervals, types 3 and 4) p.m.: REST (or 8 k recovery)
Thursday	a.m.1: 16-18 km LIT SR 20-22 a.m.2: Light weights p.m.: 18-20 km row (short intervals) RST 6 × 1' HIIT with 6-8' recovery (type 4)	a.m.: 12 km row include 7 strokes MIT-HIIT, 10 strokes LIT p.m.: 4 km recovery
Friday	a.m.: 18-20 km LIT 20-22 p.m.: 12 km row TECH	RACE DAY 1 (heat and quarter finals)
Saturday	a.m.1: 2 × 1000 (3' recovery), 2 × 750 (2' recovery), 2 × 500 HIIT (1.5') recovery) (long intervals, type 3) a.m.2: 12 km recovery	RACE DAY 2 (semifinals)
Sunday	REST	RACE DAY 3 (finals)

LIT = low-intensity training: blood lactate concentration <2.5 mmol/L, heart rate <80% HRmax.
MIT = moderate-intensity training: blood lactate concentration 2.5-4.0 mmol/L, heart rate 80%-90% HRmax.
HIIT = high-intensity interval training: blood lactate concentration >4.0 mmol/L, heart rate >90% HRmax.
TECH = Easy row, focusing on technical skills and drills.

Training Status

As mentioned, the selection of an HIIT session is not an easy one to make in the sport of rowing. As with crew boats (table 16.1), all individuals will have different physiological profiles, strengths, and weaknesses. For true individualization of HIIT to take place, sessions must either be completed in the single scull or on the indoor rowing machine. In such situations, the power continuum (whereby an athlete performs time trials on the indoor rowing machine over 10 s, 60 s, 2000 m, 6000 m, and 60 min across a 1 wk period) can be a useful test for identifying the individual characteristics of rowers so as to allow them to perform an HIIT session at an individual level. While knowledge pertaining to optimizing HIIT for individual athlete profiles is lacking, it is generally believed that the aerobic system is more malleable than the anaerobic system,

so aerobic-based HIIT intervals (types 1 and 2) generally tend to be the focus in the program.

As with other endurance-based sports, rowing coaches more often than not believe that more training is usually better, so the risk of developing overtraining is high (see chapter 7). Markers of training load include those described in the cycling (chapter 15) and triathlon (chapter 19) chapters, verbal and written training diary comments, alongside more advanced tools, including morning resting heart rate variability (17) (HRV; chapter 9).

Strategies for Structuring the Training Program Using HIIT

The typical scheduling of HIIT as competition approaches is also a critical consideration in the program (table 16.5). Early season training generally consists of mostly aerobic training with intermittent threshold work. However, as the races approach, focus tends to shift toward long and short intervals, with the final 4 wk preparatory period consisting of all three HIIT weapons (long, short, and SIT).

Within the sport of rowing (4, 20), it is generally considered best practice to separate HIIT days by ~48 h (see chapter 9). This tends to allow for appropriate recovery of the autonomic nervous system (ANS) and means each session can be completed optimally. In a recent study by Holt et al. (4), it was shown that threshold training resulted in the greatest reductions in ANS status, as assessed by HRV. This was followed by long and SIT intervals. Conversely, performance (30 s Wingate on the rowing ergometer) was most affected (i.e., time taken to return to baseline) by long intervals (followed by threshold work and SIT, respectively). This suggests that long intervals should perhaps be avoided during a taper period close to competition, while continuous days of threshold work may lead to excessive fatigue and should therefore be appropriately placed within the program.

Controllable and Uncontrollable Factors

Rowers will compete on several occasions per year. However, for elite rowers, the domestic season (typically three or four regattas) is purely a preparatory phase for the international rowing season. The international season (FISA World Rowing Cups) consists of three World Cups and a World Championship event. During each regatta, crews will compete in two to four races (heats, quarterfinals, semifinals, and a final). The number of races performed in depends on the number of entries. The World Cup events normally take place from May to late July, with the World Championship occurring in late August or early September.

Unlike several other elite sports (i.e., cycling, soccer, basketball, ice hockey), where competition frequency is high, the lower frequency of competition (if appropriately planned) enables sufficient recovery to enable the scheduling of HIIT. Smaller domestic rowing regattas are however used as a training stimulus leading into major events, to gain experience in more technical areas such as starts, pacing, race tactics, and competition environment experience.

Travel demands add another challenge to the training program that must be considered. International regattas are generally performed in Europe and are reasonably close in terms of successive proximity to one another. Thus, recovery for and from travel (i.e., rest periods before and after travel) as well as time for circadian adaptation to the time zone need to be considered (18).

Program Structure and Progression

There are several different approaches to the planning and preparation of rowing training that can be made. Generally the training planning models in rowing follow traditional theories such as classic periodization models, block periodization models, and numerous other formats (6). As the competition program is to some degree similar every year, the training program should focus on individual and crew needs, aiming at training the primary determinants of performance physiology (chapter 3; figures 16.5 and 16.6, table 16.2) needed for the key event of the year (World Championship or Olympic Games). This means that the training programs of rowers are highly unique and specific to each boat. Nevertheless, some general observations can be made across the macro-, meso-, and microcycles observed in most rowing training programs.

Macrocycle

A rower's seasons are typically periodized around a small number of key racing objectives, requiring three or four periods of maximal performance. As mentioned, for international rowers, the key events are the FISA World Rowing Cups. Every year, there are three FISA World Rowing Cups, which take place over the period from May to late July. The championship race (Olympics or World Championship) takes place around 4 to 5 wk after the final World Cup event of the season. Domestic regattas generally take place earlier in the year, and while part of the training process, are seldom a major goal for most elite rowers. These events create the general structure of the training program from a macrocycle perspective.

Mesocycle

A typical basic or preparatory mesocycle in rowing follows the traditional 4 wk approach, with three loading weeks and one recovery week. However, this will vary depending on the available time between races, and can include precompetition or transition mesocycles (~2 to 4 wk), competition mesocycles (~3 to 6 wk), and recovery mesocycles (~1 to 4 wk).

Microcycle

The microcycles of a rower's training program can be variable, but mostly occur over a 7 d weekly period. When working within crews and groups of people, 7 d microcycles allow for routine and therefore make planning for a group relatively easy. Most microcycles in rowing consist of one full day of rest per week.

Periodized Nutrition

As outlined in chapter 4, periodized nutrition can also play an important role in the training program of some rowers. Nutrition is important not only for controlling a rower's weight (particularly for lightweight rowers; see also chapter 7), but also for affecting the adaptations achieved from a training session (14). Specifically, manipulating carbohydrate consumption and either performing sessions after an overnight fast or performing multiple sessions in a day to force the rower to train with low-glycogen stores (popularly termed *training low*; chapter 4). However, in my experience, open-class rowers, who typically consume large amounts of food that are mainly carbohydrate based, seldom achieve this. Indeed, most rowers, but not all, generally fuel for every session (before, during, and after) and follow a high-carbohydrate diet. Training fasted in the morning is also seldom carried out in the present day elite rowing environment.

Sample Training Programs

Training programs for preparation and competition phases are shown in tables 16.5 and 16.6.

For the 2014 World Rowing Championships held in Amsterdam, I was fortunate to work closely alongside a top coach in the New Zealand Olympic program. The coach was coaching an athlete who was racing in the female single scull (W1x). Together, we formulated a plan that we believed could help her be successful in her event.

After the initial aerobic training preparatory period, beginning 11 mo before the World Championships, training progressed to include threshold training twice per week, including once per week of longer intervals, involving a specific race target stroke rate (100% of WBT). These intervals were progressed during the season, with one of the threshold sessions replaced with repeated sprint intervals as the race season approached (long intervals remained). HIIT was kept to a minimum during the first part of the competition season overseas, with the priority aim in this period being the maintenance of health, fitness, and recovery from racing.

We knew the final 4 wk of training prior to the last 10 taper days before the World Championships would be critical. This period consisted of sprint (5×60 s with 6 min recovery), long (e.g., 4×3.5 min on, 4 min recovery), and short intervals (e.g., 10×1 min on, 1 min recovery) during most weeks. The long intervals (considered most important for performance for this rower) were rolled through every 5 days. The rolling through of long intervals every 5 d was a particularly successful programming strategy. However, the training content between was critical to allow each long interval session to be performed optimally. We learned this the first time the athlete attempted to perform a second long-interval session just 5 d later (suboptimally). We found that the best recipe was (if the first long interval day was day 1) day 2 would be recovery, day 3 would be high intensity (either sprint of short intervals rotating each time), day 4 would be all aerobic low-intensity training, and then day 5 would be back to long intervals. This was a great mix. With five being an odd number, the programming puzzle had to be continuously adjusted, but this also meant the program was very dynamic and interesting for the athlete. Full rest days would be included somewhere within the 10 d mesocycles when it felt appropriate. This was often determined by the training responses, subjective metrics, and heart rate variability scores.

As a team, we believed in our process. The athlete responded by getting progressively better in nearly every session, and we were elated when she ultimately went on to win her first world title in the single scull.

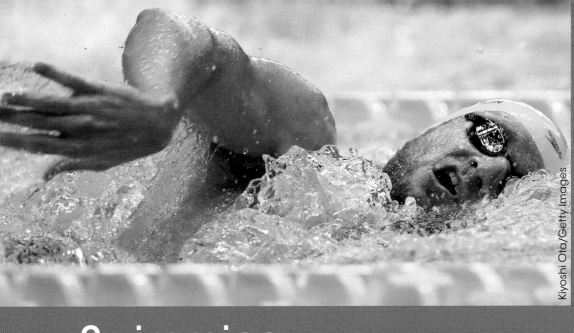

17

Swimming

• • • • • •

Tom Vandenbogaerde, Wim Derave, and Philippe Hellard

Humans are better built for walking and running than for swimming. If we compare the top speeds attained by the fastest running animal (the cheetah at 120 km/h) and swimming animal (the sailfish at 110 km/h), our fastest humans to date have reached 38% of that speed in running (Usain Bolt at 45 km/h with the 100 m track world record) and only 8% in swimming (Cesar Cielo at 8.6 km/h with the 50 m freestyle world record). Despite this fact, some anatomical and physiological adaptations suggest that human evolution has been more (semi-) aquatic than originally thought (14). In more modern times, swimming has developed into a popular recreational activity, becoming a competitive sport in Great Britain in the 19th century and part of the first modern Olympic Games in Athens in 1896.

This chapter outlines performance factors of the sport, the role that high-intensity interval training (HIIT) plays in developing athletes, snapshots of training schedules of swimmers who have won medals at the Olympic Games and/or World Championships, and practical methods to structure, plan, and monitor swim training.

Sport Description

The most obvious difference between swimming and land-based sports is that swimming is performed in the water medium, where reducing drag becomes critical for success. (The drag on the human body moving in water is about 780 times greater than the drag involved with moving through air.) Toward minimizing drag, swimming is performed with as much streamline as possible, in the horizontal position, where propulsion comes through a continuous movement of the arms, in coordinated combination with the kick.

The competition frequency for an elite swimmer is not as regular as in most popular sports (e.g., weekly for soccer, several grand slams each year for tennis, two or three competitions per week for basketball and ice hockey). For swimmers, the highest level of competition is the Olympic Games, held every 4 yr in a long-course pool (50 m). Figure 17.1 shows an overview of the individual pool-swimming events of the 2020 Tokyo Olympic program, with respective world records (updated August 2018). Pool-event durations range from ~21 s in the men's 50 m freestyle to ~15 min in the 1500 m freestyle. Events not listed in the figure are the 10 km open-water race, which takes ~2 h, and the team relays (4 × 100 m medley, 4 × 100 m freestyle, 4 × 200 m freestyle, and mixed women/men 4 × 100 m medley relay). Each event comes with rules and regulations that are published at www.fina.org.

The competition environment at major championships is generally well controlled. The pool is always exactly 50 m for long-course competitions and exactly 25 m for short-course competitions; the

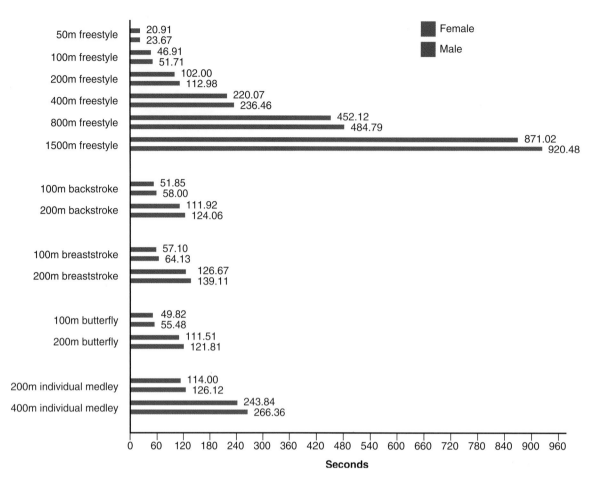

Figure 17.1 Individual pool events of the 2020 Tokyo Olympic program, with respective world records (updated August 2018) in male and female athletes. Record times are shown in seconds.

water temperature is standardized at ~27°C; and pools used for Olympic Games or World Championship events have a minimum depth of 2.0 m. Olympic Games and World Championships are always held indoors; the last Olympic Games and World Championships that were held outdoors were in Athens in 2004 and Rome in 2009, respectively. Open-water events are clearly less controlled, with differences in weather, water current, water temperature, and swimming course.

At the World Championships and Olympic Games, the 16 best performances from heat swims in each event go through to semifinals, from which the eight best performances go through to the final, where the medals are won. Exceptions include the 400 m, 800 m, 1500 m, and relay events, where there are no semifinals, and the open-water events, where there is a single mass start in a straight final.

There are strict regulations regarding swimsuits. In 2008 and 2009, technologically advanced polyurethane swimsuits appeared in the sport, which made a

swimmer's body more buoyant and streamlined. Twenty world records were set at the 2009 World Championships in Rome as a result. In 2010, the polyurethane swimsuits were banned, after an American proposal to return to textile-only suits was passed with 180 nations voting for the ban and only 7 against it.

Physical Contributors to Performance in Swimming

Performance is multifaceted in any sport. When it comes to winning medals at major championships, superior physical fitness and technical skills must go hand in hand with confidence, belief, and the ability to perform under pressure. Training the mental side of performance and appropriate daily decision-making (e.g., appropriate rest, sleep, nutrition) is equally important as training the physical side.

Figure 17.2 places swimming among other sports in terms of different proportions of physical requirements of speed, strength, and endurance. Note the

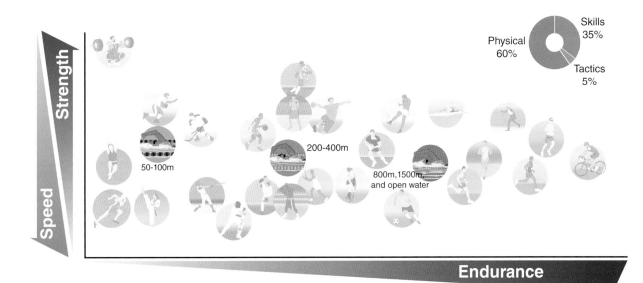

Figure 17.2 The position of the swimmer on the three axes will vary depending on the specificity of the event, with longer events naturally requiring more endurance, though other variables such as technique and propulsive efficiency may be even more important in the sport of swimming. Note the distinct position placement on the figure of swimmers specializing in the sprint (50-100 m), middle distance (200-400 m), and distance (800-1500 m and open-water) events.

Adapted from G.A. Nader, "Concurrent Strength and Endurance Training: From Molecules to Man," *Medicine & Science in Sports & Exercise* 38, no. 11 (2006): 1965-1970.

distinct position placement on the figure of swimmers specializing in the sprint (50-100 m) middle distance (200-400 m), and distance (800-1500 m and open-water) events. However, other factors such as technique, propulsive efficiency, and the ability to repeat performance under pressure are also important, demonstrated by the fact that some elite athletes win across a range of events (strokes and distances). The most prominent example is one of history's most successful Olympians, Michael Phelps (USA), who has won 23 Olympic gold medals and has set world records in backstroke, freestyle, individual medley, and butterfly events across different distances.

The physiological demands of swimming are different for each event, due to the large range in duration between them (figure 17.1). Figure 17.3 shows computer-simulated percentage energy contributions of the three energy systems involved in Olympic pool freestyle events in elite male athletes (39). The three relevant energy systems include the phosphagen system (anaerobic alactic), the glycolytic system (anaerobic lactic), and the aerobic oxidative system (see chapter 3). As shown in the figure and explained in chapter 4, the longer the duration of the event, the larger the contribution of the oxidative system; the shorter the duration of the event, the higher the

contribution of the glycolytic system. For simulations of metabolic responses during high-intensity interval training, we refer to the work of Hellard and colleagues (22).

Coaches will aim to maximize and balance the capacities of the energy systems, building those metabolic capacities with effective swim technique and neuromuscular patterns. We refer to chapters 3, 4, and 5, and specifically for the sport of swimming, to the work of coach/coach scientists Forbes Carlile (7), James Counsilman (10), Ernest Maglischo (28), Iñigo Mujika (31, 32), and Brent Rushall (40), and of scientists David Costill (9), Philippe Hellard (18, 19, 21, 22), Jan Olbrecht (33), and David Pyne (35, 37).

In addition to muscular metabolic capacities and neuromuscular patterns, the cardiac output, discussed in chapter 3, may be a discriminating factor. Many muscles are used during whole-body swimming exercise, resulting in a competition for blood flow (42). An increase in blood volume is therefore a desired training adaptation, as well as an increase in muscle blood flow capacity (26).

Anthropometric variables and body composition affect performance. While a swimmer's anthropometric characteristics are somewhat fixed after maturation (i.e., stature), body composition will

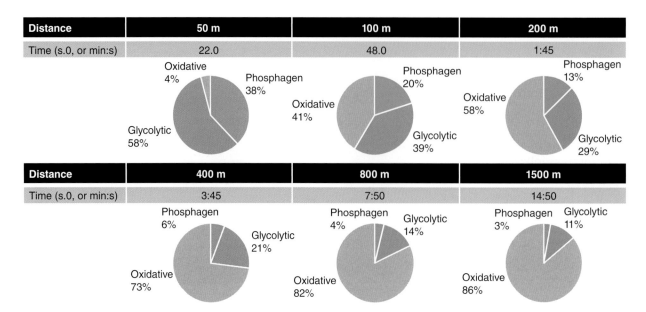

Figure 17.3 Share of energy system contribution during competitive freestyle swimming events in top-level swimmers using computer simulation.

Data from F.A. Rodriguez and A. Mader, "Energy Systems in Swimming," in *World Book of Swimming: From Science to Performance*, edited by L. Seifert, D. Chollet, and I. Mujika (New York: Nova Science, 2011): 225-240.

change according to manipulation of training load and nutritional intake. For example, as training load increases, female middle-distance swimmers generally lose total body mass and body fat (skinfolds) with minimal changes in lean mass, while male middle-distance swimmers generally gain body mass and lean mass, but show minimal changes in skinfolds (3). Anderson and colleagues also observed a decrease in body fat (skinfolds) in the taper phase in female swimmers from one season to the next, which correlated strongly with improved competition performance. For male swimmers, increased proportional lean mass occurred during several phases of the training season, which also correlated strongly to improved end-of-season competition performance time (2).

Technical changes in swimming often result in larger performance gains compared to increases in metabolic power (12, 45). The coach's experienced eye is an important vehicle used to drive such change. Technical demands vary by event, and breaststroke is a highly specialized event in this regard. Certain skills are also relatively more important in specific events. For example, the start is far more important in the 50 m freestyle than in the 1500 m freestyle. Other strategies that reduce drag include the use of different swimsuits (8), swim caps (to remove drag from head hair), and shaving (which in top male

swimmers is generally done only at major competitions and their selection events).

Another important performance factor in swimming is pacing. Athletes must pace themselves to get the best outcome, which is one of the more difficult aspects of competitive swimming, and is of importance in all swim events. For example, going out too fast in the first 50 m lap of a 100 m event can cost excessive amounts of energy, leading to a reduction in speed in the latter part of the race. Alternatively, not going out fast enough can leave a swimmer out of the race. An example in the 100 m freestyle may be that of Kyle Chalmers at the 2016 Rio Games. Kyle sat in seventh place with a 23.14 s split time at the 50 m turn, and was able to maintain velocity more effectively, returning in a 24.44 s split to win gold.

Pacing profiles do vary by event distance and by stroke (30). Swimmers typically adopt a *positive* pacing profile in all 100 m events, whereby lap time increases from the first to the second lap, which is largely due to the rapid acceleration obtained from the dive start. The most successful 100 m swimmers are able to maintain their speed more effectively in the final lap (38). In events 200 m and above, the most commonly used pacing strategies are called *fast-start even*, where laps are evenly paced after a fast first lap, and *parabolic*, which is similar but with a fast end-spurt in the final lap(s) (25, 29). Slight differences have been observed in 200 m breaststroke and butterfly events with a positive pacing profile due to the unique characteristics of these strokes (38).

Targets of Physical Performance in Swimming

Coaches generally tend to categorize swimmers into four groups as follows:

1. Sprint swimmers, who train for 50 and 100 m events,
2. Middle-distance swimmers, who train for 200 and 400 m events,
3. Distance swimmers, who train for 800 and 1500 m events, and
4. Open-water swimmers, for those racing in 5, 10, and 25 km events in lakes, rivers, seas, and oceans.

To visualize the common differences in training between groups, a case-study snapshot is shown of a mid-season training week in an athlete who has won a medal in the respective event at the Olympic Games and/or World Championships. The reader will need to place these week snapshots in perspective, bearing in mind that

1. snapshots show the overall session mileage and training focus, not the actual HIIT content or the way (technique) the athlete executed the HIIT,
2. the athletes completing such training will have been training consistently for many years,
3. training weeks, mileage, focus, and HIIT content will change substantially according to the time of season and from one season to the next,
4. different training strategies may have impacted performance positively or negatively, and
5. other medal-winning athletes may have been through very different training strategies.

The training focus of sessions in these single-week snapshots are shown simply as low aerobic, high aerobic, anaerobic, race-specific, speed, and recovery, defined as follows:

- Low aerobic: swimming at speeds ~70 to 40 beats below maximum heart rate, or at ~75% to 85% of the maximum 400 m swimming speed;
- High aerobic: longer volume sets of swimming at ~85% to 110% of the maximum 400 m swimming speed;

- Anaerobic: training sets that usually consist of ~25 to 50 m repetitions swum very fast with appropriate passive rest to ensure a high contribution of anaerobic glycolysis;
- Race-specific: a speed specific to the individual's main event;
- Speed: very fast swimming up to ~20 m;
- Recovery: a session aimed at recovery, usually following a previous session involving a high training load. This session will consist of very easy swimming, generally no longer than 45 min.

Focus categories will be explained further with examples of training sets in the HIIT Weapons and Their Manipulations section.

Sprint

The sprint group trains to perform in 50 m and 100 m events.

50 m Events

For 50 m events, the competition performance duration is between ~21 s for elite male freestylers and ~29 s for elite female breaststrokers.

There are not many programs that specialize in 50 m events because (currently) the only Olympic event at this distance is the 50 m freestyle. At the 2016 Olympic Games in Rio, the performance difference between the 50 m freestyle Olympic champion and silver medalist was 0.01 s (or 0.05%) and 0.02 s (0.08%), respectively, for male and female athletes. Conversely, the 2017 World Championships showed an average 1.0% difference between gold and silver in 50 m events (in freestyle, backstroke, breaststroke, and butterfly, which are currently part of the World Championships programs). This higher percent difference is mainly explained by the exceptional performances of Great Britain's Adam Peaty and Sweden's Sarah Sjöström, who were 0.52 s (2.0%) and 0.78 s (3.2%) ahead of the silver medalists in the 50 m breaststroke and 50 m butterfly, respectively.

To be successful in 50 m events, a swimmer needs explosive power, with superior swim-specific power and skill. Although a small share of the energy delivery during a 50 m event is provided through the oxidative system (figure 17.3), most swimmers specializing in this event follow a combination of speed, anaerobic and aerobic training, and a larger volume than would be expected in comparison with similar-duration land-based events (e.g., track running).

	Monday	Tuesday	Wednesday	Thursday	Friday	Saturday	Sunday
6–8 AM	Aerobic and speed 4000 m	Off	Technique 4000 m	Off	Max speed and easy speed Type 5 3000 m	Aerobic hypoxic 4000 m	Off
9–10 AM	Weights	Land training	Weights	Land training	Weights	Land training	
4–6 PM	Kick and transfer Type 2 4500 m	Aerobic hypoxic 4500 m	Speed range Type 5 3000 m	Aerobic hypoxic 4500 m	Kick and resistance Type 2 3400 m	Off	Off
						Total ~35,000 m	

Figure 17.4 Mid-season training week snapshot including swim-training focus and session distance of the program of an elite 50 m freestyle swimmer.

Figure 17.4 shows an example of a mid-season training week in a swimmer who has won an Olympic medal in the 50 m freestyle. The overall swimming volume of this particular week was 35 km. The week included six land-based training sessions, of which three were weight-training sessions; there is traditionally a relatively large emphasis on strength training in 50 m specialist programs.

100 m Events

In 100 m events, the event duration is between ~47 s for elite male freestyle and ~65 s for elite female breaststroke.

The 100 m long-course events consist of swimming two 50 m laps. While ~30% to 45% of the energy during a 100 m race is of an anaerobic glycolytic origin (19, 39), Hellard and colleagues have observed that only 5% to 8% of training is actualized and targeted as such for top French sprinters (20). Observations in Australian swimming programs are similar. The reason for this relatively low proportion of anaerobic training is twofold. First, there is a likely decrease in propulsive efficiency during high-intensity work in the water medium, where the coach will often stop the athlete when technique fails. Second, technique is considered critical to success, and such work has a relatively large aerobic component. The relatively large training volumes performed by swimmers will be discussed further in the HIIT Weapons and Their Manipulations section.

Competition performance times alongside personal observations in training indicate that some athletes may be more 50 and 100 m specialists, while others may be more 100 and 200 m specialists. The 50 and 100 m specialists usually have more speed and a need for longer recovery times from high-intensity training (if performance in the particular subsequent session is the desired outcome), while the 100 and 200 m specialists usually handle more training volume and recover faster from high-intensity work. Swim training will always consist of some combination of speed, anaerobic and aerobic work, and it is up to the coach to decide how the volume and content of interval training will be applied and how adjustments are incorporated for an individual swimmer.

Figure 17.5 provides a snapshot of a mid-season training week in an elite 100 m freestyle swimmer. For all swimmers, it is important to develop their aerobic and anaerobic capacities with good technique. As such, it is important to develop and fine-tune both speed and race-specific skills. Figure 17.5 shows three weight-training sessions in this particular week. While there is much internal debate on the content of land-based work for swimmers, there is little clarity on how strong a swimmer needs to be for success. While land-based strength work can influence swim performance greatly in certain cases, the individualization and periodization of this training component is essential.

Middle Distance

The middle-distance group includes swimmers training to perform in 200 m and 400 m events.

200 m Events

In 200 m events, the durations are between ~1:45 for elite male freestylers and ~2:20 for elite female breaststrokers.

A 200 m event consists of four 50 m laps, with three turns. An elite 200 m swimmer will need to

	Monday	Tuesday	Wednesday	Thursday	Friday	Saturday	Sunday
6–8 AM	Low aerobic 5000 m	Low aerobic 2600 m	Off	Low aerobic 3300 m	Low aerobic 3600 m	200 and 100–m race pace Type 4 4500 m	Off
9–10 AM	Weights		Weights		Weights		
4–6 PM	High aerobic Type 2 4800 m	100-m race pace and speed Type 5 4800 m	Low aerobic 5000 m	High aerobic and race pace Type 4 5000 m	Low aerobic 3400 m	Off	Off
						Total 42,000 m	

Figure 17.5 Mid-season training week snapshot including swim-training focus and session distance of the program of an elite 100 m freestyle swimmer.

maintain speed for a relatively long duration. As such, speed, anaerobic power, and aerobic power all need to be developed, maximized, and fine-tuned in training. Figure 17.6 shows the computer-simulated evolution of the metabolic contributions of the three energy systems in a real race situation for a 200 m freestyle Olympic swimmer (17). As with all forms of locomotion, the three energy systems are used simultaneously, though proportionally different, depending on the individual swimmer's system capacities, the duration and execution of the race, and the pacing strategy. Figure 17.7 shows a week snapshot of mid-season training of an elite 200 m swimmer. The schedule shows a range of focuses in training, aimed at developing aerobic and anaerobic capacities, and race-specific skills.

400 m Events

In 400 m events, the duration is between ~3:43 for elite male 400 m freestyle and ~4:30 for elite female 400 m individual medley.

The time to make a final at the 2016 Rio Olympic Games in the 400 m freestyle was 3:45.43 and 4:04.36 for male and female athletes, respectively. Very often, top 400 m swimmers are also elite in other distances, but either in the 200 and the 400 *or* in the 400, 800, and 1500 m events. This observation compares with the different aerobic versus anaerobic dominant 1500 m middle-distance running groups described in chapter 13. An exception in swimming is American Katie Ledecky, who is reigning Olympic Champion in the 200, 400, and 800 m events, and World Champion in the 1500 m (there was no female 1500 m event at the 2016 Olympics).

Figure 17.8 shows a week snapshot of mid-season training in a 400 m freestyle Olympic medalist. This

particular training week contained 10 swim sessions, of which 4 were high-aerobic training sessions, with an intended rating of perceived exertion of 8 or 9 out of 10, 4 low-aerobic sessions, and 2 recovery sessions. Land-based work consisted of 2 sessions enabling maintenance of already developed strength and a boxing session at the very end of the week.

Distance

Distance events include the 800 m and 1500 m events. Event durations are between ~7:30 in male 800 m freestyle and ~15:30 in female 1500 m freestyle.

Distance swimmers' training programs generally consist of a high training volume. Figure 17.9 shows the realized total swimming volume of an elite distance swimmer in the year leading to an Olympic Games. This figure shows volume only, which shouldn't be interpreted as training load, as training load will depend on how this mileage was realized (intensity × volume; chapter 8) with the relative physiological and psychological stress imposed (response to load; chapter 9). There are programs that keep the quality (swimming at higher intensities) relatively low and balanced, but there are also many successful programs that have a lot of quality in the majority of sessions throughout the week. Distance swimmers do not have the speed of sprinters and can't achieve the same absolute intensities as sprinters, which may make it possible for them to recover faster and to sustain more quality work for longer. The energy used during 800 and 1500 m races is mainly produced through aerobic oxidation (e.g., figure 17.6). Nevertheless, anaerobic capacities also need to be developed to be able to deal with changes in pace during competition, if the coach and athlete desire development of such a trait.

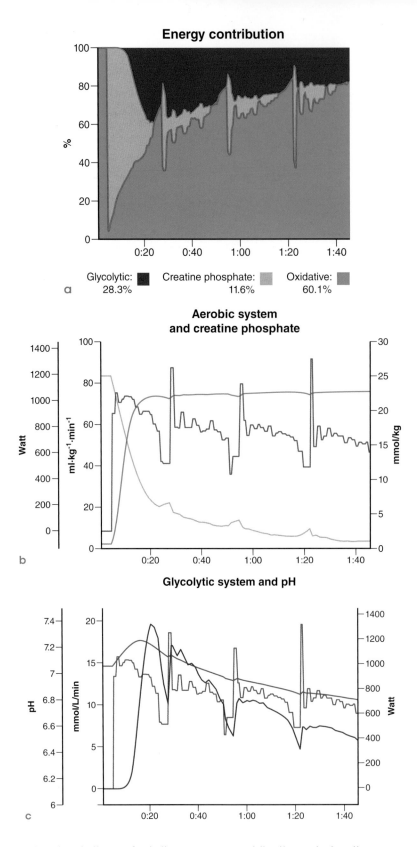

Figure 17.6 Computer simulations of relative energy contributions during the course of a 200 m race in an elite swimmer (modeled for a performance time of 1:46.99) (15). (a) % contribution of the three relevant energy systems for the duration of the race; (b) creatine phosphate (mmol/kg, gray line), $\dot{V}O_2$ (mL·kg^{-1}·min^{-1}, green line), and swim power (Watt, blue line); (c) rate of glycolysis (mmol/L/min, red line), level of pH (values below 7 indicate acidity that increases as the number decreases, orange line), and swim power (Watt, blue line).

	Monday	Tuesday	Wednesday	Thursday	Friday	Saturday	Sunday
AM	Low aerobic to threshold 6000 m	Low aerobic 6000 m	Off	Low aerobic 5200 m	Low aerobic 6000 m	Race pace Type 4 5000 m	Off
AM	Weights		Weights		Weights	Land training	
PM	High aerobic Type 2 5000 m	Anaerobic Type 5 4000 m	Low aerobic and speed 5500 m	High aerobic and race pace Type 4 5500 m	Low aerobic and speed 5000 m	Off	Off
						Total 53,200 m	

Figure 17.7 Mid-season-week snapshot including swim-training focus and session distance of the program of an elite 200 m freestyle swimmer.

	Monday	Tuesday	Wednesday	Thursday	Friday	Saturday	Sunday
AM	Low aerobic kick-pull 7000 m RPE 5	Low aerobic 7500 m RPE 4	High aerobic Type 2 7000 m RPE 8	Low aerobic kick-pull 7000 m RPE 5	Low aerobic and anaerobic set Type 5 8000 m RPE 6	High aerobic Type 2 6500 m RPE 8	Off
		Weights (maintenance)			Weights (maintenance)	Boxing session	
PM	High aerobic and speed Type 2 6000 m RPE 9	Recovery and speed 4500 m RPE 2	Off	High aerobic and speed Type 2 6000 m RPE 9	Recovery 4000 m RPE 2	Off	Off
						Total 63,500 m	

Figure 17.8 Mid-season training week snapshot with swim-training focus, session distance, and intended rating of perceived exertion (RPE) of training in an elite 400 m freestyle swimmer.

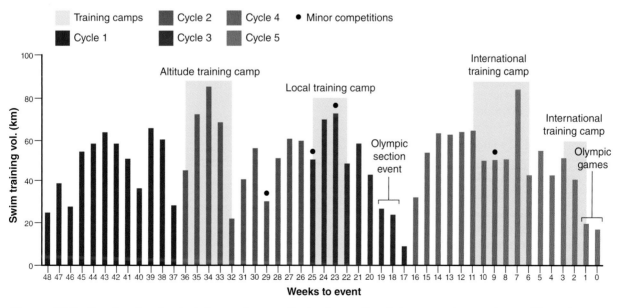

Figure 17.9 Realized swim training volumes (km) of an elite distance swimmer in an Olympic year. The X-axis shows the number of weeks until the start of the Olympic Games.

	Monday	Tuesday	Wednesday	Thursday	Friday	Saturday	Sunday
AM	Low aerobic	Low aerobic	High aerobic threshold	Low aerobic	Low aerobic and speed	High aerobic 800-m reps	Recovery
	7200 m	7000 m	7000 m	7000 m	7000 m	6000 m	3000 m
	Weights (maintenance)		Weights (maintenance)		Cardio 30 min		
PM	Low aerobic and speed	High aerobic 50-m reps	Off	800, 400, 200 race pace	Low aerobic	Off	Off
		Type 2		Type 4			
	7000 m	5500 m		6000 m	6500 m		
						Total 69,200 m	

Figure 17.10 Mid-season training week snapshot with swim-training focus and session distance of the training program of an elite distance swimmer.

Figure 17.10 shows a week snapshot of training in an elite distance swimmer. This particular week included 11 swim sessions, with four high-aerobic sessions, six low-aerobic sessions, and one session on Sunday aimed at recovery and continuity in training. The Tuesday evening session was a session with 24 × 50 m repetitions swum at high intensity, but with relatively short rest. The volume of this high-intensity work (1200 m) and the relatively short rest cycles made the overall training set high aerobic (and not anaerobic). The two weights sessions were aimed at maintaining already developed strength.

Open-Water Swimmers

The open-water Olympic event is 10 km, a race that takes about 2 h; open-water races are conducted in lakes, rivers, or seas.

At the 2016 Rio Olympic Games, Dutch swimmer Ferry Weertman touched just ahead of Greece's Spiros Gianniotis to win Olympic gold. Both touched the finish mark in a time of 1:52:59.8, separated by a few hundreds of a second. France's Marc-Antoine Olivier finished ~2 s later for bronze. This example demonstrates that open-water swimmers need endurance, but also speed and anaerobic power, as a race is very often won in the final surge or at the final touch.

Figure 17.11 shows the changes in speed during a particular open-water race in an elite athlete, measured with an accelerometer. There was substantial change in pace in this particular race, of which some can be explained by differences in current. It does demonstrate though that open-water swimmers need to be able to deliver and deal with changes in pace effectively. Other important performance factors are

orienting skills, management of water and weather conditions, and ability to navigate buoys and fence off other competitors. Swimming too wide off the buoys could result in ~10 m more swim distance, for example. The swimming conditions can be rough, with stories of goggles slammed off, ankles groped, and heads punched. Referees try to keep an eye on this, but it's often difficult for them to see it all. There are feeding stations at certain points on the course, where support staff can reach out to provide liquid foods, so deciding when to feed is part of the individual's race strategy. The drinking bottles in the figure show where the respective athlete fueled during the race.

Figure 17.12 shows a snapshot of a training week of an elite female open-water swimmer. This training-week example included a large volume of high-aerobic work with speed variations and acceleration work, to mimic intrarace speed variations. The total swim volume of the week was ~79 km, realized in 10 sessions.

Key Weapons, Manipulations, and Surveillance Tools

As throughout the book, the weapon term refers to the HIIT formats that can be used to target certain physiological responses (figure 1.5), and the surveillance tools are what is used to monitor training load (chapter 8) and individual responses (chapter 9).

HIIT Weapons and Their Manipulations

Always keep in mind that swimming is a very technical sport. Any intensity needs to be swum with

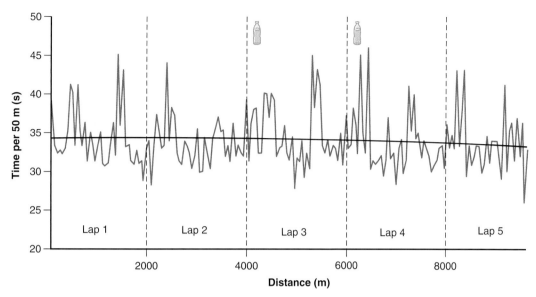

Figure 17.11 Changes in swim pace that occurred during a particular 10 km open-water race in a top athlete, measured with an accelerometer. The drinking bottles represent the timing where the athlete received food from a feeding station.

	Monday	Tuesday	Wednesday	Thursday	Friday	Saturday	Sunday
AM	High aerobic 100-m intervals Type 1 7000 m	Low and high aerobic 200 and 400-m intervals 7500 m	Anaerobic and high aerobic 50 and 300-m intervals Type 4 8800 m	Low aerobic 7400 m	Anaerobic and high aerobic 75-m intervals Type 4 6800 m	High aerobic 100 and 300-m intervals Type 4 8200 m	Off
	Weight circuit	Running		Weight circuit			
PM	Low and high aerobic 1000-m intervals 8500 m	Low and high aerobic 250-m intervals 7500 m	Off	High aerobic 800-m intervals 8500 m	Low and high aerobic 400-m intervals 8400 m	Off	Off
						Total 78,600 m	

Figure 17.12 Mid-season-week snapshot with training focus, interval distance of the main training set, and overall swim-session distance of a training program in an elite female open-water swimmer.

great technique. Energy needs to be applied effectively toward forward movement, while reducing drag is equally crucial for achieving this effect. Throughout sport, coaches often use the word *quality* to describe the intensity of a workout, but in swimming (and probably other sports as well), it should be interpreted as intensity with great technique and skill. Neuromuscular, aerobic and anaerobic adaptations for swimmers all need to be built on optimal technical skill and execution.

Swim training volumes (figures 17.4, 17.5, 17.7, 17.8, 17.10, and 17.12) are typically high relative to the duration of the competition event (figure 17.1).

Elite athletes usually swim in the pool for 2 to 6 h each day, combined with land-based work, appropriate nutrition, and rest. One possible reason for these relatively high training volumes relates to the *time on task* needed to engrain and adapt the neuromuscular blueprint that optimizes forward propulsion in the water medium. Another possible reason is that swimming is a relatively slow continuous movement. For example, male 800 m running versus 200 m swimming have comparable world records of 100.91 s and 102.00 s, respectively. The ground/water-contact time (duration of force production), however, is ~0.1 s per stride in running versus ~0.6 s per arm stroke in swimming. As a result, there is substantially more time in swimming to create propulsive force per stroke. Neuromuscular characteristics like tone, stiffness, and peak power are therefore relatively less important in swimming, while aerobic oxidative contribution to performance becomes relatively more important. Another possible factor for the higher training volumes of swimmers relates to the lower mechanical impact that swimming places on bones and joints compared to running and team sports, which makes it possible to train more.

While the large discrepancy between the physiological demands of training versus competition can be difficult to support for some physiologists, the majority of coaches observe success with these higher volumes of work, and to our knowledge, the vast majority of swimmers who have won Olympic medals have had a background of relatively large swim training volumes.

Observations in Australian and French swim programs are that some programs will avoid high-aerobic work and use a more polarized training schedule consisting of high-intensity work and predominantly low-intensity work (43), while other programs incorporate substantial volumes of high-aerobic work. Whether one strategy or another works best, or at what point in the periodized plan or career progression a specific strategy works best, largely depends on characteristics of the individual athlete, the event the athlete is training for, and the coach's specific beliefs and philosophical framework. As well, certain terms have specific meaning depending on the context; specific race-pace work for distance swimmers is high aerobic, while for sprinters it is more anaerobic.

Generally, most of the swimming volume (~60%–90%) is performed at intensities clearly below the anaerobic threshold; other volume is swum as HIIT. Paton and Hopkins (34) have published a good review on the effects of high-intensity training on performance. They classified HIIT as supramaximal, maximal, and submaximal intervals, as well as resistance exercise (including explosive, plyometrics, and weights). There are of course many ways to categorize training (see chapter 8). As already defined in this chapter, training is categorized into simple terms that include *low aerobic*, *high aerobic* (may include type 1, 2, 3, or 4 targets), *anaerobic* (type 3, 4, or 5 targets), *race-specific* (predominantly type 2 for distance swimmers, types 2 and 4 for middle-distance swimmers, and types 4 and 5 for sprint

swimmers), *speed* (type 5), and *recovery* to refer to the main areas of focus for each session. For the purposes of this chapter, the focus is on swim-specific training, omitting land-based training from discussion, although resistance and other land-based training methods form part of most successful swim training programs.

To further explain categories and swim-specific HIIT weapons, examples of training sets have been included, with indicative performance times and rest cycles of elite swimmers performing those sets in a long-course pool. Performance times will vary from swimmer to swimmer, and will depend on the current fitness and level of fatigue of the swimmer. Performance times are usually substantially faster in short-course pools, as experienced swimmers benefit from the push-off in the turns. Freestyle is the fastest stroke, followed by butterfly and backstroke; breaststroke performance times are substantially slower.

Low Aerobic

Low-aerobic training is performed at speeds ~70 to 40 beats below maximum heart rate, or at ~75% to 85% of the maximum 400 m swimming speed. This low-aerobic training intensity category is broad in swimming, with a relatively large range of heart rate intensities. Swimming longer repetitions below *threshold*, but still relatively fast, will predominantly use the aerobic system. With threshold, we refer to the anaerobic threshold, which is meant to indicate the maximal sustainable training speed without a net systemic H^+ accumulation. It is the maximum pace that a swimmer can maintain for longer distances/repetitions (see related descriptions in chapters 3 and 4). When athletes are training at threshold intensities, they induce a high stress on the oxidative system (16). The expected adaptations from performing low-aerobic work on a regular basis include metabolic and structural (enhancing $\dot{V}O_2max$ and increasing the economy of swimming at $\dot{V}O_2max$), in addition to the aforementioned neuromuscular remodeling. An example of this type of work for distance swimmers might be 6 × 800 m repetitions on a 10 min cycle. Top female distance swimmers would swim each repetition in around 9:30 min:s (~1:11/100 m) at relatively low heart rates, so they'd have about 30 s rest before starting the next 800 m repetition. Less fit or untrained swimmers would not manage this 10 min interval, and if they did, they would swim these times at much higher intensities, with higher anaerobic glycolytic engagement and overall training stress. Middle-distance swimmers do this type of work regularly as well, but usually with shorter repetitions, e.g., 6×300 m repetitions (~1:10/100 m) on a 4 min cycle, which would allow them ~30 s rest depending on the exercise intensity, or 8×200 m repetitions (~1:10/100 m) on a 2:30 cycle, which would allow them ~10 s rest. Some coaches standardize the recovery interval, e.g., a fixed 30 s rest after each repetition, but most coaches fix the interval in practice (e.g., on a 4 min cycle, meaning that each repetition starts 4 min after the previous repetition began), as programs with groups of swimmers are easier to manage this way.

High Aerobic

High-aerobic training uses longer volume sets of swimming at ~85% to 110% of the maximum 400 m swimming speed. The high-aerobic training intensity bandwidth generally consists of high-volume, short-distance, and short-rest repetitions swum at near maximum, as well as longer distance repetitions swum as fast as possible.

High Volume, Short Distance, Short Rest Training of a high volume of shorter distance repetitions, with short rest, is swum near or at maximum *best-average* pace. (Best-average means that the average time of all repetitions needs to be as fast as possible.) An example of this short-interval work would be 30×100 m freestyle repetitions at *threshold pace* on a 1:20 cycle. This threshold-pace cue translates to fast swimming, though at a sustainable pace and with good technique. Top male and female distance freestyle swimmers would swim these 100 m repetitions at ~59 s and ~63 s with about 20 or 15 s rest, respectively, before starting the next 100 m repetition. This set could also be swum at a higher intensity, e.g., 30×100 m freestyle repetitions best-average on a 1:40 cycle, where top male and female distance freestyle swimmers would swim the 100 m repetitions at ~56 s and ~60 s, respectively, so they'd have about 40 s rest before starting the next 100 m repetition (type 2). Variation of training intensity is important, and HIIT can be manipulated by changing the distance of intervals, the overall distance of the set, the rest interval, and/or the intensity of swimming (see also chapter 4).

Longer-Distance Repetitions Swum as Fast as Possible An example of this long-interval work involves 5×400 m repetitions at best-average speed on a 5 min cycle. Top male distance swimmers would

swim ~4:10 min:s for each repetition; top female distance swimmers ~4:22 min:s. That means that male distance swimmers would get ~50 s rest, and female swimmers ~38 s rest, between repetitions.

The anticipated adaptations from doing this high-aerobic work on a regular basis are also metabolic and structural (enhancing $\dot{V}O_2$max and increasing the economy of swimming at $\dot{V}O_2$max), and neuromuscular. The difference between these intensities and a swimming coach's low-aerobic intensity prescription is that there will be a higher stress on both the oxidative and glycolytic systems (types 3 and 4). This type of exercise provides a high training load, and usually warrants a relatively longer recovery time in the subsequent period.

Anaerobic

Anaerobic training consists of ~25 to 50 m repetitions swum very fast, with a high contribution of anaerobic glycolysis. An example of this work, which has aspects of repeated sprint training and sprint interval training weapons, and hits type 4 targets, is 4×25 m dive max and 4×35 m dive max with appropriate passive rest in between repetitions; top male swimmers would swim the 25 m repetitions in ~10 s and the 35 m repetitions in ~15 s.

An example of type 4 repeated sprint training targeting high-level stimulus of both anaerobic glycolysis and aerobic oxidation is 10×50 m butterfly at 100 m race-pace stroke rate, swum as fast as possible on a 2 min cycle, with passive rest between repetitions. Figure 17.13 shows the relevant physiological data of a female Australian international-level swimmer who has performed this training set. The total volume of the set, 500 m, is relatively high, which made the overall training stimulus more aerobic. Active recovery between the repetitions would also make the training set more aerobic (see chapters 4 and 5).

In the example (figure 17.13), the athlete's average 50 m performance time was 30.4 s, resulting in ~90 s rest between repetitions. This swimmer's 100 m race-pace stroke rate was 51 strokes/min, with the goal of swimming as fast as possible at this prescribed stroke rate for each 50 m repetition (see related training methods in chapter 16, rowing). As soon as the swimmer touched the wall at the finish of each repetition, a Cosmed K_4b_2 portable metabolic analyzer was worn for ~45 s to estimate $\dot{V}O_2$ during exercise using back extrapolation (11). The data showed that a $\dot{V}O_2$ peak was achieved by the 6th repetition with

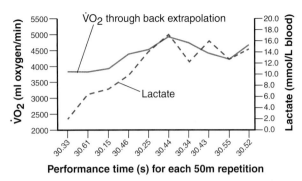

Figure 17.13 Performance data, with $\dot{V}O_2$ obtained through back extrapolation and blood lactate concentrations, of a female Australian international-level 200 m butterfly swimmer performing 10×50 m butterfly repetitions at a stroke rate of 51 cycles/min on a 2 min cycle (meaning each repetition starts 2 min after the previous repetition began). This session highlights the HIIT type 4 target.

this high-intensity work (type 4). The data have not been represented as a percentage of the swimmer's $\dot{V}O_2$max, as assessment of $\dot{V}O_2$max remains challenging in swimming.

Typical adaptations from this aerobic and anaerobic metabolic signaling during high-intensity swimming include an increase in the aerobic oxidative and anaerobic glycolytic metabolic contributions (27), an increase in buffering capacity, which translates to an improved ability to swim with the most efficient combination of stroke rate and stroke length during competition, and an increase in neuromuscular coordination at fast swim speeds. The training sets can be manipulated through changing the total number of repetitions, the rest interval, the distance of each repetition, and the stroke rate, for example (see also chapters 4 and 5). Many coaches will have the athlete stop this specific work when technique is failing, though some coaches will have the athlete push through, to challenge the swimmer to maintain good technique and fast swimming under fatigue.

Race-Specific Training

Physiologically, race-specific work for sprint swimmers could also be categorized *anaerobic* (type 4 and 5 targets), while for middle-distance swimmers it could be *anaerobic* (type 4) or *high aerobic* (type 2), and for distance and open-water swimmers *high aerobic* (predominantly type 2 targets). Training the specificity of competing in a certain event is clearly

important (figures 1.5, 17.1, and 17.2), not only for developing the necessary physiological capacities but also for the technical skills, the mental skills, the pacing, and maintenance of great technique under fatigue.

To train with specificity, some coaches and athletes work from a performance model, which typically includes target performance times for the start (usually the first 15 m of the race), the turns (usually measured from 5 m into the wall through to 10 m off the wall), the laps (50 m laps in a long-course pool), with stroke counts and rates (strokes per minute). Table 17.1 shows an example performance model for a top 200 m individual medley swimmer. Aspects of this model can then be tested and trained for.

An example of a race-specific training set for 100 m sprinters is 2× (60 m dive at 100 front-speed execution, followed by a 50 m push effort at execution of the second lap of the race), with ~40 s between the 60 m dive and the 50 m push efforts, and appropriate recovery and reactivation between the two sets. An example of a race-specific training set for a 200 m middle-distance swimmer is 2 × (75 m dive at 200 m get-out pace swim easy through to the 100 m mark, ~10 s rest, 3 × 50 m push efforts at 200 pace with ~20 s rest in between), with appropriate recovery and reactivation between the two sets. An example for 1500 m distance swimmers might be 20 × 100 m on a 1:20 cycle at 1500 m race-pace (~58 s/100 m for male swimmers). The anticipated stimulus and adaptations are similar to those described in the anaerobic work section, except are specific to the individual's race-pace motor pattern. Coaches and athletes also often use minor domestic and international competitions for training purposes, to practice very specifically for competition and to fine-tune racing skills, including the mental component.

Speed Work

Speed work consists of ~10 to 20 m repetitions at very fast speeds with relatively long rest, triggering the phosphagen system. An example of speed work in a swimmer, which resembles the repeated sprint-training weapon hitting type 5 targets, might be 4 × 20 m maximal sprint dives on a 2 min cycle. Top male freestyle athletes would swim ~8 s on each repetition, meaning they'd have ~110 s rest between repetitions. With speed work, the rate and pattern of muscle fiber stimulation by the central nervous system is increased, and the phosphagen system is triggered. This work is also aimed at developing and

Table 17.1 Individualized 200 m Individual Medley Performance Model for a Total Time of 1:56.99 (min:ss.00)

A 200 m individual medley consists of four 50 m laps, swum as butterfly, backstroke, breaststroke, and freestyle by lap.

Stroke	Segment	Segment split time (s)	Lap split time (s)	Strokes per lap (n)	SR (strokes/min)	In (s)	Out (s)	Turn (in + out, s)
Butterfly	0-15 m	5.95						
	0-25 m	11.22			52			
	25-50 m	13.58	**24.80**	18	51	2.71	5.16	7.87
Backstroke	50-75 m	14.35			42			
	75-100 m	15.10	**29.45**	34	42	3.01	5.94	8.95
Breaststroke	100-125 m	16.82			39			
	125-150 m	17.65	**34.47**	17	39	3.36	5.62	8.98
Freestyle	150-175 m	14.02			46			
	175-200 m	14.25	**28.27**	38	46	2.61		

SR: stroke rate; In: time between head passing the 5 m mark into the wall to the touch on the wall; Out: time from the touch of the wall through when the head passes the 10 m mark off the wall; Turn: sum of in and out as an overall 15 m turn time.

fine-tuning technical speed skills in individual athletes. The distance of each repetition typically ranges between 10 and 30 m, though the longer the distance and the shorter the rest, the more the anaerobic lactic and aerobic systems become involved. Manipulations can be achieved through changing the number of repetitions, rest cycles, and distance, or, for example, by including a turn off the wall.

Recovery Swimming

The most important recovery modalities for swimmers are rest, sleep, and nutrition. Discussion around recovery is beyond the scope of this chapter and is covered in chapter 7 in detail. Factors that will affect the need for recovery include the training intensity and volume, psychological stress, health and fatigue status, and the environment (e.g., temperature, humidity, altitude). A recovery swim session will generally consist of very easy swimming, which is usually no longer than 45 min or 2 km. The examples in figures 17.8 and 17.10 show recovery sessions with higher mileages (~3-4000 m), mainly because coaches usually want distance swimmers to achieve a certain mileage at the end of the week.

Load Surveillance and Monitoring Tools

The measurement and monitoring of training load, discussed in chapter 8, is an important issue for athletes, coaches, and sports scientists. A number

of informative reviews on the quantification of training have been produced (15, 24, 41). Here, we will mention a few methodologies used regularly in the sport of swimming to prescribe and monitor the external and internal training load in swimmers. As expanded on in chapter 8, the external training load involves the work completed by the individual, while the internal training load refers to the relative physiological and psychological stress imposed by the external training load.

Prescription and Monitoring of Exercise Intensity in Training Sessions

Swimming coaches often prescribe the desired training intensity based on the *heart rate* associated with submaximal efforts. In reality, however, this beats below maximum heart rate prescription in fact is a prescription of *perceived effort*. The measuring and monitoring of heart rate in swimming remains challenging, and there are also issues of validity. As discussed in chapters 2, 8, and 9, heart rate is not a valid prescription or assessment of anaerobic and speed work, or for high-intensity work swum at near maximum heart rate. There is also the issue of the validity of using heart rate to prescribe exercise intensity across individual swimmers. While heart rate shows an almost linear relationship with $\dot{V}O_2$ at submaximal intensities, this relationship is individual (1). The use of heart rate zones (chapter 8) for both prescription and monitoring of submaximal loads also needs assessment of the individual's maximum heart rate during swimming, so that beats below maximum can be both prescribed and monitored. The assessment of an individual's maximum heart rate will require a pool-based incremental and/or repeat effort test to volitional exhaustion. To our knowledge, there are no gold-standard protocols used in the literature for swimming research.

There are various devices and systems available on the market to measure heart rate in swimmers; some are used to measure heart rate at the end of each repetition, while other devices have been developed to monitor heart rate throughout exercise. The challenge with measuring heart rate at the end of a repetition includes the time lag of measurement, the time needed for the measurement (especially when there is little rest between intervals), and the effect of pacing on heart rate, when a last lap was swum faster, for example. The challenge of monitoring heart rate throughout each repetition in swimming resides in the capturing of data and ensuring its quality. Most devices capture data with a chest strap, and while this can be put underneath the swimsuit for

female swimmers, male swimmers need to swim with vests, which they find restrictive. The straps also move from time to time, especially in push-offs or dive starts. There are companies working toward capturing heart rate from the temporal vein (through integrated sensors in goggles or swim caps), but we have yet to see this properly functional. Figure 17.14 shows an example training session of a top distance swimmer, where heart rate was measured throughout using a Polar Team 2 System. The heart rate data follow the intensities according to the work in the low-aerobic training session nicely, but too often the data is not clean enough for the system to be used as a load-monitoring system in low-aerobic and high-aerobic swimming.

A method that is regularly used to prescribe training intensity is setting a *goal pace* (desired performance time) for repetitions. This pace can be in relation to any training intensity: easy aerobic swimming, race-pace swimming, maximal efforts, and speed. The advantage of using this method is that performance time can be easily measured and

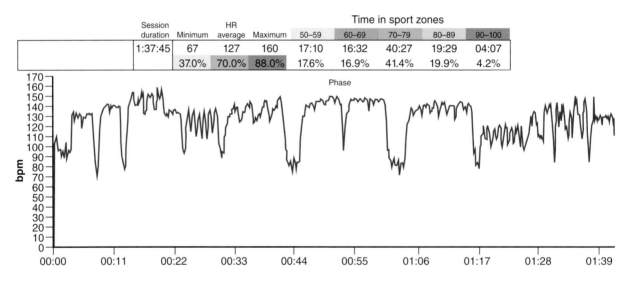

- 4 x 300-m freestyle (breathe every 3 and every 5 strokes by 50-m lap) on a 5-min cycle
- 4 x 100-m medley, change strokes at the 25-m mark on 1:45 cycle
- 1 x 200-m freestyle drill on 4-min cycle
- 6 x 50-m freestyle, work on distance per stroke, on 1-min cycle
- 4 x 200-m freestyle paddles pull on 2:45 cycle (HR 130-150)
- 2 x 400-m kick on 8-min cycle (HR < 150)
- 10 x 100-m freestyle or backstroke by 50-m lap on 1:30 cycle
- 8 x 50-m freestyle drill with fins on 1-min cycle
- 8 x 50-m medley order as (20 m fast/30 m recovery) on 1:15 cycle
- 2 x 600-m choice swim

Figure 17.14 Example of a training diary of an athlete specializing in 400 m and 800 m freestyle events. HR: heart rate; RP: race pace; Flow: how you felt moving through the water. Monitoring permits data to be shown as changes on a week-by-week basis.

monitored in the pool; the disadvantage is that the realized intensity at a certain training pace will be individualized and depends on the levels of fatigue and efficiency.

Variables that are used less frequently to prescribe intensities are the *stroke rate* and *RPE* (5). Figure 17.13 provides an example of how intensity can be prescribed using stroke rate, where the swimmer's instruction was 10 × 50 m butterfly repetitions at 51 strokes per min on a 2 min cycle. There are devices that can be used to help with standardizing a stroke rate (e.g., Finis Tempo Trainer). This tool works with some athletes, but other athletes find the beeping sound too much of a distraction to achieve good rhythm and technique. In any case, most experienced swimmers are aware of what stroke rate they swim at. The RPE method, described in chapter 2, has been validated as a robust and reliable measure for submaximal intensities (13), though many coaches prefer cues such as easy swimming, very fast swimming, race-pace swimming, maximum effort swimming, or beats below maximum heart rate, for example. Figures 17.8 and 17.14 have portions of the prescription where RPE and other cues are used to prescribe the session intensity.

Monitoring Training Load

Figure 17.9 shows the swim training volumes of an elite distance swimmer in an Olympic year. While the figure nicely describes the weekly training distances realized, it does little to describe the intensities of this work, and therefore isn't a valid measure of training load. Automated systems using inertial sensors have more recently become available to measure swimming speed, stroke rate, and mileage. While these systems have yet to properly monitor the external swim training load, good gains have been made in this area, and useful systems are predicted to be available in coming years. Currently, coaches and scientists often dissect training mileage into mileage swum at certain training intensities, which has its challenges, but provides a more accurate measurement of external training load. Monitoring tools used to assess internal training load, described in

World Championships, days to go…		93	92	91	90	89	88	87
		Mon	**Tue**	**Wed**	**Thu**	**Fri**	**Sat**	**Sun**
		22 May	**23 May**	**24 May**	**25 May**	**26 May**	**27 May**	**28 May**
Sleep	Total hours of sleep	8	8	7	8	7	8	10
	Hours of sleep during day	1	1		1			
	Quality of sleep (see scale)	7	7	7	8	7	7	8
AM training session	Low aerobic (≤ HR 155, m)	5900	6700	5900	7640	6400	4400	
	High aerobic (>HR155<RP, m)	1200	300				3000	
	800-m race pace (m)						300	
	400-m race pace (m)							
	200-m race pace (m)					150		
	100-m race pace (m)					100		
	Speed (0-25 m, m)			100	160	50		
	Total mileage (m)	7100	7000	6000	7800	6700	7700	0
	Training intensity (see scale)	6	6	4	5	7	8	
	Flow (see scale)	5	4	5	5	5	6	
Gym	AM gym training intensity			7				
PM training session	Low aerobic (≤ HR 155, m)	3280	6525		5500	6600		
	High aerobic (>HR155<RP, m)	3600			900	400		
	800-m race pace (m)							
	400-m race pace (m)							
	200-m race pace (m)		475		600			
	100-m race pace (m)							
	Speed (0-25 m, m)	120						
	Total mileage (m)	7000	7000	0	7000	7000	0	0
	Training intensity	8	8		8	6		
	Flow	7	6		6	5		
Gym	PM gym training intensity	7						

Flow (how you feel moving through the water) / **Sleep quality**
- 10 Extremely good
- 9 Very, very good
- 8 Very good
- 7 Good
- 6 Fairly good
- 5 Average
- 4 Fairly poor
- 3 Poor
- 2 Very poor
- 1 Very, very poor
- 0 None

Training intensity
- 10 Extremely hard
- 9 Very, very hard
- 8 Very hard
- 7 Hard
- 6 Fairly hard
- 5 Average
- 4 Fairly easy
- 3 Easy
- 2 Very easy
- 1 Very, very easy
- 0 No training

Figure 17.15 Example of a training diary of an athlete specializing in 400 m and 800 m freestyle events. HR: heart rate; RP: race pace; Flow: how you felt moving through the water. Monitoring permits data to be shown as changes on a weekly basis.

August 2017- August 2018

Phase band (row 1)				
Building metabolic capacities onto great technique and skill	Competition preparation	Competition preparation	Build	
Build athleticism and strength in gym	Maintain strength in gym	Maintain strength in gym		

Training calendar (days of week run Saturday → Sunday down the rows; months run across in columns). Cells with a training focus or target weekly swim mileage are noted below by date.

August (2017)
- 2 Off
- 14 build
- 19 17 km
- 21 build
- 26 32.5 km
- 28 AEC

September
- 2 36.5 km
- 4 AEC
- 9 40 km
- 11 AEC
- 16 45.5 km
- 18 REG
- 21 AEC&ANC
- 23 32 km
- 25 AEC&ANC
- 30 45 km

October
- 2 AEC&ANC
- 7 50 km
- 9 AEC&ANC
- 14 50 km
- 16 REG
- 18 AEC&ANC
- 21 32 km
- 23 AEC&ANC
- 25 travel
- 26 Minor
- 27 Competition
- 28 AEC&ANC
- 30 AEC&ANC

November
- 2 45 km
- 4 28 km
- 6 AEC&ANC
- 11 42 km
- 12 Competition
- 13 REG
- 15 AEC&ANC
- 18 Minor Comp
- 20 AEC&ANC
- 23 45 km
- 25 AEC&ANC

December
- 2 45 km
- 7 AEC&ANC
- 9 Minor
- 10 Competition
- 11 AEC&ANC
- 16 30.8 km
- 18 AEC&ANC
- 23 44.5 km
- 25 AEC&ANC
- 30 34 km

January
- 1 AEC&ANC
- 6 39.5 km
- 8 Comp Prep
- 13 35.5 km
- 17 Travel
- 19 Minor
- 20 Competition
- 21 33.9 K
- 22 Travel
- 23 REG
- 27 36 km
- 29 Comp Prep

February
- 1 Selection
- 2 Competition
- 3 35.5 km
- 4 Comp Prep
- 8 Comp Prep
- 10 35.5 km
- 12 Taper
- 17 27.5 km
- 18 Competition
- 24 22.5 km
- 28 Major-Comp

March
- 1 Selection
- 2 Competition
- 3 18.6 km
- 5 REG
- 8 Comp Prep
- 10 20 km
- 12 Comp Prep
- 17 35.5 km
- 19 Comp Prep
- 21 Taper
- 24 35.5 km
- 25 Camp
- 26 Comp Prep
- 31 Travel-21.5 K

April
- 4 Major
- 6 Competition
- 8 26.2 km
- 10 Off
- 11 Off
- 12 Off
- 14 Off - 8.3 km
- 16 build
- 21 17 km
- 23 AEC
- 28 32.5 km
- 30 AEC&ANC

May
- 5 45 km
- 7 AEC&ANC
- 12 45 km
- 14 REG
- 17 AEC&ANC
- 19 Travel
- 21 AEC&ANC
- 24 Minor
- 25 Competition
- 28 Travel
- 29 REG

June
- 3 Camp
- 4 Comp Prep
- 11 Comp Prep
- 16 travel
- 18 Taper
- 23 Comp Prep
- 25 Taper
- 27 travel

July
- 1 Major-Comp
- 2 Selection
- 3 Competition
- 5 Travel
- 7 REG
- 9 REG
- 12 Comp Prep
- 16 Comp Prep
- 21 travel
- 28 travel
- 30 Taper

August (2018)
- 4 Travel
- 6 Taper
- 9 Major
- 10 Competition

Figure 17.16 Example of three macrocycles for a sprint swimmer building toward the 2018 Commonwealth Games and Pan Pacific Games, showing mesocycles with training focus and target week swim mileage. AEC: aerobic capacity; ANC: anaerobic capacity; REG: regeneration; Comp Prep: competition preparation. The main competitions are in yellow; the minor competitions are in orange. The global structure of two of these mesocycles is expanded in detail in figure 17.17.

Regeneration

	22 Jan	23 Jan	24 Jan	25 Jan	26 Jan	27 Jan	28 Jan
Days out	37	36	35	34	33	32	31
AM	Low aerobic 4000	Low aerobic 4500	Low aerobic 4500	Low aerobic 5000	Recovery 3000	Low aerobic 5000	Off
		Land circuit	Land circuit		Land circuit	Land circuit	
PM	Off	Speed 2500	Off	Contrast Fast vs. easy 5000	Speed 2500	Off	Off

36,000

Comp Preparation

	29 Jan	30 Jan	31 Jan	1 Feb	2 Feb	3 Feb	4 Feb
Days out	30	29	28	27	26	25	24
AM	High aerobic 5000	Low aerobic 5000	Low aerobic 5000	Contrast Fast vs. easy 5000	Recovery 3000	Anaerobic 3000	Off
	Land circuit	Land circuit		Land circuit	Land circuit		
PM	Speed 2500	Anaerobic 3000	Off	Race pace 4000	Off	Off	Off

35,500

Comp Preparation

	5 Feb	6 Feb	7 Feb	8 Feb	9 Feb	10 Feb	11 Feb
Days out	23	22	21	20	19	18	17
AM	High aerobic 5000	Low aerobic 5000	Low aerobic 5000	Contrast Fast vs Easy 5000	Recovery 3000	Anaerobic 3000	Off
	Land circuit	Land circuit		Land circuit	Land circuit		
PM	Speed 2500	Anaerobic 3000	Off	Race pace 4000	Off	Off	Off

35,500

Taper

	12 Feb	13 Feb	14 Feb	15 Feb	16 Feb	17 Feb	18 Feb
Days out	16	15	14	13	12	11	10
AM	High aerobic 4000	Low aerobic 4000	Low aerobic 4000	Speed 2000	Recovery 2000	Anaerobic 3000	Off
	Land circuit	Land circuit		Land circuit	Land circuit		
PM	Speed 2000	Anaerobic 2500	Off	Race pace 4000	Off	Off	Off

27,500

Taper

	19 Feb	20 Feb	21 Feb	22 Feb	23 Feb	24 Feb	25 Feb
Days out	9	8	7	6	5	4	3
AM	High aerobic 3000	Low aerobic 3000	Low aerobic 3000	Speed 2000	Recovery 2000	Anaerobic 2500	Off
	Land circuit	Land circuit		Land circuit	Land circuit		
PM	Speed 2000	Anaerobic 2000	Off	Race pace 3000	Off	Off	Off

22,500

Competition

	26 Feb	27 Feb	28 Feb	1 Mar	2 Mar	3 Mar	4 Mar
	2	1	Major Championships Selection Event				
10:30 AM	Light swim 2000	Race prep 2500	Race prep 1600	100 free heat 2000	Recovery 2000	50 free heat 1500	Low aerobic 2000
7:30 PM	Speed 2000	Off	Off	100 free final 2000	Off	50 free final 1000	Off

18,600

Figure 17.17 Example overview of a 5 wk training block of a 100 and 50 m specialist swimmer, working toward a competition, showing overall swim training volumes and focus. This training block aligns with two of the mesocycles shown in figure 17.16. Training focus is categorized into simple terms that include *low aerobic, high aerobic* (could include type 1, 2, 3, or 4 targets), *anaerobic* (type 3, 4, or 5 targets), *race-specific* (predominantly type 2 for distance swimmers, types 2 and 4 for middle-distance swimmers, and types 4 and 5 for sprint swimmers), *speed* (type 5), and *recovery; contrast* is a session including very fast swimming and easy swimming (in line with type 4 targets).

chapter 8, include RPE and heart rate, of which session RPE may be current best practice. The use of session RPE also allows for the simultaneous monitoring of land-based training loads, which in effect add substantially to the overall load and are not included in the monitoring of swim training volumes.

Various swim squads around the world use training diaries, logbooks, or digital applications to monitor certain variables of load. Figure 17.15 shows a snapshot of an athlete's training diary, with variables of external training load (realized mileage at certain intensities per training session) and internal training load (perceived training intensity), as well as other monitoring variables such as hours and quality of sleep, and training flow (how the swimmer felt moving through the water). The challenge of the use of training diaries lies in the validity of the entered data, though they can provide good information for training and performance evaluation.

A promising method to characterize training load during high-intensity training and competition is the simulation of metabolic energy responses using mathematical models (17, 19, 22, 39). This method shows promise to help coaches and scientists better understand, visualize, and monitor the metabolic response and cost of high-intensity training and competition in individual athletes.

Strategies for Structuring the Training Program

Coaches will generally aim to have their athletes reach peak performance at major championships and major championships-selection event for their country (as dictated by the National Swimming Organization), where the athlete will need to achieve qualifying standards set by their respective organizing committee. The uncontrollable factors that the athlete and coach must navigate include the race date, venue, event order, and timing of major championship events relative to the selection trial events. Athletes and coaches will work with the competition calendar framework, using available time as effectively as possible to achieve their goals. Figure 17.16 is an example of a competition calendar that extends from August 2017 to August 2018, including competitions, training camps, and mesocycles with physiological focus and weekly target mileages. Medical checks, skinfold assessment, testing sets, training blocks, and so on can all be included within the yearly plan. Once this overview is established, the coach can then schedule the weekly microcycle training structures, deciding when and how to schedule HIIT work throughout the respective week.

Figure 17.17 shows a 5 wk training block of an athlete working toward a selection event for a major competition. This training block aligns with two of the mesocycles outlined in figure 17.16, and shows target swim volumes with individual session focuses. Examples of HIIT training sets according to the training focus have been described previously in this chapter. While the planning process is developed with the aim of reaching peak performances at certain times of the year, it unfortunately does not guarantee that maximal performance potential will be expressed in competition. As discussed previously, performance is a manifestation of many variables, which makes the pursuit of solving the performance puzzle, through coaching and the scientific support of individual athletes, a fascinating and evolving journey. It is as much an art in achieving focus on what is important in preparation for individual swimmers as it is an art for the athlete to perform when it matters most.

THINKING OUTSIDE THE BOX

Inspiration and opportunity have brought us to work with some of the world's best swimmers and their coaches, and to gain insights into training structures, HIIT content, and coach philosophies of top swim programs in Australia, France, the Netherlands, United States, New Zealand, Sweden, Denmark, and Spain.

In swimming, applied physiologists generally focus on monitoring performance in HIIT sets, including technical (e.g., stroke rate and stroke count) and physiological (e.g., RPE, lactate, heart rate) measures, to drive and assess change, and to bring individualization to training. As described in the chapter, warranted adaptations and individualization in training is mainly done through periodizing and individualizing the distance and the number of HIIT repetitions, the rest between the repetitions, the time between HIIT sessions, and the execution of HIIT.

In physiology, we also try to look within, e.g., on a muscular, cardiovascular, or hormonal level, and that's often difficult to do—more so than, for example, in biomechanics, where angles and technique can be assessed more directly through video analysis, or in anthropometry, where height, skinfolds, and bone lengths can be measured straightforwardly.

Methods to look within are, for example, the measurement of $\dot{V}O_2$ during or immediately after swimming (11, 23, 44), blood lactate profiling (33), and step tests (36). Another topical method to look within is the collaboration between radiologists and sports scientists in the Muscle Talent Scan, a method used to noninvasively estimate muscle fiber–type composition in athletes using an MRI scanning process. Here, the measurement of certain metabolites, such as carnosine concentration, can help to discriminate between fast-twitch, intermediate, and slow-twitch athletes, which may be useful for showing event-specific performance potential (4).

Wim, Philippe, and Tom have different roles in Belgium, France, and Australia, respectively, but all three are part of helping athletes and coaches achieve their goals, of helping people make more-informed decisions, and of contributing to the existing scientific knowledge. The three of us are part of a team in respective nations, and occasionally get together as a team internationally, to attempt to answer questions of coaches collectively, to address specific parts of the performance puzzle together, and in this occasion to write a book chapter. We believe our jobs are among the best in the world and are very grateful for the privilege. We hope that this chapter will help aspiring swim sport scientists and coaches think about what they do, and that it will help to structure their thinking into delivering successful training strategies. In line with the theme emphasized throughout the book, we believe our collaboration demonstrates "thinking outside the box" in applied sport science (6).

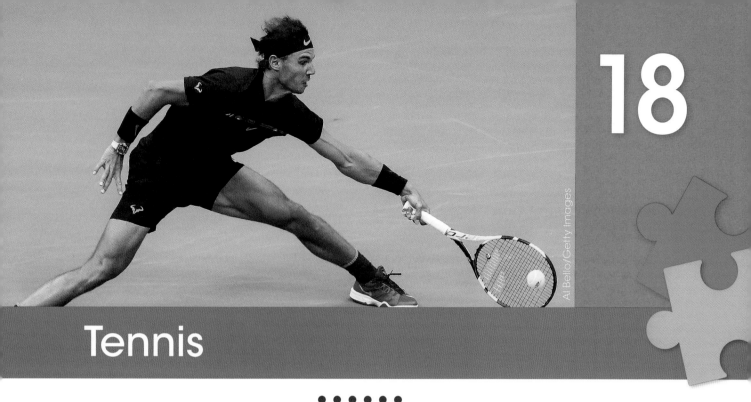

Tennis

• • • • • •

Jaime Fernandez-Fernandez

Performance Demands of Tennis

Tennis requires a complex interaction of technical, tactical, and psychological components, as well as several physical (i.e., strength, agility) and energetic demands (i.e., aerobic and anaerobic). Training is instrumental in achieving these requirements. In order to strive toward these needs, coaches and athletes must navigate a journey to optimize the various training inputs (i.e., technical, tactical, psychological) and physical conditioning content, in accordance with the most important limiting performance factors, alongside individual player needs (strengths and weaknesses).

The importance of the technical and tactical requirements for tennis performance place a key limitation on the planning of weekly physical training loads, and such needs must be placed above all others within a hierarchical model of tennis performance. Weekly training volume must be adjusted correspondingly with respective physical conditioning volume remaining comparably low. Therefore, at the elite performance level, it becomes critical for physical training to be combined with the on-court technical and tactical training, while off-court sessions should be used to address individual requirements (13).

Sport Description, Including Factors of Winning

Tennis is a game enjoyed by millions around the world who play recreationally and competitively, coupled with extremely large viewing audiences (i.e., the Australian Open 2017 men's final attracted 4.4 million viewers in Australia and 11 million across Europe). Professional tennis players travel and compete extensively year round, with more than 500 annual international tournaments available on the professional men's and women's calendars, including team events for junior, senior, and wheelchair players (34). At a basic level, tennis requires varying sequences of points, games, and sets to be won in order to win the match. Winning enough points wins a game, winning enough games wins a set, and winning enough sets wins the match. Tennis is a unique sport in that a player can be victorious in a match while winning fewer points than his opponent, who is committing more mistakes or errors.

From a physical standpoint, tennis match play is characterized by intermittent exercise, in which alternate short bouts (4 to 10 s) of high-intensity exercise and short bouts (10 to 20 s) of recovery are interrupted by several resting periods of longer duration (60 to 90 s) (33, 44). The duration of a tennis event often is greater than an hour and, in some cases, lasts for more than 5 h (e.g., Australian Open

2012 men's final was 5 h, 53 min). The typical average match time for a best of three match is 1.5 h (33), and effective playing time (percentage of the total time playing the game) amounts to approximately 20% to 30% (21, 36).

Relative Contribution of Physical Performance

The modern game of tennis evolved from a primarily technical sport in which sport-specific technical skills (e.g., racket and ball handling skills, as well as stroke skills such as serving) were the predominant winning factors to more of a dynamic and explosive sport characterized by higher stroke and serve velocities, requiring notably higher physical demands. Increasing evidence suggests that motor skills such as muscle power, strength, agility, speed, mental strength, and a highly developed neuromuscular coordinating ability correlate with tennis performance (26, 46). Moreover, if a player is not in good condition, essential characteristics in tennis, including technique, coordination, concentration, and tactics become exposed in long matches as premature fatigue impairs virtually all tennis-specific skills (27) (figure 18.1).

Targets of Physical Performance in Tennis

As previously mentioned, physical exertion during tennis involves high-intensity efforts interspersed with periods of variable duration and low-intensity activity (21). Thus, from a physiological point of view, demands alternate between energy provision for bouts of high-intensity work and replenishing energy sources and restoring homeostasis during the recovery intervals (21). The most important actions during tennis match play involve serves and strokes, accelerations, decelerations, and changes of direction, which are likely to be dependent on anaerobic energy pathways, supported largely by an aerobic metabolic background for recovery (36).

From a physiological point of view, the sport of tennis has been well defined using various portable analyzers (i.e., oxygen uptake ($\dot{V}O_2$); blood lactate ([La]); heart rate (HR)) that have described the responses during both real and simulated matches (2, 5, 45). Accordingly, mean HR during competitive matches has been shown to range from between 70% and 80% of maximum (HR_{max}), with peak values around 90% to 100% of HR_{max}. Average $\dot{V}O_2$ values correspond to approximately 50% to

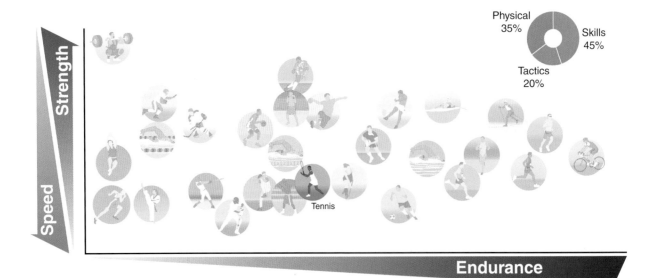

Figure 18.1 The position of the tennis player on the three axes illustrates the relative importance of the three main physical capacities for elite participation. Outside of critical psychological aspects, which are difficult to quantify, the pie chart shows the general relative importance of skills (45%), tactical awareness (20%), and physical capacities (35%) for tennis success.

Adapted from G.A. Nader, "Concurrent Strength and Endurance Training: From Molecules to Man," *Medicine & Science in Sports & Exercise* 38, no. 11 (2006): 1965-1970.

60% of $\dot{V}O_2$max, with values above 80% of $\dot{V}O_2$max recorded during intensive rallies (29). Rating of perceived exertion (RPE) has been reported as ranging from 5 to 7 arbitrary units on a scale of 1 to 10 (9, 28) and 10 to 16 arbitrary units on the Borg 20 point scale (12). Regarding [La], it has been reported to fluctuate throughout matches, increasing acutely in response to long rallies and conditions of limited recovery time, indicative of likely greater reliance on anaerobic glycolysis (12, 36). In cases where [La] has been measured during matches, samples were collected during the change of ends (14, 36), with match durations not reported, leaving results to be highly variable and inconclusive. Regardless, [La] values typically remain low during matches, with mean values reported as ranging from between 1.7 and 3.8 mmol/L (12, 33), despite some elite players reaching more than 8 mmol/L (12). With competition points lasting less than 10 s, and the inclusion of frequent rest periods, the physiological demands of match play are unlikely to lead to large accumulations of [La] where it might relate to acute fatigue during tennis matches (33).

The ability to maintain high technical efficiency during phases of high-intensity intermittent exercise is an important feature of successful tennis player performance. From an early age, tennis players spend many hours mastering their individual sport-specific skills, with technical and tactical training volumes often exceeding 15 to 20 h/wk. Moreover, although successful tennis players may not be as tall as their successful basketball or handball player counterparts, the current average height of the Women's Tennis Association (WTA) top-20 players is 176 cm (5'8"), while the average height for players in the Association of Tennis Professionals (ATP) top 50 is now 185 cm (6'1"). Thus, together with the high amount of on-court training volume, my personal belief is that it is necessary to reduce the supplementary-training volume related to running exercise (e.g., traditional interval running), as supported by the relationship shown between high training loads (i.e., on- and off-court) and several joint injuries (e.g., hip) (24, 37).

Key Weapons, Manipulations, and Surveillance Tools

In this section, the different high-intensity interval training (HIIT) weapons, their manipulations, along with ways by which we can monitor their effective-

ness (surveillance) are presented. Although tennis is a very popular sport, information concerning the effectiveness of training interventions is very scarce, and particularly absent is the impact of HIIT on tennis performance-related variables. Therefore, most of the information presented herein is based on my practical experience acquired through years in the sport and on research shown from other intermittent sports.

HIIT Weapons

As presented throughout the book, there are five different metabolic and/or neuromuscular load targets that can be applied throughout a tennis player's season (figure 1.5) by use of the five HIIT weapons (5). For tennis (figure 18.2), the large majority of these include game-based HIIT (40%, mostly in-season), followed by short intervals (30%, some preseason, but mostly in-season), repeated-sprint training (RST) (20%, in-season only), sprint interval training (SIT) (5%, in-season only), and run-based long intervals (5%, in-season only). With the exception of the run-based short and long intervals, tennis movements are mimicked during all HIIT weapon types, with greater uncertainty of play involved with game-based HIIT (figure 5.31). Of course, this breakdown is a general approach only, which should be modified based on individual player needs.

Manipulations of Interval Training Variables

The main programming strategy I implement at the beginning of a player's season is to routinely plan an appropriate volume of all HIIT weapons and target types throughout the year. Intensity of run-based HIIT is calibrated using the 30-15 IFT (chapter 2), which is conducted at the beginning of the preseason, normally after a few days of familiarization with the training routine. I usually don't change the running intensity too much during the season, which, depending on the format and needs of the player, tends to vary from 85% to 100% of V_{IFT}. Moreover, I try to vary training content as much as possible during the week, combining different HIIT formats. For the preseason of an elite junior player, for example, a possible programming combination might be as follows:

Monday, tennis-based HIIT

Wednesday, run-based short HIIT

Friday, tennis-based HIIT.

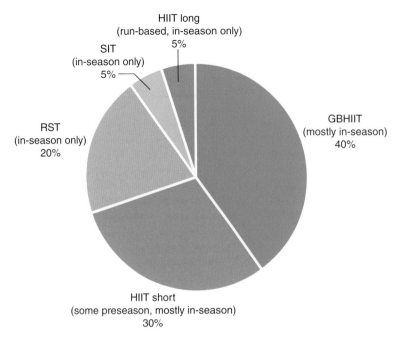

Figure 18.2 Percentage of the different HIIT weapons (formats) used throughout the annual season in elite tennis. Game-based HIIT (40%, mostly in-season), followed by short intervals (30%, some preseason, but mostly in-season), repeated-sprint training or RST (20%, in-season only), sprint interval training or SIT (5%, in-season only), and run-based long intervals (5%, in-season only). HIIT: high-intensity interval training; RST: repeated-sprint training; SIT: sprint interval training; GBHIIT: game-based HIIT.

HIIT With Long Intervals

Although I don't usually implement run-based HIIT with long intervals in tennis players, there are some exceptions. When a player has an upper-body problem (i.e., injury or overload) or low fitness, I normally implement run-based HIIT with long intervals in the outdoor environment, either on a grass pitch or in the forest (with distances marked using cones), to minimize musculoskeletal strain (5) (HIIT types 3 and 4). Generally, these sessions are performed over 800 to 1000 m efforts completed between 3 and 4 min, at intensities based on the V_{IFT} (80% to 85%), with 2 to 3 min rest, depending on the player's fitness. Normally players are grouped based on their V_{IFT} in order to complete the training sessions in individualized small groups, and typical training volumes range from 3 to 5 repetitions. Generally, these sessions are prescribed at the end of the week before a day off, so players can recover from an anticipated neuromuscular fatigue.

An example of a tennis-specific HIIT with long-interval session is shown in figure 18.3 (17, 40, 43). These involve specific groundstroke/open play from the baseline, with repeated strokes from dif-

ferent positions under pressure, but most specifically during baseline play. An experienced professional coach hand or racket feeds balls for long-HIIT drills. Irrespective of the drill, all players are instructed to move and hit with maximal effort, directing all shots to the target areas near the baseline. These tennis-specific drills differ from game-based drills (see below) due to the absence of an opponent, and in turn, the different decision-making clues and lower certainty involved with the movement patterns required (figure 18.3). Again, intensity is monitored using HR, with target zones set at 90% to 95% of HR_{max}. While overall training volume depends on the player's level, the general aim is to accumulate a minimum of 10 to 15 min of work at intensities close to $\dot{V}O_2max$, or in this case, near HR_{max} (5). It is important to acknowledge that although HR monitoring is currently the only (low-cost) method of monitoring HIIT sessions, its effectiveness is limited, as described in chapters 2, 8, and 9. It's additionally important to highlight that using HR to monitor and potentially adjust the intensity of an HIIT session may be limited, as HR cannot inform on the intensity of physical work

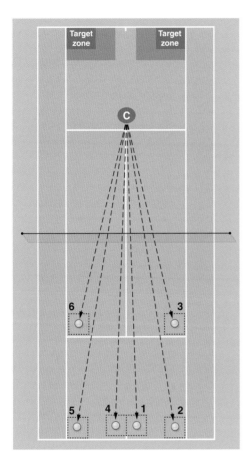

Figure 18.3 Example of tennis-specific HIIT with long intervals (1-2 min work with 45 s to 1 min 30 s rest). P: player; C: coach; 1, 2, 3: forehand strokes; 4, 5, 6: backhand strokes.

Adapted by permission from J. Fernandez-Fernandez, D. Sanz-Rivas, C. Sanchez-Munoz, J.G. de la Aleja Tellez, M. Buchheit, and A. Mendez-Villanueva, "Physiological Responses to On-Court vs Running Interval Training in Competitive Tennis Players," *Journal of Sports Science & Medicine* 10 no. 3 (2011): 540-545.

performed above the speed or power associated with $\dot{V}O_2$max (5).

HIIT With Short Intervals

My preferred HIIT weapon is the short interval, including 30 s on/30 s off, 20 s/20 s, 15 s/15 s, and 10 s/20 s (see tables 18.1 to 18.4), which target HIIT types 1, 2, 3, and 4 with exercise modality being mostly tennis-specific exercises and run-based HIIT. I have found these formats highly useful as we can fit almost all tennis drills conducted by coaches into practice sessions that integrate the conditioning goal with tennis-based skill development (42). Examples of such drills are shown in figure 18.4.

A possible training session for an elite tennis player might involve 3 sets of 10 repetitions of 30 s work and 30 s rest, with 2 min rest between sets, alternating between exercises A and B, or 4 sets of 15 repetitions of 15 s work and 15 s rest, with 90 s rest between sets of exercises C and D (see figure 18.4). Normally drills are designed to be performed in several courts, depending on the number of players training at the same time. For example, if we're working with 12 players, three tennis courts can be used, with four players on each court. Players finish the training session in about 40 min.

I usually combine these formats with run-based HIIT, as we can group players in the same facility (normally a 30 m court) based on their V_{IFT}. Thus, we organize running groups and request they run over group-based distances using cones on the court. This can be done easily using the spreadsheet developed by Martin Buchheit (https://martin-buchheit.net/) and available from the author on request. These formats are interesting due to their limited level of neuromuscular fatigue and anaerobic contribution (especially 10 s/20 s, HIIT type 2; chapter 5), which is important when players are conducting a specific training session on the same day (or session), as well as when neuromuscular-based sessions (e.g., strength) the following day are planned (5, 7).

Combinations of HIIT formats are also possible, depending on the number of players involved. For example, a group of players might perform on-court tennis drills, while another group performs sets of run-based HIIT adjacent to those players on the lateral sides of the court.

Repeated-Sprint Training

Since RST might be a time-efficient training method of enhancing aerobic adaptations relative to the lower training volume required with other HIIT formats (25), it may represent a useful training strategy for tennis players, especially during the in-season period, when busy schedules limit the number of training sessions available for fitness development. In this regard, I use the RST format (type 4 target) to implement generally 2 to 4 sets of 5 to 8 sprints across a maximum of a 20 m distance, interspersed with 14 to 25 s of passive or active (jog or sport-specific movements, e.g., side steps, crossover steps, etc.) recovery during the first part of the training session. I choose a maximum 20 m distance because relevant speed in tennis involves the ability to move at high velocity over short distances in different directions around the court (33). Indeed, initial acceleration is the key

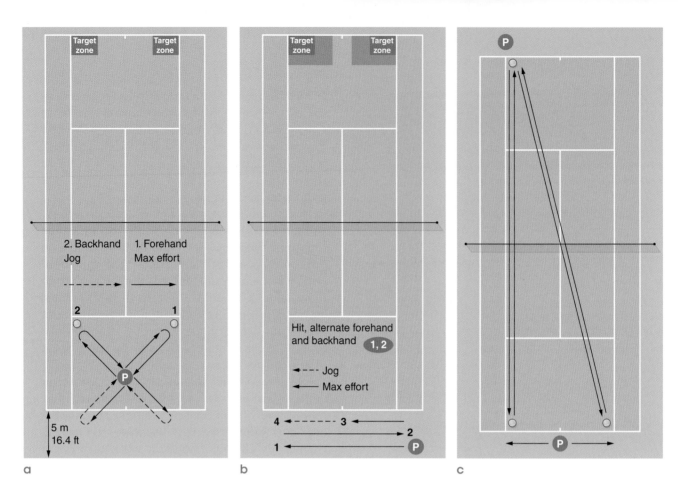

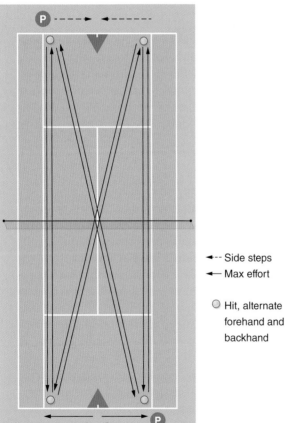

Figure 18.4 Examples of short-HIIT formats (type 3 target) conducted on the tennis court. (a) Big X: diagonal movements inside and outside the court (i.e., maximal efforts and jogging), combined with forehand and backhand strokes). (b) Suicide: movement along the baseline (i.e., maximal efforts and jogging), combined with forehand and backhand strokes). (c) Open pattern: one player remains in a corner, hits alternating (e.g., free) crosscourt strokes, then down the line while the other player must return ball to same corner. (d) Recovery/defensive: two players, both must hit crosscourt strokes, recover past the center mark after each stroke, then hit down-the-line strokes.

Reprinted by permission from J. Fernandez-Fernandez, D. Sanz-Rivas, J.M. Sarabia, and M. Moya, "Preseason Training: The Effects of a 17-Day High-Intensity Shock Microcycle in Elite Tennis Players," *Journal of Sports Science and Medicine* 14 no. 4 (2015): 783-791.

performance component, as most tennis movements occur within a 3 to 4 m radius, and rarely do players reach maximum speed (38). I also introduce short sprints with shuttles during the RST sequences, as from an injury-prevention perspective, these reduce stride length and subsequent hamstring strain risk (3). From my practical experience, a common mistake observed within training programs of tennis players around the world is using sprints greater than 20 m. With these, practitioners are often striving to obtain maximum sprinting speed. Instead, these often increase hamstring strain risk, when in reality, a tennis player rarely gets injured in this region of the body over the course of tennis matches (41).

The large neuromuscular and anaerobic responses of RST must be critically considered within a tennis player's programming puzzle (47). Such sessions should be conducted in isolation to other related content, as RST may affect the quality of subsequent sequences or sessions, as well as increase injury risk. We recently showed in top junior tennis players (16) that a combined RST and plyometrics training program, performed twice a week on top of regular tennis training sessions, led to substantial (ES = 0.56 to 1.12) improvements in sprint (−2%), jump (+2.2%), and repeated sprint performance (−1.4%). Thus, coaches can implement regular training sessions during competitive periods using a combined RST interspersed with at least 45 s of passive recovery. A sample RST program might include 3 or 4 sets of multidirectional short sprints (forward and side-to-side shuttles with one or two changes of direction, 5 or 6 × 15 to 20 m), interspersed with short (25 s) active recovery periods, and plyometric training (3 or 4 sets of 4 to 6 bodyweight exercises, bilateral and unilateral countermovement jumps [CMJ] to a 20 cm box [multidirectional], multilateral hops [hurdles], plyometric jumps [hurdles], step multilateral calf jumps, agility drills [ladders], and resisted standing start sprints [multidirectional]). Figure 18.5 shows some on-court drills I use to integrate as RST sequences conducted before the tennis-specific session.

Sprint Interval Training

Generally the anaerobic glycolytic energy system is likely to be less involved during competitive tennis match play compared to popular belief. Thus, most training drills should be designed accordingly, using short periods of maximal-intensity exercise with adequate rest between efforts to allow athletes to reproduce maximal or near-maximal performance in subsequent bouts. However, and especially at the elite level, increases in circulating [La] levels (up to 10 mmol/L) can occur under actual match play conditions during long and intense rallies, suggesting increased participation of glycolytic processes to energy supply (35, 36). Thus, SIT drills (efforts lasting 30 to 45 s; type 5 target) (23, 43) should be regularly administered to prepare a player to perform high-intensity exercise across these relevant durations. Specific on-court movements (preferably without the racket) are preferred to ensure attainment of the desired (maximal) intensities so that local muscle responses (proxy adaptations) can be fully transferred to actual match play. Due to the high anaerobic contribution and large neuromuscular fatigue associated with SIT, care of programming sessions during the week should follow a similar logic as that discussed for RST.

Game-Based HIIT

Considering that the maintenance of technical skill is a determining factor for success in tennis, and with training time always at a premium, I believe an integrated approach to conditioning and skill-based work is the most efficient training method for elite tennis players. This approach often results in the programming of game-based drills that include both technical (skills) and tactical (playing against an opponent) components as part of sport-specific conditioning (18). To facilitate this, I generally implement game-based HIIT (HIIT type 2, 3, and 4 targets, as detailed in figure 1.5 (5)). While run-based long intervals are generally associated with substantial lactate accumulation (type 3 or 4), the specific modality of tennis-specific HIIT with long intervals that includes a more intermittent neuromuscular activity (short rests between motor actions versus continuous and repeated contractions when running) likely allows for a lower anaerobic energy contribution. For that reason, some tennis-specific HIIT with long intervals can also be considered type 2 responses.

Since exercise intensity for game-based HIIT cannot be controlled precisely using percentage of V_{IFT}, opponent players are normally instructed to perform a variable number of 1 to 2 min drill-based HIIT bouts, depending on their level (e.g., pro players

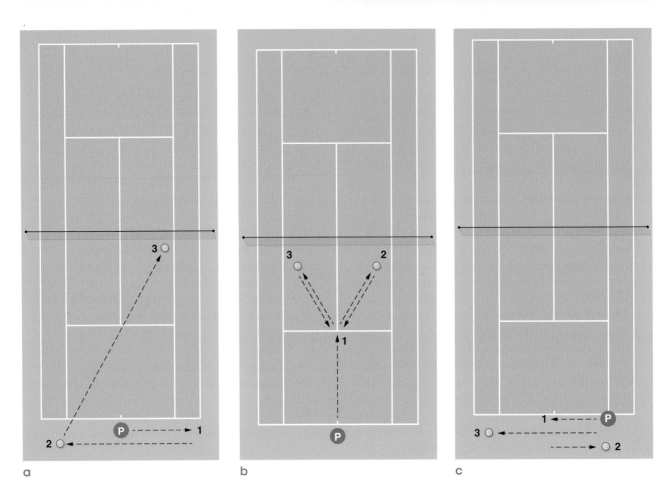

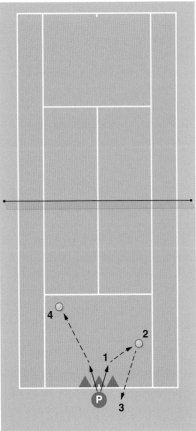

a

b

c

d

Figure 18.5 Examples of a repeated-sprint sequence format (type 4 target), in which players sprint in different directions (see number sequences), return to the center, and perform different strokes. Exercises last around 10 s, with 20 to 25 s rest, and several players can perform the exercise at the same time. P: player; 1-4: sprints.

are able to perform 8) at intensities between 90% and 95% of HR_{max} interspersed with 45 s to 90 s of passive recovery. Intensity and duration of the work bouts and recovery periods employed during these drills are selected based on prior experience, pilot studies, and previously published work (8, 31). Normally speeds are chosen individually using a trial-and-error approach to allow players to sustain the highest possible speed across all work bouts.

To ensure that all players perform at the desired intensity, we currently must rely on both HR monitoring and a player's motivation to ensure he commits to the required (likely maximum) intensity during the drills. For that reason, encouragement and scoring aims during such drills are key factors to apply, especially in professional players. It is also important to take into consideration that these drills are usually conducted with a maximum of three to four players on court, so when the number of players is higher, we need to combine training sessions (i.e., including HIIT short-interval runs at the same time using the lateral sides of the tennis court). Moreover, since players of varying fitness can train together, the relative work of the fitter players can wind up being relatively lower than that of the less fit, as happens in other intermittent sports. Therefore, the inclusion of extra tasks for fitter players can be implemented as follows:

- Before the beginning of the drill, the fittest player performs several short HIIT runs (e.g., 90% to 95% V_{IFT}) or a few short maximum sprints on the lateral side of the court.
- Before the drill commences, the fitter player performs a series of plyometric exercises.

An example of a typical on-court drill used in my training programs is shown in figure 18.6. Here players are required to perform forehand and backhand strokes in different positions for a work period of 1 to 2 min, with an experienced coach feeding balls (e.g., racket feed) outside the court. There are two different roles for both players; one is always playing inside the "defensive box," trying not to make easy mistakes and always playing in a "defensive style," while the other player must "attack" (offensive style), playing outside the defensive box. The coach feeds balls to the players when they make mistakes. Both players are required to move as fast as possible while playing their roles (i.e., defensive or offensive) until

the coach decides to change it up (i.e., normally after 45 s to 1 min). Intensity is monitored via HR monitoring, with targets set at 90% to 95% of HR_{max} (19). The number of balls played is counted as an indicator of work completed during each set. For scoring purposes, target areas can be implemented on the opposite side of the offensive player's court, and scoring points are assigned to each area. Thus, mean scores and percentage decrements for stroke accuracy can also be calculated for the drills. Training volumes rarely exceed a range of 5 to 8 repetitions, as reductions in accuracy are usually observed after the fifth set. Therefore, if the player requires more training volume, we can prescribe tennis-based HIIT with shorter exercises or run-based HIIT, using the V_{IFT} to prescribe intensity. However, in my experience, and also based on published work (17), these volumes appear optimal for obtaining improvements in markers of aerobic performance (e.g., $\dot{V}O_2max$, V_{IFT}) (5).

Longitudinal Training Effects of HIIT

Table 18.1 summarizes several studies recently conducted in nationally and internationally ranked male (junior and adult) tennis players (15-18). Overall, results showed that inclusion of HIIT programs during the preseason or in-season (2 or 3 times per wk, over 3 (shock microcycle) to 8 wk) resulted in small-to-large changes in physiological parameters (i.e., $\dot{V}O_2peak$) and performance-related variables (i.e., hit-and-turn tennis test; V_{IFT}; sprint (5-20 m); CMJ; 5-0-5 agility test). Of course, it is difficult to compare the respective effects of the different interventions due to differences in training duration, baseline performance, and player characteristics. The research examining effects on different HIIT interventions in tennis remains scarce, and further studies comparing HIIT programs in players matched for baseline physical performance are required. Currently, we can presume that supplementing tennis with different HIIT sequences is likely to improve several performance-related parameters, including $\dot{V}O_2max$, V_{IFT}, performance in tennis-specific tests such as the hit-and-turn tennis test, or RSA. However, the relationships between these test-specific improvements and tennis performance (e.g., winning more matches or having a better ranking) is difficult to estimate, as tennis performance is highly complex.

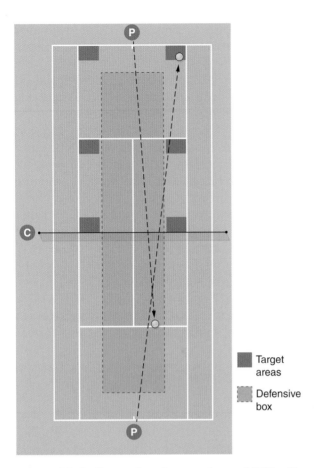

Figure 18.6 Example of game-based HIIT with long intervals (1 to 2 min work, 45 s to 1 min 30 s rest) (type 2 target). P: player; C: coach.

■ Target areas

■ Defensive box

Load Surveillance and Monitoring Tools

Despite the very recent developments of monitoring tools (e.g., GPS, tracking systems), the use of wearables and tracking technologies is still very limited in tennis and is mainly reserved for research purposes (39). In my opinion, there is little relevant research concerning training load monitoring in tennis available that is transferable into the real-life context of the daily training environment. For the last 10 years, and despite their limitations, I have been using HR monitoring in a systematic way, together with the use of session RPE, to calculate the training load associated with tennis training (39). To be more specific with training load effects, I use a local RPE scale for both upper and lower body, the OMNI Scale of perceived exertion for

young players, the total quality recovery (TQR) (6-20 Likert scale), and/or the perceived muscle and joint soreness (1-10 Likert scale) (11, 17) in order to derive more detailed information concerning a player's fatigue state.

Training Status Surveillance and Monitoring Tools

As mentioned, my basic monitoring tools in tennis involve noninvasive and low-cost measurements, including questionnaires (revised Competitive Sport Anxiety Inventory (20)), jumps (neuromuscular status) using apps (e.g., MyJump (1)), and training HR (11). Lately, we've been using a general musculoskeletal assessment protocol every 1 to 2 wk and after several matches or tournaments. This involves static measurements and clinical examinations of joint integrity (e.g., hip and shoulder), ROM tests (e.g., passive assessment), together with tests of muscular strength patterns, also in the shoulders and hips (24, 37). Additionally, we often use the HR and RPE responses to HIIT sequences as markers of adaptations (generally, the lower the better the player's fitness) (6).

Strategies for Structuring the Training Program Using HIIT

In order to structure a training program in tennis, several factors must be taken into account. These include numerous controllable and uncontrollable factors, which obviously affect the progression and periodization of a training program involving HIIT.

Controllable and Uncontrollable Factors

Tennis is a complex sport, and this makes the process of planning, programming, and periodization highly challenging for the practitioner. The main difficulty revolves around a number of uncontrollable factors. The first uncontrollable factor is the player's competitive schedule. It is not only about the number of tournaments that are played each year, or the locations of tournaments, but more the number of matches played in each tournament. Due to the nature of the sport, this is largely unpredictable, making the sport even more complex from a programming standpoint than the team sport situation. More specifically, one of the main problems we have

Table 18.1 Training Interventions Using Various HIIT Formats in Tennis Players

Reference	Participants	Training intervention	Frequency	Results
20	31 nationally ranked male players	HIIT (long intervals; type 2 target) $3 \times (3 \times 90\ s)$ level max* (90% to 95% HR_{max}), 3 min active recovery (70% of HR_{max}) between repetitions, 8 min of an on-court tennis game (i.e., 2:1 game) between sets versus RST (type 4 target) 3×10 to 20 m shuttle sprints, 20 s passive recovery between repetitions, 8 min of an on-court tennis game (i.e., 2:1 game) between sets	3 d/wk for 6 wk	For HIIT, $\dot{V}O_2$peak +4.9% (ES = 0.8), hit-and-turn test +28.9% (ES = 1.6; significantly higher than RST), no changes in RSA test. For RST, $\dot{V}O_2$peak +6% (ES = 0.7), hit-and-turn test +14.5% (ES = 1.2), RSA test mean time −3.8%.
14	16 internationally ranked competitive male junior players	Combined RST (type 5 target) 3 or 4×5 or 6 of 15 to 20 m sprints with 1 or 2 COD, 25 s active recovery plus 1 min 30 s rest with ExpS (3 or 4 sets of 4 to 6 exercises, 12 to 15 repetitions)	2 d/wk for 8 wk	Sprint (20 to 30 m) −2% to 3%, CMJ +2.2%, and RSA −1.4% were significantly improved (ES ranging from 0.56 to 1.12). No changes in V_{IFT}.
17	12 ATP-ranked male tennis players	HIIT (types 2, 3, and 4 target) shock microcycle combining on-court long intervals (7×2 min on/1 min 30 s off; 90% to 95% HR_{max}), short-interval runs (3 or 4×10 to 15 repetitions of 30 s on/30 s off; 15 s on/15 s off; 90% to 95% V_{ITF}), and on-court short and long intervals (30 s on/30 s off; 60 s on/60 s off; 90% to 95% HR_{max})	13 sessions in 17 d	V_{IFT} +6.5% (ES = 1.9), RSA mean −0.5% (ES = 0.4)
18	20 top-50 U15 nationally ranked tennis players	Mixed HIIT (type 3 and 4 targets), short intervals (15 s on/15 s off; 90% to 95% V^{ITF}) and on-court training of short and long intervals (30 s on/30 s off; 60 s on/60 s off; 90% to 95% HR_{max}) versus on-court training only (type 3 and 4 targets), short and long intervals (30 s on/30 s off; 60 s on/60 s off; 90% to 95% HR_{max})	2 d/wk for 8 wk	For mixed HIIT, $\dot{V}O_2$peak +4.2% (ES = 1.05), V_{IFT} +6.3% (ES = 0.9), 5-0-5 test −2.6% (ES = 0.8). For on-court only, $\dot{V}O_2$peak +2.4% (ES = 0,5), V_{IFT} +2.2% (ES = 0.4).

* Levelmax: maximum level reached in the hit-and-turn tennis test (22); RSA: repeated-sprint ability; $\dot{V}O_2$peak: peak oxygen uptake; ES: effect size; COD: change of direction; ExpS: explosive strength; CMJ: countermovement jump; V_{IFT}: velocity of the 30-15 intermittent fitness test; U15: under 15.

in conducting periodized programs in tennis is the lack of consistency in tournament play, as the coach–player team will constantly adjust the tournament schedule depending on results. For example, if a player loses too many first-round matches in a row, the typical reaction is to play more tournaments instead of taking a break and readjusting competition loads, conducting a proper reconditioning program, and so forth.

The most controllable situation in tennis may be the preseason, when the strength and conditioning coach is typically primarily responsible for the training program, together with the coach. However, due to the ever-increasing demands imposed on players, less and less training time tends to be devoted to preparation, with preseasons normally reduced to only 5 to 7 wk. At the highest levels of the game (i.e., ATP/WTA players or even top junior players), this preseason may be reduced further with the increase in exhibition events or team events and tournaments. Regardless, during the preseason, most tennis players prioritize fitness training during the first couple of weeks, while the maintenance of technical and tactical skills is also important. Here, all HIIT types detailed earlier fit well into the training program, alongside clear communication with the coach.

Training content is not only about HIIT weapons. Integrating strength and power training, speed and agility training, neuromuscular (e.g., injury prevention) training, as well as technical and tactical sessions is also needed. Thus, the HIIT sessions should be limited in terms of interfering with subsequent training sessions. Therefore, it is important to take into account the residual neuromuscular fatigue post-HIIT through the use of monitoring tools (see previous sections and chapters 8 and 9) (35).

For me, another uncontrollable factor is the in-season training schedule, as the match schedule will more or less dictate the training program. This creates many possible scenarios to take into account. For example, you can have a player playing qualifying rounds (2 or 3 matches, depending on the tournament), and if successful, he will play in the main draw (a week schedule, with 6 or 7 matches). When the player finishes in the tournament, the time until the next tournament dictates whether or not we have room for HIIT. Nevertheless, I tend to program 1 or 2 HIIT sessions per week when a full week between tournaments arises in the schedule.

Program Structure and Progression

As previously mentioned, and similar to other intermittent sports, very little periodization occurs in elite tennis, except during the preseason (see tables 18.2 and 18.3). The weeks available to conduct a recovery or reconditioning program dictate the periodization level of the design. In doing so, I follow some basic steps to create a tennis conditioning training program.

First, after the number of tournaments to play has been decided, select those tournaments at which the athlete needs to be in peak form and highlight them on the calendar. Players can play tournaments every week, and it is critical to schedule the tournaments appropriately to minimize the chance of injury and potential burnout (10). There are some recommendations for training and competition volume for junior tennis players that suggest that players at the junior stage of development should consider playing less than two tournaments per month, and less than 18 tournaments annually in the U18 category, in order to reduce injury risk (32). From here, I will recommend planned structures for the season (i.e., mesocycles), including specific goals. Thus, I normally suggest that coaches and players have 5 to 7 wk of preseason, and introduce 2 or 3 blocks of training (e.g., mesocycles) of 2 to 3 wk each in order to somewhat "periodize" their training. In-season, when a complete week is available to train, I attempt to keep similar weekly training loads throughout the months and focus on successive tournament preparation-match-recovery cycles. A typical example of an in-season weekly training program is shown in table 18.4.

Table 18.2 Sample Preseason Program (First Week(s) of Preseason, Typically 1 to 2 wk) of an Elite Tennis Player

Microcycle (physical emphasis)		Monday	Tuesday	Wednesday	Thursday	Friday	Saturday	Sunday
Aerobic (VO$_2$) development	AM	Injury prevention	Strength training	Injury prevention	Strength training	Injury prevention	Injury prevention	Rest
		Tennis		Tennis		Tennis	Tennis	
	PM	Type 2 HIIT long (on-court) 5 or 6×2 min at 90% to 95% HR$_{max}$, 1 min 30 s rest	Tennis	Tennis	Tennis	Type 3 HIIT short (on-court) 15 min of short and long intervals (30 s on/30 s off, 60 s on/60 s off, at 90% to 95% HR$_{max}$)	Neuromuscular training (e.g., plyometrics, speed/agility training)	
				Type 3 HIIT short (runs) 2×16×15 s on/15 s off at 90% V$_{IFT}$, 3 min rest			Tennis	

Table 18.3 Sample Preseason Program (Last Week(s) of Preseason, Typically 1 to 2 wk) of an Elite Tennis Player

Microcycle (physical emphasis)		Monday	Tuesday	Wednesday	Thursday	Friday	Saturday	Sunday
Aerobic ($\dot{V}O_2$) development	AM	Injury prevention	Strength training	Injury prevention	Tennis	Injury prevention	Neuromuscular training (e.g., plyometrics, speed/agility training)	Rest
		Tennis		Tennis		Tennis	Tennis	
	PM	Tennis	Neuromuscular training (e.g., plyometrics, speed/agility training)	Type 4 HIIT RST $3 \times$ (5 or 6×15 to 20 m with 2 or 3 shuttles), 25 s rest between repetitions, 4 min rest between sets	Strength training	Type 3 HIIT (on-court) 20 min of short and long intervals (30 s on/30 s off, 60 s on/60 s off, at 90% to 95% HR_{max})	Strength training	
		Type 3 HIIT (runs) $2 \times 22 \times 15$ s on/15 s off at 95% V_{IFT}, 3 min rest	Tennis	Tennis				

Incorporation of HIIT

During the preseason and based on testing results (e.g., 30-15 IFT (4), which I normally conduct over 28 m (30)), I include the long- and short-interval HIIT programs as part of the tennis training. Therefore, conditioning goals are integrated into the tennis practice in order to minimize the possible fatigue effects on subsequent training. If this is not possible, running-based HIIT can be conducted after tennis sessions (table 12.2).

For in-season routines, when a complete week of training is available, the HIIT sessions are incorporated into the tennis training, including more neuromuscular-demanding HIIT such as RST. The main goal of these sequences is to maintain the fitness (cardiorespiratory and neuromuscular) levels.

Sample Training Programs

Tables 18.2 and 18.3 provide examples of HIIT programming during preseason training, while table 18.4 provides an example of in-season programming in tennis.

Table 18.4 Sample Maintenance Schedule (In-season, Remainder of the Season, Through the Competitive Period, When a Full Week Is Available) of an Elite Tennis Player

Microcycle (physical emphasis)		Monday	Tuesday	Wednesday	Thursday	Friday	Saturday	Sunday
Competitive (in season)	AM	Injury prevention	Strength training	Injury prevention	Injury prevention	Injury prevention	Neuromuscular training (e.g., plyometrics, speed/agility training)	Rest
			Tennis		Tennis		Tennis	
	PM	Type 4 HIIT RST 3×5 or 6×15 to 20 m with 2 or 3 shuttles, 25 s rest between repetitions, 4 min rest between sets	Injury prevention and recovery	Neuromuscular training (e.g., plyometrics, speed/agility training)	Type 4 HIIT RST 3×5 or 6×15 to 20 m with 2 or 3 shuttles, 25 s rest between repetitions, 4 min rest between sets or Type 5 5 or 6×25 to 35 s all-out sequences, 5 min rest (low- intensity play)	Tennis	Strength training	
		Tennis		Tennis	Tennis*		Tennis	

* When the HIIT sequence conducted is type 5, the following tennis training session is normally canceled.

I've been privileged to work as a strength-and-conditioning coach, as well as a sports science consultant, for several top-100 ATP/WTA players and their coaches for the last few years. There is an interesting story about how I was able to integrate fitness into the tennis practice through the use of HIIT sequences. A few years ago, I began working with a "skeptical" coach, who for many years, defended his belief that professional tennis players needed to run and accumulate many miles of threshold-based (i.e., 80% HR_{max}) endurance runs. His view was supported by tradition and acceptance in tennis that, "Running is not only important for performance, but also for the head." Like many sports, tennis is filled with many longstanding traditions in the realm of physical training, and it can be difficult for practitioners to change these traditional preparation practices, despite what science or common sense may tell us otherwise. Related to this particular story is an old belief that, "tennis training is just tennis," and for some coaches this means no additional physical exertion during the tennis training. As you might imagine, this particular player encountered many situations in which he was doubling his training load (e.g., on- and off-court). The coach, however, continued to defend his player's need to run and accumulate the traditional endurance-based runs.

My intervention with this particular player was aimed at showing both the coach and the player that training volume could be substantially lowered with a new focus on improving injury prevention. We started by analyzing the short-term variations in the player's cardiorespiratory fitness after 6 wk of tournaments (e.g., average of 3 or 4 matches per week, plus training). The player was not allowed to conduct any endurance sessions during this time, apart from his specific tennis training (which, for the coach, was not an aerobic stimulus). We found that his $\dot{V}O_2max$ levels didn't change much (from 58 to 57 $mL{\cdot}kg^{-1}{\cdot}min^{-1}$). What I did instead was implement integrated HIIT sessions (as explained) into his regular tennis schedule for the next preseason. The player was not allowed to conduct his traditional supplemental aerobic sessions during the 7 wk period of the preseason, which can be psychologically challenging for a player due to the traditional routine he is used to, potentially leading to loss of self-confidence from a perceived fitness level perspective (i.e., "I'm not working enough"). This situation can be a challenge for the strength-and-conditioning coach to field. After 7 wk and about a 30% to 40% reduction in training volume, the player was physically better than ever. $\dot{V}O_2max$ values increased slightly (58.2 to 60.3 $mL{\cdot}kg^{-1}{\cdot}min^{-1}$), V_{IFT} improved from 20 to 21.5 km/h, and he increased HIIT work from about 40 min to more than 50 min. Moreover, the player also increased target accuracy (by about 45%) in the drills I was monitoring.

Unfortunately, the coach remained skeptical, and we ended our collaboration due to our "different visions of tennis training." Nevertheless, I felt that my aims were achieved, with physical fitness and tennis-specific performance improved. The player remained with his coach, although he recognized that his fitness level was better than ever. The player tells me that he continues running for about an hour (70% to 80% HR_{max}) three times per week.

The conclusions we can draw from this story may be that, sometimes, and especially when you're working in a high-performance sport, tradition and beliefs often trump evidence or science-based logic. However, we can continue to fight against these beliefs using our evidence-based work, with change sometimes just requiring more time and a changing of the guard. While admittedly this is difficult and challenging, it is possible to introduce coaches and players into a more-controlled training environment, using for example, monitoring tools (i.e., chapters 8 and 9). Moreover, when you're part of a strong team and the coach and player are on your side, it is possible to plan and control all the physical training loads (and also recovery schedules) in the preparation of the player. Working together and assisting the coach (e.g., using tennis-based HIIT) alongside monitoring the training loads (e.g., HR, RPE) is key.

Adam Pretty/Getty Images

19

Triathlon

• • • • • •

Daniel Plews and Paul Laursen

Performance Demands of Triathlon

This chapter describes the sport of professional triathlon, discussing the various factors of importance for success in the event, and how high-intensity interval training (HIIT) contributes to physical development in its three individual disciplines of swimming, cycling, and running.

Sport Description and Factors of Winning

Triathlon is considered by some to have its beginnings in the 1920s in France, in an annual sport called "Les trois sports." However, the first modern-day triathlon occurred at Mission Bay, San Diego, California, on September 25, 1974, and has witnessed exponential growth to the present day, where about 2.5 million competitors now compete annually in the sport of triathlon in the United States alone. The sport of triathlon is an endurance race that involves successive swimming, cycling, and running (including transition time from one event to the next), and while it can be made up of a range of competition types, distances, and durations, the majority of races are broadly categorized into four distinct race distances, termed sprint, Olympic, half-Ironman, and Ironman triathlons (table 19.1).

The varying event distances in triathlon create specific technical, physiological, and nutritional considerations for athlete and practitioner alike. A range of factors, including terrain, environmental conditions, tactics, and strategy, influence the successful outcomes in these events. However, the primary predictor of performance in any triathlon event comes down to the physical capacities of the individual triathlete. These physiological attributes that determine success in the triathlon are similar to those in each individual sport of swimming (chapter 17), cycling (chapter 15), and running (chapter 14), and include those related to mode-specific qualities of aerobic power ($\dot{V}O_2max$), economy, and fatigue resistance.

Due to the large variation in not only race distances (table 19.1) but also environment and topography,

Table 19.1   Primary Triathlon Distances for Swimming, Cycling, and Running

Event	Swim (m)	Bike (km)	Run (km)
Sprint	750	20	5
Olympic	1500	40	10
Half-Ironman	1900	90	21.1
Ironman	3800	180	42.2

there are equally subtle differences in the physiology type that can be competitive in triathlon. An example of this might be to contrast a winning sprint distance triathlete with a winning Ironman triathlete. The former athlete would be seen as generally younger, with a high $\dot{V}O_2max$, while the latter triathlete tends to be older, more experienced, and with higher levels of exercise economy and aerobic threshold levels (chapters 3 and 4). Rarely do we see athletes excelling in both distances in the spectrum at the same time of their life (i.e., winning both a sprint and Ironman triathlon in the same year). Often however we witness younger winners of sprint distance triathlons evolve to becoming successful at the Ironman distance as they age, such as 2008 Beijing Olympic champion and 2015 and 2016 Ironman champion, Jan Frodeno.

Additionally, triathlon is not without its skill requirements. Open-water swimming, although similar to pool-based swimming's physical and technical requirements (see chapter 17, swimming), has its own set of unique requirements and challenges, including a marginally adjusted technique for open-water swimming, completed often with a wetsuit versus not (depending on temperature cut-off regulations), involving the navigation and battles among other competitors, including routing around the open course taking water current and conditions into account. Cycling varies considerably in its tactics due to different rule formats generally for sprint and Olympic-based events versus half-Ironman and Ironman distance races, the former two being draft-legal at the International Triathlon Union (ITU; sprint and Olympic triathlon governing body) level, while the latter two typically are not. The draft-legal ITU formats ultimately require a similar skill and tactic base as those in road cycling, while the latter involves the aerodynamics component of the indi-

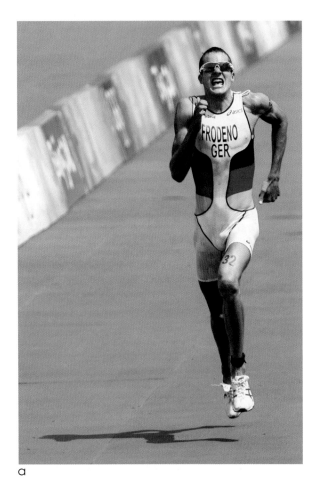

a

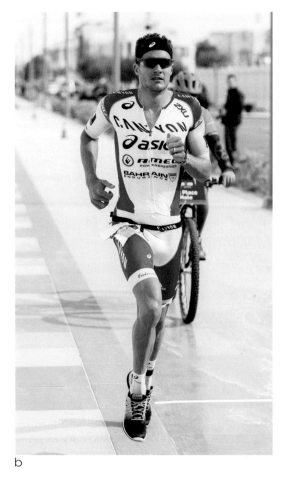

b

(a) A younger 2008 Olympic Triathlon Champion Jan Frodeno of Germany and (b) the more mature 2015 and 2016 Ironman World Champion Jan Frodeno (right).

a. Adam Pretty/Getty Images; b. Warren Little/Getty Images for Ironman.

vidual time trial (see chapter 15, road cycling). Running can also be considered a technical sport (see related chapters), and the preceding swimming and cycling phases create unique demands on a triathlete's ability to run, affecting economy, kinematics (running form), and ultimately run performance (6-8, 12, 17). Finally, the clock does not stop between individual swim, bike, and run events, so triathletes must additionally be skilled at transitioning from one event to the next (8). While sport science has to date not been able to capture the impact of transitioning on overall performance, it stands to reason that, like with F1 car racing, the transition speed and smoothness could be impactful to overall performance, when you consider that finishing time at the end of a triathlon can be separated by less than a second.

While these aspects of the sport clearly require skill, practice, and experience, compared with sports such as tennis or basketball, the requirement for skill is comparatively low, making triathlon a sport primarily about the athlete's physiology. Therefore, the successful triathlon coach is one who understands the components that maximize triathlon physiology in the individual sports of swimming, cycling,

and running, while appropriately being able to blend training for the three sports (i.e., merging swimming, cycling, and running training, allowing suitable recovery). As shown in the swimming, cycling, and running chapters, HIIT is a key component for triathletes and is used at certain times to prepare for racing in each individual discipline.

Physical Performance Contributions to Winning

Contrasting many other physical capacity–based sports completed in shorter durations of less than 10 min (rowing, athletics, swimming, running), like road cycling, triathlons are competed over much longer durations (table 19.1). Consequently, prolonged endurance capacity is a key performance indicator (figure 19.1).

As mentioned, subtle differences do exist between the ITU (sprint and Olympic) versus Ironman-type events from the bike phase standpoint, where drafting in sprint and Olympic distance events creates more variation in degree of high-intensity outputs and race tactics. While certain tactics undoubtedly occur in half-Ironman and Ironman events (i.e., getting

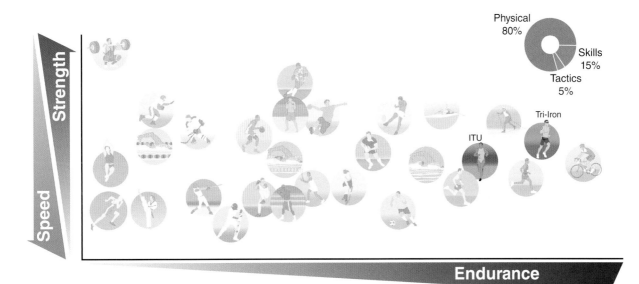

Figure 19.1 The position of the triathlete (International Triathlon Union; ITU and Iron-distance) on the three axes illustrates the relative importance of the three main physical capacities of importance for elite participation, acknowledging this varies slightly between triathlon race and across exercise modes. Outside of critical psychological aspects, which are difficult to quantify, the pie chart shows the general relative importance of skills (15%), tactical awareness (5%), and physical capacities (80%) for triathlon success.

Adapted from G.A. Nader, "Concurrent Strength and Endurance Training: From Molecules to Man," *Medicine & Science in Sports & Exercise* 38, no. 11 (2006): 1965-1970.

away on the bike), winning in these more prolonged races (3.5 to 8 h) arises more from well-paced sustained efforts (1). In contrast, winners in sprint (<1 h) and Olympic distance (<2 h) races often emerge from groups that form during the swim phase, and possibly extend their leads during the bike phase. Sometimes those who get in front during the swim phase are also highly motivated to push hard early during the bike phase to extend their leads over those who emerge later from the swim phase and may be less motivated to bridge the gap. Additionally, triathletes who have paced more appropriately from other groups can, more often than not, be seen coming from behind to catch runners who have expended substantial energy in their preceding swim and (mostly) cycling phases. Nevertheless, in these latter shorter events, the combined effect of drafting and tactics amid constantly changing terrain and course dynamics, alongside the variable energetic demands, results in critical periods of a race often dictating success (8). This implies that in the former short ITU formats, it is not always the athlete with the highest physical capacities who wins, with tactics and race execution also important.

Targets of Physical Performance in Triathlon

Undeniably, physical capacities specific to the triathlon event are important. The physiological factors of $\dot{V}O_2$max and speed/power associated with first (VT$_1$) and second threshold (VT$_2$), introduced in chapter 3 and expanded on in chapter 4, play important roles to varying extents that are specific to the event distance. While these will vary, the general contribution of these parameters to race success is shown in figure 19.2. While not exclusive and highly individual, the general trends observed with sprint and Olympic distance triathletes are high levels of speed and power associated with $\dot{V}O_2$max and VT$_2$ (8), while the older, more experienced long-distance triathletes tend to have higher speeds and power associated with VT$_1$ (11, 18).

In summary, to be competitive in triathlon, a triathlete requires physical characteristics that are specific to the race distance format, with varying degrees of speed/power associated with $\dot{V}O_2$max and VT$_1$ and VT$_2$ (8, 19). While athlete age and genetic traits are large determinants of these physiological factors, they are developed and maximized with training (22), and especially in the case of the long-

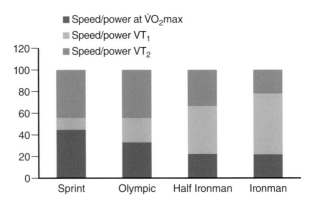

Figure 19.2 General physiological contributions to triathlon race success, including $\dot{V}O_2$max, first and second ventilatory thresholds (VT$_1$, VT$_2$) for triathletes relative to the targeted event distance (table 19.1).

distance triathlete, integrated nutrient timing (33). Running is a critical component of the triathlon (8), and the neuromuscular characteristics needed to run fast and/or prolonged under fatigue are of key importance (8). HIIT is a key tool that can be used to target these specific characteristics.

Sprint

The sprint distance triathlon, performed at maximal intensity over about 45 min for males, and 55 min for females, requires a high-aerobic capacity in swimming, cycling, and running. As the top end of the intensity spectrum ($\dot{V}O_2$max and VT$_2$; figure 19.2) are of likely key importance for this event (6), training that maximizes these capacities must be emphasized. As mentioned, successful sprint distance triathletes at the elite ITU level tend to be younger (18-30 yr), with very high sustainable capacities for short-duration swimming, cycling, and running.

Olympic

The Olympic distance triathlon, named for the format that first debuted at the Sydney 2000 Olympics, requires similar physiological characteristics as the sprint distance event (figure 19.2), and many athletes in the ITU often compete intermittently in both throughout a triathlon season. The double duration of the sprint event means that a greater emphasis is demanded on fatigue resistance and sustainable intensity. Due to the experience and time required to develop these properties, successful Olympic distance triathletes tend to be of a higher age (22-35 yr), although outliers are seen in both directions (21).

Half-Ironman

The half-Ironman distance event, from a physiological perspective considered to be ultra-endurance (16), requiring greater reliance on fat oxidation rates, carbohydrate sparing, and sustained endurance (figure 19.2), is completed in under 4 h for males and under 4.5 h for females. As with the former ITU events, specialists in half-Ironman tend to race both half-Ironman and Ironman distances, as they share similar characteristics. The half-Ironman event tends to be the first longer-distance event that an athlete graduating from ITU racing will attempt as he ages (general range of elite 27-38 years of age) and moves toward more prolonged racing. Thus, ITU athletes, with their high $\dot{V}O_2$max and VT_2 or critical power (CP) levels (chapter 4), are often immediately successful in the half-Ironman distance events (8). Present-day examples of half-Ironman winners include Olympians Alistair Brownlee (GBR) and Francisco Javier Gómez Noya (ESP).

Ironman

The Ironman event was born on February 18, 1978, off the beach of Waikiki, in Honolulu, Hawaii, when, to settle a bar bet, 15 competitors began a race to determine whether the fittest athlete was a long-distance swimmer, cyclist, or runner. The event combined three established single events in Hawaii, where the winner of all three in succession would be crowned the Ironman. It is a very long ultra-endurance event that is completed in around 8 h for top males and around 9 h for professional females. Like its half-distance counterpart, physiological attributes that enable Ironman success include high fat oxidation rates, $\dot{V}O_2$max, and sustained endurance (11). These latter characteristics are reflected in high-aerobic threshold (VT_1) levels (19) (figure 19.2), and winners tend to be older and more-experienced triathletes (age range = 30-40).

Physical attributes of successful triathletes are dominated by aerobic capacities and thresholds described before (figure 19.2), as well as neuromuscular characteristics, specifically in running. Thus, HIIT sessions for triathletes are often used to develop aerobic metabolic and neuromuscular properties.

Key Weapons, Manipulations, and Surveillance Tools

For professional triathletes, most of their training hours (12-35 h/wk) are spent accumulating large volumes of training at low exercise intensities (50%-80% of HRmax; 40%-70% $\dot{V}O_2$max) (22). This relatively unstructured part of the training is important as it develops the aerobic foundation needed to support the development of $\dot{V}O_2$max, economy, and thresholds, including high levels of fat oxidation rates (15, 16). As well as the large amounts of time training at low intensities, like cyclists (chapter 15), triathletes also complete specific pace work at medium, or mid-zone, intensities. These pieces, often performed within the middle of longer training sessions, are completed over a large range of durations that can range from 15 to 200 min at intensities of 80% to 90% HRmax or 70% to 80% $\dot{V}O_2$max, depending on the athlete's age and experience and target event.

As with other endurance sports, while HIIT contributes considerably less time to a triathlete's training program, it is no less important. Work completed during HIIT is often either specific to race intensity or building on areas around race intensity (i.e., CP) to develop these components further. HIIT is vital for developing the adaptations of the oxidative (and nonoxidative) as well as the neuromuscular/musculoskeletal properties to enable fatigue resistance over prolonged durations (chapters 3, 4, and 5). The key weapons, or HIIT formats, including their manipulations and surveillance (monitoring) tools, will be described.

HIIT Weapons, Targets, and Manipulations

The most common HIIT weapons included in triathlon training programs, and specifically in swimming, cycling, and running, are primarily long intervals, short intervals, and sprint interval training, aiming for type 1 through 5 targets, with a metabolic emphasis, depending on the mode, individual triathlete characteristics, and stage of the program. Repeated sprint training, which incorporates very short duration efforts (3-7 s), is used occasionally in swimming across all athlete groups, and sometimes in biking and running by sprint distance triathletes. The breakdown of these formats is shown in figure 19.3.

Long Intervals

Long HIIT intervals usually take the form of 1 to 8 min work durations at intensities of 85% to 95% of HRmax, 85% to 100% of p/v$\dot{V}O_2$max, generally with recovery intervals that range from 1 to 3 min

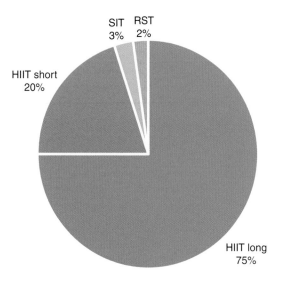

Figure 19.3 Percentage of the different HIIT formats (weapons) used throughout the annual season in professional triathlon.

(table 19.2). Total accumulated duration at these intensities during such interval sets is typically 12 to 30 min split between 1 and 5 sets. A specific long HIIT interval session (type 3 and 4 targets) for swimming might be 4×400 m in 5 min leaving on 7 min, 5×3.5 maximal maintainable power with 3 min passive (or extremely low intensity, <50 W) recovery for cycling, and 6×1000 m maximal maintainable run speed (~3 min) with 200 m recovery (passive or easy walk/jog) for running. Other good examples of long intervals specific for elite triathletes (modified appropriately) can be seen in the swimming (chapter 17), cycling (chapter 15), and running (chapter 14) chapters.

Short Intervals

Short HIIT intervals for triathletes usually take the form of 20 to 60 s work durations at intensities of 100% to 140% of v/p$\dot{V}O_2$max, generally with work:rest ratios between 1:0.5 and 1:1. Total accumulated work duration for these interval sets is between 10 and 20 min, split between 1 and 5 sets (table 19.3). An example of a short HIIT session (type 3 and 4 targets) for a triathlete would be 15×75 m completed at between 47 and 50 s per 75 m, leaving on 90 s (with a critical swim speed, CSS, of 1:13 per 100 m) for swimming, 2×(10×1 min at 110% of p$\dot{V}O_2$max with 30 s recovery), 5 min RI for cycling, and 8 to 15×200 m on 32-34 s, 100 jog leaving on 60 s for running. Short intervals tend to be more emphasized for sprint and Olympic distance athletes over long-distance triathletes.

Sprint Interval Training

SIT is used infrequently by triathletes, but can be used in certain circumstances, and particularly when a triathlete possesses low absolute speed or power in any of the three individual disciplines. SIT is composed of maximal efforts between 10 and 30 s, with recovery periods of 2 to 10 min (table 19.4). As the goal of these intervals is to reach maximal values, the number of sprints is typically low (1-5), and time between sets relatively long (>30 min). For the start of sprint and Olympic distance triathlons, all-out swim speed is critical for reaching the first 300 m marker buoy before a bottleneck that consistently occurs after about the first 10 swimmers. Thus, SIT is mostly used in swim training (type 5 target).

Manipulations of Interval Training Variables

As with the track-and-field approach to HIIT session prescription (chapter 2), competition demands pertinent to sprint, Olympic, and long-distance triathlons are often used to develop specific swim, bike, and run HIIT sessions. Thus, nearly all of the 12 HIIT vari-

Table 19.2   HIIT Long-Interval Parameter Ranges for a Triathlete's Swim, Bike, and Run Training

Mode	Work intensity	Work duration	Rest intensity	Rest duration	Rep number	Series	Between series recovery	Targets
Swim	102%-105% of CSS	200 m (~2:20-2:30)	0%-30% of CSS	90 s	4	2	100 m (2 min passive 30% CSS)	Type 4
Bike	95%-100% p$\dot{V}O_2$max	4 min	0%-30% p$\dot{V}O_2$max	3 min	5	0	Passive—40% p$\dot{V}O_2$max	Type 4
Run	95%-100% v$\dot{V}O_2$max	1000 m (3-3.5 min)	0%-30% v$\dot{V}O_2$max	200 m (90-120 s)	6	0	Passive—40% v$\dot{V}O_2$max	Type 4

CSS: critical swim speed; p$\dot{V}O_2$max: power associated with $\dot{V}O_2$max; v$\dot{V}O_2$max: velocity associated with $\dot{V}O_2$max

Table 19.3 HIIT Short Interval Parameter Ranges for a Triathlete's Swim, Bike, and Run Training

Mode	Work intensity	Work duration	Rest intensity	Rest duration	Rep number	Series	Between series recovery	Targets
Swim	108%-110% CSS	100 m (or 60-80 s)	0-30% of CSS	60 s	5	2	100 m (2 min passive 30% CSS)	Type 4
Bike	105-p$\dot{V}O_2$max	30 s	0%-30% p$\dot{V}O_2$max	30 s	10	3	5 min 40% p$\dot{V}O_2$max	Type 4
Run	103% v$\dot{V}O_2$max	30 s (or 200 m)	0%-30% v$\dot{V}O_2$max	30 s (or 100 m walk/jog)	10	2	5 min 40% v$\dot{V}O_2$max	Type 4

CSS: critical swim speed; p$\dot{V}O_2$max: power associated with $\dot{V}O_2$max; v$\dot{V}O_2$max: velocity associated with $\dot{V}O_2$max

Table 19.4 HIIT Sprint Interval Parameter Ranges for a Triathlete's Swim, Bike, and Run Training

Mode	Work intensity	Work duration	Rest intensity	Rest duration	Rep number	Series	Targets
Swim	All-out, around 114% of CSS	50 m (30-50 s)	passive	100 m or 2 min of passive recovery	6	0	Type 5 target
Bike*	All-out	15 s	passive	4 min	8	1	Type 5 target
Run*	All-out	20 s	passive	2 min	4	2	Type 5 target

* Infrequently used except potentially in particular instances of low absolute capacity (power or speed).
CSS: critical swim speed

ables (chapter 4) can be manipulated to tailor the acute physiological response (proxy adaptation).

The sprint and Olympic distance events in triathlon share some of the same issues as those outlined in the road cycling chapter (chapter 15). These shorter draft-legal formats add considerable variation to race demands, which can become unpredictable based on the dynamics and tactics of the race, and are affected by countless factors, including the outcome of the swim phase, the associated formation of varying numbers of groups, "attacks" or surges in pace to get away during the bike phase, the topography, turn number and turn type on criterium-style bike courses, as well as the effects of environment, including temperature, humidity, prevailing wind, and altitude. This array of factors, adding complexity to race outcomes, is somewhat less definitive in long-distance triathlon racing, although it can be still present to a degree. However, large surges in energy output, especially early on in a long-distance race, are often detrimental to overall performance outcomes, as the ability to sustain a high overall metabolic rate and movement speed throughout the event is reduced.

Notwithstanding these factors, the associated physiological parameters—CP, CSS, maximal lactate steady state (MLSS), functional threshold power/speed (FTP/S) (2), and ventilatory thresholds—are used to guide HIIT prescription. As with cycling, portable power meters are utilized to help guide and monitor cycling sessions, while run training sessions are often monitored using treadmill foot pods, outdoor global positioning system (GPS) or measured distances on a track, and follow the track-and-field approach to training prescription. Swimming sessions would be similar to those described in chapter 17 and are completed predominantly using measured times over set distances in the pool to determine a marker of swim specific critical power (chapter 4). These velocities can then be used to determine a CSS estimate (30), with intervals (i.e., time per 100 m) manipulated with these speeds in mind. A simple-to-use CSS estimate can be obtained from 200 and 400 m times using the following calculator (www.swimsmooth.com/training .html). The advantage to the aforementioned approaches (CSS and FTP/S) for triathletes is that strengths and weaknesses, typically evident in race performance, can be manipulated within the individual mode (swim, bike, or run) to "close gaps" to required performance standards.

As outlined in chapter 4, the most defining factors to any HIIT weapon are the intensity and duration of the work and rest periods. Generally speaking, these should be in alignment with the demands of the event (table 19.1) and the identified performance gap of the individual triathlete (figure 1.5), so that the acute response of an HIIT session partially mimics the physiological demands that will be encountered in the specific event, and adaptation occurs appropriately. To take the two extreme ends of the triathlon distance continuum as an example, and speaking generally only, shorter duration and higher intensity bike and run intervals would be more frequently used for a sprint distance athlete, while more prolonged lower intensity efforts (very long and toward mid-zone) are applied with successful Ironman athletes (8, 15). Swim training programs tend to be similar across all triathlete distance focus groups.

Additionally, the number of intervals in a series, the series duration and time between each series of HIIT, will again depend on the specific competition demands (table 19.1) and the physiological/metabolic systems being targeted by the coach. As with cyclists (chapter 15) and runners (chapter 14), the use of terrain or hills, as well as cadence in the case of bike training, can be adjusted to engage certain metabolic and neuromuscular responses (23). The impact of cadence manipulation was described in the cycling chapter (chapter 15), while the use of hill training, sometimes referred to as functional resistance training (5), is described in road running (chapter 14). The neuromuscular demands of HIIT during swim training can be manipulated using tools that include paddles, bands, fins, and snorkels (chapter 17) (28).

Finally, as training sessions tend to be relatively long in duration for the triathlete, the decision of where to implement the HIIT session can also be important (start, middle, end, or various). A triathlete lacking in absolute speed or power may benefit by completing the HIIT session at the beginning of the session, while an athlete looking to improve fatigue resistance may benefit more by having the HIIT session toward the end of training. Typically, however, the placement of HIIT across a long-duration session tends to be random, relating more to the availability of suitable terrain (hills, flat section) or perception, feel, or motivation of the day.

Surveillance and Monitoring Tools

The main surveillance and monitoring tools in professional triathlon across all codes/events include primarily GPS-integrated wristwatches that capture aspects of external and internal training load (chapter 8). These devices combine running distance, time, pace, elevation change, and heart rate; power meters that record cycling power output, cadence, elevation change, and heart rate; and swim training data that includes lap distance, lap speed, and lap pace (and optional heart rate). These integrated wristwatch systems can stream data via Bluetooth and Wi-Fi seamlessly into associated analysis software systems (chapter 8). These tools can be used extensively for many applications that advise the coach and practitioner on a triathlete's discipline-specific and overall training load and training status.

External and Internal Training Load

Conveniently, the external training load for the triathlon disciplines of swimming, cycling, and running can be both prescribed and monitored using the aforementioned tools at hand. This prescription of course will vary based on the specific event discipline being trained for and the purpose of the session (i.e., aerobic development versus HIIT). For run and bike training, prolonged submaximal periods are typically prescribed using a combination of the RPE and heart rate method (i.e., run/ride at an easy/steady pace <130 bpm or VT_1HR for 2 h), while low-intensity swim training is prescribed using pace or RPE (i.e., 500 m warm-up easy choice). The high-intensity and relatively short-duration HIIT intervals and the associated lag in HR response (see chapters 3, 8, and 9) prevent the use of HR for prescribing HIIT in any of the event disciplines. A more suitable approach is to use pace for running, using a measured track, foot pod/treadmill, or GPS-based device. Caution must be used when using such equipment, as GPS data can in our experience be variable due to a variety of environmental limitations, including cloud cover, terrain, industrialization, etc. (see chapter 8). As with road cycling (chapter 15), power output is easily measured (and viewed in real time by the athlete if desired) using power meters, with data seamlessly recorded (ANT+ or Bluetooth) and uploaded (Wi-Fi) to various software systems for immediate coach observation and analysis. Swim training mostly uses techniques described in chapter 17 where lap times are recorded across

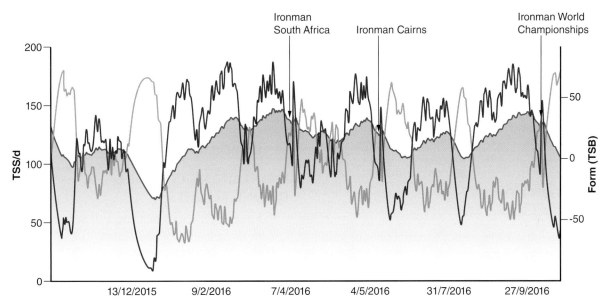

Figure 19.4 Training load monitored across one full season in an elite Ironman triathlete using the Training Stress Score available at TrainingPeaks.com. Blue shading represents the chronic training load (CTL; proxy fitness), the red line represents the acute training load (ATL; proxy training stress), while the orange line represents the training stress balance (TSB; proxy fatigue). As taught initially by Banister (4), this fitness minus fatigue equals form. Each peak in accumulated fitness (CTL) in this athlete represents the accumulation of training before a major event, finishing with the World Championships in Kona, Hawaii, in October.

known distances (either 25 m or 50 m pools). However, watch devices like Garmin are now able to record distance swum, pace, and stroke rate to give a general indication on swim training load to coaches when athletes are remote. For each of these triathlon disciplines, the training load can be estimated using various software systems that use Banister's classic fitness-fatigue modeling or training impulse (TRIMP) calculation scores in each respective discipline (3, 4, 21). Figure 19.4 shows the season-long training-load calculations for an elite Ironman triathlete.

As with other endurance-based sports, triathlon is rampant with the belief that more training is always better. Indeed, triathlon training volume, in terms of hours spent training each week, can range from as low as roughly 10 h in a starting junior sprint distance triathlete, up to reports of 40+ h in some Ironman distance triathletes. As a result, the risk of developing overtraining is high (chapter 7). The degree of training polarization, that is, the accumulation of time in an HR band associated with low intensity ($<VT_1$), mid-zone intensity (VT_1-VT_2), and high intensity ($>VT_2$) work can also give insight and raise alarm bells with respect to the appropriateness of the response to the training (see following). In our experience, we generally observe high degrees of training polarization (assessed by HR) with the accumulation of large amounts of time (>85%) below VT_1, ~10% in the mid-zone range, and <5% at high intensity.

Response to Training Load

As described in chapter 9, the body's response to the training load should also be monitored routinely to ensure the triathlete is progressing appropriately. Methods of response to training load can involve written training diary comments (13), direct face-to-face interaction (including phone/Internet conversations) with the triathlete discussing aspects of how training is feeling (feeling fast in the water, strong on the bike, light on the run as some examples), how he is sleeping, and his level of soreness. As described in chapter 9, morning resting heart rate variability (HRV; chapter 9) (24, 25) can also be used as a global assessment of the athlete's central nervous system response to training-induced stress, when assessed longitudinally against a history of morning measurements (25). A number of valid and reliable apps are now available for coaches to monitor this variable easily across groups of athletes (26).

Strategies for Structuring the Training Program Using HIIT

Implementing an HIIT program within the sport of triathlon is manageable, so long as races are scheduled to permit appropriate recovery between events. Nevertheless, there are a number of uncontrollable factors that must be managed to ensure appropriate effectiveness of the HIIT session.

Controllable and Uncontrollable Factors

Professional triathletes typically compete in 10 to 25 races each year. Such races are spread throughout the year and can depend on the personal location or home of the athlete. With key events (i.e., World Championships and Olympic Games) typically held in September or October each year, the majority of major event racing throughout the world typically is witnessed between the months of January and October.

Unlike a number of other sports (i.e., cycling, soccer, basketball, ice hockey), where competition frequency is high, the lower frequency of competition (if appropriately planned) enables sufficient recovery to enable the planned scheduling of HIIT. Smaller-level competitions are, however, used as a training stimulus leading into major events, to gain experience in more technical areas such as starts, pacing, tactics, transitions, and the competition environment experience.

Travel demands add another challenge to the training program that triathletes need to consider. Races are performed all over the world, including training camps in hot climates or at altitude (chapter 4), occasionally in difficult-to-reach places, including third-world countries that possess risk for infection from food and water sources that the triathlete may be unaccustomed to. Thus, proper planning for the location, along with recovery for and from travel (i.e., rest periods including before and after) as well as time for circadian adaptation to the time zone need to be considered (27). Here are additional strategies athletes should consider to lower the risk of illness, maintain comfort, and reduce symptoms of jet lag during long-haul travel to remote locations.

PREVENTING ILLNESS

- Avoid shaking hands or putting the hands to the eyes and nose.
- Wash hands with soap and water or an alcohol-based sanitizer (if soap and water are unavailable) before eating and after using the toilet.
- Wear a humidifying mask during flights.
- Drink plenty of fluids but avoid caffeine and alcohol.
- Be cautious of food on flights and in new destinations. Plan meals ahead, if possible.

MAINTAINING COMFORT DURING FLIGHTS

- For early flights when you will be more awake, book an aisle seat in advance so you can move around more frequently.
- For later flights during which you plan to sleep, book a window seat in advance.
- Wear compression socks and comfortable footwear during flights.
- Take regular short walks in the aisle and perform gentle stretches when possible to promote circulation.

REDUCING JET LAG BEFORE THE FLIGHT

- Be well rested before departure.
- Avoid HIIT 24 h before flying.
- Plan on-board and stop-over nutrition.
- Carry a drink bottle.

REDUCING JET LAG DURING THE FLIGHT

- Adjust to the new time zone immediately after takeoff, but still sleep when appropriate.
- If arriving early in the day, try to sleep during the second part of the flight. If arriving in the evening, sleep during the first part of the flight.
- During stopovers, sleep, walk, stretch, and shower, if time and space allow.

REDUCING JET LAG POST FLIGHT

- Perform easy aerobic training.
- Fall into your normal routine immediately, especially sleep, waking, meal patterns, and training times.
- Consume caffeine in the mornings only.
- Consider taking melatonin pills in the evening when traveling east.

Program Structure and Progression

There are a number of different approaches to triathlon training planning and preparation, and all have been used successfully at one time or another. These include classic periodization models, block periodization models, and numerous other formats (14).

The competition program for a triathlete is to some degree determined in accordance with her particular abilities/capacities and stage of development. As such, the triathlete's training program should work alongside the competition program, meaning that the training programs of triathletes are highly unique and specific to each individual athlete. Figure 19.4 shows how the training load and fitness gains in an elite Ironman triathlete fluctuate throughout the year based on the competition program, where each gain in predicted fitness corresponds with a major competition, finishing with the World Championship event at season's end. While each triathlete's program will be unique, some general observations can be made across the macro-, meso-, and microcycles.

Macrocycle

A triathlete's seasons are typically periodized around a small number of key racing objectives, requiring 2 to 8 periods of maximal performance. In ITU racing, for example, a top-level sprint or Olympic distance triathlete would typically aim to perform in 5 to 8 of the (current) nine World Triathlon Series events on offer throughout the year in order to compete in the World Series points system (cash/prize purse for most number of points in a season). In the World Triathlon Corporation (WTC), a brand that controls the majority of long-distance events, triathletes focusing on the Ironman World Championship in Kona may compete in from 2 to 5 Ironman races as well as a number of smaller-distance 70.3 events, and appropriately place emphasis on building toward those key performances, also in order to achieve entry in, and perform well in, the World Championship event (see figure 19.4). As mentioned, there are any other number of combinations of program structure that can be used that are formed appropriately to the individual athlete's goals and needs.

Mesocycle

Typical mesocycles for triathletes tend to range around 3 to 4 wk duration, with 2 to 3 loading weeks and 1 recovery wk. However, a mesocycle could be as short as 10 d or as long as 12 wk, depending on the phase of the program and the length of time between the targeted events.

Microcycle

As with most athletes, a triathlete's microcycles tend to be weekly (7 d), although they can range from as short as 4 to as long as 10 days.

Periodized Nutrition

As outlined in chapters 4 and 7, periodized nutrition can play an important role in the life of many triathletes. Nutrition philosophies and practice range considerably across a wide spectrum, from chronic diets of very high carbohydrate (low fat) (10) to very low carbohydrate (high fat) (29), and every other combination in between. As outlined in chapter 4 (nutrition), triathletes often incorporate the practice of sleeping (20) and training low (9). For athletes using the ketogenic or low-carbohydrate high-fat (LCHF) diets to enhance power and speed at VT_1, some feel that the use of HIIT is vital to allow for the appropriate metabolic machinery to be maintained and stimulated (32). Interestingly, Webster et al. (31) recently showed a 2.8% enhanced 20 km cycling time trial performance in a 2 yr LCHF-adapted elite triathlete who supplemented 8 HIIT sessions over 3 wk with 60 g/h of carbohydrate during his HIIT sessions. Indeed, the use of carbohydrate supplementation for HIIT is, in our experience, a common practice for many elite fat-adapted triathletes.

Sample Training Programs

Tables 19.5 and 19.6 offer examples of an overall year training program, an example of a preparation phase and an example of a competition phase.

Acknowledgments

For any developing coach or scientist, it's foolish to fall into the type 2 trap (chapter 10) and think we know it all. We have tried our best not to, and are grateful to have been able to learn alongside some of the best coaches in the game, including Gordon Walker, Jon Brown, Pete Pfitzinger, Greg Fraine, and the late Laurent Vidal. Thank you, gents, for sharing your knowledge.

Table 19.5 Typical Training Week of an Olympic Distance Professional Triathlete During the Preparation Period: Hard and Easy Weeks

	Hard training week	Easy training week
Monday	a.m. 1: RUN 80 min LIT a.m.2: S&C p.m. 1: SWIM 3.5 k including HIIT 8×200 m, with 100 m passive recovery (type 3) p.m.2: BIKE 2 h LIT	a.m.1: RUN 50 min LIT a.m.2: S&C p.m.1: SWIM 3.5 k including HIIT (type 1) p.m.2: BIKE 1.5 h LIT
Tuesday	a.m.1: SWIM 3 k LIT a.m.2: RUN 40 min run LIT p.m.1: BIKE 60 min LIT p.m.2: RUN track HIIT 6×1000 m with 200 m recovery (type 3)	a.m.1: SWIM 3 k LIT a.m.2: RUN 20 min run LIT p.m.: RUN track HIIT 8×800 m with 200 m recovery (type 4)
Wednesday	a.m.1: SWIM 5 k LIT a.m.2: RUN 75 min LIT p.m.: BIKE 3.5 h LIT	a.m.1: SWIM 4.5 k LIT a.m.2: RUN 60 min LIT p.m.: BIKE 2.5 h LIT
Thursday	a.m.1: SWIM 5 k include 2×(8×50 MAX) on 90 s, 100 easy between series (type 4) a.m.2: RUN 60 min LIT p.m.: BIKE 2 h including 3×20 min MIT efforts (5 min recovery)	a.m.1: SWIM 5 k including 2×(10×100 on 1:45), 200 passive recovery between series HIIT (type 3) a.m.2: RUN 60 min LIT p.m.: BIKE 2 h including 4×10 min MIT efforts (4 min recovery)
Friday	a.m.1: SWIM 4.5 k LIT a.m.2: S&C p.m.1: RUN 60 min LIT p.m.2: BIKE 60 min LIT	a.m.1: SWIM 4 k LIT a.m.2: S&C p.m.1: RUN 60 min LIT p.m.2: BIKE 60 min LIT
Saturday	a.m.1: RUN 75 min including 6×5 min HIIT (5 min recovery) (type 3) a.m.2: BIKE 3 h LIT p.m.: RUN 30 min LIT	a.m.1: RUN 75 min including 4×5 min at 90% vVO2max (5 min recovery) (type 4) a.m.2: BIKE 2.5 h LIT
Sunday	a.m.: BIKE 4 h LIT p.m.: RUN 1 h, 40 min LIT	a.m.: BIKE 3 h LIT p.m.: RUN 1 h, 15 min LIT

LIT: low-intensity training, blood lactate concentration <2.5 mmol/L, heart rate <80% HRmax; MIT: moderate-intensity training, blood lactate concentration 2.5-4.0 mmol/L, heart rate 80%-90% HRmax; HIIT: high-intensity interval training, blood lactate concentration >4.0 mmol/L, heart rate >90% HRmax; S&C: strength and conditioning

Table 19.6 Typical Training Week of an Olympic Distance Professional Triathlete During the Competition Period: Hard and Competition Weeks

	Hard training week	Competition week
Monday	a.m. 1: RUN 70 min LIT a.m. 2: S&C p.m. 1: SWIM 4 k including LIT p.m.2: BIKE 2 h LIT	a.m.: RUN 30 min run LIT p.m.1: SWIM 3.5 k including 4×200 (90 s recovery), 4×100 m (60 s recovery) (types 3 and 4) p.m.2: BIKE 2 h including 2×(10×30 s on/off) (type 3)
Tuesday	a.m. 1: SWIM 3 k LIT a.m. 2: RUN 40 min run LIT p.m.1: BIKE 60 min LIT p.m.2: RUN track 2×(10×400 m HIIT leaving on 1:45) (type 4)	a.m. 1: SWIM 3 k HIIT a.m. 2: RUN 20 min run LIT p.m.: RUN track 4×1000 m HIIT with 400 m recovery (type 4)
Wednesday	a.m. 1: SWIM 5 k LIT a.m. 2: RUN 75 min LIT including 2×20 min at MIT (10 min recovery) p.m.: BIKE 2.5 h LIT	a.m. 1: SWIM 3.5 k LIT a.m. 2: BIKE 2 h LIT p.m.: REST
Thursday	a.m. 1: SWIM 5 k including 10×200 m on 3:00 HIIT (type 3) a.m. 2: RUN 60 min LIT p.m.: BIKE 2 h, including weekly criterium racing (type 4)	a.m. 1: BIKE 90 min ride including 4×3 min HIIT with 7 min recovery (type 4) a.m. 2: RUN (off bike) 20 min including 2×3 min HIIT with 3 min recovery (type 4)
Friday	a.m. 1: SWIM 4.5 k LIT a.m. 2: S&C p.m.1: RUN 60 min LIT p.m.2: BIKE 60 min LIT	a.m. 1: SWIM 2.5 km include 6-7×100 m HIIT on 5 min (type 4) a.m. 2: BIKE 1.5 h LIT p.m.: RUN 30 min LIT
Saturday	a.m. 1: BIKE 3 h LIT a.m. 2: RUN (off bike) 75 min including 3×3 k HIIT, leaving on 15 min (type 4)	a.m. 1: SWIM 1000 m LIT a.m. 2: BIKE 60 min LIT p.m.1: RUN 15 min LIT
Sunday	a.m.: BIKE 3.5 h LIT p.m.: RUN 1 h, 30 min LIT	RACE DAY

LIT: low-intensity training, blood lactate concentration <2.5 mmol/L, heart rate <80% HRmax; MIT: moderate-intensity training, blood lactate concentration 2.5-4.0 mmol/L, heart rate 80%-90% HRmax; HIIT: high-intensity interval training, blood lactate concentration >4.0 mmol/L, heart rate >90% HRmax; S&C: strength and conditioning

Daniel Plews

While media coverage of triathlon predominantly focuses on stories of professional athletes, triathlon participation, which largely funds the sport, is predominantly made up of age-group (AG) triathletes. Here is my personal HIIT journey, the program I used to prepare for AG competition in the 2018 New Zealand Ironman triathlon.

AG triathlon competitions typically are broken into 5-year age categories (20-24, 25-29, 30-34, 35-39, etc.), which make the sport unique, permitting competition within competition as athletes strive to win their AG category. For AG athletes, who share full-time job and family commitments, training efficiency is everything. In this instance, it seemed even more important, as although I had completed four Ironman distance races previously, I had a new player in the mix, our little baby Bella, who would be 5 months old on race day. For context, the times of my previous Ironman races were 9 h 22 min (New Zealand, 2013), 9 h 08 min (New Zealand 2015), 9 h 12 min (Kona 2015), and 8 h 54 min (New Zealand, 2013).

Race day was March 3, 2018, and true preparation for IMNZ began on October 23, 2017 (19 wk). During the first 8 wk macrocycle, HIIT training was restricted to cycling only, with endurance, strength, and tempo training making up the swim, run, and other bike sessions. The first HIIT session of the week included long-interval HIIT (i.e., 3 (5×2 min at >5% critical power (CP)), 1 min recovery between reps, 4 min light spinning between sets; type 4 with type 3 short-interval HIIT (2 d later), composed of 20×60 s reps at >20% CP with 60 s recovery (light spinning). While to some in the triathlon community it might seem odd to start the training phase with such intense intervals, this is an approach I have used a number of times, where I progress from nonspecific (i.e., HIIT at powers well above IM pace) toward specific (lower intensity, longer duration) IM race pace reps. This sequencing continued for 8 wk, before the long-interval HIIT were progressed, eventually finishing with 8×4 min (>5% CP) with 2 min recovery (type 4). The follow-up short intervals were removed after 4 wk and replaced with intervals more specific to the half-Ironman distance (I was competing in half-Ironman distance races as part of my preparation). Although not technically HIIT sessions, these moderate-pace sessions consisted of longer-duration intervals (20-30 min) at an intensity ~15% below CP.

After this phase, which finished with a half-Ironman distance race, the cycle-based HIIT long intervals were reintroduced with increased durations. Sessions included 6×6 min at >5% CP and 4×8 min at >5% CP (type 4). Type 4 short-interval HIIT treadmill running immediately followed, consisting of 6 to 10×200 to 400 at 3:10 min/km pace (>15% CV). Sessions maintained throughout the entire training period included tempo runs (60 min running at around 85% HRmax) and strength sessions on the bike. These bike strength sessions, although not technically HIIT, allowed for periods at higher-power outputs and generally included 4 to 5×15 min hill ascents at 95% CP (7 min recovery).

The final 4 wk period was the most intensive period of training; all key sessions were touched on each week. To keep training as specific as possible, much time was spent performing very long intervals at moderate intensity (i.e., 4×30 min at 75% CP). HIIT was removed from the bike-training component, and the HIIT focus shifted to the run. Each week, one short (i.e., 6×200 m at 105% v$\dot{V}O_2$max, 400 m jog recovery; type 3) and one long (8×1 km with 200 m jog recovery at 100% v$\dot{V}O_2$max; type 4) interval session was completed. For me, this meant running the 1 km at 3:10/km (90 s recovery). My final "hit out" came 2 d prior to the race, an HIIT session I have done religiously before every race (I call it the Plews Primer) for as long as I can remember. This consists of 3×3 min at 102% CP with 4 min recovery (type 3). It always feels good to open the jets just before race day!

On race day, despite a small crash on the bike with 50 km to go, I couldn't have been happier with my result. My splits consisted of a 50 min swim, 4 h 47 min ride, and 2 h 52 min marathon run, resulting in an 8 h 35 min finish time, placing me 9th overall (including professionals) and first AG amateur overall by 15 min. This was also a personal best time over the Ironman distance by 20 min, and also broke the age-group course record by more than 10 min.

My actual weekly bike volume came out at only 261 km per week, which would surprise a lot of people. This is not a lot of riding relative to the time achieved. For the AG Ironman athlete, cycling is really the area that those of us who are time poor struggle with, and I certainly felt this with the demands of work and baby Bella. One of the reasons I believe I got away with such a low volume of riding was because I was very specific with the riding I was doing. HIIT was an integral part of achieving this outcome.

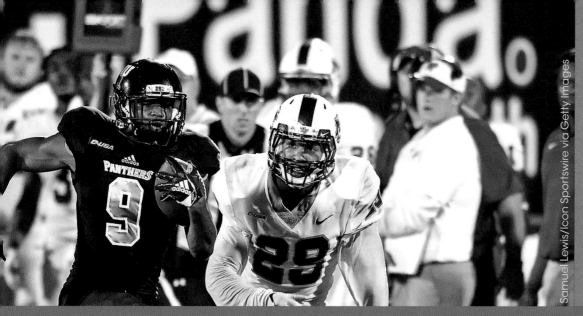

20

American Football

• • • • • •

Johann Bilsborough and Moses Cabrera

Performance Demands of American Football

In this chapter, we introduce the sport of American football (AmF) and discuss the various factors of importance for players and the relative contribution that physical performance may account for in the overall quest to win games.

Sport Description and Factors of Winning

American football (AmF), referred to as *gridiron* in some circles, is a full-contact, team-based sport played predominantly in North America. While Canada hosts a similar four-down version of the game (CFL), the main competition is known as the National Football League (NFL), made up of 32 teams interspersed throughout major cities of the United States, and is currently America's most popular sport. The NFL's final game of the year to decide the overall competition winner is famously known as the Super Bowl, and it is the largest shared event in the United States (7, 18). The 2017 NFL Super Bowl Championship was viewed by approximately 111.9 million people, placing it fourth among the most-viewed television programs in U.S. history (25). The game is played on a rectangle-shaped field (120 yd

long × 53.3 yd wide) with the last 10 yd at each end of the length of the field allocated as the scoring end zone (figure 20.1). AmF is a unique football code with respect to the fact that it has multiple specialized playing positions that are not interchangeable. Due to the specialized nature of each playing position, professional teams can have a preseason roster of up to 90 players, which is reduced to a 53-man squad once the teams are in-season.

AmF is contested between 11 players on each team (active at any one time) over four, 15 min quarters, separated by a 12 min halftime, with 2 min breaks between first and second and third and fourth quarters (15). Three specific units make up the overall AmF team: a defensive unit, an offensive unit, and a special teams unit. A specific subset of player positions are typically classified into eight groups as follows: defensive backs (DB), defensive linemen (DL), linebackers (LB), offensive linemen (OL), quarterback (QB), running back (RB), tight end (TE), wide receiver (WR), and kickers and punters (38). Each position has distinct physiological demands and activity profiles.

The offensive unit's goal is to advance down the field via running or passing the ball and has four plays (known as downs) to do so. If the offense progresses 10 yd or more in the four plays, they are awarded a new set of four plays. If unsuccessful,

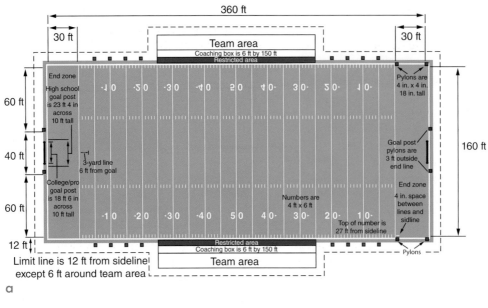

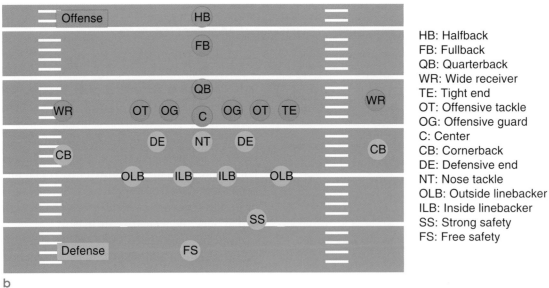

Figure 20.1 (a) American football (AmF) playing field dimensions and (b) playing positions.

then the ball and offensive play are surrendered to the other team by punting. There are two main ways to score points. A touchdown, in which the team progressively moves the ball from one end of the field to their opponent's end zone, earns the team 6 points, with the opportunity to earn an extra point by kicking the ball through the goal posts or try for a 2-point conversion by passing or running the ball into the end zone. The aim of the defensive unit is to protect the length of the field via negating the opposition advancement to score, while a special-teams player's role is to cover situations such as kickoffs, punt returns, and extra point attempts (2, 3).

Relative Contribution of Physical Performance

Despite the popularity of AmF throughout the United States at the high school, college, and professional levels, there is limited research outlining the modern physiological demands of training or games (15, 22, 30). The NFL has only recently shared privately to teams the details of their in-game player tracking via radio-frequency identification (RFID). Despite this, there is to our knowledge no peer-reviewed validation of the system in games for identification of physical demands and capacities of player positions. To the best of our knowledge, in fact, there are only two published studies that quantify game- or training-based external load in elite AmF players using global positioning systems (GPS) and accelerometers (38-41). Despite this, in-game statistics (yards covered, number of tackles, plays completed, etc.) have been reported in the NFL since 1932 (29), data that may assist practitioners to quantify game demands. This section combines the limited level of empirically based knowledge in AmF with our practical experience working in the sport.

American football players typically have well-established physical profiles of speed, power, strength, and agility (figure 20.2). Successful performers complement these physical characteristics with technical skills and tactical awareness to repeatedly carry out plays successfully during a game while adapting to changes in the environment, e.g., their opposition. The AmF research literature suggests that physical performance characteristics can discriminate between position, playing ability, draft success, and level of play (9, 32, 33, 35, 42). Unlike many other field-based football codes, AmF is often not free-flowing and sees frequent stoppages in play. Each high-intensity play lasts ~5 to

7 s, with recovery times often lasting ~25 to 40 s over a 60 min game, including frequent collisions from blocking or tackling (8, 10, 20). The larger linemen player positions require positional skill and technique plus eccentric, isometric, and concentric strength. The LB, DB, TE, RB, and QB players typically possess certain body mass and speed characteristics that allow them to run and change direction while withstanding high-impact collisions (39). The QB is the key player dictating the orchestration and structure of the team's offense. QBs are required to have high football intellect, skill, and agility plus the ability to read the play quickly and execute decisions, which often requires throwing the football with pinpoint accuracy. Athletes in AmF require the ability to complete repeated sprints (RS) and repeated high-intensity efforts (RHIE) involving accelerations and decelerations combined with tackling and impacts. Data collated from the 16-game 2017 NFL season showed that there were 63 ± 3 (mean $\pm$ SD) scrimmage plays per game, with 5.3 ± 0.5 yd covered per play (29). Certain styles of play, tactical issues, and timeouts may demand athletes to play periods of the game at a higher tempo, which in turn places additional demands on the aerobic system (10).

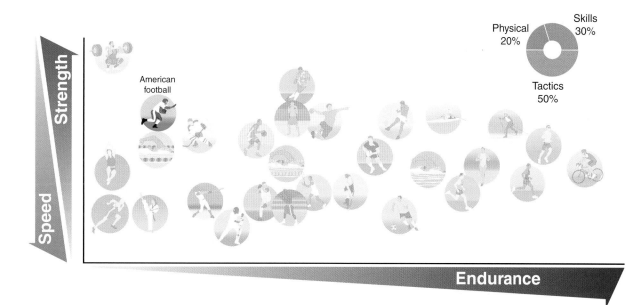

Figure 20.2 The position of the American football player on the three axes illustrates the relative importance of the three main physical capacities of importance for elite participation in the sport, acknowledging that this can vary substantially among the unique positions. Outside of critical psychological aspects and team chemistry components, which are difficult to quantify, the pie chart shows the general relative importance of skills (30%), tactical awareness (50%), and physical capacities (20%) for American football success.

Adapted from G.A. Nader, "Concurrent Strength and Endurance Training: From Molecules to Man," *Medicine & Science in Sports & Exercise* 38, no. 11 (2006): 1965-1970.

Targets of Physical Performance of American Football

The position-specific tasks required of AmF players (figure 20.1) tend to determine the physical characteristics they possess (22). Pincivero and Bompa (30) described four basic groups of established players as follows: (1) offensive and defensive linemen, (2) defensive backs and wide receivers, (3) linebackers, running backs, and tight ends, and (4) quarterbacks, punters, and kickers. Regardless of playing position, the predominant energy system of importance for all players is the anaerobic system (14). However, high-intensity interval training (HIIT) work and relief periods as determined should still be prescribed as specifically as possible for the varying positional groups that follow.

Offensive and Defensive Linemen

Typically the linemen, both offensive and defensive, are the largest athletes on the field. Players in this position exhibit higher percentages of body fat (OL, $25.3\% \pm 4.4\%$; DL $20.9\% \pm 6.5\%$) over most other positions and may weigh up to 140 kg (24, 31). The linemen positions must repeatedly apply explosive power efforts over very short distances. These athletes are characteristically stronger and more powerful than the other positions on the field, as they must possess the ability to be able to duel against opponents of similar size mirroring their position on the field (9, 30) (figure 20.1). While linemen display more physical contact with opposition players via specific blocking assignments and tackles (~4.4 per game (29)), they must nevertheless cover 200 to 600 yd per game (~7-14 yd per play; ~38-53 plays per game) including accelerations, decelerations, and changes of direction. This high-intensity work schedule in AmF players implies a high use of phosphocreatine and anaerobic glycolytic energy (15, 30). However, when such high-intensity efforts are repeated, this places additional demands on the aerobic system (see chapters 3 and 5), which are often less developed in AmF players (10, 14).

Defensive Backs and Wide Receivers

Defensive backs and wide receivers (figure 20.1) also share comparable body composition profiles. However, Bosch et al. (1) showed that WRs were slightly taller (WR 185.7 ± 3.9 cm; DB 182.2 ± 3.1 cm), slightly heavier (WR 94.0 ± 6.0 kg; DB 90.8 ± 6.1 kg), and of a similar percentage body fat (WR $12.5\% \pm 3.1\%$; DB $12.1\% \pm 3.3\%$) as DBs. These players display the greatest locomotive activity demands in AmF (39), completing the greatest volume of running (~1200 yd per game; ~24 yd per play; ~43 plays per game), with much of this being high-speed running (~16 mph). These athletes require similar energy system contributions as others on the field, with slightly more reliance on the aerobic system due to the greater active distances traveled. To meet these demands, HIIT prescription includes short intervals, repeated-sprint training (RST), sprint interval training (SIT), and game-based HIIT (GBHIIT) (see below). Tactically, WRs and DBs have more space to run, which means they reach higher peak velocities and run longer distances in a game. Hard changes of direction, accelerations, and repeated longer high-intensity efforts, implying high neuromuscular and musculoskeletal demands, are required components of performance related to success in this positional group.

Linebackers, Running Backs, and Tight Ends

An AmF team's defense is often dictated by the success of its linebackers. They are high-velocity athletes balanced with strength and skill. Reading the play and being able to respond immediately to execute a tackle is the mainstay requirement of this position. Further, linebackers provide an extra run or pass protection option.

The principal ball carrier in the offense is known as the running back (halfback or fullback; figure 20.1). He is required to receive the handoff from the quarterback for a rushing play while also being needed to catch passes and block the opposition. The successful running back can use his agility to receive handoffs from the QB to attempt a rushing play. Running backs sustain the most severe (>10G force) impacts during a match, whereas LBs endure lighter impacts (5.0-6.0G force) through collisions and tackles (39). Tight ends often are used as hybrid players who can play roles similar to those of offensive linemen, wide receivers, and running backs. They play next to the offensive linemen (figure 20.1) and often are required to block opponents on running plays. However, the TE may catch passes and be required to run the field. Players in all positions typically present with large statures (LB 109.9 ± 4.6 kg; RB 105.4 ± 8.5 kg; TE 113.9 ± 4.2 kg) and moderate percentage body fat (~16%-17%) (1). In addition, in order to accelerate and decelerate repeatedly throughout a game, TEs often must push against opponents of similar size. All three positions complete ~550 yd of high-intensity running (~16 mph) in a game (~21-24 plays per game). Accordingly, these players require exposure to RHIE that involves accelerations so they are prepared for worst-case scenarios that occur during extended game play.

Quarterback, Punters, and Kickers

When we imagine AmF, we immediately think of the quarterback, who outside the coaching staff is the leader of the team. Quarterbacks typically possess lower values of body fat and high levels of speed and agility. They require good relative upper-body explosive muscular power to repeatedly throw the football downfield, targeting teammates with high precision. Despite these necessary attributes, the main feature of the QB's performance stems from a difficult-to-quantify game intelligence, tactical prowess, and ability to read the game, making decisions with split-second reaction time. The QB may throw ~36.3 times in a game (29) and cover ~550 yd per game over 47.9 plays (7.4 yd per play), relying on short, sharp multidirectional movements, accelerations, and decelerations. While the QB controls the offensive play of the game, he still requires enough strength and fat-free soft tissue mass to withstand regular collisions and impacts. QBs perform the majority of their training using individual short-interval HIIT, alongside their lead role in GBHIIT scenarios. Such training is considered pivotal to a QB's conditioning, alongside his copious training volume spent learning and refining skills.

The role of punters and kickers is simple: kick the football to score extra points, kick the ball off a placeholder to start play, or kick the ball in play to advance it down the field. The positions are highly specialized, but teams sometimes have the same person performing both roles. The kickers may need to kick or punt the football several times per game (punter, 11.6 per game; kicker, 9.4 per game) (29) depending on the success of the offense and the tactical context of the game, and cover up to 20 yd per play. Punters and kickers do not usually take contact, nor are they typically involved in tackling or core events in the general game. Although slightly lighter than QBs (K/P 98.4 ± 5.6 kg; QB 103.6 ± 13.9 kg), kickers and punters have similar proportions of body fat (K/P 19.2% ± 4.5%; QB 19.6% ± 4.6%). Punters and kickers are specialized

positions that require high levels of skill. Due to the tactical nature of their positions, they typically endure a very low level of locomotor activity in games. Accordingly, training programs for these positions use predominantly short-interval HIIT and RST plus their involvement in GBHIIT. In addition, their role sees them performing repeated kicking scenarios under pressure to improve accuracy.

Key Weapons, Manipulations, and Surveillance Tools

The weapons we use in AmF refer to the HIIT formats applied in our programs. These weapons are chosen to ensure we are targeting the desired physiological responses and physical adaptations, while our surveillance ensures we are meeting our directives. In this section, we present the different HIIT weapons we have used in preparing professional AmF players along with their manipulations and surveillance approaches for monitoring training effectiveness.

HIIT Weapons

The general breakdown of the different HIIT weapons we use throughout the annual season in AmF are shown in figure 20.3 and include GBHIIT or small-sided games (SSGs; ~60%), short-interval HIIT (~20%), RST (~15%), and SIT (~5%). These HIIT formats and their manipulations are described below.

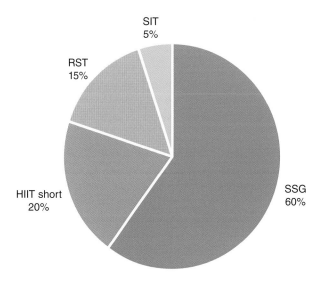

Figure 20.3 Percentage of the different HIIT formats (weapons) used throughout the annual season in American football: game-based HIIT or small-sided games (SSGs; ~60%), HIIT short intervals (~20%), RST (~15%), and SIT (~5%).

Manipulations of Interval Training Variables

Positions across the offensive and defensive roles in AmF are comparable to one another from an energetic standpoint, as they naturally mirror the movement demands. As such, training across offensive and defensive players is similar. Therefore, careful manipulation of the HIIT type, duration, intensity, and rest periods of each particular weapon are made within the weekly game cycle depending on team requirements.

Game-Based Training

While this book is about HIIT, generally defined as exercises eliciting close-to-maximal metabolic responses, for a comprehensive view of our AmF programming approach, we chose to include presentation of training from a slightly wider range of exercise intensities, including exercises performed at an intensity slightly below HIIT-specific intensities, as occurs with AmF-specific SSGs.

American football has a large training focus involving either the defensive group or the offensive group in which plays are simulated in a full and modified game format. This SSGs approach is traditional in college and professional teams and the main HIIT weapon used to build a player's conditioning. Therefore, teams will practice in their specific positional setups to optimize synchronicity of timing and strategy of plays. The combination of high-intensity running combined with specific skill involvement is seen as a favorable combination for AmF coaches over traditional running to condition the playing group. Unlike other football codes, namely soccer and Australian football in which running is more free-flowing, AmF practice sessions involve short explosive intervals with a high number of collisions. More recently, rules have been introduced by leagues to limit the number of sessions that can be completed with contact to mitigate risk of head injuries.

The breakdown of practice sees the offensive positions complete more locomotor activity by way of high-intensity running, using full-sized fields to invoke higher neuromuscular demands. This field-side modification helps to provide repeated bouts of work with increased mechanical work from accelerations, decelerations, and harder changes of direction (COD). This 5-a-side format (reduced from 11 in match play) with spatial constraints and noncontact SSG rules allows for short periods (~3 min) of play with often multiple repetitions (~6-10). This format meets the longer-duration work requirements without overloading high-intensity running volume, while hitting type 4 targets.

HIIT With Short Intervals

Due to the wide variation of physiological demands across the various positions in AmF, a key weapon used by all positions naturally becomes HIIT with short intervals. Careful prescription of short intervals allows us to hit type 1, 2, 3, or 4 HIIT targets. Prescription of slightly longer intervals (≥ 15 s) in the off-season period are used to maintain specific components of the athlete's conditioning, as preseason witnesses athletes resuming game-style play very quickly and they cannot afford to detrain. By managing the volume of this format, intensity of locomotor load, the neuromuscular fatigue, and anaerobic contribution can be manipulated accordingly, depending on the number of sessions planned for a day. This can be a useful format for rehabilitation in players who require lower neuromuscular loading (type 1) in the early phase before progressing through to type 2 and type 3 targets in preparation for type 4 short-interval work demands, involving COD running with hard decelerations. Rehabilitation players can build up to volumes of work required as percentages of their game demands calculated by known game run volume and intensity requirements. As deemed appropriate, players may complete 50% to 75% to 90% of the positional equivalent, with type 4 loading carefully controlled through prescription.

During the in-season period, there is a need for players to meet certain volumes of high-intensity running each week to lower injury risk and maintain fitness. Depending on how a game evolves, some players will not meet their demands. This may apply to both the main players and reserves, as there is no second tier competition from which players can get a game-like conditioning training load. For this situation, type 2 or 4 high-intensity running with high-grade agility and hard decelerations are required, which may serve to protect the hamstrings and mitigate deconditioning while maintaining neuromuscular loading. Such training ensures that reserve players are meeting the same game and training running loads as their senior counterparts. This training is also important for the backup kickers and punters and QB positions, who require kicking and throwing loads to match those of their game-playing counterparts.

Repeated-Sprint Training

Repeated-sprint training is a much used HIIT weapon in AmF players. The game demands of multiple positions require consistent all-out efforts that include COD and explosive efforts with short relief periods. This training replicates the intensity and frequency of game play in AmF. RST is used during both the late preseason and in the middle of the week during the in-season phase. It is commonly used in drills in which a player is required to hit tackle bags, run all out in a straight line, before changing direction in response to a stimulus, and then run again. Players may have multiple CODs requiring high levels of deceleration before applying an explosive effort again. These efforts are short (4-6 s) and based on their positional requirement. A typical format used for many positions might involve three series of 3 to 5 sprints with ~20 s of recovery over 5 to 6 min, which hits type 4 targets.

Sprint Interval Training

For the specialist positions who need to run the ball at maximum velocity down the length of the field in an attempt to score a touchdown, the SIT weapon naturally is employed as part of the periodized plan. The athletes complete this training individually when they are fresh and away from football-specific practices. The objective of this specialized session with select athletes is to be able to hit maximum velocity over ~10 repetitions over approximately 25 yd (similar to distances covered in a game per play for many positions) with extended relief periods (~2-3 min). This training forms a part of the late preseason and in-season phases and requires careful planning to prevent possible interference with other important training components and their associated neuromuscular loads (4).

Load Surveillance and Monitoring Tools

Microtechnology and the monitoring of player health have taken a longer time to gain traction in U.S. team sports, and as a result it is typically uncommon practice to see wearable technology being used in elite AmF. Over the last 5 yr, with the influence of European/UK and Australian sport scientists, both college and professional AmF have seen major advancements in this domain. The addition of complementary sport science to the area of strength and conditioning has led to the progression of understanding into the physiological demands and

responses associated with AmF (16, 17, 36). While tracking and monitoring systems still must undergo external validation, recent developments in GPS have seen embedded inertial sensors, which may be used to help understand collisions and positional differences in practice (38-41).

As discussed in chapter 8, collection of the session rating of perceived exertion (s-RPE) is a useful means to measure internal training load (13, 19), while high-definition camera systems can be useful for tracking external loads in training and games. Despite the need for validation, these systems together may be useful for quantifying overall workload to assist with alterations in weekly load distribution. This becomes important when the weekly microcycle is shortened from 7 d to 5 d during the competition phase due to scheduling (i.e., Monday night football prior to a Saturday afternoon game later in the week). Camera system limitations do arise, however, when the team is required to play an away game and train at remote locations beforehand (~6-8 games per season). Without consistent monitoring in these situations, session tracking is compromised (see related example in chapter 9). Heart rate is often monitored in non-football-related sessions, as well as in the rehabilitation setting to ensure the desired internal training load is adhered to. Such sessions may include stationary cycling, boxing, and HIIT running sessions, which are all common activities used throughout the rehabilitation phase.

Training Status Surveillance and Monitoring Tools

The training monitoring surveillance systems used in AmF are restricted to noninvasive measures to ensure compliance. With a squad that can be as high as 90 athletes in the preseason, players have many demands placed on them. For example, the preseason witnesses multiple overlaps in both position-specific and team sessions. Collectively with weight training, individual need workouts (HIIT doses for specific groups), alongside top-up conditioning for reserve players who may not have been exposed to sufficient game-time repetitions, monitoring systems must be simple, quick, and seamless for both athletes and practitioners.

The preseason period in AmF represents a discovery period for us, when we can debate and put forth what data we believe will be meaningful to collect, as surprisingly there are few longitudinal variables previously reported in either college or professional teams (21, 37). Indeed, the desire to borrow systems from other sports that have monitored athletes in other football codes (namely soccer, rugby, and Australian football; see related chapters) is tempting, but practitioners must appreciate that the embryonic stage of buy-in for any elite sport can be difficult and slow. Best practice in such a sport may be to introduce only a few systems initially, while ensuring the data is collected well, before eventually becoming a consistent aspect of the team environment. Further establishment of the data analysis must then be meaningful enough to aid in the decision-making process before introducing any other noninvasive measurements deemed necessary. Collectively, GPS and accelerometry-derived data (including both locomotor and impacts), HR, s-RPE, countermovement jump scores for neuromuscular fatigue (6), alongside simple wellness questionnaires today may represent best practice scenarios for understanding time course changes of recovery and

response to training load (12, 27) (see also chapter 9). In order to aid player compliance, many of these systems can be integrated into the program and standardized in order to change the perception that an athlete is being tested or evaluated. The use of visual analogue scales for specific issues and to aid in understanding player readiness during periods of return to sport (28) complement the other systems outlined. An example of the typical weekly team training loads experienced throughout a season are shown in figure 20.4.

Strategies for Structuring the Training Program Using HIIT

Strategies for structuring HIIT programming in AmF may be dictated partially by several controllable and uncontrollable factors, before proper progression and periodization can be appropriately implemented. This section discusses some of the

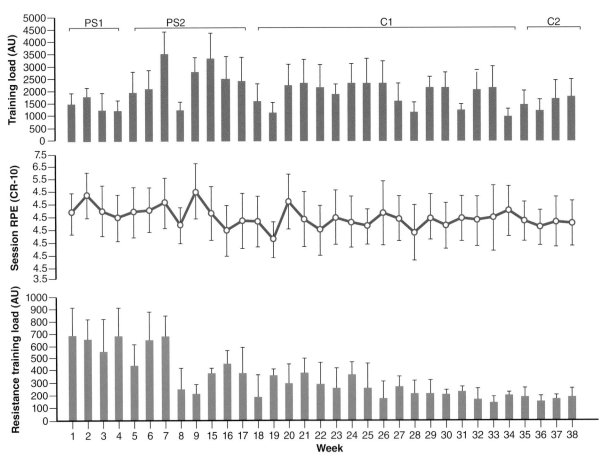

Figure 20.4 Example of seasonal weekly team training loads (AU) and session-RPE and resistance training loads (AU) during a professional American football league season. PS1: preseason phase 1; PS2: preseason phase 2; C1: competition season; C2: finals.

nuances of training program and HIIT structuring in AmF.

Controllable and Uncontrollable Factors

The uncontrollable factor in AmF at the professional level is its schedule, which determines game day, venue, and associated interstate travel (including up to three time zones in either easterly or westerly direction). The practice period, which has strict league rules regarding the amount of time players are accessible and regulations concerning the number of sessions during which contact time is permitted, is set prior to the start of the season. These aspects dictate how the program is structured in the weekly cycle and, most importantly, in accordance with the head coach's philosophies. Players and coaches are also required to partake in extensive media commitments throughout the week, both in preseason and in-season.

The planning of the preseason is carefully constructed around the technical and tactical philosophies of the head coach. For this, each group of positions outlined tends to separate and focus on individual positional roles. Indeed, practice sessions for these groups are often relatively long due to the high number of plays required to orchestrate their function without error. Therefore, completing the daily practice plans in blocks that ensure yards per minute are maintained without diluting team practice due to fundamental teaching components that may be lacking in particular athletes is a necessity. A predetermined plan of training intensity and duration is set early (chapter 8) so that drills can be established noting player availability for contact and noncontact aspects. Once the initial technical and instructional blocks are achieved, the inclusion of different HIIT components is usually blended into further tactical sessions. With live monitoring of GPS (high-intensity running and volume of running), performance staff can ensure predicted physical requirements are met. Often starters will receive appropriate training doses that include physical game outcomes, however, nonstarters will complete complementary training sessions that use additional specific HIIT work to ensure a matched training load. This load often exceeds that of consistent starters.

Program Structure and Progression

Training for professional AmF has evolved in recent years so that today it is more specific to the requirements of the individualized positions. Teams typically do not follow any specific periodized model in terms of varying training cycles during the in-season period (figure 20.4). The flexible nonlinear programming approach offers variation in training to ensure more responsive changes in the athlete (23). The off-season period begins after the Super Bowl (in February) and ends with the beginning of the next season's practices in late June, running until late July, followed by a 2 wk preseason period with lifting sessions, meetings, and limited practices. The next period of 6 wk features a weekly game factored into the cycle and progressive changes in the volume and intensity of the program. Upon completion of this phase, players ready themselves for the in-season phase in which they compete in 16 games over a 17 wk period. If successful during the regular season, the opportunity to commence post-season games may see teams play in three final high-profile playoff games.

Different aspects of the annual season can be challenging for players and performance staff. The off-season provides the biggest challenge to staff due to the inability to track and monitor players while they are away from the home training facilities. Programs are issued and many athletes complete these, but compliance is never 100%; success depends on the individual athlete's motivation. To ensure players return to the preseason in an acceptable level of physical condition, many targets are provided to players beforehand to help them avoid detraining. An adequate off-season is nevertheless important, and allows players to enter preseason with a lower risk of injury. Players must be able to perform a high volume of high-intensity work, involving slightly longer running intervals (HIIT with short intervals targeting type 4), multiple weight sessions, team technical and tactical practices without contact, and off-legs conditioning work. Work progresses carefully and involves a higher volume of straight-line running and lower-grade agility. Players involved in kicking and throwing progress in terms of intensity and volume of these activities, and the placement of these in the program is critical. There is always a desire for coaching staff to attain higher repetitions of both kicking and throwing, but this is where monitoring is essential to achieve controlled and balanced loading alongside the conditioning component of the program to ensure the incidence of injury is mitigated. Figure 20.5 shows an example of the weekly running loads experienced throughout a typical AmF season.

Preseason games start very early, and the use of wearable technology for monitoring load is still

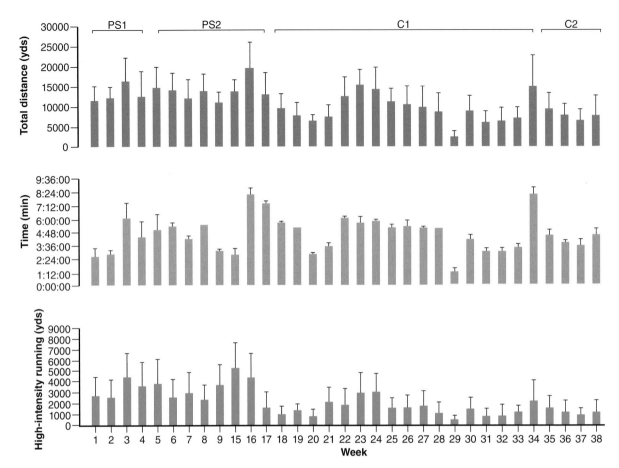

Figure 20.5 Example of seasonal weekly team running loads, total distance (yards), time (minutes), and high-intensity running (16 mph) yards during a professional American football league season. PS1: preseason phase 1; PS2: preseason phase 2; C1: competition season; C2: finals.

limited in this regard. That being said, players tend to increase RHIE and reduce rest intervals progressively, while increasing the number of harder accelerations and decelerations to replicate position-specific game-like situations. The efforts are short (4-6 s) and based on positional requirements. A typical example of training across many positions might involve three series of 3 to 5 sprints with ~20 s recovery over 5 to 6 min in which type 4 targets are reached. The priority focus is always on game 1 of the regular season, so the need to gain strength and muscle mass remains a primary focus throughout this period.

The in-season period is often the easiest phase of training to manage due to weekly training loads remaining constant over the 17 wk period to ensure optimal performance occurs at game time. Similar to most weekly football codes, there is a period of recovery that follows from the damage incurred from the weekend game (16, 17) before a buildup to the biweekly technical and tactical practices, followed

by unloading for recovery for the game. Importantly, ensuring an appropriate dose of quality high-speed running is met not only maintains fitness characteristics but also protects from injury (11, 26, 34).

Incorporation of HIIT

In AmF, planning and sequencing of HIIT between games is based on a few important aspects: the amount of work completed by the player, the level of soreness and fatigue, and, most importantly, the coach's decision. Often after a game, the coach will want to work on technical aspects to improve player and team performance. This often takes priority over most other decisions, desires, and needs of other staff. The starters and nonstarters provide an interesting scenario in this regard, as they have different loading volumes postgame. Nonstarting players are required to top up their training load as early as possible, so they follow a similar time course of training load response and recovery adaptation as their starting counterparts.

Training sessions in AmF were traditionally completed using number of repetitions or plays. For example, coaches used to use language such as "We will be running 80 plays today" instead of "We need to complete 4000 yd, 75% of which will include high-intensity running." So the shift in programming due to the inclusion of GPS/RFID tracking has markedly changed top-up session planning and execution. While this ideal scenario is now often the case, coaches still may revert back to use of more traditional language.

The higher-velocity running, sharp changes of direction, as well as accelerations and decelerations are avoided during the first 2 d after a game. We also consider the demands of other training in which HIIT is incorporated as well as the loading patterns within the weekly cycle, as these factors can influence the metabolic and neuromuscular responses to the HIIT (4, 5). The programming emphasis relies on HIIT incorporated into the main training session prior to technical and tactical training in the preseason, as the emphasis from the coach is to have players perform skills under slight fatigue. There is another portion in the form of SSG often implemented at the mid to latter end of the coach's session. The aim here is to have positional teams focus on their specific plays. The offensive and defensive linemen, for example, will complete multiple short (<3 s) efforts that involve pushing opponents off after hard, short accelerations. Ideally, the plan would be to incorporate HIIT weapons that hit type 1 and type 3 targets, to avoid the neuromuscular loading and muscle damage incurred from the full-contact game, but depending on the outcome (good or bad), there can often be running that occurs, albeit undesirable in the eyes of the performance staff.

Sample Training Programs

An example of a weekly training program structure for professional AmF for preseason and in-season phases is shown in tables 20.1 and 20.2, respectively.

Table 20.1 Sample Preseason Training Schedule

	Sunday	Monday	Tuesday	Wednesday	Thursday	Friday	Saturday
AM	Off	Rehab running group	Rehab running group	Rehab running group	Rehab running group	Rehab running group	Rehab running group
		Team meeting	Team meeting	Off	Team meeting	Team meeting	Team meeting
		Treatment physiotherapy	Treatment physiotherapy			Treatment physiotherapy	Treatment physiotherapy
		Weights for all groups				Weights, individual needs	Weights, individual needs
		Line meeting	Line meeting		Line meeting	Line meeting	Practice, tactical session
		Practice, tactical session	HIIT running		HIIT running types 1, 2	Practice, main session	Individual off-legs conditioning
			Practice, main session		Practice, main session	HIIT running types 1, 2, 3 (position specific)	
PM		HIIT running types 1, 2	Weights for all groups		Weights for all groups	Weights for all groups	Weights for all groups
		Treatment physiotherapy			Treatment physiotherapy	Treatment physiotherapy	Treatment physiotherapy

Table 20.2 Sample Competition Season Training Schedule

	Sunday	Monday	Tuesday	Wednesday	Thursday	Friday	Saturday
AM	Rehab running group	Rehab running group	Rehab running group	Rehab running group	Rehab running group	Rehab running group	Rehab running group
	Team meeting Weights for rehab group	Team meeting Treatment physiotherapy Weights for all groups	Team meeting Treatment physiotherapy		Team meeting Specialist HIIT running group types 1, 2, 3, 4 (position specific)	Team meeting Weights, individual needs	Team meeting Weights, individual needs
	Line meeting	Line meeting	Line meeting HIIT running types 2, 4 (position specific) Practice, main session	Off	Line meeting HIIT running Practice, main session	Line meeting Practice, walk through HIIT running type 4 (position specific)	Practice, walk through Individual off-legs conditioning
PM	Game	Warm up individual top-up HIIT types 1, 2 Individual off-legs conditioning Tactical overview session review Treatment physiotherapy	Weights for all groups	Treatment physiotherapy Review meeting	Treatment physiotherapy	Treatment physiotherapy Review meeting	Treatment physiotherapy

Johann Bilsborough and Moses Cabrera

This story describes how we learned to monitor and assess training more precisely and how new aspects being introduced into a high-performance culture should be well understood prior to their implementation. This is very much a "lessons learned" experience, in which the timely processing of information and understanding specificity came into play.

The start of preseason saw a new staff member added to the performance department we were part of. This skill acquisition expert was to provide the link between the coaches and the performance department. The position was to use game-based training to better prepare the players for the specific game demands. While the current staff were confident this was already being achieved, this was an upper-management hire and not one vetted by the high-performance director (HPD). At the same time, we were in the embryonic stage of microtechnology use in American football. While the technology was familiar to our sport science staff, its practical use and understanding of useful metrics were still undergoing preliminary in-house reliability and validity evaluation (see chapter 9).

During the second half of preseason, the new skill acquisition staff member was granted permission to monitor the athletes and incorporate the game-based training component of the training sessions. The coach was convinced that this was the direction to go and disregarded some of the more traditional run-based HIIT sessions in which specific loading was planned using run distances and rest intervals. Even without the microtechnology, we could still set a course and time our rest intervals to ensure prescribed and actual doses were aligned. The conditioning coach, HPD, and sport scientist observed the transition to the game-based training drills and noticed the amount of teaching required during stoppage in training. The performance group became quite frustrated when the skill acquisition staff member informed us of an issue with the GPS units and that he would get information through to the performance group when he could address the technical downloading issues. This seemed to us merely a ploy to avoid presenting his information and controlling the narrative.

Frustration grew among the performance staff and the control of training dose was lost. It was now difficult to assess the players' load being completed, and staff highlighted this issue in several subsequent meetings. But when a coach is sold that a new protocol is the right way to do things, it can be hard to sway him back. It's important to emphasize here that the concept of game-based training was not new to the current performance staff, with the sport scientist at the club just completing student supervision of a PhD in rugby-based SSG, and therefore was well-versed in how to incorporate SSG in practice. Of course, these should form part of training, and so long as they are monitored properly, can be utilized as needed (see chapter 5). Needless to say, the inability to get direct answers to the monitoring process and loading left the performance staff extremely frustrated.

Fast forward to the start of the competition season. Game 1 sees calf tears in two key starters. Game 2 sees another calf tear and a hamstring strain. Games 3 and 4 witness yet another calf tear in each game. By game 5, we had an unofficial "calf crisis" when we strained our sixth calf. Six starters were out with similar injuries. The heat was turned up on the HPD and medical department, who were questioned regarding their process. The HPD called for an external performance audit of the department to get an independent answer on the so-called "calf crisis."

In the meantime, the conditioning coach and sport scientist collected all the GPS units and conducted their own investigation. What they discovered was that many of the sessions had either not been downloaded or had not been processed. Upon completion of their report, they discovered that the early competition games were run at 157 to 164 yd per minute. The game was fast! The analysis of the preseason sessions conducted by the skill acquisition expert were shown to be high in running volume, but with the constant coaching

(continued)

stoppage and suggested spatial constraints implemented, the sessions achieved only 98 to 101 yd per minute. The in-season sessions were also of low intensity and similar volume. The new stimulus of the weekly game, however, resulted in a huge spike in yards per minute and high-intensity running. The players were not adequately prepared for these increases in intensity and high-speed running. Despite there being some peaks in work rate during some drills, the rest intervals during the game-based training were too long and the intensity not maintained. Much of the work was completed at subpar levels that did not align with the game demands.

Of course, now we were in-season, when a change in preparation is difficult. Thus, solutions required exceptionally controlled running progressions and management.

To summarize, a number of our players had detrained because the principles of training as you play were not met. Data was not processed in a timely fashion, so adjustments could not be made for subsequent sessions. This occurrence affected the season drastically, as player management was extremely difficult. The steady implementation of appropriate volumes of high-speed running helped mitigate some of the issues going forward, allowing us to survive the season. But we learned a great lesson. The need to ensure the right staff complements a department, alongside an understanding of how any planned training should be measured to be managed, is a must in elite sport.

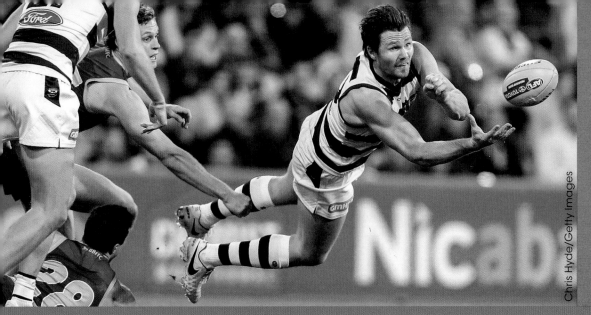

21

Australian Football

• • • • • •

Aaron Coutts, Joel Hocking, and Johann Bilsborough

Performance Demands of Australian Football

In this section, we introduce Australian football and discuss the critical factors that impact player performance and the relative contribution that physical performance makes to success.

Sport Description and Factors of Winning

Australian football (colloquially known as *Aussie rules*) is a team sport played between two teams of 22 players (18 on-field players and 4 interchange players) with an oval-shaped ball. Despite being indigenous to Australia, the major professional league, the Australian Football League (AFL), ranks among the most attended football leagues in the world. The game is played on a nonstandard-sized oval-shaped natural grass pitch 110 to 155 m wide and 135 to 185 m long with goals at each end (figure 21.1). In the AFL, each quarter is ~30 min (20 min of playing time and ~10 min of time-off), with a 6 min rest period following quarters 1 and 3, and a longer 20 min halftime period between quarters 2 and 3. Eighteen players are allowed on the field at any one time, with the remaining 4 players resting on the interchange bench. The interchange

players may be rotated onto the field to replace an existing player from the same team who leaves the field. A team is permitted to make a number of player interchanges during a match (varied number governed by the AFL).

The ultimate aim is for the team to score more points than the opposition by moving the ball through the goals at their attacking end of the field. Scoring is achieved by kicking the ball between four goal posts positioned 6.4 m apart at each end of the field, with 6 points awarded for a kick through the two middle posts and 1 point awarded for a kick through the outer posts (figure 21.1). Teams score by working collaboratively to maintain possession of the football and moving the ball to their attacking end of the field (forward line) through passing the ball, handballing, or kicking the ball to their teammates. Players are permitted to use their hands to control the ball but are not permitted to run with the ball more than 15 m without bouncing, handballing, or kicking the ball. Between-player body contact is permitted but limited. Opponents are allowed to tackle the player in possession of the ball between the shoulders and knees; push, bump, and block players within 5 m of the football (shepherding); and make contact incidental to a legitimate marking contest (i.e., where players duel to catch a ball kicked to them on the full). In contrast, the aim

393

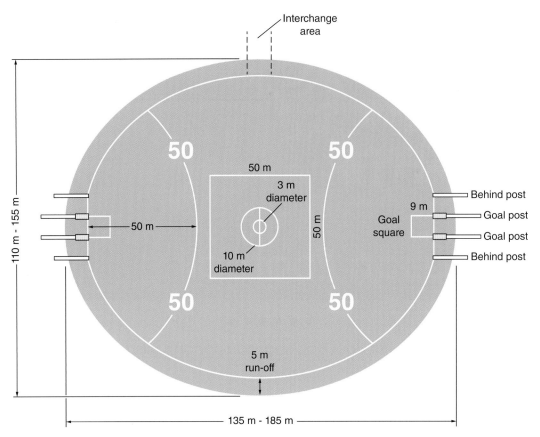

Figure 21.1 Australian football playing field dimensions.

of the team not in possession of the ball is to cause a turnover in ball possession by providing defensive pressure on the ball carrier and players who are likely to receive the ball from that player.

Playing positions have traditionally been classified by the general role that they play such as forwards, midfielders, defenders, and rucks (15, 21), but recently there has been a hybridization of these roles with many players filling many tactical positions often requiring them to rotate through the forward line, midfield, and defensive positions at different periods during a match. The number of strategic positional moves among players on the field is unlimited. This recent change has increased the need for all players to possess high-level intermittent running capacity, speed, and strength to permit them to play in multiple positions on the ground. Despite the increase in hybrid players, recent studies still show distinctive activity profiles and technical skills for various tactical roles (16). While it is important for football players to improve their physical and physiological qualities, technical skills, tactical awareness, and football intelligence are critical contributors to individual and team success (figure 21.2).

Relative Contribution of Physical Performance

Similar to other field-based team sports, individual Australian football player performance is difficult to assess. Indeed, there are innumerable constructs including physical activity capacities, tactical awareness, technical skill involvements, and skill efficiency that contribute to overall performance (figure 21.3). Certainly, high-level performance in professional Australian football relies on well-developed physical, technical, and tactical abilities (39).

It is logical that players develop fitness qualities to cope with the worst-case scenarios (i.e., repeated-sprint bouts, repeated high-intensity bouts, or short periods of intense running) that may appear in match play. It also follows that increased fitness levels are advantageous for facilitating recovery from these highly demanding efforts. Additionally, with the recent reduction and cap on the number of player interchanges permitted during games (which reduces the number of rest periods available during games), it is becoming increasingly more important to prepare highly trained players with the fitness capacities

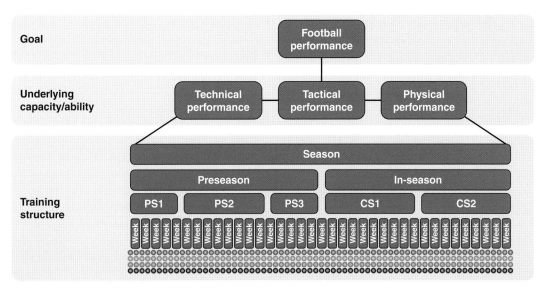

Figure 21.2 The constructs of Australian football performance and the underlying training structure that provides the basis for developing these constructs in professional Australian football. PS: preseason; CS: competition season.

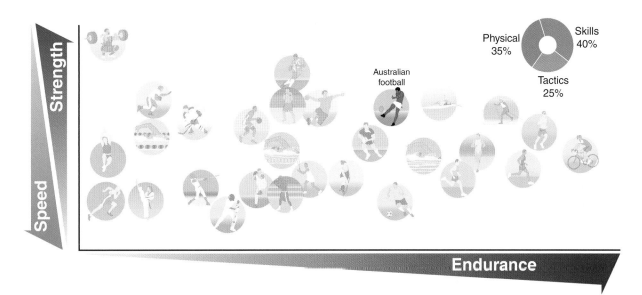

Figure 21.3 The position of the Australian football player on the three axes illustrates the relative importance of the three main physical capacities of importance for elite participation in Australian football, acknowledging that this varies slightly between positions. Outside of critical psychological aspects and team chemistry components, which are difficult to quantify, the pie chart shows the general relative importance of skills (40%), tactical awareness (25%), and physical capacities (35%) for Australian football success.

Adapted from G.A. Nader, "Concurrent Strength and Endurance Training: From Molecules to Man," *Medicine & Science in Sports & Exercise* 38, no. 11 (2006): 1965-1970.

to endure the arduous demands of match play for longer. Therefore, high-intensity interval training (HIIT) is an essential aspect of preparing Australian football players.

It is well established that players are required to travel large distances at high average speeds with significant high-speed running essential to perform well in professional Australian football (15, 16, 26, 41). Similarly, sprinting, accelerations, and repeated high-intensity efforts have also been reported to be important for Australian football performance, with increased requirements at the higher competition levels (15, 26, 41) compared to subelite (1) or youth (9) competitions. Indeed, highly trained AFL players on average complete ~29±8 sprints during match play (15, 41), which is ~1 sprint every 3 min. Notably, peak speeds achieved during match play were 29.8±1.7 km/h with peak values of 34.6 km/h. Varley et al. (41) showed that 45% of these sprint efforts were completed with >30 s recovery, showing they occur during intense periods of play and therefore may be important to performance. Professional AFL players have been shown to have a high frequency of high-speed running efforts (i.e., efforts >19.8 km/h, $0.8±0.2$ min^{-1}), which is approximately double the rate reported in professional soccer ($0.4±0.2$ min^{-1}) and rugby league players ($0.4±0.2$ min^{-1}) (41).

In addition to understanding the average demands of competition, it is also important to have insight into the most difficult periods of activity (or worst-case scenarios) in match play. A recent study reported on the duration-specific running intensities during match play and demonstrated the average speed (i.e., m/min) and peak high-speed relative distances to be greatest when data were analyzed in 1 min periods with midfielders compared to other positions, peaking at 223±35 m/min and 110±35 m/min for 1 min epochs (16). Notably, however, the acceleration and deceleration demands were similar across positions during these periods. Like most sports, these acceleration and deceleration efforts, which are metabolically demanding, occur ~4 times more frequently than sprinting. The reason for the increased frequency of acceleration and decelerations is that Australian football players are rarely provided the opportunity to reach maximal velocity due to spatial constraints imposed by field dimensions or opposing players (25). Therefore, the ability to generate speed over a short distance or duration is vital for successful moments in play (i.e., to beat an opponent or to make a break in play).

Both repeated-sprint (RS) and repeated high-intensity effort (RHIE) bouts have been used to classify intense moments in match play and have been suggested to be important for performance. A RS bout was defined as three or more sprint efforts with less than 21 s recovery between efforts (38), while RHIE bouts have been defined as consisting of three or more maximal acceleration, sprint, or collision efforts with less than 21 s recovery (2, 41). Despite general reports that RS and RHIE bouts during match play are important in Australian football performance, few studies have investigated the prevalence of these events in match play. Indeed, Varley

et al. (41) reported that professional Australian football players complete less than one RS bout in each match, suggesting that these are rare events. However, RHIE bouts were more frequent, observed once every ~9.5 min, suggesting that this classification might be a more important focus than RS bouts for training and preparation activities. This relatively high number of RHIE bouts in Australian football match play provides insight into the potential physical stress imposed on players during competition.

In summary, there are many constructs of physical performance that have been reported to be important for Australian football performance, including endurance capacity, high-intensity running, sprinting, accelerations and decelerations, as well as collisions, sport-specific skills, and RHIE. Determining the relative contribution of these to Australian football performance is difficult as recent studies highlight the complex interactions between individual players' fitness characteristics, mediating factors around match play (i.e., opponent, draw, time of season, etc.), and other match contextual factors (10, 23, 24, 35, 40, 42) on these variables in match play. Regardless, it is clear that the physical activity demands are high at greater levels of competition and are generally greater in midfielders and hybrid backs and forwards compared to tall forwards, tall backs, and rucks. It is also clear that the activity demands for professional Australian football are high, and players should prepare specifically for these so that they can perform in competitions. However, current understanding also shows that professional Australian football players do not necessarily need to be the fittest athletes, but are required to develop sufficient fitness levels (which are high) to cope with the demands of the match and their opponents and also be able to execute their tactical role and skills efficiently.

Targets of Physical Performance of Australian Football

The physical performance targets of Australian football players as a whole are similar across positions; however, subtle differences exist among midfields, talls, and ruckmen. These differences can influence our HIIT targets and therefore must be carefully considered before we choose our training weapons.

Midfield and Hybrid Players

Midfield and hybrid players—mobile forwards and backs—usually have the greatest locomotor and activity demands in professional Australian football (15, 16). This is likely a result of their nomadic role, which allows them greater pitch space to move in (midfielders) or demand to consistently lead up the ground to make space, or as a marking target before sprinting back to contests of the targeted tall players (for mobile forwards and backs). Accordingly, well-developed anthropometric characteristics, including low levels of body fat and a high proportion of muscle mass, are essential for their performance (3, 4). Similarly, high levels of speed and explosive muscular power are important physical factors for performance at the highest level (4). During match play, depending on their position and tactical strategy, professional players typically cover ~10.2 to 16.8 km (with individual reports of players traveling >17 km in a game). In addition, players execute hundreds of high-intensity actions in the form of high-speed runs (for a total of 1035 ± 385 m >19.9 km/h), accelerations and decelerations, changes of direction, collisions and tackles, and sport-specific skills such as kicking, handballing, marking, contesting with opponents, and engaging in ruck contests. Finally, since the typical playing time is 98 ± 15 min, endurance capacities are critical. Indeed, a well-developed aerobic system is likely to be beneficial, contributing not only to acute high-intensity performance but also to metabolic recovery between the explosive efforts associated with successful match performance. Accordingly, midfield and hybrid players should be exposed to sufficient training volume to develop endurance capacity and repeated bouts of higher-speed running with acceleration demands so they are best prepared for the worst-case scenarios of running requirements on match day.

Talls

Tall forwards are often used as kicking targets in attack and are often marked by similar-sized defensive players from the opposing team (backs). It is often the role of the tall backs to negate the tall forwards and to spoil their marking attempts during air duels, often resulting in jostling and intense body collisions. To counteract this, tall forwards often complete repeated leads to become marking targets during attacking plays, or alternatively move up the field to create space behind them that allows faster and often more agile forwards to run into to create scoring opportunities. Tall backs typically have lower average speed and high speeds during games, likely due to their role to maintain defensive structures

even when the ball progresses forward. Indeed, they may often zone off following a long lead from a tall forward if it is determined that the forward has run into space that is not considered dangerous for an impending attack of the opposing team. Additionally, with the recent cap in player rotations, tall backs tend to have greater match time than other positions, which may explain their lower relative speeds during matches. Due to these demands, training methods for talls should focus on developing the ability to repeat high-intensity efforts including actions such as jostling with opponents and recovering from these bouts.

Ruckmen

The rucks, usually the tallest players on any team, have the specific role of contesting any restart of play. This occurs when the ball is bounced or thrown up by an umpire and the rucks contest with the opposing ruckmen to jump palm or tip off the ball to their surrounding teammates in an attempt to clear the ball into more space. Due to their height and/or marking ability, rucks have as part of their strategic role to position themselves behind the play to become a tall target to cut off rebounding attacks from the opposing team. They also need to arrive at many contests due to their specific role in ball-ups (stoppages) and boundary throw-ins. Because of this, rucks have few rests on the interchange bench and relatively high playing times. Due to these tactical roles, rucks have lower running speeds and less higher-speed running than other positions. They are also involved in many aerial contests, which results in frequent jumping, colliding, and jostling with opponents. Accordingly, training programs should focus on developing the ability to repeatedly compete in aerial contests, including jostling and making frequent body contact. Additionally, they need to develop the capacity to repeat these efforts over long periods.

Key Weapons, Manipulations, and Surveillance Tools

The weapons we use refer to the HIIT formats applied in our programs. We use specific weapons to target the desired physiological responses and physical adaptations, while the surveillance tools refer to the system and tools that we use to monitor the individual responses to those weapons. In this section, we present the different HIIT weapons that we have used in preparing professional Australian football players along with their manipulations and our approaches for monitoring training effectiveness.

HIIT Weapons

Due to the vast demands of the competition, it is essential to target all types of HIIT sessions in Australian football (see figure 1.5; Buchheit and Laursen (6)): type 1, metabolic O_2 system; type 2, metabolic O_2 system + neuromuscular; type 3, metabolic O_2 + anaerobic system; type 4, metabolic O_2 + anaerobic and neuromuscular; and type 5, metabolic anaerobic and neuromuscular (7). Similar to most other team sports, the majority of training comes from skill-based training in the form of modified match play, open- and closed-skill training drills, and game-based HIIT (GBHIIT) or small-sided games (SSGs; ~80%, both pre- and in-season). However, short intervals (~10%, both pre- and in-season, for individual top-ups and rehabilitation), RST (~5%, both pre- and in-season, for individual top-ups and players in rehabilitation), long intervals (~5%, preseason only), and rarely SIT (<1%) are also used (figure 21.4). While the specific proportional use of the various HIIT weapons may be different across the various

groups working in Australian football, it would be highly likely that a mixed-methods approach to deploying these weapons is used in all those working at the professional level.

Manipulations of Interval Training Variables

The mode, duration, intensity, time, and recovery characteristics of each HIIT format can be manipulated to elicit desired acute physiological and locomotor responses. The careful manipulation of these variables and placement of HIIT within the physical training programs can be used to prepare professional Australian football players for performance.

HIIT With Long Intervals (Outdoor)

Longer HIIT intervals are regularly applied during the preseason period when there are requirements to develop cardiopulmonary capacity. Accordingly, there is greater emphasis in prescribing these weapons during preseason phases 1 and 2 (2× per week with ~72 h between sessions; figure 21.2). These sessions are easily conducted in a controlled manner with players using distances to control speeds. These sessions are usually conducted over interval distances of 800 to 1600 m at speeds of 90% to 100% of maximal aerobic speed (MAS), repeated 3 to 5 times with short breaks (<3 min) (type 4). Active recovery between efforts is applied to players who have greater need to develop cardiovascular fitness or when there are longer intervals between efforts. Since our squads are large (i.e., 40 to 46 players), we divide the larger group into smaller groups according to fitness levels, and these groups pace themselves so that they reach specific cones (usually coded by color) at appropriate times. These drills are usually applied at the end of training sessions once football-specific loadings have been applied, and the drills for individual players are modified for volume according to injury risk and fitness targets. This approach allows coaches to follow their tactical periodization approach and to develop technical and tactical abilities while allowing individual players to meet training load and fitness targets.

Some manipulations of longer-interval training sessions have been achieved by using similar interval work bout durations and work:rest ratios of activity requiring high-intensity intermittent running that represent worst-case scenario activity profiles observed in match play. As an example, we have used match activity data obtained from competition to

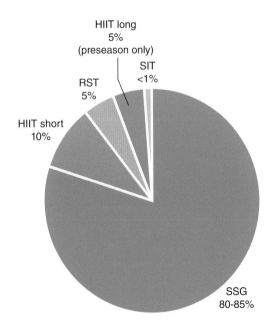

Figure 21.4 Percentage of the different HIIT formats (weapons) used throughout the annual season in Australian football. Game-based HIIT (GBHIIT) or small-sided games (SSGs) make up about 80%, short intervals about 10%, RST about 5%, long intervals about 5% (preseason only), and rarely SIT (<1%).

develop audio files that provide verbal instructions to undertake activity observed during intense periods of match play (i.e., to provide instructions to stand, walk, run, jog, run, fast run, and sprint in sequences observed during intense periods of match play). This audio file is then played over loudspeakers or with a personal iPod and players are tracked with global positioning system (GPS) devices (with heart rate [HR] monitoring). While less controllable than constant velocity HIIT, this approach provides increased movement specificity (e.g., 2 to 4 sprints with accelerations and decelerations in 4 min bouts) and high cardiovascular and anaerobic metabolic stimulus (type 4 targets).

HIIT With Short Intervals

In Australian football, short-interval HIIT is an effective training weapon. The prescriptive variables can be manipulated to carefully control the running speeds, neuromuscular load, and anaerobic contribution during the session to target specific physiologic targets. Indeed, these HIIT formats can be manipulated to meet type 1, 2, 3, or 4 targets. While we use these most regularly during the preseason, they can also be prescribed during the in-season when additional HIIT is required. These sessions are also commonly applied in rehabilitation and form much of the basis of the return-to-sport protocols following injury (depending on the nature of the injury). They are also effective for adding at the end of training sessions to help players meet individual load goals for high-speed running and neuromuscular load.

In the early phases of the preseason, short-interval HIIT sessions that meet target type 1 can be useful for reintroducing interval training after the layoff. For example, 3 sets of 5 intervals of 10 to 15 s work intervals at 100% to 110% MAS with 10 to 15 s passive recovery are well tolerated aerobic sessions. These prescriptions help players avoid reaching high peak speeds and fast accelerations and can be completed after football training without overstressing the neuromuscular system. Different formats can then be used once players adapt to training so that type 2, 3, and 4 targets are met as we move through preseason. For example, we find that once early preseason adaptations have occurred, we commonly apply short-interval HIIT weapons of 15/15 s and 20/20 s at 120% MAS. Players cope well with these interval durations but they tend to have difficulty maintaining running technique during longer-duration short-interval HIIT sessions (especially at the end of demanding skill-based sessions). Indeed, when developing speed endurance, we rarely have players run at speeds >130% MAS to assist them with maintaining form and developing movement efficiency when experiencing fatigue. We reduce work:rest ratios during short HIIT and use passive recovery to reduce anaerobic load, while increasing both work-interval intensity and the work:rest ratio to increase anaerobic contributions.

Short-interval HIIT can be modified by adding in changes of direction, ball carries and bounces, and position-specific running patterns to increase match specificity and modulate the neuromuscular loading (e.g., move from type 1 to 2 or type 3 to 4). However, careful adjustments need to be taken into account when developing the distances and duration of efforts, as when multiple changes in direction and effort durations are included in a bout, the neuromuscular load can be substantial; thus, significantly reducing the amount of higher speed running completed may be necessary in this situation. We recommend trialing new short HIIT drills on staff or smaller groups of players with stochastic work efforts or changes of direction at various angles before implementing broadly.

We also regularly apply short-interval HIIT weapons to ensure players meet higher-speed running targets during the season. For example, we have set weekly high-speed running exposure targets based on within-individual exposure history, acute:chronic workload ratio, and the period of time between match play. These factors, combined with collective experience from the sport science team and coaching staff, alongside the monitoring data, allow us to titrate training goals and manipulate the training stimulus on an individual level.

Repeated-Sprint Training

Although less common than long- and short-interval HIIT formats, RST weapons can be used in the middle and latter stages of the preseason or during the rehabilitation process in long-term injured players. RST can be useful for developing the ability to do mechanical work with changes of direction, rather than developing higher speeds. Indeed, we often implement RST using a variety of change of direction (COD) with progressions (sometimes with multiple COD in an effort to reflect match running patterns, type 5), differences in starting positions for each effort, and with varying running patterns. We also include football-specific skills in these efforts. For example, we may use stationary, rolling, and contested starts (i.e., starting while jostling with an opponent) to increase the complexity of the drill. This approach allows players to develop the ability to repeat high-intensity efforts but in a match-specific context. This type of training is completed in low volumes (i.e., 2 or 3 sets of 3 or 4 efforts) with short-effort durations (4 to 8 s). To increase anaerobic responses, sprint effort and recovery durations are increased (type 5), while shorter recovery periods between efforts are used to increase the aerobic stimulus (type 4).

Game-Based High-Intensity Interval Training

GBHIIT forms the large majority of training content in Australian football and is the central focus of any team's preparation strategy. This type of training is made up of closed- and open-skill drills including SSG training (both handball and kicking SSGs) (11, 18, 27). The main objectives of this work are to develop team strategy, optimize player positioning, develop collective cohesion and timing (in offense and defense and transition between these), and manipulate the stimulus by altering a wide range of prescriptive variables. While the prescription of GBHIIT is typically the domain of expert coaches, where the main focus is not to provide an HIIT stimulus, we like to quantify and understand the demands of these activities via GPS, HR, and skill coding to better understand the overall stimulus provided through this training. Closed-skill training drills are easy to manipulate according to traditional HIIT prescription guidelines (6, 7) and can be used to hit all targets (types 1 to 5), but match simulation and SSGs can be more complex. To overcome this, we have quantified the specific training dose and responses to each type of training drill (open and closed) and use this information as part of decision-making when selecting complementary HIIT. We also assess the duration-intensity relationship of various exercise intensity markers in these drills, which allows us to predict the stimulus provided from a training session before it is delivered. This approach allows us to assist coaches in choosing the GBHIIT exercises that meet both technical/tactical and physical goals. However, GBHIIT can be limited, and the typical responses within a group may be variable, and therefore it is not as efficient at targeting specifically desired training outcomes. As such, we complement this training with more tightly constrained HIIT training drills to ensure desired physiological and physical responses are elicited for each session. After all, a mixed-methods approach to choosing our training methods is likely the best approach for a team sport such as Australian football, as performance in matches requires a wide range of physical abilities and physiological capacities.

While generally of lower intensity than open-skill training drills, closed-skill drills involve kicking and handballing (i.e., line drills) and can also be used to elicit desired HIIT responses through manipulating the drill duration, level of coaching, distance between marker cones, number of lines (i.e., groups), players in each group, etc. For example, cone-to-cone straight-line short-kicking drills (~25 m kick distance with 35 to 45 m run distance) can be prescribed as 5 s efforts (~35 to 45 m of running) with passive rest of about 25 s when there are 5 players in each group and can be used as a form of RST training if completed at ~130% to 160% MAS. These drills can be completed in 3 to 5 sets with short active breaks between each for coaching or drink breaks. Simple alterations can be made by reducing the numbers of players in each group, increasing the work:rest ratio and anaerobic contribution to the drill. We can also modulate the targeted responses during SSGs using different prescriptions. Indeed, similar effects of manipulation of SSG design constraints that have been widely reported in soccer are also apparent in Australian football (22, 33). Specifically, in addition to typical interval bout prescription variables (6, 7), closed-drill design constraints include the player number, pitch size, the number of balls active in a drill, level or extent of opponent pressure, rule modification, as well as coaching feedback to elicit the targeted response for each session (18). In open drills, we can alter rules around the movement path of the ball, role of specific players in drills, as well as positioning or setup at specific parts of the drill. To fully understand the impact of the variation of these prescriptive variables on physical and physiological responses is difficult due to the impact of the number of degrees of freedom of these choices. Nonetheless, there are some rules of thumb that we follow when we prescribe training and fine-tune drill design.

We have found that locomotor and HR responses during match-simulation skill drills best replicate match demands when played on large-pitch areas (i.e., full-sized field drills) (type 4). Moreover, when these are completed with fewer players, the higher speed running, cardiovascular, and kicking demands increase markedly. However, when pitch area is reduced, higher speed running and sprint efforts are restricted, but accelerations and decelerations increase, resulting in high neuromechanical loading along with increased collision loads.

Match-simulation drills can be used to increase endurance capacity of players when completed in multiple (i.e., 3 to 5) shorter interval bouts (<6 min), but short rest efforts between intervals (<3 min) can alter the neuromuscular and locomotor demands through drill design. To increase the aerobic stimulus, we use longer drill bouts (>8 min) with larger field size, and locomotor demand is increased when there is no inferred pressure placed on the ball carrier. To reduce the running demands but increase acceleration and deceleration demands, we reduce the pitch size, increase player number, or increase the pressure placed on the ball carrier (e.g., handball games with shadow pressure, type 4). To meet type 3 targets, longer bouts of lower space drills at lower speeds can be prescribed. These type 3 drills are better suited to training sessions in which neuromuscular fatigue is being minimized. In contrast, training drills that have greater area available to encourage players to break defensive lines by running and carrying the ball, as well as taking longer leads, promote higher speed running, but can result in greater neuromuscular fatigue and are best suited for in-season to midweek training sessions.

Load Surveillance and Monitoring Tools

With the recent developments of wearable player tracking technologies, it is now a relatively simple task to track the training in both training and match play for all players during every session. Despite the ease of measurement, however, we still pay particular care to methods that we use to collect, treat, and interpret the data we obtain from our players. Additionally, we also aim for a simple approach to our athlete monitoring strategies so that we don't waste precious resources or time in the daily data tsunami (12). We are also careful to follow measures that have established validity, with known levels of reliability (i.e., measurement noise) and with scientific support or strong proof of concept for their use. We also take care to get advice from coaches on what information they value from our monitoring (13).

The goal of monitoring is to predict, measure, and track changes in individual daily locomotor load. We also use the acute/chronic ratio (20) as a heuristic to guide relative risk of any changes in planned training for the immediate and future training sessions. We

also monitor individual players' exposure rates to the number of sprint efforts to check that players regularly exceed >90% of their best match sprint speed during training throughout the season. Again, while this is a simple heuristic without established empirical support, the general intent is to have players achieve these speeds in two separate training sessions each week to protect against neuromuscular detraining. HR is also monitored during most training sessions that include a metabolic component (i.e., skills and football-related and HIIT-conditioning sessions), and we collect RPEs after all sessions. HR is used to track the cardiorespiratory response, and we pay specific attention to the mean heart rate but also the time spent in higher heart rate zones (i.e., >90 individual HRmax) over time. This is particularly useful in the preseason period or following a long-term injury layoff when we are aiming to develop cardiovascular fitness within individual players. The session-RPE training load is used to assess the overall load experienced by the players, and it can be analyzed by training type and assessed for temporal changes within individuals and teams (see also chapter 8). The session-RPE method has been validated for Australian football (36) and is likely the most valid measure of internal training load. The session-RPE load and intensity measures are interpreted in the context of planned training load and other measures of external training load determined from GPS (i.e., locomotor loads such as total and absolute distances and high-speed running) and other microsensors (i.e., accelerometers).

Training Status Surveillance and Monitoring Tools

Our athlete monitoring system has been developed over more than 20 years and its practical application and theoretical basis has been described elsewhere (14). We have tried most monitoring variables (including expensive and invasive blood measures, heart rate variability, a variety of neuromuscular screening measures, and countless markers derived from GPS technology) and have found that most variables were unsuitable for *our* environment, where we monitor ~46 young males daily in a time-poor environment. Following considerable trial and error (lots of time and *many errors!*), we have arrived at a simple system that includes mostly non- or low-invasive measures such as session-RPE (19), GPS-load monitoring, wellness (8, 29), exercise HR (fitness) (5, 8), and simple neuromuscular screening tests such as groin squeeze and clinical screening feedback from medical staff. The most critical aspect to the success of this system is the buy-in from players and coaching staff, and therefore we require involvement from key decision-making stakeholders, including senior coaching staff (senior coach or senior assistant coach), performance staff, and medical staff. To monitor an individual player's readiness to perform and/or to assess changes in fitness or training adaptation, we monitor the locomotor (GPS-related), HR, and RPE responses to either standardized SSGs (32), match simulations, or submaximal shuttle runs (8). In our analysis, we examine the relationship between changes in the internal:external load ratio, where the greater the load/min and lower the HR and RPE indicate an improved status. We then often use these individual responses (in conjunction with other wellness and neuromuscular screening measures) to determine future training or treatment prescription. An example of the team session-RPE loading is shown in figure 21.5.

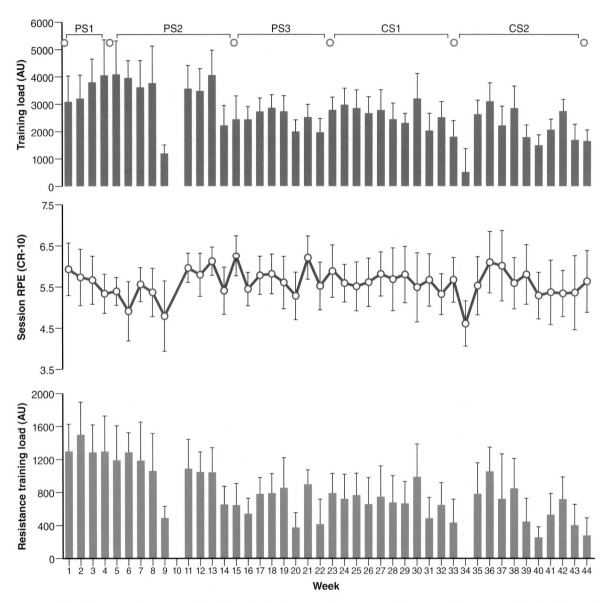

Figure 21.5 Sample team session-RPE loads for overall training (top panel), weekly training intensity (middle panel), and resistance training (bottom panel) during a professional Australian Football League season. PS: preseason; CS: competition season.

Strategies for Structuring the Training Program Using HIIT

Strategies for structuring HIIT programming in Australian football may be largely determined by various controllable and uncontrollable factors, before proper progression and periodization can be appropriately implemented. This section discusses some of the nuances of training program design and implementation of HIIT in Australian football.

Controllable and Uncontrollable Factors

In fulltime professional Australian football, there are numerous training and nontraining factors that place time constraints on training scheduling. Outside of match time and location (both uncontrollable), the strongest influence on program design is the coaching philosophy, which places a high priority on technical and tactical development. Therefore, the most viable way to introduce HIIT into a program is to add these different HIIT components to existing technical and tactical sessions. To achieve this, careful monitoring is required to understand the precise nature of these sessions. Once this is achieved, we can assist coaches with developing the timing and dosing of specific training, and then we can plan any additional HIIT requirements around these. Through this approach, coaches are able to deliver the technical and tactical training required to meet performance objectives, while also being able to provide appropriate physical training.

Program Structure and Progression

In contrast to popular theory, traditional periodization models of cyclical loading and unloading are uncommon in professional Australian football. The preseason period in professional Australian football is relatively long compared to most other team sports. The preseason period can be 15 to 19 wk (including preseason competition) and is usually divided into 2 or 3 shorter macrocycles with short rest periods between each (figure 21.2). In the first macrocycle, the focus is transitioning the players back to football training after ~2 mo of self-directed off-season training. Accordingly, caution is taken to provide progressive stimulus overload (in duration and intensity), but not to the levels that increase injury risk. We have found this to be a period of higher injury risk, especially when new technical and tactical training

drills are being introduced to the program and with an increased variation in the training status of the players returning from the off-season period (see the case study at the end of the chapter). Additionally, since players do not tend to complete a high load of intense off-line or agility training during this introductory period, we control kicking loads by manipulation of pitch size (i.e., smaller pitch area for fewer shorter kicks) and direct instruction and carefully reintroduce high-intensity actions. We also focus on type 1 HIIT targets during the early phase to avoid overloading the neuromuscular system (e.g., short intervals at 80% to 90% MAS).

In the second preseason macrocycle, the heaviest training with the greatest running volumes and resistance loads is completed (figure 21.6). Due to the lack of match play, this second phase provides the best opportunity to program increased volumes of HIIT. During this period, there is a large focus on technical and tactical training but with significant portions at high intensity. A sample weekly training schedule for the preseason period is shown in table 21.1. We aim our program to touch on all targeted qualities during the week, but with emphasis changes during the preseason. General principles are that the interval efforts should generally be reduced from longer to shorter, interval speeds increase, and the recovery time between efforts is reduced as this phase progresses. We aim to provide two sessions per week (e.g., Monday and Friday) that provide greater higher speed running distances and peak speeds (i.e., type 4 targets) and another midweek HIIT stimulus with high aerobic load but with moderate levels of higher speed running distances and lower peak speeds (type 3 targets).

An important focus for the preseason is developing a robust training base, and this is achieved by developing training continuity. Indeed, recent studies have suggested that players who complete a greater proportion of preseason training also endure higher training loads, which results in greater availability for training and selection during the competitive phase of the season (31). Finally, the third phase of preseason training is in the introduction of preseason practice matches. Clearly during this period there is a shift in programming for training to reflect the in-season training schedule, with lower training doses and decreased variability in dose; however, the emphasis for some players may be on developing physical characteristics if they have not yet been developed.

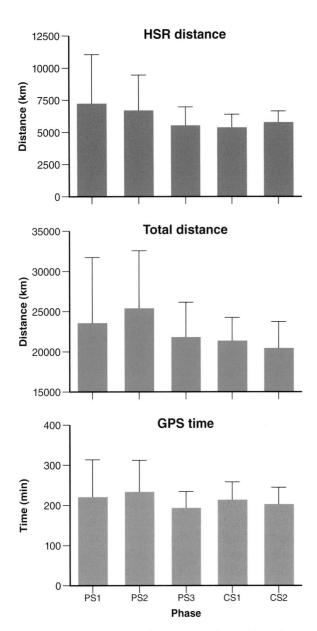

Figure 21.6 Sample GPS-derived weekly values for higher speed running (top panel), total distance (middle panel), and training duration (bottom panel) in a professional Australian Football League season. PS: preseason; CS: competition season.

During the in-season period, the periodization structure is focused on recovering from the previous match and then tapering for the next match. One priority for periodizing training during the in-season is to keep consistency in the weekly training schedule and training load. This can be challenging, especially due to the varying number of days between matches (i.e., 5 to 12 d). Accordingly, we keep a consistent structure in the weekly in-season program for the common between-match periods and this is rarely modified (table 21.2). The general goal of this structure is to allow for recovery from previous matches, to provide a stimulus between games, and then to allow for a short taper or recovery period prior to the next game. The focus of HIIT during the in-season is to complement the technical and tactical training, and we select HIIT formats that touch on the primary physiological target each week. The weekly match provides the greatest HIIT stimulus and the remainder of training is planned around this stimulus (i.e., to recover and taper before each match). Accordingly, player load management is critical and control of training dose is essential to allow for HIIT. HIIT weapons applied early in the in-season training week are targeted toward type 1 (low volume, recovery, and off-legs) and moderate volume type 3 while type 3 and 4 formats are applied ≥ 72 h after match play (i.e., midweek) after neuromuscular recovery has occurred from the previous match.

A recent case study from the AFL shows decreases in training load and intensity and increases in the proportion of recovery activities during the in-season period (30). This approach to training periodization is supported by laboratory research showing that physical performance during prolonged, high-intensity intermittent exercise is improved when lower training doses are completed between matches completed 5 d apart (37). Additionally, during the in-season, ~50% to 55% of weekly running load is obtained during games, whereas the remainder is obtained by technical and tactical training (34). These data show that there are few opportunities to add isolated HIIT sessions into a weekly schedule. This practical limitation can result in players not receiving adequate stimulus from HIIT, which may increase injury risk (17, 28). Therefore, to mitigate this risk, we ensure that adequate high-speed running and sprint efforts are completed, and we top up training with training drills (e.g., end of warm-ups or SSGs or technical and tactical drills). This approach can protect players from injury and prevent detraining these capacities.

Incorporation of HIIT

In our experience, the primary driver of training periodization and load prescription for professional

Table 21.1　Sample Preseason Training Schedule

	Monday	Tuesday	Wednesday	Thursday	Friday	Saturday	Sunday
a.m.	Warm-up Submax HR test Speed technique Skills Recovery (Hydro)	Lower weights Physio treatment/ massage	Warm-up Speed technique Skills Recovery (Hydro)	Off	Warm-up Speed technique Skills Recovery (Hydro)	Individually targeted sessions: • Cross-training • Weights • HIIT running	Off
	Lunch	Lunch	Lunch		Lunch		
p.m.	Weights Physio treatment/ massage	Off	Weights Physio treatment/ massage	Off	Weights Physio treatment/ massage	Off	Off

Table 21.2　Sample In-Season Training Schedule

	Saturday	Sunday	Monday	Tuesday	Wednesday	Thursday	Friday
a.m.	Off	Sleep in Individual recovery	Screening	Warm-up/activation/speed technique Skills	Off	Warm-up/activation/speed technique Skills	Warm-up/activation/speed technique Captain run
p.m.	Game Post-game recovery	Off	Recovery rotations (massage, hydrotherapy, mobility)	Weights Physio treatment/ massage	Off	Weights Physio treatment/ massage	Off

Australian football comes from the head coach in collaboration with high performance and medical staff. Similar to most team sports, a technical and tactical emphasis in Australian football is of most importance (figure 21.3) and is the first aspect of a training program prescribed. Once the coaches have planned the football-focused technical and tactical training sessions, we then develop team and individual player training plans that may incorporate HIIT. The session planning is done to meet the individual goals for training load (i.e., distances, high-speed running, sprinting distances, and acceleration efforts). To achieve this, we use a bespoke training database system to estimate training dose provided by the training drills planned by the coach. This is achieved by estimating loads (i.e., total distances, higher speed running, sprint number, and accelerations based on historical data) described here: https://vimeo.com/161594888. We then program additional training (i.e., HIIT) around this. If required, we usually incorporate HIIT into training sessions both at the team and individual levels at the end of the session.

When planning HIIT sessions, we consider several factors including the recent training completed, the well-being status of the athlete, the athlete's training goals, and the planned training stimulus during the weekly microcycle. Various targets are selected depending on the needs of the individual or team. We also follow several rules of thumb such as planning to avoid on-legs HIIT sessions in the first 48 hours following matches, as this may compromise recovery and subsequent performance. We also avoid programming high-speed HIIT sessions following fatiguing lower-body resistance training sessions or when players report increased levels of lower-body soreness. We also consider the demands of the other training in which HIIT is incorporated and the loading patterns within the weekly cycle, as these factors influence the metabolic and neuromuscular responses to HIIT (6, 7). In reality, the positioning of HIIT sessions within a training day or session is largely determined in consultation with coaches. With the exception of planned periods during the preseason, coaches are often reticent to train skills following heavily fatiguing HIIT, and as a consequence, isolated

HIIT sessions are mostly conducted after main skill-focused training. However, we are also careful to avoid HIIT sessions in which peak speeds are reached at the end of sessions as injury risk may be increased. However, we are also mindful of the protective effect of high-speed sessions so these are programmed around periods when players have less acute residual fatigue and muscle soreness. Indeed, we often plan higher speed days twice a week and demanding sessions with lower speed stimulus between these sessions. Carefully selecting skill-based training drills and manipulating the constraints of training drills described in the section above achieve this. Finally, when heavy HIIT sessions are programmed, these are often positioned in the weekly microcycle immediately prior to days of rest to allow players the best chance to recover from residual fatigue and soreness that may result from these sessions.

In-season programming is largely dictated by the competition draw and travel requirements. Other factors such as recent and acute training loads and expected match difficulty can also influence decision-making. Similar to preseason loading structures, we attempt to maintain a level of consistency in the nature and frequency of HIIT stimulus. During the in-season, it is vitally important to ensure players are sufficiently loaded to maintain their fitness and be prepared for performance (i.e., matches). This requires a highly individualized HIIT prescription, using a combination of different HIIT types and formats, but we avoid on-legs HIIT in the 48 to 72 h post-match.

Sample Training Programs

As discussed, we program HIIT sessions 3 or 4 times per week in preseason depending on individual needs (i.e., athlete's training age, current physical fitness, and expected competition demands). For players with nonmodified training programs, we attempt to provide some level of polarization in the HIIT stimulus within a typical week. Early in preseason, a Monday to Friday HIIT session may consist of a mixed-HIIT format running with a variety of acceleration and deceleration and speed work (as a part of warm-up); a selection of short (15 to 25 s) efforts at 100% to 120% MAS, for 5 to 10 min of work, types 3 and 4; and longer intervals (2 to 6 min efforts) for 4 to 8 bouts at 80% to 100% MAS, type 3, with ~4 to 5 km per session from high-intensity training. The interval effort durations are usually over longer distances to allow an increase in higher

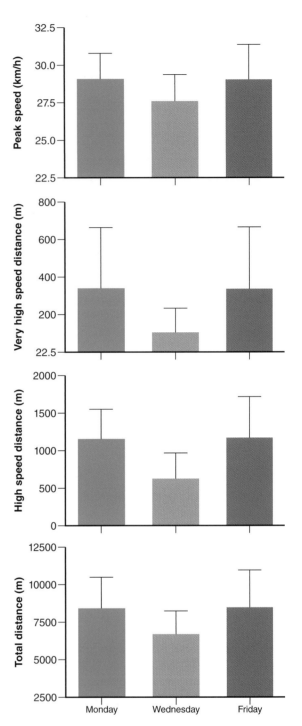

Figure 21.7 Locomotor data for main preseason sessions involving HIIT for peak speed (km/h; top panel), very high-speed running distances (>25 km/h; upper middle panel), high-speed running distance (>19.9 km/h; lower middle panel), and total distance (bottom panel).

speed running and the achievement of high peak speeds. The Wednesday session is a shorter HIIT session and may involve short-interval formats with reduced rest periods between bouts and role-specific run conditioning drills. This results in reduced higher speed running and lower peak speeds for these sessions compared with the Monday to Friday sessions (type 4 to type 3) (figure 21.7). As we move toward the season, there is a tendency to use shorter interval durations, with reduced rest periods between efforts. We also tend to develop position-specific drills that reflect position-specific running patterns. For example, hybrids, forwards, and backs develop RHIE and ability to hold high speeds, while midfields

work on repeated high-intensity efforts, but with greater focus on acceleration and deceleration with less space to move in.

While we appreciate there are a number of different ways we can skin the cat to prepare players for the season, this approach allows for HIIT to be manipulated based on the stimulus provided from technical and tactical training (i.e., the coach's main priority). During the in-season, the opportunity for HIIT is limited and is mostly achieved through specific GBHIIT. However, more generic HIIT conditioning can be used to top up high-speed running, accelerated running, and exposure to near-peak sprinting speed.

CASE STUDY

This case study is more a story about when things go wrong and the consequences of periodization errors that can arise with HIIT. The events we describe took place relatively early in our careers and, despite the negative consequences, the experience provided an invaluable learning experience for all involved.

We had just completed the first phase of preseason training and the players had returned from their two-week Christmas break in great shape and good spirits. It was the third main training day after our break, and the players looked fresh and had been performing well. They had coped well with two heavy training sessions in the past four days. The first part of the morning plan was a 2 km trial, and many players ran personal best times. We were quite bullish about the state of the players and following the great fitness test results the expectation for a good quality session was high. On the back of these results, we planned a long football-focused training session that included high-intensity technical and tactical training and match-simulation exercises. It was a hot day (93 °F/33.9 °C).

Probably due to the combined effects of residual fatigue from the time trial and the hot environmental conditions, the skill execution of the players was poor during their skills session. Our training drills weren't being completed to the expected standard (intensity and skill errors), and the coaches were becoming frustrated. As a consequence of the poor-quality session, the players were instructed to repeat the drills for longer periods of time until they met expected standards. Ultimately, the planned skills session ended up running much longer than we had planned (47% longer!). And not only that, the day wasn't finished yet.

With coaches still frustrated from the poor skills session, the players were directed to perform a character-building grappling session. This session consisted of about 30 min of technically and physically demanding grappling and body contact work. It was again a very intense session and emotions were high, to the level that one player actually fractured a clavicle! Finally, after a 1 h break for recovery and fueling, the players finished the day with their usual 45 min resistance training session.

It was obvious to the staff that the session had cooked our players. Despite this, the session was explained as being a character-building one, and we quickly moved on to plan the next session. While we were aware that we'd broken a simple rule of training, we were confident we could recover from the session and began planning the next required piece of the programming puzzle.

As might now be expected, the next day's monitoring data clearly revealed that the players hadn't recovered well. The players reported the highest soreness and fatigue levels for the preseason. Our initial plan was to have a longer type 4 HIIT interval session planned for the day, and as a result, we decided to reduce the volume and effort distance so as to reduce the loads and associated injury risk. But even this wasn't enough. Even with these modifications, two players finished the session with calf injuries, while another sprained his toe ligaments! It was a disaster.

Fundamentally, we broke a basic rule of training. We had given our players a large spike in training load, and despite being aware of this, we backed it up with an HIIT session the next day. Retrospectively, this training error is obvious, but at the time we thought we had handled it appropriately.

That training error had a significant effect on the rest of our preseason. We became extra cautious with managing player availability in the weeks following, and as a result we removed HIIT run sessions from our program for the next 3 wk. This allowed us to modify training without foregoing football-related training. We did this to ensure that we had an injury-free playing roster before the season started. But the knock-on consequence of this overly cautious approach was that we weren't able to expose our players adequately so as to prepare them for the arduous AFL season.

Again in retrospect, it is not surprising that we didn't perform as well as we had expected that year. While it is difficult to directly blame our season results on one or two training errors made 2 mo before the season actually started, we are confident that it contributed, and highlights the fall-on effects from inappropriate training in elite sport. We walk a fine line sometimes. Even to this day we regret the poor load management that occurred, as we should have known better. But we did learn a valuable lesson in that great care should be taken at all stages of the preparation process. We are now well aware that even a few small training errors and lack of thought in training delivery can have substantial long-term consequences. We learned that in elite sport, we can't take our eyes off the ball!

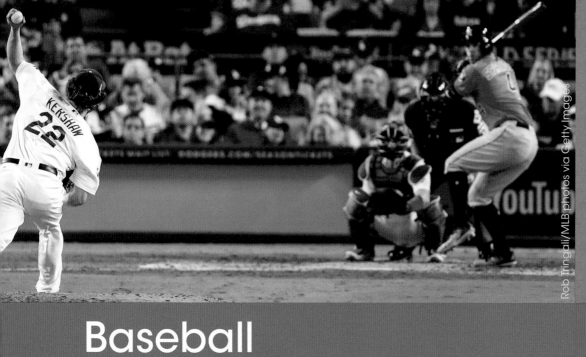

22

Baseball

• • • • • •

Robert Butler and Matt Leonard

Performance Demands of Baseball

In this chapter, we turn our focus to the sport of baseball. Beginning with the physical demands of the game that are required for success, we break down the game into its physiologic targets for practitioners, including factors that lead to sustained health and performance throughout a season, and importantly, how high-intensity interval training (HIIT) can be used to help facilitate these outcomes.

Sport Description and Factors of Winning

Baseball is a game played with a bat and a ball between two teams of nine players. The teams take turns batting the ball (offense) and fielding the ball (defense). The first professional league for the sport formed in the United States in the late 1800s, and growth of the sport has been promoted globally through the Little League World Series and the World Baseball Classic. Today it is one of the most popular sports in the United States, where as just one example, it is known that over 40 million viewers watched the seventh game final of the 2016 World Series.

The game has a fairly consistent format globally with the primary adjustment being in the number of innings. The inning is the period of play during which

each team alternates between offense and defense (3 outs). Typically the game lasts nine innings and about 3 h, however, it is often adjusted for youth games. During the Major League Baseball season, currently 162 games are played per team over 180 days, which is preceded by 27 preseason games played over the course of 29 d. An additional 20 games can be added over 30 d during the end-of-season playoffs.

The game is played on a field with two foul lines that intersect (90 degrees) at home plate. The foul lines serve as the primary boundaries of the game. There are four total bases that are 90 ft (27.4 m) apart from each other. Additional dimensions of the baseball field are illustrated in figure 22.1. The dimensions provided are for professional games, and typically these distances are scaled for youth games. The field expands from home plate forward with no official boundary limiting forward progress, however, there can be a secondary boundary in the outfield, which is required to be a minimum of 325 ft (99.1 m) from home plate on the sides and 400 ft (121.9 m) from home plate in the middle for Major League Baseball. This secondary boundary serves to designate when a home run has been hit (figure 22.1).

Players are classified into four groups depending on their location on the field. As illustrated in figure 22.2, these include outfielders, infielders, pitchers, and catchers, with the positional names indicated. Pitchers start every pitch by throwing the baseball

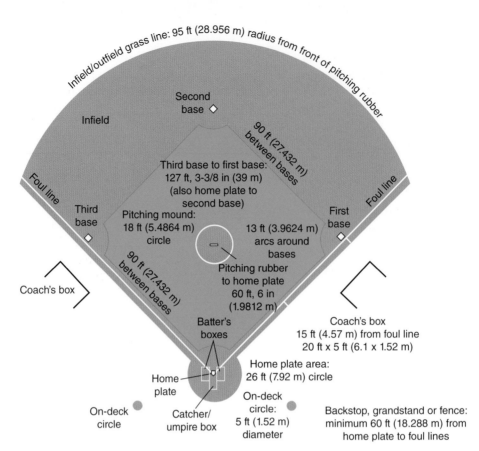

Figure 22.1 Baseball field, its dimensions, boundaries, and bases.

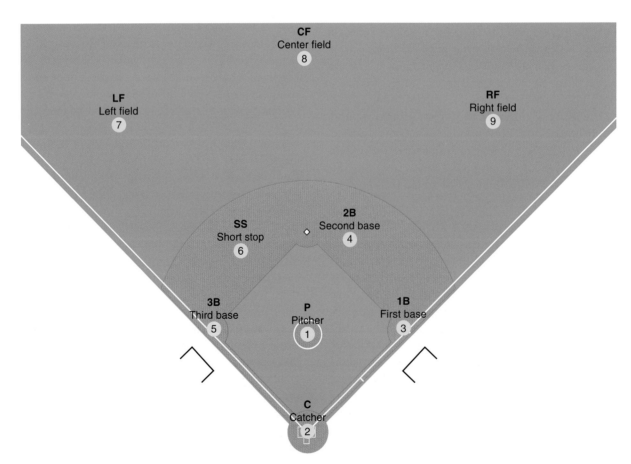

Figure 22.2 General location of the starting position of baseball player positions during most defensive situations.

from the pitching rubber to the catcher who is situated behind home plate. Traditionally the first and second basemen spread out between the space between first and second base while the shortstop and third baseman spread out in the space between second and third base (figure 22.2). There are three outfielders—left, center, and right—who typically start at a location 75% between the bases and the outfield wall in their respective areas.

When the pitcher throws the ball, a number of outcomes can occur in the game, including:

- pitch is caught by the catcher and called either a strike or a ball
- ball is hit in the air in play
- ball is hit in the air foul
- ball is hit on the ground in play
- ball is hit on the ground foul

If no contact is made between the bat and the ball during the pitching sequence, then one of two options occur: a strikeout or a walk. A strikeout occurs if three strikes are thrown by the pitcher and caught by the catcher. A strike can occur by a pitcher throwing the ball in the strike zone and not being swung at by the batter or by the batter swinging at the ball and not making contact. A walk occurs if the pitcher has four throws out of the strike zone that are not swung at by the batter. If the pitcher throws four balls before the ball is hit or three strikes are thrown, then the batter is allowed to progress to first base, or the batter is deemed "out," before the next batter comes up to bat.

If the ball is hit in the air, the fielding players can run to catch it before it hits the ground in order to record an out. If a ground ball is hit, or if a ball that is hit in the air hits the ground in fair territory before being caught, then the batter runs, without the bat, to first base and attempts to touch the base before the fielding team can gather the ball and throw it to a defensive player standing on first base. If the ball is caught at first base, or if the batter is tagged out with the ball, then the batter is out. If the batter reaches first base, or a subsequent base, prior to the ball being caught by a player touching the base, then the batter is deemed safe and the hitter remains on the base as a baserunner. During subsequent batters, the baserunners look to navigate the bases from first to second to third base to home plate in order to score a run before three outs have been recorded by the fielding team. If a ball is hit in the air that lands behind the secondary boundary, then the batter has

hit a home run and the batter is to run the bases in order along with any other baserunner who was on the bases at the time the ball was hit.

A team is at bat until recording three outs, at which point the teams switch roles to complete the inning. Full games are completed after playing nine innings. The winner of the game is determined as the team that has scored the highest number of runs at the end of nine innings. Games may go into additional innings if the teams are tied at the end of the game.

Success in the game arises from a combination of successful pitching, hitting, fielding, and situational outcomes. Particular outcomes and related factors will be described. The beginning point of each outcome starts with the ball that is thrown by the pitcher. The spin, speed, and location of pitches vary based on the pitcher's skill set as well as the tendencies of the batter he is facing. The goal is for the ball to be thrown within the strike zone (the height of the strike zone runs from the middle of the chest to just below the knees and is the width of home plate) to the catcher's glove without the batter making contact. As a result, different types of pitches with various spin patterns and speeds are used to deceive a batter as to the type of pitch being thrown to minimize the chance of being hit. If contact with the ball is made, then the goal is to keep the ball on the ground so that it has a chance to be gathered by the infielders and thrown to first base before the batter reaches the base so that an out can be recorded. To improve the chance of fielding a ground ball, adjustments are sometimes made to align the infield (known as shifting) to improve the chances of catching a ball that is hit by batters who have a greater tendency to hit the ball in specific directions. Outfielders can also be repositioned to improve the chances of catching the ball or due to situational concerns (i.e., keeping the ball in front of them). In order to improve a batter's chances to make contact with the ball, batters can vary their swing velocity as well as adjust their swing plane related to the type of pitch and the speed at which the pitch is thrown in order to maximize the chance for contact. The goal of batting typically is to hit the ball as hard as possible into a location in fair territory where a fielding player is not able to reach the ball prior to the ball hitting the ground. Once hitters make contact with the ball, they run as fast as possible around the bases until they are tagged out by an infielder holding a ball, stop at a base to prevent being tagged out, or are out at first if the ball is caught at first base by a fielder before the batter reaches first base.

Competent skill execution is imperative to game-related outcomes. The skill of pitching requires fine motor control, endurance, tactical awareness, and power to provide accurate and controlled outcomes that are coordinated with the rest of the players on the team. The average 90 mph (145 km/h) fastball takes 0.4 s to reach home plate, leaving little time for the batter and catcher to react to it. It is estimated that it takes 0.25 s to see the ball and react, which leaves 0.15 s for the motor plan to be executed regarding the type of swing to take or whether to swing at all. When the ball is struck, the average exit velocity that is produced is 86.5 mph (139.2 km/h) (MLB), giving the pitcher less than 0.5 s to react to the ball if hit back at him. As a result, reaction time is an important component of successful skill application for hitters and pitchers. In addition to reaction time, the skill of hitting requires hand–eye coordination, fine and gross motor control, rotational power, tactical awareness, and pattern recognition. When contact is made, the hitter also requires linear and curvilinear speed in navigating the base paths. Agility and change-of-direction ability are required for fielders, pitchers, and hitters under varying circumstances and greatly depend on where the ball is hit. In addition to these components, long-distance sprint ability is required for players in the outfield most often and also required by batters when balls are hit into play that allow for the hitter to advance to more than one base.

Physical Performance Contributors to Winning

Positive outcomes in baseball require a number of physical factors that span from fundamental aerobic endurance to high-level power outputs during situation-specific fielding, throwing, pitching, batting, and running. These high-level activities account for approximately 10% of the 3 h game. As a result, quick reaction times and powerful movements producing speed are a hallmark of success in the game. Figure 22.3 shows the physical requirements of positional players and the pitcher in baseball relative to other sport athletes. Between these rapid movements, there are extended periods during which focus and awareness are consistently required so that an optimal outcome can occur if a ball is hit into play. At the extreme scenario, the longest baseball game of all time took 25 innings and lasted 8 h and 6 min. With only 25 players available for a game

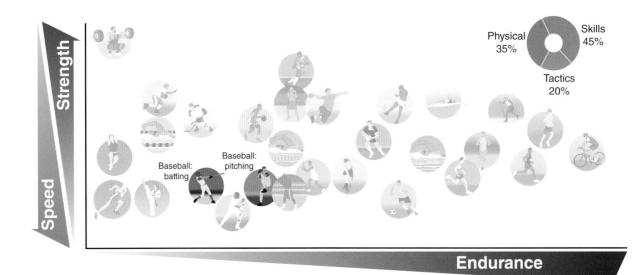

Figure 22.3 The position of baseball players (pitcher and batter) on the three axes illustrates the relative importance of the three main physical capacities of importance for elite participation, acknowledging this varies slightly between positions. Outside of critical psychological aspects and team chemistry components, which are difficult to quantify, the pie chart shows the general relative importance of skills (45%), tactical awareness (20%), and physical capacities (35%) for baseball success.

Adapted from G.A. Nader, "Concurrent Strength and Endurance Training: From Molecules to Man," *Medicine & Science in Sports & Exercise* 38, no. 11 (2006): 1965-1970.

(roughly 13 position players and 12 pitchers), the physical toll of the game can be extreme, with little time for recovery during the season (6.3 games per wk on average) and consistent travel expectations occurring every 3 or 4 d when a series of games is played away from the home stadium. The game density in professional baseball in the United States is like few other professional sports in this regard. In order to manage fatigue across the season, a high level of aerobic fitness is beneficial for minimizing the effect that the frequent playing has on performance and injury risk (7).

Targets of Physical Performance of Baseball

Due to the high game density and length of the professional season, examining the physical performance abilities of the players is important for maximizing the number of games played and in-game physical performance. Tests of grip strength, body fat percentage, vertical jump height, 10 yd (9.1 m) sprint ability, and repeated aerobic efforts using the 300 yd (274.3 m) shuttle are relevant markers used to create models that identify physical performance attributes of baseball players. Estimates of $\dot{V}O_2max$ in pitchers have been reported as being 48.1 mL·kg^{-1}·min^{-1} with typical body fat percentages of 15.3%±3.5% across all baseball positions (4, 5). Across a team of professional baseball players (pitchers and position players), similar estimates of body fat percentage (13.8%±3.0%) have been reported, while seated grip strength (111.0±16.0 kg), vertical jump height (71.9±8.2 cm), and 10 yd (9.1 m) sprint time (1.52±0.10 s) have also been recorded (5). Three-hundred-yard shuttle times tend to be around 53 s (8).

Hitters and Baserunners

The physical act of hitting during a baseball game is expected to occur within 0.15 s once the pitch has been identified as a pitch that should elicit a swing response. An effective swing requires an efficient transmission of the stabilization force from the back leg to powerful pelvic, trunk, arm, and hand rotational accelerations. During this event, the fingers must grip the bat to allow for efficient energy transmission as well as for adapting to the location where the ball was thrown by the pitcher.

Once on the bases, baserunners require quick lateral agility as well as efficient acceleration to run over a short distance. Typical runs between bases are 90 ft (27.4 m) long, however the majority of these runs begin 10% to 12% toward the base as players take a leadoff from their current base while the pitcher is completing the throwing motion. If the flight of the ball allows for the players to run to extra bases, then the runner typically completes this skill utilizing a curvilinear running approach to maximize speed around the base paths.

Because of the demands of hitting, it is beneficial for baseball players to exhibit competent lower-extremity stability, lower-extremity power, grip strength, and rotational power of the pelvis and trunk. Prior research in this area has shown that position players (hitters) in baseball display 10 yd (9.1 m) sprint values of 1.56±0.08 s, grip strength values of 108.3±13.1 kg, vertical jump values of 70.4±7.7 cm, and pro agility times of 4.48 ± 0.58 s (5). Performance in the 10 yd (9.1 m) sprint and grip strength tests appear to be two physical test areas that are positively associated with higher levels of performance in a cohort of professional baseball players from the United States (9). Differential workload demands likely exist based on at-bat results (hit versus out, etc.) that are made and the power output while on the bases, however, little published research has been completed in this area as of yet.

The majority of the benefits of HIIT training for hitters come in the form of supporting the baserunning activity. HIIT can be used to build and maintain the aerobic conditioning that is essential for health and recovery over the course of a season, while it can also provide the stimulus needed for an athlete to develop explosive power, sprint at full intensity for 20 to 30 s, and recover quickly between efforts. The health and recovery base derived from this conditioning is also presumed to support the hitter in his quest to be able to focus on the act of hitting, as opposed to being distracted from this sporting act due to lingering fatigue or soreness.

Pitchers

Each pitching event is completed in approximately 1 s from the beginning of the motion until the ball leaves the pitcher's hand. The resulting pitch has an average speed of ~92.0 mph (~148.0 km/h), and a starting pitcher will typically complete 100 pitches per start. Pitchers who come in to serve in a relief role typically throw 10 to 25 pitches at speeds up to 104 mph (167.4 km/h).

Similar to the hitting motion, the pitching motion requires full kinetic chain involvement in order to produce the consistent repetitive power necessary for successful outcomes. Pitcher peak heart rates during a game have been reported to be as high as 86.6% HRmax, and these peak heart rates typically increase during the early innings and then display a gradual reduction over later innings (82.3% HRmax in sixth inning) (2). Grip strength, lower-extremity power, and arm rotational velocity are important factors to consider in supporting successful pitching performance. Previous research has established that grip strength in pitchers tends to be similar to position players, and these values are not observed to change with age (8). However, vertical jump performance in pitchers tends to be consistently lower than position players across age groups, and pitchers observe a greater decrease with these values as they age; this change is not as large in the position players (8). An additional factor that appears to be associated with sustained musculoskeletal health is time between pitches, since it has been identified that longer periods between pitches improves recovery compared to shorter time between pitches (14). While this may be beneficial from a health standpoint, there is a potential tactical benefit of pitching faster, as well as league determinants of how much time can occur between pitches; therefore, this may be a moot point. A number of studies have also established that shoulder range of motion measure in pitchers is an important area to remain normalized in order to reduce the risk of injury to the shoulder and elbow (1, 13).

Compared to other positions, the physical demand on pitchers is the highest on the team. This workload density is the primary reason starting pitchers are on a five-player rotation to allow adequate recovery time between games. HIIT supports the development of qualities important for pitching, as pitchers are expected to produce repetitive powerful efforts (pitches) with relatively short recovery windows between successive pitches. A starting pitcher may throw 150 pitches or more over a game, including warm-up pitches before the game and between innings. Each pitch in competition must be made with similar intensity for the athlete to be successful, and the recovery period between pitches is typically 15 to 20 s. HIIT serves as a valuable conditioning tool, as properly formatted training allows pitchers to build an aerobic base, which is believed to support recovery within and between pitching appearances. HIIT sessions can be an effective means for pitchers to maintain a training effect over the course of a season, while allowing performance staff to monitor and modulate load and neuromuscular strain. In addition, HIIT creates more robust alactic and glycolytic systems, thus fueling quick recovery between pitches as well as power production in subsequent efforts.

Catchers

The catcher position is unique in its demands due to the sustained amount of time that the player is expected to hold a crouched position while still being mobile. From this position, the catcher is expected to catch the ball thrown by the pitcher, which is often traveling in a nonlinear direction and may bounce off the ground before being caught. If the catcher does not secure the ball when it is thrown, any hitter on the bases (now referred to as a baserunner) can advance to additional bases. Baserunners can also advance to other bases by stealing bases during the pitching motion. The catcher can get the runner out if he is able to receive the ball and throw it to the infield player covering the base the player is trying to steal in time for the infield player to catch the ball and tag the runner with his glove before the player touches the base. In this scenario, the catcher is required to throw the ball from the crouched position or by quickly transitioning to an upright posture (kneeling or standing) to complete a throw to the base typically within 2 s of receiving the ball. Because of these demands, catchers have specific needs related to the different postures and body motions. Based on these throwing demands, similar attributes to those that pitchers require in a posture-specific setting are relevant to assess. Due to the posture-specific nature of this position, an additional area of assessment for catchers includes thoracic and cervical spine stability as well as mobility in order to ensure that these areas can efficiently adapt to changes in the trajectory of the ball. In addition, lateral mobility and agility in the crouched position are also relevant in order to effectively catch all of the balls thrown by the pitcher. Research is lacking concerning independently examined catcher-specific metrics, with these players typically grouped as position players. Based on the needs analysis outlined, future efforts should focus on these players due to the specific demands of the position.

The benefit of HIIT for catchers is unique compared to other types of players, due to the demands of the position. Catching is one of the most physically demanding positions on the field, as the catcher is often in a squatting position for 80% to 85% of the time the team is on defense, interspersed with intermittent standing, kneeling, walking, and running over the course of a game. Catchers also typically mirror the same numbers of throws over the course of a game as the entire roster of pitchers used in the game, although each throw is performed at a much lower intensity. In addition, catchers are asked to perform the same offensive roles as other positional players on the field and thus must be prepared to meet the demands of hitting and baserunning. HIIT allows catchers to develop their aerobic and neuromuscular endurance, as well as alactic and glycolytic system power necessary for performance. Similar to pitchers, HIIT is also considered a valuable tool in managing load and neuromuscular strain in baseball players, by facilitating recovery over the course of a season.

Position Players

The infield (four players) and outfield (three players) position players have more physical demand commonalities compared to pitchers and catchers. The primary physical demand difference is due to the distance between home plate and the range of space that the players need to cover.

Infield players typically have a starting position 100 to 155 ft (30.5 to 47.2 m) away from home plate, while outfield players typically start 275 to 350 ft (83.8 to 106.7 m) away from home plate, depending on the position, game situation, and the hitting tendencies of the batter. As a result, the reaction time of the infielders needs to be faster than that of the outfielders in order to stop the ball from getting past them and reaching the outfield. Infield players typically stop these balls by quickly moving or diving laterally, which highlights the importance of lateral agility and power for infielders.

The other factor that distinguishes the physical demands of the different player groups is the distance they need to cover. The width of the outfield is almost three times as large as the width of the infield. As a result, acceleration and high-speed running ability or sprint ability over short distances is a valuable tool for an outfielder to possess. In addition, since the ball is hit off the bat with an average velocity of 86.6 mph (139.4 km/h), the outfielders have only about 2 s to get beneath a ball hit in the air, which highlights the importance of a rapid acceleration for outfield players when balls are not hit directly toward them, as usually happens. Because

of these position-specific demands, repeatable lower-extremity power is an important attribute of position players relative to pitchers and catchers. Depending on the context of a game, a position player may make multiple high-intensity efforts in the field or while on offense. However, an athlete also may participate in a game without having to produce any high-intensity efforts. Thus, an athlete must be prepared to meet the demands of a game regardless of the circumstances. HIIT is a versatile tool that can be used to build and maintain the aerobic conditioning essential for health and recovery over the course of a season, while also allowing athletes the ability to train to produce explosive power, sprint at full intensity to field their position, and recover quickly between efforts. In addition, HIIT can be applied to manage training load and neuromuscular strain as needed throughout the course of a season.

Current research into the physical attributes of infielders suggests that middle infielders (2B and SS) have similar pro agility scores (4.38 ± 0.15 s versus 4.35 ± 0.19 s, respectively) as outfielders. However, both of these groups are quicker than corner infielders (1B and 3B; 4.53 ± 0.14 s) (9). Interestingly, 10 yd (9.1 m) sprint performance was statistically faster in outfielders versus corner infielders (1.5 ± 0.1 s versus 1.6 ± 0.1 s, respectively), while middle infielders exhibited a value between these two groups. These performance times have been shown to improve with the levels of professional baseball league standards in the United States (5).

Key Weapons, Manipulations, and Surveillance Tools

This section presents a sample of the different HIIT weapons used in baseball, their manipulations, and strategies for monitoring the effectiveness of training. There exists a paucity of research literature discussing conditioning strategies for baseball performance. One issue driving this is the lack of consensus among practitioners and researchers as to the most important physical characteristics and effective training strategies needed to enhance baseball-specific performance. Traditionally, a primary conditioning strategy for pitchers has been long, slow distance training (12). Several factors made this form of training popular, including the lack of need for equipment, minimal risk of acute injury, anecdotal support of the approach by successful pitchers, and an erroneous belief that lactic acid accumulation was the source of post-pitching fatigue and soreness, with long runs used as a means of "flushing" the acid from the system. A parallel situation is also described in the ice hockey chapter, whose players share similar physical demands (figure 22.3).

Over the past 10 to 15 yr, a better understanding of the physical characteristics needed to be a successful baseball player has emerged. In turn, strategies to effectively develop these characteristics have improved. As outlined, baseball requires quick, explosive movements and repetitive expression of instantaneous power. As enhanced methods of energy system training to facilitate these characteristics have evolved, HIIT has emerged as an integral component of baseball conditioning programs. A study by Rhea et al. (10) showed significant improvements in power in college baseball players engaging in HIIT versus a group performing submaximal cardiovascular endurance training. In addition to power production, HIIT enhances skeletal muscle oxidative capacity to support cellular energetic recovery between efforts (3). Today HIIT is considered a ubiquitous component of conditioning programs throughout the training calendar for baseball players with the weapons formed in accordance to the position-related requirements and specific individual needs.

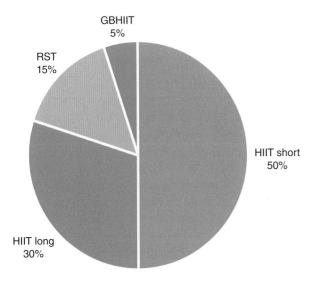

Figure 22.4 Percentage of the different HIIT weapons (formats) used throughout the annual season in elite baseball. HIIT: high-intensity interval training; RST: repeated-sprint training; GBHIIT: game-based HIIT.

HIIT Weapons

The HIIT weapons used to condition baseball players target all response types 1 to 5, as described in chapter 5, and are used at different times throughout the year, based on the time of the season, positional demands, and the individual characteristics of the player (figure 1.5). HIIT session modalities can include straight-line sprinting, sprints with changes of direction, shuttle runs, plyometric exercises, resistance-based circuit training, or conditioning exercises that use indoor stationary training equipment such as a cycle ergometer, indoor rowing machine, or VersaClimber. The very large majority of HIIT includes short intervals, followed by long intervals and repeated-sprint training (figure 22.4).

Manipulation of Interval Training Variables

HIIT programming for baseball players is systematically structured in an attempt to reach the desired acute metabolic and neuromuscular responses (i.e., physiological target types 1, 2, 3, 4, or 5), to condition the athlete appropriately throughout the season. Conditioning, just like strength training, needs to be progressed or regressed to match the desired metabolic training or recovery effect, while also providing an appropriate level of neuromuscular strain on the athlete.

Before training variables can be manipulated, a baseline level of physical performance needs to be established with each athlete, prior to routine serial testing, to ensure that the program is meeting the needs of the athlete. In some instances, testing may be performed to ensure that an athlete possesses a baseline level of a specific attribute. For example, athletes may be asked to run a certain distance in a given amount of time. They may have to repeat several efforts at this distance with established rest intervals. If an athlete is unable to satisfactorily achieve a certain standard in a test, the program will be modified to remedy the deficient attribute.

Testing might also be structured to examine an athlete's maximal capabilities. For example, an athlete may perform an activity for a set time with the instruction to produce the maximum output possible during this period. Training variables such as volume and intensity may then be modified according to this result. This allows for more precise structuring of conditioning intervals and ensures that each athlete in the team setting is given an individualized conditioning prescription, as opposed to all members of the team performing the same program with the same parameters.

Once testing is completed and a training program is established, several key variables will need to be manipulated throughout the training program. Key variables we manipulate include the training modality, intensity, work/rest intervals, and volume (see also chapter 4). Each variable is structured relative to several factors, including, but not limited to, the time of year, athlete age, anthropometry, body composition, playing position, health, and workload status.

Baseball training most often follows a relatively standard periodization schedule, with a competitive phase (CP), transition phase (TP) following the season, general physical preparation phase (GPP), and specific preparation phase (SPP). For HIIT, much like traditional strength training, it is leveraged differently during each phase of the year.

Age is an important factor to consider in the manipulation of training variables, as professional baseball players range from teenagers to individuals in their late thirties and even early forties. This highlights the importance of addressing any unique needs based on an individual's stage of development, training age, physical maturity, and injury history. As discussed by Mangine et al. (8), players who continue their careers beyond age 35 must demonstrate the ability to maintain similar levels of speed, agility, and power as they possessed earlier in their careers. The conditioning program for these athletes plays an integral role in their career longevity and should be structured with these goals in mind.

Conversely, young baseball players are often deficient in the physical attributes necessary for success at the highest level. These athletes' programs should reflect the need for systematic progression of strength, speed, and power development. In addition, the enhanced recovery ability of a young athlete means that shorter recovery times may be leveraged, although appropriate recovery needed within and between training sessions should always be assessed on an individual basis.

Body type and composition are also important factors in determining HIIT programming, with norms across positions already outlined (9, 11). HIIT can be a key tool in helping achieve body mass and composition goals, when structured appropriately. In many instances, young athletes have difficulty maintaining body mass throughout a season. Games are typically played in warm weather and the volume

of games, combined with varying dietary options, can make it difficult for athletes to consistently receive adequate nourishment (chapter 7). Conversely, some athletes have difficulty maintaining appropriate body composition during a season due to inconsistency of workload. In the off-season, strength and conditioning and nutrition are much easier to control and monitor. During the season, if an athlete is unable to maintain consistency in his conditioning and nutrition programs, body composition can reach suboptimal levels that can affect performance.

Workload is another variable that is difficult to predict and must be addressed. Throughout the season, athletes are subjected to highly variable workloads based on game schedules, individual playing time, and the nature of each competition. Athletes may be well recovered for training or may be dealing with fatigue or issues with joint and soft tissue health. HIIT must be performed in a manner so that the musculoskeletal health of the athlete is not compromised. Use of HIIT target types 1 and 3 can be an effective strategy for mitigating neuromuscular load while allowing the athlete to derive the intended metabolic training effect.

Short-Interval HIIT

As described earlier, baseball is a sport that in most instances requires some combination of acceleration, change of direction, explosive power, and reactive strength to succeed (figure 22.3). The dimensions of a baseball diamond (figure 22.1) limit the distance a player may sprint to typically no more than 270 ft (82.3 m) and more routinely 90 to 180 ft (27.4 to 54.9 m). Thus, short-interval HIIT is an integral component of baseball conditioning throughout the year.

During the general preparation phase (GPP), athletes typically use short-interval training 1 or 2 times per wk. Athletes who have an offseason training program designed to add muscle mass and strength will typically perform this type of conditioning more frequently. Athletes who have a goal of fat loss instead would be prescribed more long-interval HIIT as a foundational component of their program.

Modalities used for short-interval HIIT during GPP are straight-line sprints (types 1 and 3), shuttle runs (type 2), indoor stationary equipment (primarily type 1, e.g., treadmill, bike, VersaClimber), and body-weight strength training exercises (type 4). Work intervals are typically 10 to 45 s, with a work:rest ratio ranging from 2:1 to 1:4. Intensity is typically prescribed with a suggested rating of perceived exertion (RPE) of 0 to 10 (0 = nothing, 10 = very,

very heavy intensity; chapter 8), with proportionately higher intensities prescribed to shorter work or longer rest intervals.

As the program transitions to the baseball-SPP, a majority of HIIT involves straight-line runs (type 1) and runs with changes of direction (type 2). Change-of-direction sprinting will typically involve a 90° turn, roughly simulating the act of running bases.

During the competition phase, athletes are often observed sprinting before games as part of their warm-up routine, as well as during the game itself. Managing an athlete's load in this regard is a challenge, and it can prove difficult to compress training into a schedule that includes 5 to 7 games per wk. Thus, decreasing neuromuscular strain and mechanical load on the body is important, using predominantly type 1 (and to a lesser extent, type 3) HIIT targets. For that reason, it is common during the season to use modalities such as a stationary bike, VersaClimber, or rowing ergometer, with each modality offering individual advantages and varying levels of strain and load (see chapter 8).

Depending on the athlete, it is also possible to use reactive agility training (type 4) as a conditioning tool, with quick changes of direction in response to varied stimuli. This would be most appropriate with an athlete who has not participated in game action recently and would benefit from the increased load of the activity.

During the transition phase following the season, short-interval HIIT is incorporated in a fashion similar to its utilization during the competition phase. The goal of the transition phase is for the athlete to recover from the stress of the season, so shorter intervals using low-impact modalities (type 1) serve well in this capacity. The transition phase is typically short and should allow the athlete to prepare for the enhanced volume and intensity of the general preparation phase.

Long-Interval HIIT

Long-interval HIIT is most commonly used during the general preparation phase as a means of building aerobic capacity. During the competitive season, long-interval HIIT is leveraged less frequently, but is still used with most athletes. In particular, pitchers will often perform long-interval training throughout their recovery period between pitching appearances. High aerobic capacity has been shown to be an important attribute of starting pitchers, and long-interval HIIT supports this training goal (4). In addition, athletes who have not appeared in a game over several days may need to maintain work capacity through use of long-interval training.

The most common modalities used for long-interval HIIT are shuttle runs (type 4) and stationary cycling (type 1). These modalities are often chosen because they impart no load on the upper extremity of the throwing athlete. In addition, equipment and space is often readily available in most baseball venues. If upper-extremity load is desired, modalities such as a rower and VersaClimber can be considered.

Often during the competitive phase, strategies and training devices are incorporated that increase work performed by local muscles while decreasing the time and impact necessary to achieve the desired training effect. One example is the use of personalized blood flow restriction devices, which limit specific amounts of arterial and venous flow into and out of the limbs. The altered blood flow pattern induces local and systemic responses that produce a training effect with less training volume (6). Intervals last typically 1 to 5 min, with work:rest ratios of 2:1 to 1:2.

An additional HIIT format common throughout baseball is to use the warning track of the outfield as a running surface. Athletes will run from one foul pole to the other, with different prescriptions for distance covered and recovery intervals based on the training context and recovery variables necessary at the time of the training session. This is historically a less-structured form of training, as intensity is often self-selected and therefore can be highly variable.

Repeated-Sprint Training

RST is an important component of baseball conditioning, particularly during the general preparation and specific preparation phases. During the competitive and transition phases, repeated sprints (type 4) are less frequently used, as a primary goal is to minimize neuromuscular load and overall training volume. In addition, preservation of soft tissue health is paramount during the season, and RST carries an increased risk of acute injury.

The structure of RST during the GPP and SPP phases typically involves straight-line sprinting for distances such as 30 or 60 yd (27.4 to 54.9 m), with passive recovery periods typically ranging from 20 to 45 s, depending on the distance covered in the sprint. Volume of training is structured relative to the time of year and other training activities. Typically, athletes will complete 1 to 2 sets of 10 to 12 repetitions, with 4 to 6 min of rest between sets.

If utilized during the competitive or transition phases, volume is at the discretion of the coach. The coach must determine how much volume is necessary to provide the training effect the athlete needs based on his level of competitive activity. Most typically, this will include fewer repetitions and greater rest intervals between efforts. A common prescription of an RST session for a baseball player might be 6-8 × 30 yd (27.4 m) sprints with 45 to 60 s of rest between efforts.

Game-Based High-Intensity Interval Training

Game-based high-intensity interval training (GBHIIT) is not used as often in baseball conditioning as it is in other team sports. The nature of the game of baseball, requiring pitchers to throw at high velocities, does not lend itself to an efficient GBHIIT approach. However, activities during baseball skill practice, such as fielding outfield or infield, running the bases, and taking batting practice, often involves some degree of interval efforts. Coaches may guide athletes through situational drills, in which simulated game events are practiced in the field and while running bases. The lack of structure and predictability in this type of activity makes it difficult to classify it as any other specific type of HIIT other than GBHIIT. Examples of GBHIIT in baseball might be working on double-play routines at game speed using four groups of two middle infielders at a 1:3 work:rest ratio or working on situational baserunning during which baserunners respond to various types of hits (singles, doubles, etc.) in a simulated setting as runners cycle through the drills at appropriate work-rest intervals.

Surveillance and Monitoring Tools

In-season monitoring tools used in professional baseball are team specific and few common practices have yet to be established. A majority of player surveillance models have focused on measuring shoulder motion consistently due to the available research associating these measures with injury risk for pitchers. In looking at the position-specific needs analysis, it seems appropriate to monitor measures of upper-extremity power, lower-extremity power, rotational power, lower-extremity endurance, linear acceleration, and lateral agility. Currently, skill-based workloads are examined by charting the number of pitches thrown in a game or the number of swings taken during batting practice. While the monitoring of skill-specific workloads is beneficial, they should

be taken into context of the overall workload in order to understand if they have a meaningful effect on overuse injuries across a 6 mo season or have a deleterious effect on skill development.

Based on the game length and load density of professional baseball, questioning a player's fatigue may be of benefit in identifying a player's response to training workloads (chapters 8 and 9). Combining the physical preparation plan, alongside skill-specific training workload data and subjective workload reports, may offer the practitioner a holistic view of the training load-input response cycle in order to systematically identify how a player should modify future training workloads in order to maximize long-term development.

Strategies for Structuring the Training Program Using HIIT

Strategies for structuring HIIT programming in baseball are influenced by various controllable and uncontrollable factors. This section discusses some of the nuances regarding the integration of HIIT into the strength and conditioning program for baseball.

Controllable and Uncontrollable Factors

The schedule throughout a baseball season presents logistical challenges to maintaining a consistent strength and conditioning program. Throughout the year, some factors are consistent and relatively controllable, whereas other factors are highly variable and difficult to predict. During various phases of the off-season (GPP, SSP, TP), most training factors are controllable. Athletes are typically on predictable and modifiable skill training programs, and strength and conditioning work is of high priority during this period to build resiliency for the upcoming season. Athletes often reside in one location during the off-season and can maintain a consistent training schedule with access to necessary facilities, equipment, and coaching.

Based on the predictable nature of the offseason as opposed to the highly variable schedule during the competitive season, most significant gains in strength and conditioning metrics are achieved during the offseason training cycles. It is also more acceptable for an athlete to experience appropriate levels of soreness and fatigue from training during off-season phases, though athletes are still closely monitored and health remains the highest priority.

During the competitive season, workload and schedule present the most significant obstacles to training. Workloads for players can vary considerably from week to week and from position to position. Starting pitchers may pitch on a regular schedule, while relief pitchers' appearances may be highly variable from week to week. Starting pitchers still typically perform supplemental conditioning work throughout the season. Some of the planning is contingent on the pitcher's preference, as certain athletes desire more consistent conditioning sessions between competitive events. Relief pitchers, on the one hand, might pitch across multiple days in a row or may not pitch for several days in a row. In addition, a pitcher might throw 1 pitch or he might throw 120 pitches. The variability in workload must be met with a flexible conditioning schedule that mirrors the needs of the athlete.

Position players may also have inconsistent workloads from day to day. Some athletes are in the lineup almost daily, while other players may wait several days between game appearances. In addition, position player workloads are highly dependent on the context of the game. A position player's load is directly correlated with the number of sprint efforts he makes during the game, both in the field and on the bases. Player conditioning programs must therefore be modified to reflect the volume of sprinting performed in the days preceding the training session.

Travel presents an additional challenge during the competitive season. Athletes may be on the road (hotels, airports, and buses) for 2 wk at a time, with cross-country flights occurring several times throughout the year. The fatigue from late-night travel, shifting time zones, and altered sleep schedules can leave the athlete feeling too fatigued to follow a normal

Table 22.1 Sample Training Program for a Position Player With HIIT Targets

	Monday	Tuesday	Wednesday	Thursday	Friday	Saturday	Sunday
GPP	Lower body + short-interval HIIT (types 1, 3, 4)	Upper body	Mobility work	Lower body + long-interval HIIT (type 1 or 4)	Upper body	Short- or long-interval HIIT (types 1, 3, 4)	Recovery
SPP	Lower body + RST (type 4)	Upper body	Mobility work	Lower body + short-interval HIIT (types 1, 3, 4)	Upper body	RST (type 4)	Recovery
CP	Game	Short HIIT (type 1) + game	Game	Full-body workout	Game	Game	Full-body workout + game
TP	Short-interval HIIT (type 1 or 3)	Full-body workout	Recovery	Short HIIT (type 1 or 3)	Full-body workout	Recovery	Recovery

GPP: general physical preparation phase; SPP: specific preparation phase; CP: competitive phase; TP: transition phase; HIIT: high-intensity interval training; RST: repeated-sprint training

Table 22.2 Sample Training Program for a Starting Pitcher With HIIT Targets

	Monday	Tuesday	Wednesday	Thursday	Friday	Saturday	Sunday
GPP	Lower body + short-interval HIIT (types 1, 3, 4)	Upper body	Mobility work	Lower body + long-interval HIIT (type 1 or 4)	Upper body	Short- or long-interval HIIT (types 1, 3, 4)	Recovery
SPP	Lower body + RST (type 4)	Upper body	Mobility work	Lower body + short-interval HIIT (type 1, 3, or 4)	Upper body	RST (type 4)	Recovery
CP	Game (start)	Full-body workout	Long-interval HIIT (type 1)	Recovery	Prep work	Game (start)	Full-body workout
TP	Short-interval HIIT (type 1 or 3)	Light full-body workout	Recovery	Short-interval HIIT (type 1 or 3)	Light full-body workout	Recovery	Recovery

GPP: general physical preparation phase; SPP: specific preparation phase; CP: competitive phase; TP: transition phase; HIIT: high-intensity interval training; RST: repeated-sprint training

training schedule. Facilities on the road may also offer varying levels of accessibility and training equipment selection. It is important for the program to include training options that require minimal equipment and the ability for exercises to be performed with varying amounts of time and space.

Program Structure and Progression

As previously described, baseball strength and conditioning is often divided into some form of a standard periodization schedule, with a competitive phase, transition phase, general preparation phase, and specific preparation phase. Sample training programs for position players and starting pitchers are shown in tables 22.1 and 22.2, respectively.

The primary goals during the competitive season are health, load management and recovery, and maintenance of the physical attributes trained for performance. It is beneficial for athletes to exhibit minimal soreness or fatigue from training during the season to maximize on-field performance, which highlights the importance of types 1 and 3 HIIT in the athlete's program. Strength and conditioning is typically fit into the schedule twice per week, with the structure of each session highly context driven (tables 22.1 and 22.2).

During the competitive phase, the biggest discrepancies between the programs of pitchers and position players emerge. Pitchers, particularly starters, are on a continuous 5 d cycle (table 22.2), beginning with a pitching appearance and culminating with preparation for the next game started. During the 5 d, most pitchers have a preference for specific lifting and conditioning schedules, but in general, most pitchers try to get at least one strength training session and one conditioning session in per cycle.

During the season, the program is without significant progression or advancement in training volume or intensity, and should be designed to provide

the minimal effective dose necessary to keep athletes at or near optimal levels of physical performance.

During the off-season, there is typically a deloading period (also referred to as a transition phase), which commonly lasts 2 to 3 wk. During this phase, the focus of the strength and conditioning program is on mobility, recovery, and low volume and intensity of training. Athletes are often fatigued physically and mentally from the season, so the break in training is beneficial.

Once the athlete has had ample time to rest and recover, the program moves to the general physical preparation block, with a focus on building maximum strength, speed, and aerobic capacity, while concurrently working toward mass or strength and body composition goals. Training is structured around the basic principle of progressive overload in all facets, including conditioning. Serial testing is performed to recalibrate and progress the program each month and to ensure the program is creating the desired training effects.

As the competitive season nears, the athlete transitions from general to specific physical preparation, with the incorporation of more type 2 and 4 HIIT activities. Training during this phase is structured to more closely address key physical attributes for baseball success, including power, speed, acceleration, and agility. Players should be at peak levels of physical performance as they transition into competition.

Incorporation of HIIT

As discussed throughout the chapter, HIIT is incorporated into nearly every phase of the training calendar for professional baseball players (tables 22.1 and 22.2). Practitioners must consider each of the factors and variables discussed when determining how to best leverage HIIT to help players achieve and maintain optimal levels of physical performance throughout the season.

The importance of the targeted HIIT approach highlighted in this chapter is potentially most relevantly leveraged during long-term rehabilitation stints. For the most part, longer-term injuries tend to force the athlete to focus on the next season rather than the current season. However, due to the length of the professional baseball season, some players who sustain longer-term injuries during spring training may have the opportunity to return to activity by the end of the season and into the playoffs. In these scenarios, an a priori developed continuum of key performance indicators (KPIs) can help minimize bias due to external influences during the return-to-play decision-making process.

This case involved a right-handed starting pitcher who underwent an ACL reconstruction on his left leg (lead leg) in March. The injury occurred during spring training to which the player had reported in good physical condition. As a result, the goal was to maintain as much strength and conditioning of his body (upper-extremity and core focus due to no limitations) while his knee was given time to heal and recover from the surgery. The team had no expectation that he would return during the year.

During the early part of the rehabilitation, the focus was on restoring function to the left knee, however, equal attention was paid to make sure the rest of the body would be ready to progress with loading when the knee was ready. As with most ACL injuries, restoring knee extension precedes restoring full knee flexion, and this was the same with this surgery as well. This a priori established protocol provided some specific guidelines regarding movements that could be loaded (neutral knee extension) as opposed to movements that should resist excessive loading (full knee flexion). Priorities were established with hinging and single-leg stance movements to load as well as to utilize for training various metabolic pathways since these movements had no isolated joint limitation and remained competent with body weight load. As mentioned earlier in the chapter, a strong metabolic base is important for starting pitchers who need to have endurance as well as intermittent repeatable bouts of total-body power when pitching in the game. These movements and positions were used to identify methods to utilize HIIT to develop anaerobic power as well as maintain an aerobic fitness base.

In this specific case, the player's knee flexion did not respond well. He experienced soreness and muscle guarding with heavy sprinting or squatting. As a result, training expectations were adjusted to target sled pulls and goblet squats with heavy kettlebells to allow the incorporation of similar loading patterns in a tissue tolerant loading environment. Due to this revision in the training plan, there was minimal formal running. However, in order to efficiently test his fitness levels, it was required for him to run two 300 yd (274.3 m) shuttles (50 yd × 6) (45.7 m × 6) with a 3 min rest period between bouts. The player also completed a 5-10-5 agility test to indicate how his knee functioned under higher-level agility tasks. The times for the 300 yd (274.3 m) shuttle were a strong 53 and 51 s, respectively, and his time for the 5-10-5 would have placed him among the top performers at that year's professional football combine. While the activities were not specifically tested, it is believed that the HIIT programming likely established a solid foundation for high-level performance under these conditions. At the end of the season (5 mo since the surgery), the player was able to return to function as a starting pitcher with his team and remained in this role throughout the playoffs. This outcome was a collaboration of the player's hard work and grit as well as the staff's ability to identify multiple training pathways to achieve the relevant KPIs as efficiently as possible in order to support the players on-field goals.

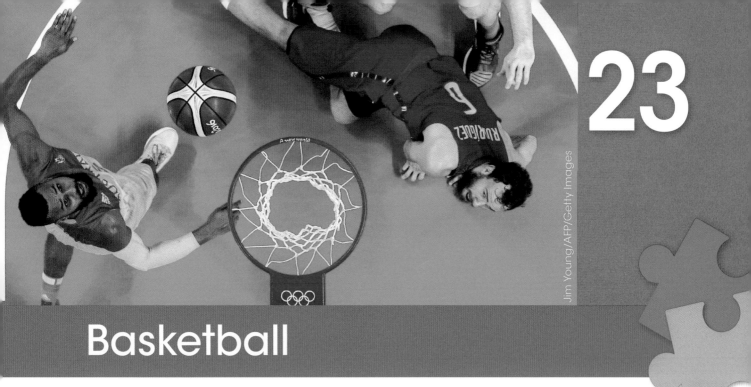

Jim Young/AFP/Getty Images

Basketball

● ● ● ● ● ●

Xavi Schelling and Lorena Torres-Ronda

Performance Demands of Basketball

In this section, we introduce the sport of basketball, and discuss the various performance factors and the relative contribution that physical performance makes toward achieving performance and winning.

Sport Description and Factors of Winning

Basketball is a stochastic, intermittent high-intensity sport characterized by periods of high aerobic oxidative and anaerobic glycolytic demands, continuous changes of direction (COD) that challenge the neuromuscular system, including accelerations and decelerations, jumps, sprints, physical contact, and sport-specific skills (7, 28). Furthermore, cognitive demands, such as perception, decision-making, and anticipatory processes are considered key winning factors in basketball (1, 7, 38, 48). The players are typically classified into five playing positions that include point guard (PG), shooting guard (SG), small forward (SF), power forward (PF), and center (C), although it is also common to pool players into just three categories of guards (G), wings (W), and bigs (B). Each of these playing positions requires specific skills, along with differing physical performance demands.

Depending on the body that regulates the competition (e.g., International Basketball Federation [FIBA], National Basketball Association [NBA], Asociación de Clubes de Baloncesto [ACB], National Collegiate Athletic Association [NCAA], etc.), there are small differences in terms of playing times and court dimensions. In the NBA, for instance, the game consists of four periods of 12 min, played on a 28.7 by 15.2 m (94 × 50 ft) indoor court. FIBA prescribes a game consisting of four periods of 10 min, with indoor court dimensions of 28 by 15 m (91.9 × 49.2 ft). The team that scores the most points by the end of regulation time is declared the winner.

Relative Contribution of Physical Performance

Basketball players require high levels of physical conditioning to elicit technical and tactical skills throughout a game (figure 23.1). Although all three aspects of speed, strength, and endurance are relevant to the player, the percentage contribution of importance for any given game will depend on the characteristics and style of the player (e.g., a tactical point guard, a three-point shooting specialist guard, a physical center) and the configuration of the roster, which may be more focused on emphasizing any three of these aspects. The desired performance-based characteristics of a basketball player are simply to:

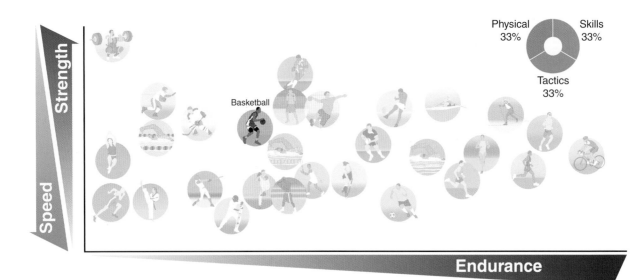

Figure 23.1 The position of the basketball player on the three axes illustrates the relative importance of the three main physical capacities of importance for elite participation in basketball, acknowledging this varies slightly between positions. Although all three aspects are relevant in the game, the percentage of participation of these aspects varies depending on the characteristics of the player and the team. The pie chart shows the balanced relative importance of skills (33%), tactical awareness (33%), and physical capacities (33%) for team success, again acknowledging the variance across positions.

Adapted from G.A. Nader, "Concurrent Strength and Endurance Training: From Molecules to Man," *Medicine & Science in Sports & Exercise* 38, no. 11 (2006): 1965-1970.

1. run faster and jump higher than the opponent,
2. have strength and balance to endure physical contact and collisions involved in the game, and
3. perform these demands with less fatigue than the opponent.

Furthermore, these tasks must be carried out optimally in relation to a specific context, that is, in coordination with teammates, against opponents, and according to ball location on the court.

Decision-making processes and expertise are additionally critical to maximize the player's overall athletic performance. A recent study (40) on game performance indicators comparing "all-star" versus "non-all-star" players in the NBA (1,230 games analyzed during the 2013-14 regular season) showed a tendency for all-star players to cover slightly less distance per game and at lower average velocities. This highlights the higher efficiency of these players versus non-all-stars, a finding that is consistent with others (55). Thus, all-star players appear to make fewer mistakes when deciding when and where to run in both offensive and defensive situations, possibly taking shorter paths to reach destinations. These fewer mistakes made could lead to lower total dis-

tances covered by these players, leading to lower energy demands during a game. In fact, research suggests that motor efficiency achieved through intensive training leads to improved perception, focus, anticipation, planning, and fast responses (57). In such specific environments, optimal actions do not necessarily require the peak potential of the player. Nevertheless, the better the potential of the individual, the greater the availability of resources, or lower relative cost of actions (44). All this together emphasizes the importance of proper exercise design, including how HIIT fits into the program.

Targets of Physical Performance in Basketball

Previous analysis of the physiological determinants of success in basketball has shown the importance of both aerobic oxidative and anaerobic glycolytic capacities (15). Due to the large number of short, high-intensity actions and basketball-specific movements, neuromuscular power capabilities, including accelerations and COD, screening, and blocking or positioning for rebounds are equally important. A proper conditioning program must allow players to obtain, maintain, or enhance these physical capabilities, which ultimately may optimize sport performance while lowering the risk of injury.

Players

In a sport where the scoring goal is at 3.05 m (10 ft), a player's height is obviously a key factor for success. Thus, in basketball, anthropometry is of great importance. The adage "one size does not fit all," despite being true across sport, is especially relevant in basketball, which has a large variance of size within any squad (36). In the NBA, the average height for PG is 1.86 m (6.1 ft), for W (SG and SF) 1.97 m (6.5 ft), and for B (PF and C) 2.06 m (6.7 ft). At the extremes, there are players as tall as 2.30 m (7.5 ft) (i.e., Manute Bol) or as short as 1.57 m (5.15 ft) (i.e., Muggsy Bogues). For most team sports, physical and physiological demands are position dependent in terms of movement patterns, distance covered, high-intensity actions, and work:rest ratios (7, 8, 45, 53). One of our group's last studies with Spanish professional basketball players (ACB league) (45) showed that guards reached the highest acceleration loads, irrespective of the drill performed. These results support two logical principles:

1. The smaller the player, the lower the body mass, with resulting easier accelerations due to less applied force (force = mass × acceleration; acceleration = force × mass^{-1}).

2. The tactical principles of basketball usually imply that the playing zones for bigger players are smaller in area than those for small players, meaning that small players usually have to cover more distance per play or possession for tactical reasons (45).

With regard to principle 1 (player size), it seems reasonable to use a scaling factor such as body mass or body mass index to minimize such inter-player differences and to obtain an individualized external load. As previously reported in other team sports, such as Australian football, the identification of position-specific acceleration profiles would assist coaches and staff members, as well as sports scientists, to develop position-specific dependent drills aimed at improving a player's conditioning (54).

Key Weapons, Manipulations, and Surveillance Tools

Our previously proposed conditioning training methodology (43, 44) is based on:

- exercise specificity progression according to the task orientation (how similar the exercise is in relation to an actual basketball game: general, directed, special, and competitive) (47),
- the approach level (0$^-$, 0$^+$, I, II, III, IV, and V; described further below) related to the orientation (31), and
- player needs.

Using this as a framework, the following high-intensity interval training (HIIT) weapons form part of the training progression (from general to specific). Based on the physical, physiological, and cognitive targets, we manipulate each of the variables defining our conditioning sessions (i.e., chapter 4), including work and rest modality, intensity, duration, number of sets and repetitions, as well as decision-making complexity, and others (10, 28, 44).

HIIT Weapons

In our opinion, well-designed general aerobic power development using long-interval HIIT (level I; types 2 and 3) should be carried out in the off-season, early in the preseason, or to address specific player needs. During the preseason, we recommend focusing on game-based HIIT (GBHIIT) or basketball-based repeated high-intensity effort ability using small-sided games (SSGs) and actual basketball games mainly (levels IV and V, respectively). Eventually, we may also want to include less cognitively demanding but neuromuscularly challenging methods such as run-based short HIIT, repeated-sprint training (RST), or sprint interval training (SIT) with COD (types 3, 4, and 5), but we would rather integrate them as part of basketball-based drills manipulating their constraints (levels II and III). The progression of volume and intensity depend on the players' characteristics and fitness levels, but ideally, we will build up the players' capability to cope with high-intensity loads throughout the preseason to prepare them for the high demands of competition. During the season, skill-based conditioning and SSGs tend to predominate (levels IV and V, types 3 and 4), but we should not lose sight of the risk involved in losing control of level V work. Thus, the periodic

Table 23.1 Conditioning Specific Training: Orientation and Approach Level Characteristics

Orientation	Approach level	Similarity	Training method	Intensity	Confrontation format	Place	Ball
Competitive	V	Basketball	Actual game	Optimal	5 v 5	On court	With ball
			Simulated game	Supra-, equal-, or infra-competitive	5 v X, 4 v 4		
Special	IV	Basketball	Small-sided games	Supra-, equal-, or infra-competitive	4 v X	On court	With ball
					3 v 3, 3 v X		
					2 v 2, 2 v X		
					(1 v 1)		
Directed	III	Basketball-based	RST (COD) (<7 s)	All-out or supra-competitive	1 v 0 (X v 0)	On court	With/without ball
			SIT (COD) (7-15 s)				
	II		Short HIIT (COD) (15-60 s)	Anaerobic speed reserve (ASR)			
General	I	Run-based/basketball-based	Short HIIT (15-60 s)	Anaerobic speed reserve (ASR)	None/X v 0	Off/ on court	With/without ball
			Long HIIT (> 60 s)	>90% $\dot{V}O_2$max			
	0⁺	Nonspecific (run-based)	Continuous or interval training	<85% $\dot{V}O_2$ max	None	Off court	Without ball
	0⁻	Nonspecific					

/: optional; ( ): optional but normally unused; X: a number smaller than the first number (e.g., 3 v X = 3 v 1 and 3 v 2, but not 3 v 3 or 3 v 4); ASR: anaerobic speed reserve, faster than $\dot{V}O_2$max speed and slower than maximum sprint speed; $\dot{V}O_2$max: maximal oxygen uptake; min: minutes. Here are shown just a few examples; there are myriad options.

* As defined by Buchheit and Laursen, 2013.

Adapted by permission from X. Schelling and L. Torres-Ronda, "Conditioning for Basketball: Quality and Quantity of Training," *Strength and Conditioning Journal* 35 no. 6 (2013): 89-94.

Orientation	Type 1 HIIT* Metabolic (O_2)	Type 2 HIIT* Metabolic (O_2) + neuromuscular	Type 3 HIIT* Metabolic (O_2) + La^+	Type 4 HIIT* Metabolic (O_2) + La^+ + neuromuscular	Type 5 HIIT* Metabolic (peripheral O_2) + La^+ + neuromuscular
Competitive	The characteristics of an actual game imply all five types of physiological demands depending on the player's playing position and pacing strategy and the context of the game (schedule, score, remaining time, opponent characteristics, etc.)				
		4v4-4v4-4v4 in <15 s, (3 courts, ~40+40 s), 3 groups, 2:1	4v4-4v4-4v4 in < 15 s, (3 courts, ~40 s), 3 groups + speech, 1:1	5 v 4(+1) in < 10 s, (3 courts, ~30 s), 2 groups + speech, 1:2	
Special		4v3-3v2-2v1 (3 courts, ~30+30 s), 3 groups, 2:1	4v3-3v2-2v1 (3 courts, ~30 s), 3 groups + speech, 1:1	4v3-3v2-2v1 (3 courts, ~30 s), 3 groups + speech, 1:2	
		3 v 3 full court (2 courts, ~20+20 s), 4 groups, 2:1	3 v 3 (6 v 6) (2 courts, ~20 s), 2 groups, 1:1	Fast break 3v2-2v1 (2 courts, ~15 s), 3 groups + speech, 1:3	
		2 v 2(+2p) (2 courts, ~15+15 s), 3 groups, 2:1	2 v 2(+2p) (2 courts, ~15 s), 3 groups + speech, 1:1	Fast break 2v1-3v0 (2 courts, ~20 s), 4 groups of 3, 1:3	
		2-way 1 v 1 defense, (2 courts, ~8+8 s), 6 groups, 2:1	1 v 1 defense, (1 court, ~8 s), 6 groups + speech, 1:1	1 v 1 full court defense, (1/2 court, ~5 s), 6 groups of 2, 1:4	
Directed				All-out or supra-competitive skill-based session (1 v 0), 2-5 s with incomplete recovery	All-out or supra-competitive skill-based session (1 v 0), 2-5 s with complete recovery
					All-out or supra-competitive skill-based session (1 v 0), 10-15 s with complete recovery
		Fast break 3 v 0 (3 courts, ~20 s), 2 groups of 6, 2:1	Fast break 4 v 0 (3 courts, ~20 s), 2 groups of 4, 1:1	Fast break 3 v 0 (3 courts, ~20 s), 4 groups of 3, 1:3	
General		2×[8×(15 s on/15 s off)] at ASR+ or 2×[8×(30 s on/30 s off)] at ASR+	2×[8×(15 s on/30 s off)] at ASR++ or 2×[8×(30 s on/60 s off)] at ASR++	2×[8×(15 s on/45 s off)] at ASR+++ or 2×[8×(30s on/90 s off)] at ASR+++	
			6×2 min at 90%-95% $\dot{V}O_2$max, 1 min rest	6×2 min at 95%-100% $\dot{V}O_2$max, 2 min rest	
	Not necessarily involving HIIT, but it has to be run-based (e.g., 3-4×8 min at 75%-80% $\dot{V}O_2$max, 2 min rest)				
	Not necessarily involving HIIT. This level is meant for non-sport-specific, low-intensity, longer sessions such as long riding, rowing, or swimming at low-moderate intensity (e.g., 30 min at 65%-70% $\dot{V}O_2$max).				

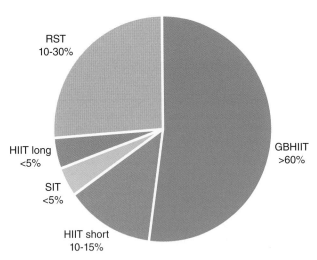

Figure 23.2 Percentage of the different HIIT weapons (formats) used throughout the annual season in elite basketball. HIIT: high-intensity interval training; RST: repeated-sprint training; SIT: sprint interval training; GBHIIT: game-based HIIT. If we consider all individual development sessions skill focused, as SIT and RST with change of direction, the percentage of this HIIT weapon would be on the top range (30%), since the players tend to do these types of sessions almost every day (please see table 23.1). GBHIIT in the form of small-sided and official games are the main technical, tactical, and physical resources.

implementation of level II and/or level III work is important (e.g., once a wk or every 2 to 3 wk), especially with the players not playing minutes (table 23.1).

Training Manipulation

As discussed above, we approach the conditioning training (obtain, maintain, or enhance) based on the principles of sport specificity, task orientation, and player needs. Once we know the needs of the individual player and the main goals of the team, the main aim of the training session (metabolic, neuromuscular, cognitive) becomes established, and the principle of specificity guides us in choosing the best weapon to implement (i.e., SIT, RST, short HIIT, long HIIT, SSG, or scrimmage; figure 23.2). The periodization, either at a weekly or monthly level, of each of these weapons is not discriminant nor conducted in isolation, but is more an overlap of the different training levels desired, while respecting the much needed recovery processes, high-intensity tolerance, and workload variety. Hereafter we describe our training orientation model, including its general, directed, special, and competitive appli-

cations, alongside the HIIT weapons and target types referred to throughout the book.

General Orientation (Levels 0⁻, 0⁺, and I)

The general orientation levels are associated with aerobic and anaerobic responses. Unless a player has special needs (e.g., limiting injuries, joint or tendon pain, etc.), continuous moderate intensity run, bike, and swim training is not a priority conditioning task for basketball players. In fact, we prefer using HIIT as soon as possible. The levels 0^- and 0^+ can be performed across any exercise mode (running, cycling, swimming, rowing, etc.) and the maximum training volume is determined either by a player's distance covered in a game (<2000-5500 m (<1.24-3.42 mi (8, 40))) or total game duration (<42 min of game time or <2 h of real time). The intensity varies depending on physiological targets (aerobic efficiency, aerobic capacity, or aerobic power). In our opinion, the most important goal is to improve the maximal oxygen uptake ($\dot{V}O_2max$) characterized by lower volume and higher training intensities (see chapter 3). It is important to consider that team sport athletes require a fairly high level of aerobic fitness in order to generate and maintain power output during repeated high-intensity efforts and to optimize their recovery (49). At this level, physical activity can be either sport specific or not, including varying surface types such as grass, the basketball court, with or without the ball, with or without specific movement patterns or specific skills, etc. The only critical aspect that should be respected is that the proposed exercises (movement patterns, technical skills, etc.) should not limit the required metabolic responses needed to target the training goal.

- **Level 0⁻:** Non-sport-specific physical activity. Decision-making does not appear at this level. Here, we suggest using different activities that do not involve specific movement patterns, such as cycling, swimming, rowing, etc., enabling low joint impact, and not necessarily involving HIIT (e.g., as a recovery workout (50) or conditioning injured players (11)).

- **Level 0⁺:** Non-sport-specific physical activity but using similar locomotor responses as basketball. While movement patterns here are not sport specific, activities are primarily run based. Decision-making does not come into play, but intensity is higher than level 0⁻ and HIIT with long intervals is recommended (type 2), although continuous methods can also be used at this level.

- **Level I:** Actions and movement patterns replicate those seen in basketball. Decision-making does not come into play or is very simple and nonspecific and not a limiting factor to attaining the metabolic and neuromuscular targets. Here, we can work with basketball skill-based drills, using already consolidated skills (e.g., shooting drills or X v 0 half or full court; note: X implies any number of players, 0 implies no opposition, v implies versus). If the player's basketball skills are not yet well developed (e.g., junior players), it may be better to use generic drills (running based with basic basketball-movement patterns), either on or off the court. Intensity should range from 90% to 100% of $\dot{V}O_2max$ (29), generally using long-interval HIIT, >60 s (type 3) (4, 10, 16, 41).

Directed Orientation (Levels II and III)

These orientation levels refer to all-out efforts, including RST and SIT, as well as very-high but not all-out short efforts (short HIIT), aiming for type 4 and 5 targets (10). These drills are performed on court and include COD and basketball-specific formats, taking into account playing-position characteristics. For us, useful drills include tactical situations with specific pathways, involving offensive or defensive plays, etc. We also recommend performing these exercises without opposition (1 v 0, 2 v 0, 3 v 0), to allow maximal intensity. The two directed orientation levels are described:

- **Level II:** Drills simulate basketball movement patterns and context. Decision-making is simple and basketball based or it is absent (e.g., X v 0). The intensity of the effort is very high but not maximal (within anaerobic speed reserve (ASR) (10)). This level is physiologically associated with high anaerobic metabolic and neuromuscular contributions. Drills are performed on court, using HIIT with short intervals (e.g., 15 s on/40 s off, ASR efforts interspersed with 2 to 4 min passive recovery periods; work:rest ratio of 1:3).
- **Level III:** Drills simulate basketball movement patterns and context. Decision-making is simple and basketball based, although it may be absent (e.g., X v 0). Drills must allow maximal effort. This level targets acceleration and deceleration abilities using RST or SIT methods, defined by

the recovery type (complete or incomplete) and the duration of the effort (<7 s or 7-15 s) (see table 23.1 for examples). Due to the court dimensions, linear maximal efforts longer than 5 or 6 s are rare in basketball, hence including specific COD and jumps helps lengthen efforts more appropriately.

Special Orientation (Level IV)

We consider the special orientation level essential for skill-based conditioning, in the form of SSGs (2 v 2, 2 v X, 3 v 3, 3 v X, and 4 v X) (types 2, 3, or 4; see table 23.1 for examples). Decision-making is complex and basketball specific. Several authors have argued that SSGs are as efficient as other forms of HIIT to develop specific aerobic and anaerobic characteristics for team sport players (2, 23, 25, 49), with benefits that include:

1. better transfer of physiological adaptations when the exercise simulates sport-specific movement patterns,
2. athletes simultaneously develop technical and tactical skills under high physical loads, and
3. motivation is higher for athletes performing sport-specific rather than traditional conditioning (2, 19, 27).

As described in chapters 2 and 5, however, controlling the overall load cannot be precisely standardized or, in our opinion, can be more complex. However, new technologies and tracking systems are allowing us to have a much better understating and control of these drills (45). Careful consideration of a player's skill levels, current fitness, number of players involved in the task, court dimensions, game rules, work:rest ratios, and availability of player encouragement is required (27, 35, 49). By manipulating these constraints, we can influence the overall physiological and cognitive workload (2). While somewhat described already in chapters 2 and 5, we would like to highlight the following training variables that are important for basketball SSGs:

1. **Number of players:** Reducing the number of players over the same court size results in increases in physiological demands (14). The 3 v 3 and 2 v 2 full-court (5) drills represent great formats for aerobic and anaerobic training stresses, when higher than (supra-) actual game conditions are desired (see table 23.1 for examples).

2. Court dimensions: Exercises can be classified by the number of courts required: half court (1/2; the drill is carried out only in half court), half court plus one court (1/2 + 1; the drill is carried out in half court, but includes a fast break or transition to the opposite basket), half court plus two courts (1/2 + 2; the drill is carried out in half court, but includes a fast break to the opposite basket, followed again by a transition finishing back to the same basket where the drill started), and open court (X courts; drills with more than two transitions or fast breaks such as 3, 4, 5, etc.). The topic of court dimensions is expanded on below.

3. Work:rest ratios: When we are designing any training exercise, it is important to know the characteristics of our sport and, accordingly, to propose training that is higher than (supra-), equal to (equal-) or less than (infra-), the actual game conditions. If the mean work:rest ratio for an actual game is about 1:4 (actually 1:3.6 (8)), we can manipulate this in training using player rotations (i.e., number of players playing on court and number of players resting off court) and modifying game rules (reducing or increasing the stop time by using fouls, out of bounds, free throws, etc.) (2, 20, 35). Within any drill design, we can use two different resting periods, termed intra-set and inter-set pauses. Intra-set pauses refer to the time that the drill design allows the player to rest within a set. Inter-set pauses refer to the time that the coach gives to the player to rest between different sets of the same exercise. These pauses, which determine the work:rest ratio, affect both the total and the relative load or intensity. For instance, with longer rests we can make the drill less lactic (change from HIIT type 4 to 2). Thus, when considering SSG drills, the workload, intensity, and its metabolic and neuromuscular responses must be considered, not only with the game format (1 v 1, 2 v 2, 3 v 3, 4 v 4, or 5 v 5) and playing space (half court, full court, open court), but also with rotations and associated intra- and inter-set pauses (45).

4. Coach encouragement: The external motivation provided by coach supervision has been shown to achieve greater gains and training adherence for SSGs and should be used as required (2, 35).

In light of these highlighted points, a good high-intensity exercise level in basketball tends to be achieved with 2 v X or 3 v X full-court drills, with coach encouragement throughout the drills. Limiting dribbling or possession time is also a useful means of increasing intensity.

Competitive Orientation (Level V)

The competitive orientation level is the most specific conditioning format, involving the most realistic physical, physiological, and cognitive requirements. The decision-making is complex and basketball specific. Exercises involve 4 v 4, 5 v X, and 5 v 5. The value of involving a larger number of players in these SSGs lies in enhancing team-specific decision-making skills: more teammates and adversaries are involved in the decision-making processes (17). We believe that in team sports, conditioning training is a way to improve player capabilities (fitness, cognition, technique, tactic, teamwork, etc.) but is never an exclusive goal. Players must be better at level V (playing actual basketball), and not, for example, at level 0⁺ or level III orientations. Nonetheless, training exclusively at levels IV and V is risky, because tasks are open, and some players might not receive enough of a needed training response/stimuli (due to insufficient effort or requirement in the level IV/V task), and as a result, lose fitness. In this sense, the topic "play as you train and train as you play" is crucial, meaning if your goal is that your team runs every fast break as fast as they can, fights for every ball, or collects every rebound, you must demand the same in every action of every drill to instill the desired attitude in your players. If not, their fitness level will be the least of your concerns. The design of drills at this level should follow the considerations discussed in the special orientation, which are common to SSGs. In this level it is usual to use game incentives (e.g., points) or modify other rules.

Metabolic Responses to Changes in Court Dimensions Several studies have shown that with the same number of players, increasing the court dimensions results in incremental physiological demands (i.e., full-court games produce significantly higher physiological responses than half-court games (5, 30, 45, 53), so that type 2 exercises become type 4. However, a smaller playing space entails significantly higher frequency of technical actions, and, consequently, more COD, accelerations and decelerations, etc. (12, 13, 38, 41).

In one of our recent studies with professional basketball players from the Spanish 1st division (ACB league) (53), the manipulation of court dimensions (half court, full court, and more than one court with different drills across X v 0, 1 v 1, 2 v X, 2 v 2, 3 v X, 3 v 3, 4 v X, 4 v 4, 5 v X, 5 v 5) showed that larger sizes led to a greater increase in HR, with the more-than-one court drills showing the higher HR values, ranging from moderate to large effects. Previous studies have also shown that the fewer the players involved in the exercise within the same court size, the greater the HR_{avg} (14, 18, 39). Nevertheless, in order to properly assess the metabolic and neuromuscular demands of SSGs, research using a portable gas analyzer and EMG is needed due to the limitations that the HR response alone presents across variable and short high-intensity actions (9, 42).

Locomotor Responses to Changes in Court Dimensions In a recent time-motion study on our group of professional basketball players, we found that even though there was a tendency for more frequency of movement per minute when the court was smaller (full-court versus half-court drills) these results were not constant across positions (G, W, and B), with each position showing different trends (53).

In another of our studies with professional basketball players (45), where we analyzed workloads with accelerometers, results showed that full-court 3 v 3 and 5 v 5 had the highest acceleration load per minute compared to other traditional balanced

basketball drills (2 v 2 and 4 v 4). Consistent with previous studies, 3 v 3 full-court drills seem to be a good drill choice for developing a higher game pace (supra-competitive drill), due to the smaller player number (13, 52). Interestingly, half-court 5 v 5 also showed high acceleration loads per minute, which may be due to its ecological validity, since the cognitive and physical requirements are closer to an actual basketball game, and the smaller size of the court may imply more interventions per player (37).

The following SSG examples (figures 23.3 to 23.8) run across different court sizes and confrontation formats for basketball. The drills include work:rest ratios and associated HIIT type. For more examples, and their acceleration loads, see Schelling and Torres-Ronda (45).

Load Surveillance and Monitoring Tools

It is important to take into account that, as of September 2018, in basketball, the use of wearables is not permitted during official games. Thus, as described

2 v 2 Fast break (6 v 6)

Number of players: 2 v 2
Space: full court (2 courts)
Bout duration (approximately): 15 to 20 s
Work:rest ratio (approximately): 1:2
HIIT type: type 4

Description
Player A attacks to player B and defends player C. Player B gets the rebound and passes to player C, who runs a fast break against player A. Rotation: A to B to C to A.

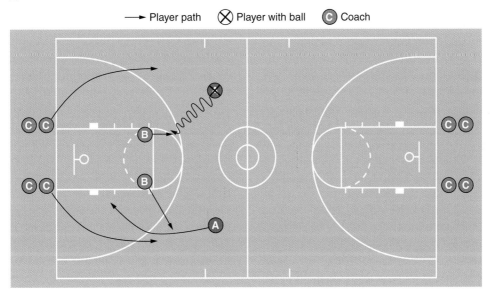

Figure 23.3 2 v 2 fast break (6 v 6).

3 v 3 Fast break (6 v 6)

Number of players: 3 v 3

Space: full court (2 courts)

Bout duration (approximately): 20 to 30 s

Work:rest ratio (approximately): 1:1

HIIT type: type 3

Description

Player B attacks to player A and defends player D. Player A gets the rebound and passes to player D who runs a fast break against player B.

Rotation: offense to defense to rest.

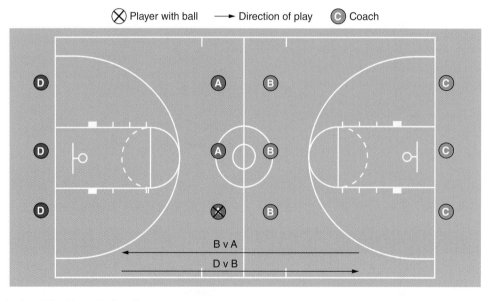

Figure 23.4   3 v 3 fast break (6 v 6).

in chapter 9, a disconnect is inevitable when assessing training and competition external and internal loads with the various monitoring tools at our disposal.

Nowadays, there is a large array of tools we can use to assess both the internal response and the external loads, both through subjective and objective measurements (chapters 8 and 9). Undoubtedly, the use of technology presents a great opportunity to obtain data in real time using devices that are less invasive, lighter, more precise, smaller, safer, and cheaper. The challenge for technology companies is to provide multiple, integrative, and synchronized sources of information that describe both the external and internal load of the athlete using the least invasive manner possible (51).

One of the most recent advances in assessing in-game basketball performance is through the use of optical player-tracking technology. This technology uses computer vision systems designed with algorithms capable of measuring the positions of players with a sampling rate of around 25 frames per second (34). Of course, kinematic variables such as distance, velocity, or acceleration may be derived from these data, and sampling frequencies might improve in the future. Another approach that has gained acceptance within the area of indoor player tracking are the devices that incorporate microelectromechanical systems, gyroscopes, magnetometers, and accelerometers into a single player-worn unit (12). The devices utilize triaxial accelerometers that are not positional based, but movement based (anterior-posterior, medial-lateral, and vertical) (3). In recent times, there has been an increase in radio frequency identification-based technology for assessing indoor positional data. With these systems (only allowed in practice, not in official games) we can obtain descriptors of sport-specific activities, such as the type, frequency, and intensity of player movements (33, 45, 56). These performance variables represent duality of the performer and the environment in

4 v 4/4 v 4/4 v 4

Number of players: 4 v 4

Space: full court (2.5 courts)

Bout duration (approximately): 30 to 40 s

Work:rest ratio (approximately): 2:1

HIIT type: type 2

Description

Player A attacks to player B on half court and defends player B on transition defense. After player B's fast break, player A counterattacks player B once more and player B performs transition defense. When player A versus player B is finished, player A stays in as a defender and player C comes in as the attacker.

Rotation: starting in offense to starting in defense to rest. Rotation work:rest ratio is 2:1.

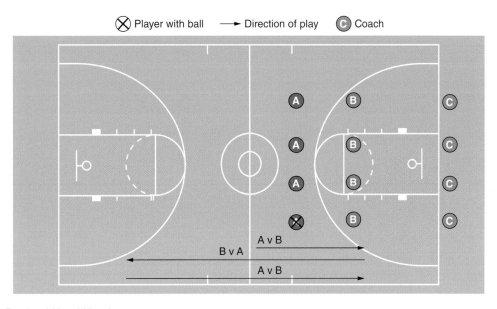

Figure 23.5   4 v 4/4 v 4/4 v 4.

order to understand how players engage with others alongside the resulting performance (21). In this sense, game- or practice-related statistics can provide insight into the function of the players as a successful unit. These measures of coadaptation describe the way that players function as part of a larger system (the team), coadapting to small but important changes in each other's structure and function (26).

For internal load, monitoring the HR response during training is the most common practice, but the use of small patches or wearables capable of measuring sweat composition, hydration level, glucose or lactate levels, among others, is also becoming more popular. As for subjective measurements such as rating of perceived exertion, they are affordable and practical tools, but we also must keep in mind their limitations and validity (6, 32).

Training Status Surveillance and Monitoring Tools

Assuming that the total workload is the result of the combined psychological and biological demands (actual load) produced by training and/or competition (prescribed load) (22), which is additionally a function of the individual player characteristics (24), we must do our best to control the load appropriately to the actual state of our players. To do so, we recommend incorporating a variety of assessments, e.g., perceived effort or fatigue, specific biomarker levels, neuromuscular and power profiles, and HR response

5 v 5 (Half Court)

Number of players: 5 v 5

Space: half court

Bout duration (approximately): 10 to 24 s

Work:rest ratio (approximately): depends on coach's explanation

HIIT type: type 2 to 4; at higher pace with reduced rest, higher LA+; at lower pace with reduced rest, higher O_2

Description

Player A attacks to player B (figure 23.6).

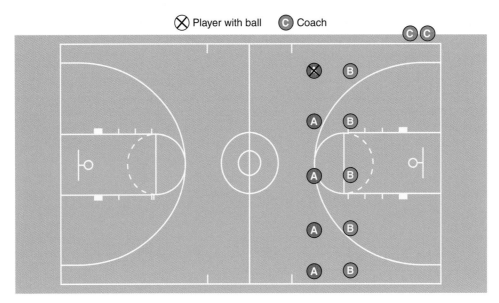

Figure 23.6 5 v 5 (half court).

to a standardized load, to track the acute and long-term adaptations to training and competition loads. Our personal experience with professional basketball teams has led us to perform daily, weekly, and monthly assessments that include self-reported wellness; maximal countermovement jump; specific biomarkers in blood, sweat, and saliva; heart rate response and recovery index in a submaximal test; and body composition. On top of this, additional assessments might be performed based on individual needs (acute or previous injuries, body composition, or basketball performance).

Strategies for Structuring the Training Program Using HIIT

In the following section we will outline the strategies we adhere to for structuring the training programming using HIIT, including the controllable and uncontrollable factors, the program structure and progression, alongside example programs.

Controllable and Uncontrollable Factors

As with most team sports, multiple games occur every week (1-5 games per wk). This schedule dictates the training and recovery prescription. This factor is uncontrollable, since it depends on the official body that organizes the competition (locally and internationally), and the only option is to adjust the training and recovery sessions accordingly.

A more controllable factor that can be managed is the minutes played per game (MPG). There are teams where the athletic performance department, with its sports scientists, doctors, physiotherapists, strength-and-conditioning coaches, etc., has some influence over in-competition player participation based on the individual accumulation and variance of external and internal loads. This scenario allows for a better periodization of training and recovery individually. On the contrary, some teams prescribe the in-game minutes only or base their decisions on

5 v 5/5 v 5/5 v 5

Number of players: 5 v 5

Space: full court (2.5 courts)

Bout duration (approximately): 30 to 40 s

Work:rest ratio (approximately): depends on coach's explanation

HIIT type: type 2 to 4; at higher pace with reduced rest, higher LA+; at lower pace with reduced rest, higher O_2

Description

Player A attacks to player B on half court and defends player B on transition defense (figure 23.7). After player B's fast break, player A counterattacks player B once more and player B goes into transition defense. When player A versus player B is finished, the resting time between sets depend on the coach's post-play feedback.

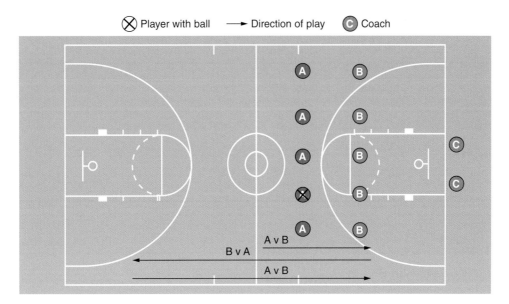

Figure 23.7 5 v 5/5 v 5/5 v 5.

a player's acute performance. The latter scenario requires one to compensate for the competition demands of each player. For example, some players play 35 min per game, three times a week, while other players play less than 10 min per game, once a week. Both groups of players require different strategies; one group needs adjustment for the lack of competitive stimuli, while the other group needs recovery for being exposed to very high workloads. This differentiated internal response, depending on the MPG throughout the season, was shown in a four-year study with professional basketball players that our group published in 2015 (46). This particular study clustered the players into three groups—less than 12 MPG, 13 to 25 MPG, and more than 26 MPG—with those players with less than 12 MPG and those with more than 26 MPG requiring special interventions; players with 13 to 25 MPG demon-

strated a pro-anabolic hormonal profile throughout the season.

Program Structure and Progression

From a periodization point of view, we divide the season into three main phases: off-season, preseason (open gym and training camp), and in-season. Off-season can range from several weeks to several months depending on the team. Thus, depending on individual player needs, this is the ideal, if not the only time, to apply training to maintain or enhance aerobic and/or anaerobic needs using more traditional training. During the preseason, we focus on improving the ability to repeat high-intensity efforts, interspersed with SSGs, actual basketball (levels IV and V), and official friendly games. During the in-season, the competition (in the NBA and for

5 v 5 Scrimmage

Number of players: 5 v 5

Space: full court (open court)

Bout duration (approximately): usually based on time (e.g., 3, 5, 6, 10 min)

Work:rest ratio (approximately): depends on coach's explanation

HIIT type: type 2 to 4; at higher pace with reduced rest, higher LA⁺; at lower pace with reduced rest, higher O_2

Description

Players play a 5-on-5 game simulation (figure 23.8).

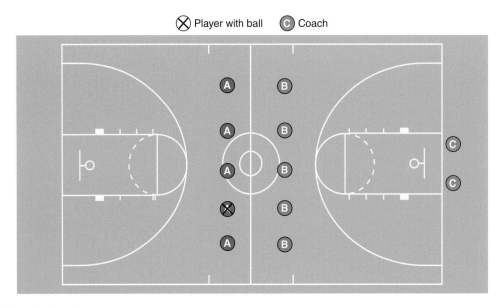

Figure 23.8   5 v 5 scrimmage.

the very-top European teams) consists of 82 games in 25 wk (plus playoff games when applicable), which means an average of 3.5 games per week (with a range of 3-5), leaving the teams little room for practicing, with the competition itself optimizing and maintaining the fitness level of the players. Thus, skill-based conditioning and SSGs will dominate (levels IV and V) in-season. However, we recommend performing level II or level III workouts once a week or every 2 to 3 wk, depending on individual needs (e.g., players not playing, playing less than 15 min, players with body composition goals, or injured players) (44) (see table 23.1 for examples of HIIT types and approaching levels).

Incorporation of HIIT

Ideally, the necessary training is integrated into the basketball sessions themselves, and the drills are designed according to the technical and tactical needs, as well as the physical needs (levels IV and V).

Level III is skill based, usually integrated into the player's individual development sessions with the player development coach and with the presence and support of the strength-and-conditioning coach. Then, unless a player has special needs (e.g., to decrease percentage of body fat, to improve recovery HR, and so on, in which case we may do off-court extra sessions at level 0⁻, 0⁺, I, or II), the HIIT training is part of the basketball practice, where we modulate the load-defining variables, including number of sets, drill duration, work:rest ratios (and rotations), number of teammates and opponents, court size, decision-making complexity, etc.

Sample Training Programs

Table 23.2 provides a typical 3 wk outline of the training routine performed by a professional basketball team, based on the number of games played in a week as well as for different player groups that have different amounts of minutes played per game.

Table 23.2 Sample 21-Day In-Season Schedule, Based on Number of Games per Week and Minutes Played per Game (MP)

This schedule does not show pregame activation or corrective routines, team shoot-around sessions on the morning of game days (no shoot-around during back-to-backs), or strength sessions.

	Monday	Tuesday	Wednesday	Thursday	Friday	Saturday	Sunday
Game	Away			Home		Away	Home
< 15 MP	None	SSGs: level III, type 5 and level IV, types 2 and 4	Team practice: level III, type 5 and level IV, types 2 and 4	None	SSGs: level III, type 5 and level IV, types 2 and 4	None	Postgame: level I, types 2 or 3, based on need
15-25 MP	Postgame recovery	Optional skill based 1 v 0 session (level III, ≤ competitive)		Postgame recovery	Recovery	Postgame recovery	Postgame recovery
>25 MP	Postgame recovery	Recovery		Postgame recovery	Recovery	Postgame recovery	Postgame recovery
Game		Home		Home	Away		Home
< 15 MP	Skill-based 1 v 0 session (level III, type 5)	None	SSGs: level III, type 5 and level IV, types 2 and 4	None	Pregame (AM) short skill-based 1 v 0 (level III, type 5)	Day off	None
15-25 MP	Recovery	Postgame recovery	Recovery	Postgame recovery	Postgame recovery	Day off	Postgame recovery
>25 MP	Recovery	Postgame recovery	Recovery	Postgame recovery	Postgame recovery	Day off	Postgame recovery
Game		Home		Home			Away
< 15 MP	SSGs: level III, type 5 and level IV, types 2 and 4	None	SSGs: level III, type 5 and level IV, types 2 and 4	None	Skill-based 1 v 0 session (level III, type 5)	Team practice: level III, type 5 and level 4, types 2 and 4	None
15-25 MP	Recovery	Postgame recovery	Recovery	Postgame recovery	Recovery		Postgame recovery
>25 MP	Recovery	Postgame recovery	Recovery	Postgame recovery	Recovery		Postgame recovery

Xavi Schelling

To implement any sort of training methodology as a sports scientist, it is necessary to have complete buy-in from the head coach and the assistant coaches. The development process of the players has to be integrative and oriented to make the player better on court, as well as to maximize the player's durability throughout the season and his or her career. To achieve this buy-in, the proposed methodology must be based on basketball needs. It can't just be focused on physiological principles, but must be aligned with the tactical and technical requirements of the sport.

Each basketball coach has his or her own way of periodizing the implementation of different tactical structures, usually based on a hierarchy of goals. The development of the team's and players' fitness should serve to emphasize these tactical principles as much as possible from a physiological demand perspective while maintaining ecological validity.

The more you get to know the head coach's philosophy, the easier it becomes to periodize and integrate the athletic performance content into the team development program. The following is an example of an integrative methodology I (X. Schelling) experienced, where I integrated conditioning as part of the basketball program.

I was lucky enough to work for 8 yr with the same head coach and friend, Jaume Ponsarnau. We worked together in Bàsquet Manresa (Spanish 1st Division, aka ACB League) and with the Spanish U20 National Team. A mutual understanding allowed us to have a very integrative methodology, by considering each drill as a different aspect of the development process. This meant designing every session together, not considering a type of session to be basketball, conditioning, strength, etc., but more along the lines of what the team needed for that cycle or day or what we wanted to emphasize (i.e., recovery, tactics, conditioning, skills, competition). Each week we had tactical, conditional, and social goals to achieve. Nothing was worked on in isolation, but instead, a continued overlapping of areas was present in each drill.

In 2014, I worked as a sports scientist and strength-and-conditioning coach for the U20 Spanish National team at the European Championship in Crete. We ended up winning the silver medal after a very tight final against Turkey.

The preparation phase with a national team is typically very short (3 or 4 wk). Here we have to make sure the team learns the rules, plays together, and gets in shape. In 2014, we had 3 wk to achieve this. Our main goals in those 3 wk were to maximize the time we spent on court to develop tactical concepts, build team chemistry, and prepare the team to cope with the schedule of the competition (3 games in 3 nights to start the championship).

The key factor we consider when we are preparing for maximal exposure (volume of training load) is taking into account the necessary recovery. To do so, we try to optimize the recovery window (i.e., logistics, treatments, and nutrition), while also managing the intensity of the sessions. In order to quantify the volume and intensity of the sessions, the entire preparation phase was monitored using accelerometers and heart rate monitors (see total acceleration loads per session, in arbitrary units, in figure 23.9).

Conditioning wise, we must keep in mind that the physiological adaptations over 3 wk are going to be limited, and we really rely on the player joining us on the first day with an already developed good level of fitness. Without this, the overload in intensity, frequency, and/or volume could temporarily fatigue the player (chapter 7), which can affect his performance throughout the competition. Thus, the preparation of a national team must start well before the first day of the preparation phase. For this, we communicated with players during the season, and once the season was over, typically 4 to 8 wk before the start of the preparation phase, we contact the players, and their team's strength-and-conditioning coaches, to provide them with the program we want to see that allows the player to recover appropriately from the season but also allows him to prepare for the national team.

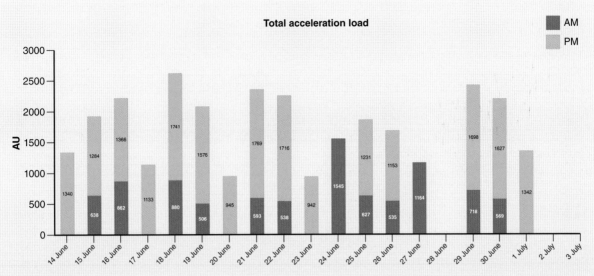

Figure 23.9 Training load as a function of total acceleration load throughout the 3 wk build-up to a major championship (see text for details). AM: morning practice; PM: afternoon practice; AU: arbitrary units.

The program the players completed before joining the team focused on the player's aerobic capacity through long HIIT (levels 0+ and I, type 2) and progressed to develop aerobic power through long- and short-HIIT (level II, types 2 and 3) and skill-based sessions on court (level III, types 4 and 5). The strength program focused on specific weaknesses or injuries the players had during the season (level 0−, 0+, I).

Once the preparation phase in Spain started, we did as much conditioning as we could on court, unless a specific need or injury advised us otherwise (e.g., one of the players came with a mild hamstring strain, and we had him doing an individualized program for 7 d). For the first 3 d of camp, the team progressively increased training volume, but training was without all-out exercises. The drills were mainly half court (level III and IV, types 3 and 4), and on the third day we introduced full-court drills (level IV, types 4 and 5). Since the hardest challenge of the championship was to mentally and physically cope with three straight games of competition, our subcycles within the microcycle were 3 d long, with the fourth day off, emphasizing recovery or very light training (half court with no opposition at low intensity, walk-through or shooting). For the second subcycle of 3 d in the first week, we increased the number of full-court exercises (level IV, types 2-4) and introduced 4 v 4 and 5 v 5 scrimmages (level IV and V, types 2-4).

For the second week, we played a friendly tournament in Spain, which mimicked the 3-games-in-3-nights scenario we knew we'd have to endure (level V). In this tournament, we spread the minutes played evenly among the players, and the stints on court were shorter than the ones we would actually do in the official championship.

In the third week of preparation, we had another friendly tournament (level V), this one in Crete, which also had a 3-in-3 structure. The minutes played and the stints in this event were closer to the ones we had planned to do in the official championship.

Throughout the build-up and competition, we had no injuries to speak of. The talent and desire of the players to provide the best defense in the championship led us to the championship finals after a very tough classification phase. The finals witnessed a beautiful game for all, with good rhythm, tough defense, and a tight score, which, unfortunately for us, ended with a Turkish win. Irrespective of this final score, we had a plan, we executed it as best as we could, and we enjoyed doing it. As one of the assistant coaches said, "Silver medal, golden memories."

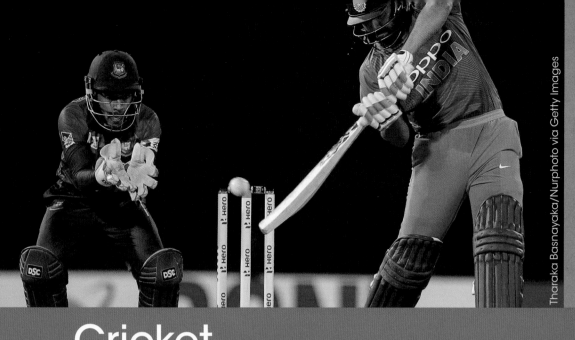

24

Cricket

• • • • • •

Carl Petersen and Aaron Kellett

Performance Demands of Cricket

In this section, we introduce the sport of cricket and discuss the various positional demands within the game and the factors that contribute to successful performance. We also look at the relative contribution that physical performance makes toward sustaining long-term performance and winning.

Sport Description and Factors of Winning

Cricket is a bat-and-ball sport played between two teams of 11 players. Globally it is played in more than 125 countries, and it is particularly popular in the Asian subcontinent where it is the most popular sport in five countries and enjoyed by a combined population of over 1.4 billion people. Three different game formats are played at the elite level: Twenty20 (T20) is a three-hour game consisting of 20 overs per side, where an over is a set of six balls bowled by the same bowler. The One Day International format (ODI) consists of a maximum of 50 overs per side and takes ~7 h. These first two formats are also categorized as *limited overs cricket*. Last, the most traditional format is termed Test Match Cricket, which is played over 5 d, taking ~30 h. The sport is played on an oval field (minimum diameter of 137 m

[150 yd]) with a central 20.1 m (22 yd) grass pitch with wickets (a set of three wooden stumps planted in the ground with two smaller pieces of wood [bails] sitting on top of them) located at each end (figure 24.1).

Player positions are typically classified into primary skill disciplines within the game. These are described as batters, bowlers (fast, medium, spin), fielders (with a multitude of different positional names), and a wicketkeeper (see figure 24.1). The object of the game is to score runs by running between the two crease lines marked ~17.7 m (19.4 yd) apart on the pitch. To score a run a batter must generally hit the ball away from the fielders to allow enough time for the batting pair to complete one or more runs. Other methods of scoring runs include hitting the ball past the boundary line after bouncing (4 runs) or over the boundary on the full without bouncing (6 runs). The fielding side tries to end the batting team's innings early by dismissing 10 of the opposing team's batters. The most common dismissal methods are to hit the batter's wickets when bowling (bowled); to catch the ball on the full after the batter has hit it (caught out); or to field and throw the ball to hit the wickets before a batter has made his ground (within the safety of the crease zone) when attempting a run (run out). The team that accumulates the highest number of runs after both teams have either batted once (limited over formats) or twice (test format) wins.

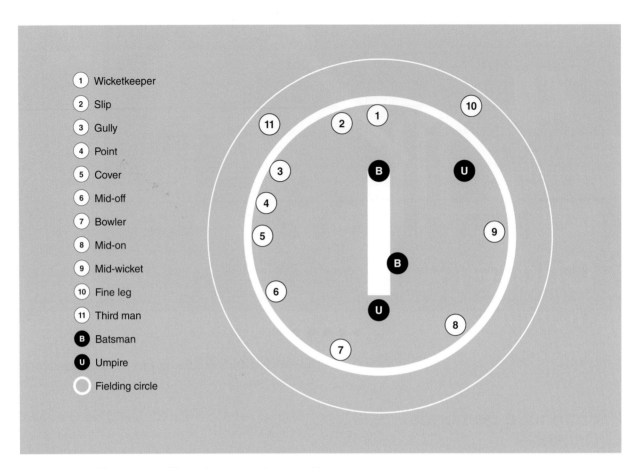

Figure 24.1 Fielding positions for a right-handed batsman.

To understand the factors that underpin team success in cricket, one must consider the tactical elements involved. Cricket is a very tactical game and revolves around how aggressively (amount of risk taking) to bat to either *set* or *chase* a total number of runs. Coaches often use performance analysis to map an innings, determining where a team should be reaching certain scores by at each stage of an inning to enhance probability of winning the game (27). Different types of hits (shots) carry different levels of risk. Key performance indicators have been used to distinguish between winning and nonwinning teams (16), and to identify times during an innings when it is better for the fielding team to take a wicket (3, 14) or for the batting team to score a higher percentage of boundaries (9). The captain (often in consultation with his bowlers) is responsible for all of the tactical decisions made on the field and has the important role of determining where the nine fielding players (excluding the bowler and wicketkeeper) are spread (placed) around the field to both maximize the chances of taking wickets and restrict the opportunities for opposing batters to score

runs. To limit players scoring runs, the bowlers on the fielding team will try to disguise the type of delivery they are bowling using movement pattern similarity (23) or by bouncing the ball in areas of the pitch from which the batter will find it hardest to score. The direction and placement of a bowler's pitch of the ball determines where on the field a batter is more likely to hit the ball (4). Captains develop knowledge of these likely hit placement locations through years of playing experience, talking to coaches and other players, consulting coaching resources, or using technology tools such as CricketPlaybook app (13).

Like so many sports, skill plays an important role in cricket success. The skill of cricket bowling is being able to execute the intended type of delivery with a high degree of accuracy and consistency, thereby allowing the captain to set his planned field placements. A bowler strives to deceive a batter into missing the ball, or playing a mistimed shot, and different types of bowlers specialize in special forms of deception. Fast bowlers may use extreme speed, while slower spin bowlers impart a large number of sideways revolutions on the ball to induce lateral movement after the ball bounces. Bowlers can also make the ball move laterally (swing) in the air. NASA aerodynamics scientist Rabindra Mehta (8) explains that there are three types of swing (conventional, reverse, contrast), and bowlers devote many practice hours trying to maximize their swing, speed, or spin. The batting challenge is exacerbated by the limits of human reaction time with studies showing that any ball that makes an unpredictable movement less than 170 to 200 ms from the batter is physically unplayable (2, 7). Batters develop technique strategies to deal with this challenge (soft hands, closer foot placement to the ball bounce location) to reduce their likelihood of getting dismissed (28). Batters refine their technique with hours of practice to enhance their ability to judge the line and length of deliveries from different types of bowlers in different types of conditions.

Physical Performance Contributors to Winning

Coaches often describe the ultimate cricket performance as the interaction of four key factors: technical, tactical, psychological, and physical. Cricket is described as an interceptive action sport, with batting skill heavily reliant on hand-eye coordination or reaction time. Elite batters need to move quick enough to hit a ball moving up to 160 km/h (100 mph). Cricket also requires the ability to concentrate over extended time periods and remain tactically aware of the present game situation. As an extreme example, Test batter Hanif Mohammad holds the record for the longest time spent at the crease (over 16 h, scoring 337 runs in 1958). The fact that a typical day of Test cricket consists of three sessions of 2 h each, with breaks of 40 min for lunch and 20 min for tea, Hanif would have batted for more than 2.5 d! Common to all the different game formats, and from a physical standpoint, cricket is interspersed with numerous brief explosive moments of action.

As illustrated by its central placement in figure 24.2, cricket is, above all else, a game requiring inordinate physical characteristics and mental aptitude, including the ability to concentrate intensely for very prolonged periods. However, displaying high levels of physical features cannot, on its own, fully compensate for any lack of ability of the other key factors (10). Maintaining a high level of physical fitness is increasingly important to both maximize

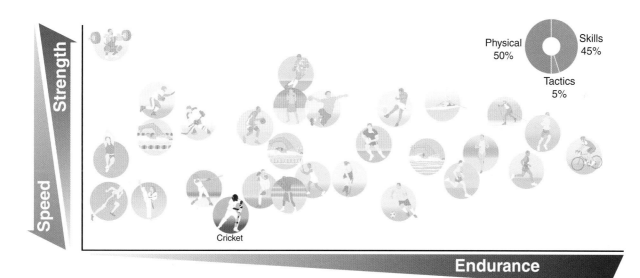

Figure 24.2 The position of the cricket player on the three axes illustrates the relative importance of the three main physical capacities of importance for elite participation, acknowledging this varies slightly between specialist positions (batters, fast bowlers, wicketkeeper). Outside of critical psychological and team chemistry components, which are difficult to quantify, the pie chart shows the general relative importance of skills (45%), tactical awareness (5%), and physical capacities (50%) for cricket fast bowling success.

Adapted from G.A. Nader, "Concurrent Strength and Endurance Training: From Molecules to Man," *Medicine & Science in Sports & Exercise* 38, no. 11 (2006): 1965-1970.

performance but also to cope with high workloads in order to minimize injury risk. Modern elite cricket players can expect to tour for up to 11 mo and play a high volume of matches (n = 100 d approximately) in a calendar year. The injury prevalence is higher in international players as they play for most of the year without a substantial off-season (11). Therefore, enhanced physical fitness may help a player to be physically more resilient to injuries and thereby be in a position to contribute to the team for a greater number of matches throughout the season.

Targets of Physical Performance in Cricket

Given the length of the international cricket season and touring demands, superior aerobic fitness is thought to assist players to recover and sustain elite performance. Body composition measures with tests of vertical jump; sprint split times over 5, 10, and 20 m (5, 11, 22 yd) (from a stationary start); and an aerobic field test are the most commonly used testing battery for elite cricketers. Mean data from Australian national level cricketers (20) shows running performance in the Yo-Yo intermittent recovery test (IRT) of 18.1 ± 1.8 levels (1863 ± 444 m; 2037 ± 486 yd) for males and 15.8 ± 1.2 levels (970 ± 385 m; 1061 ± 421 yd) for females, with countermovement vertical jump scores of 60 ± 9 cm (24 ± 4 in.) and 44 ± 6 cm (17 ± 2 in.), and 20 m (22 yd) sprint times of 3.06 ± 0.11 s and 3.43 ± 0.15 s (male and female international data, respectively) also reported.

Batters

All players are required to bat, so successful physical performance attributes apply to all players. Batters must judge how quickly they can complete a run compared to how quickly the fielding team can return the ball. Being a quicker sprinter between the wickets will allow for a greater number of potential run-scoring opportunities. Turning, or change of direction (COD) ability, is another important attribute and is commonly measured for each leg separately with a 5-0-5 test. Elite 5-0-5 scores of 2.27 ± 0.13 s (males, same scores for both legs); 2.49 ± 0.36 s and 2.45 ± 0.09 s (female left and right leg turn, respectively) have been reported (20). It has been postulated that the repeated eccentric muscle contractions that occur in acceleration, deceleration, and the COD required in running between the wickets is likely to encompass a large neuromuscu-

lar demand, inducing muscle damage, and hence the best way to prepare the body for these demands is to substantially increase the eccentric muscle strength of the involved musculature (28). During a 30 min innings, T20 batters have been shown to cover ~2.5 km (1.6 mi), while sprinting 12 ± 5 times, with a mean sprint distance of 14 ± 3 m (15 ± 3 yd), and a total sprint distance of 160 ± 80 m (175 ± 87 yd) (15). The demands of batting also require a high level of aerobic fitness in order to play for up to 6 h a day. Higher aerobic fitness also helps with better thermoregulation responses and faster adaptations when playing in hot and humid climatic conditions, which is especially important due to the protective equipment that batters choose to wear (19).

Bowlers (Fast, Medium, Spin)

Bowlers are primarily classified by their ball release speed, but we will only focus here on fast bowlers as they have the greatest physical demands. Fast bowlers generally have 15 to 30 m (16 ± 33 yd) run-ups, with those running in from the longer 30 m (33 yd) length needing to be nearly as aerobically fit as a triathlete to sustain this for 30 overs a day (28). On average, a fast bowler's run-up lasts about 4 s from when he hits his stride cruising intensity. The run-up culminates in the explosive delivery stride, when the bowler absorbs high ground-contact forces and the momentum is transferred to the 156 g (0.34 lb) ball to bowl it quickly. Global positioning system (GPS)–based time-motion analyses have shown fast bowlers during multiday matches will cover ~22.6 ± 4.0 km (14 ± 2.5 mi) total distance in a day with 1.4 ± 0.9 km (0.9 ± 0.6 mi) at sprinting intensities (17). In comparison, ~13 km (8 mi) and ~5.5 km (3.4 mi) total distance are covered in One Day and T20 matches, respectively (17). In T20 cricket, a fast bowler can expect to sprint 42 ± 8 times, with a mean and maximal sprint distance of 17 ± 2 m (18.6 ± 2 yd) and 51 ± 20 m (56 ± 22 yd), respectively (15). Woolmer describes bowling fast "as one of the most demanding activities in the world of sport: to reach the pinnacle of the game, and prosper there, modern fast bowlers must be among the most athletic of humans" (28).

Most injury research has been undertaken on fast bowlers as this position has the greatest injury prevalence. Orchard et al. (12) found high acute workload (more than 50 overs in a match) may lead to a somewhat delayed increased risk of injury up to 3 to 4 wk after the acute overload, possibly via a mechanism of damaging immature (repair) tissue.

The most common injury is hamstring strain (seasonal incidence 8.7 injuries/100 players per season), but the most costly injury is a lumbar stress fracture, with 1.9% of players unavailable at all times owing to these injuries, representing 15% of all missed playing time (11).

Wicketkeeper

The wicketkeeper is a specialist fielding position. A wicketkeeper must catch and stop fast-moving balls, which requires anticipation, agility, speed, quick acceleration, and often diving laterally or jumping vertically. The wicketkeeper is potentially involved in every single delivery during the fielding innings and will run to the stumps in anticipation of a run-out opportunity or to catch the ball being thrown in by the fielders, with wicketkeepers taking ~41 catches from the field per 50 over innings (6). Interestingly, wicketkeepers rarely sprint long distances despite still covering a daily distance of 16.6 ± 2.1 km (10.3 ± 1.3 mi) in multiday cricket (17) and 6.4 ± 0.7 km (4 ± .4 mi) in T20 (15). A vital conditioning requirement for wicketkeepers is repetitive, multiplanar, low-intensity exercise with intermittent bouts of explosive movement (6).

Fielders

All other players are required to field and can be classified as either infielders or outfielders based on how close to the central wicket area they are positioned. Outfielders will often have longer sprints, while infielders tend to have shorter sprint activity. Some specialist catching fielding positions, like slips fielders, are virtually stationary. But generally, fielders should be agile and fast to catch and stop fast-moving balls. Ideally, fielders should have a fast, strong, accurate throw that can be used to run a batter out. Fielders have been shown to cover 8.1 ± 1.3 km (5 ± .8 mi) total distance in an 80 min T20 innings, with sprinting accounting for 554 ± 353 m (595 ± 386 yd) (15). A fielding player can expect to sprint 31 ± 18 times with a mean and maximal sprint distance of 17 ± 4 m (19 ± 4 yd) and 54 ± 23 m (59 ± 25 yd), respectively (15).

Key Weapons, Manipulations, and Surveillance Tools

Recall that weapons refer to the high-intensity interval training (HIIT) formats we can use to target the physiological responses of importance (chapters 4 and 5), while the surveillance tools (chapters 8 and 9) are what we use to describe and monitor the individual responses to those weapons. In this section, we present the different HIIT weapons we use in cricket, their manipulations, along with ways to monitor their effectiveness (surveillance).

Often the full spectrum of training activities undertaken across the year is not reported in cricket research. However, one study of elite academy cricketers over a 14 wk preseason preparation phase has defined 28 distinct training drills (18). These were then classified into four more general drill categories (high- and low-intensity conditioning drills, game simulations, and skill-based drills). Of the high-intensity sessions, most were running-based variations, including the square running-based drill that involved varied duration agility efforts over 20 to 60 m (22 ± 66 yd) (HIIT type 2), but Tabata-like bike sessions (HIIT type 4) were also used. One limitation of this study was the failure to account for the strength-based sessions (see chapter 6). Indeed, nonspecific gym-based HIIT drills can account for a significant proportion of training in elite programs, making up ~15% of training (24).

By far, the most common and traditional form of training for cricketers is cricket net-based training with bowlers bowling to a batter in an enclosed net. The number of bowlers sharing a net will influence the intensity of the session for each bowler. It is quite common for bowlers to bowl in a pair to mimic the time between balls in a match (20 to 30 s), and after a pair of bowlers has each bowled their six deliveries, they will often swap with another pair to replicate the between-over rest period. Batters will often utilize a bowling machine instead of bowlers in order to gain a greater volume of work or to practice against a particular type of delivery. While repeated sprints (type 5) are sometimes programmed into a net session, traditionally batters have generally tended to remain stationary. More recently, consequence (batter dismissed) shuttle sprints (of repeated 2 and 3 s = 40 to 60 m [44 ± 66 yd]) have become popular in net sessions at the international level.

HIIT Weapons

In our experience, we typically target three main HIIT types throughout the season (figure 24.3). As cricket consists of numerous brief explosive moments of action (<10 s), the most popular HIIT sessions implemented are short-interval HIIT and repeated-sprint training (RST) sessions (types 2 to 4, 5 targets).

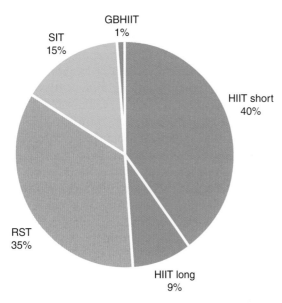

Figure 24.3 Percentage of the different HIIT weapons (formats) used throughout the annual season in elite cricket. HIIT: high-intensity interval training; RST: repeated-sprint training; SIT: sprint interval training; GBHIIT: game-based HIIT.

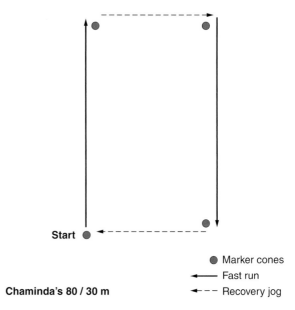

Chaminda's 80 / 30 m

Figure 24.4 Example of an HIIT short running-based activity used for bowlers (HIIT type 1).

Additionally, prescribed year-round for their injury protective qualities, in addition to their development of speed abilities, sprint interval training (SIT) sessions (type 5 target) are becoming increasingly popular across elite teams. Finally, as building aerobic fitness is important, long-interval HIIT sessions tend to be implemented occasionally in the pre-season (type 3 and 4 targets). Game-based HIIT sessions (type 2 and 4 targets) are used infrequently and tend to be of more interest to researchers.

Short-Interval HIIT

Conditioning intervals for aerobic power and repeat effort ability have become increasingly popular with strength and conditioning coaches across elite cricket. These are programmed using a cricketer's calculated maximal aerobic speed (MAS), and commonly the prescription ranges from 10 to 30 s work bouts, using a 1:1 to 1:3 work:rest ratio (HIIT type 4). With the increasing use of GPS data across cricket, conditioning intervals are also prescribed to target specific mechanical and physiological qualities. These can be used to overload training time within specific zones according to individual need or can be used to top-up players who are not exposed to desired stimuli from match play alone.

Despite their lack of cricket specificity, other sessions employed at the elite level include Tabata cycling protocols with 20 s on/10 s off (HIIT type 4). These sessions are particularly useful when trying to acclimate players before traveling to more challenging environmental conditions, and are occasionally performed inside a heat tent. Treadmill sprints using 20 s efforts with 40 s recovery periods at ~18 km/h (11 mi) are also a favorite method for providing a quick recovery-type workout (HIIT type 1) as is Chaminda's 80/30 m drill (HIIT type 1; figure 24.4).

Repeated Sprint Training

In our experience, RST is the most commonly used HIIT type in cricket. Coaches design interval sprints to simulate the run-up approach of fast bowlers, fielding drills to work on accelerations and handling skills, and running between the wickets for batters. Pyke and Davis (22) in their book *Cutting Edge Cricket* recommend that fast bowlers complete a series of 25 to 30 m (27 ± 33 yd) sprints at about 90% of top speed with 15 s recovery periods between them and sets of 6 to 8 sprints should be interspersed with 60 to 90 s breaks between sets (HIIT type 4). During the preseason, coaches will progressively increase these bowl-throughs to simulate the expected bowling loads (number of overs) that the bowler is expected to experience in a game. It is prudent for bowlers to undertake these on similar surfaces to what they will be bowling on. Often bowlers may build up their RST volumes on softer winter grounds and make the mistake of failing to adjust their RST training volume when they travel to their preseason training camp and start training on summer-hardened foreign pitches, the progression of neuromuscular loading suddenly becoming inappropriate. In-season RST is often used for individual top-ups.

Using published cricket-specific time-motion data, Houghton et al. (5) released an app (BATEX) that simulates scoring a one-day cricket century through verbal instructions and audio beeps. The BATEX app develops fitness in batsmen by adding realistic running to net sessions, by controlling the number of runs and the pace of running through six different stages. The BATEX app has been utilized to compare batting skill performance between different competitive levels. The findings from this study showed a 12% better percentage of good bat–ball contacts were made by higher-grade compared to the lower-grade batsmen (5), which may indicate a possible relationship between fitness, concentration, and skilled performance.

Simulated batting innings have been a common training methodology employed by conditioning coaches, especially in the preseason. Armed with a stopwatch and yelling a predetermined number of runs (from 1 to 4) players are conditioned to the specific demands of accelerating and decelerating and working on the technique of quickly turning between the wickets. Progressively increasing the cumulative number of runs undertaken in a session adjusts volume. To add a competitive element, the drill is often completed in pairs or even within a group setting. A required target time completion incentive for these run repetitions is also often provided. Using the BATEX protocol of scoring a simulated century, 17 university-level male batters were found to have heart rates of 124 ± 15 to 159 ± 14 beats/min, with measured oxygen uptakes of 29.3 ± 6.1 to 43.4 ± 6.3 mL·kg^{-1}·min^{-1} and core temperature readings of 37.7 ± 0.3 °C (32 °F) to 38.7 ± 0.4 °C (33 °F) (21). Yet, generally practitioners will only use performance times and occasionally heart rate to gauge progress.

Numerous fielding drills can additionally be classified as RST. The intensity and recovery periods depend on the number of players involved in the drill, the throwing intensity being employed, and the execution of the involved skills. A common fielding drill is around the world, which involves players taking turns to stop an incoming ball, shy (throw accurately and quickly) at the stumps, sprint to the next cone, and back up the incoming throw (HIIT type 5; figure 24.5). Another drill we use particularly in-season during the warm-up is the Southern Cross Energizer (figure 24.6). This drill involves two players simultaneously performing a quick 5 s agility run with either one or two catches or one-handed ground pickups, and encourages quickness of movement and accuracy of fielding skill execution. Fielding high ball catches and boundary ground fielding can be manipulated via the use of both acceleration

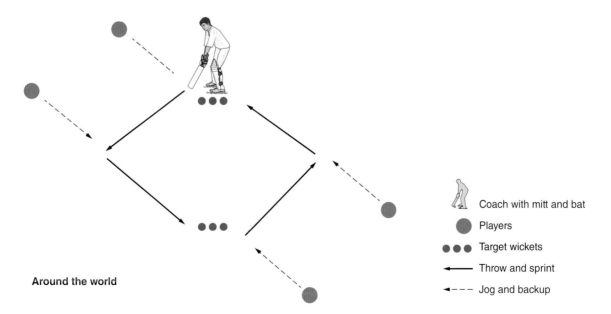

Around the world

Coach with mitt and bat

Players

● ● ● Target wickets

⟵ Throw and sprint

◀--- Jog and backup

Figure 24.5 Example of an HIIT fielding activity incorporating shying at the wickets, sprinting, and rotating around the field to back up the throws (HIIT type 4).

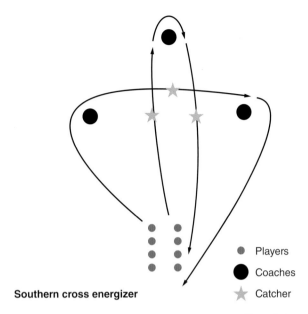

Southern cross energizer

• Players

● Coaches

★ Catcher

Figure 24.6 Example of a pregame HIIT activity incorporating fielding, catching, and/or ground fielding (HIIT type 4).

zones and/or strategic feeding of balls to challenge an individual's ability to make the catch or ground ball at a desired sprint speed. These can be done with specific work:rest ratios to elicit targeted physiological responses.

Long-Interval HIIT

Using the circumference of the playing oval (~500 m) (547 yd), conditioners often prescribe long-interval HIIT using full repetitions of this distance (~90 to 95 s for elites) in the preseason period, primarily because of their important neuromuscular load. The intensity is normally at a bowler's striding pace and sometimes monitored using heart rate. However, more commonly used instructions are to maintain a set RPE or to try to replicate the last repetition (recovery time of 1 to 2 min). The number of repetitions is increased up to 10 as the preseason progresses. On-field high-intensity running sessions (for example, colored cones indicating varied intensity and distances of sprints and recoveries) are also employed in the team environment during the in-season to provide a fitness top-up (HIIT type 4).

Gym-based cycling (HIIT type 1) is also commonly used to provide a cardiovascular top-up, especially for players who need to limit lower-body impact. Long-interval HIIT is also used for muscular endurance (HIIT type 4) across a variety of exercises such as weighted chin-ups and bodyweight

exercises such as press-ups and burpees. These exercises are rotated through with each exercise performed for 60 s in 3×10 min training blocks with 3 min between blocks.

Game-Based Training

Often coaches will give scenario-based instructions to practice particular components of a game. However, in our experience, it is hard to replicate match intensities using open-wicket simulation sessions for all positions. Previously we have recommended that conditioning drills are interspersed within the simulation drills to exceed the match demands. Players can then execute their skills under a higher level of physical demand than actually is required in a game. Researcher Will Vickery has coined the term *battlezone* to describe using an open-wicket training practice with a modified smaller field and with fewer fielders, which is similar to the small-sided games approach used in other sports. This game-based training helps to provide a similar physical and technical match-specific training response (26). Through experimentation it has been found that the physical demands of cricket-specific training can be increased via rule variations, including hit-and-run activities, more so than field size or player number (25).

Manipulations of Interval Training Variables

The running intensity and modality of each HIIT format is systematically adjusted to reach the acute metabolic or locomotor response desired. Examples of adjustment methods include adjusting speeds and distances for straight-line intervals using GPS zones, MAS data, bowler run-up speeds, or increasing sprint zone speeds. For COD intervals, using shuttles with repeat runs between wickets on set times (using testing data and/or MAS calculations) is a commonly employed manipulation method.

Surveillance and Monitoring Tools

The monitoring tools that we've used in cricket are generally limited to player-friendly measures with comparisons made to historical data. Measures include bowling loads, time on feet or session durations, and sessional RPE responses, while neuromuscular-related fatigue is often assessed with countermovement jump protocols and gym-based power monitoring. GPS (distances and speeds) and accelerometry-acquired data have emerged from the research domain and are now used extensively across the majority of first-class and international teams in the major cricket-playing countries. While logistically challenging in many instances, the use of real-time data capture and in-session feedback is increasing. This is beginning to enhance the quality and accuracy of interval training methods, particularly in the skill domain where the interval training variables are less easily standardized. Finally, we often use the individual responses compared to an individual's history to tailor a player's subsequent training with top-up HIIT training in the case of insufficient fitness.

Strategies for Structuring the Training Program Using HIIT

Strategies for structuring HIIT programming in cricket may be confined by various controllable and uncontrollable factors before progression and periodization can be implemented. This next section discusses some of the nuances of training program and HIIT structuring in cricket.

Controllable and Uncontrollable Factors

The real uncontrollable factor within the training program design is the actual physical stimuli of the match based on the influence of performance to the magnitude of load. As an example, a batter making 100 runs in an ODI match has a very large load compared to the player who is dismissed early in a test match and doesn't do anything for 3 d. Other factors important in programming decisions include the match schedule, traveling requirements, and match locations. As highlighted previously, the congested playing schedule with three different game formats, in addition to the fact that players may be playing for several different teams within a calendar year, makes it challenging to program and keep tabs on what players are doing, especially when they are involved with different professional teams around the globe and may or may not be playing different games. Preseason periods are often completed with smaller squad numbers and with other players joining later for a reduced preseason due to their other playing commitments. Another factor to consider when programming sessions is that elite cricket squads often display a large age range, with some players breaking into the squad in their late teens, whereas others are still playing the game professionally into their late thirties and even early forties.

During the in-season period, training programming needs to be flexible, making the most of opportunities when presented (rain days, early finishes) and adjusted based on players' prior match workloads, while factoring in anticipated upcoming game involvement based on the likely squad rotations. Communication between the medical, conditioning, and coaching staff is crucial to the success of any training program, especially during the in-season period. Being a largely skill-based game, the time allocated to HIIT conditioning will always be much lower in priority than obtaining the required volume of skill-based training. Running-based SIT may be incorporated into an extended warm-up to target speed qualities and provide a stimulus for prevention of hamstring injuries at high speeds. HIIT sessions are sometimes incorporated into the skilled sessions in order to increase the physiological loading and allow players to perform skills with more challenge. An example would be to use a run-based HIIT between two skill sequences, and often this is used with wicketkeepers (HIIT type 3).

Program Structure and Progression

In cricket, there is actually very little periodization in terms of the training cycles, except during the preseason. In-season, the preparation-match-recovery cycles are dictated by the match schedule, however, even players experiencing the same matches will experience very different match involvement and physical loading. The periodization model is more condensed, where the training days between matches are often manipulated and adjusted with the short-, medium-, and longer-term objectives in mind. For these reasons, training prescription needs to be highly flexible and individualized, and to do so requires a sound monitoring program, using the principles outlined in chapters 8 and 9.

Incorporation of HIIT

In the earlier preseason program, strengthening and conditioning often take precedence over the technical training, whereas in the later part of the preseason, the technical and skill-based sessions are prioritized. In the later preseason, HIIT is occasionally combined and incorporated into game-based training and open-wicket practices, whereas in the earlier preseason, HIIT sessions are often programmed as stand-alone conditioning sessions. HIIT sessions, particularly RST, are gradually progressed to prepare players for the expected playing demands in the early season (bowling overs, number of runs between the wickets). Once into the in-season (which is most of the training year), HIIT prescription is less team based and more individualized.

In-season, when match schedules dictate the training program, there are likely to be numerous combinations of match days within a week ranging from 1 to 6 d. The amount of weekly HIIT prescribed is therefore player dependent and takes into account individual overall playing time and loading history over the recent past and expected short-term future volume. The HIIT prescription is highly individualized and can be achieved through a combination of different HIIT types and formats. Batters are extremely challenging to program for due to the

unknown factor of when and for how long they will bat, and a conservative approach is nearly always used. It is somewhat easier to predict bowlers' expected future bowling loads; however, again, it is unknown how long a player will be required to be in the field (can be multiple days). Conditioning coaches will therefore often prescribe extra strength and HIIT sessions for the 12th man (reserve fielder) on match days.

Sample Training Programs

Figures 24.7 to 24.9 provide examples of HIIT programming during different phases of training, i.e., preseason and in-season. Figures 24.4 to 24.6 show types of HIIT drills incorporated into fielding sessions.

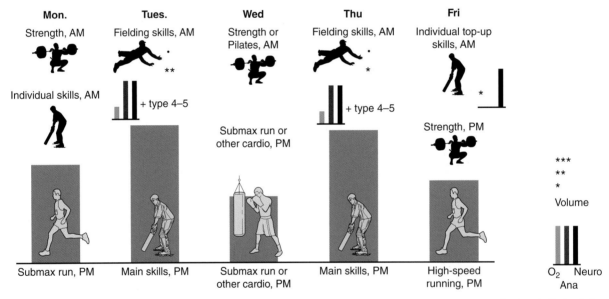

Figure 24.7 Example of preseason programming in an elite team. The blue bars refer to daily training volume (includes technical and tactical in different forms). High-speed running consists of maximal sprint work. HIIT RST is incorporated within fielding drills.

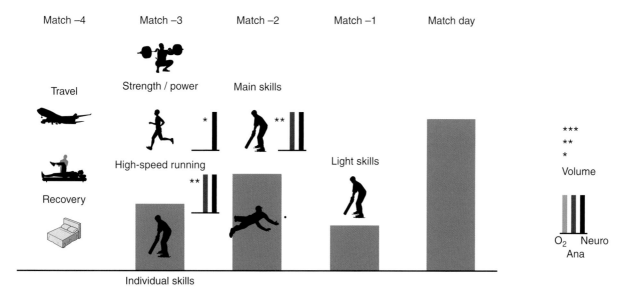

Figure 24.8 Example of in-season programming with one match day for an international team. Training times at international level are determined by home cricket boards, whereby one team will have facility access in the a.m. and the other in the p.m. This will generally be geared toward the home team enjoying the best training times for key days. Interval training is aligned with skill sessions, whereby the timing of strength and recovery modalities will take into account the strength facility access and availability. The blue bars refer to all technical and tactical training volume in different forms. High-speed running consists of maximal sprint work.

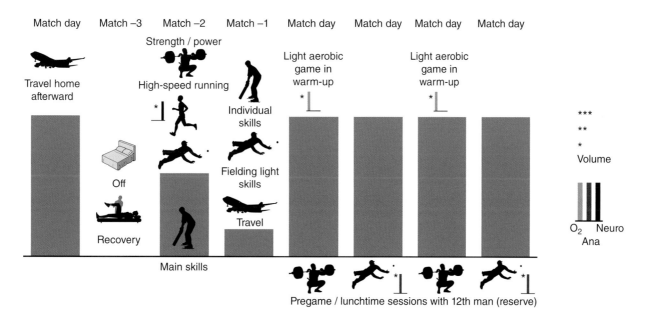

Figure 24.9 Example of in-season programming for a 4 d match for a domestic team. Note, in reality scheduling is not consistent with random numbers of days between matches. The 12th man is decided on the first match day and may or may not stay for the whole 4 d game, depending on where and when the second X1 team is playing. Travel time will vary from 1 to 6 h.

The game location and year of occurrence for the following story won't be revealed in the name of confidentiality, but it did occur. Postseason, it is common in a number of countries including Australia, England, and New Zealand for the domestic and national conditioning coaches to get together with the team physiotherapists to discuss best practice, check the annual injury audit data, and hear from invited international experts. In one of these settings, I attended a presentation from Dr. Raphael Brandon, who had recently written his thesis (1) on the neuromuscular response to elite training. The presentation included data and suggestions for the prevention of lower-limb injuries, especially the hamstrings, with the primary recommendation being that in addition to gym-based strengthening, athletes needed to regularly sprint to reduce injury risk.

Injury prevention is a key aspect of any cricket program. Having any player sitting on the sideline injured reduces the overall squad strength and impacts the chance of team success, especially in smaller squads. So in building the annual plan for the upcoming year, we took on-board the recommendations and dutifully prioritized RST both throughout the preseason and for in-season phases. The athletes were easily sold on the idea, and everyone enjoyed the quick sharp sprint session (5 to 8 sprints of 40 to 70 m [44 to 77 yd], with intensity at 90% to 100% with slow walk-back recoveries), which were incorporated into the program at least once a week. However, one particular player was very reluctant to push himself to the required sprinting intensity and would clearly hold back, running at around 70% intensity. Through discussions with the player it became clear that he held a psychological fear about a previous injury from a few years earlier, which he believed might recur if he sprinted. Despite being informed of the rationale for the exercise and consulting with the physiotherapist who also informed him that it was in his best interest to sprint, the player decided that he would prefer to take the chance and risk the consequences rather than push himself to the required 90% to 100% sprint intensities requested to build resiliency. As the player predominantly fielded stationary catching positions, he only infrequently needed to sprint in a game. Privately, the physiotherapist and I considered the athlete's injury risk to be a ticking time bomb.

It was only a few months later, when unfortunately, the athlete's gamble did not pay off. As it happens in cricket, the great unknown for any batter is when he will need to bat, which often can be a substantial time after the warm-up. For this reason, players will often use ladders or perform other activities to keep the body warm and ready while waiting to bat. The other confounding factor is that even during summer, the weather can often be cold, damp, and at times miserable, which it was on this occasion. The player was waiting for a relatively extended time to bat before having to appear in the crease. He started at the nonstriker's end, and literally the first ball bowled was hit, and he was called to sprint through. With the fielder attempting to throw the stumps down at the wicketkeeper's end, our player had to sprint, stretch to slide his bat into the crease, and . . . bang—injured. Of course, we will never actually know if the requested RST conditioning done at the proper intensities would have prevented the injury, but anecdotally speaking, as a squad that year, we had reduced lower-limb injuries in those who followed the prescription properly, and my feeling is that the RST conditioning was an important component of that result.

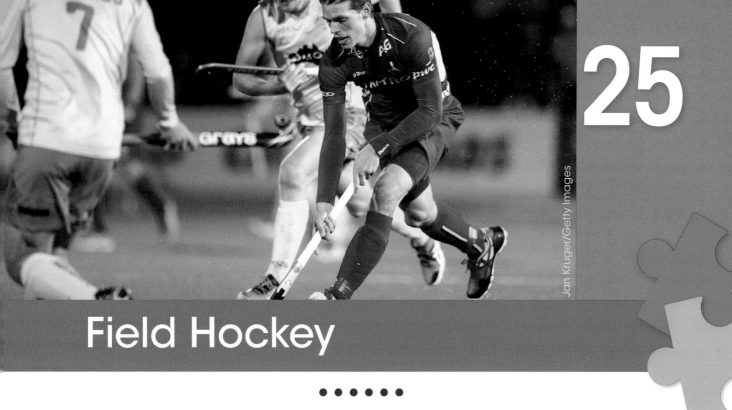

Jan Kruger/Getty Images

25

Field Hockey

• • • • • •

Dave Hamilton

Performance Demands of Field Hockey

First played in 19th century Great Britain, the sport of field hockey is now enjoyed in both indoor and outdoor settings. The latter format is far more popular and became a permanent Olympic staple in 1928. Field hockey is similar to many field-based team sports in that it requires a blend of technical, tactical, and physical variables to perform well and be successful. This section will introduce the sport of field hockey with focused discussion on performance variables at the competitive level.

Sport Description and Factors of Winning

Field hockey is a team sport played by both men and women. The game has indoor and outdoor formats, but it is the traditional outdoor format that draws the biggest audiences with the two largest tournament-based competitions being the Olympic Games and World Cup. The outdoor teams are made up of 11 players, normally 10 field players and 1 goalkeeper. The field dimensions are not dissimilar to those of other field sport cousins (soccer, rugby, lacrosse), with the dimensions being 91×55 m (100×60 yd) (figure 25.1). The modern game is played on a synthetic water-based pitch with artifi-

cial grass, which serves to reduce friction between all stick-to-turf and ball-to-turf activities. This water-based feature has facilitated a faster game and increased the finer motor skill demands of the athletes as it pertains to stick-and-ball control through hand dexterity and hand-eye coordination.

The 11 players on a team can typically be classified into four categories that include forwards, midfielders, backs, and goalkeepers (figure 25.1). While each position requires slightly different skillsets, all players are free to roam the entire field, with no offside rule ever called during play. Scoring can occur only when players strike the ball within the opponent's shooting circle, called the D. Rolling substitutions with the 11 on-field players and the 7 benched players are a defining component of the game, as there is no limit to the number of substitution rotations that can be completed. This creates the opportunity to maintain intermittent levels of high intensity throughout the game, much like a high-intensity interval training (HIIT) format. In 2014, the International Hockey Federation game format was changed from 2×35 min halves with a 10 min halftime, into 4×15 min quarters, with 2 min rest periods and one 10 min halftime. In simple terms, today's format consists of a 60 min game that includes four 15 min quarters.

Field hockey is a highly demanding intermittent effort sport requiring myriad high-intensity actions.

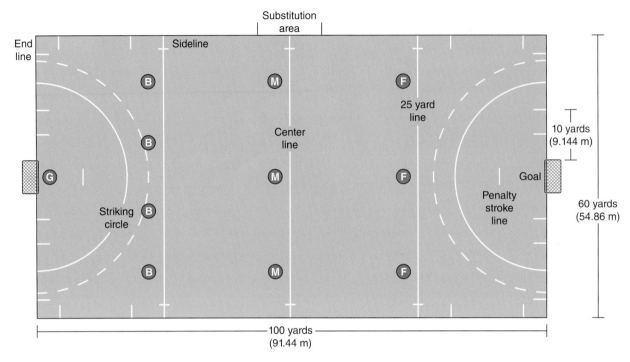

Figure 25.1 Field hockey field diagram, including dimensions and positions. F: forwards; M: midfielders; B: backs; G: goalkeepers.

Global positioning system (GPS) analysis has shown that outfield players can cover up to 5 to 9 km per game. It is therefore appropriate to view field hockey as an aerobically demanding sport, with frequent although brief superimposed anaerobic efforts. High-intensity actions contribute to a significant percentage of match activities (12% to 26%), and it is the successful completion of these high-intensity actions that can often determine the outcome of a field hockey match (6). It is clear that hockey by nature requires a high level of aerobic fitness, a quality that when well developed will facilitate an athlete's ability to cover greater distances during a match and recover effectively between repeated high-intensity efforts.

Relative Contribution of Physical Performance

The demands of field hockey match play and intensity are typically higher than those described in other field-based sports, an outcome inherently created through the rulings of unlimited rolling substitutions, no offside, and the self-pass rule from free hits (5). The purpose of such rule modifications was to improve the spectacle of the game for the audience by reducing stoppages and increasing the relative time the ball was in play. As a result, the modern game has created a greater reliance on not only

technical and tactical capabilities but physical qualities as well that underpin an athlete's ability to repeat these high-intensity activities throughout a game (figure 25.2). Having athletes who can endure and tolerate repeated bouts of low-to-ground actions, high-speed running, rapid changes of direction, and forceful accelerations and decelerations is paramount for success. Indeed, the ability to display these speed, strength, and power qualities throughout the game, while mitigating excessive fatigue, has been shown to play a crucial role alongside endurance as key determinants of field hockey success (7, 10). Like many field or court-based sports, successful outcomes and winning can heavily depend on the ability to sustain these actions consistently throughout a game and/or season.

It's clear that an athlete who is physically strong and aerobically fit offers the coach a springboard from which to develop an impactful player, but the demands of international hockey are very specific. With club and league hockey systems, 1 or 2 games are played each week over a 20 to 30 wk season. Group games, back-to-back games, knockout stages, shoot-outs, and the need to perform for 8 games in 12 d during Olympic and World Championship tournaments are the keys to success at the international level. The physical resilience and conditioning levels required for these specific competition stresses

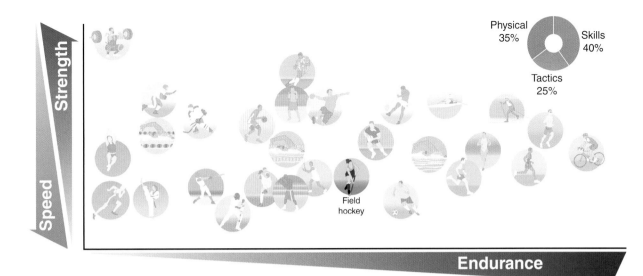

Figure 25.2 The position of the field hockey player on the three axes illustrates the relative importance of the three main physical capacities of importance for elite participation in field hockey, acknowledging this varies slightly between positions. Outside of critical psychological aspects and team chemistry components, which are difficult to quantify, the pie chart shows the general relative importance of skills (40%), tactical awareness (25%), and physical capacities (35%) for field hockey success.

Adapted from G.A. Nader, "Concurrent Strength and Endurance Training: From Molecules to Man," *Medicine & Science in Sports & Exercise* 38, no. 11 (2006): 1965-1970.

undoubtedly bring unique challenges to the way we prepare athletes. With this in mind, the goal of any physical preparation program should be to develop an athlete who can tolerate high workloads and is robust and durable enough to endure the rigors of tournament field hockey. The focus then shifts to developing a training approach that systematically improves tolerance levels, so that athletes can endure the high training volumes required to succeed in competitions such as the Olympic Games.

Repeating high-intensity actions and having the ability to express high-force outputs is crucial and underpins the opportunity for improved success. We know that athletes who possess high relative strength are capable of expressing higher forces and superior levels of speed and power. Field hockey is a sport in which success depends on players winning individual battles. The ability to accelerate effectively and perform rapid unilateral movements in and out of low-to-ground positions are key characteristics that may help shape successful outcomes against counterparts.

Benchmarking

Benchmarking is the process of identifying the key physical performance characteristic needed to be successful in your sport, as well as offering insight into the type of athlete you have at your disposal.

It additionally provides your athlete with clear guidelines on her physical development as it relates to her sport. It is imperative that the tests chosen for benchmarking are valid, standardized, and reflect the physical performance characteristics deemed conducive for success in field hockey, thus allowing for the amalgamation of normative data, future cross comparisons, and the highlighting of key performance indicators. An example of my benchmarking is shown in table 25.1.

Figure 25.3 shows the benchmarking of physical qualities identified as important in elite female field hockey players. These standards are based on normative data collected from a number of elite female athlete populations across a variety of field and court-based sports (rugby, soccer, netball, tennis, and lacrosse). For more unique assessments with limited data sets, the use of the standard deviation (SD) away from the mean can be a useful process to help clarify benchmarking categories. The physical tests outlined in table 25.1 and figure 25.3 are designed to highlight an athlete's current level of development as it relates to elite-level counterparts.

Benchmarking also gives the athlete clear objective goals for which to strive. These chosen tests allow for a simplified overview of all the physical qualities deemed essential for athletic prowess in

Table 25.1 Benchmarking Tests and the Variables Assessed

Physical quality	Test	Variable assessed
Gym-based strength	Back squat, bench press, wide chins, and jump squat profiling	2 to 5 RMs
Strength	Isometric mid-thigh pull	Rate of force development Absolute and relative strength
Power	Countermovement jump squat jump	Dynamic force qualities Eccentric utilization ratio
Speed	10, 20, 40 m	Acceleration, peak velocity
Anaerobic endurance	6×40 m (20 m shuttle)	Fatigability
Aerobic power	30-15 intermittent fitness test (30-15 IFT)	High-intensity intermittent performance $\dot{V}O_2$max (predicted) Max heart rate
Movement quality	Movement assessment	Flexibility control through ROM Kinetic chain efficiency and neuromuscular system
Anaerobic speed reserve	30-15 intermittent fitness test (30-15 IFT)	Anaerobic speed reserve (peak velocity attained in 30-15 IFT)

	Speed			Strength				Conditioning	
	5 m	10 m	40 m	ISO pull	Back sq	Bench press	Wide pull-ups	Mean RSA	30-15$_{IFT}$
Elite and 2012	0.99	1.75	5.4	3.75	2	1.05	12	7.2	21
Green	1.04	1.8	5.65	3	1.75	0.9	9	7.45	20
Amber	1.1	1.87	5.85	2.4	1.5	0.75	6	7.7	19.5
Red	1.15	1.93	6	2	1.25	0.6	3	7.9	19

Figure 25.3 Athlete profile traffic light, showing the benchmarking of physical qualities identified as important for elite female field hockey players. Speed 5, 10, 40 m=time (s); strength back squat and bench=relative strength (× body mass); pull-up=repetitions; repeated sprint ability (RSA)=average time across 6 sprints; 30-15 IFT=level reached.

field hockey. This traffic light system (figure 25.3) has been put together so that athletes understand where they are and how much they need to develop when competing at the world-class elite level. Figure 25.3 shows the physical level and expectation of field hockey athletes leading into an Olympic campaign. Typically these tests are performed preseason, mid-season, and 6 wk prior to the first major international competition, allowing sufficient time for any prescriptive changes to address specific physical qualities.

Field Tests and Order Performed

DAY 1

Speed: 10, 20, 30, 40 m; acceleration qualities and peak velocity established

Aerobic power: 30-15 IFT (2); establish an athlete's aerobic and anaerobic power, recovery, and change of direction (COD) abilities

DAY 2

Anaerobic power and agility: Hamilton 6 × 40 m RSA (see drill protocol and figure 25.4); highlight anaerobic qualities and fatigability of the athletes

Strength test: power (countermovement jump [CMJ] and squat jump [SJ]); relative power and dynamic force qualities analyzed; eccentric utilization ratio (EUR) can also be established (8)

The schematic shown in figure 25.2 offers a perceptual guide as to where field hockey demands sit in regard to their physiological demands and where

Hamilton RSA Protocol for Field Hockey Players

The Hamilton RSA protocol for field hockey players consists of a 20-20 shuttle with an active 20 m recovery. It uses a rolling 30 s clock for each 40 m effort.

Protocol

- The athlete starts 0.5 m behind the timing gate.
- The athlete's foot must touch the line at the end of the 20 m turning point. Failure to do so means the test is stopped, the athlete rests 5 min, and the test is repeated.
- During the recovery phase, it is essential that the athlete complete the 20 m recovery, going around the cone set 10 m behind the starting line.

Pre-Test

- The athlete starts 0.5 m behind the timing gate. On the tester's call, the athlete performs a maximal 40 (20 m shuttle) sprint.

- The athlete must ensure that a maximal effort is achieved. The tester is responsible for providing verbal encouragement.
- The time is recorded and the athlete is given an additional 5 min recovery before the RSA test begins. This score is used to ensure all sprints are of maximal effort.

RSA Test

- The athlete performs 6 repeated 40 m efforts on a rolling 30 s clock.
- The time taken for the sprint dictates the recovery time available within the rolling 30 s.
- All times should be recorded for the 6 sprints with verbal encouragement given throughout.
- For the active recovery, the athlete completes a 10 m shuttle (total 20 m) in the recovery period.

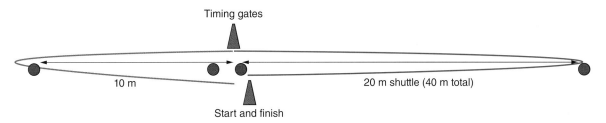

Figure 25.4 Setup for the Hamilton RSA protocol for field hockey players. Red line: sprint; blue line: active recovery.

training should be focused. The substitution component of field hockey allows us to maximize output and facilitate a higher intensity of work on the field. Players typically have multiple playing spells lasting 3 to 12 min (position dependent). Figures 25.5 and 25.6 represent in-house data collected by teams from over 60 international matches. Figure 25.5 shows the expected relationship between player work rate speed and spell length, while figure 25.6 similarly shows the correlation between work rate and total playing time during international field hockey matches. These data show the expected reduction in work rate speed as either shift length or total playing duration increases.

Clearly, having athletes play for longer durations results in lowered work rates, high-intensity actions and work output. Figure 25.7 highlights how the combination of physiological benchmarking and profiling can be incorporated to target the conditioning areas needed to develop field hockey athletes.

Targets of Physical Performance

The unique movement patterns required by field hockey players may be attributed (at least in part) to the right-handed-only sticks players use to

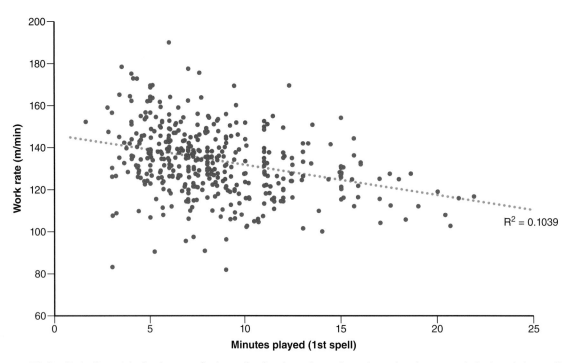

Figure 25.5 Relationship between first spell minutes played and work rate speed during international field hockey match play. Note the expected general decline in work rate speed with increased first spell duration.

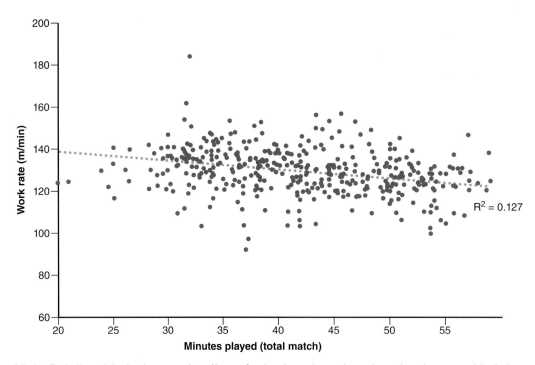

Figure 25.6 Relationship between duration of minutes played and work rate speed in international field hockey matches. Note the expected general decline in work rate speed with increased minutes played.

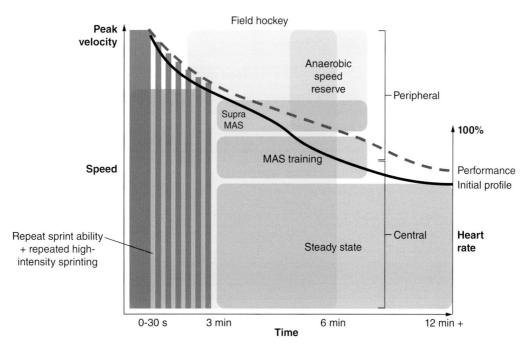

Figure 25.7 The Hamilton field hockey physiology profile used for benchmarking and training targets. MAS: maximal aerobic speed.

control the ball. Holding the stick with the left hand at the top and the right hand closer to the bottom half of the stick has led to a number of predetermined movement patterns associated with tackling, running with the ball, striking the ball, and free running without the ball. Inevitably, such skill sets can create unilateral asymmetries as players consistently become exposed to repetitive asymmetrical musculoskeletal loads. The left leg is often the preferred and functionally more proficient leg adopted during the forward lunge when tackling (left hand to the ground) and when striking the ball as a plant leg. High deceleration loads are placed on the left leg compared to the right, and programming will often need to reflect these demands to appropriately prepare the players. The highly explosive rotational actions performed in deep-flexed positions bring about other stresses as they pertain to muscle function around the hip and spine. Additionally, the sport requires these actions to be performed for 60 min while covering significant distances (5 to 9 km) up and down the field while enduring all the physical qualities needed to be a successful athlete in an evasion-based sport. At a club level, fixtures will take place once a week and weekly training is scheduled in such a manner as to help players recover early in the week, subject them to loading midweek, before tapering or unloading appropriately toward the end of the week and the next game. Internationally, the

demands on players are different again. In this environment, where the game is even faster (1), players are required to play on consecutive days and often over an 8 to 12 d period in the Olympic Games and World Cup, a competition schedule unlike any other. Understandably, preparation approaches between club and country commitments will differ substantially due to the constraints of the environment and the type of competition schedule being prepared for.

Time-motion studies reveal that athletes typically cover 5 to 9 km over the course of a game, with 12% to 26% of that time spent performing high-intensity running or sprinting. For the purpose of this chapter, high-intensity actions (HIA) have been assessed using GPS data and are classified as any running volume above 15 km/h (9 mph). GPS systems have become invaluable tools in more recent times for helping coaches and practitioners better quantify the work being completed during training and in competition. This numerical understanding of physical workload has assisted us to refine training methodologies, to manipulate training through drills and small-sided game strategies, as well as make position-specific modifications, work:rest interval adjustments, and understand a player's training load (see chapter 8). GPS technology allows us to set our own metrics to describe the relevant work being completed, including speed zones, number of accelerations, and types of accelerations (easy, hard, etc.). The

Table 25.2 Time-Motion Analysis and GPS Speed Zones (km/h) for Male and Female Hockey Players

	Speed km/h						
	Zone 1 standing	Zone 2 walking	Zone 3 jogging	Zone 4 running	Zone 5 striding	Zone 6 sprinting	Zone 7*
Male	0-0.6	0.6-6	6-11	11-15	15-19	19-21	21+
Female	0-0.6	0.6-6	6-11	11-15	15-19	19+	

* Zone 7 sprinting used only for men as an additional sprinting metric.

Table 25.3 Average Time-Motion Data for International Male and Female Hockey Players (120+ Games), 2009-2016

	Total distance (m)	Work rate (m/min)	HIA distance >15 km/h	% HIA	Average playing time (min)
Female	5700	128	1050	18	44
Male	6000	136	1240	19.5	44

Table 25.4 Average Positional Data, Including Total Distance, Work Rate, High-Speed Running, and Average Spell Length From International Field Hockey Play Across Forwards, Midfielders, and Defenders

Position	Total distance (m)	Work rate (m/min)	High-speed running (> 15 km/h)	Average spell length (min)
Forward	4544	130	1000	6.5
Midfielder	5511	128	1117	8.6
Defender	5783	115	605	14.7

downside of such flexibility with this technology arises from the difficulty that then transpires when trying to compare data sets between teams and across sports. Table 25.2 highlights the speed zones used by the Great Britain and US Olympic field hockey teams during the 2009 to 2016 quadrennial cycles. As a means to understand and quantify training and game loads for athletes, time-motion data (GPS) was used to quantify exactly how far athletes were running at different speeds during a game. These zones were chosen to reflect game impact and describe the type of work being completed.

As shown in figure 25.2, the aerobically demanding, intermittent anaerobic nature of field hockey is not dissimilar to that of many sports detailed in this book, including soccer or Australian rules football (9). Therefore, a well-developed aerobic system is integral to field hockey performance, not only for the consistent active nature of field hockey but also for the metabolic recovery needed between high-

intensity efforts. While there is consensus on the overall physical demands of field hockey, there is some variability and differences across genders and positions, as highlighted in table 25.3.

Outfield Players

As previously mentioned, there is a wide range of physical performance requirements and countless high-intensity actions superimposed on the aerobically demanding game that is field hockey. Developing the aerobic system, a favorable body composition, and high relative strength levels is paramount for players to be able to sustain high-velocity actions and recover effectively between the multiple bouts of low-to-ground activities that can shape the outcome of a game. Outfield players can be broken down into the positional groups of forwards, midfielders, and defenders (or screens), with positional data shown in table 25.4.

Goalkeepers

Goalkeepers have the most unique demands of any position in field hockey. For starters, keepers wear far more equipment than any field player, with large leg guards typically measuring 24 to 28 in. tall by 10 to 11 in. wide, padded shoes called *kickers*, large blocking gloves on each hand, a chest protector, padded pants or girdles, a helmet with full face protection, and a specialized goalkeeping stick. Furthermore, the physical requirements are substantially different from those of the outfield players.

There are many physical attributes thought to be important for success in the position. A keeper should be kinesthetically aware of her limb positions, possess high levels of power-to-weight due to the additional equipment loads she must bear, have strong lateral and linear speeds, alongside high rates of force development (RFD) as they pertain to mitigating movement lag toward the ball or players as required. Reactive qualities highly depend on high relative strength levels, RFD, and neural drive. Goalkeepers must develop and embed these characteristics within both lower- and upper-limb movements.

The ability of a goalkeeper to track game play and position in or around the goal in such a manner as to manipulate an advantage in the goal space is critical to making scoring a goal as difficult as possible for the attacker. With this skill comes the necessity to perform both linear and lateral movements, both of which need to be performed in an optimal athletic posture that allows key reactive movements to be performed.

Often during shot attempts on goal, goalkeepers will commit to a fully extended ground position to block the shot attempt. Unfortunately, such positions can leave the goalkeeper and goal vulnerable should a deflection occur. It is crucial therefore that a goalkeeper possess sufficient strength and power qualities to react and return to her feet as quickly as possible. This ability requires excellent overall body strength, power, and limb coordination. Additionally, shoulder strength and arthrokinematics (movement at joint surfaces) are thought to be important for goalkeeper success.

Impact of Game Format Change: Halves Versus Quarters

In 2014, the game format at the international level changed substantially, shifting from two halves of 35 min to a four-quarter format involving 4 × 15 min

periods of faster play (1). Play is separated by 2 min rest periods between quarters 1 and 2 and between quarters 3 and 4, with a 10 min halftime stoppage between quarters 2 and 3. This format was introduced to complement TV formats at the Olympic Games, in the hopes of improving viewer interest by providing an even faster and more explosive brand of international field hockey. Figure 25.8 shows a GPS data set comparing an international team across the transition from one international season playing halves into the new international quarter format. These data highlight the substantial impact of the format change as it relates to the physical demands of the athletes, with 5% to 10% increases in overall work rate and high-intensity work rates generally shown across all outfield playing groups.

It is apparent from this data that the change in game format (halves to quarters) has had a meaningful impact on the positional lines at the international level (figure 25.8). With average total playing time being reduced to accommodate the 10 min game length reduction, all playing lines have had reductions in their average playing spell length times. Additionally, this reduction in field playing time has facilitated an increase in work rate (meters per minute) and HIA (distance covered over 15 km/h) in the new 60 min game compared to its 70 min counterpart. While there is no observable change in total distance covered per game, players must work harder to cover a similar total distance in a shorter time. This has implications as to how teams should prepare and train players, and hence the importance of prescribing the most appropriate HIIT weapon for hitting these aforementioned targets.

Key Weapons, Manipulations, and Surveillance Tools

In this section, I present the different HIIT weapons used in field hockey, their manipulations, along with ways we can use surveillance to help keep us on track throughout an international field hockey season.

HIIT Weapons

Different times within a training cycle or season call for bespoke changes in training priorities. Understanding how and when to make these adjustments is paramount to running a successful program. The ultimate goal must be to develop athletes who are capable of withstanding the demands of the

Position	Game type	Total distance	Work rate m/min	Total distance sprinting	% HIA	Total playing minutes	Average spell
Defender	Half	5783	115	605	10.8	51	14.7
Defender	Quarter	5978	122	651	11.2	48	10.5
Percentage difference		3	6	8	4	-6	-29

Position	Game type	Total distance	Work rate m/min	Total distance sprinting	% HIA	Total playing minutes	Average spell
Forwards	Half	4544	130	1000	21.7	36	6.5
Forwards	Quarter	4622	135	1174	23.5	32	5.5
Percentage difference		2	4	17	8	-11	-15

Position	Game type	Total distance	Work rate m/min	Total distance sprinting	% HIA	Total playing minutes	Average spell
Midfields	Half	5511	128	1117	20.1	42.6	8.6
Midfields	Quarter	5528	134	1231	22.2	41.4	6.7
Percentage difference		0	5	10	10	-3	-22

Position	Game type	Total distance	Work rate m/min	Total distance sprinting	% HIA	Total playing minutes	Average spell
Screens	Half	5918	124	885	15.3	48	10.9
Screens	Quarter	6003	131	1095	18.2	45	7.7
Percentage difference		1	6	24	19	-6	-29

Figure 25.8 Half versus quarter comparison in key GPS markers across international field hockey time-motion data for all positional groups.

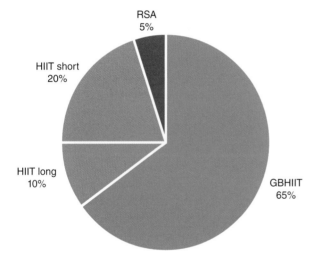

Figure 25.9 Percentage of the different HIIT formats (weapons) used throughout the annual season in elite field hockey: GBHIIT 65%, HIIT with long intervals 10%, HIIT with short intervals 20%, RSA 5%.

sport, allowing them to perform to their potential. Ultimately, we need to develop athletes who are resilient to the asymmetrical stresses of the sport and the demands of a competitive schedule. Using HIIT appropriately is key in this regard. The percentage breakdown of the different HIIT weapons pre-dominantly used to prepare field hockey players is shown in figure 25.9.

Manipulations of Interval Training Variables

The initial focus of any training program will be dictated by the phase of the training year. Being in season or out of season will heavily determine the focus of the physical qualities we address and the structure of training to prioritize the desired outcomes. Out of season for a club team often refers to any period outside of the competitive league fixture list. However, for the international teams the out-of-season tag is slightly more fluid in order to accommodate changing annual schedules and rotation into major events, alongside the different locations and qualification processes. The international fixtures typically occur from October to August, although there may be opportunities for breaks between international competitions. Generally, there is a break from all international fixtures during September and October, and often this follows the last major event in the international calendar (World Championships, Continental Championships, or the Olympic Games).

Immediately postseason offers a great opportunity for regeneration of the body and mind following extended exposures to the demands of the game. Like anything, however, a balanced approach to recovery and training is paramount for continued success. Returning too soon to training can lead to the resurgence of soft tissue issues, if injuries aren't fully recovered, whereas returning too late can result in inappropriate loading relative to the level of resiliency. As a result of this, and in order to progress the physical development of the athletes, it is paramount that physical demands accumulated during the season are not altogether lost due to inactivity. Neuromuscular aspects (type 2, 4, and 5 targets), including changes of direction and the high mechanical stress associated with low-to-ground actions, evasive activities, and the stop-start nature of the running patterns, mean that these need to be accommodated for during training when out of season. Repeated sprint activities, shuttles, and interval-based work should be present, as should customized

agility drills that allow athletes to train with their stick in hand. Adding the stick provides a training stimulus that facilitates additional loads and more-specific movement patterns. Similar to a monkey using its tail for balance, a stick in the hand will allow for sport-specific foot patterning and loading patterns, thus improving musculoskeletal tissue tolerance levels for future hockey demands. A 6 wk out-of-season RSA drill program is shown in table 25.5 and figure 25.10, while the Hamilton RSA protocol is described earlier in the chapter and in figure 25.4.

The positive side effect of these types of RSA and shuttle activities is that they facilitate higher neuromuscular stress (type 2, 4, and 5 targets) and develop the tissue tolerance levels needed to prepare athletes for the demands of on-field activities when

Table 25.5 Six Week Out-of-Season Repeated Sprint Ability (RSA) Drills for Field Hockey

Session	Week 1	Week 2	Week 3	Week 4	Week 5	Week 6
Dynamic warm-up	15 exercises × 15 m (16 yd)	15 exercises × 15 m	15 exercises × 15 m	15 exercises × 15 m	15 exercises × 15 m	15 exercises × 15 m
RSA (40 m) always on a rolling 30 s cycle			3 × 6 sprints (2.5 min rest between sets)	3 × 7 sprints (3 min rest between sets)	2 × 6 sprints (1 drill), 2 × 6 sprints (another drill), 5 min between drills, 3 min between sets	2 × 6 sprints (1 drill), 2 × 6 sprints (another drill), 5 min between drills, 2.5 min rest between sets

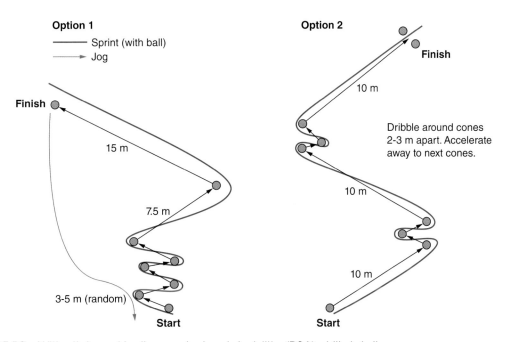

Figure 25.10   With stick and ball repeated sprint ability (RSA) drill details.

Table 25.6 Six Week Out-of-Season Field Hockey Speed and Conditioning Plan

Week	Monday	Tuesday	Wednesday
1			Conditioning 4 mile (6.4 km) run at self-selected pace Focus: central adaptation
2	Recovery: bike 30 min at 60 to 80 rpm Low resistance Type 1		Conditioning 4 mile run at target sub 30 min Focus: central adaptation Type 1
3	Speed session	Conditioning treadmill 5×3 min at 85% (30-15 V_{IFT}), 3 min rest between sets Focus: central adaptation Type 3	
4	Speed session	Conditioning treadmill 5×3 min at 88% (30-15 V_{IFT}), 3 min rest between sets Focus: central adaptation Type 3	Speed session
5		Conditioning treadmill 6×3 min at 85% (30-15 V_{IFT}), 3 min rest between sets Focus: central adaptation Type 3	
6	Speed session	Conditioning 4 mile run at sub 28 min Type 3	

out of season. However, the negative aspect or challenge to these activities is that they facilitate higher neuromuscular stress. Therefore it is critical to have a well thought out plan and weekly structure to ensure the volume of work completed is actualized in a manner favorable to long-term athlete development. Understanding the recovery needs following any training stress is also important and will depend on the system trained, load of the activity performed (chapter 8), training history, and individual aspects. We know that a *physical poke* results in some kind of metabolic or neuromuscular response and the degree of that response depends on the individual athlete, their fitness level and prior training history, along with the intensity, duration, and mode of activity (see chapter 9).

During the off-season and preseason phases, we should look to take direction from what is learned from training load monitoring in season and around the constraints of competition. By quantifying and periodizing these training loads, we can strategically prescribe training that accurately replicates the in-season load demands. Replicating exactly the in-season training load is not the solution. However, progressive exposure to competition load levels is more the goal. Using the HIIT weapons appropriately is key in this regard. Table 25.6 shows an example of a 6 wk out-of-season field hockey speed and conditioning plan, while figure 25.11 provides conditioning drill details.

Maximal aerobic speed (MAS) prescriptions, or long intervals (greater than 3 min exposures of

Week	Thursday	Friday	Saturday	Sunday
1				Conditioning treadmill: 4×4 at 82% (30-15 vIFT) Focus: central adaptation Type 3
2	Speed session		Conditioning hockey match or 3×10 15:15 shuttle at 95% (30-15 vIFT), 3 min rest between sets Focus: introduce COD and peripheral adaptation Type 4	
3	Conditioning repeat sprint (see options in figure 25.11) Focus: peripheral adaptation Type 5		Conditioning hockey match 3×14/12/12 at 95% 15:15 straight, 3 min rest between sets Focus: peripheral adaptation Type 4	
4	Conditioning repeat sprint (see options in figure 25.11) Focus: peripheral adaptation Type 5		Conditioning 3×12 at 100% 15:15 straight, 3 min rest between sets Focus: peripheral adaptation Type 4	
5	Conditioning repeat sprint (see options in figure 25.11) Focus: peripheral adaptation Type 5		Conditioning 3×14 at 95% 10:10 straight, 3 min rest between sets Focus: peripheral adaptation Type 1	
6	Conditioning repeat sprint (see options in figure 25.11) Focus: peripheral adaptation Type 5		Conditioning 3×12 at 100% 10:10 straight, 3 min rest between sets Focus: peripheral adaptation Type 1	

running), are an excellent training methodology to elicit a physiological poke guaranteed to promote adaptation. This type of training prescription is multifaceted when it comes to effectiveness, as it is simple to prescribe and individualize and can be performed in multiple training environments (gym treadmill, courts, fields, tracks, etc.). It offers an appropriate volume and intensity of training with a high physiological adaptation response to facilitate central adaptations (type 3 and 4 targets), while mitigating the excessive running, sometimes referred to as junk miles, associated with long slow runs (LSR) or traditional fartlek approaches. Both LSR and fartlek work have their place in off-season training, but more as a means of amplifying running volume in the week when accurate prescriptions of distances and time are not possible, such as during a vacation where facilities may be limited.

Periods of training at or near $\dot{V}O_2max$ for sustained periods of time will provide the necessary training stimulus to promote central and peripheral adaptations within the aerobic system (chapter 3). Therefore the maximal aerobic speed (MAS) sessions described across a 4 wk block of training are an excellent means of ensuring that sufficient training intensity and duration are achieved. In this weekly structure, we have a balanced approach to the management and development of the aerobic system, while controlling for the high neuromuscular demand of small-sided game (SSG) and hockey match play throughout the week. Straight-line MAS is the preferred training methodology during the

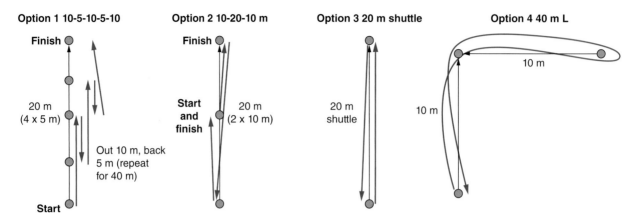

Figure 25.11 Without stick-and-ball drills.

Table 25.7 Seasonal Prescription Loads for MAS (Using 30-15V$_{IFT}$ Values for Prescription) During a Training Week

	Week 1	Week 2	Week 3	Week 4	Week 5	Week 6
MAS 1 (straight)	3×12 at 95% 15:15	3×12/10/10 at 100% 15:15	3×12/10/8 at 103% 15:15	3×14 at 95% 10:10	3×12 at 100% 10:10	3×12/10/10 at 105% 10:10
HIIT type	Type 2	Type 3	Type 4	Type 2	Type 3	Type 4
MAS 2 (shuttle)	3×9 at 95% 15:15 shuttle	3×8 at 98% 15:15 shuttle	3×7 at 100% 15:15 shuttle	3×9 at 95% 10:10 shuttle	3×8 at 100% 10:10 shuttle	3×8/8/6 at 102% 10:10 shuttle
HIIT type	Type 2	Type 4	Type 5	Type 4	Type 5	Type 5

in-season training week. This type of straight-line prescription allows for controlled exposure to the training intensities required to elicit an appropriate dose of aerobic responses, while mitigating the unnecessary mileage and high neuromuscular loads associated with the mechanical loading of musculature during shuttles and changes of direction. A 6 wk prescription of training using 30-15V$_{IFT}$ values for prescription is shown in table 25.7.

During the training week in season, I prioritize 1 or 2 additional MAS sessions to help facilitate improvements to this system. Game-based HIIT or small-sided games (SSGs) are fantastic for developing myriad physical attributes (speed, COD, lactate profiling, anaerobic and aerobic processes) through the manipulation of player numbers, pitch size, playing duration, and rest. However, despite the high level of variety possible in game structure, we are unable to guarantee total development to all players uniformly during these sessions. SSGs can offer an opportunity for individuals to hide, control effort lengths, and even limit their development and improvement opportunities.

As the off-season progresses and the season approaches, the run volume (distance/time) prescription within the repetitions is lowered. This small tweak in repetition volume allows for a higher number of total repetitions to be performed, along with a larger volume of accelerations and decelerations and higher running speeds. This change in prescription allows for transition from the centrally focused adaptations more toward the peripherally focused ones (figure 25.7; see also chapter 3). This is a training adaptation unique to the prescription and a key quality that will help underpin high-intensity actions throughout a game. I recommend performing such long intervals 2 to 4 times a week, separated by 24 to 48 h of recovery.

Load Surveillance and Monitoring Tools

Successful training prescription is most effective when we adopt an athlete-centered approach and develop our understanding of both training load (chapter 8) and the individual athlete response (chapter 9). It is important that we create a training environment that is rich in information to remove subjectivity around our loading and unloading strategies. The ultimate goal for athlete management has to be having our athletes arrive at their competitive peak in a predictable way. This requires a thorough needs analysis of the athlete and an integrated approach to assessing the components that will positively impact on performance by developing unique and bespoke monitoring systems.

As with any athlete who strives to improve performance, there is often a systematic increase in training frequency, volume, and intensity of training. This increase in training load is often successful and represented as a performance improvement. However, athletes will also experience varying severe levels of fatigue during such challenges, and since performance and training can be compromised during such periods, it is paramount that effective monitoring strategies are put in place. It is the role of the support staff to effectively monitor and assess fatigue to facilitate optimal recovery and prevent abnormal fatigue states or overtraining from occurring (see chapter 7).

As described in chapters 8 and 9, the physical stress that forms the training load creates a physiological response, and the extent of the response will vary depending on the individual and their reaction to the intensity, volume, and type of activity performed. A performance program rich in information will allow you to more effectively understand the individuals on the team. Monitoring should involve a set of activities designed to help establish the acute training status of the athlete, so that appropriate and timely training adjustments can take place that ensure ongoing performance targets are attained. Essentially, the outcome from a monitoring system should be to produce a training environment that facilitates the greatest amount of development and ensures optimal performance around the competition program. Once we have the information, we can be well situated to make accurate and timely decisions around recovery interventions, physical development, and competition strategies.

Training Status Surveillance and Monitoring Tools

The primary training status surveillance and monitoring tools we use in field hockey include GPS for external load and session rating of perceived exertion (RPE) for internal load, with wellness questionnaires and drop jumps to assess the response to loading.

GPS Systems (External Training Load)

As discussed throughout the chapter, GPS systems are used extensively by international hockey squads to measure external training load. GPS systems have become invaluable tools for helping coaches and practitioners better quantify the work being completed during training and in competition. This numerical understanding of physical workload has helped us refine training methodologies, manipulate training through drills and SSG strategies, and make position-specific modifications and work:rest interval adjustments, and understand a player's training load (see chapter 8). As a means to understand and quantify training and game loads for athletes, time-motion data (GPS) can be used to quantify exactly how far athletes are running at different speeds during a game. Zones can be chosen to reflect game impact and describe the type of work being completed (see tables 25.2 to 25.4 and figure 25.8).

Session RPE (Internal Load)

Session RPE is an excellent way for the field hockey coach and athlete to monitor training intensity without equipment (see chapter 8). Numerous studies have shown that session RPE is an excellent way to assess globally an athlete's perception of internal training load (4) and this has proven effective for a variety of resistance and conditioning session types (11). RPE is extremely useful in the context of field hockey player monitoring across the large variety of training modes players undergo during a typical training week. An example of a session RPE load capture across 4 wk is shown in figure 25.12.

Wellness Questionnaires

It is generally accepted that excessive training stress can be associated with psychological disturbances and changes in disposition as well as marked changes to both cognitive and somatic markers in the body (chapter 7). In order to address such factors, we use wellness questionnaires to assess daily wellness scores and extensively monitor these varying manifestations of stress. It is important to realize that for a wellness tool to be a truly effective indicator of physical performance, there is a need for it to be used in conjunction with other physical performance

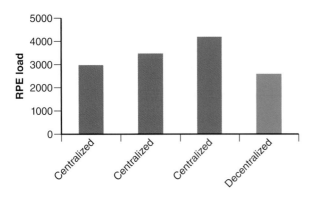

Figure 25.12 A four-week linear model of loading measured using session rating of perceived exertion (RPE).

tests that offer insight into the mechanistic changes that may be impacting the athlete.

Neuromuscular Assessment

When considering the impact of field hockey on an athlete and trying to understand the implication of training and competition on performance, it is important to look beyond the metabolic cost of energy systems and to also consider the mechanical cost of low-to-ground actions, high decelerations, and multiple changes of direction. Fatigue will manifest in different facets of the body's functionality, and an area often overlooked due to feasibility of assessment and resourcing is the neuromuscular system (chapters 3, 4, and 5). A compromised neuromuscular system has an effect on force, velocity, and power qualities and ultimately performance potential (3). Assessment of neuromuscular fatigue, including drop jumps and the reactive strength index, is described in chapters 3 and 8.

Strategies for Structuring the Training Program Using HIIT

I use a number of strategies in field hockey to structure the training program and HIIT prescription, which must be made alongside the context of the program, and its controllable and uncontrollable factors.

Controllable and Uncontrollable Factors

Time availability for training specific physical qualities can become limited during the season and during the training week. It is fundamental that we understand what truly underpins and impacts success in our sports. Experience, mastery, and exposure to the event are key to long-term success within our chosen fields. Learning from situational play, repeated exposure to game-specific situations, and developing mastery of our skills form the backbone philosophy of our program. Our main goal then is to give our international athletes back to our club coaches as often as we can. Nevertheless, having the ability to compromise is imperative for success, and the ability to pick the training tools to invoke the largest and most appropriate training response in a timely fashion is what separates the great teams from the good ones.

Program Structure and Progression

Due to the length of an international season and the extended preparation time required, it is important to build an intelligent program that provides resiliency in the athletes through appropriately progressed training loads and adequate recovery. With an international field hockey program that is often full time and centralized (athletes train out of the same facility), a 4 wk linear periodization model has been proven to be an effective means by which athletes may achieve this outcome (i.e., figure 25.12). The 4 wk linear model is structured in such a way as to facilitate an increase in hockey training frequency and volume each week. The program is built around a 4 wk mesocycle consisting of 3 wk of progressive hockey and physical development loading and 1 wk of unloading when no mandatory team hockey sessions are completed. Instead, physical qualities are targeted and off-feet conditioning becomes a priority. This 4 wk loading pattern facilitates an accumulation of hockey-specific training load, while also allowing for a regeneration week and a hockey-specific stress unloading period from the asymmetric demands of the game.

The advantage of this type of periodized model is that it develops most athletes' ability to tolerate multiple training sessions in a day and across consecutive days of hockey match play, while establishing timely recovery windows to support the regeneration of tissue from hockey-specific overload. This model involving 3 wk of hockey load complements and appropriately prepares the players for the demands of tournament hockey, where they are typically required

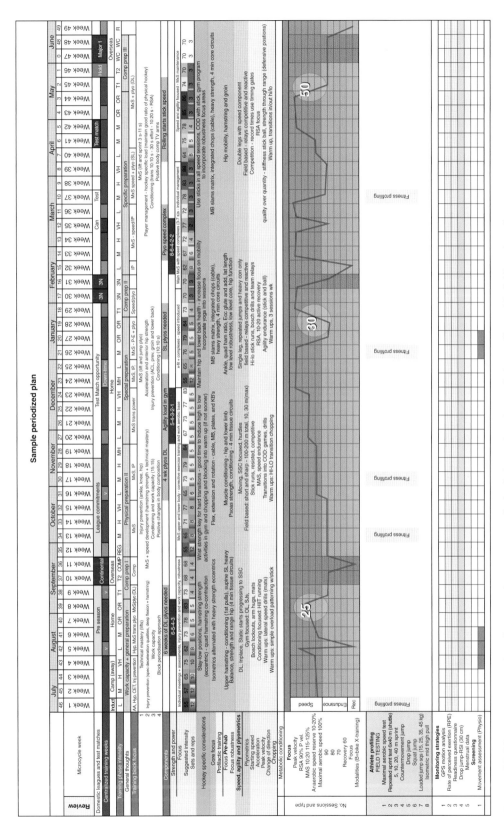

Figure 25.13   An example of a yearly macrocycle training plan in an international field hockey team.

Training phase	Comp schedule	Week	Monday	Tuesday	Wednesday	Thursday	Friday	Saturday	Sunday	Gym	Cond	Rob	Sp&ag	Reps	Gym intensity	Physical load 1 low 5-very high
Physical preparation ii	Regeneration	35	Rest	Bike recovery	Bike-interval	Circuit	Conditioning	Rest	Rest	2	2	1	0	12	55	1
			Rest	Upper body	Robustness	Rest	Rest	Rest	Rest							
	Centralized	34	Gym	Hockey	Gym-upper	Hockey	Gym	Conditioning	Rest	3	2	1	1	8	65	3
			Hockey	Hockey	Rest	Hockey	Rest	Rest	Rest							
	Centralized	33	Gym	Hockey	Gym-upper	Hockey	Gym	Conditioning	Rest	3	2	1	1	6	79	4
			Hockey	Hockey	Rest	Hockey	Rest	Rest	Rest							
	Centralized	32	Gym-testing	Hockey	Gym-upper	Hockey	Gym	Conditioning	Rest	3	2	1	1	3	85	5
			Hockey	Hockey	Rest	Hockey	Rest	Rest	Rest							
	Regeneration	31	Bike recovery	Gym-speed	Bike-interval	Gym	Speed* conditioning	Rest	Rest	3	4	0	2	5	65	2
			Gym-upper	Rest	Mobility	Rest	Rest	Rest	Rest							
	Centralized	30	30-15 + speed	RSA	Gym	Hockey	Hockey	Gym	Rest	3	2	1	1	5	72	3
			Gym-upper	Hockey	Rest	Hockey	Rest	Rest	Rest							
	Centralized	29	Gym	Hockey	Gym-upper	Hockey	Gym	Speed* conditioning	Rest	3	2	1	1	5	77	4
			Hockey	Hockey	Rest	Hockey	Rest	Rest	Rest							
	Centralized	28	Gym	Hockey	Gym-upper	Hockey	Gym	Conditioning	Rest	3	2	1	1	5	82	4
			Hockey	Hockey	Rest	Hockey	Rest	Rest	Rest							
	Regeneration	27	Bike recovery	Gym-speed	Bike-interval	Circuit	Speed* conditioning	Bike-RSA	Rest	3	2	1	2	4	74	2
			Gym-upper	Rest	Mobility	Rest	Rest	Rest	Rest							

Figure 25.14 A sample mesocycle bimonthly training plan in an international field hockey team.

Table 25.8   Sample Microcycle (One Week) Training Plan of an International Field Hockey Team

Monday	Tuesday	Wednesday	Thursday	Friday	Saturday	Sunday
Hockey	Hockey	Gym	Hockey	Hybrid: gym and hockey	Conditioning: MAS 2	OFF
Gym	Hockey + MAS 1		Hockey + SSG			OFF

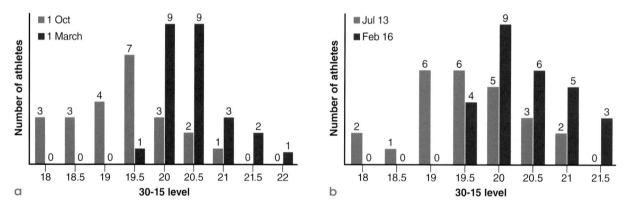

Figure 25.15 The impact of MAS prescription and changes in 30-15 IFT performance in two international field hockey teams across two quadrennial cycles, (a) 2012 and (b) 2016 Games. Pre-value levels in blue, post-value levels in red, with numbers representing the number of team members achieving that level.

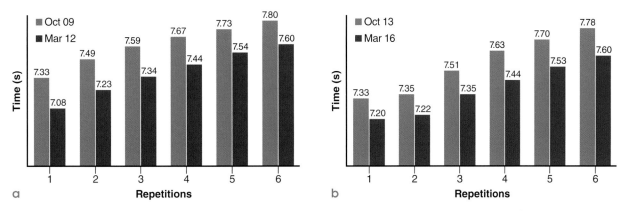

Figure 25.16 The impact of repeated sprint ability (RSA) prescription on changes in RSA performance in two international field hockey teams across two quadrennial cycles: (a) 2012 and (b) 2016 Games. Pre-value levels in blue, post-value levels in red, with numbers representing the number of 40 m sprint repetitions achieved.

Table 25.9 Physical and Performance Markers in Two Separate Teams Across Two Olympic Cycles

Measures include body weight, relative back squat and bench press performance, as well as 5 m, 10 m, mean repeated sprint ability performance(s), and 30-15 intermittent fitness test (30-15) level.

Team	Date	Body weight (kg)	Relative back squat	Relative bench press	5 m (s)	10 m (s)	Mean RSA 6×40 m shuttle (s)	30-15 level (km/h)
2012 Olympic team	Late 2009	65.6	1.29	0.68	1.11	1.85	7.87	19.2
	Early 2010	67.3	1.58	0.80	1.05	1.82	7.62	20.1
	Late 2010	64.5	1.35	0.76	1.07	1.85	7.68	19.4
	Early 2011	64.4	1.52	0.86	1.00	1.78	7.54	19.7
	Late 2011	63.2	1.55	0.89	1.07	1.81	7.54	20.2
	Early 2012	63.2	1.59	0.95	1.00	1.77	7.40	20.5
2016 Olympic team	Late 2013	61.0	1.55	0.91	1.02	1.79	7.54	19.4
	Early 2014	60.7	1.58	0.95	1.01	1.77	7.47	20.0
	Early 2015	60.4	1.65	0.90	0.97	1.76	7.43	20.2
	Late 2015	60.0	1.76	0.99	0.97	1.72	7.37	20.3
	Early 2016	59.8	1.70	0.96	0.97	1.74	7.42	20.4

to compete on consecutive days. In fact, during the major events of international field hockey—Champions Trophy, Continental Cups, World Cups, and the Olympic Games—teams are expected to complete 7 games in 12 d. Ultimately, this model of 3 wk on and 1 wk off will allow for the development of athlete robustness and resilience alongside a training structure that promotes longevity.

Specifically, we look to develop three qualities that underpin field hockey performance in our athletes, including:

1. **Durability:** ability to withstand the daily wear and tear that a prolonged central program delivers, while avoiding the potential injury risks associated with repetitive movements.

2. **Robustness:** development of strong and tough tissue that has adapted to the demands of hockey-specific overload and can tolerate a high frequency of repetitive movements.

3. **Recoverability:** an innate resilience to fatigue, with efficient movement skill and an ability to maintain postures and positions for prolonged periods.

Having clear goals and training objectives established throughout a training year is important, but understanding how to structure the training week (microcycle) will form the foundation and key building block needed to make the goals achievable.

Sample Training Programs

Macrocycle, mesocycle, and microcycle examples of international field hockey teams are shown in figures 25.13 and 25.14 and table 25.8, respectively.

Longitudinal Training Effects

Figure 25.15 represents the impact of MAS prescription and positive changes in 30-15 IFT performance in two international field hockey teams across two quadrennial cycles, while figure 25.16 shows related outcomes of RSA training and Hamilton RSA performance along a similar time course in the same teams. Table 25.9 shows the longitudinal physical and performance markers measured across two Olympic cycles in two separate teams.

Acknowledgments

I would like to thank Bobby Lucas for his assistance with data collection and analysis. The experiences had with players and staff involved throughout the two Olympic campaigns described herein are also greatly valued.

It was a brisk Tuesday afternoon at the Olympic park in Stratford, London. Our Team GB hockey team was still 5 mo from the Olympic Games, but as host nation, we had the ability to gain brief access to the Olympic venue. This was an edge we believed we couldn't pass up, even if it meant we would have to endure a 2 h bus journey through London traffic, countless nights in hotels, eating our lunch pitch side, and meeting in cold porta-cabins sitting on the floor. No stadium was built at this point—just the pink and blue turfs, surrounded by scaffolding and heavy-duty construction trucks. While not the ideal training venue, the opportunity to increase familiarity with the Olympic turf, see our Olympic pitch develop, and be a part of the process could offer us the advantage we were after. As the rewards of playing at the unfinished Olympic turf far outweighed the logistical and administrative difficulties of getting there, we made systematic trips to the Olympic park over the 12 mo lead-in period to the Games, each time developing familiarity with the turf.

We felt our preparations for the London Games were on track and going well. We had witnessed some exciting changes within the group physically, both on and off the field. Our world ranking status was steadily improving since 2010, and we had medaled at all but one major event since the team centralized at Bisham Abbey (October 2009). Our team was now reaping the rewards of our preparation, ensuring we left nothing on the field during the quadrennial plan in our search of a podium finish in our home Olympic Games. Visiting the partially constructed Olympic park regularly was one of the important decisions.

On this particular Tuesday afternoon at the Olympic park, training was to have a surprise element to it, a calculated and planned element that none of the athletes were aware of. The content of the session had been devised 1 wk earlier as a means of rectifying a small glitch in the system. The team was coming off a couple of favorable training weeks and into the decentralized week, during which athletes had no national hockey team commitments and a light centralized training week (figure 25.12). However, on this particular occasion, we were unexpectedly not seeing as positive a response in the group's recovery as we were more accustomed to seeing. Players were tired, complaining of a lack of rest in the session content, as well as with the session's difficulty levels. Warm-ups were taking longer, and the staff had to work to motivate the team in exercises, and post-training conditioning runs were perceived as difficult. As a staff, we did what most coaches and support staff would do. We looked inward on ourselves and asked the obvious questions:

- Are we doing too much?
- Are we overtraining them?
- Do we have the timing all wrong?

But our performance metrics told us differently. By taking ourselves from Google Street View to Google Earth perspective, the disconnect was clear. There was no apparent reason for excessive fatigue. Perhaps it wasn't about overtraining, but more about the monotony of training. Could the repetitive nature of our training program, which requires athletes to rinse and repeat every 4 wk, have actually created a false fatigue response, manifesting more as mental, not physical, fatigue? Indeed, we too as staff had similar feelings.

But being 5 mo out from the Games was not the time to take the foot off the gas and risk losing the adaptations we had worked so hard to create. So instead, we decided that this was exactly the time to throw the rope around ourselves as a team, to refocus on our purpose, as well as the goals, commitment, and promise we had set as a team in October 2009. The Tuesday would provide the opportunity to take this group of aspiring Olympians to a place they had never been before. It would be an opportunity to show themselves as a group just how far they had come in their journey, and the level of robustness and resilience they had developed as a team. Fundamentally, the purpose of the session was to help the athletes reset their understanding of what *hard* actually is. While we know training monotony is undesirable from an injury perspective, it can also create a numbness or lack of feel to

(continued)

training load. This following planned exposure would potentially help reset the monotony cycle. At least that was our belief.

The Tuesday afternoon session at the Olympic pitch contained the usual content, finishing with 3 v 2 SSG toward the goal. The 2 h on the pitch was now up, and the team looked to be wrapping up the session, beginning to debrief with coaches. As was normal during this stage of the sessions, players started looking for me. Where was Dave? Was he setting up cones for the conditioning component of the sessions that typically followed the session? Smiles ensued, as they saw no cones out. "Yes, today we have no running," you could hear being whispered among the group.

"OK, cool down," I shouted. The girls started the two-lap cooldown that preempted team stretching. We wanted the athletes to feel relaxed, happy, safe, and comfortable in their environment. We wanted them to believe this was the end of training. Only three or four athletes had made it back to the bench before the head coach blew the whistle, sending all the players to the goal line, where I was waiting. The staff rapidly set up the cones. We had caught the team off guard, as planned. Questions ensued from the player group, demanding to know what was up. As agreed by the coaching staff, no information was to be given to the team pertaining to session details, except for the prescription of the run format, which was 10:10 at 102% straight, with a straight repetition followed by a shuttle, repeat until we say stop.

The athletes set themselves up into their respective 30-15 IFT groups for the conditioning (level 19.5, 20, 20.5, etc.) so the correct running distances were assigned. "How many are we doing?" a couple of athletes demanded.

Ignoring all questions, I simply shouted, "Ready?" The whistle went and the dislocation of expectation session began. I could still hear the players talking among themselves. "He normally does 12 reps of this, so worst case 14," was one comment.

The group was well conditioned and at this stage in our Olympic prep, the average 30-15 IFT score for the women's Olympic team was 20.8. This was an aerobically gifted group of athletes and I was unsure how many repetitions and sets of 10:10 at 102% it was going to take. It was the one unknown about this session experience that we couldn't account for. I suggested 15 to 17 repetitions would be uncomfortable, and that we would start to see substantial lagging in 20% to 30% of the group by then. I could not have been more wrong, and we as a staff could not have hoped for a better response and showing of resolve by the team.

After 22 repetitions, athletes started to fall to their knees during the rest periods, with players trying to motivate one another, yet barely getting more than one or two syllables out. Despite that, I counted down from 5. The athletes dragged themselves and each other off their knees to their feet for number 23. Their resolve and intent to not give up was impressive, but that was enough for that series. I faked the whistle and shouted, "Stop." The players collapsed to the ground.

That is it, it is over, they must have thought. "Three minutes rest," I shouted.

The staff was looking at each other and the players to see their response. Within 2 min, they were back to their feet and ready to go again. The mental strength and physical resilience to put themselves back on the line was the sole purpose of the session, and not the associated type 4 stimulus it had. That ability to go beyond what would be considered normal (12 to 14 repetitions in this case) and into a much darker place, a place they didn't think possible (22 repetitions), was the real aim. Perhaps this is such a place an athlete might find herself in during an Olympic match with a medal on the line. How much resolve can be found in the last 2 or 3 min, when you've already given everything and feel exhausted? What do you really have left to give for your team? Do you really know if you have it in you? As staff, we now knew that they really did.

I blew the whistle and we started again. But we had seen what we wanted. I stopped the session at 8 repetitions, and the players crumbled to the floor a second time. This time nothing was actually next. Just home on the bus, but with a new sense of what was now possible, and with a greater understanding of what hard really is.

The team medaled at the Olympics, achieving the first field hockey team medal in 20 years.

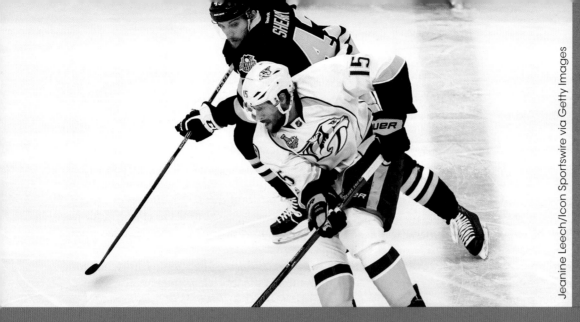

26

Ice Hockey

• • • • • •

Matt Nichol

Performance Demands of Ice Hockey

While every sport has its own intricacies, I would argue that no sport requires such a robust combination of highly specific skills, variable energy system demands, and physical resiliency as the sport of ice hockey. The playing surface alone creates truly unique demands on the body unlike any other team sport.

In this section, the sport of ice hockey is described, including the various physical demands that it imposes on its participants. Additionally, we'll examine the role of the unique playing surface as well as the equipment and rules of play, which impact the way we need to prepare ice hockey players to be successful.

Sport Description and Factors of Winning

There are currently two distinct versions of the game of ice hockey: the International or Olympic version and the North American or National Hockey League (NHL) version. For the purposes of this chapter, we will be mostly referring to the North American or NHL version of ice hockey. Although there are very obvious differences with respect to the size of the playing surface and some slight variations in the rules, the energy system demands are similar. The most

significant difference between the two formats is the larger playing surface in Olympic-style ice hockey. This allows for a greater number of tactical options for coaches and requires its players to be more proficient skaters, or perhaps more accurately, exposes those players whose skating insufficiencies might be covered up through above-average size and strength or stickhandling abilities. The Olympic version of the game may require a slightly larger anaerobic fitness component, but the reader can extrapolate from the suggestions made herein and apply these to the international game as needed.

Ice hockey is played on a hockey rink, which is an oval sheet of ice contained within a perimeter of high-density composite plastic walls referred to as the boards. The playing surface is 61 m × 26 m (67 × 28 yd), with a corner radius of 8.5 m (9.3 yd), and the distance from the end boards to the nearest goal line is 3.4 m (3.7 yd). The boards surrounding the playing surface prevent the players from going out of bounds at any time; however, play is immediately stopped if the puck exits the playing surface (entering either the player's bench or the spectator seating area). The playing surface is made entirely of ice, which imposes unique physical demands on the players from both a biomechanical and physiological standpoint (see following).

A game consists of three periods of 20 min each, played with stop time, with the clock running only when the puck is in play. An 18 min intermission occurs after the first and second periods, and the total average time of an NHL hockey game is 2 h and 30 min. Games are played between two teams of six players per side, including five skaters and one goaltender. The goaltender is able to play the puck offensively from directly in front of his net or inside the trapezoid area directly behind his net. Typically, the goaltender does not leave the immediate area of the goal or net. The five skaters on the ice are divided into three forwards and two defensemen. The forward positions consist of a center and two wingers: a left wing and a right wing. The defensemen play together as a pair and are divided into left and right depending on their dominant shooting sides. Forwards play together as units or lines, with the same three forwards consistently playing together. Teams will generally play each game with four lines of forwards and three pairings of defensemen and two goaltenders (starter and backup), for a total of 20 players dressed each game.

A substitution of an entire unit at once is called a line change. To achieve this, teams typically employ alternate sets of forward lines and defensive pairings when shorthanded or on a power play (down a man due typically to a penalty). Substitutions are permit-

ted at any time during the game. When players are substituted during play, it is called changing on the fly. When a team substitutes a player on the fly, the defensemen are forced to remain on the ice longer to protect against any scoring opportunities by the opposition while the team is momentarily outnumbered. As a result of this tactic, the defensemen end up having fewer opportunities to change and spend a greater amount of time on the ice. This point is important with respect to the time-motion analysis of the game and the subsequent additional conditioning demands for defensemen.

Relative Contribution of Physical Performance

Although ice hockey is a physically demanding sport, the primary differentiating factor between elite performers is not one specific measure of strength or fitness but rather high levels of technical skill with the puck, elite-level skating ability, and tactical awareness (commonly referred to as *hockey sense*). While it would be expected that all players at the professional level would exhibit levels of strength and fitness that would be superior to the amateur population, it is not uncommon to find elite performers in the sport who

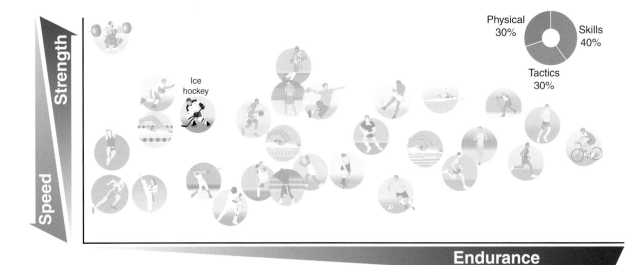

Figure 26.1 The position of the ice hockey player on the three axes illustrates the relative importance of the three main physical capacities of importance for elite participation in ice hockey, acknowledging that this varies slightly between positions. Outside of critical psychological and team chemistry components, which are difficult to quantify, the pie chart shows the general relative importance of skills (40%), tactical awareness (30%), and physical capacities (30%) for ice hockey success.

Adapted from G.A. Nader, "Concurrent Strength and Endurance Training: From Molecules to Man," *Medicine & Science in Sports & Exercise* 38, no. 11 (2006): 1965-1970.

have average or even below-average levels of strength or fitness compared to their cohorts. Figure 26.1 illustrates the relative importance of these factors in relation to other common sports found in this book.

Common markers of physical fitness do play a role in team success, but like many team sports, there is no direct correlation (11). While it stands to reason that faster and better-conditioned teams pose a greater chance of success, due to a lack of standardized testing across teams and the confidential nature of such tests for most teams, it is hard to quantify this with any degree of certainty. One longitudinal study published on an NHL team, however, showed that markers related to team success included peak 5 s anaerobic power performed during a 30 s Wingate power test, team average percent body fat, and lean body mass (12).

While the purpose of this section of the chapter is to discuss the physical preparation of ice hockey players and specifically to examine methods for developing the relevant energy systems, it must be stated that the number one determinant for success is hockey-specific skill. This is an important consideration for those responsible for the physical preparation of elite ice hockey players, as we must never lose sight of the relative importance of specific on-ice training for the athletes.

The literature available with respect to the anthropometric and physiological profiles of professional hockey players reveals that while these athletes are superior to the average recreational player, their profiles are not as strikingly dissimilar as might be seen in a professional basketball player, American football player, or elite track-and-field athlete. What sets the elite in ice hockey apart is their ability to technically apply their physical attributes on a surface of sheer ice balancing on a blade less than 1/8th of an inch thick. The act of skating on ice is a very unnatural movement and expert performance requires thousands of hours of technical training. Likewise, the ability to control the puck and make offensive plays with it (passing, scoring) requires incredible dexterity, exceptional visual processing skills, hand-eye coordination, and functional strength that is difficult to develop outside of playing the sport itself.

Ice hockey is generally regarded as the fastest team sport in the world. The players themselves can achieve speeds on their skates in excess of 40 km/h (25 mph). When shot, the puck can travel up to 180 km/h (112 mph) and punish players brave enough to place their bodies between the shooter and their goal. For goaltenders to successfully save such a shot requires lightning-quick reactive abilities. The lack of friction on the ice surface coupled with the high speed of movement necessitates great eccentric strength to execute the repeated rapid stops and starts and changes of direction of travel that occur during each shift. Such movements additionally require high metabolic rates.

Low body fat percentage, high lean body mass, high relative strength (squat, chin- or pull-up) and power (Wingate peak and mean power, vertical and broad jump) have all shown high correlation with on-ice accelerative ability, but not necessarily individual point production or team winning (11). It is also important to note that ice hockey is a high-speed collision sport that incurs an extremely high incidence of injury during play. Those responsible for the physical preparation of elite-level ice hockey players must take this aspect into consideration when designing the annual training plan, by including posture-specific balancing exercises, skating strength, power, and agility exercises (9).

Targets of Physical Performance in Ice Hockey

As I've touched on, ice hockey is a high-speed, discontinuous, repeated-sprint sport. The play on the ice is characterized by rapid and irregular changes in movement patterns, accelerations and decelerations, as well as alternations between extremely high- and relatively low-intensity movements over a short time period (5). It is a sport that involves high-speed collisions and high-speed projectiles (pucks, sticks, and skate blades), and thus involves a large degree of potential for injury and bodily harm.

While some requisite level of aerobic fitness is likely to be beneficial for ice hockey performance, I don't believe you need to achieve this through traditional aerobic training that you might see in some of the other sports presented in this book. In my experience, athletes are prepared using almost no traditional aerobic training (outside of occasional walks in nature), yet these players can achieve some of the highest scores in their team's fitness testing rounds, play some of the most minutes on their teams, and in excess of 1000 NHL games over a career. While such outcomes are believed to be unachievable without a good level of aerobic fitness, I believe these results can be achieved using more unconventional but highly effective ways (see HIIT Weapons).

Forwards and Defensemen

Shift players may play for as long as 90 s or as short as 10 s, depending on a multitude of factors (penalties, poor line changes, coach decisions, official time interruptions, etc.). However, the average length of a shift for a forward in the NHL is 46 s, with a total time on the ice averaged at 16 min. The average shift length for a defenseman in the NHL is 55 s with an average total time on the ice of 20 min. The recovery time between shifts is 3 to 5 min for forwards and 2 to 4 min for defensemen. Clearly, the nature of the game of modern ice hockey itself resembles a high-intensity interval training (HIIT) format, specifically the repeated-sprint training (RST) format. A time-motion analysis study by Jackson (7) suggests that the average intra-shift work:rest (W:R) ratio (purposeful medium- to high-intensity movement versus nonpurposeful or stationary to low-intensity movement) across all players during even-strength play was 1:1.6, and the game W:R (time on ice versus time on bench) was 1:3.7 (7). Each on-ice shift is composed of a series of rapid accelerations and decelerations of only 1 to 3 s, interspersed with low- to medium-intensity gliding and occasional physical struggles with an opponent for possession of the puck. Thus, the ability to perform a multitude of short explosive bouts of work with little recovery, known as repeated-sprint ability (6), and described within the book as RSS, or repeated-sprint sequences, is a critical requirement for ice hockey. This form of training (i.e., RST, chapters 4 and 5), and specifically type 4 and 5 targets,

needs to be the predominant training applied in an ice hockey player's program.

Time-motion analysis by Bracko et al. (3), illustrated in figure 26.2, shows that, contrary to popular belief, the majority of the time a player is on the ice, he is engaged in very low-intensity movements, such as gliding, low- to medium-intensity forward skating, and stationary play, both with and without the puck (3, 7). Thus, regardless of the position played, all skaters spend the majority of their time on the ice (up to 55%) performing low-intensity work. This time is important to allow the replenishment of energy stores required for subsequent high-intensity moments of play (see also chapter 4 (10)). As described by Montgomery (10), a typical player performs for 15 to 20 min of a 60 min game, where each shift lasts from 30 to 80 s, and there is typically 4 to 5 min of recovery between shifts.

Due to the lack of friction on ice, players continue moving after they stop active locomotion, and are able to glide with little to no work once their momentum is generated, making this sport low demand relative to others from an endurance context (figure 26.1). Conversely, stopping completely or making a 180-degree change of direction creates large mechanical costs relative to similar movements executed in land-based sport surfaces of high friction (court, field-turf, etc.). This aspect creates large neuromuscular demands on both forwards and defensemen, however, these demands may be greater on the defensemen as their movements also require a large reactive component.

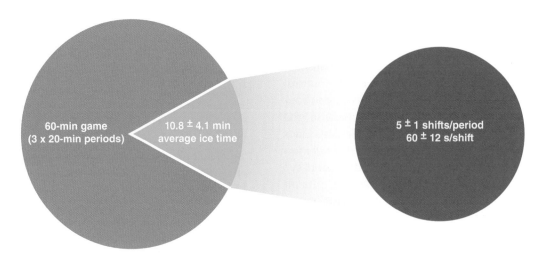

Figure 26.2 Time-motion analysis data showing both the mean ice hockey shift interval alongside the typical skating characteristics of the first 30 s of each shift period.

Adapted from M.R. Bracko, G.W. Fellingham, L.T. Hall, et al., "Performance Skating Characteristics of Professional Ice Hockey Forwards," *Sports Medicine, Training and Rehabilitation* 8(3): 251-263.

Nevertheless, the aerobic oxidative system is certainly active during ice hockey. With respect to its metabolic requirements, while direct $\dot{V}O_2$ data is limited, Bell and colleagues (1) reported that male forwards showed mean and peak heart rate (HR) values of 96% and 100% HRmax during competition, respectively, which recovered to 75% HRmax between shifts. Defensemen were similar, with work values of 92% and 96% HRmax, respectively, and recoveries to 71% HRmax between shifts. This data highlights the maximal intensity nature of the sport for forwards and defensemen.

The anaerobic glycolytic system is also engaged during ice hockey, although perhaps not to the degree that most in the sport believe it to be. For example, Nichol and McNeely (unpublished observations) measured lactates during a regular season game across periods in 10 male professional American Hockey League players (25 ± 2 yr, 90 ± 5 kg) (198 ± 11 lb) with NHL experience. Blood lactate increased from 2.4 ± 0.5 to 6.4 ± 3.7 mmol/L in period 1, from 3.4 ± 3.1 to 7.5 ± 2.8 mmol/L in period 2, and from 3.4 ± 1.9 to 7.1 ± 3.1 mmol/L in period 3. While lactate likely increased to a greater value than that measured during play (due to the lag time between exercise and measurement), it nevertheless recovered to homeostatic levels from one period to the next without any evidence of carryover effect.

Goaltenders

There is relatively little research published on the physiological demands of goaltenders. Each team generally has two goaltenders dressed to perform, and barring an unforeseen injury or substandard play, only one of these goaltenders will typically play during the match. Other than during complete stoppages of play (team or official time-outs, TV time-outs, or intermissions), the goaltenders do not have the luxury of a passive recovery period on the bench like their teammates do. Goaltenders must then have the ability to remain calm and focused for long periods of time, before displaying fast reaction speeds and explosive power at a moment's notice. Goaltenders are truly aerobic/alactic, or RST-type athletes, with the majority of their time on ice spent standing in their crease waiting for play to develop. When required, however, a split-second reaction followed by an explosive and dynamic movement is needed to stop a shot. Goaltenders additionally require high levels of flexibility and, in particular, hip mobility, as well as high levels of core stability

and specific endurance of postural muscles to endure the ready position, with a flexed torso, for a substantial time. Goaltenders also must be able to play from a kneeling position.

Key Weapons, Manipulations, and Surveillance Tools

In this section, I present the different HIIT weapons used in ice hockey, their manipulations, along with ways we can monitor their effectiveness (surveillance). The breakdown of the different HIIT weapons used in elite ice hockey is shown in figure 26.3.

HIIT Weapons

The principle of specificity within sport is well documented. The more similar the movement patterns and work:rest ratios of the training exercises to the actual sport, the greater the transfer effect may be. Anyone who has experience playing hockey or training those who do will tell you that there is simply no substitute for on-ice work. Therefore, my belief is that the following components should form the majority of weapons involved with training ice hockey players:

- High-intensity alactic-dominant efforts (short-duration maximal efforts)

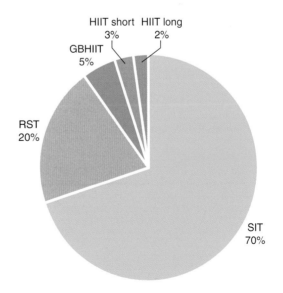

Figure 26.3 Percentage of the different HIIT weapons (formats) used throughout the annual season in elite ice hockey. HIIT: high-intensity interval training; RST: repeated-sprint training; SIT: sprint interval training; GBHIIT: game-based HIIT.

- Closed kinetic chain and weight-bearing exercises
- Repeated rapid accelerations and decelerations
- Unplanned and reactive movements
- On-ice specific exercise where possible
- Movements both with and without the puck
- Work:rest ratios of 1:2 to 1:3 for defensemen and 1:3 to 1:5 for forwards

Using these principles, the predominant weapons that form in ice hockey (figure 26.3) would be described as RST, SIT, and short-interval HIIT, mostly all done in a sport-specific format. Off the ice, long-interval HIIT is done occasionally, for specific situations described later, but rarely if at all for most players. As my study and practice in this sport has progressed over the years, I have realized long-interval HIIT is much less specific and beneficial than many believe it to be. While such training might provide benefit with regard to mental strength and cardiovascular endurance, by pushing a player to build a certain level of grit by accomplishing difficult and nonenjoyable tasks, I believe such training has a low carryover effect to game performance. The majority of our long-interval HIIT work is devoted to preparing our players for the training camp fitness testing that they will have to perform with their teams rather than for performance in the actual sport itself. Regardless of whether or not I agree with the specificity of the tests that these teams select, I do have an obligation to prepare my players so that they can perform well in these tests. Some of my more veteran and well-established players do not concern themselves with this type of training, for they know that they will not be judged on their performances at training camp. For younger players, however, or those who are less established, there is still a need to perform well on the team testing so as to make a statement to the coaches and management that they are hard-working, fit players.

Manipulations of Interval Training Variables

In the following section, I describe in detail the primary HIIT weapons used to train ice hockey players, as well as their manipulations. As mentioned, these include sport-specific RST, SIT, and short-interval HIIT. Long-interval HIIT is used sparingly in the preseason for certain isolated situations, and as these are so infrequently used for training ice hockey

players, they will not be elaborated on. Note that nearly all HIIT weapons are on-ice operations, and generally involve handling the puck, shooting the puck on goal, and tracking the opposing player. However, as there is no real play element involving decision-making, these are not classified as GBHIIT or SSG.

Sprint Interval Training

As shown in figure 26.3, SIT is the predominant form of HIIT used in elite ice hockey preparation in my experience. SIT for ice hockey can take many forms, but the predominant variations of SIT that I use involve five different drill formats that include cross-ice tracking, long-pass tracking, and chase-the-rabbit tracking drills.

Note that all ice-based drills are a collaboration between myself and Steve Spott of the San Jose Sharks. Steve is a good friend and is one of my on-ice coaches for the NHL off-season camp that I run.

Repeated-Sprint Training

In a discontinuous repeat sprint sport such as ice hockey, high-intensity maximal power might not be the only quality that you need to train, but it is certainly most important. Nobody cares how long you can skate if your skating is slow and your play ineffective. My philosophy for developing a player's capacity here is as follows:

1. Develop a high level of relative strength and power in the weight room.
2. Develop a high rate of acceleration power and deceleration strength on the track and on the ice.
3. Increase repeat sprint ability and repeated sprint ability on the ice.

In layman's terms, I believe we have to improve ability to accelerate explosively and decelerate rapidly, and do this over and over and over again. I believe that RST is instrumental in achieving this (i.e., HIIT type 4). Like many of the sport-specific SIT drills already discussed, the four-corner tracking drill is similar in terms of sport specificity, but in the RST format, the emphasis for this drill is really on explosive-quality skating.

HIIT With Short Intervals

On- and off-ice short-interval HIIT work is used more for warm-up purposes using the assault 10/20, the fox and rabbit off-ice tag game, and the on-ice fly

30-15 INTERMITTENT ICE TEST

Martin Buchheit

While yet to be adopted across NHL teams, one of the tests that has recently emerged is that of the 30-15 intermittent ice test (30-15$_{IIT}$) (2, 4). Modeled after the running-based 30-15 intermittent fitness test (https://30-15ift.com; see chapter 2), the 30-15$_{IIT}$ has a similar duration of exercise and recovery period (i.e., 30/15 s for exercise/recovery) and shuttle distances (i.e., 40 m, figure 26.4), which can be used for assessing both cardiovascular fitness and anaerobic speed reserve specific to ice hockey. Starting speeds of 10.8 km/h (6.7 mph) for the first 30 s stage, together with a speed increment of 0.63 km/h (0.39 mph), is generally considered appropriate for reaching both a high HR and a fast skating velocity, while at the same time enabling exercise to last at least 5 to 6 min. The 30-15$_{IIT}$ can be set up in less than 5 min, and requires a measuring tape (2×20 m) (2×22 yd), 9 cones, a sound system with the 30-15$_{IIT}$ audio track, and at least two observers.

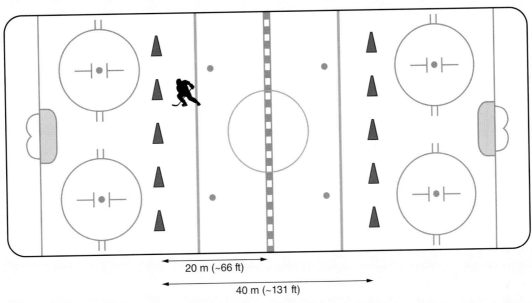

20 m (~66 ft)

40 m (~131 ft)

Figure 26.4 Area prepared for the 30-15 intermittent ice test (30-15$_{IIT}$) (4).

As with the 30-15 IFT, an audio signal sounds at appropriate intervals for players to adjust their skating speed. At the start of each stage, players rest upright with their front skate parallel to the starting line of the 40 m shuttle course. At the first audible signal, the player begins skating while holding the hockey stick with the preferred hand. Skating velocity is adapted to meet the midpoint of the course (20 m) in synchrony with the second audible signal. Without stopping, and if necessary adjusting skating velocity, the player continues skating to reach the end of the course in synchrony with the third auditory signal. At the 40 m (44 yd) end, the player immediately changes direction and starts skating in the opposite direction (stop and go) to reach the midpoint in time with the fourth audible signal, and so on until the end of the 30 s stage.

As with the running version of the test, attention is paid to the change of direction on the extremity lines, with players needing to decelerate, cross the line with at least one foot, turn, and recommence skating. At the end of the 30 s stage, players are instructed to either glide or skate slowly to the closest line (either on the end of the 40 m [44 yd] shuttle course or on the midpoint line) for a 15 s rest period, before beginning the next stage. Similar criteria are used to determine the maximal skating speed (VS$_{IIT}$). The test has been shown to be valid (i.e., final velocity on ice very largely correlated with the velocity reached during the off-ice test version, r = 0.72) and reliable (CV <2%) (4), and may provide a more specific assessment of the anaerobic and neuromuscular demands of ice hockey, as evidenced by the higher blood lactate response in the 30-15$_{IIT}$ compared to the 30-15 IFT (2).

On-Ice 45 s Shift Length Conditioning Drill

The setup for the 45 s on-ice shift conditioning drill involves dividing the team into four groups. Players start on the bench, before jumping onto the ice to skate easy/relaxed around for 30 s. On the coach's whistle, players perform 15 s of position-specific all-out sprinting (figure 26.5), followed by a hard line change on a finishing whistle, whereby the next group exits the bench to commence the start of the drill. The goaltenders will work with their goalie coach during the 15 s phase to perform their position-specific movements. This is an all-out SIT drill with an effort-to-pause ratio of ~20 s on to ~3.5 min off, aiming for type 5 targets.

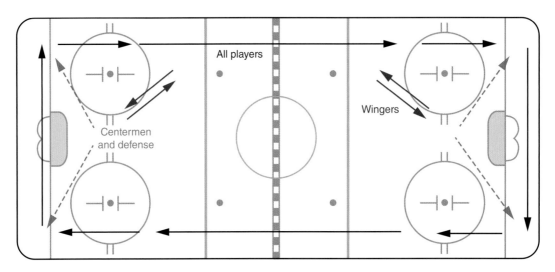

Figure 26.5 On-ice 45 s shift length conditioning.

drill. These are used sparingly in the off-season for specific players. The frequency can increase for some athletes whose fitness levels are subpar, for players who are not receiving regular shifts (those who are scratched from the lineup or playing a limited role on the fourth line), or players returning from a prolonged injury. In these latter cases, these short intervals can be used 3 to 5 times per month in-season to maintain conditioning levels.

HIIT With Long Intervals

Like short intervals, long intervals are used sparingly and really mostly in isolated cases when athletes have clear high-intensity aerobic conditioning deficiencies that require a solution or might have an injury and still require conditioning. The modality for HIIT with long intervals is generally nonspecific, including bike ergometer in the form of long-interval sets. One example of a long-interval session that I occasionally use in these isolated instances might be 3 min easy (RPE = 10), 2 min moderately hard

(RPE = 16), and 1 min maximal (RPE = 18 to 20), repeated 4 to 6 times.

Additional Strength and Conditioning Exercises for Ice Hockey Players

Most people (athletes and coaches combined) separate the work done in the weight room with barbells, dumbbells, cables, and so forth from any other work done. We tend to think of any work done with weighted implements as being solely strength or power training and assume that *metabolic conditioning* refers only to the training performed without weighted implements for specified periods of time or with specific heart rate goals. I do not believe this should be the case. As I've described, ice hockey consists of very short-duration bouts of explosive power and relies on the ability to rapidly accelerate and decelerate, regardless of the manner in which this occurs. Thus, I try to create similar demands on the athletes from the strength and power work we do in the gym.

Cross-Ice Tracking Drill

The cross-ice tracking drill is an ice hockey–specific SIT drill set up as shown in figure 26.6. Here, roughly five players begin in each of the four corners of the rink. Starting at one end and one side of the ice, on the coach's whistle, the player with the puck skates straight down the ice to shoot on net. An opposing player from the other side of the ice crosses over to the opposite player on the whistle to track against him. For this drill, we ask for all-out speed and explosiveness and full energy, from both the puck carriers and trackers, with each player going through about four times, making an effort-to-pause ratio of about 20 s on, 2 min off, aiming for type 5 targets.

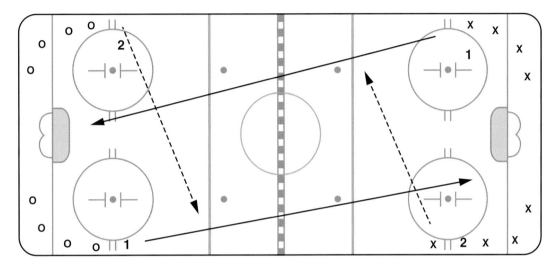

Figure 26.6 Cross-ice tracking drill.

When coaches think about the best methods of developing power in the gym, it is often the Olympic lifts and their variations that come to mind. Although Olympic-style weightlifting can be considered a sport unto itself, the exercises and their variations have been used by a wide variety of athletes outside of weightlifting to improve sport performance. Although the exercises do not mimic the specific actions seen on the ice, they do incorporate some of the more important aspects, such as being performed in a closed kinetic chain environment as total body lifts. With respect to the hang variations of the snatch and clean, the lifts begin and end in an athletic posture that is common to most team sports including ice hockey. Training these lifts can improve strength, rate of force development, and movement velocity. Another equally important benefit (or arguably more important) is the improvement of eccentric strength and rate of force development, which greatly enhance the ability to decelerate and change direction at high speeds during game play.

Although there are tremendous benefits to the use of Olympic-style weightlifting, there are also many inherent problems for ice hockey players. Many ice hockey players lack the requisite joint mobility to perform the lifts properly. The nature of the sport of ice hockey requires players to be in a flexed-torso position, which affects both hip and thoracic spine posture over time and leads to difficulty with overhead lifting. Many ice hockey players at the professional level also have difficulty with the catch position of the lift as it places tremendous strain on the wrists. Stickhandling in ice hockey is a highly specific skill and induces repetitive strain of the wrists in a flexion pattern. Injuries to the wrist are highly problematic at the elite level, since hockey players require sound wrists for stick handling, passing, and shooting of the puck, and such fine-motor skill can be disrupted by even the smallest interruptions in feel. As such, players are normally very tentative about performing any nonspecific activities that they believe might cause excessive

Long-Pass Tracking Drill

With the long-pass tracking drill (figure 26.7), players start at one end on opposite corners, with roughly five players in each of the four corners. On the coach's whistle, players make two long passes (one each) before (again on the coach's whistle) taking a shot on net, then turning hard to track back against another player. For this sport-specific SIT drill, we ask for all-out speed and energy, and each player goes four times. The defending tracker of the puck carrier must track back through the middle of the ice with good stick position, and players must execute long passes, working on pass accuracy and receiving. All-out speed and explosiveness here is emphasized for both trackers and puck carriers, making an effort-to-pause ratio of about 20 s on, 2 min off, aiming for type 5 targets.

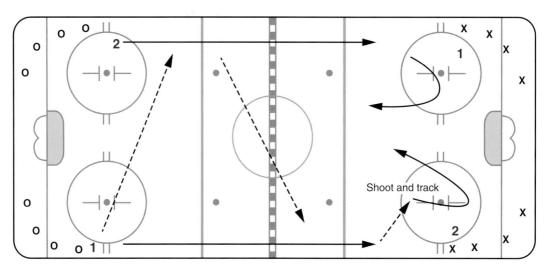

Figure 26.7 Long-pass tracking drill.

strain at this joint. For athletes who find the Olympic lifts and their variations to be problematic, alternate exercises include the second pull of the Olympic lifts without a catch, the use of loaded jumps, resisted sprints, and structuring our training program using conjugated periodization or a modified "Westside" style of conjugated periodization programming.

Additional conditioning exercises I use for ice hockey players are described in table 26.1. The skipping complex is done daily, but only as a warm-up with 2 repetitions. The slideboard exercise is done once a week in June when we are not skating, but more as prehabilitation or part of a rehabilitation program for any injured athletes. For this, we focus on controlled movement, not all-out conditioning. The sled work is done once per week in late June and early July, while the medicine ball toss and chase drill is done a couple times a summer as a fun finishing exercise or as a punishment to incentivize athletes to work hard and focus on a previous drill.

Recovery Programming and Adjunct Training

There are additional activities that I feel are important to support the high-intensity nature of the on- and off-ice training applied in ice hockey players. These include walking meditation, yoga, Qigong, and Pilates. All of these activities are quite different, but the common denominator is that they teach the athletes to connect proper breathing patterns with movement and, when done properly, will stimulate the parasympathetic nervous system, which is beneficial for recovery.

Load Surveillance and Monitoring Tools

When I worked with the NHL's Toronto Maple Leafs hockey team, we used heart rate monitoring during every practice and discovered that many of the drills described (figures 26.5 to 26.10) achieved much

Chase-the-Rabbit Tracking Drill

With this ice hockey–specific SIT drill, shown in figure 26.8, we start with roughly six forwards and four defensemen at opposite ends. On the coach's whistle, players skate all out (full energy) down the ice, 2 on 1, with a puck to pass and shoot on net before turning hard back to track against the opposing players performing the same action. Each player goes four times before switching sides and repeating. The game ele- ment of chase the rabbit is mostly for the defending player who is tracking the puck carrier. The defending player should be holding a good gap between the 2 on 1 against him, knowing he has a tracker applying backpressure. We ask for all-out speed and explosiveness for both the puck carriers and trackers, and this drill tends to result in an effort-to-pause ratio of about 20 s on and 2 min off, aiming for type 5 targets.

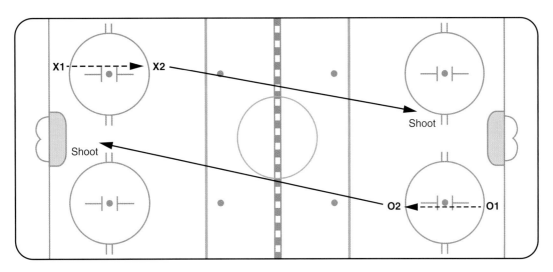

Figure 26.8 Chase-the-rabbit tracking drill.

Table 26.1 Additional Conditioning Exercises Used for Off-Ice Hockey Player Strength and Conditioning

Drill/exercise	Description	Repetitions
Slideboard intervals	15 to 30 s work, 30 to 60 s rest	6 to 10 reps
Sled push/pull	15 s reverse sled walk, 15 s forward sled push, 30 to 60 s rest	4 to 8 reps
Skipping complex	20 double leg jumps, 20 alternate leg double contact jumps (left, left, right, right), 20 hip twists, 20 high knees, 30 s rest	Repeat 5 to 8 times. If athlete can perform 8 sets of 20 reps each, increase to 5 sets of 30 reps each.
Medicine ball toss and chase exercise	Explosive medicine ball chest toss then sprint after the ball, two-foot stop at the ball and repeat. Upon reaching 100 m (109 yd), collect the ball and sprint back to the start. Rest 30 to 60 s.	Repeat 2 or 3 times.

higher heart rates than expected. My guess is this might be due to the higher neuromuscular demand imposed. I would also measure the player's heart rate variability (HRV; chapter 9) following each game and the morning after each game to assess their recovery and readiness to train. My team also performed comprehensive blood and urine analyses before, during, and after the season to examine effects on the player's biochemistry. While the data collection was very rudimentary, it was still informative. Today

With the four-corner tracking drill, shown in figure 26.9, players on all four corners of the rink (shown as Xs and Os, 1 to 4) skate down the ice with a puck and on the coach's whistle take a shot on net before making a tight turn to track back against another player. Roughly five players begin in each of the four corners, and each player goes through the drill three times.

For this drill, we demand full all-out speed and energy from the players. While we ask for an accurate shot on goal by the offensive player and purposeful tracking by the opposing player, we are really looking for speed and explosiveness. The effort-to-pause ratio for this drill is roughly 12 to 15 s all-out, 45 s rest, aiming for type 4 targets.

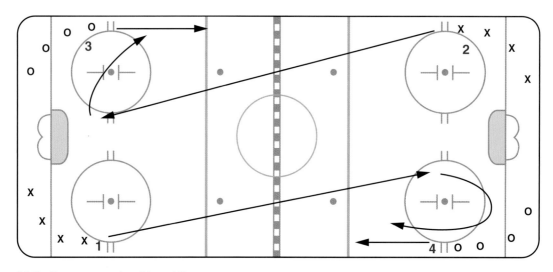

Figure 26.9 Four-corner tracking drill.

Assault 10/20

The assault bike is a stationary bike that uses wind resistance by means of a large fan wheel that matches the athlete's power output with an equal amount of resistance. This enables athletes to easily perform HIIT work without having to fumble around with buttons or dials, as the machine automatically scales the workload according to the player's capacity as needed on that particular day. Our go-to HIIT cycling sprint workout involves a 4 min bout of 10 s hard (RPE starting at 15 and building to 20) interspersed with 20 s of recovery (passive spinning). Objectively the heart rate data that we collect shows that this hits type 1 targets and can improve Wingate peak and mean power scores. Subjectively, players will routinely

tell us that this test mimics the physical feeling they get from a preseason conditioning skate practice.

We typically use the assault 10/20 once per week in the second phase of the off-season training period (late June to mid-July) to build a player's fitness. In the final phase of the off-season (late July to late August), we require the athletes to successfully complete a certain amount of work on this test on at least two occasions before we trust them to maintain their fitness in the off-season, and thereafter we no longer test them. For the assault 10/20, which would be considered a short-interval format, we aim for 5 to 8 min of total work time broken down into 1 min sets with 3 to 4 min recovery between series.

Fox and Rabbit Off-Ice Tag Game

We use a variety of methods to incorporate vision, reaction, coordination, and high-speed decision-making into our drills, which include but are not limited to visual and auditory cues by the coach and reactive light devices (fusion sport, Fit-Lights, etc.). None of these are as effective, as fun, or as efficient for team training as a good old-fashioned game of tag. Tag does not require any expensive equipment and can be administered to very large groups by a single coach with little more than a stopwatch and a whistle. We use a variety of different formats depending on the size of the group or the primary objective of the workout.

One example of a particularly effective version that we use for groups of 12 to 20 athletes is described. Note that when there are fewer athletes you can reduce the size of the playing area or use only one active chaser (fox). In a

30×30 m² (33×33 yd²) area marked off by pylons, two players are designated as being foxes while the remaining athletes are rabbits. The goal of the foxes is to attempt to tag as many rabbits as possible in 30 to 45 s, thus resembling the short-interval HIIT format (types 3, 4). When players are tagged, they immediately stop where they are and perform an isometric push-up. Players who have not been tagged by the fox can free a rabbit who is holding an isometric push-up by jumping over the rabbit. The drill continues for 30 to 45 s and then the players have 30 to 45 s of active rest during which they must keep walking. Players get no early warning of when the next work bout will begin, so they must keep their wits about them during the rest period and be prepared to react. The two foxes with the greatest number of rabbits in an isometric push-up at the end of the active time are the winners.

Fly Drill

For the fly drill, illustrated in figure 26.10, players on opposite sides (shown as Xs and Os) skate hard down the ice with a puck and shoot on goal. On the coach's whistle, the player returns by tracking back the opposing player. For this drill, we have roughly 8 to 10 players in each opposite corner, and have each player go through this three times before switching sides and repeating the drill. The fly drill is done at

about 3/4 maximal skating speed effort, and is done continuously without stopping once the drill has commenced. With the exception of taking a shot on an empty net, there's not really any game element to this drill. The effort-to-pause ratio is about 10 s on (3/4 maximal skating speed effort), 20 s off, and the fly drill is typically used as a warm-up drill, hitting type 2 targets.

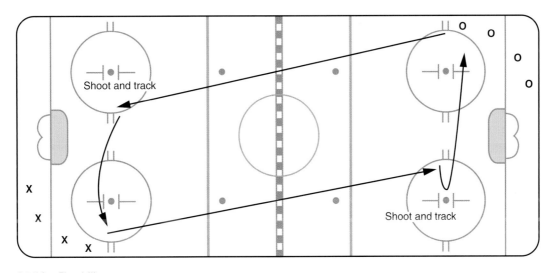

Figure 26.10 Fly drill.

Walking Meditations

There is a great abundance of research that shows that a regular meditation practice can improve focus and concentration, reduce stress, enhance sleep, and improve overall well-being. There is research to show that even as little as 10 minutes per day can be effective. Despite this, many athletes are reluctant to make this a structured part of their training regimen.

I encourage all of my athletes to incorporate meditation into their daily routines, and I have found that one of the most effective ways to do this is with walking meditations.

I encourage all of my athletes to walk at least one day per week for a minimum of 40 min. They are asked to walk at a comfortable pace and focus on controlled-breathing patterns. I never track these sessions with regard to intensity or look for a specific effect, but I certainly feel that this is important to control stress and restore the player (see chapter 7).

Yoga and Qigong

In the second phase of our off-season (middle of the off-season), our yoga and Qigong work becomes more flow-based, with less rest between postures. Most of our athletes will average around 50% to 60% HR_{max} during these sessions, but less-conditioned athletes or those with particularly poor posture and mobility can display even higher values.

my surveillance tends to focus more on direct observation of the athlete's behaviors, alongside direct communication with the athlete, although we do regularly use the following pieces of technology to monitor progress:

- Heart rate monitoring
- Accelerometers to measure bar speed velocity in the weight room
- Nord Board to assess both hamstring strength and pelvic asymmetries
- Laser timers to test acceleration and speed both on and off the ice
- Complex Electrical Muscle Stimulation to assist with recovery from training and injury rehabilitation

Strategies for Structuring the Training Program Using HIIT

The following section outlines strategies for structuring the HIIT aspect of the training program for elite ice hockey players.

Controllable and Uncontrollable Factors

As with most of the professional sports highlighted in the book, ice hockey conditioning is mostly limited to the work that can be done in the preseason to prepare for team testing. Once the season commences, we are at the mercy of the 82-game regular season schedule, which generally means playing 2 to 4 times per week throughout an 8 mo period, before a similar rate of game playing when an athlete's team makes the playoffs. For the regular season then, alongside the significant travel aspect (41 away games throughout North America), the emphasis is on recovery for the key players and conditioning maintenance for benched, injured, or less-used players. A general program structure is shown in tables 26.2 and 26.3.

Sample Training Programs

The final section in this chapter details the yearly structure and progressions of the HIIT work across the season in elite ice hockey players. An example of a weekly training microcycle used during the general preparation phase is shown in table 26.2. For an NHL player this is typically in late June or early July. Note in this example how the program-

Table 26.2 Example of a Weekly Training Microcycle During the General Preparation Phase

	Monday	Tuesday	Wednesday	Thursday	Friday	Saturday	Sunday
Focus	Dynamic effort lower-body strength training and RST	Max effort upper-body strength training and short intervals	Short intervals and recovery	Max effort lower-body strength training and RST	Torso and strength endurance	General aerobic	Rest
HIIT	RST contrast sprints: 5-7 × 14-23 m) (5-8 × 15-25 yd loaded/20-30 yd unloaded, 30 s rest between loaded and unloaded phases (type 5) RST change of direction/agility drills: 3-6 s on, 15-30 s off × 10 (type 5)	Short intervals assault bike 10/20 test (type 1)	Tempo run warm-up 10 min easy. MS: 10 × 90 yd in ~15 s, 30-45 s rest (type 1)	RST 20 yd prowler push forward/reverse, 10 s on/60 s off × 5 each (type 5)	Short intervals assault bike 10/20 test (type 1)		
Strength	Dynamic box squat 8-12 sets of 2-3 repetitions, 55%-70% 1RM at >0.8 m/s, 3 min rest between sets	A1) Single-arm DB snatch, 4 × 3 at >1.0 m/s B1) Incline DB press, 4 × 4-6 B2) Dynamic cable wood chop 4 × 6-8 B3) Single-arm DB row 4 × 6-8 C1) Isometric neck strengthening, 3 × 6-10 × 6 s per position C2) Rolling side bridge and prone bridge and reach, 2 × 2	Yoga	A1) Trap bar DL, 4 × 4 A2) Band resisted standing long jump, 4 × 3 A3) Nordic hamstring curl, 4 × 3-5 B1) Single-leg skater squats, 3 × 6-10 reps B2) Single-leg RDL, 3 × 6-10 reps B3) Slideboard lateral lunge, 3 × 6-10 reps C1) Side bridge, 2 × 6 × 6 s	A1) Half kneeling cable chop, 3 × 7-10 A2) Half kneeling cable lift, 3 × 7-10 A3) Parallel grip chin-up, 3 × 7-10 B1) Swiss ball mountain climber, 3 × 40-60 s B2) Swiss ball stir the pot, 3 × 40-60 s B3) Swiss ball oblique lateral flexion, 3 × 8-12 C1) Wrist roller, 3 × 40-60 s C2) Isometric neck strengthening, 3 × 6-10 × 6 s per position		

Note the programming of the different HIIT types across the week to maximize adaptation, minimize interference, and accommodate for the neuromuscular demands. The consecutive type 1 HIIT on Tuesday and Wednesday would be likely to limit neuromuscular overload (Tuesday) and facilitate recovery (Wednesday), allowing the hardest work (type 5) to be performed on Thursday.

ming of the different HIIT types across the week are placed so as to maximize adaptation, minimize interference, and accommodate for the neuromuscular demands of the training. As shown in this example, the consecutive type 1 targets on Tuesday and Wednesday would be likely to limit neuromuscular stress (Tuesday) and facilitate recovery (Wednesday), allowing the hardest work (type 5) to be performed Thursday after the recovery day.

During the NHL season, as with many of the other high-performance team sports, the microcycle is vastly different (table 26.3). Here, it is important to note that due to the frequency of games (nearly every other day) combined with the travel schedule, it is very challenging to achieve much in the way of quality off-ice training.

For players who are below their time on ice (TOI) thresholds during a home game (forwards 14 to 17 min, defensemen 18 to 22 min), we have them complete additional HIIT work on top of any strength training that may be prescribed on that specific day.

Table 26.3 Example of a Weekly Training Microcycle During the Regular Season

	Sat	Sun	Mon	Tues	Wed	Thurs	Fri	Sat	Sun
Focus	Home game	Technical and tactical training on-ice Low-neuro and -metabolic demand Individualized corrective exercise/rehab off-ice	Prepractice strength	Home game	Prepractice individualized corrective exercise/rehab off-ice	Away game	Practice day on the road	Away game On-ice SIT (type 5) in a.m. of game day for players not in lineup that night	Day off
HIIT	SIT (type 5) for players with insufficient TOI			SIT (type 5) for players with insufficient TOI			SIT (Type 5) for players with insufficient TOI in previous game and expected to play insufficient minutes		
Strength	Postgame strength A1) Front squat or trap bar deadlift, work up to 2×3-5 at 70%-80% 1RM A2) Horizontal row, 3×8-12 B1) Single-leg squat, 2×5-7 B2) Single-leg deadlift, 2×5-7 B3) Alternating single-leg push-ups, 2×max		A1) Hang power clean and front squat, 4×1+2 at 1.1 m/s (50%-65% 1RM) or trap bar deadlift jumps, 4×3 at 1.0 m/s A1) Dynamic box squat, 6×3 at 1.1 m/s (55%-65% 1RM+bands) B1) Split stance med ball ballistic throws on wall, 3×5 B2) Glute-ham raise, 3×5	Postgame strength A1) Parallel grip chins, 2-3×4-6 A2) Incline DB press, 2-3×4-6 A3) Rear delt lateral raise, 2-3×8-12 A4) Side bridge, 2-3×5×5 s+30 s isometric					

When I initially began training professional ice hockey players in 1998, I had very little experience with the sport. I had never played ice hockey and was only a casual fan. I ran a business training American football players in their off-season, and my training style was heavily influenced by my own personal background competing in American football, powerlifting, and track and field. I slowly began attracting more and more ice hockey players and more or less trained them in the same fashion as I did my football players. I restricted my work solely to the gym assuming (incorrectly) that their coaches would be doing specific conditioning on the ice in addition to their technical and tactical drills. I was always pleasantly surprised at the fact that the athletes I trained would perform at the top of their groups in their team fitness testing despite not having done any of the traditional conditioning that their teammates claimed to have been doing.

I trained my private hockey clients at a track-and-field center that did not have stationary bikes, treadmills, or popular strength-training machines. What we did have was lots of open space, free weights, and medicine balls. We did our strength training with free weights (Olympic lifting and powerlifting), alongside ballistic work with medicine balls and considerable speed and power work on the track.

In 2002, I accepted a position as head strength-and-conditioning coach for the NHL's Toronto Maple Leafs. In addition to being my first full-time strength-and-conditioning position with a high-profile professional team, the position was arguably the most prestigious position in my industry in my country. While I was honored to get the job, I was equally very nervous, as the responsibility came with pressure and scrutiny. In addition to being the youngest person performing this job in the NHL at the time, I was also the least experienced in terms of working with hockey players compared to others in the industry.

The culture of hockey at the time was for teams to perform conditioning programs on the stationary bike after practice to improve their fitness. For example, long slow-duration aerobic rides after games to "clear lactic acid" were the staple prescription (see chapter 3 for discussion on this topic). Most of the weight training that was done was in the form of circuit training, primarily with higher volume and lower intensity protocols. Since everyone was doing this type of training, and I was the least experienced guy in the business, I assumed that I was the one who was ignorant, and that I'd better hedge my bets and get on board with the program.

I spoke with several other strength coaches around the NHL to get the stationary bike programs that they were using; however, after receiving these, the practice still never sat right with me. I could understand the need for "conditioning" in addition to our regular strength training, but could not understand why everyone was performing long- or even medium-length intervals. I heard arguments such as "if shift lengths were 45 s then we should do 45 s intervals," and my favorite was, "if shifts were 45 s long then we should be doing 90 s intervals so that the 45 s shifts feel easy by comparison."

I decided to take it upon myself to study the science of ice hockey. I wanted to really understand the demands of the sport with respect to the underpinning biomechanics and physiology. I began to measure heart rate data during every practice and every game, as well as the players' heart rate variability (HRV; chapter 9) following each game, and the morning following each game, to assess their recovery and readiness to train. We performed comprehensive blood analysis and urinalysis before, during, and after the season to examine measurable effects on the players' biochemistry. While the data collection was very rudimentary, it was still informative. And most importantly, I watched A LOT of hockey.

When I began my investigation in 2002, no available technology provided a reliable way to track the movements and velocities of the players on the ice. This was long before the days of GPS tracking. Our technology was limited to stopwatches and the careful eyes of some volunteer testers, but this was still an extremely useful practice. It did not take long to determine that although a shift may be 45 to 60 s long in total duration, this did not

(continued)

consist of 45 to 60 s of consistent work, but rather several very short bouts of explosive movements, including accelerations, decelerations, collisions, and shots, interspersed with longer periods of relative inactivity, such as gliding and rest during stoppages in play. This analysis allowed me the confidence to do something drastic and change my practice, going against the grain.

The following season, after some discussion, our coaching staff allowed me to replace our traditional cycle ergometer fitness tests with on-ice tests of speed and endurance, the things that mattered. We chose to test on-ice acceleration and speed with timing gates set up at 0, 20, 35, and 55 m intervals, and the modified Reed repeat sprint skating test (8) to test both speed and recovery ability (and consequently the anaerobic power and aerobic fitness). In addition to timing the athletes, we also collected blood samples from each athlete immediately following the test at specific intervals to determine blood lactate levels (described earlier). Based on the data collected, we were able to create a profile on each player and conduct a needs analysis based on whether they would benefit most from an increased concentration on acceleration, speed, or speed endurance training. The coaching staff also allowed me to replace our traditional steady state aerobic work and long-interval training with more sport-specific sprint interval work. Perhaps an important lesson for future practitioners entering into a new program would be as follows—just because things have always been done a certain way doesn't mean they are right. Make relevant observations, test assumptions, and have the courage to trust not only your data but also your gut and make changes that you truly believe will help your players.

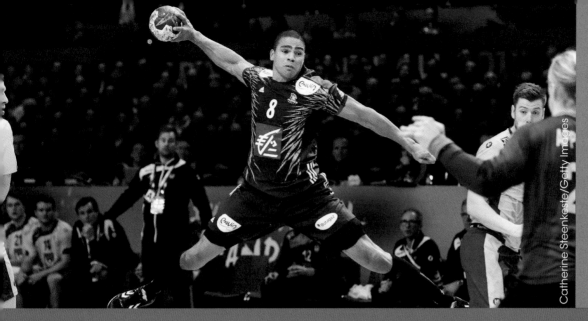

27

Handball

• • • • • •

Martin Buchheit

Performance Demands of Handball

Every sport is unique in terms of how it's played, how it's won, and the associated demands. Handball is no exception. In this section, we introduce the sport and discuss the various performance factors for outfield players and the relative contribution that physical performance makes toward achieving team performance and winning.

Sport Description and Factors of Winning

Handball, also known as team handball or Olympic handball, is a team sport played by ~20 million players throughout the world involving two teams of seven players (six outfield players and a goal-keeper), which hand-pass a ball toward the aim of eventually throwing it into the other team's goal. A standard match consists of two periods of 30 min on a 40 × 20 m indoor court. The team that scores the most goals wins. Handball is referred to as a *transition game* because players frequently switch between defensive and offensive play, and the game is characterized by frequent high-intensity body contacts, along with intermittent running and sprinting.

Relative Contribution of Physical Performance

As for all ball-based team sports, technical skills, tactical awareness, and game intelligence are without doubt the main contributors of success. Players with limited ability to pass the ball precisely, shoot, or make the right decisions in the moment will never become champions, irrespective of the physical fitness attributes they may possess or develop. Fitness is, however, important to support the development of technical performance on the field. While physical fitness will never guarantee success, a lack of any given physical attribute can be the cause of failure (figure 27.1).

Targets of Physical Performance in Handball

Anthropometric characteristics, as well as high levels of strength, muscle power, and throwing velocity, are the most important generalized physical factors needed for gaining an advantage in handball that would translate into an improved probability of success at the elite level (21, 27). Additionally, as in most team sports, physical demands are clearly position dependent in terms of movement patterns, volume of high-intensity actions, and associated work:recovery

495

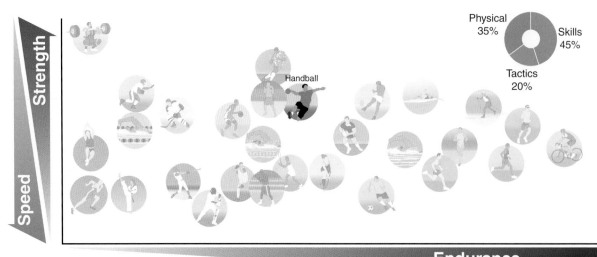

Figure 27.1 The position of the handball player on the three axes illustrates the relative importance of the three main physical capacities of importance for elite participation in handball, acknowledging this varies between outfield positions (24) except the goalkeeper, who is a different beast and does not require much high-intensity interval training. Outside of critical psychological and team chemistry components, which are difficult to quantify, the pie chart shows the general relative importance of skills, tactical awareness, and physical capacities for handball success.

Adapted from G.A. Nader, "Concurrent Strength and Endurance Training: From Molecules to Man," *Medicine & Science in Sports & Exercise* 38, no. 11 (2006): 1965-1970.

ratios (24), which require further levels of individualization when it comes to conditioning players. As player demands are clearly position dependent, the following discussion describes the specific physical attributes and needs of the different player positions.

Outfield Players

In addition to the general physical targets, development of aerobic power should not be underestimated. During match play, players run from 4 to 6 km (24) at a mean intensity of roughly 80% to 90% of maximal heart rate (HRmax) (25). Significant associations between maximal oxygen uptake ($\dot{V}O_2max$) and playing level have also been shown (21, 27). In fact, elite players have been shown to repeat more than 120 high-intensity actions during a game (24). Thus, a well-developed aerobic system is likely to be beneficial for metabolic recovery between the explosive efforts associated with successful handball match performance (29, 31).

Goalkeepers

For the goalkeepers, there is no need to generate excessive neuromuscular fatigue from running, so the better strategy is to remove them from the run

conditioning exercises and have them do some general aerobic conditioning on a stationary cycle ergometer or perform goalkeeper-specific training exercises.

Key Weapons, Manipulations, and Surveillance Tools

Recall that weapons refer to the high-intensity interval training (HIIT) formats we can use to target the physiological responses of importance, while the surveillance tools are what we are using to monitor the individual responses to those weapons. In this section, we present the different HIIT weapons, their manipulations, along with ways that we can monitor their effectiveness (surveillance).

HIIT Weapons

As outlined, there are five different metabolic and/ or neuromuscular load targets I aim for throughout the season (see figure 1.5 (7)):

Type 1: metabolic O_2 system

Type 2: metabolic O_2 system + neuromuscular

Type 3: metabolic O_2 + anaerobic systems

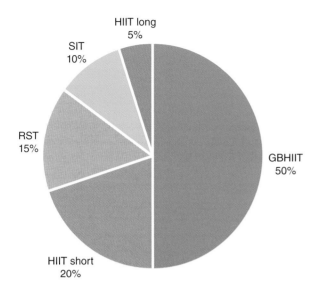

Figure 27.2 Percentage of the different HIIT weapons (formats) used throughout the annual season in elite handball. HIIT: high-intensity interval training; RST: repeated-sprint training; SIT: sprint interval training; GBHIIT: game-based HIIT.

Type 4: metabolic O_2 + anaerobic systems and neuro-muscular

Type 5: metabolic anaerobic system and neuro-muscular

The five HIIT weapons used to hit these targets were detailed earlier in chapters 4 and 5 (8). For handball (figure 27.2), the large majority of these are game-based HIIT, i.e., small-sided games (SSGs) (50%, essentially in-season), followed next by short intervals (20%, some preseason, but mostly in-season), repeated-sprint training (RST) (15%, in-season only), sprint interval training (SIT) (10%, in season only), and long intervals (5%, preseason exclusively).

Manipulations of Interval Training Variables

The running intensity for each HIIT weapon I've used has tended to be almost fixed for each format; rather, adjustments are achieved through programming variations between the different days/weeks. For example, if a short-interval HIIT weapon is programmed to target type 1 on a given day/week, RST, SIT, or SGGs formats might be used to target types 3 and 4 for the next day/week, which also adds variation to the training content.

HIIT With Long Intervals (Outdoor)

I generally implement HIIT with long intervals in the outdoor environment, either on a track, on a

soccer pitch (grass), or in the forest (with distances marked on the path), so as to minimize the musculo-skeletal strain (7) (avoiding HIIT type 5, and possibly type 4 targets (7)). These typical long-interval weapons are generally performed over 3 to 4 min at 90% of $V_{Inc.Test}$ or 85% V_{IFT}. This represents 750 to 950 m efforts completed over 3 min, depending on a player's fitness, with athletes running 3 to 5 repetitions interspersed by 2 min of passive recovery. Players are generally spread across 4 or 5 groups (15 km/h, 16 km/h, 17 km/h, 18 km/h, and >18 km/h for $V_{Inc.Test}$ or 17 km/h, 18 km/h, 19 km/h, 20 km/h, and >21 km/h for V_{IFT}) and are requested to reach group-specific cones set across the running track at appropriate times. These sessions are generally prescribed at the end of the week, before a day off, so that players can recover from an anticipated neuro-muscular fatigue (see the example in table 27.1 at the end of the chapter). Additionally, I try to schedule these at the end of the day so that athletes may benefit from a greater $\dot{V}O_2$ slow component, i.e., higher $\dot{V}O_2$ for a similar or lower running speed due to muscle fatigue and loss of metabolic efficiency (8).

HIIT With Short Intervals

My preferred HIIT short-interval weapon formats include 15 s on/15 s off, 20 s/20 s, and more often 10 s/20 s (see tables 27.1 to 27.4 at the end of the chapter), which can be used to target almost all HIIT types (1, 2, 3, and 4). I chose these formats as they can be associated with a limited level of neuromuscular fatigue and anaerobic contribution (especially 10 s/20 s, HIIT type 1), which helps preserve the quality of the conjoined handball sequences (same session) as well as the strength/speed sessions planned the following day (12, 13). We generally spread our players into 5 groups (17 km/h, 18 km/h, 19 km/h, 20 km/h, and >21 km/h for V_{IFT}), and we request that they run over group-based distances using cones on the court. For example, for players with a V_{IFT} of 19 km/h, and for a 15 s/15 s HIIT format run at 95% of V_{IFT} (relief interval: passive), the target distance will be (19/3.6) × 0.95 × 15 = 75 m (19 is divided by 3.6 to convert the speed from km/h to m/s, for convenience) (3). However, since most runs must be performed with changes of direction (CODs) to fit in the 40 m handball court, the time needed for COD must be considered when calculating the target run distance in order to ensure a similar cardiorespiratory load compared with straight-line runs, while remaining close to type 1 target loading (or in the worst-case scenario, type 2 but at the lower

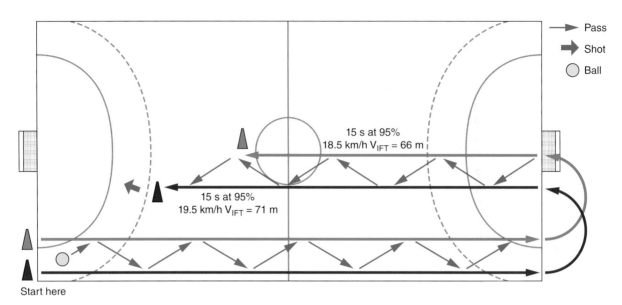

Figure 27.3 Example of handball-specific high-intensity interval training with short intervals (15 s/15 s format, type 3 target) based on V_{IFT}. The exercise consists of two players passing the ball continuously while running at a set speed and finishes with a shot on goal. The exercise is easier if players with similar V_{IFT} run together, but can also be implemented using individualized distances. In this example, the player on the red course is fitter than the player on the green course, so he must cover 5 m more within the same time period.

Reprinted by permission from M. Buchheit, "Programming High-Intensity Training in Handball," *Aspetar Sports Medicine Journal* 3, Targeted Topic: Sports Medicine in Handball (April 2014): 120-128.

end of neuromuscular constraint for this target type). Therefore, in relation to the estimated energetic cost of COD during HIIT (see chapter 2, V_{IFT} section), if the players have to run over a 40 m shuttle, they would instead cover 71 m. If the shuttle length is divided in half (i.e., a 20 m shuttle), the distance to cover drops to 65 m (3). A spreadsheet that completes this calculation for 15 players at a time is available from the author on request.

To make HIIT with short intervals more handball specific, we often integrate the ball into the activity on different occasions. For example, the players can run together and continuously pass the ball to one another, before the last player with the ball at the end shoots at the goal (figure 27.3). Another way to individualize HIIT with short intervals is to use the position-specific work:rest ratio and/or game-specific effort distribution (24). Under this situation, wingers need to perform HIIT with more intense runs interspersed by longer rest periods (for example, 10 s (110% of V_{IFT})/ 20 s (passive)), compared with backs (20 s (95%)/ 20 s (jog) or 30 s (90%)/ 30 s (jog)) (24).

Finally, merging specific defensive action maneuvers into short intervals is also possible; however, at least two important aspects must be considered. First, repeating such actions for the entire duration of the work bout (i.e., 10 to 20 s) reduces game specificity. That is, in a game, a defender generally only reaches an attacker once or twice per defensive action before the game is either stopped (technical fault) or continues on across other players. Performing defensive actions throughout the 10 to 20 s period and accumulating a number of repetitions would amount to an inappropriate number of defensive maneuvers. Second, only using defensive movements does not allow control over the exercise interval intensity, as it does with run-based drills. Thus, an attractive option is to combine the defensive actions for 5 s with individualized running tasks occurring for the remaining 10 or 15 s of the interval (figure 27.4).

Repeated-Sprint Training

For the RST format (type 4 target), I generally implement 2 to 4 sets of 5 to 8 sprints across 15 to 30 m distances, interspersed with 14 to 25 s of passive or active (jog or ~45% V_{IFT}) recovery (7) during the first part of the training session. I intersperse these between two training sequences. For example, I might implement the following: warm-up, 10 to 20 min technical sequences, RST, prior to the

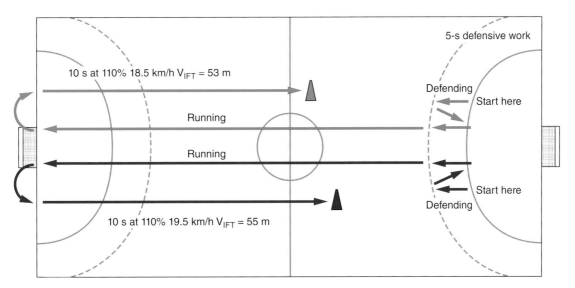

Figure 27.4 Defensive actions performed for 5 s are combined with an individualized running task for the remaining 10 s of the 15 s interval (short interval; type 3 and 4 targets). This allows control of the exercise intensity (running section) while preserving the specificity of the defensive task (players generally do not defend continuously for 15 to 20 s).

Reprinted by permission from M. Buchheit, "Programming High-Intensity Training in Handball," *Aspetar Sports Medicine Journal* 3, Targeted Topic: Sports Medicine in Handball (April 2014): 120-128.

remainder of the training day (12). See, for example, the video at https://www.youtube.com/watch?v =nb4Ft9cyW6M. The RST weapon is well suited for team relays and when it comes to implementing position-specific sequences, such as counterstrike work for wingers (figure 27.5). Sprints can also be performed in shuttle format, which would, from an injury-prevention perspective, lower stride length and subsequently hamstring strain risk (8). As with short-interval HIIT weapons, game demands of sprinting can be used to design position-specific repeated-sprint sequences (24), such as 20 to 30 m sprints and 10 to 15 m sprints for wingers and backs, respectively. The programming of these sequences (see table 27.4) should be well considered due to the associated very large anaerobic contribution and neuromuscular fatigue that may impact the quality of the strength, speed, and tactical work performed during subsequent sequences or sessions. It is also important to discontinue programming RST at the end of a demanding session, when fatigue may acutely increase injury risk.

Sprint Interval Training

I've used SIT weapons in the form of 3 to 6 all-out 30 s shuttle sprints over 40 m, interspersed with 2 to 4 min of passive recovery (type 5 target) (7, 10). Given the intensity and duration of the format, it is difficult to involve ball work during these drills; however, it can nevertheless be added at the end of the runs. Due to the high anaerobic contribution and large neuromuscular fatigue associated with SIT, its programming during the sessions and during the week is similar to that discussed above for RST (see table 27.3).

Game-Based HIIT Training

As with most team sports, and described in depth in chapters 2 and 5, I tend to organize game-based training in the format of small-sided games (SSGs, figure 27.6) involving a varying number of players, generally less than during official competitions, https://www.youtube.com/watch?v=26VKke RDTMM, over various field dimensions (e.g., 12×24 m, 30×15 m, 32×16 m, or 40×20 m, figures 27.7 and 27.8 (17)). In regional-to-national level players, we've shown that 4 versus 4 handball SSGs (+ 2 goalkeepers, 40×20 m, full handball court) are an effective means of achieving and maintaining a high percentage of $\dot{V}O_2$max during training, despite lower blood lactate levels compared to run-based HIIT (14) (type 2 target). In addition, players tend to perceive SSGs as less painful (https://www.youtube .com/watch?v=X8kuZ4I0B6A).

In my experience, I have tended to simplify or modify typical handball rules with the aim of

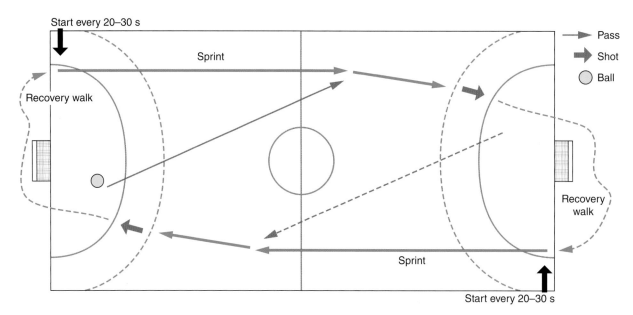

Figure 27.5 Example of a repeated-sprint sequence format (type 4 target) in which players sprint, receive the ball from the goalkeeper, and shoot before preparing to start again on the other side of the court (6 repetitions). With mean exercise time around 6 s per effort, up to 5 players can play at the same time (player rotation ~30 s).

Reprinted by permission from M. Buchheit, "Programming High-Intensity Training in Handball," *Aspetar Sports Medicine Journal* 3, Targeted Topic: Sports Medicine in Handball (April 2014): 120-128.

maximizing physiological responses for the following reasons.

To avoid game breaks that would unnecessarily reduce exercise intensity:

1. dribbling and defense contacts are not allowed; infringement of minor technical rules (such as walking) are not sanctioned;

2. throw-on after a goal is immediately made by goalkeepers from their 6 m area;

3. coaches are always available to immediately replace the ball when it is kicked away from the playing area; and

4. all four players must be in the opponent's half of the court for a goal to be validated (9).

To ensure that all players perform at the desired intensity, since exercise intensity cannot be controlled during SSGs—as with run-based drills—we must rely on player motivation to ensure that all players commit to the required (likely maximum) intensity during the drills. For that reason, encouragement and winning objectives between the teams are key. However, since players of varying fitness levels must play together (to preserve game-specific relationships between players), the relative work of the fitter players can wind up being relatively lower than that of the less fit. Indeed, a negative correlation ($r = -0.88$) has been shown between relative exercise intensity during a 4 versus 4 SSG (% of $\dot{V}O_2max$ maintained during the SSG) and a player's $\dot{V}O_2max$ as measured during the 30-15 IFT (14). This suggests that, over time, fitter players might not benefit enough from these drills to improve their aerobic power/endurance capacity. To overcome these limitations, additional rules can be implemented, including:

- whenever an identified fitter player releases the ball, he performs two push-ups (which increases overall energy demands);

- whenever an identified fitter player releases the ball, he has to place one foot on the court's sidelines before coming back into the game (which increases his overall running demands);

- one identified fitter player is always involved in the attacking team, so that his volume of play is increased.

While there are infinite ways to modulate exercise intensity during a run-based HIIT (7), little data is available to guide training manipulation based on physiological loading during handball SSGs. Simple modification of rules, such as permission for player

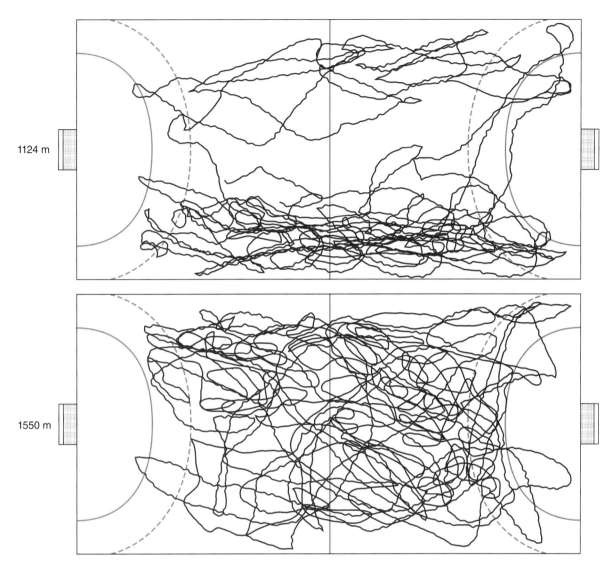

Figure 27.6 Distance covered by two different players (a, $V_{IFT} = 18.5$ km/h; b, $V_{IFT} = 20.5$ km/h) during an 8 min, 4 versus 4 small-sided handball game over the full court (12).

Reprinted by permission from M. Buchheit, "Programming High-Intensity Training in Handball," *Aspetar Sports Medicine Journal* 3, Targeted Topic: Sports Medicine in Handball (April 2014): 120-128.

contact or not, is probably the first alteration that I use in practice. For example, in national junior players, noncontact 3-a-side SSGs were shown to be associated with increased rating of perceived exertion (RPE) and a 50% greater sprinting distance despite similar HR responses than contact-based games (19). We also often alter court dimensions, as in other team sports, to manipulate the acute physiological demands of handball games (17).

Metabolic Responses to Changes in Court Dimensions

An increase in playing area has shown no predictable effect on HR responses during SSGs (figure 27.7) (14, 17). This is likely related to the fact

that, over smaller playing areas, the number of changes in velocity, COD, and contacts increases, compared to larger pitches (17), which compensates for the lower running-only demands (14, 17). It is also worth noting that, because of the static phases and handball-specific muscular contractions, which increase HR independently of muscle O_2 demands, HR responses during SSGs tend to become dissociated from $\dot{V}O_2$ values. Therefore, extrapolating metabolic responses from HR is limited in this special situation (15).

Locomotor Responses to Changes in Court Dimensions

In contrast to HR, we tend to see a linear relationship between running demands and

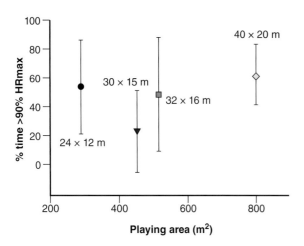

Figure 27.7 Time spent above 90% of maximal heart rate (HRmax, 90% confidence intervals) during 3 versus 3 small-sided games with different playing areas.

Reprinted by permission from M. Buchheit, "Programming High-Intensity Training in Handball," *Aspetar Sports Medicine Journal* 3, Targeted Topic: Sports Medicine in Handball (April 2014): 120-128.

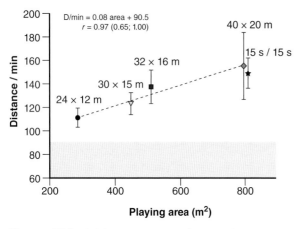

Figure 27.8 Distance covered per minute as a function of playing area during 3 versus 3 small-sided handball games (90% confidence intervals). The gray area represents distance per minute during games (24). The distance per minute covered during the short-interval exercise format (15 s/15 s) is also provided for comparison.

Reprinted by permission from M. Buchheit, "Programming High-Intensity Training in Handball," *Aspetar Sports Medicine Journal* 3, Targeted Topic: Sports Medicine in Handball (April 2014): 120-128.

playing area (figure 27.8). Additionally, the running pace reached during four different SSGs (17) has actually been shown to be higher than that during a match (24). Thus, SSGs represent an appropriate overload for the locomotor and likely the metabolic (peripheral at least) systems (figure 27.8). Interestingly,

playing 4 versus 4 on the full handball pitch allows players to reach the same running pace as during short-interval HIIT (figure 27.8), which is ~50% greater than game demands (see chapter 30 for a similar training approach).

In summary, changes in court dimensions or game rules can be used, as with other team sports, to manipulate the acute physiological demands of handball games, where the larger the playing area, the greater the running pace, but not necessarily the HR. Further research is needed to improve SSG programming, including research into best duration, repetitions, number of players, rules, and playing position-specific formats. If some specific rules are implemented to increase the relative exercise intensity of the fitter players, SSGs represent an interesting alternative to traditional HIIT, especially for in-season training content (see table 27.4).

The main advantages of SSGs include:

1. lower anaerobic contribution in training (type 2 targeting),
2. perceived as less painful by the majority of players,
3. time with the ball is maximized,
4. training interest and enjoyment is improved, and
5. the format allows work under fatigue to develop important handball components, such as agility, reaction time, and hand-eye coordination.

The only disadvantage of SSGs compared to run-based short-interval HIIT is the likely greater neuromuscular work that may impact the quality of the strength, speed, and tactical work performed during subsequent training sessions, but this would be very likely less than RSS and SIT by comparison.

Longitudinal Training Effects of HIIT

Figure 27.9 summarizes the effects of different HIIT interventions that I conducted in highly trained young players over several years in France in the late 2000s (National Talent Programs) (10, 12, 13). It shows that both high-intensity running capacity (V_{IFT}) and repeated-sprint performance (average time of six repeated sprints) can be improved during the season after 4 to 10 wk of HIIT supplementation (~2 sessions per wk, in addition to usual training) in highly trained players (~10 hours of training + 1 competitive game

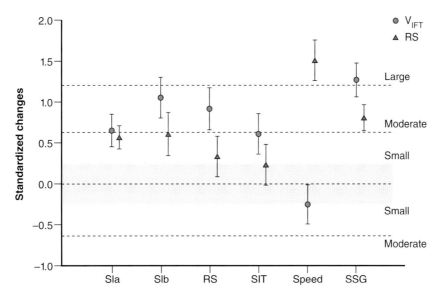

Figure 27.9 Standardized changes in the peak speed reached in the 30-15 intermittent fitness test (V_{IFT}) and mean repeated-sprint time following different training interventions based on short intervals (SI), repeated-sprint sequences (RS), sprint interval sessions (SIT), speed agility (Speed), and small-sided games (SSG) in highly trained young handball players. The gray area represents trivial changes. The short-interval (SIa) program consisted of 2 sessions per week involving 6 to 12 min of intermittent running for 15 s (95% V_{IFT}) interspersed with 15 s of passive recovery for 10 consecutive weeks (13). The short-interval (SIb) program consisted of 2 sessions per week involving 6 to 12 min of intermittent running for 15 s (95% V_{IFT}) to 20 s (90% V_{IFT}) interspersed with 15 to 20 s of passive recovery for 9 consecutive weeks (12). The repeated-sprint training program occurred across 9 consecutive weeks and consisted of 2 to 3 sets of 5 to 6×15 to 20 m shuttle sprints interspersed with 14 s of passive or 23 s of active recovery (45% V_{IFT}) (12). The SIT, conducted over 4 consecutive weeks, involved 3 to 6 repetitions of 30 s all-out shuttle sprints over 40 m, interspersed with 2 min of passive recovery (10). Speed training took place over 4 consecutive weeks and consisted of 4 to 6 series of 4 to 6 exercises (e.g., agility drills, standing start, and very short shuttle sprints, all of <5 s duration); each repetition and series was interspersed with at least 30 s and 3 min of passive recovery, respectively (10). SSG training consisted of small handball games (2 to 4×2 min 30 s to 4 min games) for 10 consecutive weeks (13).

Reprinted by permission from M. Buchheit, "Programming High-Intensity Training in Handball," *Aspetar Sports Medicine Journal* 3, Targeted Topic: Sports Medicine in Handball (April 2014): 120-128.

per week). Importantly, all changes reported in figure 27.9 (irrespective of the HIIT weapon format) can be considered substantial because they were all small to large in magnitude and clearly greater than their smallest worthwhile change (22) (the gray area represents trivial to nonsubstantial changes). Interestingly, the magnitude of improvement in both V_{IFT} (r=0.56) and mean repeated-sprint time (r=−0.75) after HIIT training (excluding speed) was linearly related to training duration (number of weeks). In addition, the magnitude of improvement in the average repeated-sprint time after HIIT training (excluding speed) was inversely related to baseline performance (r=−0.68); however, this relationship was unclear for V_{IFT}. The magnitude of improvement in mean repeated-sprint time (excluding speed) and

V_{IFT} was also largely correlated (−0.73). Therefore, while it is difficult to compare the respective effects of the different interventions because of the differences in training duration and baseline performance, the 10 wk SSG program was the only training method associated with large and moderate improvements in V_{IFT} and repeated-sprint performance, respectively (13). In all the aforementioned experimental training phases, only one type of HIIT was used (for study design purposes). Of course, the optimal physical conditioning scenario likely involves a combination of all types of HIIT supplementation (see table 27.5). Further studies comparing these HIIT programs over a similar duration in players matched for baseline physical performance are required to draw definitive conclusions.

Load Surveillance and Monitoring Tools

Despite some very recent developments of inertial sensors (26, 32) and semiautomatic video systems (16), the use of wearables and tracking technologies is still very limited in handball and is mainly reserved for research purposes. To our knowledge, a noninvasive practical tracking device has yet to be produced that can be used during training sessions, as might be implemented in other sports such as soccer or rugby. For this reason, despite its limitations (see above), I generally monitor HR during some training sessions, including the various HIIT formats, and collect RPEs after each session (see chapter 8). Training load can then be calculated via the popular session-RPE method (23).

Training Status Surveillance and Monitoring Tools

As described in chapter 9, the training status monitoring tools that I've used in handball are generally limited to noninvasive and low-cost measurements and include wellness questionnaires (overall well-being (28)), jumps (neuromuscular status (8)), exercise HR (fitness (6)), and resting heart rate variability (HRV, overall training status (6)). Since the early 2000s, we have been using HRV to track Sélestat (Senior French First League) player adaptation to intense preseason training cycles. Figure 27.10 shows how heterogeneous the training response can be between players exposed to the same training stimulus, but with large differences in volume (see story at the end of the chapter). We used this individual response to tailor each player's subsequent training. Additionally, we often use the HR and RPE responses to HIIT sequences as markers of adaptations (the lower, the better the player's fitness when comparing all similar sequences between players) (11).

Strategies for Structuring the Training Program Using HIIT

Strategies for structuring HIIT programming in handball may be confined by various controllable and uncontrollable factors before proper progression and periodization can be appropriately implemented. This section discusses some of the nuances of the training program and HIIT structuring in handball.

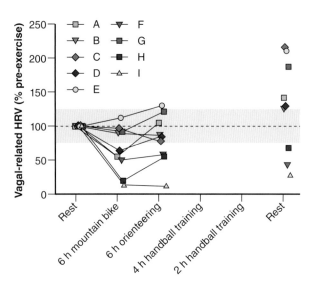

Figure 27.10 Individual cardiac parasympathetic responses of elite handball players during 4 consecutive days of training. The heart rate variability (HRV) values correspond to the measurement taken in the morning (5 min, supine at home) after a rest day, mountain biking, orienteering (running), or handball-specific training including SSGs. Shaded area represents the coefficient of variation for vagal-related HRV indices under resting conditions (1).

Reprinted by permission of Springer Nature from J. Stanley, J.M. Peake, and M. Buchheit, "Cardiac Parasympathetic Reactivation Following Exercise: Implications for Training Prescription," *Sports Medicine* 43, no. 12 (2013): 1259-1277.

Controllable and Uncontrollable Factors

In my experience, the only truly uncontrollable factors within my training program design are the match locations and game schedule timing, which are controlled by the sport federation. Minor to this is the constant requirement for gym-based work (strength and power) combined with high-quality technical sessions, which together constrain the timing, volume, and objective of the HIIT sequences within a given training week. Thus, the chosen HIIT session must induce the least possible subsequent level of fatigue. In fact, I believe that residual neuromuscular fatigue post-HIIT can reduce a player's attention and technical proficiency during tactical sessions, as well as his force production capacity and rate of force application during subsequent (strength/speed) sessions, which likely impairs the learning process and attenuates the training stimuli needed for optimal neuromuscular adaptation (2, 20).

In-season, when match schedules dictate the training programming, there are likely to be only two weekly scenarios, with 1 or 2 matches per week. In the latter case, there winds up being no room for HIIT. In contrast, I generally program 1 or 2 HIIT sequences in the week when we have a full week between matches (see table 27.4).

Program Structure and Progression

In handball, as with many team sports, there actually is very little periodization that occurs, except during the preseason (see table 27.5). In-season, I try to keep the weekly training load almost constant throughout the months and focus on the successive match preparation-match-recovery cycles, with a short emphasis on development during midweek days when possible (18). For these reasons, the skeleton of the weekly program (see table 27.4) and the program objectives remains similar across the season.

Incorporation of HIIT

In the off-season, I often program heavy-loading run-based HIIT sessions using long intervals after handball sessions (and not during), mainly due to the fact that these need to be implemented outdoors

(forest, field, track). These can be achieved in the off-season relative to the in-season, as the level of exhaustion created is substantial and affects subsequent training.

In-season, the HIIT sequences become fully incorporated into technical handball sessions over 1 or 2 d in the middle of the week (see table 27.4), and as such are performed in between technical and tactical drills during the main session. The objective of these low-volume, mainly handball-specific HIIT sequences is mostly maintenance of cardiorespiratory fitness, while limiting anaerobic contribution, neuromuscular stress, and fatigue before subsequent day gym sessions. It is worth noting, however, that in some scenarios, like substitute players who lack competitive time, a high neuromuscular load during HIIT might be desired. Thus, neuromuscular-demanding HIIT (e.g., RST) may help such players prepare best for specific match demands (24).

Sample Training Programs

The following tables provide examples of HIIT programming during different phases of training, i.e., preseason (tables 27.1 to 27.3) and in-season (table 27.4). Note the distribution of the different HIIT types in relation to the microcycle's objectives.

Table 27.1 $\dot{V}O_2$ Development Cycle (First Week[s] of Preseason; Typically, 1 to 2 Week Duration) (8)

Microcycle (physical emphasis)		Monday	Tuesday	Wednesday	Thursday	Friday	Saturday	Sunday
$\dot{V}O_2$ development++	AM	Rest	Handball	Generic strength/ injury prevention	Handball	Rest	Handball	Rest
	PM	Handball	Handball	Handball	Handball	Handball	Handball	
		Type 3 HIIT with long intervals (grass) 5×3 min (85% $V_{Inc.Test}$)/ 2 min (0) or type 3 HIIT with short intervals (grass) 2×12 min 30 s (85% V_{IFT})/ 30 s (40% V_{IFT})			Type 1 HIIT with short intervals (grass) 2×12 min 15 s (95% V_{IFT})/ 15 s (40% V_{IFT})		Type 4 HIIT with long intervals (soft outdoor track) 5×3 min (90% $V_{Inc. Test}$)/ 2 min (0) HIIT	

Note that 2 d are allowed after the lactic session (30 s/30 s) and that the long-bout HIIT (greater speed and performed on a slightly harder outdoor surface) is programmed prior to the day off. Type refers to the physiological target.

Table 27.2 $\dot{V}O_2$ and Strength/Speed Development Cycle (Generic Phase, Preseason; Typically 2 Weeks Duration) (8)

Microcycle (physical emphasis)		Monday	Tuesday	Wednesday	Thursday	Friday	Saturday	Sunday
$\dot{V}O_2$+strength/ speed development (generic)	AM	Generic strength/ speed/ injury prevention	Rest	Generic power/speed	Rest	Generic strength/ speed	Handball Type 3 HIIT with short intervals (grass) 2×10 min 20 s (95% V_{IFT})/20 s (0)	Rest
	PM	Handball	Handball Type 1 HIIT with short intervals (grass) 2×10 min 10 s (110% V_{IFT})/20 s (0)	Handball	Handball	Handball	Rest	

Note the de-emphasis of lactic work in Tuesday's HIIT session. Both HIIT sessions have limited neuromuscular demands to allow leg freshness for the strength/speed development. Type refers to the physiological target.

Table 27.3 $\dot{V}O_2$ and Strength/Speed Development Cycle (Specific Phase, Preseason; Typically 2 Weeks Duration) (8)

Microcycle (physical emphasis)		Monday	Tuesday	Wednesday	Thursday	Friday	Saturday	Sunday
$\dot{V}O_2$+strength/ speed development (specific)	AM	Specific strength/ speed/ injury prevention	Rest	Type 2 GBHIIT 2×3 min (SSG) 4 vs. 4 RPE 6 + Type 1 6 min 10 s (100% V_{IFT} shuttle)/10 s (0)	Rest	Specific power/ speed	Handball	Rest
	PM	Handball	Handball	Handball	Handball	Rest	Handball Type 5 SIT 6×30 s (all-out shuttle)/4 min (0)	

Note that the lactic session is programmed before the day off. Type refers to the physiological target.

Table 27.4 Maintenance (In-Season; Remainder of the Season, Typically 9 to 10 Months) (8)

Microcycle (physical emphasis)		Monday	Tuesday	Wednesday	Thursday	Friday	Saturday	Sunday
Competitive (in season)	AM	Recovery/ strength/ injury prevention	Rest	Rest	Strength/ power/ speed	Rest	Rest	Rest
	PM	Handball	Handball	Handball	Handball	Handball	Game	
			Type 1	Type 2				
			HIIT with short intervals	GBHIIT				
			1 × 10 min	3 × 4 min (SSG)				
			10 s (110% V$_{IFT}$ shuttle)/20 s (0)	4 vs. 4				
			For substitutes or if the power/speed session of Thursday is canceled:	RPE 7				
			Type 4					
			2 × RST					
			6 × 20 m-90° COD/25 s (0) with 15 min (handball) between RSS					

Note that the RST session is performed with 90° COD to reduce glycolytic anaerobic energy release and is performed only by substitutes or when the speed/power session is missed (to partially compensate for the neuromuscular work at high intensity). SSGs can also be selected for their specificity, to lower the anaerobic glycolytic energy contribution 3 d before the game. Type refers to the physiological target.

I was privileged to be in the position charged with preparing the First French League Hand-ball Team of Sélestat in 2004-2005 for a season that would become one of the best in its history. It was my second season at the club, and I had gained the benefit of my experience from the first year, along with knowing the players and staff better, knowing their individual needs, and gaining their trust. Additionally, through some trial and error, I had developed a better understanding of what worked and what didn't; that is, I knew the training stimulus (load) that was triggering adaptation for certain players versus others. Together with Francois Berthier, the head coach, our strategy was to increase the aerobic conditioning of the team using a greater training volume in the first 2 weeks. Our plan involved using a challenging 4 d camp in the mountains to permit some team integration for a few new players who had joined the squad over the summer. The training involved some epic mountain biking tours as well as a short 6 h mountaineering session in the hilly forest of the Voges, not to mention evening handball practice alongside a few run-based HIITs.

The rules of the mountaineering race were relatively simple: players were given a map when they woke (without breakfast) along with the key checkpoints that had to be reached to obtain their food and drink for the day; the winning team needed to reach all locations in the minimum amount of time. To be sure the players provided their best effort and were motivated, the volume of HIIT applied in the remainder of the week (table 27.5) was to be inversely related to the mountaineering results shown from the eight different pairs of players. The first team would do what was planned, the second team would perform an additional 3 min effort, and so forth.

On the morning of the race, the faces of certain players said it all. A social night at the hotel got carried away, creating the unfortunate state we were seeing in front of us (hang-overs; little sleep). In return for this, the coaching staff opted to lengthen the orienteering course out a ways to provide a statement and indicate intent for the year. At the same time, unbeknownst to us, a few team leaders had already in fact moved checkpoints of their fellow teammates to challenge them further.

At the end of the day, the players' return times ranged from late in the afternoon to very late at night. Nevertheless, the deep levels of fatigue, mental and physical challenge, along with the necessary cooperation to achieve the tasks caused strong team bonds to be formed that I feel brought us together as a team from very early on. From that point, however, I told the players that their attitude to our camp and subsequent consequence had compromised my plan, and that I wasn't sure how to best adapt their training load in the following days. Some had been in the forest for 12 h, while others for only 4. The predicament could not have played into my hands any better, and I was able to then suggest to the team that I could try using HRV to adjust their training load accordingly. Desperate that the sugges-tion might work in their favor, the guys bought in, and you can view the data from this story in figure 27.10 (notice the massive effect in some players from the mountaineering event). Importantly, most guys continued to make the effort to take the morning measurement throughout the remainder of the year.

The preseason went on as planned, with successful friendly games and no major injuries. At the end of 6 wk, the boys were doing fine on the court, but many were complaining of heavy legs. While there is no direct link between a player's physical capacities and game outcomes, the team had the worst start to the season in years. After many stressful nights, chats with colleagues and mentors and comparisons with past year training plans, I attributed the reported heavy legs to an overreliance on RST during the last 3 wk of the preparation. After a few weeks into the season, I changed the programming toward handball-specific but isolated speed and HIIT training sessions (short interval and SSGs, table 27.4) (4), and neuromuscular freshness returned, in line with noticeable team freshness and success. We went on to make some big wins and made the quarterfinals of the French Cup, losing in the match by a few points. Nevertheless, it was a year in my sporting life that as a practitioner

Table 27.5 Focus on the HIIT Prescription of the 6 Week Preseason Conditioning Program Used in July 2004 With Sélestat Handball Team (First French League)

Type refers to the physiological target of the HIIT format.

	HIIT	Repeated-sprint training	Sprint interval training	Small-sided games	Total HIIT time (T at $\dot{V}O_2$max)
Week 1	(1) Short Type 1 2×6 min 15 s [95%] / 15 s [jog] + (2) Short Type 3 2×6 min 20 s [95%] / 20 s [passive]				~24 min (15-18 min)
Week 2	(1) Short Type 3 2×6 min 30 s [90%] / 30 s [jog] + (2) Long Type 4 4×3 min [80%] / 2 min [passive]			(3) Type 2 3×3 min 4 vs. 4	~33 min (18-21 min)
Week 3	(1) Short Type 3 10 min 15 s [100%] / 15 s [passive] + (2) Long Type 4 5×3 min [80%] / 2 min [passive]			(3) Type 2 3×4 min 4 vs. 4	~37 min (20-24 min)
Week 4	(1) Short Type 1 6 min 10 s [95%] / 10 s [passive]		(2) Type 5 6×30 s every 2 min (40 m shuttles)	(3) Type 2 4×4 min 4 vs. 4	~35 min (12-15 min)
Week 5		(1) Type 4 3×(6×15+15 m shuttle every 30 s) (2) Type 4 3×(4×20+20 m shuttle every 30 s)		(3) Type 2 3×3 min 4 vs. 4	~26 min (10-12 min)
Week 6	(1) Short Type 1 6 min 10 s [105%] / 20 s [passive]	(1) Type 4 2×(4×15+15 m shuttle every 30 s)		(2) Type 2 3×4 min 4 vs. 4	~22 min (10-14 min)

The numbers in parentheses indicate the number of separate days when the different HIIT formats were implemented. The numbers in brackets refer to running intensity as either a percentage of V_{IFT} or recovery jog. Number of players for small-sided games refers to field players. Note the distribution of HIIT-type targets. For example, when a type 4 target is introduced week 2, a type 3 target is replaced by a type 2 target to compensate for the overall anaerobic contribution. When a type 5 target is introduced week 4, the other session targets are limited to type 1 and 2 to limit weekly neuromuscular and anaerobic participation. Note also the overreliance on RST the last 3 weeks (as discussed in the text).

(continued)

I was proud to contribute to. I made mistakes, which drove me harder toward understanding the reasons for them, and I learned and gained experience as a result. As a team, we came together to achieve something special for a little club with the league's second smallest budget. The experience showed me the importance of training monitoring (HRV) to better manage (sometimes unplanned) variations in load, as well as how to program and solve the training program puzzle to use the different HIIT formats in relation to an ever-evolving context.

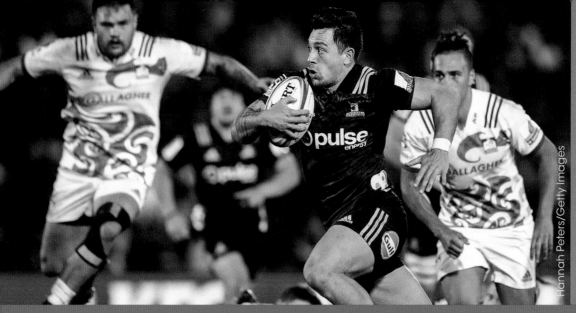

Peters/Getty Images

Rugby Union

● ● ● ● ● ●

Nic Gill and Martyn Beaven

Performance Demands of Rugby Union

In this section, we introduce the sport of Rugby Union and discuss the various factors of importance for players (and individual positions) and the relative contributions that physical performance characteristics make to winning games.

Sport Description and Factors of Winning

Rugby Union, commonly known as rugby, is a contact team sport that originated in England in the first half of the 19th century. Rugby Union is an invasion sport that requires mostly running with ball in hand with the game objective of scoring more points than the opposition. Points can be scored in several ways. A try, scored by grounding the ball over the try-line in the in-goal area of the opposition (between the try-line and the dead-ball line), is worth 5 points and a subsequent conversion kick scores 2 points. A successful penalty kick or a drop goal each scores 3 points. Kicks are required to pass between two goalposts and over a connecting crossbar. Rugby is a game of territory and possession with players allowed to pass or kick the ball. The most common form of rugby is a game between two teams

of 15 players using an oval-shaped ball on a rectangular field (100 m long and 70 m wide) with H-shaped goalposts situated centrally on each try-line. Rugby is a global sport with about 9 million players registered in 2016 and over 100 ranked and accredited nations. Rugby boasts the second most lucrative and most attended sporting World Cup, with the 2015 Rugby World Cup selling 2.47 million tickets and generating ~$500 million in revenue.

The player positions are shown in figure 28.1. Positions typically are classified into two main groups, the forwards and backs. Forwards consist of front rowers (props and hooker; numbers 1 to 3), second row (locks; numbers 4 and 5), and the back row (or loose forwards; numbers 6 to 8). The backs consist of inside backs (halfback, also called a Scrum-half, first 5/8, second 5/8; numbers 9 to 12) and outside backs (center, wings, and fullback; numbers 13 to 15).

Rugby Union games are divided into 40 min halves, separated by a 10 to 15 min half-time break. Stoppages for injury or to allow the referee to take disciplinary action do not count as part of the playing time, so that the elapsed time is usually longer than 80 min (often approximately 100 min). Rugby Union is an intermittent sport characterized by periods of intense activity such as sprints, tackles, accelerations, decelerations, rucks, mauls, and scrums, interspersed with low-intensity periods

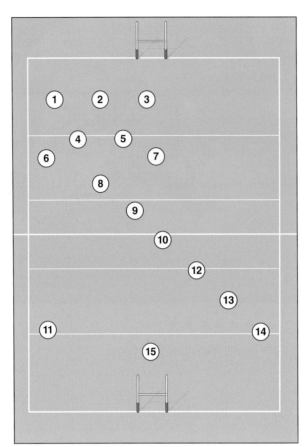

Figure 28.1 The positions of Rugby Union.

1. Loosehead prop
2. Hooker
3. Tighthead prop
4. Second row
5. Second row
6. Blindside flanker
7. Openside flanker
8. Number 8
9. Scrum-half
10. Fly-half
11. Left wing
12. Inside centre
13. Outside centre
14. Right wing
15. Full-back

primarily consisting of walking and jogging (5, 7, 28). Research using time-motion analysis and wearable tracking technology such as a global positioning system (GPS) shows activity profiles that vary between playing positions (15, 21). Like many sports, intensity is typically shown to increase as the competition standard rises (5, 21). As well, during match play, backs tend to cover a greater total distance, more high-intensity running distance (6 to 8 m/s), and very high-speed running distance (>8 m/s) than forwards (1, 21, 25). The positional requirements of forward play require that these players perform higher volumes of high-intensity activity (22), repeated high-intensity efforts (15), and contact loads (21) than backs.

Passing and Kicking

The ball in rugby can be passed laterally or backward but not forward. The ball tends to be moved forward in three ways including by kicking, by having a player run with it, or by moving the ball within a scrum or maul (see below). Only players in possession of the ball may be tackled.

Any player may kick the ball forward in an attempt to gain territory. When a player anywhere in the playing area kicks the ball into touch (across the sideline), a lineout is taken. Here, the opposite team that kicked the ball into touch gets to throw the ball into a lineout (see below).

Breakdowns

Tackles in rugby must be below the neck, with the aim of impeding or grounding the player with the ball. The aim of the defending side is to stop the player with the ball, either by bringing him to the ground (termed a *ruck*) or by contesting for possession with the ballcarrier on his feet (termed a *maul*). Such a circumstance is called a breakdown, and specific laws govern each situation.

Tackling

A player can tackle an opposing player who has the ball by holding him while bringing him to the ground. However, it is illegal to push, shoulder-charge, or trip a player using the feet or legs, although hands can be used.

Lineout

As mentioned before, when the ball leaves the side of the field (either through a kick, pass, or a player being tackled out across the sideline), a lineout is awarded against the team that last touched the ball. Forward players from each team line up a meter apart, perpendicular to the touchline and between 5 m and 15 m from the touchline. The team's hooker will use an overhead throw to toss the ball down the middle of the lines created by the two teams. One or more players from each team will be lifted by their teammates in order to try to gain possession of the ball from the air (24). Both sides compete for the ball and players have the option of lifting their teammates. A jumping player cannot be tackled until he lands, and only shoulder-to-shoulder contact is allowed.

Scrum

A scrum is a way of restarting the game safely and fairly after a minor infringement. Scrums are awarded when the ball has been knocked or passed forward, if a player takes the ball over his own try-line and puts the ball down, when a player is accidentally offside, or when the ball is trapped in a ruck or maul with no realistic chance of being retrieved. A team may also opt for a scrum if awarded a penalty.

A scrum is formed by the eight forwards from each team (see figure 28.1) binding together in three rows. The front row consists of the two props and a hooker. The second row consists of two locks and the back row consists of two flankers and a number 8. Once a scrum is formed, the scrum-half from the team awarded the scrum rolls the ball into the gap between the two opposing front rows. The two hookers then compete for possession by hooking the ball backward with their feet, while each pack tries to push the opposing pack backward to help gain possession.

Relative Contribution of Physical Performance

Possessing certain physical attributes is important for Rugby Union players, but is of limited value if the athlete does not possess the specific positional skills and game understanding, which are fundamental to performance. In conjunction with time-motion analysis, a parallel stream of research within Rugby Union has been the use of notational analysis to quantify the physical and skill requirements of competition. Notational analysis provides objective feedback of games and player actions through the frequencies of key performance indicators (9, 16). Specifically, notational analysis has been used to determine differences in playing patterns between teams and individuals and assist in understanding what leads to successful performance (10, 14, 16). It is clear from existing data that as the level of competition gets higher, the positional skills and understanding of the game improves. In saying this, however, so too do the physical capabilities of the athletes.

When it comes to the match, the team that is likely to win tends to be the team that can execute the game plan at the highest intensity level for the game duration. This means the positional skills need to be accurate, the understanding of the game plan needs to be sound, and players must have the physical capacity to execute all required tasks at a high intensity for 80 minutes. At the very least, rugby players need to be fit enough to tolerate the requirements of their positions and have the ability to execute their roles under fatigue, under pressure, and within many dynamic and fast-changing situations. Notwithstanding the varying requirements of the multiple Rugby Union positions shown (figure 28.1; described below), a rugby player generally requires very high levels of strength and the ability to repeatedly and effectively express that strength and power over the entire game duration (figure 28.2). Players maintain heart rates close to 90% of maximum (4), and hence, HIIT becomes a vital component in the arsenal of the conditioning program designed to enhance metabolic aspects and repeated high-intensity requirements vital to Rugby Union success.

Targets of Physical Performance in Rugby Union

The physical characteristics of Rugby Union players and the differences between positions and playing levels are well documented. Essentially, forwards are typically heavier and stronger than backs, while backs are faster and more agile than forwards (19). The differences between positions are related to the differences in the position-specific tasks performed during a match. For example, time-motion analysis and the use of GPS have shown backs travel farther, sprint farther and more frequently, and have lower work:rest ratios than forwards (1, 4, 6, 7).

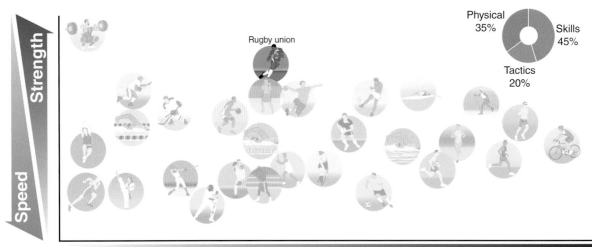

Figure 28.2 The position of the Rugby Union player on the three axes illustrates the relative importance of the three main physical capacities of importance for elite participation, acknowledging that this will vary between positions. Outside of critical psychological aspects and team chemistry components, which are difficult to quantify, the pie chart shows the general relative importance of skills (45%), tactical awareness (20%), and physical capacities (35%) for Rugby Union success.

Adapted from G.A. Nader, "Concurrent Strength and Endurance Training: From Molecules to Man," *Medicine & Science in Sports & Exercise* 38, no. 11 (2006): 1965-1970.

Tight Forwards

The front row and second row play vital roles in securing possession of the ball in the restarts, lineouts, and scrum situations during the game. Due to the required tasks of these players, strength and power are very important assets for pushing, jumping, and tackling. While these players are also typically the heaviest members of the team, the need for aerobic fitness is also important, as they will typically cover 4 to 6 km in a game. Offensively and defensively these players are in the closer channels to the high-contact ruck and maul situations and can make between 10 and 30 tackles a game. Lean muscle mass, strength, and power are therefore crucial physical attributes for these players to perform their core roles.

Back Row

Back row players are typically involved in running with the ball and tackling in slightly wider channels than tight forwards. While these players still have an important role in the restarts, lineouts, and scrums, they also have a role in linking the tight forwards with the backs and getting into a number of positions quickly to have influence on the game. Turning over the ball (stealing from the opposition)

and supporting line breaks are an important role and requires speed, power, and a high level of anaerobic and aerobic metabolic conditioning.

Inside Backs

Numbers 9, 10, and 12 (figure 28.1) are typically smaller than most other players and typically are the kickers of the team. Their tactical nous and game understanding is typically very high as they are called on to drive the team around the field. Due to the natural link between the forwards and the outside backs, these players must normally possess a balance of speed, power, endurance, and agility.

Outside Backs

As the outside backs have a major role in finishing plays, counterattacking, and chasing kicks, these players are typically explosive and very fast runners of the ball. Typically the leanest players on the field, they often cover the most distance in a game (especially the fullback). Often distances of sprints for these players are longer than all other players on the field.

Match Demands

Austin et al. (1) found that the work:rest ratios of Super 14 Rugby Union players were 1:4, 1:5, and 1:6

for front row and back row forwards, inside backs, and outside backs, respectively. During game play, players cover substantial distance and are involved in multiple high-intensity running and nonrunning activities (1, 11, 13, 20). The demands of professional Rugby Union matches between the years 2008 and 2015 were recently reported by Hogarth and colleagues (13), who showed that the distance covered by players during a match ranged from 4662 to 7227 m, depending on playing position and the level of competition. The 33 to 39 min ball-in-play duration of a match and the total distance covered by players suggest that there is a significant demand on a player's aerobic system to provide the required energy to perform the necessary activities over this period of time (8). During most competition matches, the duration of each play (whistle to whistle) typically depends on the level of competition, but lasts for 35 s on average, although some periods of play can last up to 6 min.

In addition to requiring a well-conditioned aerobic system, a significant demand is placed on the player's anaerobic system due to the intermittent short high-intensity running and nonrunning activities that occur throughout a match (4, 6, 8). Austin et al. (1) found that the passive:high-intensity task work ratio (nonrunning:scrum, ruck, maul) varied the most between the forwards and backs, with front rowers and back rowers performing the most of these tasks (62 ± 13 and 68 ± 15, respectively) and the inside and outside backs completing only one-third of this type of work (17 ± 7 and 14 ± 5), respectively.

Key Weapons, Manipulations, and Surveillance Tools

Developing and monitoring both endurance and high-intensity running abilities are important considerations for many team sport athletes. The enhancement of these qualities can positively impact performance during the repeated bouts of high-intensity activity that occur in professional Rugby Union competition (2, 17, 27). For example, a moderate correlation (r = −0.38) has been shown between match activity rate (tasks/min) and repeated sprint ability (23), while increased aerobic capacity, as determined by maximal aerobic running speed, is correlated (r = 0.746) to increased match running distance in professional Rugby Union players (25). This evidence supports strategies aimed at enhance-

ment of aerobic endurance and high-intensity running capacity in professional rugby players. However, it is important to acknowledge the complex interplay of physical, technical, tactical, environmental, and cognitive factors that influence competitive match performance (figure 28.2), which makes it difficult to directly relate match performance to specific outcomes on physical tests.

HIIT Weapons

We typically target a range and combination of HIIT weapons throughout the year depending on the individual needs, training phase (preseason, in-season, etc.), turnaround time between games, technical and tactical training load, and intensity, training surface, weather, and travel factors. Game-based high-intensity interval training (GBHIIT), generally broken down into small-sided games (SSGs) and skill-based games (SBGs), as well as short and long intervals (on-feet and off-feet) and mixed-fuel circuits, form the basis of conditioning content for Rugby Union players. The general percentage breakdown of our HIIT weapons over the course of a season is shown in figure 28.3.

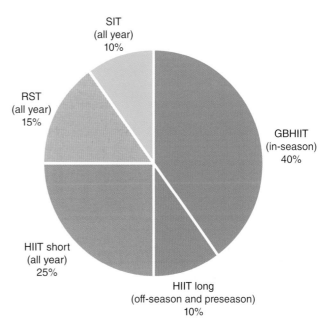

Figure 28.3 Percentage of the different HIIT formats (weapons) used throughout the annual season in elite Rugby Union preparation. Note that a 12 mo cycle consists of approximately 30 games, and the exact breakdown depends on the level of competition encountered, the duration of competition, and the positional and individual needs.

Manipulations of Interval Training Variables

The running intensity, inclusion of static work, duration of effort, and work:rest ratios are the main variables manipulated to achieve the desired stress for the particular purpose of any given HIIT session in Rugby Union player preparation. Positional needs, individual needs, and specific metabolic and neuromuscular focus are considered for each session, each week, and during each macrocycle.

GBHIIT

Due to the overall importance of skill and game understanding in Rugby Union, it is vital to incorporate these game-based factors into the conditioning program. For many teams, GBHIIT is the main HIIT weapon of choice! Essentially, this incorporation is due to a number of reasons, but the fact that skill- or game-based conditioning can be an efficient way to improve game-specific skill and understanding for groups or teams, while also requiring periods of high-intensity work, makes it a staple weapon for most teams (12), although it is acknowledged that GBHIIT may not always adequately mimic the demands of competitive matches (26). Rugby Union players, like most athletes, are highly competitive,

so utilizing this competitive drive helps to ensure that athletes work hard when there is a ball involved. Get them individually or in a line to do some tough intervals, and the motivation for many athletes is not quite the same. In addition, the benefit of having a bit of fun while working hard together cannot be underestimated in terms of interpersonal relationships and team building.

SSGs are an effective training modality and are increasingly used across team sports in an attempt to elicit a physiological response, while simultaneously challenging technical, tactical, and decision-making aspects of performance. For example, analysis of various soccer-specific SSGs showed these to be reliable and effective training measures across sessions in terms of running output, and they can be manipulated through alterations in various constraints such as field size and number of players (3, 18). With regard to alterations in GBHIIT, volume, and intensities, it typically comes down to the purpose of the session and training or competition phase, but adjustments in field size, player numbers, rules, and so forth enable us to deliver the running load, metabolic load, and skill acquisition aspects required to challenge and progressively load athletes. To be clear, we don't necessarily want to be hitting match intensity all the time (see also

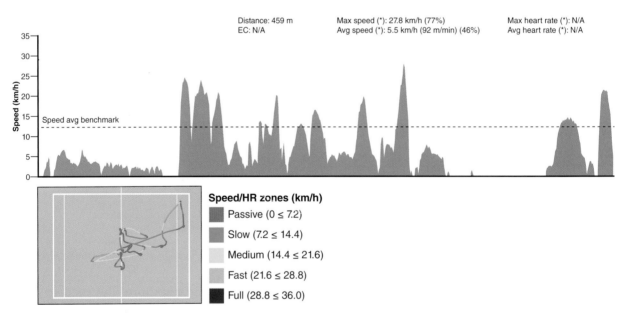

Figure 28.4 International Women's Rugby Match. The diagram illustrates what was identified as a very high 5 min period in a women's international rugby player's workload. In isolation, this speed profile tells us only part of the picture in determining overall workload. However, it does provide a valuable insight into what we can use to prescribe relevant bouts of high-speed running, repeated efforts, and their relationship to game-related skills. Finding the hardest and most intense periods in your sport can greatly assist the design of SSGs and other conditioning activities.

SSG 1: Modified Rugby League

Each SSG in its own right can be valuable when managing or replicating match intensity in training, along with the integration of core skills. For our modified Rugby League SSG (figure 28.5), we play 3 versus 3 across a 35×10 m area (from sideline to halfway across and halfway to 10 m line). The player must touch the sideline after making a tackle. Each side is allowed 6 tackles only, as per Rugby League rules. Players must rise to their feet after being tackled to tap the ball, and no kicking is allowed. The idea is to keep the games moving, and there are no stoppages. When a try is scored, the team is to immediately play on. The high neuromuscular loads experienced in this SSG, due to the changes of direc-

tion, short work durations, and short recovery periods, align with a type 4 HIIT target.

Correlation to Match Metrics

- Distance = low
- HI distance = low
- HI duration = low
- Sprints = moderate
- Impacts = high

Here we identified a high relationship between SSG impacts and game demands with a moderate relationship to in-game sprint metrics but a low relationship to high-intensity distance and durations.

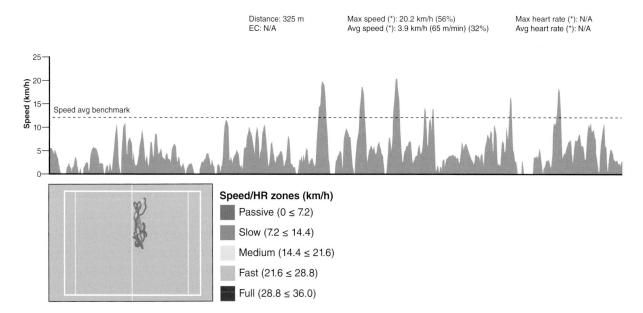

Distance: 325 m
EC: N/A

Max speed (*): 20.2 km/h (56%)
Avg speed (*): 3.9 km/h (65 m/min) (32%)

Max heart rate (*): N/A
Avg heart rate (*): N/A

Speed avg benchmark

Speed/HR zones (km/h)
- Passive (0 ≤ 7.2)
- Slow (7.2 ≤ 14.4)
- Medium (14.4 ≤ 21.6)
- Fast (21.6 ≤ 28.8)
- Full (28.8 ≤ 36.0)

Figure 28.5 Modified 3 versus 3 Rugby League on a 35×10 m playing field.

chapters 29 and 30), so subtle manipulations in GBHIIT factors (see chapter 5) can help you achieve the stimulus you desire.

It is important to understand the game demands for the positional groups you are working with (figure 28.1). Figure 28.4 illustrates a GPS-derived game demand example and how simple GBHIIT sessions (figures 28.5 to 28.7) can be manipulated to achieve the appropriate training response at, below, or above the match demands as required. In these

examples, the metrics to determine game demands included:

- Distance covered (m)
- High-intensity (HI) distance covered (m over 15 km/h)
- Duration at high intensity (HI) (min:s over 15 km/h)
- Sprints (quantity over 20 km/h)
- High-intensity impacts (#)

SSG 2: Follow Me, Modified Rugby Union

With this SSG, we identified its large relationship with match demands for high-intensity distance, duration, repeated high-intensity efforts, and sprint metrics. Follow me (figure 28.6) is played 12 versus 12 across the field on a 70×28 m area from sideline to sideline and halfway to the 22 m line. The rules are like Rugby Union, but you can tackle only your allocated opposite number (figure 28.1), although blocking is allowed. No kicking, tackles are unlimited, and rucks are uncontested (i.e., when the ballcarrier releases the ball, the opposition cannot touch it). When tackled, players pop off the ground, with defenders moving 5 m back. No stoppages occur to keep the game moving, and when a try is scored, play immediately moves on. Coaches encourage all players to work back behind the ball. This game is closest to match demands when considering the number of repeated high-intensity efforts (RHIEs), and by adding an interchange rule it can be narrowed further. The game's high neuromuscular and metabolic loads associated with its changes of direction, extended work durations, and short recovery periods allow this SSG weapon to hit the type 4 HIIT target.

Correlation to Match Metrics

- Distance = high
- HI distance = high
- HI duration = high
- Sprints = high
- Impacts = high

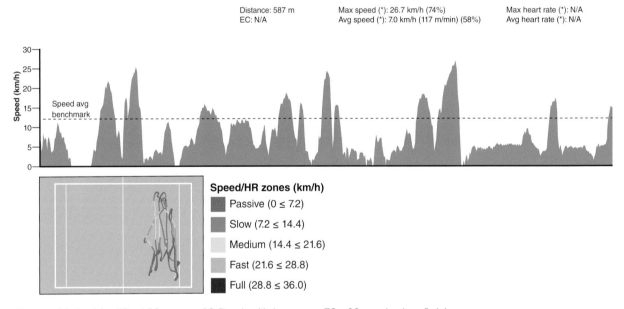

Distance: 587 m
EC: N/A

Max speed (*): 26.7 km/h (74%)
Avg speed (*): 7.0 km/h (117 m/min) (58%)

Max heart rate (*): N/A
Avg heart rate (*): N/A

Speed/HR zones (km/h)
Passive (0 ≤ 7.2)
Slow (7.2 ≤ 14.4)
Medium (14.4 ≤ 21.6)
Fast (21.6 ≤ 28.8)
Full (28.8 ≤ 36.0)

Figure 28.6 Modified 12 versus 12 Rugby Union on a 70×28 m playing field.

HIIT With Short Intervals

Throughout the world of high-performance sport, there seems to be good awareness of the importance of achieving certain volumes of high-speed running. Short intervals that include changes in direction (type 2 and 4 targets) are a good way to manage this need for high-intensity work while still managing the training stress. We prefer to keep the duration of our efforts short, using short-interval weapons of 10 s to 20 s efforts on a 1:1 to 1:4 work:rest ratio (see figure 28.8).

Such intervals are used regularly during the season to provide extra work to individuals who need to maintain their levels of aerobic oxidative and anaerobic glycolytic power. In others, short intervals are used as top-ups at the end of training sessions

SSG 3: Down and Up, Modified Touch Rugby

This SSG we call down and up (figure 28.7) is played 12 versus 12 across the field on a 70×100 m area, from sideline to sideline and full field length. The game follows the basic rules of touch rugby, but as the name implies, all players must go to ground before returning to the opposition try-line after making a touch or being touched. All touches must be two-handed, and only six total are allowed. Kicks are allowed to hand only, with no bounce to regather. No stoppages are used to keep the game moving, and when a try is scored, play immediately moves on. For this SSG, we identified a moderate relationship with match demands for high-intensity distance, duration, and sprint metrics, but a low relationship to impacts. Again, there is high neuromuscular loading associated with changes of direction, work durations are extended, with short recovery periods aligning this SSG as a type 4 HIIT weapon. Importantly, impacts and the associated neuromuscular burden are low, so it can be used to facilitate recovery.

Correlation to Match Metrics

- Distance = high
- HI distance = moderate
- HI duration = moderate
- Sprints = moderate
- Impacts = low

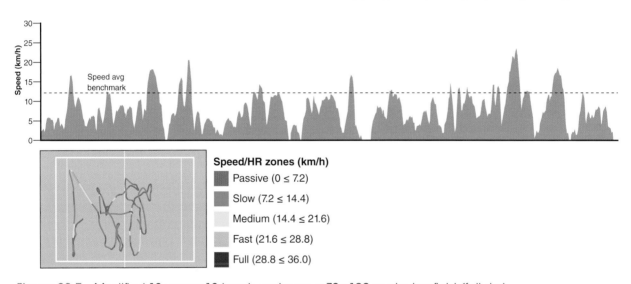

Distance: 558 m
EC: N/A

Max speed (*): 23.4 km/h (65%)
Avg speed (*): 6.7 km/h (112 m/min) (56%)

Max heart rate (*): N/A
Avg heart rate (*): N/A

Speed avg benchmark

Speed/HR zones (km/h)
Passive (0 ≤ 7.2)
Slow (7.2 ≤ 14.4)
Medium (14.4 ≤ 21.6)
Fast (21.6 ≤ 28.8)
Full (28.8 ≤ 36.0)

Figure 28.7 Modified 12 versus 12 touch rugby on a 70×100 m playing field (full size).

to provide additional volume to players who may be lacking fitness, have been exposed to minimal game time, or (due to injury, illness, or selection pressures) are training fully with the team but just not playing.

Typically we use a number of methods to determine the health and fitness of our squad. One such method is benchmarking, or monitoring, that occurs in-season, such as with timed shuttles or intervals, where we have acceptable position-related targets. For example, we might use a 150 m shuttle in 25 s

for outside backs with one turn (100 m then 50 m). Likewise, an intermittent bouncing to feet 88 m for tight forwards is used: the player starts on the ground, bounces to his feet, sprints 22 m, hits the ground, bounces to his feet again, and repeats for 88 m (4×22 m), which must be performed in less than 20 s.

The issue with doing large amounts of straight-line running and shuttles is of course the lack of specificity related to game performance and the resulting weak transference of such training, e.g.,

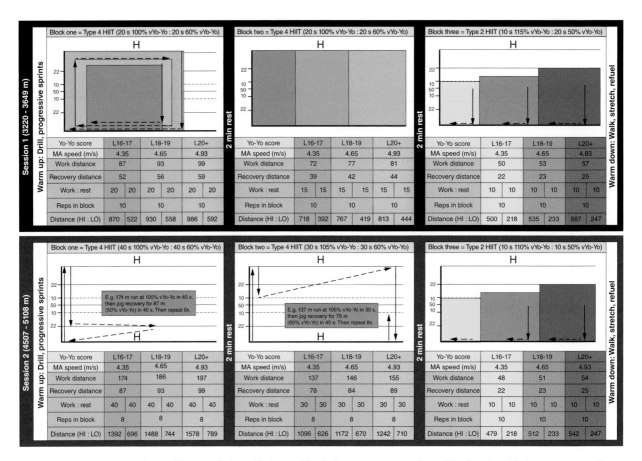

Figure 28.8 Examples of typical short-interval training weapons for elite Rugby Union preparation. Note the individualized approach based on vYo-Yo. Here specific conditioning targets (type 2, 3, etc.) are addressed by utilizing the range of interval training weapons shown.

the best shuttle runner does not necessarily translate to being the best player. To continue to improve relevance and transference, the inclusion of position-specific tasks, skills, and movements is often applied. For example, we may ask a player to complete a shuttle before having him work on some rugby-specific ball skill, or complete a taxing static task before, during, or after the running effort, e.g., ball wrestle, four consecutive tackles, and so forth.

While the optimal combination of high-speed running, deceleration, acceleration, static tasks, skills, metabolic, and locomotor stress is difficult to quantify, the guiding principle we use is to obtain certain target percentage levels of game stress for varied durations and volumes, e.g., 10 min of work for top-up or 45 to 60 min of work if a player is returning to play from a lengthy time on the sidelines.

Repeated Sprint Training

The use of repeated sprint training (RST) or repeated speed is highly relevant for backs and loose forwards.

The need to run fast during the game occurs often for these players and therefore developing speed, and repeated speed, with only short to moderate recovery is important. Typically this should be kept as game specific as possible, across distances of between 5 and 70 m, with rest periods of 3 to 4 times the duration of the effort. For these weapons, aiming for type 5 targets, the number of repetitions depends on the duration of the effort, such that if we are focused on training or improving speed off the mark (e.g., maximal acceleration) in a manner similar to a defensive line coming forward quickly (e.g., line speed), then we may have blocks of 6 to 10 efforts of 10 m with 15 to 20 s rest periods. Completing 3 to 6 blocks of this exercise can occur depending on what else needs to be included in the day's training. For example, this acceleration focus may then lead on to an attack focus in which we are now interested in working on 30 to 40 m efforts, the wing or full-back has a ball in hand, and is running fast but at the same time trying to beat a defender (1 versus 1).

This exercise might involve 5 to 8 repetitions on attack and defense to ensure adequate rest between attacking efforts.

In addition to RST on-feet, we also use metabolic training with similar work:rest intervals and intensities, but in off-feet type situations, e.g., using a rowing or bike ergometer. In this way we can add cardiovascular and metabolic stress (i.e., type 3 targets) but not necessarily add neuromuscular and locomotor stress associated with types 2, 4, and 5 targets, thus helping reduce the likelihood of injury that can occur with excessive high-speed running volume.

HIIT With Long Intervals

We believe that long-interval HIIT is important for all Rugby Union playing positions during the preseason, as well as sometimes during the competition season for certain players (particularly for backs and loose forwards). Typically, these efforts are made up of 300 to 1200 m shuttles. Due again to the importance and regularity of deceleration and acceleration, these long intervals have a lot of turns involved, forming type 4 HIIT targets for us. During some parts of the season, these turns may require the player to go to ground and/or bounce to feet before continuing with the effort. Such modifications are made based on the individual's needs or requirements and current game load. These intervals will usually be on a varied work:rest ratio of 2:1 to 1:1.

Maximal aerobic speed (MAS) blocks are often prescribed in Rugby Union using many different formats (e.g., shuttles, field loops, etc.). Essentially, we prescribe targets using percentages of the vYo-Yo (calculated from YoYo test results; see figure 28.8). This method allows for target speeds to be prescribed around MAS, ensuring the appropriate stimulus is prescribed relative to the desired outcome.

Another common long-interval shuttle is the Bronco (1.2 km shuttle; 20 m, 40 m, 60 m out-and-back shuttle completed 5 times without rest), which is an effective and practical benchmarking run with applications in rehabilitation and return to play, hitting type 4 targets.

Depending on the athlete and the session priority, this type of long-interval session could be prescribed first (while fresh and to maximize running speed and performance) with other sessions (e.g., strength and power) scheduled after. However, if strength and power are the priorities for the individual, the priority session will occur in the morning and the session of secondary importance performed later in the day

(for further expansion on this issue, refer to chapter 6). The contents of each session, the purpose of each session, and the focus for the individual need constant consideration. Sequencing is vital to ensure desired adaptations occur and injury risk is reduced.

Sprint Interval Training

As Rugby Union players, it is important to be able to run fast! Line breaks and speed are one physical attribute that has been correlated with scoring tries; so it does appear that speed is king. To develop speed and sprint ability, it is common for us to use SIT to hit type 5 targets, with all-out sprints over 20 to 150 m (up to 30 s) at maximal effort and velocity, with long rests to ensure sufficient recovery and quality repeats (3 to 4 min; 1:8 work:rest). Depending on the positional group, the tight forwards are likely to not complete efforts longer than 20 m, but as we work through the loose forwards, inside backs, and outside backs, the distances (and ranges) increase.

Load Surveillance and Monitoring Tools

As already discussed, it is common practice to use GPS to track training load in elite Rugby Union. We find this to be a sound method of tracking locomotor load (e.g., distance, intensity, acceleration, deceleration, collisions, etc.) and predicting metabolic load. Many systems also allow for the simultaneous collection of heart rate data, and many elite teams use this information to inform their conditioning practices. While other aspects of load need consideration (see chapter 8), GPS data does offer insight into what is actually happening on the field and is our main marker of external training load. RPE is also an important consideration we use to assess the internal training load of the program.

There is a range of prescription ratios, percentages, and performance targets that are set within a team environment, but, while we believe that there is a place for the data, there is equally a requirement for common sense. The blend of the two is crucial. For example, hitting stable acute-to-chronic loading ratios is one thing, but not keeping an eye on how your players move so as to pick up obvious signs of movement competency, or lack thereof, is pure neglect. There is obviously the physical load of playing and training that needs consideration, but there are equally other stressors involved of importance, such as travel (and associated sleep deprivation), individual game load, training age, positional stressors, and home life, on top of the psychological load experienced by players, including monotony, team meetings, media scrutiny, and, of course, the game.

Balancing stress (e.g., metabolic, psychological, performance, selection, etc.; see chapter 7) with recovery and relaxation strategies should always be prioritized to ensure optimal performance. Looking at one or two variables in isolation or becoming fixated on data over player well-being can be a dangerous practice. Time and energy must be directed toward practices that make a meaningful difference to athlete wellness that will translate into sharpness, as well as training and performance readiness.

Training Status Surveillance and Monitoring Tools

The training status monitoring tools that we've used in Rugby Union are generally limited to noninvasive measures and include wellness questionnaires and GPS/accelerometer-derived data, HR, and RPE responses to sessions. From a physical perspective (figure 28.2), it is common practice that players will undergo monitoring of strength, power, speed, and acceleration ability during certain times of the season. If an athlete is not strong enough relative to his history, ability, age, or position, then a strength focus may be implemented for the subsequent cycle. Similarly, if a player is carrying too much body fat, then extra work may be prescribed and nutrition habits addressed (see chapter 7). Similarly, if a player is not hitting the speed and acceleration numbers desired or expected, then there may be a shift toward more explosive movement focus in the program. From a fitness perspective, and specifically related to HIIT, the 1.2 km shuttle run (the Bronco mentioned previously) is often used to assess a player's fitness level. If fitness is not where it needs to be, then various HIIT weapons are prescribed accordingly to address identified deficiencies, depending on the time of the year, training cycle, as well as individual and positional needs.

Strategies for Structuring the Training Program Using HIIT

The inclusion of HIIT weapons into a rugby program can occur in many different ways for many different reasons. Within a season, there are numerous variables that we must balance to achieve consistent high-level performance. Considering all of the important variables, not just a couple, ensures greater likelihood of success. In Rugby Union, we believe that traditional periodization approaches across all aspects of physical preparation can be unrealistic to achieve. The complexities of getting a 120 kg athlete lean, strong, powerful, light-footed, and fit with good ball skills and game understanding means that plans and periodization must be agile and adaptable. This flexible prescription implies considering the individual and team with respect to how workloads build toward peak targeted performance. The following section addresses some of the subtleties of a Rugby Union training program, specifically in relation to HIIT weapons.

Controllable and Uncontrollable Factors

Well in advance of most rugby seasons, we have a clear idea about who our opposition will be, when we will play them, where, and at what time. This schedule is locked in concrete and allows us to put our structures in place. However, once we have commenced our season, the balance between gym time, field time, meeting time, recovery time, travel time, home life, and relaxation becomes a moving beast and hence agile and adaptable programming and periodization becomes a necessity. In addition to this, the performance of the individual and the team requires the flexibility to adjust technical and tactical input if, and when, required.

Typically, the best way to ensure we are getting the metabolic, neuromuscular, and mechanical load we require for the team is to allow each individual to adapt and adjust often. If a game for a given player was very physical, with a relatively high number of tackles but relatively low high-intensity running distance meters, then our approach for the following week will immediately adapt from a preplanned program to accommodate the game exposure. Likewise, if we have traveled for 24 hours, the physical load of the subsequent week may change slightly to accommodate for individual differences in responses to the travel stress. Either way, it is important to ensure that each athlete is achieving a sufficient stimulus each week to maintain or improve physical capabilities.

Program Structure and Progression

In Rugby Union, the off-season and preseason typically follow a structured and periodized program mixing physical, technical, and tactical training focuses, as there is no game to taper for nor is there a game to recover from. These phases are very easy to manipulate to target the desired mix of HIIT weapons. Bearing in mind we are preparing for upcoming matches, the need to introduce collisions becomes an important consideration during this phase.

During competition, the training week structure often becomes a reflection of how the team is performing and relates to player energy levels. Usually the training week becomes a balance between the need to recover from the game and to taper for the next game, and this is dramatically impacted by the turnaround time. Sometimes there may be as few as 3 or 4 d between matches and very little ability to complete physical work, so the emphasis must be on technical and tactical aspects. This constraint is not an issue for players involved in the games, but over time, can become an issue for those players not getting sufficient game exposure to enable them to be physically prepared as, and when, required.

To program and select the most appropriate HIIT target type for each player, we first must understand the landscape, that is, what has the player been exposed to from an overall stress perspective (physical, mental, etc.) and what is the next week likely to look like for him or her? It is important to understand the load experienced in skills, drills, and training each day, and each week, to then be able to implement the right weapon, in the right amount, and at the right time! The physiological load of each individual session/day is generally easy to define, as we have planned in advance and we understand what it is we need. If there is a need to get more technical work completed on a specific day, then the ability to include somewhere in the day the appropriate weapon for each person is important. Some players who have high game exposure may simply have a recovery focus, while those players light on game exposure may be required to complete a variety of HIIT weapons on any given day.

Incorporation of HIIT

There are numerous ways to incorporate HIIT sequences into preparation weeks for Rugby Union, whether they occur within a technical or tactical session, at the end of a field-based session, or as a stand-alone session. Similarly, off-feet HIIT sessions before, during, or after strength and power work is common practice. The important consideration is whether individuals or the team require the stimulus and selection of the right weapon to address each player's moving target. This consideration ensures that the delivery of specific HIIT weapons is based on who needs what and when.

Nic Gill

While preparing a rugby team for a pinnacle game in the rugby calendar, we were required to travel 30 h 6 d before the away match. The match was to be played in front of 80,000 people supporting our opposition and we were to play in conditions 7 °C warmer than home and at altitude.

Six months earlier, we were informed of the challenge ahead, so the structures were put in place to allow us to do the impossible. In the 8 wk prior, while playing five other matches, we had planned to ensure our aerobic and anaerobic conditioning was reaching higher levels than previously. This required the prescription during bye weeks to include a range of HIIT weapons (see above) that ensured we had our bases covered. Rugby Union is about strength, power, speed, endurance, skill, and decision-making under pressure, so the need for the weapons to target long periods of play, as well as short intense periods of work, repetitively, with varied recovery times, was crucial to arm us with the arsenal needed to combat the enemy. We needed to ensure the physical stress of playing in the heat, and at altitude, did not inhibit our players' ability to perform their skills, execute their game plan, and make good decisions under pressure.

While the training load in the weeks between games was significant, we needed to ensure that we also dealt with the travel and environmental concerns. We did the work, gained confidence from the work, and dealt with what we were to experience. The need to recover from the matches, while improving our physical fitness over the 8 wk build, was a process of balancing on a knife's edge at times.

While the entire staff and players were put under enormous physical and technical pressure, we survived the battle to come out on top!

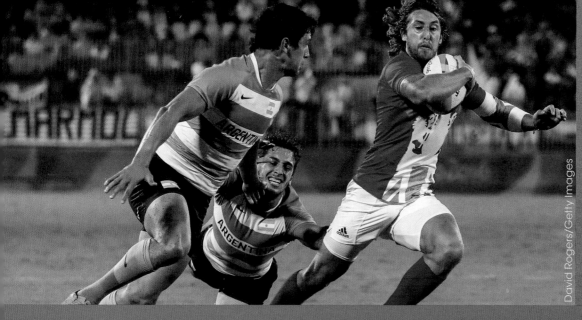

David Rogers/Getty Images

Rugby Sevens

• • • • • •

Nick Poulos

Performance Demands of Rugby Sevens

In this chapter, we introduce the sport of Rugby Sevens, which is unique from Rugby Union (chapter 28), the 15-a-side game, and discuss the various performance factors and relative contribution that physical attributes contribute toward achieving performance and winning games, with particular emphasis on repeated performances over the typical tournament format.

Sport Description and Factors of Winning

Rugby Union Sevens (7s), also known as Rugby Sevens or Sevens Rugby, is a new Olympic sport that debuted at the 2016 Summer Olympic Games in Rio de Janeiro. Rugby 7s is a contact sport and considered a high-intensity variant of the traditional 15-a-side game. In 7s, teams are allowed seven players on the field at any time, with five players available for interchange. Elite international male teams compete across 10 tournaments between December and May each year as part of the Sevens World Series, in addition to major event tournaments (Olympic Games, Commonwealth Games, Rugby Sevens World Cup, each held every 4 yr). Games are typically played over a 2 d tournament, and occasionally over a 3 d tournament. Matches consist of two 7 min halves, plus stoppage times, with a 2 min halftime interval on a full-dimension rugby field (maximum length of playing area = 100 m; maximum width of playing area = 70 m). Pool matches are held on day 1 to determine seedings for day 2, where teams compete for World Series points (20). The tournament usually consists of three group stage matches on the first day, each separated by ~2 to 4 h, and depending on results, up to 3 games on the second day of competition. The World Series is generally scheduled as sets of 2 tournaments in a row, in relative close proximity to one another, with sets separated by 4 to 6 wk, and with tournaments held in different countries, often on opposite sides of the world (20). Rugby 7s player positions are generally categorized into two distinct playing groups: forwards and backs. Recently, however, specific players often classified as hybrid players possess the ability to perform either position. Like Rugby Union (chapter 28), the object of the game is to score a try (5 points) by placing the ball across the opposition goal line and/or kicking the ball over a regulation Rugby Union goal post as a conversion following a try (2 points), penalty (3 points), or in general play (3 points). Basic rules mimic Rugby Union also, where players may use their hands or feet to move the ball, may pass the ball only in line or backward, and may not lose the ball forward while in motion.

Relative Contribution of Physical Performance

As with all team-based sports, especially those that are combative in nature or involve collisions, technical skills, tactical awareness, game knowledge, and experience are the main contributors to successful outcomes. Players with limited ability to pass the ball accurately, tackle, compete at the ruck contest or breakdown, or execute technical ability in a scrum or lineout will never compete at the elite level of Rugby 7s. In addition, circumstantial factors inherent with the game of Rugby 7s can prevent highly trained players the opportunity to exploit their physical qualities. Nevertheless, physical conditioning is extremely important in Rugby 7s to support the technical and tactical performance on the field, especially when under fatigue (figure 29.1). Physical conditioning, done properly, will support technical proficiency on the field. However, specific physical attributes are not always the difference between success and failure in Rugby 7s.

Given the ~45% greater relative game running distance/volume and ~135% greater high-velocity (>5 m/s) running demands than the 15-player rugby game, international level Rugby 7s players are likely to have higher levels of endurance, lower levels of body fat, and higher lean mass profiles than 15-a-side Rugby Union players (15). While it is often proposed that additional body fat may act as a protective buffer in contact situations, excess fat will reduce a player's power-to-weight ratio, lower his ability to accelerate, and increase energy expenditure (12). Elite-level male Rugby 7s players have been reported to possess average skinfolds (sum of 7 sites) of 54.5 ± 11.6 mm. At the time of writing, our current squad skinfold average in late preseason is 40.5 ± 5.8 mm.

Elite-level Rugby 7s players are often selected based on their superior running speed and endurance qualities compared to 15-a-side players. Rugby 7s players have been reported to cover between 113 and 120 m/min, 45% more than Rugby Union players, and with a higher portion of that distance run at high velocity (>6 or 6.7 m/s) (15, 19, 24, 31). These running demands (speed and work:rest ratio) are higher than those previously recorded in Rugby Union (84 m/min with a work:rest ratio of 1.7:1) and rugby league (66 m/min with a work:rest ratio of 1.3:1) (11, 18, 29, 32). While caution is needed when

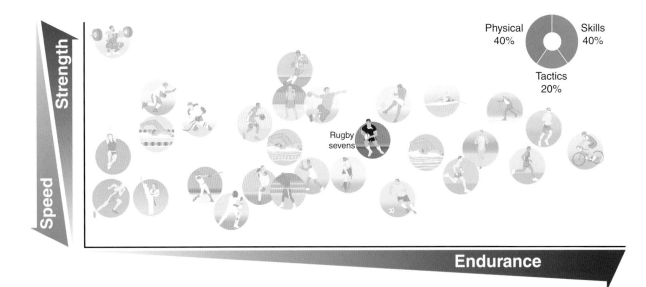

Figure 29.1 The position of the Rugby 7s player on the three axes illustrates the relative importance of the three main physical capacities of importance for elite participation, acknowledging this varies slightly between positions (forwards, backs, hybrids). Outside of critical psychological aspects and team chemistry components, which are difficult to quantify, the pie chart shows the general relative importance of skills (40%), tactical awareness (20%), and physical capacities (40%) for Rugby 7s success.

Adapted from G.A. Nader, "Concurrent Strength and Endurance Training: From Molecules to Man," *Medicine & Science in Sports & Exercise* 38, no. 11 (2006): 1965-1970.

comparing studies across different global positioning system (GPS) technologies (chapter 8), a 2012 study (15) of international players showed relative running intensities of 117 m/min with a work:rest ratio of ~1.8:1, while trained Spanish domestic Rugby 7s players have been reported as running at 107 m/min for backs and 98 m/min for forwards with a work:rest ratio of 1.7:1 (29). In comparing international against domestic matches in male 7s players, while total distance covered is similar, international matches are more intense, as shown by greater distances covered at higher velocities, along with more accelerations and decelerations (15). Higher distances at medium and sprinting speeds are also observed in backs relative to forwards in Rugby 7s (29). While Rugby 7s athletes are traditionally separated into forward and back positions, recently a hybrid profile athlete has emerged due to the specific skills and tactical elements required of the game. Indeed, players able to play a combination of both roles throughout a tournament may be important factors that enable Rugby 7s player success.

When comparing positions, game analysis suggests that Rugby 7s forwards spend 19% more time jogging, with backs spending 8% more time running (21, 23), while some have shown no clear delineation between positions (16, 24). Rugby 7s backs have been reported to cover more total distance and distance at medium (>14 km/h) and high speeds (>20 km/h) than forwards (30). However, forwards are involved in a higher number of scrums, tackles, and time spent at heart rate intensities >90% of maximum (HRmax).

In a World Rugby Sevens Series tournament, it is of note that team starters cover approximately 51% greater total distance and receive approximately 40% more contact efforts over the course of a tournament compared to backs in an 80 min 15-a-side Rugby Union match, despite similar playing durations (24, 28).

Basic anthropometric characteristics of Rugby 7s players have been reported as being substantially different than 15-a-side rugby players. International Rugby 7s backs tend to be ~2 cm shorter and ~6 kg lighter than international 15-a-side backs, with forwards ~1 cm shorter and ~13 kg lighter (16). Forwards are typically slightly larger and stronger than backs, possibly due to set-piece requirements, although the differences are not as significant as in 15-a-side rugby (19). International players have been reported as having greater upper-body strength and lower-body power and perform better during maximal

aerobic testing (effect size, 0.26 to 2.26) compared to provincial players, with mostly trivial-to-small differences between backs and forwards (25, 26). In addition, only trivial-to-small differences in physical match actions have been shown between forwards and backs, with forwards engaging in more contact situations and backs performing more passes, ball handles, and high-speed movements (28).

Rugby 7s players are often required to play a variety of positions during a match or tournament, with the exception of the scrum, performed by the half or hooker (28). Thus, Rugby 7s players as a team can generally be trained for similar match demands, with adjustments for individual player plans made based on individual physical capacities and requirements (28).

Targets of Physical Performance in Rugby 7s

The key targets of physical performance in Rugby 7s, illustrated relative to other sports in figure 29.1, include speed and metabolic conditioning (endurance).

Speed

Measures of speed have shown moderate and large relationships with attack-specific tasks within a match in international and provincial-level Rugby 7s players (26). Large relationships between 40 m sprint time ($r = 0.70$) and number of line breaks and defenders beaten per match suggest that maximal speed is important to possess for elite Rugby 7s success. Similar relationships ($r = 0.87$) have been shown with 10 m sprint times, suggesting that acceleration is also an important component of Rugby 7s players. Previous research (26) in international Rugby 7s players also showed that defensive and contact-specific match activities were related to sprint distance performances (5 m, 10 m, and 40 m), with all sprint distances showing moderate negative relationships with tackle score ($r = -0.32$ to 0.38) and missed tackles ($r = 0.43$ and 0.47, for 10 m and 40 m, respectively). In addition, sprint momentum at 10 m (body weight [kg] multiplied by sprint velocity [m/s]) also appeared to be a greater indicator of performance effectiveness than 10 m sprint time alone in contact situations, as evidenced by the stronger relationships shown between 10 m sprint momentum and effective defensive rucks ($r = 0.36$ versus -0.09, respectively) and dominant tackles (r = 0.31 versus −0.14, respectively) (26). In addition, a strong relationship (r = −0.59) was previously demonstrated between tackle score and repeat sprint (10 × 40 m) performance (26), suggesting the importance of being able to maintain speed under fatigue to consistently tackle effectively.

Metabolic Conditioning

Rugby 7s players at the elite level additionally require well-developed aerobic capacity and power to permit the repeating of these high-velocity actions over the course of a game and a tournament (30). Indeed, the ability to recover from high-intensity activities is especially important in Rugby 7s, as it is with many team sports (17). In addition, the ability to sustain very high-intensity activity over the duration of a match and tournament suggests that factors affecting fatigue and recovery are important considerations for performance (15). By way of illustration, international male Rugby 7s players have been reported to run an average of 1452 ± 243 m per match with an average of 252 ± 103 m accumulated at or above 5 m/s, with a mean peak velocity over 8 m/s (28). International Rugby 7s players have similar speed characteristics to 15-a-side backs across distances of 10 to 30 m. However Rugby 7s players possess superior aerobic endurance (24). As already outlined, Rugby 7s is characterized by relatively high running demands (speed, accelerations, changes of direction) with only short recovery periods between running bouts (15, 31). In addition, contacts encountered elicit greater internal loads (i.e., amplified HR responses) than just running alone (29). At the elite international level, match score line, opposition, and substitute timing have all been shown to influence the activity profile, with Rugby 7s players more likely to run hard against higher-ranked opponents and when the score line is close (20).

Key Weapons, Manipulations, and Surveillance Tools

Recall that weapons refer to the high-intensity interval training (HIIT) formats we can use to target the physiological responses of importance, while the surveillance tools are what we use to monitor the individual responses to those weapons, to tell us whether or not we achieved our target. In this section, the different HIIT weapons, their manipulations, along with ways to monitor their effectiveness (surveillance) in Rugby 7s are offered.

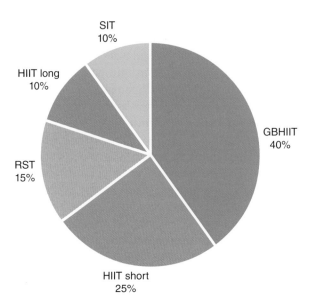

Figure 29.2 Percentage breakdown of the different HIIT formats (weapons) used throughout the annual season in elite international Rugby 7s.

HIIT Weapons

Recall that weapons refer to the HIIT formats we can use to target the physiological responses or target types. In the preparation of our national team, as previously outlined, we target all five HIIT types presented in figure 1.5 (5). For Rugby 7s, the large majority of these are opposed games, or game-based HIIT (GBHIIT), with rule variations or manipulation of attack and defense numbers, essentially variations of small-sided games (SSGs). This HIIT format is sometimes better known as manipulated numbers and/or rules (MNRs), and is completed on a full field or modified field size (40% both pre- and in season). The other weapons we use are short intervals (25%, some preseason but mostly in season), repeated-sprint training (RST) (15%, both pre- and in season), sprint interval training (SIT) (10%, mostly in season, some preseason, and for player rehabilitation or in-season conditioning top-up), and long intervals (10%, mostly preseason, some in season, some during specific stages of player rehabilitation, and some for in season top-up conditioning). The general breakdown of the HIIT formats used across a season for Rugby 7s is shown in figure 29.2.

Manipulations of Interval Training Variables

The running intensity and modality of each HIIT format we use is systematically manipulated to reach desired acute metabolic and locomotor responses on specific days throughout the training week, which may vary between preseason and in-season periods. The unique nature of international World Series Rugby 7s tournaments (i.e., 3 to 4 wk turnaround between back-to-back tournaments) offers a unique programming puzzle we must aim to solve on a weekly basis. Adjustments in training are achieved through programming variations within and between the different days/weeks and cycles between tournaments. For example, if a high-intensity SSG or MNR rugby session is prescribed with speed injections (repeated all-out short sprints) targeting type 4, then a type 1 short-interval segment may be prescribed within or at the end of the training session, often in a straight line with slight 45° turns, as opposed to sharp change-of-direction repetitions to avoid overloading an already taxed neuromuscular system. This is particularly important as vital strength sessions are typically prescribed later in the training day. Alternatively, should a high-intensity SSG or MNR rugby session be prescribed, with no subsequent training session in the afternoon (e.g., a half day off) alongside recovery/rest days following, then a type 5 session may be prescribed within or upon completion of the session (e.g., 3 to 6 × all-out 30 s with 2 to 4 min recovery).

HIIT With Long Intervals (Outdoor)

We generally implement HIIT with long intervals during the off-season or very early preseason, usually on a rugby pitch (grass) or on a track, so as to minimize musculoskeletal strain (HIIT type 1 or 3 targets (6)). These typical HIIT sessions are generally performed over 2 to 3 min at ~85% to 93% of maximal aerobic speed (MAS), calculated from the average velocity attained over a 2 km time trial (1). This represents 490 to 580 m efforts completed over 2 min, depending on a player's fitness, with athletes running 3 to 6 repetitions interspersed by 2 min of passive recovery. For these, players are generally spread across 4 or 5 groups depending on their MAS. Sessions are generally prescribed 1 or 2 times per week, increasing to a frequency of 2 or 3 times prior to official preseason training. Such sessions also tend to be prescribed prior to a rest or recovery day, so that players can recover from an anticipated neuromuscular fatigue (see example in table 29.1). Importantly, this HIIT format is beneficial in that it evokes a large cardiopulmonary system response without reaching very high running speeds (<18 to 19 km/h). This is of primary importance in the context of the

weekly high-speed running load management, especially as a weekly high-speed running dose is prescribed and periodized in the final few weeks of the off-season in preparation for official preseason training. The prescription of such long-interval HIIT sessions lowers the locomotor and musculoskeletal overload, allowing other sessions to target this response with less risk of injury (14). We also use long-interval HIIT with players returning from rehabilitation or transitioning to structured training to ensure controlled straight-line running volumes and intensity. Here, our aim is to increase the chronic training load in a periodized or controlled manner to progressively enable return to play. Often, we may incorporate a ball (e.g., working in pairs or passing a specific set width) to allow players to practice their passing under the altered perception of load, as opposed to just straight-line long-interval running (see figure 29.3).

HIIT With Short Intervals

Our preferred short-interval HIIT weapons in Rugby 7s includes 10 s on/10 s off, 15 s/15 s, 20 s/20 s, and occasionally 10 s/20 s (e.g., figures 29.4 and 29.5), the latter format being low with respect to acute neuromuscular fatigue (figure 5.42 (5)). We often prescribe such HIIT short-interval sessions toward the end of a high-intensity rugby skills or tactical session. These repeated speed injections are used to add volume and intensity of locomotor load (i.e., high-speed running and mechanical work) so that neuromuscular load and anaerobic contribution can be carefully manipulated in consideration of future training sessions. Thus, type 1 short-interval HIIT is often used. In the latter stages of preseason, HIIT short intervals may include 20 s on/20 s off or 30 s on/30 s off (type 3), mostly straight line, with gradual introduction of change of direction or shuttles, again depending on the running and mechanical work that was part of the main rugby session.

Type 1, 2, 3, or 4 targets can all be hit with short intervals for Rugby 7s training. We use a number of these HIIT formats during the preseason within the training session, or at the end of the session, as stand-alone running. While we occasionally use short-interval HIIT formats during the preseason, these intervals are most often used in season for both team-based supplementary running or for players requiring specific individualized locomotor loads. A classic example of their use is in rehabilitating players or transitioning players from rehabilitation into the main high-intensity rugby drills or training sessions.

Table 29.1 $\dot{V}O_2$ and Strength/Speed Development Cycle (General Phase, Earlier Preseason; Typically 3-4 Weeks Duration)

Microcycle		Monday	Tuesday	Wednesday
$\dot{V}O_2$ + strength/ speed development (generic)++	a.m.	Speed qualities	Strength: UB core lifts	Speed qualities
		Rugby: includes type 1 or 2; 7v7, 7v6; 4-8 sets×60 s to 2 min, 1 min rest depending on volume and periodization; gradual increase in COD (monitor) throughout preseason and transition between tournaments	Contact conditioning	Rugby (contact): low-volume running load
		Conditioning: RST type 4 or 5; 3-6×30-40 m with 12-25 s recovery (1-2 sets throughout session) based on loading and careful periodization of VHIR (team and individual); mostly straight line, hamstring load		Conditioning: repeat effort off-ground conditioning with repeat acceleration over 10-20 m (type 4)
		HIR short interval: type 2 (20 s/20 s) and type 3 (30 s/30 s) mostly straight line or gradual introduction of COD/ shuttle into next phase of preseason		
	p.m.	Rugby: craft session or low-intensity/ low running-volume skills	Rest	Speed qualities (acceleration): careful consideration to volume and type of type 4; repeat effort/ acceleration in the morning session and time between morning field session and after-noon session
		Strength: LB or WB core lifts		Strength: LB complexes with acceleration sprints (10-20 m indoor, 3-6 repetitions)

Note that two days are allowed after the lactic session Friday and that the long-bout HIIT is programmed before the day off. Type refers to the physiological target.

COD: change of direction; core lifts LB=squat variations, trap bar variations; core lifts WB=whole-body clean variations, snatch variations, deadlift variations, selected posterior chain exercises; core lifts UB=bench press variations, overhead pressing variations, vertical or horizontal pulling variations; HIR=high-intensity running (>5 m/s); VHIR=very high-intensity running (>6.7 m/s); contact conditioning=rugby-specific contact skills (e.g., wrestling variations); SSC=stretch shortening cycle.

Here, collective GBHIIT may not be either recommended or the players may not be ready to undertake such high-speed running or mechanical work. For rehabilitation players or transitioning players, we may also start with type 1 HIIT before progressing, depending on the type of injury, toward hitting type 2 targets (tailored toward either more high-speed running versus mechanical work), followed by type 3 targets, and finally, type 4.

In practice, we generally divide our players into 4 or 5 groups (19 km, 19.5 km, 20 km, 20.5 km, and >21 km for V_{IFT}) and request they run over group-based distances using cones on the rugby field. For example, for players with a V_{IFT} of 20 km/h, and for a 20 s/20 s HIIT run at 95% of V_{IFT} (relief interval: passive), the goal distance would be $(20/3.6) \times 0.95 \times 20 = 106$ m (20 is divided by 3.6 to convert the speed from km/h to m/s, for convenience) (3). When we plan runs with changes of directions (CODs) to lower the volume of high-speed running and associated mechanical work, the time needed for COD must be considered when setting the goal run distance to ensure a related cardiorespiratory load compared to straight-line runs.

To make HIIT with short intervals more appealing to players and a bit more rugby specific in terms of movement patterns and locomotor loading, the ball is often integrated within the conditioning set in a variety of ways and often with a rugby-specific drill included within the set of the short-interval HIIT. For example, players run following position-specific running patterns for the required duration while reproducing position-specific technical sequences, including passes or defensive patterns or structures

Thursday	Friday	Saturday	Sunday
Rest	Speed qualities	Rugby: low speed clarity	Rest
	Rugby: includes type 1 or 2; 7v7, 7v6; 4-8 sets×60 s to 2 min, 1 min rest depending on volume and periodization; gradual increase in COD (monitor) throughout preseason and transition between tournaments	Strength/cross training: individual specific needs	
	Conditioning: RST type 4 or 5; 3-6×30-40 m with 12-25 s recovery (1-2 sets throughout session) based on loading and careful periodization of VHIR (team and individual); mostly straight line, hamstring load		
	HIR short interval: type 2 (20 s/20 s) and type 3 (30 s/30 s) mostly straight line or gradual introduction of COD/shuttle into next phase of preseason		
	Rugby: craft session or low intensity/low running-volume skills	Rest	
	Strength: WB or LB power or complexes/plyometrics; fast SSC activity (late preseason and lower volume)		

(e.g., figures 29.4 and 29.5). Merging specific offensive or defensive movement patterns into short intervals is also an addition to our HIIT short intervals.

We also often insert an HIIT short-interval block between sets of rugby-specific defense attack drills. For example, 2×2 min periods of a 7 versus 7 attack defense drill may be followed by a 4 to 6 min HIIT short-interval segment of 15 s on/15 s off before another 2×2 min period of 7 versus 7 occurs. Often this is undertaken in straight-line format to avoid increased mechanical work or with a 45° turn to reduce neuromuscular load (type 1), unless sharper turns (90° to 180°) have been prescribed (increased neuromuscular requirements associated with deceleration and acceleration phases, increasing mechanical work, shifting to type 2 or 4 targets). Alternatively, an HIIT short-interval session can be given at the

end of the session for select individuals or the group (mostly type 1 for reasons previously stated) depending on periodized volumes (total volume, high-intensity or very high-intensity running volumes) or to ensure some players have received the appropriate dose after feedback using live GPS throughout the training session (see surveillance section below).

Repeated-Sprint Training

For our RST (type 4 target), we usually implement 1 or 2 sets of 3 to 6×30 to 40 m sprints, with 12 to 25 s of passive or active (jog or ~45% V_{IFT}) recovery (6) during the session, depending on load and periodization of very high-intensity running (VHIR), aiming to achieve >6.7 m/s (team and individual targets). Another variation of RST blocks is often

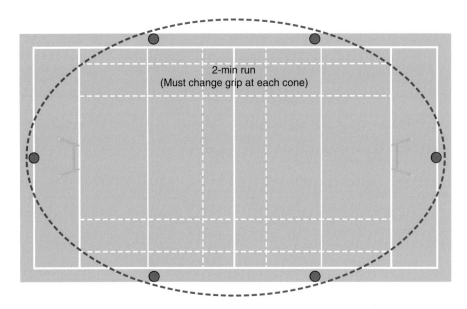

Figure 29.3 Example of a 2 min long-interval HIIT (type 3 target) with 2 min passive rest using the ball. For this session, we perform 2 min of straight-line running with the ball (individual distances based on 85% to 93% MAS from 2 km time trial). After passing each cone, grip is changed as follows: right arm (RA) with ball on chest, left arm (LA) with ball on chest, RA with ball on wrist, LA with ball on wrist, RA with ball in hand, LA with ball in hand. Following 2 min of passive rest, we repeat for 3 to 6 repetitions, depending on a number of variables.

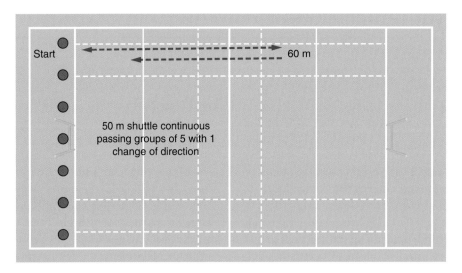

Figure 29.4 For this short-interval HIIT drill, we use a 20 s run over individual distances at 95% of the peak velocity achieved in the 30-15 IFT (see text, V_{IFT}). For a player with a V_{IFT} of 20 km/h, distance covered would be 1×60 m shuttle plus 42 m (102 m) as an example. It should be noted that this short-interval drill is placed within or at the end of a training session. V_{IFT} intensity may need to be adjusted (e.g., reduced to 92%-93%) due to accumulated fatigue in the training session. To begin the drill, players start to spread out across the field (approximately 5-8 m apart), use 20 s rest intervals, and use continuous passing for 50 m, including coach variations of 5 to 15 m passing widths with one shuttle run at ~92% V_{IFT}. This short-interval type 2 HIIT sequence is repeated for 6 to 12 min, depending on planned volumes, periodization, and placement within the training session. Sequence would be (i) Passing shuttle 50 m out and back; (ii) 20 s rest; (iii) 20 s run (1×60 m shuttle plus 42 m back using this example; (iv) 20 s rest; Repeat.

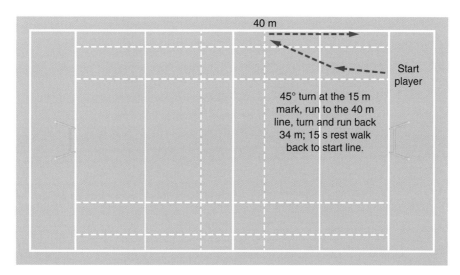

Figure 29.5 This short-interval sequence uses 15 s shuttle runs with 15 s passive (walk to target) recovery. During the 15 s shuttle, we simulate a press to shape the defense (running at ~45°) to the 40 m mark (before turning and running back toward the start). We run these at 92% to 97% V_{IFT} (adjusting individual %V_{IFT} from 95% V_{IFT} for 45° angle and 180° shuttle). For someone running at 93% V_{IFT} (20 km/h), the player starts on the goal line, runs to the 15 m mark before turning ~45° and running until the 40 m marker, before shuttling and running back to about the 34 m mark, to walk or jog for 15 s to the start. The short-interval type 4 HIIT sequence is repeated for 5 to 8 min depending on planned volumes, periodization, and placement in the training session.

implemented as 2 sets of 5 s efforts/15 s active recovery over 4 min (figure 29.6) (5). We run these between the 22 m and halfway line, with a 15 s active recovery jog to the opposite 22 m line) (https://www.youtube.com/watch?v=7aQb9M7ky7k). These speed injections are mostly performed in the straight-line format, which come with the associated high hamstring load to be mindful of. We also implement an RST format of progressive rolling 30 m sprints or flys (10-20 m roll into 30 or 40 m fly) at progressive intensities early in the session following an adequate warm-up with the aim of reaching speeds >9 to 9.3 m/s, typical of speeds attained in a match but undertaken in a controlled manner in a nonfatigued state during the session. This allows an adequate dose of high-speed exposure (as an injury prevention tool) prior to commencing the main very high-intensity rugby drills throughout the forthcoming session.

As mentioned, we often intersperse these RST blocks between two training sequences as follows: warm-up; 5 min of technical work, speed technique, or speed efficiency; 5 to 10 min of another technical session; RST 1, which might include 20 m rolls progressing to 30 m fly sprints (>9 m/s), followed by walk recoveries (60-90 s) before 10 to 20 min of technical sequences; speed injection 1; 10 min of another technical sequence, followed by an HIIT

short interval block of 4 to 6 min (i.e., figure 29.5); finishing with another technical sequence. The programming of RST blocks should be carefully considered and executed with respect to forthcoming sequences or training sessions due to their substantial anaerobic and neuromuscular contributions (see tables 29.2 and 29.3 for more detail).

Sprint Interval Training

We typically use SIT in the form of 3 to 6 × all-out 20 to 30 s efforts with 2 to 4 min of passive recovery (type 5 target) (6, 8). As previously mentioned, SIT weapons are considered applicable when we have a clear afternoon schedule without a strength session planned and usually when a rest or recovery day follows. We may also insert the SIT weapon within a planned rugby-specific session. The SIT weapon is prescribed mostly in the final preparation period in our preseason once an adequate tolerance to high-speed running volume is attained. Given the intensity and duration of the format, it is difficult to intersperse rugby-specific work during these drills. Nevertheless, these can be added to the end of a session. Due to the high anaerobic contribution of SIT, strongly engaging the anaerobic glycolytic pathway alongside a large neuromuscular load and subsequent fatigue (22), its programming logic

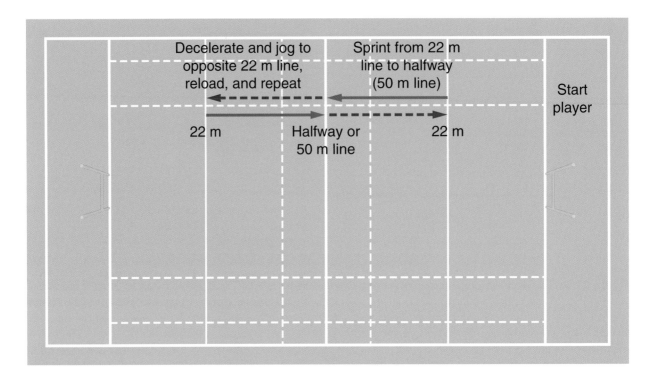

	A grid	B grid	C grid	D grid	E grid
Distance	25 m	28 m (22-m line)	31 m	34 m	37 m
+ 1 (plus 1 stride more than the marker)	A + (26 m)	B + (29 m)	C + (32 m)	D + (35 m)	E + (38 m)
− 1 (minus 1 stride less than the marker)	A − (24 m)	B − (27 m)	C − (30 m)	D − (33 m)	E − (36 m)

Figure 29.6 As adapted from the work of John Pryor, SpeedPowerPlay (https://www.youtube.com /watch?v=7aQb9M7ky7k), this sequence of speed injections, which hits type 4 targets, involves 5 s sprints from the 22 m line to the halfway line, followed by 15 s active jogging to the opposite 22 m line. Players perform 4 to 6 repetitions depending on planned high-intensity running volumes, periodization, and placement within the training session. Note: faster or slower players can be grouped based on the four distance variations shown, which can be used to manipulate the training dose between sessions or even sets according to the situation. The field diagram illustrates a typical B grid.

applied during the sessions and during the week is similar to that described above for RST (see tables 29.2 and 29.3).

Game-Based High-Intensity Interval Training

We tend to plan and design GBHIIT in the form of opposed drills involving a varied number of players, with more or less numbers in attack or defense depending on the tactical purpose of the session or the target type of the drill. Most opposed sessions involve variations of 7 versus 7 or 7 versus 6 (7 attackers versus 6 defenders), in which defenders are required to cover greater distances at consequently a high (>5 m/s) or very high running intensity (>6.7 m/s) in a full-field scenario. Other variations may include 10 versus 7 (10 attackers versus 7 defenders), in which players are required to defend a 100 m width within only 70 m of attacking territory.

While many practitioners in Rugby 7s use a variety of conditioning games or SSGs in their programming, we prefer to use mainly one common drill, termed offside touch, in which physiological and locomotor loading can be adjusted using variations of field dimensions and player number rules (as above). Another specific example of a GBHIIT we use is based on an unstructured random game-based defensive situation in which 4 players must continuously defend against 7 or 8 attackers for 60 or 90 s. For this GBHIIT, defenders are required to plug random defensive holes of the attacking wave, immediately reset within a grid (see table 29.4 for variations in dimensions and associated impact on physical parameters) before another attacking wave is launched from another random side of a grid. The number of times the defenders are able to plug and prevent an attacking wave from scoring within the allocated time is counted as the competition element for the teams/sides.

Figure 29.7 provides a comparison between a typical SSG (offside touch) and tactical drill (7v7) in comparison to typical HIIT sessions and specific game demands. Such a comparison allows us to plan and periodize specific elements of our training over multiple weeks. As shown, the SSG and tactical drill provide lower accelerations and decelerations per minute compared to the tactical 7v7 drill and peak periods during a typical match.

Load Surveillance and Monitoring Tools

With the recent advent of GPS, inertial sensors, and semiautomatic video systems, the use of wearables and tracking technologies is common in Rugby 7s, during both training and matches (10, 24, 30). In our practice, we measure individual daily locomotor load tracking potential changes over time (i.e., acute/chronic ratio (14)). Despite their known limitations (chapter 8), we also tend to monitor HR during most training sessions that include a metabolic component, like HIIT.

Training Status Surveillance and Monitoring Tools

In alignment with the recommendations in chapter 9, the training status monitoring tools that we use in Rugby 7s generally involve simple, noninvasive, and inexpensive measurements, including overall well-being (27), jumps (neuromuscular status (5)), exercise HR (fitness (4) using a submaximal [12 km/h] HR test (9)), and GPS/accelerometer-derived data (including both locomotor loads and mechanical work (7)).

We have more recently used HR responses to HIIT sequences as general relevant markers of training adaptation (the lower, the better the player's fitness when comparing similar individual sequences) (9). We also use the training responses to assist us with decisions regarding an individual player's subsequent top-up HIIT training or cross-training, as required.

Strategies for Structuring the Training Program Using HIIT

Strategies for structuring HIIT programming in Rugby 7s may be confined by various controllable and uncontrollable factors, before proper progression and periodization can be appropriately implemented. This section discusses some of the nuances of training prescription and HIIT structuring in Rugby 7s.

Controllable and Uncontrollable Factors

In our experience, the only truly uncontrollable factors within the planning and design of the Rugby 7s training program are the tournament locations and game schedule timing, which are controlled by World Rugby. In addition, gym-based strength and power training, in addition to high-quality technical sessions (e.g., handling drills, scrum and lineout technical and tactical sessions) together can constrain the timing, volume, and objective (HIIT type) of the HIIT sequences within a given week, as well as between tournaments. The chosen HIIT sessions within or at the end of a high-intensity Rugby 7s training session need careful consideration, with the aim of minimizing any neuromuscular strain post-HIIT and potential interference effects (chapter 6) should the subsequent strength and power session be performed on the same day, as can occur in our program. For example, some HIIT sequences require a large amount of mechanical work (i.e., types 2 and 4) on top of high-intensity rugby sessions, which may include the previously mentioned speed injections. Therefore, any undertaken HIIT training should be prescribed with the aim of minimizing subsequent neuromuscular strain (i.e., type 1), given a strength and power session and possibly a low-volume tactical running or technical session may be completed several hours later in the day. In addition, just as with the sport of elite soccer (chapter 30), the performance of a high-intensity rugby training session that incorporates HIIT can lower a player's attention to detail

Table 29.2 $\dot{V}O_2$ and Strength/Speed Development Cycle (Specific Phase 1, Late Preseason; Typically 4 Weeks During or Occasionally as a Heavier Preparation Week Between Tournaments)

Microcycle		Monday	Tuesday	Wednesday
$\dot{V}O_2$ + strength/ speed development (specific)++	a.m.	Speed qualities	Strength: UB core lifts	Speed qualities
		Rugby: includes type 1 or 2; 7v7, 7v6; 4-8 sets × 60 s to 2 min, 1 min rest depending on volume and peri-odization; gradual increase in COD (monitor) throughout preseason and transition between tournaments	Contact conditioning	Rugby (contact): low-volume running load
		Conditioning: RST type 4 or 5; 3-6 × 30-40 m with 12-25 s recovery (1-2 sets throughout session) based on loading and careful periodization of VHIR (team and individual); mostly straight line, hamstring load		Conditioning: repeat effort off-ground conditioning with repeat acceleration over 10, 20, or 30 m (type 4); consider lactate**
		HIR short interval: straight line (type 1) or COD (type 2) 10 s/10 s or 15 s/15 s/ shuttle depending on focus for strength session in p.m. (avoid mechanical load); mostly straight line as neuromuscular already overloaded in high-intensity game simulated segments during training		
	p.m.	Rugby: craft session or low intensity/ low running-volume skills	Rest	Speed qualities (accelera-tion): careful consideration to volume and type of type 4; repeat effort/accelera-tion in the morning session and time between morning field session and afternoon session
		Strength: LB or WB core lifts		Strength: LB complexes with acceleration sprints (10-20 m indoor, 3-6 repetitions)

Note that two days are allowed after the lactic session Friday and that the long-bout HIIT is programmed before the day off. Type refers to the physiological target.

COD: change of direction; core lifts LB = squat variations, trap bar variations; core lifts WB = whole body clean variations, snatch variations, deadlift variations, selected posterior chain exercises; core lifts UB = bench press variations, overhead pressing variations, vertical or horizontal pulling variations; HIR = high-intensity running (>5 m/s); VHIR = very high-intensity running (>6.7 m/s); contact conditioning = rugby-specific contact skills (e.g., wrestling variations); SSC = stretch shortening cycle.

and technical proficiency in a subsequent afternoon session, while additionally lowering force production, capacity, and rate of force application during a poten-tial afternoon strength and power session (refer to chapter 6). The latter aspect may occur due to the potential impairment of the learning process along-side a lessening of the training stimuli needed for maximal neuromuscular adaptation (2, 13).

During back-to-back tournaments, which often have a 6 d turnaround time where match schedules dictate the training programming, there may be minimal time for HIIT. In contrast, we generally program 1 or 2 HIIT sequences during weeks where a full training week is permitted between tourna-ments (see table 29.5).

Program Structure and Progression

In Rugby 7s, as with most team sports, there is little periodization that occurs during tournament weeks.

Thursday	Friday	Saturday	Sunday
Rest	Speed qualities	Rugby: low speed clarity	Rest
	Rugby: includes type 1 or 2; 7v7, 7v6; 4-8 sets×60 s to 2 min, 1 min rest depending on volume and periodization; gradual increase in COD (monitor) throughout preseason and transition between tournaments	Strength/cross training: individual specific needs	
	Conditioning: RST type 4 or 5; 3-6×30-40 m with 12-25 s recovery (1-2 sets throughout session) based on loading and careful periodization of VHIR (team and individual); mostly straight line, hamstring load		
	(1) Type 5: 3-6×all-out 30 s with 2-4 min recovery (consider mostly when no afternoon strength session), possibly interspersed within rugby session; (2) HIIT short interval: type 1; 10 s/10 s, 15 s/15 s, straight line or selected periodized COD/shuttle depending on strength focus for p.m. session (avoid mechanical load); mostly straight line as neuromuscular already overloaded in high-intensity game simulated segments during training.		
	Rugby: craft session or low intensity/low running-volume skills	Rest	
	Strength: WB or LB power or complexes/plyometrics; fast SSC activity (late preseason and lower volume)		

In season, we aim to keep the weekly training contents consistent in terms of a structured taper into tournament weeks (table 29.6). During tournament weeks, we aim to keep the weekly training load nearly constant, with a slightly lower volume during week 2 throughout the World Series and focus on successive tournament preparation. Simply put, the cycle runs as tournament, recovery, preparation, taper, tournament, and so forth. There is a small emphasis on physical development with increases in training volume and intensity during preparation periods between back-to-back tournaments with careful consideration given to individual player and group monitoring (fitness and fatigue monitoring; e.g., wellness, groin squeeze, neuromuscular, HR) as well as the monitoring of acute and chronic workloads (i.e., acute/chronic ratio (14)).

The format of within- and between-tournament programs (see table 29.5) and program objectives remain similar across the season, with the exception of preparation for stand-alone tournaments such as the Olympic Games or Rugby Sevens World Cup, with a longer and more structured periodization and associated taper.

Table 29.3 $\dot{V}O_2$ and Strength/Speed Development Cycle (Specific Phase 2, Preparation Phase Between Tournaments; Typically 1-2 Weeks Duration)

Microcycle		Monday	Tuesday	Wednesday
$\dot{V}O_2$ + strength/ speed development (specific)++	a.m.	Speed qualities	Strength: UB core lifts	Speed qualities
		Rugby: includes type 1 or 2; 7v7, 7v6; 4-8 sets×60 s to 2 min, 1 min rest depending on volume and periodization; gradual increase in COD (monitor) throughout preseason and transition between tournaments	Contact conditioning	Rugby (contact): low-volume running load
		Conditioning: RST type 4 or 5; 3-6×30-40 m with 12-25 s recovery (1-2 sets throughout session) based on loading and careful periodization of VHIR (team and individual); mostly straight line, hamstring load		Conditioning: repeat effort off-ground conditioning with repeat acceleration over 10, 20, or 30 m (type 4); consider lactate**
		HIR short interval: straight line (type 1) or COD (type 2) 10 s/10 s or 15 s/15 s or shuttle depending on week and periodization		
	p.m.	Rugby: craft session or low intensity/ low running-volume skills	Rest	Speed qualities (acceleration): careful consideration to volume and type of type 4 repeat effort/ acceleration in the morning session and time between morning field session and afternoon session
		Strength: LB core lifts		Strength: LB complexes with acceleration sprints (10-20 m indoor, 3-6 repetitions)

Note that two days are allowed after the lactic session Friday and that the long-bout HIIT is programmed before the day off. Type refers to the physiological target.

COD: change of direction; core lifts LB = squat variations, trap bar variations; core lifts WB = whole body clean variations, snatch variations, deadlift variations, selected posterior chain exercises; core lifts UB = bench press variations, overhead pressing variations, vertical or horizontal pulling variations; HIR = high-intensity running (>5 m/s); VHIR = very high-intensity running (>6.7 m/s); contact conditioning = rugby-specific contact skills (e.g., wrestling variations); SSC = stretch shortening cycle.

Incorporation of HIIT

In the off-season, we often prescribe a heavy loading run-based HIIT program, with the aim of enhancing aerobic capacity and aerobic power prior to the commencement of the preseason. During the preseason, we incorporate HIIT sequences into training sessions either in between technical and tactical sets or repetitions (mostly SSGs or MNRs) or at the end of the session with group or individual modifications made based on fitness and fatigue monitoring or individual load management. The two most important considerations made with respect to selecting the desired types of metabolic and neuromuscular responses to the HIIT sequences during the training week within our program are

1. the demands of the other training components in which HIIT is incorporated, and

2. the individual locomotor loading patterns over the weekly cycle so HIIT can be used to complement or compensate the load arising from training while lessening as much fatigue accumulation as possible to promote subsequent session quality (e.g., afternoon or following day).

It should also be noted that while more optimal within-day programming may exist, our program works within the constraints of coach priorities as well as logistical challenges (e.g., access to fields during visits to foreign countries; see the case study at the end of the chapter), not to mention team and train-

Thursday	Friday	Saturday	Sunday
Rest	Speed qualities	Rugby: low speed clarity	Rest
	Rugby: includes type 1 or 2; 7v7, 7v6; 4-8 sets×60 s to min, 1 min rest depending on volume and periodization; gradual increase in COD (monitor) throughout preseason and transition between tournaments	Strength/cross training: individual specific needs	
	Conditioning: RST type 4 or 5; 3-6×30-40 m with 12-25 s recovery (1-2 sets throughout session) based on loading and careful periodization of VHIR (team and individual); mostly straight line, hamstring load		
	Usually a half day before departing for travel, no afternoon training sessions. Key posterior strength exercises or injury prevention exercises may be undertaken at completion of the main field session.		
	Rugby: craft session or low-intensity/low running-volume skills	Rest	
	Strength: WB or LB power or complexes/plyometrics; fast SSC activity (late preseason and lower volume)		

ing culture. Therefore, the type of additional HIIT sequences within or at the completion of a rugby training session is given careful consideration, alongside awareness that HIIT sequences can be included in the morning prior to an afternoon strength and power session, often twice a week during the preseason, or in preparation weeks between tournaments. In addition, more challenging HIIT sequences are typically prescribed before a day off or before an off-legs training day to allow for more appropriate recovery. Consideration is therefore given to minimize possible interference effects to maximize adaptation (see chapter 6).

In season or during preparation weeks between tournaments, the amount of weekly HIIT prescribed takes into account individual overall playing volume and loading history over the previous few days and weeks. In Rugby 7s, our priority is to ensure all players are sufficiently loaded so as to maintain fitness and be prepared for the required intensity during match play across a tournament, and in particular the high-intensity running and acceleration, deceleration, and change of direction volumes (mechanical work), as well as tapering enough to feel fresh entering a tournament. This requires a highly individualized HIIT prescription that can be achieved using a combination of different HIIT types and formats.

Sample Training Programs

Tables 29.1, 29.2, 29.3, and 29.5 provide examples of HIIT programming during different phases of training, i.e., preseason (tables 29.1 to 29.3) and in season (table 29.5). Note the distribution of the different HIIT types and loading in relation to the microcycle's objectives (table 29.6).

Table 29.4 Example Small-Sided Games (SSGs) or Manipulated Numbers and Rules (MNRs)

Drill	Field size (m)	Number of players	Duration of set (min)	m/min	HIR	VHIR	VHIR%	Average HR (% of max)	Max HR (% of max)	Accelerations/min (>2.5 m/s)	Decelerations/min (<2.5 m/s)
Contested plug defense drill	55×55	6v3	1	191.1	48	11	5.0	88.6	94.5	3.7	2.8
		6v4	1.5	186.7	74	17	5.6	90.0	94.8	2.4	1.7
	60×60	7v4	1.5	204.2	98	26	7.6	91	96	2.1	1.6
SSG offside touch	100×70	6v6	3	196.5	205	29	5.3	175	95.5	0.4	0.4
		7v7	2	182.5	97	19	4.9	174	94.4	0.8	0.2
			2.5	188.6	111	12	2.8	175	92.4	0.4	0.3
			3	187.8	196	25	4.2	169	92.8	0.3	0.3
			3.5	167.9	210	36	6.4	171	92.6	0.8	0.5
	50×70	3v3	2.5	154.9	53	7	2.0	168	93.2	1.4	0.9
			3	157.5	68	1	1.0	164	90.6	2.7	1.4
		4v4	4	155.4	68	3	0.5	N/A	N/A	1.4	0.7
	60×38	4v4	2	185.7	100	15	4.2	174	93.8	0.8	0.4
			2.5	174.9	105	15	3.3	169	94.2	0.8	0.6
	70×30	4v4	2	176.9	137	41	11.4	160	89.8	0.9	1.3
			2.5	150.0	91	30	8.4	168	91.1	0.7	0.8
	70×50	5v5	2	176.5	130	20	5.1	182	96.4	0.8	0.5
			2.5	177.8	102	12	2.8	176	96.3	0.9	0.6

HIR: high-intensity running >5 m/s; VHIR: very high-intensity running >6.7 m/s; VHIR%: % very high-intensity running >6.7 m/s in relation to volume; average HR: average heart rate; N/A: not available

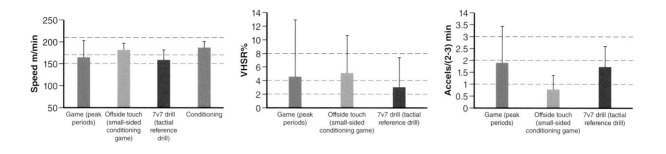

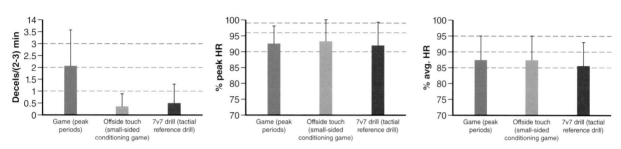

Figure 29.7 Comparison of physiological and performance demands between a typical game, a SSG (offside touch), a tactical drill (7v7), and HIIT conditioning sessions. Offside touch = 2 min duration; 7v7 drill = 2 min duration; game (peak periods) and worst case scenarios calculated from comparison of GPS and time-stamped video files; conditioning = average m/min for conditioning drills undertaken (e.g., 15 s on/15 s off, 20 s/20 s, 30 s/30 s, 45 s/15 s); red line indicates highest values seen with regular frequency in match play. Green lines indicate range of most peak activity occurring. Analysis determined through visual inspection of histograms. VHSR% = percentage high-speed running (>6.7 m/s) in relation to total volume. Accels/min = accelerations per minute (>2.5 m/s). Decels/min = decelerations per minute (<-2.5 m/s). Peak and avg HR = peak and average heart rate reached during the different drills.

Table 29.5 Maintenance (In Season; Tournament Week 1, Typically Follows Long-Haul Travel)

Microcycle (physical emphasis)		Monday	Tuesday	Wednesday	Thursday	Friday	Saturday	Sunday
Competitive (in-season tournament week 1)	a.m.	Travel, arrive	Flush session	Speed qualities	Rest	Game preparation	Tournament	Tournament
		Recovery or flush session	Submaximal HRR test: 3-4×3-4 min submaximal run intervals at increasing intensity; 3-4 strides over 40-50 m (maximum 70% maximum velocity), light skills or game with low running volume, HIR, and VHIR	Rugby: includes type 1 or 2; 7v7, 7v6; 4-8 sets×60 s to 2 min; 1 min rest depending on volume or periodization; gradual increase in COD (monitor) throughout preseason and transition between tournaments		Rugby: low-volume rugby skills with approximately 10 min of lower-intensity tactical sequences		
			Strength: UB core lifts			Strength: UB×30 min priming session		
	p.m.	Recovery + mobility, trigger, or roll session throughout the day depending on travel schedule; continue adjustment to time zone changes and associated strategies to minimize jet lag especially after long-haul travel	Rest	Strength: WB or LB power or complexes or plyometrics; fast SSC activity; some exposure to core LB exercises in week 1		Rest		

Note that two days are allowed after the lactic session Friday and that the long-bout HIIT is programmed before the day off. Type refers to the physiological target.

COD: change of direction; core lifts LB = squat variations, trap bar variations; core lifts WB = whole body clean variations, snatch variations, deadlift variations, selected posterior chain exercises; core lifts UB = bench press variations, overhead pressing variations, vertical or horizontal pulling variations; HIR = high-intensity running (>5 m/s); VHIR = very high-intensity running (>6.7 m/s); contact conditioning = rugby-specific contact skills (e.g., wrestling variations); SSC = stretch shortening cycle; HRR = submaximal heart rate response test that involves 4 min continuous running at 12 km/h with 50 m intervals undertaken every 15 s.

Table 29.6 Example of Typical Periodization Between Tournaments

Week	Periodized load		Total distance (m)	HIR (m)	VHIR (m)
Week 3	Medium to high volume	Mean±SD	19216±1719	3097±1072	512±48
		Range	17563-21345	1663-4491	451-581
Week 2	High volume	Mean±SD	15581±2134	2461±581	746±153
		Range	13681-18714	1594-3090	553-917
Week 1	Medium volume	Mean±SD	13015±576	1788±243	463±59
		Range	12525-14015	1566-2193	386-526
T1	Tournament	Mean±SD	17505±1912	2278±496	578±145
		Range	15139-19536	1588-2802	374-752
T2	Tournament	Mean±SD	15840±3462	1911±583	477±181
		Range	11031-19791	1136-2469	244-671

HIR=>5 m/s; VHIR=>6.7 m/s

The following story describes a series of events that led to a minor hamstring injury and subsequent scenarios leading to the return of a key player to competition only 2 wk later. To provide some background for this story, we begin mid-season following our Las Vegas World Series tournament, where this particular player had been given an individual session to undertake between this tournament and Vancouver (March 12-14, 2016; see story timeline in figure 29.8). We had not been able to obtain GPS data from the Vancouver tournament due to its indoor nature, nevertheless the player was required to undertake an easy progressive running session that included some strides over 50 m to a self-regulated intensity of approximately 80%. This typical flush session involves about 3 to 4 km in total running volume, with about 30 to 50 m of high-intensity running (>6.7 m/s) gained while undertaking a series of strides over 50 m. On this occasion, the player did not complete the individual flush session for reasons unknown to us, further highlighting the challenges of even professional athletes taking responsibility for the undertaking of individual external training themselves.

The following week, upon commencement of our main preparation week for the Hong Kong Sevens, the player produced far more high-intensity running during selected drills in the first session than was planned or as drill predictions had indicated. This meant a significant spike in high-intensity run load following the previous tournament week in Vancouver (which had been completed 8 d earlier). The player also missed the following few days of training with illness. Upon returning 4 d later, the player was required to undertake a supervised extended flush session, including a type 2 targeted short-interval HIIT session involving 10 min of 30 s running at 95% VIFT with 30 s passive recovery over an 80 m shuttle, in order to progress run volume prior to returning to the main squad and performing in a high-intensity rugby session.

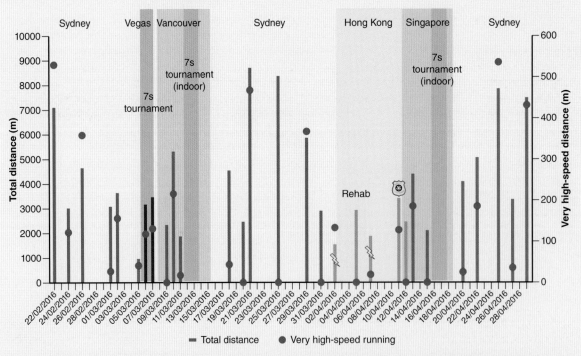

Figure 29.8 Total and very high-speed distance (>6.7 m/s) shown. No GPS data available for both indoor tournaments. Session of injury and reinjury occurrence (slipping during rehab) are shown in yellow. Rehab sessions in green. The session in Hong Kong seeking access to fields to undertake progression of volume and exposure to speed or high-intensity running is shown by the badge.

In the final preparation week prior to departure for Hong Kong, the player completed the normal main Rugby 7s training session earlier in the week, typical of a session in the week prior to a tournament (5-6 km total distance; 350-400 m of high-intensity running [>6.7 m/s]). In our final main training session prior to departure for the Hong Kong Sevens tournament (a marquee tournament on the World Series Sevens circuit), the player experienced a minor hamstring aggravation during his final set of high-speed flys (20 m roll to 30 m sprint).

Following clinical testing and assessment, it was decided that although the strain was minor, he would still travel and complete his rehabilitation and return-to-play protocol alongside myself and our head physiotherapist while we were in Hong Kong, in order to give him the best opportunity to play in the following tournament in Singapore (6 d after the completion of the Hong Kong Sevens tournament). As a performance and medical team, we acknowledged that even with the diagnosis of a minor hamstring strain, time wasn't on our side to get our player ready to perform in the Singapore tournament, but collectively decided that his best chance would be to travel with the team. With a carefully planned progression of volume, high-intensity running, and gradual increases in mechanical load over the 2 wk, we felt the player could potentially be ready to play in the Singapore tournament, even if it meant having him available for day 2 of the tournament with controlled game time on day 1 if required.

The day following arrival in Hong Kong, the player completed a normal flush session as described above, which also served as a controlled assessment of hamstring function and pain. Two days later, a planned progression of volume and high-intensity running was interrupted when the player slipped and felt a small degree of pain at the hamstring injury site during a short footwork warm-up progression drill (low mechanical load). As one can imagine, we were extremely concerned. However, the player was reassessed 24 hours later, presented well clinically, and following recalibration of our high-speed running, changes of direction, and mechanical load progressions, the player remained on track and abreast of all technical and tactical requirements for the upcoming tournament. On the Monday prior to the Singapore tournament, with the remainder of the squad undertaking a recovery session in Hong Kong prior to our Singapore flight, the injured player and I were forced to search for a field or open space in Hong Kong to ensure our targeted progression of volume and high-intensity running stayed on track. This was a crucial session to prepare for the main training session for the week on the Wednesday in Singapore (2 d later) prior to the Saturday tournament. We caught a taxi from the hotel to a proposed available and prebooked field that was supposed to be available for us, but when we arrived, we were unable to find the pitch. After unsuccessfully searching for another 20 min, we jumped a fence into a closed private sports club, commenced a basic warm-up and agility progression and into our pre-scribed HIIT program, set up at the far end of the field away from the clubhouse and entrance in case we were disturbed. As expected, a staff member at the sports club approached me, at which time I told the player to continue the HIIT set (another 4 min) while I pleaded ignorance to the staff member and kept him occupied. While we were kindly asked to leave the premises, it was not until the player completed a good portion of his prescribed HIIT set. However, with some volume, reactive agility, footwork, strides, and further progression of VHIR still required, we embarked on another venture to source field space to complete the remainder of the planned session. Fortunately, we were able to find another enclosed sports stadium, and given our time restraints, made the decision to jump yet another fence to complete the remainder of the training session. Our player immediately commenced the remainder of the session himself, knowing that I would continue to provide interference and distraction for incoming security guards and groundskeepers. Following a second encounter, the session was completed and we quickly hailed a taxi back to the hotel before flying out to Singapore. The player was subsequently able to complete the main training session of the

(continued)

week 2 days later with the team and performed well during the Singapore Sevens World Series tournament.

I was extremely relieved that the player could compete at the tournament after I and our performance and medical team encouraged the travel decision. However, I was disappointed in myself for not minimizing player risk during his rehabilitation progressions. I had set the warm-up and reactive agility station in an area of the ground that presented as a wet and uneven surface, and missed seeing the player perform this part of the session in runners and not boots. The experience not only reminded me of the importance of paying attention to detail required when undertaking a crucial rehabilitation session with time restraints, but also the importance of monitoring progressions of training load and VHIR at any time in the program. Each day and each session becomes more and more critical as a tournament or major competition looms.

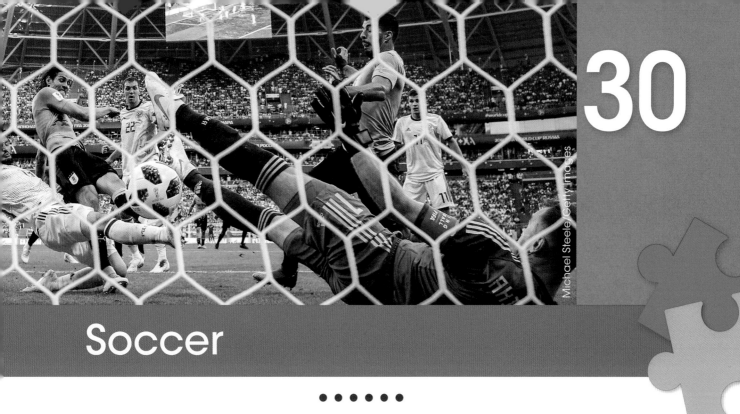

30

Soccer

● ● ● ● ● ●

Martin Buchheit, Mathieu Lacome, and Ben Simpson

Performance Demands of Soccer

In this chapter, we introduce the sport of soccer (called football in most of the world outside of the United States) and discuss the various factors of importance for outfield players and the relative contribution that physical performance makes to winning games.

Sport Description and Factors of Winning

Association football, more commonly known as football or soccer, and nicknamed "the beautiful game," is a team sport played between two teams of 11 players with a spherical ball. It is considered the world's most popular sport and is played by more than 250 million players in 200 countries and dependencies globally. The game is played on a 105 × 70 m outdoor (grass) pitch with a goal at each end. Player positions are typically classified as strikers (forward), midfielders (midfield), defenders (back toward the goal), and the goalkeeper. The object of the game is to score by directing the ball into the opposing goal. Players are not allowed to touch the ball with their hands or arms while the ball is in play, unless they are goalkeepers (and then only when within their penalty area). Other players mainly use their feet to strike or pass the ball, but may also use other areas of their legs, head, and torso. The team that scores the most goals by the end of the match wins.

Relative Contribution of Physical Performance

While it is important for football players to have well-developed physical and physiological qualities, technical skills, tactical awareness, and game intelligence are without doubt the main contributors of success (figure 30.1). Importantly also, contextual factors inherent in a match often prevent highly trained players from fully utilizing their physical potential during matches. Indeed, between-match high-intensity running varies greatly, irrespective of the game outcome (13). In the case of an early player dismissal, the nine outfield players remaining on the pitch generally increase their individual running demands during the match as necessary to maintain overall team running performance (14). Additionally, elite young central midfielders and strikers have been reported to reach only ~85% to ~94% of their maximal sprinting speed during matches, respectively (31). The current understanding is that elite football players do not necessarily need to be the fittest athletes, but at least fit enough to cope with the demands of the match and execute their tactical roles efficiently.

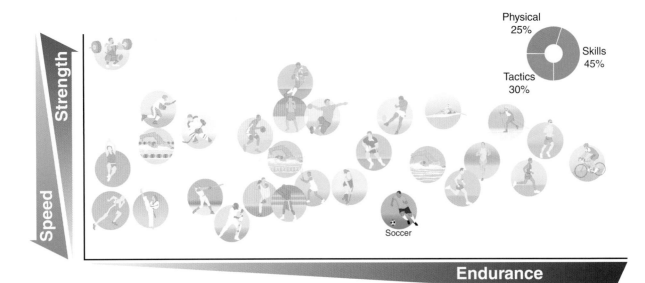

Figure 30.1 The position of the soccer player on the three axes illustrates the relative importance of the three main physical capacities of importance for elite participation in soccer, acknowledging this varies slightly between positions (10, 30). Outside of critical psychological aspects and team chemistry components, which are difficult to quantify, the pie chart shows the general relative importance of skills (45%), tactical awareness (30%), and physical capacities (25%) for soccer success.

Adapted from G.A. Nader, "Concurrent Strength and Endurance Training: From Molecules to Man," *Medicine & Science in Sports & Exercise* 38, no. 11 (2006): 1965-1970.

Targets of Physical Performance in Soccer

Targets of physical performance in soccer depend on the playing position of the individual and can be broken down simply to that of outfield players and goalkeepers. While it may be possible to detail specific targets for each position, the brevity of the present chapter already prevents such elaboration here, and the focus will be on the main two position categories.

Outfield Players

Varying anthropometric characteristics, including a low percentage of body fat, as well as high levels of speed and explosive muscular power, are the most important physical factors needed for outfield players to gain an advantage in soccer that would translate into an improved probability of success at the elite level (36) (figure 30.1). Notwithstanding these critical factors, focused development of aerobic power and endurance should not be ignored. During match play, besides the 10 to 12 km typically covered at the professional level, players will repeat a minimum of 200 high-intensity efforts in the form of high-

speed runs (for a total of 500-1300 m >19.8 km/h), accelerations, decelerations, and changes of direction (2). Thus, a well-developed aerobic system is likely to contribute not only to the acute high-intensity performance but also to metabolic recovery between the explosive efforts associated with successful soccer match performance (38, 39).

Goalkeepers

For the goalkeepers, there is no need to generate excessive neuromuscular fatigue from running, so the better strategy is to remove them from the majority of running-based conditioning exercises and have them do general aerobic conditioning on a stationary cycle, ergometer/rowing machine or, more often, perform goalkeeper-specific training exercises.

Key Weapons, Manipulations, and Surveillance Tools

Recall that weapons refer to the high-intensity interval training (HIIT) formats we can use to target the physiological responses of importance, while the surveillance tools are what we are using to monitor

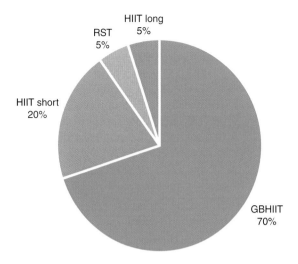

Figure 30.2 Percentage of the different HIIT formats (weapons) used throughout the annual season in elite soccer.

the individual responses to those weapons (figure 1.5). In this section, we present the different HIIT weapons, their manipulations, along with ways to monitor their effectiveness (surveillance).

HIIT Weapons

In our experience, we typically target throughout the season all HIIT target types (see figure 1.5), with the exception of type 5 (type 1: metabolic O_2 system; type 2: metabolic O_2 system + neuromuscular; type 3: metabolic O_2 + anaerobic systems; type 4: metabolic O_2 + anaerobic systems and neuromuscular) (6). As shown in figure 30.2, the very large majority of the weapons used to reach these targets are game-based HIIT, with the majority of them being in the format of small-sided games (SSGs) (70%, both pre- and in-season), followed next by short intervals (20%, both pre- and in-season, essentially for individual top-ups and rehabilitation), repeated-sprint training (RST) (5%, both pre- and in-season, essentially for individual top-ups), and long intervals (5%, preseason exclusively).

Manipulations of Interval Training Variables

The running intensity and modality of each HIIT format is systematically modulated to reach the desired acute metabolic and locomotor responses (i.e., physiological targets, types 1, 2, 3, or 4), which, in turn, solves the programming puzzle on a weekly basis for us.

Factors to consider when choosing an HIIT session type for soccer include match-play demands, player profile, desired long-term adaptations, and training periodization. Together, these factors determine the desired physiological response target type, including type 1 aerobic metabolic, with large demands placed on the oxygen (O_2) transport and utilization systems (cardiopulmonary system and oxidative muscle fibers); type 2 metabolic as per type 1 but with a greater degree of neuromuscular strain; type 3 metabolic as per type 1 with a large anaerobic glycolytic energy contribution but limited neuromuscular strain; type 4 metabolic as with type 3 but with a high neuromuscular strain. The type 5 target, a session with limited aerobic demands but with a large anaerobic glycolytic energy contribution and high neuromuscular strain, is rarely if ever used in our context. The type 6 response (not considered HIIT) refers to typical speed and strength training with a high neuromuscular strain only. Note that for all HIIT types that involve a high neuromuscular strain, possible variations of the strain include more high-speed running (HS, likely associated with a greater strain on hamstring muscles) oriented work or mechanical work (MW, accelerations, decelerations, and changes of direction, likely associated with a greater strain of quadriceps and gluteus muscles).

HIIT With Long Intervals (Outdoor)

Because of their important (but less soccer locomotor-specific) neuromuscular load and anaerobic contribution (type 4), we generally implement HIIT with long intervals exclusively during the preseason over a 300 m loop designed around the pitch. These typical HIIT exercise bouts are generally performed over 3 to 4 min at 90%-95% $V_{IncTest}$ or 80% V_{IFT} (see chapter 2). This represents 800 to 1000 m efforts completed over 3 min, depending on player fitness, with athletes running 3 to 5 repetitions interspersed by 2 min of passive recovery. Players are generally spread across 4 groups (16 km/h, 17 km/h, 18 km/h, and >18 km/h for $V_{incTest}$ or 18 km/h, 19 km/h, 20 km/h, and >21 km/h for V_{IFT}) and are requested to reach group-specific cones set across the running loop at appropriate times. These sessions are generally prescribed at the end of the day, so that athletes may benefit from a greater $\dot{V}O_2$ slow component, i.e., higher $\dot{V}O_2$ for a similar or lower running speed due to muscle fatigue and loss in metabolic efficiency (6)), which may help in limiting overall musculoskeletal strain and fatigue. Importantly, this HIIT format also has an advantage in that it stresses the cardiopulmonary system at high rates without the need for reaching high running speeds (<18-19 km/h). This is of primary importance for the weekly high-speed running load management, since it leaves room for the other sessions to target this locomotor component with less risk of locomotor or musculoskeletal overload (20).

HIIT With Short Intervals

Our preferred HIIT short-interval weapons include 10 s on/10 s off, 15 s/15 s, 20 s/20 s, and more often 10 s/20 s (figures 30.3 and 30.4) since this latter format has been shown to be low with respect to acute neuromuscular fatigue (figure 5.41 (6)). We implement these HIIT formats for the main reason that both the volume and intensity of the locomotor load (i.e., high-speed running and mechanical work), and in turn, the associated neuromuscular load and fatigue and anaerobic contribution, can be tightly manipulated. For example, type 1, 2, 3, or 4 targets can all be hit with short intervals. While we may sometimes use these HIIT formats in the preseason during a few collective team training sessions, HIIT with short intervals is of greater use to us in-season for individual players requiring well-tailored locomotor loads, i.e., rehabilitating players or conditioning substitute players, for which collective game-based training may not be recommended or fulfill their needs completely. In fact, programming HIIT with low levels of neuromuscular load (type 1) may be required during the preseason to assist with preserving the quality of the conjoined soccer sequences (same session) as well as the type 6 strength and speed sessions planned the following day (see chapter 6). Similarly, during rehab, it may be prudent to start with type 1 HIIT before progressing, depending on the type of injury, toward hitting type 2 targets (tailored toward either more high-speed running versus mechanical work, figure 30.3), followed by type 3 targets, and finally, type 4 targets. For substitute players, HIIT with short intervals is generally the only weapon available as a top-up to compensate for the high-speed running load that players miss while not playing, since the large majority of SSGs in which they participate (figure 30.5) fail to over-

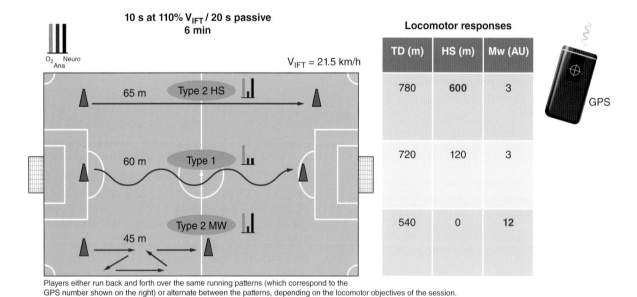

Players either run back and forth over the same running patterns (which correspond to the GPS number shown on the right) or alternate between the patterns, depending on the locomotor objectives of the session.

Figure 30.3 Example of three HIIT sequences with short intervals (10 s run/20 s passive recovery periods) including or not including turns at different angles to modulate the neuromuscular responses (type 1 versus type 2). The associated locomotor responses analyzed by global positioning system (GPS) are provided for each run. Run type (e.g., straight line and zig-zag runs) can be alternated to create hybrid locomotor loads that include both high-speed and mechanical work responses. Note that for longer intervals, the anaerobic participation is greater, for type 3 and 4 targeting. TD: total distance; HS: high-speed running >19.8 km/h; MW: mechanical work (>2 ms^2 accelerations, decelerations, and changes of directions); V_{IFT}: velocity achieved during the 30-15 intermittent fitness test (see chapter 2). Degree of contribution from oxidative (O_2), anaerobic (Ana), and neuromuscular (Neuro) systems is shown by the degree of green, red, and black bars.

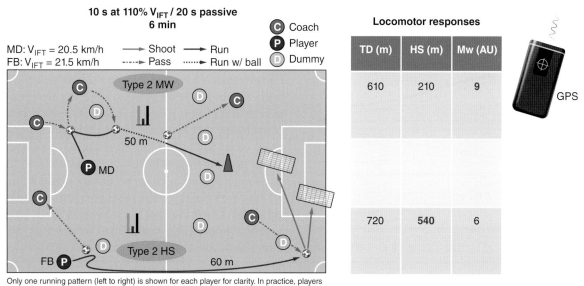

Only one running pattern (left to right) is shown for each player for clarity. In practice, players would have to run over a similar course from right to left and alternate those two runs for the entire HIIT duration.

Figure 30.4 Example of two position-specific (midfielder, MD, and fullback, FB) HIIT with short intervals (10 s/20 s format, type 2) based on V_{IFT}. The associated locomotor responses analyzed by GPS are provided for each run. HS: high-speed running >19.8 km/h. The FB can't progress because of an opponent (dummy), so he passes the ball to a coach playing as a central defender, then runs along the sideline to receive from a second coach another ball close to the box where he shoots into one of two mini-goals (as if he were crossing). The MD comes close to the central defender to receive the ball, then to eliminate a defender, passes and receives to/from a second coach situated on the sideline as an FB, before running forward with the ball where he passes to a third coach and finishes his run toward the box. Note the large differences in terms of high-speed running and mechanical work between the two position-specific efforts, which likely equal their match-specific loading targets (28). TD: total distance; HS: high-speed running >19.8 km/h; MW: mechanical work (>2 ms^2 accelerations, decelerations, and changes of directions); V_{IFT}: velocity achieved during the 30-15 intermittent fitness test (see chapter 2). Degree of contribution from oxidative (O_2), anaerobic (Ana), and neuromuscular (Neuro) systems are shown by the degree of green, red, and black bars (figure 30.3).

load this locomotor component respective to match demands.

In practice, we generally spread the players into 5 groups (17 km/h, 18 km/h, 19 km/h, 20 km/h, and >21 km/h for V_{IFT}) and request they run over group-based distances using cones on the pitch. For example, for players with a V_{IFT} of 19 km/h, and for a 15 s/15 s HIIT run at 95% V_{IFT} (relief interval: passive), the target distance will be $(19/3.6) \times 0.95 \times 15 = 75$ m (19 is divided by 3.6 to convert the speed from km/h to m/s, for convenience) (3). When we plan runs with changes of directions (CODs) to decrease the amount of high-speed running and modulate mechanical work, the time needed for COD must also be considered when setting the target run distance in order to ensure a similar cardiorespiratory load compared to straight-line runs. Therefore, in relation to the estimated energetic cost of COD during HIIT (see chapter 2, V_{IFT} section), if

the players have to run over a 40 m shuttle, for example, they would instead cover 71 m. If the shuttle length is divided in half (i.e., 20 m shuttle), the distance they must cover drops to 65 m (3). (A spreadsheet that completes this calculation for 180° CODs for 15 players at a time is available through the 30-15 IFT App: https://30-15ift.com/.) Finally, to further modulate the locomotor demands and, in turn, the neuromuscular load of these runs, we use turns at different angles that can either decrease or increase braking and acceleration demands. In fact, using research technology that included measures of ground impacts and muscle activity and oxygenation during (repeated) high-intensity runs (8, 21, 22) (https://www.youtube.com/watch?v=KFL8STOyaB0), we showed that while straight-line runs promote stride work (and hamstring loading) via increased high-speed running (HS, type 2 or 4), sharp turns (90°-180°) rather increase thigh work (quads and

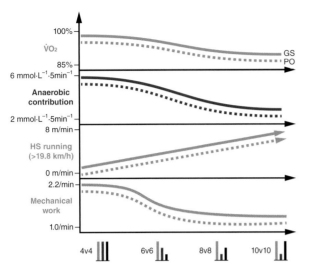

Figure 30.5 Schematic effect of increasing player number (and relative pitch size) on metabolic and locomotor responses to SSGs (personal data) with (game simulation, GS) or without (possession, PO, dotted lines) goalkeepers. Possession tends to systematically be associated with lower locomotor and metabolic responses compared with GS (18). Note that 6v6 to 10v10 may not be considered as HIIT due to their relatively lower metabolic responses. Degree of contribution from oxidative (O_2), anaerobic (Ana), and neuromuscular (Neuro) systems is shown by the degree of green, red, and black bars. $\dot{V}O_2$: oxygen uptake.

glutes) via the increased neuromuscular requirements associated with deceleration and acceleration phases (i.e., increased mechanical work, type 2 or 4). Interestingly, we also showed that 45° turns were likely associated with the lowest neuromuscular load, since neither high-speed nor sharp decelerations and accelerations are involved within this condition (8, 22) (type 1).

To make HIIT with short intervals more appealing to players and a bit more specific in terms of movement patterns and locomotor loading, the ball is often integrated into the activity on different occasions. For example, players run following position-specific running patterns for the required duration while reproducing position-specific technical sequences including passes, receptions, and/or shots on mini-goals at the end of the run (figure 30.3).

Finally, while the optimal loading in terms of HIIT volume and, in turn, high-speed running distance and mechanical work is difficult to define, we often use match demands as targets. For example, we

progressively build up locomotor loads during rehab to reach the match-play distance equivalent of 45, 60, and 90 min or sometimes more. We also use within-player load modeling such as the acute/chronic ratio (20) (and associated predictions) for both rehab and healthy players to define volume targets at different times of the week. For example, considering that a competitive match requires players to cover 600 to 1300 m >19.8 km/h (2), compensation training the day following the match including a 6 min HIIT (in which series duration and volume are based on player's profile and position) may allow substitutes to maintain their weekly high-speed running volume at a stable level, which may limit injury risk before the next match (20).

Repeated-Sprint Training

We implement RST (type 4 target) with the overall team at some very specific moments during the last stages of the preseason, with substitute players in-season, or with rehabilitation players at the end of their return-to-play process. We tend to implement RST formats that involve large amounts of mechanical work rather than straight-line running, so as not to overload high-speed running while still stressing the ability to repeat high-intensity efforts. Our RST blocks are generally implemented as 5 s efforts with 15 to 25 s passive recovery periods over 4 min (2 sets) (6), or less commonly as 6 s efforts with 6 s rest over 1 min (2 to 4 sets), with the same approach as described for HIIT with short intervals (i.e., modulation of mechanical work with varying COD angles, and using position-specific running patterns and technical sequences, figure 30.3).

Game-Based Training

As in many sports, we organize the majority of game-based training in the format of SSGs (24, 34), which we consider to be the main HIIT weapon when it comes to conditioning the overall group of players. Despite the fact that players and the global soccer culture today tend to disregard run-based types of conditioning in the name of training specificity (15), the science-informed coaches we are finally were convinced to embrace and implement this particular HIIT format in light of the near-to-maximal HRs and high blood lactate levels reached during some types of SSGs (24, 34). Additionally, training programs of several weeks using SSGs have also reported improvements in various match winning-related factors including speed, strength, and endurance performance, but also, and probably more importantly, technical proficiency and tactical awareness (17, 23, 26), confirming the potential of this approach as a strong alternative to run-based HIIT. The final argument for the use of SSGs as an HIIT weapon is that they are similar to the different strategies available to modulate exercise intensity during a run-based HIIT, and in turn, metabolic and locomotor responses (5). Physiological and locomotor loading during SSGs can be adjusted using, among others (see chapter 5), manipulations in pitch dimensions, number of players, and rules (24, 34).

In practice, using SSGs based on the expected metabolic, locomotor, and neuromuscular responses (figures 30.5 and 30.6) is appropriate, but can we do even better? If we compare the locomotor responses to match demands, this might help ensure optimal loading (not too much, not too little) and a more manageable work/recovery balance from one day to the next (figure 30.7). One of the challenges of assessing match demands, however, is that the intensity and density of actions is likely time dependent, i.e., the longer the period of play, the lower the average intensity of that period. For this reason, it is difficult to compare the locomotor intensity of different SSG formats of various durations with the demands of a 90 min game. To examine the extent that different SSG formats could be used to either under- or overload the running and/or mechanical demands of competitive matches, we recently used power law modeling (figure 30.7) to compare the peak locomotor intensity of different typical SSGs with those of official matches in terms of running demands and mechanical work over different rolling average durations (28). We found that match simulations (10v10 SSG, 102 × 67 m) were the only games that allowed players to reach similar running intensities compared to official matches (total distance and HS running). However, 4v4 was the only SSG that allowed players to reach a greater mechanical work intensity than during official games (from 50% to 100% more than during matches over 1 to 5 min, respectively) and was strongly associated with much less running above 14.4 km/h (from 30% to 40% less over 1 to 5 min, respectively) (figure 30.7). The other SSG formats (6v6 or 8v8) were not shown to overload mechanical work or high-speed running (28).

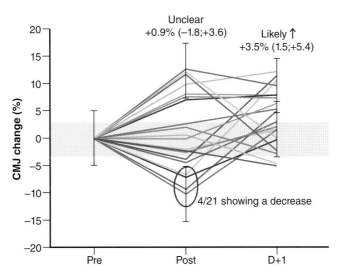

CMJ responses to SSGs : 4v4 PO

Figure 30.6 Changes in countermovement jump (CMJ) immediately (post) and 24 h after a session including 4 × 3 min, 4 versus 4 SSGs (40 m × 16.5 m, possession (PO) without goalkeeper, free touch) in highly trained U14 soccer players from an elite academy (29). Despite the limitation of CMJ height to assess neuromuscular fatigue per se, these data suggest that the level of neuromuscular fatigue associated with such SSGs may be limited. The following day (D+1), all players (including the 4 individuals showing a performance decrement immediately after the session) had at minimum recovered or even showed small to large improvements. The gray zone represents the smallest worthwhile change (SWC, 3%). Error bars representing the error of the measurement (TE, 5%) have been added to the two extreme individual player responses at post. This data revealed that only 4 players out of 21 were affected with likely substantial changes, i.e., greater than TE+SWC.

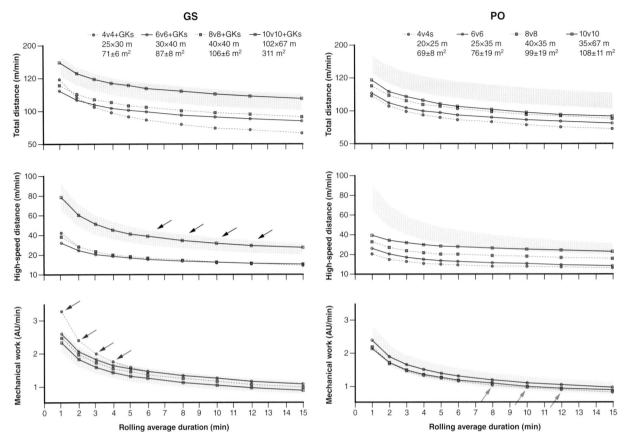

Figure 30.7 Peak locomotor intensity during typical small-sided games (SSGs) including two additional goalkeepers (game simulation, GS) or not (possession game, PO), compared with match demands as a function of each rolling average period in a group of 25 professional soccer players (gray zones stand for match average ± standard deviation) (28). Red arrows highlight how mechanical work can be overloaded compared to match demands using short periods of 4v4 GS. Black arrows highlight how match high-speed running intensity can be replicated using 10v10 GS. Finally, green arrows highlight how match mechanical work can be underloaded or at least matched using various periods of 8v8 PO. High-speed running: >14.4 km/h.

USE OF THE DIFFERENT SSG FORMATS

• Based on these modeling data (figure 30.7) and others (figure 30.5), we often use 4 to 6×3 to 4 min bouts of 4v4 SSGs as our primary HIIT weapons. These SSGs are generally implemented on days when we are targeting strength and high levels of metabolic power (high V̇O₂ and blood lactate values), when most of the training sequences tend to overload the neuromuscular system at high levels, both in terms of intensity (mechanical work per min) and volume (see Program Structure and Progression). Interestingly, despite this intense neuromuscular load (as inferred from the high mechanical work values), CMJ (figure 30.6 (29)), sprint performance (35), and stride kinematic (vertical stiffness (11)) data collected immediately after

such sessions and the following day suggest that these sessions are associated with a limited amount of neuromuscular fatigue. In fact, the neuromuscular responses to 4v4 SSGs are likely individual (some players, but not all, may experience a temporary decrease in performance immediately after the session, figure 30.6) and more importantly for our programming purpose, overall performance tends to fully recover for the majority of players the following day. Note that the metabolic responses to such SSGs are also almost near to maximal (24), which shows us again that during such soccer-specific drills, it is unlikely that we can train physical capacities in complete isolation (resulting in HIIT type 4 targeting). These formats are likely suited to develop maximal aerobic power rather than endurance per se, which explains why this SSG format fits better into locomotor "strength" than endurance-oriented conditioning sessions.

- We use 6v6 and 8v8 SSGs for the so-called "endurance days" (type 1 and 2 targets). Despite the lower running pace compared to matches (figure 30.7), the high but not maximal metabolic responses (high heart rate responses, moderate lactate levels (24)) help to improve a player's ability to maintain high work rates over time (i.e., endurance) when programmed over prolonged durations (e.g., >8 min for 6v6 and >15 min for 8v8). Importantly, these formats allow players to train at the same mechanical work intensity (i.e., game simulation including goalkeepers, GS) or at lower work intensity (i.e., possession game without goalkeepers, PO) than during matches (figure 30.7) resulting in relative recovery compared to a "strength day," while at the same time limiting the volume of high-speed running. With these constrained locomotor demands, large volumes of work can be accumulated without excessive (at least acute) neuromuscular fatigue. This likely allows a more complete recovery from the session of the day(s) before (often a strength day), and may help to promote freshness for the following days and lower overall injury risk.

- For "speed days," we use 10v10 (type 1 and 2) and variations in the forms of possession games over large spaces (especially field length >60 m, systematically greater than field width), often using specific rules (e.g., players need to receive the ball behind the goal line while respecting the offside rule (11)), that leads players to sprint more often and/or over longer distances. Additionally, most of the tactical sequences over at least half of a pitch (building up, crossing, finishing) tend to promote high-speed running, which nicely complements the large SSGs used.

Finally, in addition to variations in player number and pitch area (figure 30.6), there are many simple options available to modulate the intensity of the mechanical work, for example, as shown in figure 30.5, using possession games (without GK) instead of game simulations (with GK) or adding wide players to the sides of the playing area who can serve as relay targets to decrease mechanical work intensity. Similarly, the greater the number of individual touches (or ball contacts) allowed per possession, the lower the metabolic and locomotor demands (16)). While it has received less research interest to date, the shape of the playing area (i.e., length and width for a similar playing area) is an important factor to consider to modulate high-speed running. For example, a longer pitch length favors sprinting distance while allowing deeper runs toward an opponent's scoring area; in contrast, pitches of larger width constrain high-speed running and favor wider (laterally) passing sequences. When it comes to modulating an individual player's responses, which is always challenging within a team training setting without compromising the overall game dynamics and preserving specificity, using individual players as a joker (or floater) is an easy option to substantially decrease a player's locomotor demands (27), but less likely to affect his metabolic responses as inferred from HR (although not without limitations (5)) (figure 30.8).

Longitudinal Training Effects of HIIT

We completed an important study in young elite players in Iran (33), in which we compared the performance effects of a biweekly training supplementation of run-based HIIT with long intervals (3 sets of 3 min 30 s), the difference being the way exercise intensity was prescribed, i.e., 65% to 70% V_{IFT} versus 90% to 95% HR_{max}. Interestingly, the group for which HIIT was prescribed using the %V_{IFT} approach showed an 86% greater weekly improvement than the other group (figure 30.9) (33).

With the large majority of the professional players we have worked with, however, we were unable to implement training interventions that would appropriately isolate the effect of HIIT per se and realize physiological or performance testing to actually monitor the effect of these potential interventions. Therefore, for a better understanding of the possible training effects of the other HIIT formats that we also use routinely, and especially SSGs, the reader is referred to the following publications: (17, 23, 26).

Load Surveillance and Monitoring Tools

Chapters 8 and 9 outline our general approach to load surveillance and individual response monitoring. With the recent developments of global positioning systems, inertial sensors, and semiautomatic video systems, the use of wearables and tracking technologies is very common in soccer, during both training and matches (1, 7). In our practice, we compute individual daily locomotor

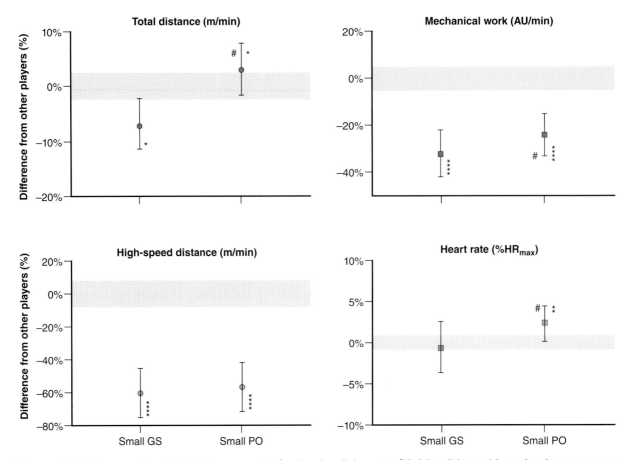

Figure 30.8 Locomotor (with high-speed referring to distance >14.4 km/h) and heart rate responses of joker players (i.e., playing with both teams but not allowed to shoot) compared to the rest of the group during small and large SSGs (with two additional goalkeepers, game simulation, GS, or without goalkeepers, possession game, PO). *: possible difference vs. other players; **: likely difference vs. other players; ***: very likely difference vs. other players; ****: almost certain difference vs. other players; #: between game (GS vs. PO) difference.

Data from M. Lacome, B.M. Simpson, Y. Cholley, and M. Buchheit, "Locomotor and Heart Rate Responses of Floaters During Small-Sided Games in Elite Soccer Players: Effect of Pitch Size and Inclusion of Goalkeepers," *International Journal of Sports Physiology and Performance* 13 no. 5 (2018): 668-671.

load and track potential changes over time (20). Despite their limitations (see chapters 3, 8, and 9), we also generally monitor HR during most training sessions that include a metabolic component (and hence, HIIT) and collect RPE after each session. Perceived training load can then be calculated via the popular session RPE method (25), to be considered alongside the locomotor load.

Training Status Surveillance and Monitoring Tools

The training status monitoring tools that we've used in soccer are generally limited to noninvasive and player-friendly measures and include wellness questionnaires (overall well-being (37)), exercise HR (fitness (4)), and GPS/accelerometer-derived data (including both locomotor loads and mechanical work (7)). More specifically, we use the locomotor (GPS-related), HR, and RPE responses to either standardized SSGs (figure 30.10 (7)), HIIT (12), or submaximal runs (9) (figure 30.11) as markers of readiness to perform or adaptation. More precisely, the greater the activity/min and lower the HR and RPE, the better we consider a player's readiness or fitness level in comparison to the player's historical data. We then often use these individual responses to tailor a player's subsequent training (top-up HIIT training in the case of insufficient fitness or physio interventions when imbalances are detected, figure 30.11).

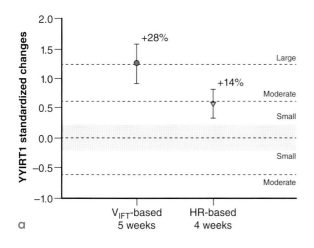

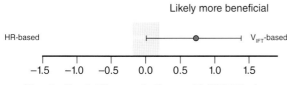

Figure 30.9 Standardized changes following the two high-intensity interval training (HIIT) approaches: (a) within-group changes; (b) difference in weekly improvements. The shaded areas represent trivial changes/differences (0.2×pooled standard deviation). YYIRT1: Yo-Yo intermittent recovery interval level 1.

Reprinted from A. Rabbani and M. Buchheit, "Heart Rate-Based Versus Speed-Based High-Intensity Interval Training in Young Soccer Players." In *International Research in Science and Soccer II*, edited by T. Favero, B. Drust, and B. Dawson (New York: Routledge, 2015).

Strategies for Structuring the Training Program Using HIIT

Strategies for structuring HIIT programming in soccer may be confined by various controllable and uncontrollable factors before proper progression and periodization can be appropriately implemented. This section discusses some of the nuances of training program and HIIT structuring in soccer.

Controllable and Uncontrollable Factors

In our experience, the only truly uncontrollable factors within our training program design are the game schedule timing and match locations, which are controlled by the sport federation and media.

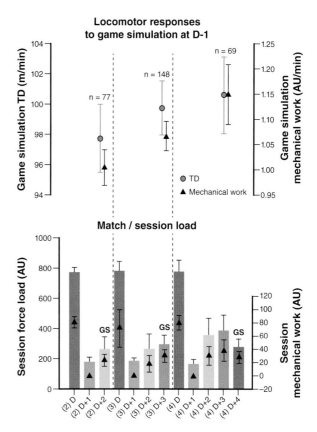

Figure 30.10 Locomotor responses (total distance covered (circles) and mechanical work (triangles) per minute) during game simulation drills (MS) the day before a game (D-1), as a function of the number of days between two consecutive matches in professional soccer players from an elite French team (upper panel). Sessions/match force load (bars) and mechanical work (triangles) as a function of the number of days between two consecutive matches (lower panel). Game simulations: 9 vs. 9 players (2 goalkeepers), 50×55 m, free touches, 2×8 min. Mechanical work is a variable provided by the ADI analyzer (7) as a compound measure of accelerations, decelerations, and changes of direction.

Reprinted by permission from M. Buchheit and B.M. Simpson, "Player-Tracking Technology: Half-Full or Half-Empty Glass?" *International Journal of Sports Physiology and Performance* 12 Suppl 2 (2017): S35-S41.

Next is the constant requirement for high-quality technical sessions often including strength and speed components, which together constrain the timing, volume, and objective (HIIT type) of the HIIT sequences within a given training week. For example, some HIIT sequences require a large amount of mechanical work (i.e., strength sessions, types 2 and 4), while with others, we want these

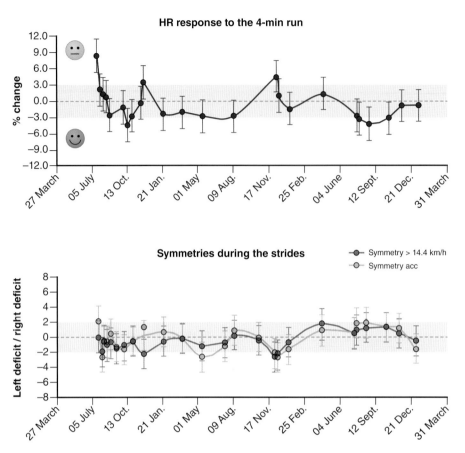

Figure 30.11 Individual report showing both the changes in HR response to a 4 min submaximal run (12 km/h) and the right versus left force load balance during stride runs (4×60 m high-speed runs) (personal data).

components as low as possible to minimize the subsequent level of neuromuscular fatigue (i.e., recovery or endurance sessions, type 1). Finally, with soccer being a skill and tactical sport (figure 30.1), the time allocated to HIIT will never be more than that permitted for team tactics, for example, and high levels of specificity are often expected, which constrains further the HIIT formats available. Therefore, these must be short and with ball integration. This shows that it's not only the physiological objectives of the HIIT sequences that determine its format, but more importantly, the contextual considerations.

Program Structure and Progression

In soccer, as with many team sports, there actually is very little periodization in terms of training cycles, except during the preseason. In-season, we try to keep the weekly training load almost constant throughout the months and focus on the successive

match preparation–match recovery cycles, with a short emphasis on development during the midweek days when possible (15). For these reasons, the skeleton of the weekly program and the program objectives remains similar across the season. The only differences arise from the different macrocycles possible, which depend directly on the number of days of recovery and training between two consecutive matches (generally from 2 to 7).

To program and select the most appropriate HIIT type (and, in turn, format) and solve the puzzle during the training week, we first define the physiological targets of the sequence (5) and then use the anticipated acute metabolic and locomotor and neuromuscular responses to each HIIT weapon to make the decision (figures 30.5 and 30.12). The physiological goal of the session or day is generally easy to define, since we tend to orient as much as possible the training stimuli toward a given physical quality on a given day, i.e., strength and high metabolic power, endurance, and speed days. While we know many roads lead to Rome (chapter 4), the training approach that we have embraced so far follows the main orientations of the tactical periodization training paradigm, in which daily training components are not only structured in relation to technical and tactical objectives but also in line with the physical capacities to be targeted ("Physiological dimensions provide the biological framework where the soccer-specific training/recovery continuum lies" (15)). Focusing on the successive development and maintenance of the main three physical capacities on separate (often consecutive) days likely allows the training stimulus to be maximized when the other qualities recover, which may decrease physiological interferences (19) and, in turn, lead to greater adaptations (6). Practically, we organize all within-session training sequences toward the same quality. For example, a strength-conditioned session would include a strength-oriented warm-up (e.g., light plyometric drills, single-leg horizontal hops), locomotor-based strength work (e.g., accelerations, changes of direction, sled pulling), and game-play sequences, including, irrespective of the actual technical and tactical requirements, high and qualitative neuromuscular demands (e.g., high number of player-to-playing area ratio, maximal intensity of actions with adequate rest periods).

Incorporation of HIIT

We incorporate HIIT sequences into training sessions both at the team and individual levels either between two other technical and tactical sequences (mostly SSGs) or at the end of the session (mostly run-based HIIT). As shown in figure 30.12, the two most important aspects to consider when selecting the desired types of metabolic and neuromuscular responses to the HIIT sequences are (1) the demands of the other sequences of the training (or day) in which HIIT is incorporated and (2) the individual locomotor loading patterns over the actual weekly cycle. By doing so, HIIT can be used to compensate or complement the load arising from training and matches played or missed, while minimizing as much as possible fatigue accumulation to promote the quality of the adjacent sessions.

The optimal within-session (HIIT at the start versus at the end of the session) and within-day (HIIT included in the morning versus afternoon session) programming of the different HIIT sequences is often defined by the overall training dynamics (e.g., coaches and players often reluctant to train skills after run-based HIIT, harder HIIT sequences better programmed before a day off to allow recovery) rather than on a purely scientific

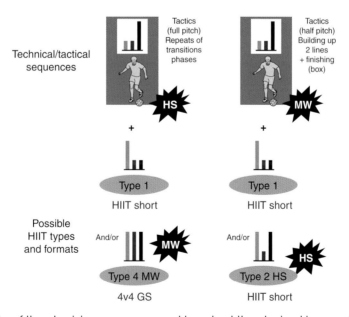

Figure 30.12 Example of the decision process used to select the desired types of metabolic and locomotor (and in turn neuromuscular) responses to HIIT, when this latter aspect is programmed alongside tactical and technical sequences during a given training session. The simple idea is that the added HIIT demands should compensate or complement those of the tactical and technical sequences. HS: high-speed running >19.8 km/h; MW: mechanical work (>2 ms² accelerations, decelerations, and changes of directions).

basis in terms of adaptations, mechanisms, and interferences. For more details about this fascinating topic, the reader is referred to the work of Jackson Fyfe in chapter 6.

In-season, when match schedules dictate the training program, there are likely to be only two weekly scenarios, with 1 (figure 30.14) or 2 (figure 30.15) matches per week, although the actual number of days between the games may be used to fine-tune the programming, especially for substitutes (figure 30.16). The amount of weekly HIIT prescribed is therefore player dependent and takes into account individual overall playing volume and loading history over the past few days and weeks. Our goal is to make sure all players are sufficiently loaded to maintain their fitness and be prepared for possible increases in load during congested periods of matches, while still remaining fresh to compete on a weekly to biweekly basis. This requires a highly individualized HIIT prescription that can be achieved through a combination of different HIIT types and formats (figures 30.14 and 30.15). For example, during a week with 2 games (figure 30.15), while the starters of the first match will only complete recovery (D+1) and light (D+2/D+3) sessions

during the days following their match, substitutes will likely complete a combination of HIIT formats at D+1 (compensation session), targeting both mechanical work (type 4 via SSG, 4v4) and high-speed running (types 2 or 4 via HIIT with short intervals, often with the ball under the form of finishing drills) that may help to maintain a stable weekly locomotor load and balance their overall fitness and freshness (28). The neuromuscular load of these compensation sessions may also play an important role in preserving substitutes' muscle power, as recently highlighted (32). In practice, a D+1 session (with a minimum of 3 d between matches) for substitutes that aims to compensate for a ~60 min match (TD: ~6000 m; HS: ~1200 m, mechanical work (MW): ~50) could include the following (not including warm-up) (28):

1. 8v8 (possession), 2 sets of 10 min (1920 m with 260 m at HS, MW: 11)

2. Type 4 MW HIIT in the form of an SSG: 4v4 (+ 2 GK), 4 sets of 4 min (1660 m, 290 m at HS, MW: 28)

3. Type 4 run-based HIIT (15 s on/15 s off), 1 set of 6 min (1020 m, 850 m at HS, MW: 2)

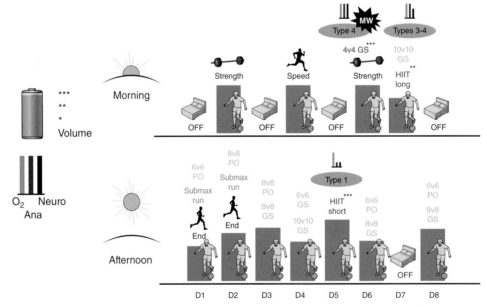

Figure 30.13 Example of preseason programming in an elite team (typically 1-2 wk duration, but there is likely a friendly match during the second week that may replace the HIIT sequence with long intervals). The physical orientation of some of the sessions is given. Those with no indication have only technical and tactical objectives. Red: HIIT; orange: submaximal intensity exercises. The blue bars refer to all technical and tactical training content in forms other than SSGs. The programming principle follows the principle shown in figure 30.12 and is based on the metabolic and locomotor responses summarized in figures 30.5 and 30.7. Run-based HIITs are always performed at the end of the session. MW: mechanical work (>2 ms² accelerations, decelerations, and changes of directions).

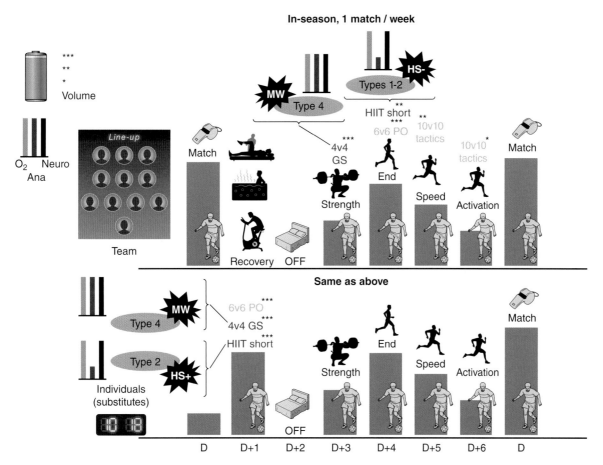

Figure 30.14 Example of in-season programming with one game per week. Red: HIIT; orange: sub-maximal intensity exercises. The blue bars refer to all technical and tactical training content in forms other than SSGs. The programming principle follows the principle shown in figure 30.12 and is based on the metabolic and locomotor responses summarized in figures 30.5 and 30.7. Run-based HIITs are always performed at the end of the session. HS: high-speed running >19.8 km/h, MW: mechanical work (>2 ms^2 accelerations, decelerations, and changes of directions).

resulting in a total of ~60 min training duration, ~4600 m covered with ~1400 m at HS and an MW of 41. Note that the individual tailoring of locomotor loads can be maximized during the latter compensation session when using the variations shown in figure 30.3.

When there are only 2 d between matches, the same substitutes may in contrast perform lower dose, type 1 run-based HIIT, with high running speeds reached via progressive (and safer) type 6 exercise (low metabolic demands) rather than HIIT (figure 30.15).

Sample Training Programs

During the preseason (figure 30.13), we tend to restrict locomotor load and high neuromuscular load during the first few days, using the most applicable SSG formats (6v6 and 8v8, PO) and type 1 HIIT with short intervals. On specific days, however, type 4

HIIT may be programmed, such as 4v4 GS during a strength-oriented session and HIIT with long intervals before 24 h of rest.

In-season, as detailed in Manipulations of Interval Training Variables, we program 4v4 SSG (GS) during strength-oriented sessions, which may be the major HIIT format used with starters. For substitutes, however, these 4v4 GS are often complemented with run-based HIIT including various levels of neuromuscular constraints, depending on the timing of the following match, with greater emphasis on locomotor load with one (figure 30.14, type 2 HS) versus two (figure 30.15, types 1 or 2) games a week. Finally, note also that the overall training volume of work for the substitutes is adjusted based on their playing time the preceding day (i.e., they generally played for 5 to 40 min or didn't play at all, figure 30.16).

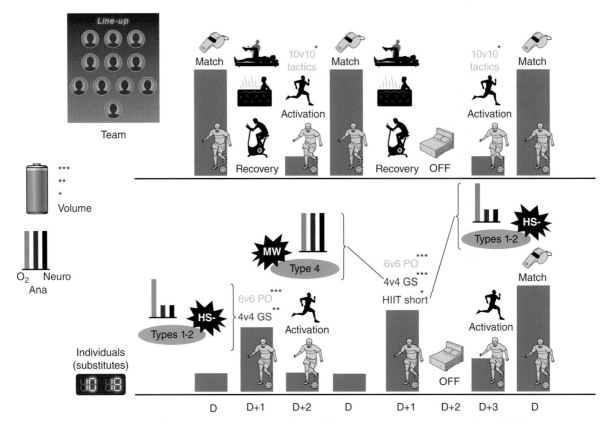

Figure 30.15 Example of in-season programming with two games per week. Red: HIIT; orange: sub-maximal intensity exercises. The blue bars refer to all technical and tactical training contents in forms other than SSGs. The programming principle follows the standard shown in figure 30.12 and is based on the metabolic and locomotor responses summarized in figures 30.5 and 30.7. Run-based HIITs are always performed at the end of the session. MW: mechanical work (>2 ms² accelerations, decelerations, and changes of directions).

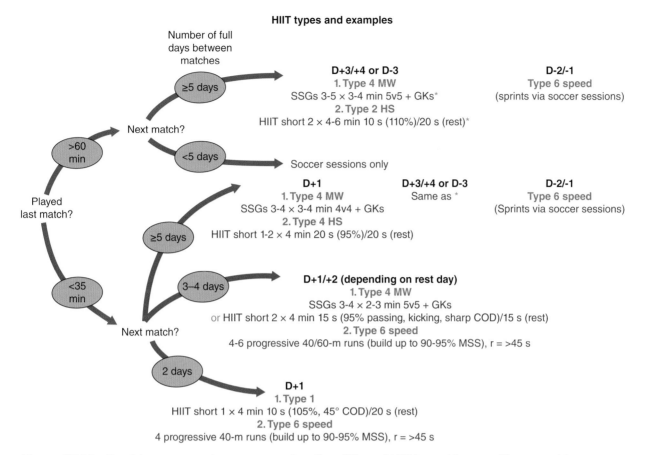

HIIT types and examples

Number of full
days between
matches

≥5 days

Next match?

>60
min

<5 days

Played
last match?

≥5 days

<35
min

3–4 days

Next match?

2 days

D+3/+4 or D-3
1. Type 4 MW
SSGs 3-5 × 3-4 min 5v5 + GKs*
2. Type 2 HS
HIIT short 2 × 4-6 min 10 s (110%)/20 s (rest)*

D-2/-1
Type 6 speed
(sprints via soccer sessions)

Soccer sessions only

D+1
1. Type 4 MW
SSGs 3-4 × 3-4 min 4v4 + GKs
2. Type 4 HS
HIIT short 1-2 × 4 min 20 s (95%)/20 s (rest)

D+3/+4 or D-3
Same as *

D-2/-1
Type 6 speed
(Sprints via soccer sessions)

D+1/+2 (depending on rest day)
1. Type 4 MW
SSGs 3-4 × 2-3 min 5v5 + GKs
or HIIT short 2 × 4 min 15 s (95% passing, kicking, sharp COD)/15 s (rest)
2. Type 6 speed
4-6 progressive 40/60-m runs (build up to 90-95% MSS), r = >45 s

D+1
1. Type 1
HIIT short 1 × 4 min 10 s (105%, 45° COD)/20 s (rest)
2. Type 6 speed
4 progressive 40-m runs (build up to 90-95% MSS), r = >45 s

Figure 30.16 Decision process for programming the different HIIT target types with respect to competition/match participation. SSGs: small-sided games; MW: mechanical work (>2 ms² accelerations, decelerations, and changes of directions); HS: high-speed running (>19.8 km/h).

CASE STUDY

Martin Buchheit

The location and year of occurrence for the following story can't be revealed in the name of confidentiality, but it did occur. The team I was with was back in training after a 5 wk break. It may be the fact that the previous season had been very successful (winning nearly all possible titles), but regardless, the feeling I had, which was shared by the coaching staff, was that the players might have taken it a bit easier than usual during their break. In fact, players had for the most part spent their entire holidays at the beach. With the exception of a few beach soccer matches, they had been very likely sedentary during their (well-deserved) holidays. The HR responses to the 4 min run (see surveillance section) confirmed our fears—many players were greatly out of shape compared to historical data. We had 6 wk to get them fit again for the first official game, but we had never before started from such a low level of fitness. We were rightly concerned.

Because of the integration of new players and slight changes in our coaching approach, we dived straight into high-intensity soccer-specific exercises during the first sessions (small-sided games, finishing work including some high-speed running), which at first glance surprised most of the players, who expected a more gradual increase in soccer-specific and speed loading. At the same time, we needed to fil some conditioning work within the puzzle, and in fact, more than usual in response to the poor fitness levels highlighted at the start of the preseason.

Admittedly, I had never been so happy to be using GPS to monitor soccer-specific content than during these first weeks. Due to the high-intensity demands of the technical sessions (both metabolic and neuromuscular), I realized that we would have to dramatically adapt our usual HIIT programming. Programming the most appropriate HIIT doses and formats is never easy, but needs to be tailored around the technical sessions (and not the other way around, figure 30.12). One of the first adjustments we made was to change our HIIT targets from type 3 and 4 targets, including some important volume at high speed such as HIIT with short intervals (e.g., using 15 s/15 s or 30 s/30 s in a straight line at 90%-100% V_{IFT} as weapons), to type 1 targets (e.g., using 10 s at 90% V_{IFT}/10 s (passive) with 45° angles or 20 s at 85% V_{IFT}/10 s (passive) in a straight line as weapons) to avoid overloading the neuromuscular system, which was already highly taxed during the technical sequences. We also tried to implement as much as possible some submaximal run-based intervals at the end of the training days (i.e., 3 min runs at 90%-95% $V_{incTest}$) to make the most of the increased energetic cost of running when fatigued while decreasing locomotor load. These changes in conditioning formats were initially challenging for everyone, players and coaches included. As we had all seen the benefits from the previous year, no one understood why anything should be changed. Additionally, with longer intervals and little ball integration, the formats we used that year were definitely less appealing for the players. Most players complained, which increased further the pressure on the conditioning staff to explain why suddenly everything had changed. "What for?" they would ask. While we did our best to explain the situation to the players, our reasoning appeared to fall on deaf ears.

Fortunately, a few weeks later, players and staff started to feel more reassured. In fact, the new approach had allowed us to reach the start of the preseason with the large majority of the group remaining injury free, and more importantly, with players getting their fitness back to or above the levels of the previous years (4 min run). We easily won our first official match against one of our direct rivals for the league and left a great impression of both fitness and freshness, as emphasized by the media. Moreover, we learned that despite the natural tendency to go back to what worked previously, the start to every season needs to be challenged. Indeed, a flexible approach and willingness to adapt content to fit the overall context can highly affect the efficacy of a program, rather than the contents per se.

The authors thank Philippe Lambert and Julen Mirena Masach Urrestilla for their valuable contributions to the work presented, and strength and conditioning coach Nicolas Mayer for his helpful collaboration.

References

Chapter 1

1. Gerschler de Fribourg W. "Distance Running." Paper presented at International Running Day conference, March 30, 1958, Karlsruhe, Germany.

2. Åstrand I, Åstrand PO, Christensen EH, Hedman R. Intermittent muscular work. *Acta Physiol Scand*. 1960;48:448-53.

3. Bangsbo J. *Fitness Training in Soccer: A Scientific Approach*. Spring City, PA: Reedswain Publishing; 1994.

4. Billat LV. Interval training for performance: A scientific and empirical practice. Special recommendations for middle- and long-distance running. Part I: Aerobic interval training. *Sports Med*. 2001;31(1):13-31.

5. Billat LV. Interval training for performance: A scientific and empirical practice. Part II: Anaerobic interval training. *Sports Med*. 2001;31(2):75-90.

6. Buchheit M, Laursen PB. High-intensity interval training, solutions to the programming puzzle. Part I: Cardiopulmonary emphasis. *Sports Med*. 2013;43(5):313-38.

7. Buchheit M, Laursen PB. High-intensity interval training, solutions to the programming puzzle. Part II: Anaerobic energy, neuromuscular load and practical applications. *Sports Med*. 2013;43(10):927-54.

8. Buchheit M, Laursen PB, Kuhnle J, Ruch D, Renaud C, Ahmaidi S. Game-based training in young elite handball players. *Int Sports Med*. 2009;30(4):251-8.

9. Castagna C, Belardinelli R, Impellizzeri FM, Abt GA, Coutts AJ, D'Ottavio S. Cardiovascular responses during recreational 5-a-side indoor-soccer. *J Sci Med Sport*. 2007;10(2):89-95.

10. Christensen EH, Hedman R, Saltin B. Intermittent and continuous running. (A further contribution to the physiology of intermittent work.) *Acta Physiol Scand*. 1960;50:269-86.

11. Cipryan L, Tschakert G, Hofman P. Acute and post-exercise physiological responses to high-intensity interval training in endurance and sprint athletes. *J Sports Sci and Med*. 2017;17:219-29.

12. Daniels J. *Jacks Daniels Formula*. Champaign, IL: Human Kinetics; 1998.

13. Ettema JH. Limits of human performance and energy production. *Int Z Angew Physiol*. 1966;22:45-54.

14. Fox EL, Robinson S, Wiegman DL. Metabolic energy sources during continuous and interval running. *J Appl Physiol*. 1969;27(2):174-8.

15. Hill-Haas SV, Dawson B, Impellizzeri FM, Coutts AJ. Physiology of small-sided games training in football: A systematic review. *Sports Med*. 2011;41(3):199-220.

16. Laursen PB. Training for intense exercise performance: High-intensity or high-volume training? *Scandinavian Journal of Medicine & Science in Sports*. 2010;20 Suppl 2:1-10.

17. Laursen PB, Jenkins DG. The scientific basis for high-intensity interval training: Optimising training programmes and maximising performance in highly trained endurance athletes. *Sports Med*. 2002;32(1):53-73.

18. Lydiard A. *Running to the top*. Indianapolis, IN: Cardinal Publishers Group; 2011.

19. MacInnis MJ, Gibala MJ. Physiological adaptations to interval training and the role of exercise intensity. *J Physiol*. 2017;595(9):2915-30.

20. Nader GA. Concurrent strength and endurance training: From molecules to man. *Med Sci Sports Exerc*. 2006;38(11):1965-70.

21. Noakes TD. *The Lore of Running.* Champaign, IL: Leisure Press; 1991.

22. Rampinini E, Impellizzeri FM, Castagna C, Abt G, Chamari K, Sassi A, et al. Factors influencing physiological responses to small-sided soccer games. *J Sports Sci.* 2007;25(6):659-66.

23. Reindell H, Roskamm H. Ein Beitrag zu den physiologischen Grundlagen des Intervall training unter besonderer Berück- sichtigung des Kreilaufes. *Schweiz Z Sportmed.* 1959;7:1-8.

24. Seiler S. What is best practice for training intensity and duration distribution in endurance athletes? *Int J Sports Physiol Perform.* 2010;5(3):276-91.

25. Thompson WR. Worldwide survey of fitness trends for 2018: The CREP Edition. *ACSM's Health & Fitness Journal.* 2017;21(6):10-9.

26. Wilt F. *How They Train: Half Mile to Six Mile.* Los Altos, CA: Track and Field News; 1959.

Chapter 2

1. Bangsbo J, Iaia FM, Krustrup P. The Yo-Yo intermittent recovery test: A useful tool for evaluation of physical performance in intermittent sports. *Sports Med.* 2008;38(1):37-51.

2. Barbero-Alvarez JC, Coutts A, Granda J, Barbero-Alvarez V, Castagna C. The validity and reliability of a global positioning satellite system device to assess speed and repeated sprint ability (RSA) in athletes. *J Sci Med Sport.* 2010;13(2):232-5.

3. Bentley DJ, McNaughton LR. Comparison of W(peak), VO2(peak) and the ventilation threshold from two different incremental exercise tests: Relationship to endurance performance. *J Sci Med Sport.* 2003;6(4):422-35.

4. Berthon P, Fellmann N. General review of maximal aerobic velocity measurement at laboratory. Proposition of a new simplified protocol for maximal aerobic velocity assessment. *J Sports Med Phys Fitness.* 2002;42(3):257-66.

5. Berthon P, Fellmann N, Bedu M, Beaune B, Dabonneville M, Coudert J, et al. A 5-min running field test as a measurement of maximal aerobic velocity. *Eur J Appl Physiol Occup Physiol.* 1997;3(75):233-8.

6. Billat LV. Interval training for performance: A scientific and empirical practice. Special recommendations for middle- and long-distance running. Part II: Anaerobic interval training. *Sports Med.* 2001;31(2):75-90.

7. Billat LV. Interval training for performance: A scientific and empirical practice. Special recommendations for middle- and long-distance running. Part I: Aerobic interval training. *Sports Med* 2001;1(31):13-31.

8. Billat LV, Koralsztein JP. Significance of the velocity at VO2max and time to exhaustion at this velocity. *Sports Med.* 1996;22(2):90-108.

9. Billat V, Renoux JC, Pinoteau J, Petit B, Koralsztein JP. Reproducibility of running time to exhaustion at VO2max in subelite runners. *Med Sci Sports Exerc.* 1994;26(2):254-7.

10. Blondel N, Berthoin S, Billat V, Lensel G. Relationship between run times to exhaustion at 90, 100, 120, and 140% of vVO2max and velocity expressed relatively to critical velocity and maximal velocity. *Int J Sports Med.* 2001;22(1):27-33.

11. Bosquet L, Leger L, Legros P. Methods to determine aerobic endurance. *Sports Med.* 2002;32(11):675-700.

12. Boullosa DA, Tuimil JL, Alegre LM, Iglesias E, Lusquinos F. Concurrent fatigue and potentiation in endurance athletes. *Int J Sports Physiol Perform.* 2011;6(1):82-93.

13. Buchheit M. [The 30-15 Intermittent Fitness Test: A new intermittent running field test for intermittent sport players - Part 1. *Approches du Handball.* 2005;87:27-34.

14. Buchheit M, ed. The 30-15 intermittent fitness test: Reliability and implication for interval training of intermittent sport players. 10th European Congress of Sport Science; July 2005; Belgrade, Serbia.

15. Buchheit M. 30-15 Intermittent Fitness Test and repeated sprint ability. *Science & Sports.* 2008;23(1):26-8.

16. Buchheit M. The 30-15 intermittent fitness test: Accuracy for individualizing interval training of young intermittent sport players. *J Strength Cond Res.* 2008;22(2):365-74.

17. Buchheit M. The 30-15 Intermittent Fitness Test: 10 year review. *Myorobie Journal* 2010; 1(September):http://www.martin-buchheit.net

18. Buchheit M. Individualizing high-intensity interval training in intermittent sport athletes with the 30-15 Intermittent Fitness Test. *NSCA Hot Topic Series wwwnsca-liftorg.* 2011;November.

19. Buchheit M. Monitoring training status with HR measures: Do all roads lead to Rome? *Front Physiol.* 2014;5:73.

20. Buchheit M, Mendez-Villaneuva A. Supramaximal intermittent running performance in relation to age and locomotor profile in highly-trained young soccer players. *J Sports Sci.* 2013;31(13):1402-11.

21. Buchheit M, Laursen PB. High-intensity interval training, solutions to the programming puzzle: Part I: Cardiopulmonary emphasis. *Sports Med.* 2013;43(5):313-38.

22. Buchheit M, Mendez-Villanueva A. Reliability and stability of anthropometric and performance measures in highly-trained young soccer players: Effect of age and maturation. *J Sports Sci.* 2013;31(12):1332-43.

23. Buchheit M, Mendez-Villanueva A. Changes in repeated-sprint performance in relation to change in locomotor profile in highly-trained young soccer players. *J Sports Sci.* 2014;32(13):1309-17.

24. Buchheit M, Hader K, Mendez-Villanueva A. Tolerance to high-intensity intermittent running exercise: Do oxygen uptake kinetics really matter? *Front Physiol.* 2012;3:406.

25. Buchheit M, Mendez-Villanueva A, Simpson BM, Bourdon PC. Match running performance and fitness in youth soccer. *Int J Sports Med.* 2010;31(11):818-25.

26. Buchheit M, Abbiss CR, Peiffer JJ, Laursen PB. Performance and physiological responses during a sprint interval training session: Relationships with muscle oxygenation and pulmonary oxygen uptake kinetics. *European Journal of Applied Physiology.* 2012;112(2):767-79.

27. Buchheit M, Simpson BM, Peltola E, Mendez-Villanueva A. Assessing maximal sprinting speed in highly-trained young soccer players. *Int J Sports Physiol Perform.* 2012;7(1):76-8.

28. Buchheit M, Laursen PB, Millet GP, Pactat F, Ahmaidi S. Predicting intermittent running performance: critical velocity versus endurance index. *Int J Sports Med.* 2007;29(4):307-15.

29. Buchheit M, Haydar B, Hader K, Ufland P, Ahmaidi S. Assessing running economy during field running with changes of direction: Application to 20-m shuttle-runs. *Int J Sports Physiol Perform.* 2011;6(3):380-95.

30. Buchheit M, Morgan W, Wallace J, Bode M, Poulos N. Physiological, psychometric, and performance effects of the Christmas break in Australian football. *Int J Sports Physiol Perform.* 2015;10(1):120-3.

31. Buchheit M, Laursen PB, Kuhnle J, Ruch D, Renaud C, Ahmaidi S. Game-based training in young elite handball players. *Int J Sports Med.* 2009;30(4):251-8.

32. Buchheit M, Al Haddad H, Leprêtre PM, Millet G, Newton M, Ahmaidi S. Cardiorespiratory and cardiac autonomic responses to 30-15 intermittent fitness test. *J Strength Cond Res.* 2009;23(1):93-100.

33. Buchheit M, Lepretre PM, Behaegel AL, Millet GP, Cuvelier G, Ahmaidi S. Cardiorespiratory responses during running and sport-specific exercises in handball players. *J Sci Med Sport.* 2009;12(3):399-405.

34. Buchheit M, Kuitunen S, Voss SC, Williams BK, Mendez-Villanueva A, Bourdon PC. Physiological strain associated with high-intensity hypoxic intervals in highly trained young runners. *J Strength Cond Res.* 2012;26(1):94-105.

35. Bundle MW, Hoyt RW, Weyand PG. High-speed running performance: A new approach to assessment and prediction. *J Appl Physiol.* 2003;95(5):1955-62.

36. Casamichana D, Castellano J, Castagna C. Comparing the physical demands of friendly matches and small-sided games in semiprofessional soccer players. *J Strength Cond Res.* 2012;26(3):837-43.

37. Castagna C, Impellizzeri FM, Chaouachi A, Ben Abdelkrim N, Manzi V. Physiological responses to ball-drills in regional level male basketball players. *J Sports Sci.* 2011;29(12):1329-36.

38. Castagna C, Belardinelli R, Impellizzeri FM, Abt GA, Coutts AJ, D'Ottavio S. Cardiovascular responses during recreational 5-a-side indoor-soccer. *J Sci Med Sport.* 2006.

39. Cataldo A, Cerasola D, Russo G, Zangla D, Traina M. Mean power during 20 sec all-out test to predict 2000 m rowing ergometer performance in national level young rowers. *J Sports Med Phys Fitness.* 2015;55(9):872-7.

40. Cazorla G, ed. Test de terrain pour évaluer la capacité aérobie et la vitesse aérobie maximale. Actes du colloque international de la Guadeloupe; 1990.

41. Celine CG, Monnier-Benoit P, Groslambert A, Tordi N, Perrey S, Rouillon JD. The perceived exertion to regulate a training program in young women. *J Strength Cond Res.* 2011;25(1):220-4.

42. Cerretelli P, Di Prampero PE. Kinetics of respiratory gas exchange and cardiac output at the onset of exercise. *Scand J Respir Dis.* 1971;Suppl(77):35a-g.

43. Cosgrove MJ, Wilson J, Watt D, Grant SF. The relationship between selected physiological variables of rowers and rowing performance as determined by a 2000 m ergometer test. *J Sports Sci.* 1999;17(11):845-52.

44. Coutts AJ, Rampinini E, Marcora SM, Castagna C, Impellizzeri FM. Heart rate and blood lactate correlates of perceived exertion during small-sided soccer games. *J Sci Med Sport.* 2009;12(1):79-84.

45. Dabonneville M, Berthon P, Vaslin P, Fellmann N. The 5 min running field test: Test and retest reliability on trained men and women. *Eur J Appl Physiol.* 2003;88(4-5):353-60.

46. Daniels J. *Jacks Daniels formula.* Champaign (IL): Human Kinetics; 1998.

47. Daniels J, Scardina N, Hayes J, Foley P. Elite and subelite female middle- and long-distance runners. In Landers DM, ed. *Sport and Elite Performers: The 1984 Olympic Scientific Congress Proceedings, Vol 3.* Champaign, IL: Human Kinetics; 1984:57-72.

48. Daussin FN, Ponsot E, Dufour SP, Lonsdorfer-Wolf E, Doutreleau S, Geny B, et al. Improvement of Da-vO2 by cardiac output and oxygen extraction adaptation during intermittent versus continuous endurance training. *Eur J Appl Physiol.* 2007;101(3):377-83.

49. Dellal A, Hill-Haas S, Lago-Penas C, Chamari K. Small-sided games in soccer: Amateur vs. professional players' physiological responses, physical, and technical activities. *J Strength Cond Res.* 2011;25(9):2371-81.

50. Dellal A, Lago-Penas C, Wong del P, Chamari K. Effect of the number of ball contacts within bouts of 4 vs. 4 small-sided soccer games. *Int J Sports Physiol Perform.* 2011;6(3):322-33.

51. Dellal A, Varliette C, Owen A, Chirico EN, Pialoux V. Small-sided games versus interval training in amateur soccer players: Effects on the aerobic capacity and the ability to perform intermittent exercises with changes of direction. *J Strength Cond Res.* 2012;26(10):2712-20.

52. Dellal A, Keller D, Carling C, Chaouachi A, Wong DP, Chamari K. Physiologic effects of directional changes in intermittent exercise in soccer players. *J Strength Cond Res.* 2010;24(12):3219-26.

53. di Prampero PE, Atchou G, Bruckner JC, Moia C. The energetics of endurance running. *Eur J Appl Physiol Occup Physiol.* 1986;55(3):259-66.

54. Di Salvo V, Baron R, Gonzalez-Haro C, Gormasz C, Pigozzi F, Bachl N. Sprinting analysis of elite soccer players during European Champions League and UEFA Cup matches. *J Sports Sci.* 2010;28(14):1489-94.

55. Dishman RK, Patton RW, Smith J, Weinberg R, Jackson A. Using perceived exertion to prescribe and monitor exercise training heart rate. *Int J Sports Med.* 1987;8(3):208-13.

56. Dupont G, Akakpo K, Berthoin S. The effect of in-season, high-intensity interval training in soccer players. *J Strength Cond Res.* 2004;18(3):584-9.

57. Dupont G, Blondel N, Lensel G, Berthoin S. Critical velocity and time spent at a high level of VO2 for short intermittent runs at supramaximal velocities. *Can J Appl Physiol.* 2002;27(2):103-15.

58. Dupont G, Defontaine M, Bosquet L, Blondel N, Moalla W, Berthoin S. Yo-Yo intermittent recovery test versus the Université de Montreal Track Test: Relation with a high-intensity intermittent exercise. *J Sci Med Sport.* 2010;13(1):146-50.

59. Fernandez-Fernandez J, Sanz-Rivas D, Sanchez-Muñoz C, Gonzalez de la Aleja Tellez J, Buchheit M, Mendez-Villanueva A. Physiological responses to on-court vs running interval training in competitive tennis players. *Journal of Sports Science and Medicine* 2011;10:540-5.

60. Gabbett TJ. Skill-based conditioning games as an alternative to traditional conditioning for rugby league players. *J Strength Cond Res.* 2006;20(2):309-15.

61. Gibala MJ, McGee SL. Metabolic adaptations to short-term high-intensity interval training: A little pain for a lot of gain? *Exerc Sport Sci Rev.* 2008;36(2):58-63.

62. Harling SA, Tong RJ, Mickleborough TD. The oxygen uptake response running to exhaustion at peak treadmill speed. *Med Sci Sports Exerc.* 2003;35(4):663-8.

63. Hawley JA, Noakes TD. Peak power output predicts maximal oxygen uptake and performance in trained cyclists. *Eur J Appl Physiol.* 1992;65:79-83.

64. Helgerud J, Hoydal K, Wang E, Karlsen T, Berg P, Bjerkaas M, et al. Aerobic high-intensity intervals improve VO2max more than moderate training. *Med Sci Sports Exerc.* 2007;39(4):665-71.

65. Hill-Haas S, Coutts A, Rowsell G, Dawson B. Variability of acute physiological responses and performance profiles of youth soccer players in small-sided games. *J Sci Med Sport.* 2008;11(5):487-90.

66. Hill-Haas S, Rowsell G, Coutts A, Dawson B. The reproducibility of physiological responses and performance profiles of youth soccer players in small-sided games. *Int J Sports Physiol Perform.* 2008;3(3):393-6.

67. Hill-Haas SV, Coutts AJ, Rowsell GJ, Dawson BT. Generic versus small-sided game training in soccer. *Int J Sports Med.* 2009;30(9):636-42.

68. Hill-Haas SV, Dawson B, Impellizzeri FM, Coutts AJ. Physiology of small-sided games training in football: A systematic review. *Sports Med.* 2011;41(3):199-220.

69. Hill DW, Rowell AL. Running velocity at VO2max. *Med Sci Sports Exerc.* 1996;28(1):114-9.

70. Hill DW, Rowell AL. Significance of time to exhaustion during exercise at the velocity associated with VO2max. *Eur J Appl Physiol Occup Physiol.* 1996;72(4):383-6.

71. Hoff J, Wisloff U, Engen LC, Kemi OJ, Helgerud J. Soccer specific aerobic endurance training. *Br J Sports Med.* 2002;36(3):218-21.

72. Iaia FM, Bangsbo J. Speed endurance training is a powerful stimulus for physiological adaptations and performance improvements of athletes. *Scand J Med Sci Sports.* 2010; 20 Suppl 2:11-23.

73. Impellizzeri FM, Marcora SM, Castagna C, Reilly T, Sassi A, Iaia FM, et al. Physiological and performance effects of generic versus specific aerobic training in soccer players. *Int J Sports Med.* 2006;27(6):483-92.

74. Lacour JR, Padilla-Magunacelaya S, Barthelemy JC, Dormois D. The energetics of middle-distance running. *Eur J Appl Physiol Occup Physiol.* 1990;60(1):38-43.

75. Laursen PB, Shing CM, Jenkins DG. Reproducibility of the cycling time to exhaustion at . VO2peak in highly trained cyclists. *Canadian*

Journal of Applied Physiology (Revue Canadienne de Physiologie Appliquee). 2003;28(4):605-15.

76. Laursen PB, Rhodes EC, Langill RH, McKenzie DC, Taunton JE. Relationship of exercise test variables to cycling performance in an Ironman triathlon. *European Journal of Applied Physiology.* 2002;87:433-40.

77. Laursen PB, Shing CM, Peake JM, Coombes JS, Jenkins DG. Interval training program optimization in highly trained endurance cyclists. *Med Sci Sports Exerc.* 2002;34(11): 1801-7.

78. Laursen PB, Shing CM, Peake JM, Coombes JS, Jenkins DG. Interval training program optimization in highly trained endurance cyclists. *Medicine and Science in Sports and Exercise.* 2002;34(11):1801-7.

79. Leger LA, Boucher R. An indirect continuous running multistage field test: The Université de Montreal track test. *Can J Appl Sport Sci.* 1980;5(2):77-84.

80. Manoel F, Da Silva DF, de Lima J, Machado FA. Peak velocity and its time limit are as good as the velocity associated with VO2max for training prescription in runners. *Sports Medicine International Open.* 2017;1(1):E8–E15.

81. Marcora S. Perception of effort during exercise is independent of afferent feedback from skeletal muscles, heart, and lungs. *J Appl Physiol.* 2009;106(6):2060-2.

82. Marcora SM. Role of feedback from Group III and IV muscle afferents in perception of effort, muscle pain, and discomfort. *J Appl Physiol.* 2011;110(5):1499; author reply 500.

83. Marcora SM, Staiano W, Manning V. Mental fatigue impairs physical performance in humans. *J Appl Physiol.* 2009;106(3):857-64.

84. Mendez-Villanueva A, Bishop D, Hamer P. Reproducibility of a 6-s maximal cycling sprint test. *J Sci Med Sport.* 2007;10(5):323-6.

85. Mendez-Villanueva A, Hamer P, Bishop D. Fatigue in repeated-sprint exercise is related to muscle power factors and reduced neuromuscular activity. *Eur J Appl Physiol.* 2008;103(4):411-9.

86. Mendez-Villanueva A, Buchheit M, Simpson B, Bourdon PC. Match play intensity distribution in youth soccer. *Int J Sports Med.* 2013;34(2):101-10.

87. Mendez-Villanueva A, Buchheit M, Simpson BM, Bourdon PC. Match play intensity distribution in youth soccer. *Int J Sport Med.* 2013;34(2):101-10.

88. Mendez-Villanueva A, Buchheit M, Simpson B, Peltola E, Bourdon P. Does on-field sprinting performance in young soccer players depend on how fast they can run or how fast they do run? *J Strength Cond Res.* 2011;25(9):2634-8.

89. Mendez-Villanueva A, Buchheit M, Kuitunen S, Poon TK, Simpson B, Peltola E. Is the relationship between sprinting and maximal aerobic speeds in young soccer players affected by maturation? *Ped Exerc Sci.* 2010;4(22):497-510.

90. Midgley AW, McNaughton LR, Wilkinson M. Is there an optimal training intensity for enhancing the maximal oxygen uptake of distance runners?: Empirical research findings, current opinions, physiological rationale and practical recommendations. *Sports Med.* 2006;36(2):117-32.

91. Midgley AW, McNaughton LR, Carroll S. Time at VO2max during intermittent treadmill running: Test protocol dependent or methodological artefact? *Int J Sports Med.* 2007;28(11): 934-9.

92. Midgley AW, McNaughton LR, Carroll S. Reproducibility of time at or near VO2max during intermittent treadmill running. *Int J Sports Med.* 2007;28(1): 40-7.

93. Mosey T. High intensity interval training in youth soccer players - using fitness testing results practically. *J Aust Strength Cond.* 2009;17(4):49-51.

94. Noakes TD. Implications of exercise testing for prediction of athletic performance: A contemporary perspective. *Med Sci Sports Exerc.* 1988;20(4):319-30.

95. Noakes TD. Time to move beyond a brainless exercise physiology: The evidence for complex regulation of human exercise performance. *Applied Physiology, Nutrition, and Metabolism (Physiologie Appliquee, Nutrition et Metabolisme).* 2011;36(1):23-35.

96. Nummela AT, Heath KA, Paavolainen LM, Lambert MI, St Clair Gibson A, Rusko HK, et al. Fatigue during a 5-km running time trial. *Int J Sports Med.* 2008;29(9):738-45.

97. Pirie G. *Running Fast and Injury Free.* Dr. John S. Gilbody; 1996.

98. Pugh LG. The influence of wind resistance in running and walking and the mechanical efficiency of work against horizontal or vertical forces. *J Physiol.* 1971;213(2):255-76.

99. Quod MJ, Martin DT, Martin JC, Laursen PB. The power profile predicts road cycling MMP. *International Journal of Sports Medicine.* 2010;31(6):397-401.

100. Rabbini A, Buchheit M. Heart rate-based versus speed-based high-intensity interval training in young soccer players. *International Research in Science and Soccer II.* 2015: 119-30.

101. Rampinini E, Impellizzeri F, Castagna C, Abt G, Chamari K, Sassi A, et al. Factors influencing physiological responses to small-sided soccer games. *J Sports Sci.* 2007;6(25):659-66.

102. Saltin B, Blomqvist G, Mitchell JH, Johnson RL, Jr., Wildenthal K, Chapman CB. Response to exercise after bed rest and after training. *Circulation.* 1968;38(5 Suppl):VII1-78.

103. Sandford GN, Pearson S, Allen SV, Malcata RM, Kilding AE, Ross A, et al. Tactical Behaviours in Men's 800m Olympic and World Championship Medallists: A Changing of the Guard. *Int J Sports Physiol Perform.* 2017:1-13.

104. Saunders PU, Cox AJ, Hopkins WG, Pyne DB. Physiological measures tracking seasonal changes in peak running speed. *Int J Sports Physiol Perform.* 2010;5(2):230-8.

105. Seiler S, Sjursen JE. Effect of work duration on physiological and rating scale of perceived exertion responses during self-paced interval training. *Scand J Med Sci Sports.* 2004;14(5):318-25.

106. Seiler S, Hetlelid KJ. The impact of rest duration on work intensity and RPE during interval training. *Med Sci Sports Exerc.* 2005;37(9):1601-7.

107. Seiler S, Sylta O. How does interval training prescription impact physiological and perceptual responses? *Int J Sports Physiol Perform.* 2017:1-22.

108. Sheppard JM, Borgeaud R. Skill based conditioning: A perspective from elite volleyball. *NSCA Hot Topic Series.* Dec 2009. www.nsca-lift.org.

109. Ufland P, Ahmaidi S, Buchheit M. Repeated-sprint performance, locomotor profile and muscle oxygen uptake recovery. *Int J sport Med.* 2013;34(10):924-30.

110. Ulmer HV. Concept of an extracellular regulation of muscular metabolic rate during heavy exercise in humans by psychophysiological feedback. *Experientia.* 1996;52(5):416-20.

111. Weyand PG, Bundle MW. Energetics of high-speed running: Integrating classical theory and contemporary observations. *Am J Physiol Regul Integr Comp Physiol*. 2005;288(4):R956-65.

112. Weyand PG, Lin JE, Bundle MW. Sprint performance-duration relationships are set by the fractional duration of external force application. *Am J Physiol Regul Integr Comp Physiol*. 2006;290(3):R758-65.

113. Whipp BJ, Higgenbotham MB, Cobb FC. Estimating exercise stroke volume from asymptotic oxygen pulse in humans. *J Appl Physiol*. 1996;81(6):2674-9.

114. Wisloff U, Helgerud J. Methods for evaluating peak oxygen uptake and anaerobic threshold in upper body of cross-country skiers. *Med Sci Sports Exerc*. 1998;30(6):963-70.

Chapter 3

1. Acevedo EO, Goldfarb AH. Increased training intensity effects on plasma lactate, ventilatory threshold, and endurance. *Med Sci Sports Exerc*. 1989;21(5):563-8.

2. Altenburg TM, Degens H, van Mechelen W, Sargeant AJ, de Haan A. Recruitment of single muscle fibers during submaximal cycling exercise. *J Appl Physiol*. 2007;103(5):1752-6.

3. Andersson H, Raastad T, Nilsson J, Paulsen G, Garthe I, Kadi F. Neuromuscular fatigue and recovery in elite female soccer: Effects of active recovery. *Med Sci Sports Exerc*. 2008;40(2):372-80.

4. Astrand PO, Rodhal K. *Textbook of Work Physiology: Physiological Bases of Exercise*. Champaign, IL: Human Kinetics, MacGraw-Hill Series in Health Education, Physical Education, and Recreation; 2003.

5. Baar K. Nutrition and the adaptation to endurance training. *Sports Med*. 2014;44(Suppl 1):S5-12.

6. Bae SY, Hamaoka T, Katsumura T, Shiga T, Ohno H, Haga S. Comparison of muscle oxygen consumption measured by near infrared continuous wave spectroscopy during supra-maximal and intermittent pedalling exercise. *Int J Sports Med*. 2000;21(3):168-74.

7. Bangsbo J. Quantification of anaerobic energy production during intense exercise. *Med Sci Sports Exerc*. 1998;30(1):47-52.

8. Barclay CJ. Mechanical efficiency and fatigue of fast and slow muscles of the mouse. *J Physiol*. 1996;497(Pt 3):781-94.

9. Belardinelli R, Barstow TJ, Porszasz J, Wasserman K. Changes in skeletal muscle oxygenation during incremental exercise measured with near infrared spectroscopy. *Eur J Appl Physiol Occup Physiol*. 1995;70(6):487-92.

10. Beneke R, Leithauser RM, Ochentel O. Blood lactate diagnostics in exercise testing and training. *Int J Sports Physiol Perform*. 2011;6(1):8-24.

11. Bergman BC, Wolfel EE, Butterfield GE, Lopaschuk GD, Casazza GA, Horning MA, et al. Active muscle and whole body lactate kinetics after endurance training in men. *J Appl Physiol*. 1999;87(5):1684-96.

12. Billat LV. Interval training for performance: A scientific and empirical practice. Special recommendations for middle- and long-distance running. Part I: Aerobic interval training. *Sports Med* 2001;1(31):13-31.

13. Billat LV, Koralsztein JP. Significance of the velocity at VO2max and time to exhaustion at this velocity. *Sports Med*. 1996;22(2):90-108.

14. Billat LV, Slawinksi J, Bocquet V, Chassaing P, Demarle A, Koralsztein JP. Very short (15s–15s) interval-training around the critical velocity allows middle-aged runners to maintain VO2 max for 14 minutes. *Int J Sports Med*. 2001;22(3):201-8.

15. Billaut F, Davis JM, Smith KJ, Marino FE, Noakes TD. Cerebral oxygenation decreases but does not impair performance during self-paced, strenuous exercise. *Acta Physiol (Oxf)*. 2010;198(4):477-86

16. Binnie MJ, Peeling P, Pinnington H, Landers G, Dawson B. Effect of training surface on acute physiological responses following interval training. *J Strength Cond Res*. 2013;27(4):1047-56.

17. Binnie MJ, Dawson B, Pinnington H, Landers G, Peeling P. Effect of training surface on acute physiological responses after interval training. *J Strength Cond Res*. 2013;27(4):1047-56.

18. Bishop D, Spencer M. Determinants of repeated-sprint ability in well-trained team-sport athletes and endurance-trained athletes. *J Sports Med Phys Fitness*. 2004;44(1):1-7.

19. Bompa TO, Haff GG. *Periodization*, 5th Edition. Chicago, IL: Human Kinetics; 2009.

20. Bonacci J, Chapman A, Blanch P, Vicenzino B. Neuromuscular adaptations to training, injury and passive interventions: Implications for running economy. *Sports Med.* 2009;39(11):903-21.

21. Bouchard C, Rankinen T. Individual differences in response to regular physical activity. *Med Sci Sports Exerc.* 2001;33:S446-51.

22. Buchheit M. Performance and physiological responses to repeated-sprint and jump sequences. *Eur J Appl Physiol.* 2010;110(5):1007-18.

23. Buchheit M. Performance and physiological responses to repeated-sprint and jump sequences. *Eur J Appl Physiol.* 2010;101(5):1007-18.

24. Buchheit M. Should we be recommending repeated sprints to improve repeated-sprint performance? *Sports Med.* 2012;42(2):169-72; author reply 72-3.

25. Buchheit M, Ufland P. Effect of endurance training on performance and muscle reoxygenation rate during repeated-sprint running. *Eur J Appl Physiol.* 2011;111(2):293-301.

26. Buchheit M, Laursen PB. High-intensity interval training, solutions to the programming puzzle: Part I: Cardiopulmonary emphasis. *Sports Med.* 2013;43(5):313-38.

27. Buchheit M, Laursen PB. High-intensity interval training, solutions to the programming puzzle: Part I: Cardiopulmonary emphasis. *Sports Med.* 2013;43(5):313-38.

28. Buchheit M, Laursen PB. High-intensity interval training, solutions to the programming puzzle. Part II: Anaerobic energy, neuromuscular load and practical applications. *Sports Med.* 2013;43(10):927-54.

29. Buchheit M, Spencer M, Ahmaidi S. Reliability, usefulness, and validity of a repeated sprint and jump ability test. *Int J Sports Physiol Perform.* 2010;5(1):3-17.

30. Buchheit M, Abbiss CR, Peiffer JJ, Laursen PB. Performance and physiological responses during a sprint interval training session: Relationships with muscle oxygenation and pulmonary oxygen uptake kinetics. *Eur J Appl Physiol.* 2012;112(2):767-79.

31. Buchheit M, Mendez-Villanueva A, Quod MJ, Quesnel T, Ahmaidi S. Improving acceleration and repeated sprint ability in well-trained adolescent handball players: Speed vs. sprint interval training. *Int J Sports Physiol Perform.* 2010;5(2):152-64.

32. Buchheit M, Al Haddad H, Mendez-Villanueva A, Quod MJ, Bourdon PC. Effect of maturation on hemodynamic and autonomic control recovery following maximal running exercise in highly trained young soccer players. *Front Physiol.* 2011;2:69.

33. Buchheit M, Cormie P, Abbiss CR, Ahmaidi S, Nosaka KK, Laursen PB. Muscle deoxygenation during repeated sprint running: Effect of active vs. passive recovery. *Int J Sports Med.* 2009;30(6):418-25.

34. Buchheit M, Kuitunen S, Voss SC, Williams BK, Mendez-Villanueva A, Bourdon PC. Physiological strain associated with high-intensity hypoxic intervals in highly trained young runners. *J Strength Cond Res.* 2012;26(1):94-105.

35. Burgomaster KA, Hughes SC, Heigenhauser GJ, Bradwell SN, Gibala MJ. Six sessions of sprint interval training increases muscle oxidative potential and cycle endurance capacity in humans. *J Appl Physiol.* 2005;98(6):1985-90.

36. Burnley M. Found in translation: The dependence of oxygen uptake kinetics on O2 delivery and O2 utilization. *J Appl Physiol.* 2008;105(5):1387-8.

37. Cettolo V, Ferrari M, Biasini V, Quaresima V. Vastus lateralis O2 desaturation in response to fast and short maximal contraction. *Med Sci Sports Exerc.* 2007;39(11):1949-59.

38. Charloux A, Lonsdorfer-Wolf E, Richard R, Lampert E, Oswald-Mammosser M, Mettauer B, et al. A new impedance cardiograph device for the non-invasive evaluation of cardiac output at rest and during exercise: Comparison with the "direct" Fick method. *Eur J Appl Physiol.* 2000;82(4):313-20.

39. Christmass MA, Dawson B, Arthur PG. Effect of work and recovery duration on skeletal muscle oxygenation and fuel use during sustained intermittent exercise. *Eur J Appl Physiol Occup Physiol.* 1999;80(5):436-47.

40. Christmass MA, Dawson B, Passeretto P, Arthur PG. A comparison of skeletal muscle oxygenation and fuel use in sustained continuous and intermittent exercise. *Eur J Appl Physiol.* 1999;80(5):423-35.

41. Cooper Gt. Basic determinants of myocardial hypertrophy: A review of molecular mechanisms. *Annu Rev Med.* 1997;48:13-23.

42. Cotter JD, Thornton SN, Lee JK, Laursen PB. Are we being drowned in hydration advice? Thirsty for more? *Extrem Physiol Med.* 2014;3:18.

43. Coyle EF. Physical activity as a metabolic stressor. *Am J Clin Nutr.* 2000;72(2 Suppl):512S–20S.

44. Coyle EF, Trinity JD. The stroke volume response during or throughout 4-8 min of constant-power exercise that elicits VO2max. *J Appl Physiol.* 2008;104(1):282-3; author reply 4-5.

45. Cumming GR. Stroke volume during recovery from supine bicycle exercise. *J Appl Physiol.* 1972;32(5):575-8.

46. Daussin FN, Ponsot E, Dufour SP, Lonsdorfer-Wolf E, Doutreleau S, Geny B, et al. Improvement of Da-vO2 by cardiac output and oxygen extraction adaptation during intermittent versus continuous endurance training. *Eur J Appl Physiol.* 2007;101(3):377-83.

47. Daussin FN, Zoll J, Dufour SP, Ponsot E, Lonsdorfer-Wolf E, Doutreleau S, et al. Effect of interval versus continuous training on cardiorespiratory and mitochondrial functions: Relationship to aerobic performance improvements in sedentary subjects. *Am J Physiol Regul Integr Comp Physiol.* 2008;295(1):R264-72.

48. Daussin FN, Zoll J, Ponsot E, Dufour SP, Doutreleau S, Lonsdorfer E, et al. Training at high exercise intensity promotes qualitative adaptations of mitochondrial function in human skeletal muscle. *J Appl Physiol.* 2008;104(5):1436-41.

49. Dempsey JA, Wagner PD. Exercise-induced arterial hypoxemia. *J Appl Physiol.* 1999;87(6):1997-2006.

50. Di Michele R, Del Curto L, Merni F. Mechanical and metabolic responses during a high-intensity circuit training workout in competitive runners. *J Sports Med Phys Fitness.* 2012;52(1):33-9.

51. Dupont G, Berthoin S. Time spent at a high percentage of VO2max for short intermittent runs: Active versus passive recovery. *Can J Appl Physiol.* 2004;29(Suppl):S3–S16.

52. Dupont G, Moalla W, Guinhouya C, Ahmaidi S, Berthoin S. Passive versus active recovery during high-intensity intermittent exercises. *Med Sci Sports Exerc.* 2004;36(2):302-8.

53. Ekblom J, Hermansen L. Cardiac output in athletes. *J Appl Physiol.* 1968;25:619-25.

54. Enoka RM. *Neuromechanics of Human Movement, 4th ed.* Champaign, IL: Human Kinetics; 2008.

55. Essen B, Hagenfeldt L, Kaijser L. Utilization of blood-borne and intramuscular substrates during continuous and intermittent exercise in man. *J Physiol.* 1977;265(2):489-506.

56. Faisal A, Beavers KR, Robertson AD, Hughson RL. Prior moderate and heavy exercise accelerate oxygen uptake and cardiac output kinetics in endurance athletes. *J Appl Physiol.* 2009;106(5):1553-63.

57. Fernandez-del-Olmo M, Rodriguez FA, Marquez G, Iglesias X, Marina M, Benitez A, et al. Isometric knee extensor fatigue following a Wingate test: Peripheral and central mechanisms. *Scand J Med Sci Sports.* 2013;23(1):57-65.

58. Fontana P, Betschon K, Boutellier U, Toigo M. Cardiac output but not stroke volume is similar in a Wingate and VO2peak test in young men. *Eur J Appl Physiol.* 2011;111(1):155-8.

59. Fox EL, Mathews DK. *Interval Training: Conditioning for Sports and General Fitness.* Orlando, FL: Saunders College Publishing; 1974.

60. Fyfe JJ, Bishop DJ, Stepto NK. Interference between concurrent resistance and endurance exercise: Molecular bases and the role of individual training variables. *Sports Med.* 2014;44(6):743-62.

61. Fyfe JJ, Bishop DJ, Zacharewicz E, Russell AP, Stepto NK. Concurrent exercise incorporating high-intensity interval or continuous training modulates mTORC1 signaling and microRNA expression in human skeletal muscle. *Am J Physiol Regul Integr Comp Physiol.* 2016;310(11):R1297-311.

62. Gajer B, Hanon C, Lehenaff D, Vollmer JC. Analyse comparée de différentes séances de développement de $\dot{V}O_2$max. *Expertise et sport de haut niveau: actes des Entretiens de l'INSEP, Novembre 2002.* Paris: Institut National du Sport et de l'éducation physique; 2002.

63. Garrandes F, Colson SS, Pensini M, Seynnes O, Legros P. Neuromuscular fatigue profile in endurance-trained and power-trained athletes. *Med Sci Sports Exerc.* 2007;39(1):149-58.

64. Gastin PB. Energy system interaction and relative contribution during maximal exercise. *Sports Med.* 2001;31(10):725-41.

65. Gathercole R, Sporer B, Stellingwerff T. Counter-movement jump performance with increased training loads in elite female rugby athletes. *Int J Sports Med*. 2015;36(9):722-8.

66. Girard O, Mendez-Villanueva A, Bishop D. Repeated-sprint ability - Part I: Factors contributing to fatigue. *Sports Med*. 2011;41(8):673-94.

67. Girard O, Micallef JP, Millet GP. Changes in spring-mass model characteristics during repeated running sprints. *Eur J Appl Physiol*. 2011;111(1):125-34.

68. Gollnick PD, Piehl K, Saltin B. Selective glycogen depletion pattern in human muscle fibres after exercise of varying intensity and at varying pedalling rates. *J Physiol*. 1974;241(1):45-57.

69. Gonzalez-Alonso J. Point: Stroke volume does/does not decline during exercise at maximal effort in healthy individuals. *J Appl Physiol*. 2008;104(1):275-6; discussion 9-80.

70. Gonzalez-Alonso J, Calbet JA. Reductions in systemic and skeletal muscle blood flow and oxygen delivery limit maximal aerobic capacity in humans. *Circulation*. 2003;107(6):824-30.

71. Gorostiaga EM, Asiain X, Izquierdo M, Postigo A, Aguado R, Alonso JM, et al. Vertical jump performance and blood ammonia and lactate levels during typical training sessions in elite 400-m runners. *J Strength Cond Res*. 2010;24(4):1138-49.

72. Grassi B. Skeletal muscle VO2 on-kinetics: Set by O2 delivery or by O2 utilization? New insights into an old issue. *Med Sci Sports Exerc*. 2000;32(1):108-16.

73. Green H, Tupling R, Roy B, O'Toole D, Burnett M, Grant S. Adaptations in skeletal muscle exercise metabolism to a sustained session of heavy intermittent exercise. *Am J Physiol Endocrinol Metab*. 2000;278(1):E118-26.

74. Hamaoka T, McCully KK, Quaresima V, Yamamoto K, Chance B. Near-infrared spectroscopy/imaging for monitoring muscle oxygenation and oxidative metabolism in healthy and diseased humans. *J Biomed Opt*. 2007;12(6):062105.

75. Hamaoka T, Iwane H, Shimomitsu T, Katsumura T, Murase N, Nishio S, et al. Noninvasive measures of oxidative metabolism on working human muscles by near-infrared spectroscopy. *J Appl Physiol*. 1996;81(3):1410-7.

76. Harmer AR, McKenna MJ, Sutton JR, Snow RJ, Ruell PA, Booth J, et al. Skeletal muscle metabolic and ionic adaptations during intense exercise following sprint training in humans. *J Appl Physiol*. 2000;89(5):1793-803.

77. Heck H, Mader A, Hess G, Mucke S, Muller R, Hollmann W. Justification of the 4-mmol/l lactate threshold. *Int J Sports Med*. 1985;6(3):117-30.

78. Helgerud J, Engen LC, Wisloff U, Hoff J. Aerobic endurance training improves soccer performance. *Med Sci Sports Exerc*. 2001;33(11):1925-31.

79. Helgerud J, Hoydal K, Wang E, Karlsen T, Berg P, Bjerkaas M, et al. Aerobic high-intensity intervals improve VO2max more than moderate training. *Med Sci Sports Exerc*. 2007;39(4):665-71.

80. Henriksson J, Reitman JS. Time course of changes in human skeletal muscle succinate dehydrogenase and cytochrome oxidase activities and maximal oxygen uptake with physical activity and inactivity. *Acta Physiol Scand*. 1977;99(1):91-7.

81. Hill-Haas SV, Dawson B, Impellizzeri FM, Coutts AJ. Physiology of small-sided games training in football: A systematic review. *Sports Med*. 2011;41(3):199-220.

82. Hill DW, Rowell AL. Significance of time to exhaustion during exercise at the velocity associated with VO2max. *Eur J Appl Physiol Occup Physiol*. 1996;72(4):383-6.

83. Hodgson M, Docherty D, Robbins D. Post-activation potentiation: Underlying physiology and implications for motor performance. *Sports Med*. 2005;35(7):585-95.

84. Hoff J, Wisloff U, Engen LC, Kemi OJ, Helgerud J. Soccer specific aerobic endurance training. *Br J Sports Med*. 2002;36(3):218-21.

85. Hoier B, Hellsten Y. Exercise-induced capillary growth in human skeletal muscle and the dynamics of VEGF. *Microcirculation*. 2014;21(4):301-14.

86. Holloszy JO, Coyle EF. Adaptations of skeletal muscle to endurance exercise and their metabolic consequences. *J Appl Physiol*. 1984;56(4):831-8.

87. Hoppeler H, Vogt M, Weibel ER, Fluck M. Response of skeletal muscle mitochondria to hypoxia. *Exp Physiol*. 2003;88(1):109-19.

88. Iaia FM, Bangsbo J. Speed endurance training is a powerful stimulus for physiological adapta-

tions and performance improvements of athletes. *Scand J Med Sci Sports.* 2010;20(Suppl 2):11-23.

89. Illi SK, Held U, Frank I, Spengler CM. Effect of respiratory muscle training on exercise performance in healthy individuals: A systematic review and meta-analysis. *Sports Med.* 2012;42(8):707-24.

90. Impellizzeri FM, Marcora SM, Castagna C, Reilly T, Sassi A, Iaia FM, et al. Physiological and performance effects of generic versus specific aerobic training in soccer players. *Int J Sports Med.* 2006;27(6):483-92.

91. Ispirlidis I, Fatouros IG, Jamurtas AZ, Nikolaidis MG, Michailidis I, Douroudos I, et al. Time-course of changes in inflammatory and performance responses following a soccer game. *Clin J Sport Med.* 2008;18(5):423-31.

92. Jacobs I. Lactate, muscle glycogen and exercise performance in man. *Acta Physiol Scand Suppl.* 1981;495:1-35.

93. Jacobs I, Kaiser P. Lactate in blood, mixed skeletal muscle, and FT or ST fibres during cycle exercise in man. *Acta Physiol Scand.* 1982;114(3):461-6.

94. Jeukendrup AE. Periodized nutrition for athletes. *Sports Med.* 2017;47(Suppl 1):51-63.

95. Jones AM, Poole DC. *Oxygen Uptake Kinetics in Sport, Exercise and Medicine.* London: Routledge; 2005.

96. Joyner MJ, Coyle EF. Endurance exercise performance: The physiology of champions. *J Physiol.* 2008;586(1):35-44.

97. Kilding A, Wood M, Sequira G, Bonetti D. Effect of hyperoxic-supplemented interval training on endurance performance in trained cyclists *Int J Sports Med.* 2012;33(5):359-63

98. Komiyama T, Quaresima V, Shigematsu H, Ferrari M. Comparison of two spatially resolved near-infrared photometers in the detection of tissue oxygen saturation: Poor reliability at very low oxygen saturation. *Clin Sci (Lond).* 2001;101(6):715-18.

99. Krustrup P, Mohr M, Steensberg A, Bencke J, Kjaer M, Bangsbo J. Muscle and blood metabolites during a soccer game: Implications for sprint performance. *Med Sci Sports Exerc.* 2006;38(6):1165-74.

100. Krustrup P, Ortenblad N, Nielsen J, Nybo L, Gunnarsson TP, Iaia FM, et al. Maximal voluntary contraction force, SR function and glycogen resynthesis during the first 72 h after a high-level competitive soccer game. *Eur J Appl Physiol.* 2011;111(12):2987-95.

101. Lattier G, Millet GY, Martin A, Martin V. Fatigue and recovery after high-intensity exercise. Part I: Neuromuscular fatigue. *Int J Sports Med.* 2004;25(6):450-6.

102. Laursen PB. Training for intense exercise performance: High-intensity or high-volume training? *Scand J Med Sci Sports.* 2010;20(Suppl 2):1-10.

103. Laursen PB, Shing CM, Peake JM, Coombes JS, Jenkins DG. Interval training program optimization in highly trained endurance cyclists. *Med Sci Sports Exerc.* 2002 Nov;34(11):1801-7.

104. Lepretre PM, Koralsztein JP, Billat VL. Effect of exercise intensity on relationship between VO2max and cardiac output. *Med Sci Sports Exerc.* 2004;36(8):1357-63.

105. Lepretre PM, Foster C, Koralsztein JP, Billat VL. Heart rate deflection point as a strategy to defend stroke volume during incremental exercise. *J Appl Physiol.* 2005;98(5):1660-5.

106. Lepretre PM, Lopes P, Koralsztein JP, Billat V. Fatigue responses in exercise under control of VO2. *Int J Sports Med.* 2008;29(3):199-205.

107. Linossier MT, Dennis C, Dormois D, Geyssant A, Lacour JR. Ergometric and metabolic adaptation to a 5-s sprint training programe. *Eur J Appl Physiol.* 1993;67:408-14.

108. Lopez-Otin C, Galluzzi L, Freije JM, Madeo F, Kroemer G. Metabolic control of longevity. *Cell.* 2016;166(4):802-21.

109. Lucia A, Hoyos J, Perez M, Chicharro JL. Heart rate and performance parameters in elite cyclists: A longitudinal study. *Med Sci Sports Exerc.* 2000;32(10):1777-82.

110. MacDougall JD, Hicks AL, MacDonald JR, McKelvie RS, Green HJ, Smith KM. Muscle performance and enzymatic adaptations to sprint interval training. *J Appl Physiol.* 1998;84(6):2138-42.

111. MacInnis MJ, Gibala MJ. Physiological adaptations to interval training and the role of exercise intensity. *J Physiol.* 2017;595(9):2915-30.

112. Margaria R, Edwards H, Dill DB. The possible mechanisms of contracting and paying the oxygen debt and the role of lactic acid in muscular contraction. *Am J Physiol.* 1933(106):689-715.

113. Maron BJ, Pelliccia A. The heart of trained athletes: Cardiac remodeling and the risks of sports, including sudden death. *Circulation.* 2006;114(15):1633-44.

114. Marrier B, Le Meur Y, Robineau J, Lacome M, Couderc A, Hausswirth C, et al. Quantifying neuromuscular fatigue induced by an intense training session in Rugby Sevens. *Int J Sports Physiol Perform.* 2017;12(2):218-23.

115. McCole SD, Davis AM, Fueger PT. Is there a disassociation of maximal oxygen consumption and maximal cardiac output? *Med Sci Sports Exerc.* 2001;33(8):1265-9.

116. Medbo JI, Mohn AC, Tabata I, Bahr R, Vaage O, Sejersted OM. Anaerobic capacity determined by maximal accumulated O2 deficit. *J Appl Physiol.* 1988;64(1):50-60.

117. Midgley AW, Mc Naughton LR. Time at or near VO2max during continuous and intermittent running. A review with special reference to considerations for the optimisation of training protocols to elicit the longest time at or near VO2max. *J Sports Med Phys Fitness.* 2006;46(1):1-14.

118. Midgley AW, McNaughton LR, Wilkinson M. Is there an optimal training intensity for enhancing the maximal oxygen uptake of distance runners? Empirical research findings, current opinions, physiological rationale and practical recommendations. *Sports Med.* 2006;36(2):117-32.

119. Midgley AW, McNaughton LR, Jones AM. Training to enhance the physiological determinants of long-distance running performance: Can valid recommendations be given to runners and coaches based on current scientific knowledge? *Sports Med.* 2007;37(10):857-80.

120. Millet GY, Muthalib M, Jubeau M, Laursen PB, Nosaka K. Severe hypoxia affects exercise performance independently of afferent feedback and peripheral fatigue. *J Appl Physiol (1985).* 2012;112(8):1335-44.

121. Mortensen SP, Damsgaard R, Dawson EA, Secher NH, Gonzalez-Alonso J. Restrictions in systemic and locomotor skeletal muscle perfusion, oxygen supply and VO2 during high-intensity whole-body exercise in humans. *J Physiol.* 2008;586(10):2621-35.

122. Mucci P, Blondel N, Fabre C, Nourry C, Berthoin S. Evidence of exercise-induced O2 arterial desaturation in non-elite sportsmen and sportswomen following high-intensity interval-training. *Int J Sports Med.* 2004;25(1):6-13.

123. Newton RU, Laursen PB, Young W. Clinical exercise testing and assessment of athletes. In Schwellnus MP, ed. *Olympic Textbook of Medicine in Sport.* XIV. Oxford, UK: Blackwell Publishing; 2008:160-99.

124. Nielsen HB, Bredmose PP, Stromstad M, Volianitis S, Quistorff B, Secher NH. Bicarbonate attenuates arterial desaturation during maximal exercise in humans. *J Appl Physiol (1985).* 2002;93(2):724-31.

125. Nioka S, Moser D, Lech G, Evengelisti M, Verde T, Chance B, et al. Muscle deoxygenation in aerobic and anaerobic exercise. *Adv Exp Med Biol.* 1998;454:63-70.

126. Noordhof DA, de Koning JJ, Foster C. The maximal accumulated oxygen deficit method: A valid and reliable measure of anaerobic capacity? *Sports Med.* 2010;40(4):285-302.

127. Opar DA, Williams MD, Shield AJ. Hamstring strain injuries: Factors that lead to injury and re-injury. *Sports Med.* 2012;42(3):209-26.

128. Paavolainen L, Hakkinen K, Nummela A, Rusko H. Neuromuscular characteristics and fatigue in endurance and sprint athletes during a new anaerobic power test. *Eur J Appl Physiol Occup Physiol.* 1994;69(2):119-26.

129. Palmer CD, Sleivert GG. Running economy is impaired following a single bout of resistance exercise. *J Sci Med Sport.* 2001;4(4):447-59.

130. Parra J, Cadefau JA, Rodas G, Amigo N, Cusso R. The distribution of rest periods affects performance and adaptations of energy metabolism induced by high-intensity training in human muscle. *Acta Physiol Scand.* 2000;169(2):157-65.

131. Paton CD, Hopkins WG, Cook C. Effects of low- vs. high-cadence interval training on cycling performance. *J Strength Cond Res.* 2009;23(6):1758-63.

132. Perrey S, Racinais S, Saimouaa K, Girard O. Neural and muscular adjustments following repeated running sprints. *Eur J Appl Physiol.* 2010;109(6):1027-36.

133. Powers SK, Dodd S, Lawler J, Landry G, Kirtley M, McKnight T, et al. Incidence of exercise induced hypoxemia in elite endurance athletes

at sea level. *Eur J Appl Physiol Occup Physiol.* 1988;58(3):298-302.

134. Rampinini E, Sassi A, Azzalin A, Castagna C, Menaspa P, Carlomagno D, et al. Physiological determinants of Yo-Yo intermittent recovery tests in male soccer players. *Eur J Appl Physiol.* 2008;108(2):401-9.

135. Richard R, Lonsdorfer-Wolf E, Dufour S, Doutreleau S, Oswald-Mammosser M, Billat VL, et al. Cardiac output and oxygen release during very high-intensity exercise performed until exhaustion. *Eur J Appl Physiol.* 2004;93(1-2):9-18.

136. Richard R, Lonsdorfer-Wolf E, Charloux A, Doutreleau S, Buchheit M, Oswald-Mammosser M, et al. Non-invasive cardiac output evaluation during a maximal progressive exercise test, using a new impedance cardiograph device. *Eur J Appl Physiol.* 2001;85(3-4):202-7.

137. Rodas G, Ventura JL, Cadefau JA, Cusso R, Parra J. A short training programme for the rapid improvement of both aerobic and anaerobic metabolism. *Eur J Appl Physiol.* 2000;82(5-6):480-6.

138. Rolf C. Overuse injuries of the lower extremity in runners. *Scand J Med Sci Sports.* 1995;5(4):181-90.

139. Rooks CR, Thom NJ, McCully KK, Dishman RK. Effects of incremental exercise on cerebral oxygenation measured by near-infrared spectroscopy: A systematic review. *Prog Neurobiol.* 2010;92(2):134-50.

140. Ross A, Leveritt M. Long-term metabolic and skeletal muscle adaptations to short-sprint training: implications for sprint training and tapering. *Sports Med.* 2001;31(15):1063-82.

141. Ross A, Leveritt M, Riek S. Neural influences on sprint running: training adaptations and acute responses. *Sports Med.* 2001;31(6):409-25.

142. Rowell LB. *Human Cardiovascular Control.* New York: Oxford University Press; 1993.

143. Rusko H, Nummela A, Mero A. A new method for the evaluation of anaerobic running power in athletes. *Eur J Appl Physiol Occup Physiol.* 1993;66(2):97-101.

144. Seiler S. What is best practice for training intensity and duration distribution in endurance athletes? *Int J Sports Physiol Perform.* 2010;5(3):276-91.

145. Seiler S, Hetlelid KJ. The impact of rest duration on work intensity and RPE during interval training. *Med Sci Sports Exerc.* 2005;37(9):1601-7.

146. Shibuya K, Tanaka J, Ogaki T. Muscle oxygenation kinetics at the onset of exercise do not depend on exercise intensity. *Eur J Appl Physiol.* 2004;91(5-6):712-5.

147. Shibuya K, Tanaka J, Kuboyama N, Ogaki T. Cerebral oxygenation during intermittent supramaximal exercise. *Respir Physiol Neurobiol.* 2004;140(2):165-72.

148. Shibuya K, Tanaka J, Kuboyama N, Murai S, Ogaki T. Cerebral cortex activity during supramaximal exhaustive exercise. *J Sports Med Phys Fitness.* 2004;44(2):215-9.

149. Simoneau JA, Lortie G, Boulay MR, Marcotte M, Thibault MC, Bouchard C. Effects of two high-intensity intermittent training programs interspaced by detraining on human skeletal muscle and performance. *Eur J Appl Physiol Occup Physiol.* 1987;56(5):516-21.

150. Skof B, Strojnik V. Neuro-muscular fatigue and recovery dynamics following anaerobic interval workload. *Int J Sports Med.* 2006;27(3):220-5.

151. Small K, McNaughton LR, Greig M, Lohkamp M, Lovell R. Soccer fatigue, sprinting and hamstring injury risk. *Int J Sports Med.* 2009;30(8):573-8.

152. Smith KJ, Billaut F. Influence of cerebral and muscle oxygenation on repeated-sprint ability. *Eur J Appl Physiol.* 2010;109(2):989-99.

153. Sobhani S, Dekker R, Postema K, Dijkstra PU. Epidemiology of ankle and foot overuse injuries in sports: A systematic review. *Scand J Med Sci Sports.* 2013;23(6):669-86.

154. Stanley J, Buchheit M. Moderate recovery unnecessary to sustain high stroke volume during interval training. A brief report. *J Sports Sci Med.* 2014;13(2):393-6.

155. Stapelfeldt B, Mornieux G, Oberheim R, Belli A, Gollhofer A. Development and evaluation of a new bicycle instrument for measurements of pedal forces and power output in cycling. *Int J Sports Med.* 2007;28(4):326-32.

156. Tabata I, Irisawa K, Kouzaki M, Nishimura K, Ogita F, Miyachi M. Metabolic profile of high intensity intermittent exercises. *Med Sci Sports Exerc.* 1997;29(3):390-5.

157. Takahashi T, Hayano J, Okada A, Saitoh T, Kamiya A. Effects of the muscle pump and body posture on cardiovascular responses during recovery from cycle exercise. *Eur J Appl Physiol.* 2005;94(5-6):576-83.

158. Turner AP, Cathcart AJ, Parker ME, Butterworth C, Wilson J, Ward SA. Oxygen uptake and muscle desaturation kinetics during intermittent cycling. *Med Sci Sports Exerc.* 2006;38(3):492-503.

159. Twomey R, Aboodarda SJ, Kruger R, Culos-Reed SN, Temesi J, Millet GY. Neuromuscular fatigue during exercise: Methodological considerations, etiology and potential role in chronic fatigue. *Neurophysiol Clin.* 2017;47(2):95-110.

160. Verges S, Rupp T, Jubeau M, Wuyam B, Esteve F, Levy P, et al. Invited review: Cerebral perturbations during exercise in hypoxia. *Am J Physiol Regul Integr Comp Physiol.* 2012;302(8):R903-16.

161. Volek JS, Noakes T, Phinney SD. Rethinking fat as a fuel for endurance exercise. *Eur J Sport Sci.* 2015;15(1):13-20.

162. Vollaard NB, Constantin-Teodosiu D, Fredriksson K, Rooyackers O, Jansson E, Greenhaff PL, et al. Systematic analysis of adaptations in aerobic capacity and submaximal energy metabolism provides a unique insight into determinants of human aerobic performance. *J Appl Physiol.* 2009;106(5):1479-86.

163. Vuorimaa T, Vasankari T, Rusko H. Comparison of physiological strain and muscular performance of athletes during two intermittent running exercises at the velocity associated with VO2max. *Int J Sports Med.* 2000;21(2):96-101.

164. Vuorimaa T, Hakkinen K, Vahasoyrinki P, Rusko H. Comparison of three maximal anaerobic running test protocols in marathon runners, middle-distance runners and sprinters. *Int J Sports Med.* 1996;17 Suppl 2:S109-13.

165. Vuorimaa T, Virlander R, Kurkilahti P, Vasankari T, Hakkinen K. Acute changes in muscle activation and leg extension performance after different running exercises in elite long distance runners. *Eur J Appl Physiol.* 2006;96(3):282-91.

166. Warburton DE, Gledhill N. Counterpoint: Stroke volume does not decline during exercise at maximal effort in healthy individuals. *J Appl Physiol.* 2008;104(1):276-8; discussion 8-9.

167. Weston AR, Myburgh KH, Lindsay FH, Dennis SC, Noakes TD, Hawley JA. Skeletal muscle buffering capacity and endurance performance after high-intensity interval training by well-trained cyclists. *Eur J Appl Physiol Occup Physiol.* 1997;75(1):7-13.

168. Wu HC, Hsu WH, Chen T. Complete recovery time after exhaustion in high-intensity work. *Ergonomics.* 2005;48(6):668-79.

169. Yeo WK, Paton CD, Garnham AP, Burke LM, Carey AL, Hawley JA. Skeletal muscle adaptation and performance responses to once a day versus twice every second day endurance training regimens. *J Appl Physiol.* 2008;105(5):1462-70.

170. Yeo WK, McGee SL, Carey AL, Paton CD, Garnham AP, Hargreaves M, et al. Acute signalling responses to intense endurance training commenced with low or normal muscle glycogen. *Exp Physiol.* 2010;95(2):351-8.

171. Yoshida T. Effect of dietary modifications on lactate threshold and onset of blood lactate accumulation during incremental exercise. *Eur J Appl Physiol Occup Physiol.* 1984;53(3):200-5.

172. Zoladz JA, Gladden LB, Hogan MC, Nieckarz Z, Grassi B. Progressive recruitment of muscle fibers is not necessary for the slow component of VO2 kinetics. *J Appl Physiol.* 2008;105(2):575-80.

Chapter 4

1. Abbiss CR, Burnett A, Nosaka K, Green JP, Foster JK, Laursen PB. Effect of hot versus cold climates on power output, muscle activation, and perceived fatigue during a dynamic 100-km cycling trial. *J Sports Sci.* 2010;28(2):117-25.

2. Abbiss CR, Peiffer JJ, Peake JM, Nosaka K, Suzuki K, Martin DT, et al. Effect of carbohydrate ingestion and ambient temperature on muscle fatigue development in endurance-trained male cyclists. *J Appl Physiol (1985).* 2008;104(4):1021-8.

3. Ahmaidi S, Granier P, Taoutaou Z, Mercier J, Dubouchaud H, Prefaut C. Effects of active recovery on plasma lactate and anaerobic power following repeated intensive exercise. *Med Sci Sports Exerc.* 1996;28(4):450-6.

4. Astrand I, Astrand PO, Christensen EH, Hedman R. Intermittent muscular work. *Acta Physiol Scand.* 1960;48:448-53.

5. Baar K. Nutrition and the adaptation to endurance training. *Sports Med*. 2014;44(Suppl 1):S5-12.

6. Belcastro AN, Bonen A. Lactic acid removal rates during controlled and uncontrolled recovery exercise. *J Appl Physiol*. 1975;39(6):932-6.

7. Billat LV. Interval training for performance: A scientific and empirical practice. Special recommendations for middle- and long-distance running. Part I: Aerobic interval training. *Sports Med* 2001;1(31):13-31.

8. Bogdanis GC, Nevill ME, Lakomy HK, Graham CM, Louis G. Effects of active recovery on power output during repeated maximal sprint cycling. *Eur J Appl Physiol Occup Physiol*. 1996;74(5):461-9.

9. Bompa TO, Haff GG. *Periodization*, 5th ed. Chicago, IL: Human Kinetics; 2009.

10. Brocherie F, Girard O, Faiss R, Millet GP. Effects of repeated-sprint training in hypoxia on sea-level performance: A meta-analysis. *Sports Med*. 2017;47(8):1651-60.

11. Buchheit M. The 30-15 Intermittent Fitness Test: A new intermittent running field test for intermittent sport players - Part 1. *Approches du Handball*. 2005;87:27-34.

12. Buchheit M. The 30-15 Intermittent Fitness Test: 10 year review. *Myorobie Journal*. Sep 2010;1:http://www.martin-buchheit.net.

13. Buchheit M. Should we be recommending repeated sprints to improve repeated-sprint performance? *Sports Med*. 2012;42(2):169-72; author reply 72-3.

14. Buchheit M, Al Haddad H, Mendez-Villanueva A, Quod MJ, Bourdon PC. Effect of maturation on hemodynamic and autonomic control recovery following maximal running exercise in highly trained young soccer players. *Front Physiol*. 2011;2:69.

15. Buchheit M, Cormie P, Abbiss CR, Ahmaidi S, Nosaka KK, Laursen PB. Muscle deoxygenation during repeated sprint running: Effect of active vs. passive recovery. *Int J Sports Med*. 2009;30(6):418-25.

16. Casadio JR, Kilding AE, Cotter JD, Laursen PB. From lab to real world: Heat acclimation considerations for elite athletes. *Sports Med*. 2017;47(8):1467-76.

17. Christensen EH, Hedman R, Saltin B. Intermittent and continuous running. (A further contribution to the physiology of intermittent work.) *Acta Physiol Scand*. 1960;50:269-86.

18. Cipryan L, Plews DJ, Ferretti A, Maffetone P, Laursen PB. Effects of a 4-week very low carbohydrate diet on high-intensity interval training responses. *J Sport Sci Med*. 2018;17(2):259-68.

19. Connolly DAJ, Brennan KM, Lauzon CD. Effects of active versus passive recovery on power output during repeated bouts of short term, high intensity exercise. *J Sports Sci Med*. 2003(2):47-51.

20. Cotter JD, Thornton SN, Lee JK, Laursen PB. Are we being drowned in hydration advice? Thirsty for more? *Extrem Physiol Med*. 2014;3:18.

21. Dorado C, Sanchis-Moysi J, Calbet JA. Effects of recovery mode on performance, O2 uptake, and O2 deficit during high-intensity intermittent exercise. *Can J Appl Physiol*. 2004;29(3):227-44.

22. Dupont G, Moalla W, Matran R, Berthoin S. Effect of short recovery intensities on the performance during two Wingate tests. *Med Sci Sports Exerc*. 2007;39(7):1170-6.

23. Dupont G, Moalla W, Guinhouya C, Ahmaidi S, Berthoin S. Passive versus active recovery during high-intensity intermittent exercises. *Med Sci Sports Exerc*. 2004;36(2):302-8.

24. Faiss R, Girard O, Millet GP. Advancing hypoxic training in team sports: From intermittent hypoxic training to repeated sprint training in hypoxia. *Br J Sports Med*. 2013;47 Suppl 1:i45-50.

25. Favier FB, Britto FA, Freyssenet DG, Bigard XA, Benoit H. HIF-1-driven skeletal muscle adaptations to chronic hypoxia: Molecular insights into muscle physiology. *Cell Mol Life Sci*. 2015;72(24):4681-96.

26. Febbraio MA, Snow RJ, Stathis CG, Hargreaves M, Carey MF. Effect of heat stress on muscle energy metabolism during exercise. *J Appl Physiol*. 1994;77(6):2827-31.

27. Febbraio MA, Snow RJ, Hargreaves M, Stathis CG, Martin IK, Carey MF. Muscle metabolism during exercise and heat stress in trained men: Effect of acclimation. *J Appl Physiol*. 1994;76(2):589-97.

28. Gandevia SC. Spinal and supraspinal factors in human muscle fatigue. *Physiol Rev*. 2001;81(4):1725-89.

29. Garrett AT, Goosens NG, Rehrer NJ, Patterson MJ, Harrison J, Sammut I, et al. Short-term heat

acclimation is effective and may be enhanced rather than impaired by dehydration. *Am J Hum Biol.* 2014;26(3):311-20.

30. Gibson OR, Taylor L, Watt PW, Maxwell NS. Cross-adaptation: Heat and cold adaptation to improve physiological and cellular responses to hypoxia. *Sports Med.* 2017;47(9):1751-68.

31. Girard O, Brocherie F, Millet GP. Effects of altitude/hypoxia on single- and multiple-sprint performance: A comprehensive review. *Sports Med.* 2017;47(10):1931-49.

32. Girard O, Brocherie F, Morin JB, Millet GP. Running mechanical alterations during repeated treadmill sprints in hot versus hypoxic environments. A pilot study. *J Sports Sci.* 2016;34(12):1190-8.

33. Girard O, Brocherie F, Morin JB, Racinais S, Millet GP, Periard JD. Mechanical alterations associated with repeated treadmill sprinting under heat stress. *PLoS One.* 2017;12(2):e0170679.

34. Gorostiaga EM, Asiain X, Izquierdo M, Postigo A, Aguado R, Alonso JM, et al. Vertical jump performance and blood ammonia and lactate levels during typical training sessions in elite 400-m runners. *J Strength Cond Res.* 2010;24(4):1138-49.

35. Havemann L, West SJ, Goedecke JH, Macdonald IA, St Clair Gibson A, Noakes TD, et al. Fat adaptation followed by carbohydrate loading compromises high-intensity sprint performance. *J Appl Physiol.* 2006;100(1):194-202.

36. Henstridge DC, Febbraio MA, Hargreaves M. Heat shock proteins and exercise adaptations. Our knowledge thus far and the road still ahead. *J Appl Physiol (1985).* 2016;120(6):683-91.

37. Hetlelid KJ, Plews DJ, Herold E, Laursen PB, Sieler S. Rethinking the role of fat oxidation: Substrate utilisation during high-intensity interval training in well-trained and recreationally trained runners. *BMJ Open Sport & Exercise Medicine* 2015;1(1).

38. Hill AV. The physiological basis of athletic records. *Nature.* 1925;116:544-8.

39. Hill AV. The dimensions of animals and their muscular dynamics. *Sci Prog.* 1950;38:209.

40. Krustrup P, Mohr M, Steensberg A, Bencke J, Kjaer M, Bangsbo J. Muscle and blood metabolites during a soccer game: Implications for sprint performance. *Med Sci Sports Exerc.* 2006;38(6):1165-74.

41. Lane SC, Areta JL, Bird SR, Coffey VG, Burke LM, Desbrow B, et al. Caffeine ingestion and cycling power output in a low or normal muscle glycogen state. *Med Sci Sports Exerc.* 2013;45(8):1577-84.

42. Laursen PB, Shing CM, Peake JM, Coombes JS, Jenkins DG. Interval training program optimization in highly trained endurance cyclists. *Med Sci Sports Exer.* 2002;34(11):1801-7.

43. Marquet LA, Hausswirth C, Molle O, Hawley JA, Burke LM, Tiollier E, et al. Periodization of carbohydrate intake: Short-term effect on performance. *Nutrients.* 2016;8(12).

44. Midgley AW, Mc Naughton LR. Time at or near VO2max during continuous and intermittent running. A review with special reference to considerations for the optimisation of training protocols to elicit the longest time at or near VO2max. *J Sports Med Phys Fitness.* 2006;46(1):1-14.

45. Muller EA. The physiological basis of rest pauses in heavy work. *Q J Exp Physiol Cogn Med Sci.* 1953;38(4):205-15.

46. Munoz-Martinez FA, Rubio-Arias JA, Ramos-Campo DJ, Alcaraz PE. Effectiveness of resistance circuit-based training for maximum oxygen uptake and upper-body one-repetition maximum improvements: A systematic review and meta-analysis. *Sports Med.* 2017;47(12):2553-68.

47. Nedeljkovic A, Mirkov DM, Bozic P, Jaric S. Tests of muscle power output: The role of body size. *Int J Sports Med.* 2009;30(2):100-6.

48. Rowell LB. *Human Cardiovascular Control.* New York: Oxford University Press; 1993.

49. Seiler S, Hetlelid KJ. The impact of rest duration on work intensity and RPE during interval training. *Med Sci Sports Exerc.* 2005;37(9):1601-7.

50. Spencer M, Bishop D, Dawson B, Goodman C, Duffield R. Metabolism and performance in repeated cycle sprints: Active versus passive recovery. *Med Sci Sports Exerc.* 2006;38(8):1492-9.

51. Spencer M, Dawson B, Goodman C, Dascombe B, Bishop D. Performance and metabolism in repeated sprint exercise: Effect of recovery intensity. *Eur J Appl Physiol.* 2008;103(5):545-52.

52. Stanley J, Buchheit M. Moderate recovery unnecessary to sustain high stroke volume during interval training. A brief report. *J Sports Sci Med.* 2014;13(2):393-6.

53. Stanley J, Halliday A, D'Auria S, Buchheit M, Leicht AS. Effect of sauna-based heat acclimation on plasma volume and heart rate variability. *Eur J Appl Physiol*. 2015;115(4):785-94.

54. Stellingwerff T. Contemporary nutrition approaches to optimize elite marathon performance. *Int J Sports Physiol Perform*. 2013;8(5):573-8.

55. Stepto NK, Hawley JA, Dennis SC, Hopkins WG. Effects of different interval-training programs on cycling time-trial performance. *Med Sci Sports Exer*. 1999;31(5):736-41.

56. Trincat L, Woorons X, Millet GP. Repeated-sprint training in hypoxia induced by voluntary hypoventilation in swimming. *Int J Sports Physiol Perform*. 2017;12(3):329-35.

57. Volek JS, Noakes T, Phinney SD. Rethinking fat as a fuel for endurance exercise. *Eur J Sport Sci*. 2015;15(1):13-20.

58. Weltman A, Stamford BA, Fulco C. Recovery from maximal effort exercise: Lactate disappearance and subsequent performance. *J Appl Physiol*. 1979;47(4):677-82.

59. Wu HC, Hsu WH, Chen T. Complete recovery time after exhaustion in high-intensity work. *Ergonomics*. 2005;48(6):668-79.

60. Yeo WK, Paton CD, Garnham AP, Burke LM, Carey AL, Hawley JA. Skeletal muscle adaptation and performance responses to once a day versus twice every second day endurance training regimens. *J Appl Physiol*. 2008;105(5):1462-70.

61. Yeo WK, Paton CD, Garnham AP, Burke LM, Carey AL, Hawley JA. Skeletal muscle adaptation and performance responses to once a day versus twice every second day endurance training regimens. *J Appl Physiol*. 2008;105(5):1462-70.

62. Yeo WK, McGee SL, Carey AL, Paton CD, Garnham AP, Hargreaves M, et al. Acute signalling responses to intense endurance training commenced with low or normal muscle glycogen. *Exper Physiol*. 2010;95(2):351-8.

63. Yeo WK, Lessard SJ, Chen ZP, Garnham AP, Burke LM, Rivas DA, et al. Fat adaptation followed by carbohydrate restoration increases AMPK activity in skeletal muscle from trained humans. *J Appl Physiol*. 2008;105(5):1519-26.

64. Zeevi D, Korem T, Zmora N, Israeli D, Rothschild D, Weinberger A, et al. Personalized nutrition by prediction of glycemic responses. *Cell*. 2015;163(5):1079-94.

Chapter 5

1. Abt G, Siegler JC, Akubat I, Castagna C. The effects of a constant sprint-to-rest ratio and recovery mode on repeated sprint performance. *J Strength Cond Res*. 2011;25:1695-1702.

2. Ahmaidi S, Collomp K, Prefaut C. The effect of shuttle test protocol and the resulting lactacidaemia on maximal velocity and maximal oxygen uptake during the shuttle exercise test. *Eur J Appl Physiol*. 1992;65:475-9.

3. Ahmaidi S, Granier P, Taoutaou Z, Mercier J, Dubouchaud H, Prefaut C. Effects of active recovery on plasma lactate and anaerobic power following repeated intensive exercise. *Med Sci Sports Exerc*. 1996;28:450-6.

4. Altenburg TM, Degens H, van Mechelen W, Sargeant AJ, de Haan A. Recruitment of single muscle fibers during submaximal cycling exercise. *J Appl Physiol*. 2007;103:1752-6.

5. Astrand I, Astrand PO, Christensen EH, Hedman R. Intermittent muscular work. *Acta Physiol Scand*. 1960;48:448-53.

6. Astrand I, Astrand PO, Christensen EH, Hedman R. Myohemoglobin as an oxygen-store in man. *Acta Physiol Scand*.1960;48:454-60.

7. Astrand PO, Rodahl K. *Texbook for Work Physiology*. New York, NY: McGraw-Hill; 1977.

8. Balsom PD, Seger JY, Sjodin B, Ekblom B. Maximal-intensity intermittent exercise: Effect of recovery duration. *Int J Sports Med*.1992;13:528-33.

9. Balsom PD, Seger JY, Sjodin B, Ekblom B. Physiological responses to maximal intensity intermittent exercise. *Eur J Appl Physiol Occup Physiol*.1992;65:144-9.

10. Barnes KR, Hopkins WG, McGuigan MR, Kilding AE. Effects of different uphill interval-training programs on running economy and performance. *Int J Sports Physiol Perform*. 2013;8:639-47.

11. Barstow TJ, Jones AM, Nguyen PH, Casaburi R. Influence of muscle fiber type and pedal frequency on oxygen uptake kinetics of heavy exercise. *J Appl Physiol*. 1996;81:1642-50.

12. Belcastro AN, Bonen A. Lactic acid removal rates during controlled and uncontrolled recovery exercise. *J Appl Physiol*. 1975;39:932-6.

13. Belfry GR, Paterson DH, Murias JM, Thomas SG. The effects of short recovery duration on VO2

and muscle deoxygenation during intermittent exercise. *Eur J Appl Physiol.* 2012;112:1907-15.

14. Bergman BC, Wolfel EE, Butterfield GE, Lopaschuk GD, Casazza GA, Horning MA, et al. Active muscle and whole body lactate kinetics after endurance training in men. *J Appl Physiol.* 1999;87:1684-96.

15. Billat LV. Interval training for performance: A scientific and empirical practice. Special recommendations for middle- and long-distance running. Part I: Aerobic interval training. *Sports Med.* 2001;1:13-31.

16. Billat LV. Interval training for performance: A scientific and empirical practice. Special recommendations for middle- and long-distance running. Part II: Anaerobic interval training. *Sports Med.* 2001;31:75-90.

17. Billat LV, Renoux J, Pinoteau J, Petit B, Koralsztein JP. Validation d'une épreuve maximale de temps limiteà VMA (vitesse maximale aérobie) et à V̇O2max. *Sci Sports.* 1994;9:3-12.

18. Billat LV, Slawinksi J, Bocquet V, Chassaing P, Demarle A, Koralsztein JP. Very short (15s-15s) interval-training around the critical velocity allows middle-aged runners to maintain VO2 max for 14 minutes. *Int J Sports Med.* 2001;22:201-8.

19. Billat V. *L'entraînement en pleine nature - Conseils de préparation aux sports outdoor.* Paris: De Boeck; 2005.

20. Billat V, Binsse V, Petit B, Koralsztein JP. High level runners are able to maintain a VO2 steady-state below VO2max in an all-out run over their critical velocity. *Arch Physiol Biochem.* 1998;106:38-45.

21. Billat V, Petit B, Koralsztein J. Calibration de la durée des répétition d'une séance d'interval training à la vitesse associée à VO2max en référence au temps limite continu: Effet sur les réponses physiologiques et la distance parcourue. *Sci Mot.* 1996;28:13-20.

22. Billat V, Renoux JC, Pinoteau J, Petit B, Koralsztein JP. Reproducibility of running time to exhaustion at VO2max in subelite runners. *Med Sci Sports Exerc.* 1994;26:254-7.

23. Billat VL, Blondel N, Berthoin S. Determination of the velocity associated with the longest time to exhaustion at maximal oxygen uptake. *Eur J Appl Physiol Occup Physiol.* 1999;80:159-61.

24. Billat VL, Slawinski J, Bocquet V, Demarle A, Lafitte L, Chassaing P, et al. Intermittent runs at

the velocity associated with maximal oxygen uptake enables subjects to remain at maximal oxygen uptake for a longer time than intense but submaximal runs. *Eur J Appl Physiol.* 2000;81:188-96.

25. Binnie MJ, Peeling P, Pinnington H, Landers G, Dawson B. Effect of training surface on acute physiological responses following interval training. *J Strength Cond Res.* 2013;27(4):1047-56.

26. Bisciotti GN. L'incidenza fisiologica dei parametri di durata, intensità e recupero nell'ambito dell'allenamento intermittente. *Sienza di Sport.* 2004;60:90-6.

27. Bogdanis GC, Nevill ME, Boobis LH, Lakomy HK. Contribution of phosphocreatine and aerobic metabolism to energy supply during repeated sprint exercise. *J Appl Physiol.* 1996;80:876-84.

28. Bogdanis GC, Nevill ME, Lakomy HK, Graham CM, Louis G. Effects of active recovery on power output during repeated maximal sprint cycling. *Eur J Appl Physiol Occup Physiol.* 1996;74:461-9.

29. Bravo DF, Impellizzeri FM, Rampinini E, Castagna C, Bishop D, Wisloff U. Sprint vs. interval training in football. *Int J Sports Med.* 2008;29:668-74.

30. Brito J, Krustrup P, Rebelo A. The influence of the playing surface on the exercise intensity of small-sided recreational soccer games. *Human movement science.* 2012;31:946-56.

31. Brooks GA. Current concepts in lactate exchange. *Med Sci Sports Exerc.* 1991;23:895-906.

32. Brughelli M, Cronin J, Levin G, Chaouachi A. Understanding change of direction ability in sport: A review of resistance training studies. *Sports Med.* 2008;38:1045-63.

33. Buchheit M. [The 30-15 Intermittent Fitness Test: A new intermittent running field test for intermittent sport players - Part 1]. *Approches du Handball.* 2005;87:27-34.

34. Buchheit M. The 30-15 intermittent fitness test: Accuracy for individualizing interval training of young intermittent sport players. *J Strength Cond Res.* 2008;22:365-74.

35. Buchheit M. The 30-15 Intermittent Fitness Test: 10 year review. *Myorobie Journal.* 2010;1: http://www.martin-buchheit.net.

36. Buchheit M. Performance and physiological responses to repeated- sprint and jump sequences. *Eur J Appl Physiol.* 2010;101:1007-18.

37. Buchheit M. Individualizing high-intensity interval training in intermittent sport athletes with the 30-15 Intermittent Fitness Test. *NSCA Hot Topic Series wwwnsca-liftorg* November, 2011.

38. Buchheit M. Should we be recommending repeated sprints to improve repeated-sprint performance? *Sports Med.* 2012;42:169-72.

39. Buchheit M. Programming high intensity training in handball. *Aspetar Sports Medicine Journal.* 2014;3:120-8.

40. Buchheit M. Programming high-intensity training in handball. *Aspetar Sports Medicine Journal.* 2014;3:120-8.

41. Buchheit M, Abbiss C, Peiffer JJ, Laursen PB. Performance and physiological responses during a sprint interval training session: Relationships with muscle oxygenation and pulmonary oxygen uptake kinetics. *Eur J Appl Physiol.* 2012;111:767-79.

42. Buchheit M, Abbiss CR, Peiffer JJ, Laursen PB. Performance and physiological responses during a sprint interval training session: Relationships with muscle oxygenation and pulmonary oxygen uptake kinetics. *Eur J Appl Physiol.* 2012;112:767-79.

43. Buchheit M, Bishop D, Haydar B, Nakamura F, Ahmaidi S. Physiological responses to shuttle repeated-sprint running. *Int J Sports Med.* 2010;31:402-9.

44. Buchheit M, Cormie P, Abbiss CR, Ahmaidi S, Nosaka KK, Laursen PB. Muscle deoxygenation during repeated sprint running: Effect of active vs. passive recovery. *Int J Sports Med.* 2009;30:418-25.

45. Buchheit M, Duthie G, Ahmaidi S. Increasing passive recovery duration leads to greater performance despite higher blood lactate accumulation and physiological strain during repeated shuttle 30-s sprints. Presented at 14th European Congress of Sport Science, Olso, Norway, 2009.

46. Buchheit M, Haydar B, Ahmaidi S. Repeated sprints with directional changes: Do angles matter? *J Sports Sci.* 2012;30:555-62.

47. Buchheit M, Haydar B, Hader K, Ufland P, Ahmaidi S. Assessing running economy during field running with changes of direction: Application to 20-m shuttle-runs. *Int J Sports Physiol Perform.* 2011;6:380-95.

48. Buchheit M, Kuitunen S, Voss SC, Williams BK, Mendez-Villanueva A, Bourdon PC. Physiological strain associated with high-intensity hypoxic intervals in highly trained young runners. *J Strength Cond Res.* 2012;26:94-105.

49. Buchheit M, Laursen PB. High-intensity interval training, solutions to the programming puzzle: Part I: Cardiopulmonary emphasis. *Sports Med.* 2013;43:313-38.

50. Buchheit M, Laursen PB. High-intensity interval training, solutions to the programming puzzle: Part I: Cardiopulmonary emphasis. *Sports Med.* 2013;43:313-38.

51. Buchheit M, Laursen PB. High-intensity interval training, solutions to the programming puzzle. Part II: Anaerobic energy, neuromuscular load and practical applications. *Sports Med.* 2013;43:927-54.

52. Buchheit M, Laursen PB, Ahmaidi S. Parasympathetic reactivation after repeated sprint exercise. *Am J Physiol Heart Circ Physiol.* 2007;293:H133–H141.

53. Buchheit M, Laursen PB, Ahmaidi S. Effect of prior exercise on pulmonary O2 uptake and estimated muscle capillary blood flow kinetics during moderate-intensity field running in men. *J Appl Physiol.* 2009;107:460-70.

54. Buchheit M, Laursen PB, Kuhnle J, Ruch D, Renaud C, Ahmaidi S. Game-based training in young elite handball players. *Int J Sports Med.* 2009;30:251-8.

55. Buchheit M, Laursen PB, Millet GP, Pactat F, Ahmaidi S. Predicting intermittent running performance: Critical velocity versus endurance index. *Int J Sports Med.* 2007;29:307-15.

56. Buchheit M, Lepretre PM, Behaegel AL, Millet GP, Cuvelier G, Ahmaidi S. Cardiorespiratory responses during running and sport-specific exercises in handball players. *J Sci Med Sport.* 2009;12:399-405.

57. Buchheit M, Mendez-Villanueva A, Delhomel G, Brughelli M, Ahmaidi S. Improving repeated sprint ability in young elite soccer players: Repeated sprints vs. explosive strength training. *J Strength Cond Res.* 2010;24:2715-22.

58. Buchheit M, Mendez-Villanueva A, Quod MJ, Quesnel T, Ahmaidi S. Improving acceleration and repeated sprint ability in well-trained adolescent handball players: speed vs. sprint

interval training. *Int J Sports Physiol Perform.* 2010;5:152-64.

59. Buchheit M, Mendez-Villanueva A, Simpson BM, Bourdon PC. Match running performance and fitness in youth soccer. *Int J Sports Med.* 2010;31:818-25.

60. Buchheit M, Millet GP, Parisy A, Pourchez S, Laursen PB, Ahmaidi S. Supramaximal training and post-exercise parasympathetic reactivation in adolescents. *Med Sci Sports Exerc.* 2008;40:362-71.

61. Buchheit M, Simpson BM, Mendez-Villaneuva A. Repeated high-speed activities during youth soccer games in relation to changes in maximal sprinting and aerobic speeds. *Int J sport Med.* 2012;34:40-8.

62. Burnley M, Doust JH, Ball D, Jones AM. Effects of prior heavy exercise on VO(2) kinetics during heavy exercise are related to changes in muscle activity. *J Appl Physiol (1985).* 2002;93:167-74.

63. Byrnes WC, Clarkson PM, White JS, Hsieh SS, Frykman PN, Maughan RJ. Delayed onset muscle soreness following repeated bouts of downhill running. *J Appl Physiol.* 1985;59:710-15.

64. Castagna C, Abt G, Manzi V, Annino G, Padua E, D'Ottavio S. Effect of recovery mode on repeated sprint ability in young basketball players. *J Strength Cond Res.* 2008;22:923-29.

65. Castagna C, Belardinelli R, Impellizzeri FM, Abt GA, Coutts AJ, D'Ottavio S. Cardiovascular responses during recreational 5-a-side indoor-soccer. *J Sci Med Sport.* 2007;10:89-95.

66. Castagna C, D'Ottavio S, Granda Vera J, Barbero Alvarez JC. Match demands of professional Futsal: A case study. *J Sci Med Sport.* 2009;12:490-4.

67. Castagna C, Impellizzeri FM, Chaouachi A, Ben Abdelkrim N, Manzi V. Physiological responses to ball-drills in regional level male basketball players. *J Sports Sci.* 2011;29:1329-36.

68. Christensen EH, Hedman R, Saltin B. Intermittent and continuous running. (A further contribution to the physiology of intermittent work.) *Acta Physiol Scand.* 1960;50:269-86.

69. Christmass MA, Dawson B, Arthur PG. Effect of work and recovery duration on skeletal muscle oxygenation and fuel use during sustained intermittent exercise. *Eur J Appl Physiol Occup Physiol.* 1999;80:436-47.

70. Christmass MA, Dawson B, Passeretto P, Arthur PG. A comparison of skeletal muscle oxygenation and fuel use in sustained continuous and intermittent exercise. *Eur J Appl Physiol.* 1999;80:423-35.

71. Clemente FM, Martins FM, Mendes RS. Developing aerobic and anaerobic fitness using small-sided soccer games: Methodological proposals. *Strength Cond J.* 2014;36:76-87.

72. http://expertise-performance.u-bourgogne.fr/pdf/lactate.pdf. Accessed January 19, 2012.

73. Corvino M, Tessitore A, Minganti C, Šibila M. Effect of court dimensions on players' external and internal load during small-sided handball games *J Sports Sci & Med.* 2014;13:297-303.

74. Dellal A, Keller D, Carling C, Chaouachi A, Wong DP, Chamari K. Physiologic effects of directional changes in intermittent exercise in soccer players. *J Strength Cond Res.* 2010;24:3219-26.

75. Dellal A, Lago-Penas C, Wong del P, Chamari K. Effect of the number of ball contacts within bouts of 4 vs. 4 small-sided soccer games. *Int J Sports Physiol Perform.* 2011;6:322-33.

76. Demarie S, Koralsztein JP, Billat V. Time limit and time at VO2max during a continuous and an intermittent run. *J Sports Med Phys Fitness.* 2000;40:96-102.

77. Di Michele R, Del Curto L, Merni F. Mechanical and metabolic responses during a high-intensity circuit training workout in competitive runners. *J Sports Med Phys Fitness.* 2012;52:33-9.

78. di Prampero PE, Fusi S, Sepulcri L, Morin JB, Belli A, Antonutto G. Sprint running: A new energetic approach. *J Exp Biol.* 2005;208:2809-16.

79. Dorado C, Sanchis-Moysi J, Calbet JA. Effects of recovery mode on performance, O2 uptake, and O2 deficit during high-intensity intermittent exercise. *Can J Appl Physiol.* 2004;29:227-44.

80. Dupont G, Akakpo K, Berthoin S. The effect of in-season, high-intensity interval training in soccer players. *J Strength Cond Res.* 2004;18:584-9.

81. Dupont G, Berthoin S. Time spent at a high percentage of VO2max for short intermittent runs: Active versus passive recovery. *Can J Appl Physiol.* 2004;29(Suppl):S3–S16.

82. Dupont G, Blondel N, Berthoin S. Performance for short intermittent runs: Active recovery vs. passive recovery. *Eur J Appl Physiol*. 2003;89:548-54.

83. Dupont G, Blondel N, Lensel G, Berthoin S. Critical velocity and time spent at a high level of VO2 for short intermittent runs at supramaximal velocities. *Can J Appl Physiol*. 2002;27:103-15.

84. Dupont G, Millet GP, Guinhouya C, Berthoin S. Relationship between oxygen uptake kinetics and performance in repeated running sprints. *Eur J Appl Physiol*. 2005;95:27-34.

85. Dupont G, Moalla W, Guinhouya C, Ahmaidi S, Berthoin S. Passive versus active recovery during high-intensity intermittent exercises. *Med Sci Sports Exerc*. 2004;36:302-8.

86. Enoka RM, Stuart DG. Neurobiology of muscle fatigue. *J Appl Physiol*. 1992;72:1631-48.

87. Fernandez-Del-Olmo M, Rodriguez FA, Marquez G, Iglesias X, Marina M, Benitez A, et al. Isometric knee extensor fatigue following a Wingate test: Peripheral and central mechanisms. *Scand J Med Sci Sports*. 2013;23(1):57-65

88. Gabbett TJ, Ullah S. Relationship between running loads and soft-tissue injury in elite team sport athletes. *J Strength Cond Res*. 2012;26(4):953-60.

89. Gaitanos GC, Williams C, Boobis LH, Brooks S. Human muscle metabolism during intermittent maximal exercise. *J Appl Physiol*. 1993;75:712-19.

90. Gajer B, Hanon C, Lehenaff D, Vollmer JC. Analyse comparée de différentes séances de développement de V̇O₂max. In *Expertise et sport de haut niveau: actes des Entretiens de l'INSEP, Novembre 2002*. Paris: Institut national du sport et d l'éducation pysique; 2002.

91. Gastin PB. Energy system interaction and relative contribution during maximal exercise. *Sports Med*. 2001;31:725-41.

92. Gaudino P, Gaudino C, Alberti G, Minetti AE. Biomechanics and predicted energetics of sprinting on sand: Hints for soccer training. *J Sci Med Sport*. 2013;16:271-5.

93. Gerbino A, Ward SA, Whipp BJ. Effects of prior exercise on pulmonary gas-exchange kinetics during high-intensity exercise in humans. *J Appl Physiol*. 1996;80:99-107.

94. Gibala MJ, McGee SL. Metabolic adaptations to short-term high-intensity interval training: a little pain for a lot of gain? *Exerc Sport Sci Rev*. 2008;36:58-63.

95. Girard O, Mendez-Villanueva A, Bishop D. Repeated-sprint ability. Part I: Factors contributing to fatigue. *Sports Med*. 2011;41:673-94.

96. Girard O, Micallef JP, Millet GP. Changes in spring-mass model characteristics during repeated running sprints. *Eur J Appl Physiol*. 2011;111:125-34.

97. Gollnick PD, Piehl K, Saltin B. Selective glycogen depletion pattern in human muscle fibres after exercise of varying intensity and at varying pedalling rates. *J Physiol*. 1974;241:45-57.

98. Gollnick PD, Piehl K, Saltin B. Selective glycogen depletion pattern in human muscle fibres after exercise of varying intensity and at varying pedalling rates. *J Physiol*. 1974;241:45-57.

99. Gorostiaga EM, Asiain X, Izquierdo M, Postigo A, Aguado R, Alonso JM, et al. Vertical jump performance and blood ammonia and lactate levels during typical training sessions in elite 400-m runners. *J Strength Cond Res*. 2010;24:1138-49.

100. Gottschall JS, Kram R. Ground reaction forces during downhill and uphill running. *J Biomech*. 2005;38:445-52.

101. Hader K, Mendez-Villanueva A, Williams B, Ahmaidi S, Buchheit M. Changes of direction during high-intensity intermittent runs: Neuromuscular and metabolic responses. *BMC Sports Sci Med Rehabil*. 2014;6:2.

102. Harling SA, Tong RJ, Mickleborough TD. The oxygen uptake response running to exhaustion at peak treadmill speed. *Med Sci Sports Exerc*. 2003;35:663-8.

103. Harris RC, Edwards RH, Hultman E, Nordesjo LO, Nylind B, Sahlin K. The time course of phosphorylcreatine resynthesis during recovery of the quadriceps muscle in man. *Pflugers Arch*. 1976;367:137-42.

104. Haydar B, Al Haddad H, Buchheit M. Assessing inter-efforts recovery and change of direction abilities with the 30-15 Intermittent Fitness Test. *J Sports Sci Med*. 2011;10:346-54.

105. Hetlelid KJ, Plews DJ, Herold E, Laursen PB, Sieler S. Rethinking the role of fat oxidation: Substrate utilisation during high-intensity

interval training in well-trained and recreationally trained runners. *BMJ Open Sport & Exercise Medicine.* 2015;1(1):e000047.

106. Higashihara A, Ono T, Kubota J, Okuwaki T, Fukubayashi T. Functional differences in the activity of the hamstring muscles with increasing running speed. *J Sports Sci.* 2010;28:1085-92.

107. Hill DW, Halcomb JN, Stevens EC. Oxygen uptake kinetics during severe intensity running and cycling. *Eur J Appl Physiol.* 2003;89:612-18.

108. Hill DW, Rowell AL. Responses to exercise at the velocity associated with VO2max. *Med Sci Sports Exerc.* 1997;29:113-16.

109. Hill DW, Stevens EC. VO2 response profiles in severe intensity exercise. *J Sports Med Phys Fitness.* 2005;45:239-47.

110. Hill DW, Williams CS, Burt SE. Responses to exercise at 92% and 100% of the velocity associated with VO2max. *Int J Sports Med.* 1997;18:325-9.

111. Hill-Haas SV, Coutts AJ, Dawson BT, Rowsell GJ. Time-motion characteristics and physiological responses of small-sided games in elite youth players: The influence of player number and rule changes. *J Strength Cond Res.* 2010;24:2149-56.

112. Hill-Haas SV, Dawson B, Impellizzeri FM, Coutts AJ. Physiology of small-sided games training in football: A systematic review. *Sports Med.* 2011;41:199-220.

113. Hodgson M, Docherty D, Robbins D. Postactivation potentiation: Underlying physiology and implications for motor performance. *Sports Med.* 2005;35:585-95.

114. Hughson RL, O'Leary DD, Betik AC, Hebestreit H. Kinetics of oxygen uptake at the onset of exercise near or above peak oxygen uptake. *J Appl Physiol.* 2000;88:1812-19.

115. Iaia FM, Bangsbo J. Speed endurance training is a powerful stimulus for physiological adaptations and performance improvements of athletes. *Scand J Med Sci Sports.* 2010;20(Suppl 2):11-23.

116. Impellizzeri FM, Marcora SM, Castagna C, Reilly T, Sassi A, Iaia FM, et al. Physiological and performance effects of generic versus specific aerobic training in soccer players. *Int J Sports Med.* 2006;27:483-92.

117. Karcher C, Buchheit M. On-court demands of elite handball, with special reference to playing positions. *Sports Med.* 2014;44:797-814.

118. Kilding AE, Winter EM, Fysh M. A comparison of pulmonary oxygen uptake kinetics in middle- and long-distance runners. *Int J Sports Med.* 2006;27:419-26.

119. Lakomy J, Haydon DT. The effects of enforced, rapid deceleration on performance in a multiple sprint test. *J Strength Cond Res.* 2004;18:579-83.

120. Lattier G, Millet GY, Martin A, Martin V. Fatigue and recovery after high-intensity exercise. Part I: Neuromuscular fatigue. *Int J Sports Med.* 2004;25:450-6.

121. Laursen PB, Jenkins DG. The scientific basis for high-intensity interval training: Optimising training programmes and maximising performance in highly trained endurance athletes. *Sports Med.* 2002;32:53-73.

122. Laursen PB, Rhodes EC, Langill RH, McKenzie DC, Taunton JE. Relationship of exercise test variables to cycling performance in an Ironman triathlon. *Eur J Appl Physiol.* 2002;87:433-40.

123. Laursen PB, Shing CM, Jenkins DG. Temporal aspects of the VO2 response at the power output associated with VO2peak in well trained cyclists–implications for interval training prescription. *Res Q Exerc Sport.* 2004;75:423-8.

124. Little T. Optimizing the use of soccer drills for physiological development. *Strength Cond J.* 2009;31:67-74.

125. Little T, Williams AG. Effects of sprint duration and exercise: Rest ratio on repeated sprint performance and physiological responses in professional soccer players. *J Strength Cond Res.* 2007;21:646-8.

126. Little T, Williams AG. Measures of exercise intensity during soccer training drills with professional soccer players. *J Strength Cond Res.* 2007;21:367-71.

127. McCartney N, Spriet LL, Heigenhauser GJ, Kowalchuk JM, Sutton JR, Jones NL. Muscle power and metabolism in maximal intermittent exercise. *J Appl Physiol.* 1986;60:1164-9.

128. McCartney N, Spriet LL, Heigenhauser GJ, Kowalchuk JM, Sutton JR, Jones NL. Muscle power and metabolism in maximal intermittent exercise. *J Appl Physiol (1985).* 1986;60:1164-9.

129. Medbo JI, Mohn AC, Tabata I, Bahr R, Vaage O, Sejersted OM. Anaerobic capacity determined

by maximal accumulated O2 deficit. *J Appl Physiol.* 1988;64:50-60.

130. Mendez-Villanueva A, Buchheit M, Simpson BM, Bourdon PC. Match play intensity distribution in youth soccer. *Int J Sport Med.* 2012;34(2):101-10.

131. Mendez-Villanueva A, Hamer P, Bishop D. Fatigue responses during repeated sprints matched for initial mechanical output. *Med Sci Sports Exerc.* 2007;39:2219-25.

132. Midgley AW, Mc Naughton LR. Time at or near VO2max during continuous and intermittent running. A review with special reference to considerations for the optimisation of training protocols to elicit the longest time at or near VO2max. *J Sports Med Phys Fitness.* 2006;46:1-14.

133. Midgley AW, McNaughton LR, Carroll S. Physiological determinants of time to exhaustion during intermittent treadmill running at vV̇O(2max). *Int J Sports Med.* 2007;28:273-80.

134. Midgley AW, McNaughton LR, Carroll S. Reproducibility of time at or near VO2max during intermittent treadmill running. *Int J Sports Med.* 2007;28:40-7.

135. Midgley AW, McNaughton LR, Carroll S. Time at VO2max during intermittent treadmill running: Test protocol dependent or methodological artefact? *Int J Sports Med.* 2007;28:934-9.

136. Millet GP, Candau R, Fattori P, Bignet F, Varray A. VO$_2$ responses to different intermittent runs at velocity associated with VO2max. *Can J Appl Physiol.* 2003;28:410-23.

137. Millet GP, Libicz S, Borrani F, Fattori P, Bignet F, Candau R. Effects of increased intensity of intermittent training in runners with differing VO2 kinetics. *Eur J Appl Physiol.* 2003;90:50-7.

138. Minetti AE, Moia C, Roi GS, Susta D, Ferretti G. Energy cost of walking and running at extreme uphill and downhill slopes. *J Appl Physiol.* 2002;93:1039-46.

139. Mooney M, O'Brien B, Cormack S, Coutts A, Berry J, Young W. The relationship between physical capacity and match performance in elite Australian football: A mediation approach. *J Sci Med Sport.* 2011;14:447-52.

140. Nakamura FY, Soares-Caldeira LF, Laursen PB, Polito MD, Leme LC, Buchheit M. Cardiac autonomic responses to repeated shuttle sprints. *Int J Sports Med.* 2009;30:808-13.

141. Ngo JK, Tsui MC, Smith AW, Carling C, Chan GS, Wong del P. The effects of man-marking on work intensity in small-sided soccer games. *J Sports Sci Med.* 2012;11:109-14.

142. Nimmerichter A, Eston R, Bachl N, Williams C. Effects of low and high cadence interval training on power output in flat and uphill cycling time-trials. *Eur J Appl Physiol.* 2012;112:69-78.

143. Norris SR, Petersen SR. Effects of endurance training on transient oxygen uptake responses in cyclists. *J Sports Sci.* 1998;16:733-8.

144. Nummela A, Vuorimaa T, Rusko H. Changes in force production, blood lactate and EMG activity in the 400-m sprint. *J Sports Sci.* 1992;10:217-28.

145. Oliver JL. Is a fatigue index a worthwhile measure of repeated sprint ability? *J Sci Med Sport.* 2009;12:20-3.

146. Omeyer C, Buchheit M. Vertical jump performance in response to different high-intensity running sessions. In: *Faculté des sciences du sport (STAPS)*. Strasbourg, 2002.

147. Opar DA, Williams MD, and Shield AJ. Hamstring strain injuries: Factors that lead to injury and re-injury. *Sports Med.* 2012;42:209-26.

148. Osgnach C, Poser S, Bernardini R, Rinaldo R, di Prampero PE. Energy cost and metabolic power in elite soccer: A new match analysis approach. *Med Sci Sports Exerc.* 2010;42:170-8.

149. Paavolainen L, Nummela A, Rusko H. Muscle power factors and VO2max as determinants of horizontal and uphill running performance. *Scand J Med Sci Sports.* 2000;10:286-91.

150. Parolin ML, Chesley A, Matsos MP, Spriet LL, Jones NL, Heigenhauser GJ. Regulation of skeletal muscle glycogen phosphorylase and PDH during maximal intermittent exercise. *Am J Physiol.* 1999;277:E890-900.

151. Perrey S, Racinais S, Saimouaa K, Girard O. Neural and muscular adjustments following repeated running sprints. *Eur J Appl Physiol.* 2010;109(6):1027-36.

152. Pringle JS, Carter H, Doust JH, Jones AM. Oxygen uptake kinetics during horizontal and uphill treadmill running in humans. *Eur J Appl Physiol.* 2002;88:163-9.

153. Pringle JS, Doust JH, Carter H, Tolfrey K, Campbell IT, Sakkas GK, et al. Oxygen uptake kinetics during moderate, heavy and severe intensity "submaximal" exercise in humans: the

influence of muscle fibre type and capillarisation. *Eur J Appl Physiol.* 2003;89:289-300.

154. Pugh LG. The influence of wind resistance in running and walking and the mechanical efficiency of work against horizontal or vertical forces. *J Physiol.* 1971;213:255-76.

155. Putman CT, Jones NL, Lands LC, Bragg TM, Hollidge-Horvat MG, Heigenhauser GJ. Skeletal muscle pyruvate dehydrogenase activity during maximal exercise in humans. *Am J Physiol.* 1995;269:E458-68.

156. Rampinini E, Impellizzeri FM, Castagna C, Abt G, Chamari K, Sassi A, et al. Factors influencing physiological responses to small-sided soccer games. *J Sports Sci.* 2007;25:659-66.

157. Rebelo AN, Silva P, Rago V, Barreira D, Krustrup P. Differences in strength and speed demands between 4v4 and 8v8 small-sided football games. *J Sports Sci.* 2016;34:2246-54.

158. Ross A, Leveritt M, Riek S. Neural influences on sprint running: Training adaptations and acute responses. *Sports Med.* 2001;31:409-25.

159. Rozenek R, Funato K, Kubo J, Hoshikawa M, Matsuo A. Physiological responses to interval training sessions at velocities associated with VO2max. *J Strength Cond Res.* 2007;21:188-92.

160. Rusko H, Nummela A, Mero A. A new method for the evaluation of anaerobic running power in athletes. *Eur J Appl Physiol.* 1993;66:97-101.

161. Rusko HK, Tikkanen HO, Peltonen JE. Altitude and endurance training. *J Sports Sci.* 2004;22:928-44; discussion 945.

162. Seiler S, Hetlelid KJ. The impact of rest duration on work intensity and RPE during interval training. *Med Sci Sports Exerc.* 2005;37:1601-7.

163. Seiler S, Sjursen JE. Effect of work duration on physiological and rating scale of perceived exertion responses during self-paced interval training. *Scand J Med Sci Sports.* 2004;14:318-25.

164. Skof B, Strojnik V. Neuro-muscular fatigue and recovery dynamics following anaerobic interval workload. *Int J Sports Med.* 2006;27:220-5.

165. Slawinski J, Dorel S, Hug F, Couturier A, Fournel V, Morin JB, et al. Elite long sprint running: A comparison between incline and level training sessions. *Med Sci Sports Exerc.* 2008;40:1155-62.

166. Small K, McNaughton LR, Greig M, Lohkamp M, Lovell R. Soccer fatigue, sprinting and hamstring injury risk. *Int J Sports Med.* 2009;30:573-8.

167. Smith TP, Coombes JS, Geraghty DP. Optimising high-intensity treadmill training using the running speed at maximal O(2) uptake and the time for which this can be maintained. *Eur J Appl Physiol.* 2003;89:337-43.

168. Smith TP, McNaughton LR, Marshall KJ. Effects of 4-wk training using Vmax/Tmax on VO2max and performance in athletes. *Med Sci Sports Exerc.* 1999;31:892-6.

169. Stepto NK, Hawley JA, Dennis SC, Hopkins WG. Effects of different interval-training programs on cycling time-trial performance. *Med Sci Sports Exerc.* 1998;31:736-41.

170. Stepto NK, Martin DT, Fallon KE, Hawley JA. Metabolic demands of intense aerobic interval training in competitive cyclists. *Med Sci Sports Exerc.* 2001;33:303-10.

171. Stratton G, Reilly T, Williams AM, Richardson D. *Youth Soccer: From Science to Performance.* London: Routledge; 2004.

172. Tabata I, Irisawa K, Kouzaki M, Nishimura K, Ogita F, Miyachi M. Metabolic profile of high intensity intermittent exercises. *Med Sci Sports Exerc.* 1997;29:390-5.

173. Tardieu-Berger M, Thevenet D, Zouhal H, Prioux J. Effects of active recovery between series on performance during an intermittent exercise model in young endurance athletes. *Eur J Appl Physiol.* 2004;93:145-52.

174. Thevenet D, Leclair E, Tardieu-Berger M, Berthoin S, Regueme S, and Prioux J. Influence of recovery intensity on time spent at maximal oxygen uptake during an intermittent session in young, endurance-trained athletes. *J Sports Sci.* 2008;26:1313-21.

175. Thevenet D, Tardieu M, Zouhal H, Jacob C, Abderrahman BA, Prioux J. Influence of exercise intensity on time spent at high percentage of maximal oxygen uptake during an intermittent session in young endurance-trained athletes. *Eur J Appl Physiol.* 2007;102:19-26.

176. Thevenet D, Tardieu-Berger M, Berthoin S, Prioux J. Influence of recovery mode (passive vs. active) on time spent at maximal oxygen uptake during an intermittent session in young and endurance-trained athletes. *Eur J Appl Physiol.* 2007;99:133-42.

177. Tomazin K, Morin JB, Strojnik V, Podpecan A, Millet GY. Fatigue after short (100-m), medium (200-m) and long (400-m) treadmill sprints. *Eur J Appl Physiol*: [Epub ahead of print], 2011.

178. van Beijsterveldt AM, van de Port IG, Vereijken AJ, Backx FJ. Risk factors for hamstring injuries in male soccer players: A systematic review of prospective studies. *Scand J Med Sci Sports*. 2013;23(3):253-62.

179. Vuorimaa T, Hakkinen K, Vahasoyrinki P, Rusko H. Comparison of three maximal anaerobic running test protocols in marathon runners, middle-distance runners and sprinters. *Int J Sports Med*. 1996;17(Suppl 2): S109-13.

180. Vuorimaa T, Vasankari T, Rusko H. Comparison of physiological strain and muscular performance of athletes during two intermittent running exercises at the velocity associated with VO2max. *Int J Sports Med*. 2000;21:96-101.

181. Wakefield BR, Glaister M. Influence of work-interval intensity and duration on time spent at a high percentage of VO2max during intermittent supramaximal exercise. *J Strength Cond Res*. 2009;23:2548-54.

182. Clemente FM, Lourenco Martins FM, Mendes RS. Developing aerobic and anaerobic fitness using small-sided soccer games methodological proposals. *Strength Cond J*. 2014;36(3):76-87.

183. Impey SG, Hammond KM, Shepherd SO, Sharples AP, Stewart C, Limb M, et al. Fuel for the work required: A practical approach to amalgamating train-low paradigms for endurance athletes. *Physiol Rep*. 2016;4(10).

184. Impey SG, Hearris MA, Hammond KM, Bartlett JD, Louis J, Close GL, et al. Fuel for the work required: A theoretical framework for carbohydrate periodization and the glycogen threshold hypothesis. *Sports Med*. 2018;48(5):1031-48.

185. Vernillo G, Giandolini M, Edwards WB, Morin JB, Samozino P, Horvais N, et al. Biomechanics and physiology of uphill and downhill running. *Sports Med*. 2017;47(4):615-29.

Chapter 6

1. Aagaard P, Andersen JL. Effects of strength training on endurance capacity in top-level endurance athletes. *Scand J Med Sci Sports*. 2010;20(Suppl 2):39-47.

2. Abernethy PJ. Influence of acute endurance activity on isokinetic strength. *J Strength Cond Res*. 1993;7:141-6.

3. Apro W, Moberg M, Hamilton DL, Ekblom B, van Hall G, Holmberg HC, et al. Resistance exercise-induced S6K1 kinase activity is not inhibited in human skeletal muscle despite prior activation of AMPK by high-intensity interval cycling. *Am J Physiol Endocrinol Metab*. 2015;308(6):E470-81.

4. Areta JL, Burke LM, Ross ML, Camera DM, West DW, Broad EM, et al. Timing and distribution of protein ingestion during prolonged recovery from resistance exercise alters myofibrillar protein synthesis. *J Physiol*. 2013;591(Pt 9):2319-31.

5. Atherton PJ, Babraj J, Smith K, Singh J, Rennie MJ, Wackerhage H. Selective activation of AMPK-PGC-1alpha or PKB-TSC2-mTOR signaling can explain specific adaptive responses to endurance or resistance training-like electrical muscle stimulation. *FASEB J*. 2005;19(7):786-8.

6. Baar K. Using molecular biology to maximize concurrent training. *Sports Med*. 2014;44(Suppl 2):S117-25.

7. Balabinis CP, Psarakis CH, Moukas M, Vassiliou MP, Behrakis PK. Early phase changes by concurrent endurance and strength training. *J Strength Cond Res*. 2003;17(2):393-401.

8. Bartlett JD, Hawley JA, Morton JP. Carbohydrate availability and exercise training adaptation: Too much of a good thing? *Eur J Sport Sci*. 2015;15(1):3-12.

9. Bell GJ, Syrotuik D, Martin TP, Burnham R, Quinney HA. Effect of concurrent strength and endurance training on skeletal muscle properties and hormone concentrations in humans. *Eur J Appl Physiol*. 2000;81(5):418-27.

10. Bentley DJ, Zhou S, Davie AJ. The effect of endurance exercise on muscle force generating capacity of the lower limbs. *J Sci Med Sport*. 1998;1(3):179-88.

11. Bentley DJ, Smith PA, Davie AJ, Zhou S. Muscle activation of the knee extensors following high intensity endurance exercise in cyclists. *Eur J Appl Physiol*. 2000;81(4):297-302.

12. Bergstrom J, Hermansen L, Hultman E, Saltin B. Diet, muscle glycogen and physical performance. *Acta Physiol Scand*. 1967;71(2):140-50.

13. Buchheit M, Laursen PB. High-intensity interval training, solutions to the programming puzzle: Part II: Anaerobic energy, neuromuscular load

and practical applications. *Sports Med.* 2013;43(10):927-54.

14. Buchheit M, Kuitunen S, Voss SC, Williams BK, Mendez-Villanueva A, Bourdon PC. Physiological strain associated with high-intensity hypoxic intervals in highly trained young runners. *J Strength Cond Res.* 2012;26(1):94-105.

15. Buckner SL, Dankel SJ, Mattocks KT, Jessee MB, Mouser JG, Counts BR, et al. The problem of muscle hypertrophy: revisited. *Muscle Nerve.* 2016;54(6):1012-14.

16. Burke LM, Hawley JA, Wong SH, Jeukendrup AE. Carbohydrates for training and competition. *J Sports Sci.* 2011;29(Suppl 1):S17-27.

17. Burt DG, Twist C. The effects of exercise-induced muscle damage on cycling time-trial performance. *J Strength Cond Res.* 2011;25(8):2185-92.

18. Bush JE, Plews DJ, Kilding AE, Olsen R, Laursen PB. Cardiac autonomic recovery and high-intensity interval training performance following strength training in elite sprint endurance athletes: implications for concurrent training. SPort INnovation (SPIN) Summit; October 4-6; Richmond, British Columbia, 2017.

19. Camera DM, West DW, Burd NA, Phillips SM, Garnham AP, Hawley JA, et al. Low muscle glycogen concentration does not suppress the anabolic response to resistance exercise. *J Appl Physiol.* 2012;113(2):206-14.

20. Cantrell GS, Schilling BK, Paquette MR, Murlasits Z. Maximal strength, power, and aerobic endurance adaptations to concurrent strength and sprint interval training. *Eur J Appl Physiol.* 2014;114(4):763-71.

21. Chtara M, Chamari K, Chaouachi M, Chaouachi A, Koubaa D, Feki Y, et al. Effects of intra-session concurrent endurance and strength training sequence on aerobic performance and capacity. *Br J Sports Med.* 2005;39(8):555-60.

22. Coffey VG, Hawley JA. Concurrent exercise training: do opposites distract? *J Physiol.* 2016;595(9):2883-96.

23. Cormie P, McGuigan MR, Newton RU. Developing maximal neuromuscular power: Part 1: Biological basis of maximal power production. *Sports Med.* 2011;41(1):17-38.

24. Craig B, Lucas J, Pohlman R. Effects of running, weightlifting and a combination of both on

growth hormone release. *J Appl Sport Sci Res.* 1991;5:198-203.

25. Davis JK, Green JM. Caffeine and anaerobic performance: Ergogenic value and mechanisms of action. *Sports Med.* 2009;39(10):813-32.

26. Davis WJ, Wood DT, Andrews RG, Elkind LM, Davis WB. Concurrent training enhances athletes' strength, muscle endurance, and other measures. *J Strength Cond Res.* 2008;22(5):1487-502.

27. de Salles Painelli V, Alves VT, Ugrinowitsch C, Benatti FB, Artioli GG, Lancha AH, Jr., et al. Creatine supplementation prevents acute strength loss induced by concurrent exercise. *Eur J Appl Physiol.* 2014;114(8):1749-55.

28. de Souza EO, Tricoli V, Franchini E, Paulo AC, Regazzini M, Ugrinowitsch C. Acute effect of two aerobic exercise modes on maximum strength and strength endurance. *J Strength Cond Res.* 2007;21(4):1286-90.

29. Di Donato DM, West DW, Churchward-Venne TA, Breen L, Baker SK, Phillips SM. Influence of aerobic exercise intensity on myofibrillar and mitochondrial protein synthesis in young men during early and late postexercise recovery. *Am J Physiol Endocrinol Metab.* 2014;306(9):E1025-32.

30. Dolezal BA, Potteiger JA. Concurrent resistance and endurance training influence basal metabolic rate in nondieting individuals. *J Appl Physiol.* 1998;85(2):695-700.

31. Doma K, Deakin GB. The effects of combined strength and endurance training on running performance the following day. *Int J Sport Health Sci.* 2013;11:1-9.

32. Doma K, Deakin GB, Bentley DJ. Implications of impaired endurance performance following single bouts of resistance training: An alternate concurrent training perspective. *Sports Med.* 2017;47(11): 2187-200.

33. Doncaster GG, Twist C. Exercise-induced muscle damage from bench press exercise impairs arm cranking endurance performance. *Eur J Appl Physiol.* 2012;112(12):4135-42.

34. Dudley GA, Djamil R. Incompatibility of endurance- and strength-training modes of exercise. *J Appl Physiol.* 1985;59(5):1446-51.

35. Egan B, Zierath JR. Exercise metabolism and the molecular regulation of skeletal muscle adaptation. *Cell Metab.* 2013;17(2):162-84.

36. Fyfe JJ, Bishop DJ, Stepto NK. Interference between concurrent resistance and endurance exercise: Molecular bases and the role of individual training variables. *Sports Med.* 2014;44(6):743-62.

37. Fyfe JJ, Bishop DJ, Zacharewicz E, Russell AP, Stepto NK. Concurrent exercise incorporating high-intensity interval or continuous training modulates mTORC1 signalling and microRNA expression in human skeletal muscle. *Am J Physiol Regul Integr Comp Physiol.* 2016;310(11):R1297-311.

38. Fyfe JJ, Bartlett JD, Hanson ED, Stepto NK, Bishop DJ. Endurance training intensity does not mediate interference to maximal lower-body strength gain during short-term concurrent training. *Front Physiol.* 2016;Nov 3;7(487).

39. Glowacki SP, Martin SE, Maurer A, Baek W, Green JS, Crouse SF. Effects of resistance, endurance, and concurrent exercise on training outcomes in men. *Med Sci Sports Exerc.* 2004;36(12):2119-27.

40. Glynn EL, Fry CS, Drummond MJ, Dreyer HC, Dhanani S, Volpi E, et al. Muscle protein breakdown has a minor role in the protein anabolic response to essential amino acid and carbohydrate intake following resistance exercise. *Am J Physiol Regul Integr Comp Physiol.* 2010;299(2):R533-40.

41. Häkkinen K, Alen M, Kraemer WJ, Gorostiaga E, Izquierdo M, Rusko H, et al. Neuromuscular adaptations during concurrent strength and endurance training versus strength training. *Eur J Appl Physiol.* 2003;89(1):42-52.

42. Hamilton DL, Philp A. Can AMPK mediated suppression of mTORC1 explain the concurrent training effect? *Cel Mol Ex Physiol.* 2013;2(1).

43. Harber MP, Konopka AR, Douglass MD, Minchev K, Kaminsky LA, Trappe TA, et al. Aerobic exercise training improves whole muscle and single myofiber size and function in older women. *Am J Physiol Regul Integr Comp Physiol.* 2009;297(5):R1452-9.

44. Harber MP, Konopka AR, Undem MK, Hinkley JM, Minchev K, Kaminsky LA, et al. Aerobic exercise training induces skeletal muscle hypertrophy and age-dependent adaptations in myofiber function in young and older men. *J Appl Physiol (1985).* 2012;113(9):1495-504.

45. Hawley JA. Molecular responses to strength and endurance training: Are they incompatible? *Appl Physiol Nutr Metab.* 2009;34(3):355-61.

46. Hennessy L, Watson A. The interference effects of training for strength and endurance simultaneously. *J Strength Cond Res.* 1994;12:9-12.

47. Hickson RC. Interference of strength development by simultaneously training for strength and endurance. *Eur J Appl Physiol Occup Physiol.* 1980;45(2-3):255-63.

48. Hickson RC, Rosenkoetter MA, Brown MM. Strength training effects on aerobic power and short-term endurance. *Med Sci Sports Exerc.* 1980;12(5):336-9.

49. Hodgson M, Docherty D, Robbins D. Post-activation potentiation: Underlying physiology and implications for motor performance. *Sports Med.* 2005;35(7):585-95.

50. Hoff J, Helgerud J. Endurance and strength training for soccer players: Physiological considerations. *Sports Med.* 2004;34(3):165-80.

51. Hood DA, Tryon LD, Carter HN, Kim Y, Chen CC. Unravelling the mechanisms regulating muscle mitochondrial biogenesis. *Biochem J.* 2016;473(15):2295-314.

52. Howarth KR, Phillips SM, MacDonald MJ, Richards D, Moreau NA, Gibala MJ. Effect of glycogen availability on human skeletal muscle protein turnover during exercise and recovery. *J Appl Physiol (1985).* 2010;109(2):431-8.

53. Hunter G, Demment R, Miller D. Development of strength and maximum oxygen uptake during simultaneous training for strength and endurance. *J Sports Med Phys Fitness.* 1987;27:269-75.

54. Inoki K, Zhu T, Guan KL. TSC2 mediates cellular energy response to control cell growth and survival. *Cell.* 2003;115(5):577-90.

55. Jones TW, Howatson G, Russell M, French DN. Performance and neuromuscular adaptations following differing ratios of concurrent strength and endurance training. *J Strength Cond Res.* 2013;27(12):3342-51.

56. Kazior Z, Willis SJ, Moberg M, Apro W, Calbet JA, Holmberg HC, et al. Endurance exercise enhances the effect of strength training on muscle fiber size and protein expression of Akt and mTOR. *PLoS One.* 2016;11(2):e0149082.

57. Kraemer WJ, Patton JF, Gordon SE, Harman EA, Deschenes MR, Reynolds K, et al. Compatibility of high-intensity strength and endurance training on hormonal and skeletal muscle adaptations. *J Appl Physiol (1985)*. 1995;78(3):976-89.

58. Kreider RB, Kalman DS, Antonio J, Ziegenfuss TN, Wildman R, Collins R, et al. International Society of Sports Nutrition position stand: Safety and efficacy of creatine supplementation in exercise, sport, and medicine. *J Int Soc Sports Nutr*. 2017;14:18.

59. Lemos A, Simao R, Polito M, Salles B, Rhea MR, Alexander J. The acute influence of two intensities of aerobic exercise on strength training performance in elderly women. *J Strength Cond Res*. 2009;23(4):1252-7.

60. Lepers R, Hausswirth C, Maffiuletti N, Brisswalter J, van Hoecke J. Evidence of neuromuscular fatigue after prolonged cycling exercise. *Med Sci Sports Exerc*. 2000;32(11):1880-6.

61. Leveritt M, Abernethy P. Acute effects of high-intensity endurance exercise on subsequent resistance activity. *J Strength Cond Res*. 1999;13:47-51.

62. Leveritt M, MacLaughlin H, Abernethy PJ. Changes in leg strength 8 and 32 h after endurance exercise. *J Sports Sci*. 2000;18(11):865-71.

63. Leveritt M, Abernethy PJ, Barry BK, Logan PA. Concurrent strength and endurance training. A review. *Sports Med*. 1999;28(6):413-27.

64. Lovell R, Siegler JC, Knox M, Brennan S, Marshall PW. Acute neuromuscular and performance responses to Nordic hamstring exercises completed before or after football training. *J Sports Sci*. 2016;34(24):2286-94.

65. Lundberg TR, Fernandez-Gonzalo R, Gustafsson T, Tesch PA. Aerobic exercise alters skeletal muscle molecular responses to resistance exercise. *Med Sci Sports Exerc*. 2012;44(9):1680-8.

66. Lundberg TR, Fernandez-Gonzalo R, Gustafsson T, Tesch PA. Aerobic exercise does not compromise muscle hypertrophy response to short-term resistance training. *J Appl Physiol (1985)*. 2013;114(1):81-9.

67. Macnaughton LS, Wardle SL, Witard OC, McGlory C, Hamilton DL, Jeromson S, et al. The response of muscle protein synthesis following whole-body resistance exercise is greater following 40 g than 20 g of ingested whey protein. *Physiol Rep*. 2016;4(15).

68. Marcotte GR, West DW, Baar K. The molecular basis for load-induced skeletal muscle hypertrophy. *Calcif Tissue Int*. 2015;96(3):196-210.

69. Mascher H, Ekblom B, Rooyackers O, Blomstrand E. Enhanced rates of muscle protein synthesis and elevated mTOR signalling following endurance exercise in human subjects. *Acta Physiol (Oxf)*. 2011;202(2):175-84.

70. McCarthy JP, Pozniak MA, Agre JC. Neuromuscular adaptations to concurrent strength and endurance training. *Med Sci Sports Exerc*. 2002;34(3):511-9.

71. Millet GY, Lepers R. Alterations of neuromuscular function after prolonged running, cycling and skiing exercises. *Sports Med*. 2004;34(2):105-16.

72. Millward DJ, Bowtell JL, Pacy P, Rennie MJ. Physical activity, protein metabolism and protein requirements. *Proc Nutr Soc*. 1994;53(1):223-40.

73. Moore DR, Camera DM, Areta JL, Hawley JA. Beyond muscle hypertrophy: Why dietary protein is important for endurance athletes. *Appl Physiol Nutr Metab*. 2014;39(9):987-97.

74. Moritani T, deVries HA. Neural factors versus hypertrophy in the time course of muscle strength gain. *Am J Phys Med*. 1979;58(3):115-30.

75. Morton RW, Murphy KT, McKellar SR, Schoenfeld BJ, Henselmans M, Helms E, et al. A systematic review, meta-analysis and meta-regression of the effect of protein supplementation on resistance training-induced gains in muscle mass and strength in healthy adults. *Br J Sports Med*. 2018;52(6):376-84.

76. Murlasits Z, Kneffel Z, Thalib L. The physiological effects of concurrent strength and endurance training sequence: A systematic review and meta-analysis. *J Sports Sci*. 2018;36(11):1212-19.

77. Nader GA. Concurrent strength and endurance training: From molecules to man. *Med Sci Sports Exerc*. 2006;38(11):1965-70.

78. Nelson AG, Arnall DA, Loy SF, Silvester LJ, Conlee RK. Consequences of combining strength and endurance training regimens. *Phys Ther*. 1990;70(5):287-94.

79. Panissa VL, Tricoli VA, Julio UF, Ribeiro N, de Azevedo Neto RM, Carmo EC, et al. Acute effect of high-intensity aerobic exercise performed on treadmill and cycle ergometer on strength

performance. *J Strength Cond Res.* 2015;29(4):1077-82.

80. Perez-Schindler J, Hamilton DL, Moore DR, Baar K, Philp A. Nutritional strategies to support concurrent training. *Eur J Sport Sci.* 2015;15(1):41-52.

81. Perry CG, Lally J, Holloway GP, Heigenhauser GJ, Bonen A, Spriet LL. Repeated transient mRNA bursts precede increases in transcriptional and mitochondrial proteins during training in human skeletal muscle. *J Physiol.* 2010;588(Pt 23):4795-810.

82. Putman CT, Xu X, Gillies E, MacLean IM, Bell GJ. Effects of strength, endurance and combined training on myosin heavy chain content and fibre-type distribution in humans. *Eur J Appl Physiol.* 2004;92(4-5):376-84.

83. Ratamess NA, Kang J, Porfido TM, Ismaili CP, Selamie SN, Williams BD, et al. Acute resistance exercise performance is negatively impacted by prior aerobic endurance exercise. *J Strength Cond Res.* 2016;30(10):2667-81.

84. Res PT, Groen B, Pennings B, Beelen M, Wallis GA, Gijsen AP, et al. Protein ingestion before sleep improves postexercise overnight recovery. *Med Sci Sports Exerc.* 2012;44(8):1560-9.

85. Roberts LA, Raastad T, Markworth JF, Figueiredo VC, Egner IM, Shield A, et al. Post-exercise cold water immersion attenuates acute anabolic signalling and long-term adaptations in muscle to strength training. *J Physiol.* 2015;593(18):4285-301.

86. Robineau J, Babault N, Piscione J, Lacome M, Bigard AX. Specific training effects of concurrent aerobic and strength exercises depend on recovery duration. *J Strength Cond Res.* 2016;30(3):672-83.

87. Ronnestad BR, Mujika I. Optimizing strength training for running and cycling endurance performance: A review. *Scand J Med Sci Sports.* 2014;24(4):603-12.

88. Ronnestad BR, Hansen EA, Raastad T. High volume of endurance training impairs adaptations to 12 weeks of strength training in well-trained endurance athletes. *Eur J Appl Physiol.* 2012;112(4):1457-66.

89. Sale DG, Jacobs I, MacDougall JD, Garner S. Comparison of two regimens of concurrent strength and endurance training. *Med Sci Sports Exerc.* 1990;22(3):348-56.

90. Sands WA, McNeal JR, Murray SR, Stone MH. Dynamic compression enhances pressure-to-pain threshold in elite athlete recovery: Exploratory study. *J Strength Cond Res.* 2015;29(5):1263-72.

91. Snijders T, Res PT, Smeets JS, van Vliet S, van Kranenburg J, Maase K, et al. Protein ingestion before sleep increases muscle mass and strength gains during prolonged resistance-type exercise training in healthy young men. *J Nutr.* 2015;145(6):1178-84.

92. Sporer BC, Wenger HA. Effects of aerobic exercise on strength performance following various periods of recovery. *J Strength Cond Res.* 2003;17(4):638-44.

93. Staples AW, Burd NA, West DW, Currie KD, Atherton PJ, Moore DR, et al. Carbohydrate does not augment exercise-induced protein accretion versus protein alone. *Med Sci Sports Exerc.* 2011;43(7):1154-61.

94. Stephens JM, Halson S, Miller J, Slater GJ, Askew CD. Cold-water immersion for athletic recovery: One size does not fit all. *Int J Sports Physiol Perform.* 2017;12(1):2-9.

95. Suchomel TJ, Nimphius S, Stone MH. The importance of muscular strength in athletic performance. *Sports Med.* 2016;46(10):1419-49.

96. Tan JG, Coburn JW, Brown LE, Judelson DA. Effects of a single bout of lower-body aerobic exercise on muscle activation and performance during subsequent lower- and upper-body resistance exercise workouts. *J Strength Cond Res.* 2014;28(5):1235-40.

97. Tipton KD, Ferrando AA, Phillips SM, Doyle D, Jr., Wolfe RR. Postexercise net protein synthesis in human muscle from orally administered amino acids. *Am J Physiol.* 1999;276(4 Pt 1):E628-34.

98. van Wessel T, de Haan A, van der Laarse WJ, Jaspers RT. The muscle fiber type-fiber size paradox: Hypertrophy or oxidative metabolism? *Eur J Appl Physiol.* 2010;110(4):665-94.

99. Wilkinson SB, Phillips SM, Atherton PJ, Patel R, Yarasheski KE, Tarnopolsky MA, et al. Differential effects of resistance and endurance exercise in the fed state on signalling molecule phosphorylation and protein synthesis in human muscle. *J Physiol.* 2008;586(Pt 15):3701-17.

100. Wilson JM, Marin PJ, Rhea MR, Wilson SM, Loenneke JP, Anderson JC. Concurrent train-

ing: A meta-analysis examining interference of aerobic and resistance exercises. *J Strength Cond Res.* 2012;26(8):2293-307.

101. Zourdos MC, Dolan C, Quiles JM, Klemp A, Jo E, Loenneke JP, et al. Efficacy of daily one-repetition maximum training in well-trained powerlifters and weightlifters: A case series. *Nutricion Hospitalaria.* 2016;33(2):437-43.

Chapter 7

1. *Dietary Reference Intakes for Thiamin, Riboflavin, Niacin, Vitamin B6, Folate, Vitamin B12, Pantothenic Acid, Biotin, and Choline.* The National Academies Collection: Reports funded by National Institutes of Health. Washington, DC; 1998.

2. Ackland TR, Lohman TG, Sundgot-Borgen J, Maughan RJ, Meyer NL, Stewart AD, et al. Current status of body composition assessment in sport: Review and position statement on behalf of the ad hoc research working group on body composition health and performance, under the auspices of the I.O.C. Medical Commission. *Sports Med.* 2012;42(3):227-49.

3. Alaranta A, Alaranta H, Heliovaara M, Airaksinen M, Helenius I. Ample use of physician-prescribed medications in Finnish elite athletes. *Int J Sports Med.* 2006;27(11):919-25.

4. Alentorn-Geli E, Myer GD, Silvers HJ, Samitier G, Romero D, Lazaro-Haro C, et al. Prevention of non-contact anterior cruciate ligament injuries in soccer players. Part 1: Mechanisms of injury and underlying risk factors. *Knee Surg Sports Traumatol Arthrosc.* 2009;17(7):705-29.

5. Alshahrani F, Aljohani N. Vitamin D: Deficiency, sufficiency and toxicity. *Nutrients.* 2013;5(9):3605-16.

6. American Dietetic A, Dietitians of C, American College of Sports M, Rodriguez NR, Di Marco NM, Langley S. American College of Sports Medicine position stand. Nutrition and athletic performance. *Med Sci Sports Exerc.* 2009;41(3):709-31.

7. Angeli A, Minetto M, Dovio A, Paccotti P. The overtraining syndrome in athletes: A stress-related disorder. *J Endocrinol Invest.* 2004;27(6):603-12.

8. Aragon AA, Schoenfeld BJ, Wildman R, Kleiner S, VanDusseldorp T, Taylor L, et al. International society of sports nutrition position stand: Diets and body composition. *J Int Soc Sports Nutr.* 2017;14:16.

9. Armas LA, Hollis BW, Heaney RP. Vitamin D2 is much less effective than vitamin D3 in humans. *J Clin Endocrinol Metab.* 2004;89(11):5387-91.

10. Armstrong LE, Johnson EC, Kunces LJ, Ganio MS, Judelson DA, Kupchak BR, et al. Drinking to thirst versus drinking ad libitum during road cycling. *J Athl Train.* 2014;49(5):624-31.

11. Ashwell M, Hsieh SD. Six reasons why the waist-to-height ratio is a rapid and effective global indicator for health risks of obesity and how its use could simplify the international public health message on obesity. *Int J Food Sci Nutr.* 2005;56(5):303-7.

12. Asif IM, Harmon KG. Incidence and etiology of sudden cardiac death: New updates for athletic departments. *Sports Health.* 2017;9(3):268-79.

13. Aubry A, Hausswirth C, Louis J, Coutts AJ, Buchheit M, Le Meur Y. The development of functional overreaching is associated with a faster heart rate recovery in endurance athletes. *PLoS One.* 2015;10(10):e0139754.

14. Baguley B, Zilujko J, Leveritt MD, Desbrow B, Irwin C. The effect of ad libitum consumption of a milk-based liquid meal supplement vs. a traditional sports drink on fluid balance after exercise. *Int J Sport Nutr Exerc Metab.* 2016;26(4):347-55.

15. Bandegan A, Courtney-Martin G, Rafii M, Pencharz PB, Lemon PW. Indicator amino acid-derived estimate of dietary protein requirement for male bodybuilders on a nontraining day is several-fold greater than the current recommended dietary allowance. *J Nutr.* 2017;147(5):850-7.

16. Bartlett JD, Hawley JA, Morton JP. Carbohydrate availability and exercise training adaptation: Too much of a good thing? *Eur J Sport Sci.* 2015;15(1):3-12.

17. Bartolotto C. Does consuming sugar and artificial sweeteners change taste preferences? *Perm J.* 2015;19(3):81-4.

18. Beard J, Tobin B. Iron status and exercise. *Am J Clin Nutr.* 2000;72(Suppl 2):594S-7S.

19. Bernardis LL, Bellinger LL. The lateral hypothalamic area revisited: Ingestive behavior. *Neurosci Biobehav Rev.* 1996;20(2):189-287.

20. Bezard J, Blond JP, Bernard A, Clouet P. The metabolism and availability of essential fatty acids in animal and human tissues. *Reprod Nutr Dev.* 1994;34(6):539-68.

21. Bjelakovic G, Gluud LL, Nikolova D, Whitfield K, Wetterslev J, Simonetti RG, et al. Vitamin D supplementation for prevention of mortality in adults. *Cochrane Database Syst Rev.* 2014(1):CD007470.

22. Bonnavion P, Mickelsen LE, Fujita A, de Lecea L, Jackson AC. Hubs and spokes of the lateral hypothalamus: Cell types, circuits and behaviour. *J Physiol.* 2016;594(22):6443-62.

23. Brenna JT. Efficiency of conversion of alpha-linolenic acid to long chain n-3 fatty acids in man. *Curr Opin Clin Nutr Metab Care.* 2002;5(2):127-32.

24. Brooks KA, Carter JG. Overtraining, exercise and adrenal Insufficiency. *Novel Physiotherapies.* 2013;3(1).

25. Buchheit M. Monitoring training status with HR measures: Do all roads lead to Rome? *Front Physiol.* 2014;5:73.

26. Buchheit M, Simpson MB, Al Haddad H, Bourdon PC, Mendez-Villanueva A. Monitoring changes in physical performance with heart rate measures in young soccer players. *Eur J Appl Physiol.* 2012;112(2):711-23.

27. Buchheit M, Chivot A, Parouty J, Mercier D, Al Haddad H, Laursen PB, et al. Monitoring endurance running performance using cardiac parasympathetic function. *Eur J Appl Physiol.* 2010;108(6):1153-67.

28. Bueno NB, de Melo IS, de Oliveira SL, da Rocha Ataide T. Very-low-carbohydrate ketogenic diet v. low-fat diet for long-term weight loss: A meta-analysis of randomised controlled trials. *Br J Nutr.* 2013;110(7):1178-87.

29. Burke LM, Hawley JA, Wong SH, Jeukendrup AE. Carbohydrates for training and competition. *J Sports Sci.* 2011;29(Suppl 1):S17-27.

30. Burke LM, Slater G, Broad EM, Haukka J, Modulon S, Hopkins WG. Eating patterns and meal frequency of elite Australian athletes. *Int J Sport Nutr Exerc Metab.* 2003;13(4):521-38.

31. Campagnolo N, Iudakhina E, Irwin C, Schubert M, Cox GR, Leveritt M, et al. Fluid, energy and nutrient recovery via ad libitum intake of different fluids and food. *Physiol Behav.* 2017;171:228-35.

32. Cannell JJ, Hollis BW, Sorenson MB, Taft TN, Anderson JJ. Athletic performance and vitamin D. *Med Sci Sports Exerc.* 2009;41(5):1102-10.

33. Carbone A, D'Andrea A, Riegler L, Scarafile R, Pezzullo E, Martone F, et al. Cardiac damage in athlete's heart: When the "supernormal" heart fails! *World J Cardiol.* 2017;9(6):470-80.

34. Chang CH, Shau WY, Kuo CW, Chen ST, Lai MS. Increased risk of stroke associated with nonsteroidal anti-inflammatory drugs: A nationwide case-crossover study. *Stroke.* 2010;41(9):1884-90.

35. Chang CK, Borer K, Lin PJ. Low-carbohydrate-high-fat diet: Can it help exercise performance? *J Hum Kinet.* 2017;56:81-92.

36. Chazaud B. Inflammation during skeletal muscle regeneration and tissue remodeling: Application to exercise-induced muscle damage management. *Immunol Cell Biol.* 2016;94(2):140-5.

37. Cheung SS, McGarr GW, Mallette MM, Wallace PJ, Watson CL, Kim IM, et al. Separate and combined effects of dehydration and thirst sensation on exercise performance in the heat. *Scand J Med Sci Sports.* 2015;25(Suppl 1):104-11.

38. Chmura J, Nazar K. Parallel changes in the onset of blood lactate accumulation (OBLA) and threshold of psychomotor performance deterioration during incremental exercise after training in athletes. *Int J Psychophysiol.* 2010;75(3):287-90.

39. Cillard J, Cillard P. Prooxidant effect of alpha-tocopherol on essential fatty acids in aqueous media. *Ann Nutr Aliment.* 1980;34(3):579-91.

40. Clark A, Mach N. Exercise-induced stress behavior, gut-microbiota-brain axis and diet: A systematic review for athletes. *J Int Soc Sports Nutr.* 2016;13:43.

41. Coleman LS. Stress repair mechanism activity explains inflammation and apoptosis. *Advances in Bioscience and Biotechnology.* 2012;3:459-503.

42. Collins SM, Silberlicht M, Perzinski C, Smith SP, Davidson PW. The relationship between body composition and preseason performance tests of collegiate male lacrosse players. *J Strength Cond Res.* 2014;28(9):2673-9.

43. Cordain L, Eaton SB, Sebastian A, Mann N, Lindeberg S, Watkins BA, et al. Origins and evolution of the Western diet: Health implications for the 21st century. *Am J Clin Nutr.* 2005;81(2):341-54.

44. Corrado D, Basso C, Thiene G. Letter by Corrado et al. regarding article, "Sudden deaths in young competitive athletes: analysis of 1866 deaths in the United States, 1980-2006." *Circulation.* 2009;120(16):e143; author reply e4.

45. Corrado D, Basso C, Rizzoli G, Schiavon M, Thiene G. Does sports activity enhance the risk of sudden death in adolescents and young adults? *J Am Coll Cardiol.* 2003;42(11):1959-63.

46. Corrigan B, Kazlauskas R. Medication use in athletes selected for doping control at the Sydney Olympics (2000). *Clin J Sport Med.* 2003;13(1):33-40.

47. Cotter JD, Thornton SN, Lee JK, Laursen PB. Are we being drowned in hydration advice? Thirsty for more? *Extrem Physiol Med.* 2014;3:18.

48. Cox PJ, Kirk T, Ashmore T, Willerton K, Evans R, Smith A, et al. Nutritional ketosis alters fuel preference and thereby endurance performance in athletes. *Cell Metab.* 2016;24(2):256-68.

49. Databases UFC. 2017. Available from: https://ndb.nal.usda.gov/ndb/

50. Dattilo M, Antunes HK, Medeiros A, Monico Neto M, Souza HS, Tufik S, et al. Sleep and muscle recovery: Endocrinological and molecular basis for a new and promising hypothesis. *Med Hypotheses.* 2011;77(2):220-2.

51. de Oliveira EP, Burini RC, Jeukendrup A. Gastrointestinal complaints during exercise: Prevalence, etiology, and nutritional recommendations. *Sports Med.* 2014;44(Suppl 1):S79-85.

52. Decroix L, Lamberts RP, Meeusen R. Can the Lamberts Submaximal Cycle Test reflect overreaching in professional cyclists? *Int J Sports Physiol Perform.* 2018;13(1):23-8.

53. DePalma MT, Koszewski WM, Romani W, Case JG, Zuiderhof NJ, McCoy PM. Identifying college athletes at risk for pathogenic eating. *Br J Sports Med.* 2002;36(1):45-50.

54. Dupuy O, Renaud M, Bherer L, Bosquet L. Effect of functional overreaching on executive functions. *Int J Sports Med.* 2010;31(9):617-23.

55. Elliott KR, Harmatz JS, Zhao Y, Greenblatt DJ. Body size changes among National Collegiate Athletic Association New England Division III football players, 1956-2014: Comparison with age-matched population controls. *J Athl Train.* 2016;51(5):373-81.

56. Emerson DM, Torres-McGehee TM, Emerson CC, LaSalle TL. Individual fluid plans versus ad libitum on hydration status in minor professional ice hockey players. *J Int Soc Sports Nutr.* 2017;14:25.

57. Enoka RM, Stuart DG. Neurobiology of muscle fatigue. *J Appl Physiol (1985).* 1992;72(5):1631-48.

58. Faraut B, Boudjeltia KZ, Dyzma M, Rousseau A, David E, Stenuit P, et al. Benefits of napping and an extended duration of recovery sleep on alertness and immune cells after acute sleep restriction. *Brain Behav Immun.* 2011;25(1):16-24.

59. Feinman RD, Pogozelski WK, Astrup A, Bernstein RK, Fine EJ, Westman EC, et al. Dietary carbohydrate restriction as the first approach in diabetes management: Critical review and evidence base. *Nutrition.* 2015;31(1):1-13.

60. Flegal KM, Carroll MD, Kit BK, Ogden CL. Prevalence of obesity and trends in the distribution of body mass index among US adults, 1999-2010. *JAMA.* 2012;307(5):491-7.

61. Fondell E, Axelsson J, Franck K, Ploner A, Lekander M, Balter K, et al. Short natural sleep is associated with higher T cell and lower NK cell activities. *Brain Behav Immun.* 2011;25(7):1367-75.

62. Fretts AM, Howard BV, Siscovick DS, Best LG, Beresford SA, Mete M, et al. Processed meat, but not unprocessed red meat, is inversely associated with leukocyte telomere length in the strong heart family study. *J Nutr.* 2016;146(10):2013-18.

63. Friedman JE, Lemon PW. Effect of chronic endurance exercise on retention of dietary protein. *Int J Sports Med.* 1989;10(2):118-23.

64. Fritsch P, Dalla Pozza R, Ehringer-Schetitska D, Jokinen E, Herceg V, Hidvegi E, et al. Cardiovascular pre-participation screening in young athletes: Recommendations of the Association of European Paediatric Cardiology. *Cardiol Young.* 2017;27(9):1655-60.

65. Fry AC, Kraemer WJ, Ramsey LT. Pituitary-adrenal-gonadal responses to high-intensity resistance exercise overtraining. *J Appl Physiol (1985).* 1998;85(6):2352-9.

66. Fry RW, Morton AR, Keast D. Overtraining in athletes. An update. *Sports Med.* 1991;12(1):32-65.

67. Fuller JT, Bellenger CR, Thewlis D, Arnold J, Thomson RL, Tsiros MD, et al. Tracking performance changes with running-stride variability when athletes are functionally overreached. *Int J Sports Physiol Perform.* 2017;12(3):357-63.

68. Garber CE, Blissmer B, Deschenes MR, Franklin BA, Lamonte MJ, Lee IM, et al. American College of Sports Medicine position stand. Quantity and quality of exercise for developing and maintaining cardiorespiratory, musculoskeletal, and

neuromotor fitness in apparently healthy adults: Guidance for prescribing exercise. *Med Sci Sports Exerc.* 2011;43(7):1334-59.

69. Garrett AT, Goosens NG, Rehrer NJ, Patterson MJ, Harrison J, Sammut I, et al. Short-term heat acclimation is effective and may be enhanced rather than impaired by dehydration. *Am J Hum Biol.* 2014;26(3):311-20.

70. Garth AK, Burke LM. What do athletes drink during competitive sporting activities? *Sports Med.* 2013;43(7):539-64.

71. Gibson AL, Heyward VH, Mermier CM, Janot JM, Wilmerding MV. Comparison of DXA, Siri's 2C, and Lohman's Db-mineral models for estimating the body fat of physically active adults. *Int J Sport Nutr Exerc Metab.* 2004;14(6):657-72.

72. Gillen JB, Trommelen J, Wardenaar FC, Brinkmans NY, Versteegen JJ, Jonvik KL, et al. Dietary protein intake and distribution patterns of well-trained Dutch athletes. *Int J Sport Nutr Exerc Metab.* 2017;27(2):105-14.

73. Gorski T, Cadore EL, Pinto SS, da Silva EM, Correa CS, Beltrami FG, et al. Use of NSAIDs in triathletes: Prevalence, level of awareness and reasons for use. *Br J Sports Med.* 2011;45(2):85-90.

74. Guellich A, Seiler S, Emrich E. Training methods and intensity distribution of young world-class rowers. *Int J Sports Physiol Perform.* 2009;4(4):448-60.

75. Hackney AC, Kallman A, Hosick KP, Rubin DA, Battaglini CL. Thyroid hormonal responses to intensive interval versus steady-state endurance exercise sessions. *Hormones (Athens).* 2012;11(1):54-60.

76. Halson SL. Sleep in elite athletes and nutritional interventions to enhance sleep. *Sports Med.* 2014;44(Suppl 1):S13-23.

77. Halson SL, Jeukendrup AE. Does overtraining exist? An analysis of overreaching and overtraining research. *Sports Med.* 2004;34(14):967-81.

78. Halton TL, Hu FB. The effects of high protein diets on thermogenesis, satiety and weight loss: A critical review. *J Am Coll Nutr.* 2004;23(5):373-85.

79. Harray AJ, Boushey CJ, Pollard CM, Panizza CE, Delp EJ, Dhaliwal SS, et al. Perception v. actual intakes of junk food and sugar-sweetened beverages in Australian young adults: Assessed using the mobile food record. *Public Health Nutr.* 2017:1-8.

80. Heikura IA, Burke LM, Mero AA, Uusitalo ALT, Stellingwerff T. Dietary microperiodization in elite female and male runners and race walkers during a block of high intensity precompetition training. *Int J Sport Nutr Exerc Metab.* 2017;27(4):297-304.

81. Hetlelid KJ, Plews DJ, Herold E, Laursen PB, Sieler S. Rethinking the role of fat oxidation: Substrate utilisation during high-intensity interval training in well-trained and recreationally trained runners. *BMJ Open Sport & Exercise Medicine* 2015;1(1):e000047.

82. Holick MF. Vitamin D deficiency. *N Engl J Med.* 2007;357(3):266-81.

83. Holmes MV, Newcombe P, Hubacek JA, Sofat R, Ricketts SL, Cooper J, et al. Effect modification by population dietary folate on the association between MTHFR genotype, homocysteine, and stroke risk: A meta-analysis of genetic studies and randomised trials. *Lancet.* 2011;378(9791):584-94.

84. Holmes N, Cronholm PF, Duffy AJ, 3rd, Webner D. Nonsteroidal anti-inflammatory drug use in collegiate football players. *Clin J Sport Med.* 2013;23(4):283-6.

85. Hu FB. Resolved: There is sufficient scientific evidence that decreasing sugar-sweetened beverage consumption will reduce the prevalence of obesity and obesity-related diseases. *Obes Rev.* 2013;14(8):606-19.

86. Hynynen E, Uusitalo A, Konttinen N, Rusko H. Cardiac autonomic responses to standing up and cognitive task in overtrained athletes. *Int J Sports Med.* 2008;29(7):552-8.

87. Iellamo F, Legramante JM, Pigozzi F, Spataro A, Norbiato G, Lucini D, et al. Conversion from vagal to sympathetic predominance with strenuous training in high-performance world class athletes. *Circulation.* 2002;105(23):2719-24.

88. Institute of Medicine FaNB. *Dietary Reference Intakes for Energy, Carbohydrate, Fiber, Fat, Fatty Acids, Cholesterol, Protein, and Amino Acids.* Washington, DC: National Academies Press; 2005.

89. Jensen RK, Fletcher P. Distribution of mass to the segments of elderly males and females. *J Biomech.* 1994;27(1):89-96.

90. Jerome SP, Sticka KD, Schnurr TM, Mangum SJ, Reynolds AJ, Dunlap KL. 25(OH)D levels in trained versus sedentary university students at 64 degrees north. *Int J Circumpolar Health.* 2017;76(1):1314414.

91. Jordan TR, Khubchandani J, Wiblishauser M. The impact of perceived stress and coping adequacy on the health of nurses: A pilot investigation. *Nurs Res Pract.* 2016;2016:5843256.

92. Juanola-Falgarona M, Salas-Salvado J, Ibarrola-Jurado N, Rabassa-Soler A, Diaz-Lopez A, Guasch-Ferre M, et al. Effect of the glycemic index of the diet on weight loss, modulation of satiety, inflammation, and other metabolic risk factors: A randomized controlled trial. *Am J Clin Nutr.* 2014;100(1):27-35.

93. Kaur N, Chugh V, Gupta AK. Essential fatty acids as functional components of foods: A review. *J Food Sci Technol.* 2014;51(10):2289-303.

94. Kavazis AN. Exercise preconditioning of the myocardium. *Sports Med.* 2009;39(11):923-35.

95. Kentta G, Hassmen P. Overtraining and recovery. A conceptual model. *Sports Med.* 1998;26(1):1-16.

96. Keteyian SJ, Hibner BA, Bronsteen K, Kerrigan D, Aldred HA, Reasons LM, et al. Greater improvement in cardiorespiratory fitness using higher-intensity interval training in the standard cardiac rehabilitation setting. *J Cardiopulm Rehabil Prev.* 2014;34(2):98-105.

97. Khodaee M, Olewinski L, Shadgan B, Kiningham RR. Rapid weight loss in sports with weight classes. *Curr Sports Med Rep.* 2015;14(6):435-41.

98. Kilian Y, Engel F, Wahl P, Achtzehn S, Sperlich B, Mester J. Markers of biological stress in response to a single session of high-intensity interval training and high-volume training in young athletes. *Eur J Appl Physiol.* 2016;116(11-12):2177-86.

99. Knutson KL, Spiegel K, Penev P, Van Cauter E. The metabolic consequences of sleep deprivation. *Sleep Med Rev.* 2007;11(3):163-78.

100. Konig D, Berg A, Weinstock C, Keul J, Northoff H. Essential fatty acids, immune function, and exercise. *Exerc Immunol Rev.* 1997;3:1-31.

101. Koundourakis NE, Avgoustinaki PD, Malliaraki N, Margioris AN. Muscular effects of vitamin D in young athletes and non-athletes and in the elderly. *Hormones (Athens).* 2016;15(4):471-88.

102. Kraemer WJ, French DN, Paxton NJ, Hakkinen K, Volek JS, Sebastianelli WJ, et al. Changes in exercise performance and hormonal concentrations over a Big Ten soccer season in starters and nonstarters. *J Strength Cond Res.* 2004;18(1):121-8.

103. Kreher JB. Diagnosis and prevention of overtraining syndrome: An opinion on education strategies. *Open Access J Sports Med.* 2016;7:115-22.

104. Kreher JB, Schwartz JB. Overtraining syndrome: A practical guide. *Sports Health.* 2012;4(2):128-38.

105. Kreider RB, Wilborn CD, Taylor L, Campbell B, Almada AL, Collins R, et al. ISSN exercise & sport nutrition review: Research & recommendations. *J Int Soc Sports Nutr.* 2010;7:7.

106. Kuipers H, Keizer HA. Overtraining in elite athletes. Review and directions for the future. *Sports Med.* 1988;6(2):79-92.

107. Kuster M, Renner B, Oppel P, Niederweis U, Brune K. Consumption of analgesics before a marathon and the incidence of cardiovascular, gastrointestinal and renal problems: A cohort study. *BMJ Open.* 2013;3(4).

108. Landsberg L. Feast or famine: The sympathetic nervous system response to nutrient intake. *Cell Mol Neurobiol.* 2006;26(4-6):497-508.

109. Langfort J, Pilis W, Zarzeczny R, Nazar K, Kaciuba-Uscilko H. Effect of low-carbohydrate-ketogenic diet on metabolic and hormonal responses to graded exercise in men. *J Physiol Pharmacol.* 1996;47(2):361-71.

110. Larson-Meyer DE, Willis KS. Vitamin D and athletes. *Curr Sports Med Rep.* 2010;9(4):220-6.

111. Lautenbacher S, Kundermann B, Krieg JC. Sleep deprivation and pain perception. *Sleep Med Rev.* 2006;10(5):357-69.

112. Layman DK, Evans E, Baum JI, Seyler J, Erickson DJ, Boileau RA. Dietary protein and exercise have additive effects on body composition during weight loss in adult women. *J Nutr.* 2005;135(8):1903-10.

113. Le Meur Y, Buchheit M, Aubry A, Coutts AJ, Hausswirth C. Assessing overreaching with heart-rate recovery: What is the minimal exercise intensity required? *Int J Sports Physiol Perform.* 2017;12(4):569-73.

114. Le Meur Y, Hausswirth C, Natta F, Couturier A, Bignet F, Vidal PP. A multidisciplinary approach to overreaching detection in endurance trained athletes. *J Appl Physiol (1985).* 2013;114(3):411-20.

115. Le Meur Y, Louis J, Aubry A, Gueneron J, Pichon A, Schaal K, et al. Maximal exercise limitation in functionally overreached triathletes: Role of cardiac adrenergic stimulation. *J Appl Physiol (1985)*. 2014;117(3):214-22.

116. Leeder J, Glaister M, Pizzoferro K, Dawson J, Pedlar C. Sleep duration and quality in elite athletes measured using wristwatch actigraphy. *J Sports Sci*. 2012;30(6):541-5.

117. Lewis NA, Collins D, Pedlar CR, Rogers JP. Can clinicians and scientists explain and prevent unexplained underperformance syndrome in elite athletes: An interdisciplinary perspective and 2016 update. *BMJ Open Sport Exerc Med*. 2015;1(1):e000063.

118. Longland TM, Oikawa SY, Mitchell CJ, Devries MC, Phillips SM. Higher compared with lower dietary protein during an energy deficit combined with intense exercise promotes greater lean mass gain and fat mass loss: A randomized trial. *Am J Clin Nutr*. 2016;103(3):738-46.

119. Luden N, Hayes E, Galpin A, Minchev K, Jemiolo B, Raue U, et al. Myocellular basis for tapering in competitive distance runners. *J Appl Physiol (1985)*. 2010;108(6):1501-9.

120. Luger A, Deuster PA, Kyle SB, Gallucci WT, Montgomery LC, Gold PW, et al. Acute hypothalamic-pituitary-adrenal responses to the stress of treadmill exercise. Physiologic adaptations to physical training. *N Engl J Med*. 1987;316(21):1309-15.

121. Lukaski HC. Vitamin and mineral status: Effects on physical performance. *Nutrition*. 2004;20(7-8):632-44.

122. Lukaski HC, Penland JG. Functional changes appropriate for determining mineral element requirements. *J Nutr*. 1996;126(Suppl 9):2354S-64S.

123. Maffetone P. *Complementary Sports Medicine*. Champaign, IL: Human Kinetics; 1999.

124. Maffetone P, Laursen PB. Athletes: Fit but unhealthy? *Sports Med*. 2015;2(24).

125. Maffetone PB, Laursen PB. Reductions in training load and dietary carbohydrates help restore health and improve performance in an Ironman triathlete. *Int J Sports Sci Coach*. 2017;12(4):514-19.

126. Maffetone PB, Rivera-Dominguez I, Laursen PB. Overfat and underfat: New terms and definitions long overdue. *Front Public Health*. 2016;4:279.

127. Maffetone PB, Rivera-Dominguez I, Laursen PB. Overfat adults and children in developed countries: The public health importance of identifying excess body fat. *Front Public Health*. 2017;5:190.

128. Mah CD, editor. Annual Meeting of the Associated Professional Sleep Societies; June 9, 2008; Baltimore MD.

129. Mah CD, Mah KE, Kezirian EJ, Dement WC. The effects of sleep extension on the athletic performance of collegiate basketball players. *Sleep*. 2011;34(7):943-50.

130. Manore MM. Exercise and the Institute of Medicine recommendations for nutrition. *Curr Sports Med Rep*. 2005;4(4):193-8.

131. Maron BJ, Zipes DP, Kovacs RJ. Eligibility and disqualification recommendations for competitive athletes with cardiovascular abnormalities: Preamble, principles, and general considerations: A scientific statement from the American Heart Association and American College of Cardiology. *J Am Coll Cardiol*. 2015;66(21):2343-9.

132. Maron BJ, Doerer JJ, Haas TS, Tierney DM, Mueller FO. Sudden deaths in young competitive athletes: Analysis of 1866 deaths in the United States, 1980-2006. *Circulation*. 2009;119(8):1085-92.

133. Maron BJ, Haas TS, Murphy CJ, Ahluwalia A, Rutten-Ramos S. Incidence and causes of sudden death in U.S. college athletes. *J Am Coll Cardiol*. 2014;63(16):1636-43.

134. Matava MJ. Ethical considerations for analgesic use in sports medicine. *Clin Sports Med*. 2016;35(2):227-43.

135. Mathur N, Pedersen BK. Exercise as a means to control low-grade systemic inflammation. *Mediators Inflamm*. 2008;2008:109502.

136. Matthews MJ, Green D, Matthews H, Swanwick E. The effects of swimming fatigue on shoulder strength, range of motion, joint control, and performance in swimmers. *Phys Ther Sport*. 2017;23:118-22.

137. McArdle A, Pattwell D, Vasilaki A, Griffiths RD, Jackson MJ. Contractile activity-induced oxidative stress: Cellular origin and adaptive responses. *Am J Physiol Cell Physiol*. 2001;280(3):C621-7.

138. McGinnis GR, Ballmann C, Peters B, Nanayak-kara G, Roberts M, Amin R, et al. Interleukin-6 mediates exercise preconditioning against myocardial ischemia reperfusion injury. *Am J Physiol Heart Circ Physiol.* 2015;308(11):H1423-33.

139. McKay JM, Selig SE, Carlson JS, Morris T. Psychophysiological stress in elite golfers during practice and competition. *Aust J Sci Med Sport.* 1997;29(2):55-61.

140. McLeay Y, Stannard S, Houltham S, Starck C. Dietary thiols in exercise: Oxidative stress defence, exercise performance, and adaptation. *J Int Soc Sports Nutr.* 2017;14:12.

141. Meardon SA, Hamill J, Derrick TR. Running injury and stride time variability over a prolonged run. *Gait Posture.* 2011;33(1):36-40.

142. Medicine ACoS. *ACSM's Health-Related Physical Fitness Assessment, 4th Ed.* Philadelphia: Wolters Kluwer Health/Lippincott Williams & Wilkins health; 2013.

143. Meerlo P, Sgoifo A, Suchecki D. Restricted and disrupted sleep: Effects on autonomic function, neuroendocrine stress systems and stress responsivity. *Sleep Med Rev.* 2008;12(3):197-210.

144. Meeusen R, Duclos M, Foster C, Fry A, Gleeson M, Nieman D, et al. Prevention, diagnosis, and treatment of the overtraining syndrome: Joint consensus statement of the European College of Sport Science and the American College of Sports Medicine. *Med Sci Sports Exerc.* 2013;45(1):186-205.

145. Miyajima H, Sakamoto M, Takahashi Y, Mizo-guchi K, Nishimura Y. [Muscle carnitine deficiency associated with myalgia and rhabdo-myolysis following exercise]. *Rinsho Shinkeigaku.* 1989;29(1):93-7.

146. Mohammadi F, Roozdar A. Effects of fatigue due to contraction of evertor muscles on the ankle joint position sense in male soccer players. *Am J Sports Med.* 2010;38(4):824-8.

147. Monteiro CA. Nutrition and health. The issue is not food, nor nutrients, so much as processing. *Public Health Nutr.* 2009;12(5):729-31.

148. Morales-Alamo D, Ponce-Gonzalez JG, Guadalupe-Grau A, Rodriguez-Garcia L, Santana A, Cusso MR, et al. Increased oxidative stress and anaerobic energy release, but blunted Thr172-AMPKalpha phosphorylation, in response to sprint exercise in severe acute hypoxia in humans. *J Appl Physiol (1985).* 2012;113(6):917-28.

149. Morelli KM, Brown LB, Warren GL. Effect of NSAIDs on recovery from acute skeletal muscle injury: A systematic review and meta-analysis. *Am J Sports Med.* 2018;46(1):224-33.

150. Mountjoy M, Sundgot-Borgen J, Burke L, Carter S, Constantini N, Lebrun C, et al. The IOC consensus statement: Beyond the female athlete triad—relative energy deficiency in sport (RED-S). *Br J Sports Med.* 2014;48(7):491-7.

151. Mullington JM, Simpson NS, Meier-Ewert HK, Haack M. Sleep loss and inflammation. *Best Pract Res Clin Endocrinol Metab.* 2010;24(5):775-84.

152. Murach K, Raue U, Wilkerson B, Minchev K, Jemiolo B, Bagley J, et al. Single muscle fiber gene expression with run taper. *PLoS One.* 2014;9(9):e108547.

153. Murphy MH, Breslin G, Trinick T, McClean C, Moore W, Duly E, et al. The biochemical, physiological and psychological consequences of a "1,000 miles in 1,000 hours" walking challenge. *Eur J Appl Physiol.* 2012;112(2):781-8.

154. National Institutes of Health NH, Lung and Blood Institute. 2017 [Available from: https://www.nhlbi.nih.gov/health/health-topics/topics/ida/diagnosis.]

155. Neary JP, Martin TP, Quinney HA. Effects of taper on endurance cycling capacity and single muscle fiber properties. *Med Sci Sports Exerc.* 2003;35(11):1875-81.

156. Noakes T, Volek JS, Phinney SD. Low-carbohydrate diets for athletes: What evidence? *Br J Sports Med.* 2014;48(14):1077-8.

157. Noakes TD. Changes in body mass alone explain almost all of the variance in the serum sodium concentrations during prolonged exercise. Has commercial influence impeded scientific endeavour? *Br J Sports Med.* 2011;45(6):475-7.

158. Noakes TD, Windt J. Evidence that supports the prescription of low-carbohydrate high-fat diets: A narrative review. *Br J Sports Med.* 2017;51(2):133-9.

159. Noakes TD, St Clair Gibson A, Lambert EV. From catastrophe to complexity: A novel model of integrative central neural regulation of effort and fatigue during exercise in humans. *Br J Sports Med.* 2004;38(4):511-4.

160. Noakes TD, Sharwood K, Speedy D, Hew T, Reid S, Dugas J, et al. Three independent biological mechanisms cause exercise-associated hyponatremia: Evidence from 2,135 weighed competitive athletic performances. *Proc Natl Acad Sci USA*. 2005;102(51):18550-5.

161. O'Donnell S, Driller MW. Sleep-hygiene education improves sleep indices in elite female athletes. *Int J Exerc Sci*. 2017;10(4):522-30.

162. O'Keefe JH, Franklin B, Lavie CJ. Exercising for health and longevity vs peak performance: Different regimens for different goals. *Mayo Clin Proc*. 2014;89(9):1171-5.

163. Ohlund I, Silfverdal SA, Hernell O, Lind T. Serum 25-hydroxyvitamin D levels in preschool-age children in northern Sweden are inadequate after summer and diminish further during winter. *J Pediatr Gastroenterol Nutr*. 2013;56(5):551-5.

164. Owens DJ, Sharples AP, Polydorou I, Alwan N, Donovan T, Tang J, et al. A systems-based investigation into vitamin D and skeletal muscle repair, regeneration, and hypertrophy. *Am J Physiol Endocrinol Metab*. 2015;309(12):E1019-31.

165. Page AJ, Reid SA, Speedy DB, Mulligan GP, Thompson J. Exercise-associated hyponatremia, renal function, and nonsteroidal antiinflammatory drug use in an ultraendurance mountain run. *Clin J Sport Med*. 2007;17(1):43-8.

166. Paoli A, Bianco A, Grimaldi KA. The ketogenic diet and sport: A possible marriage? *Exerc Sport Sci Rev*. 2015;43(3):153-62.

167. Paoli A, Grimaldi K, D'Agostino D, Cenci L, Moro T, Bianco A, et al. Ketogenic diet does not affect strength performance in elite artistic gymnasts. *J Int Soc Sports Nutr*. 2012;9(1):34.

168. Paoloni JA, Milne C, Orchard J, Hamilton B. Non-steroidal anti-inflammatory drugs in sports medicine: Guidelines for practical but sensible use. *Br J Sports Med*. 2009;43(11):863-5.

169. Parijat P, Lockhart TE. Effects of quadriceps fatigue on the biomechanics of gait and slip propensity. *Gait Posture*. 2008;28(4):568-73.

170. Park SW, Son SM, Lee NK. Exercise-induced muscle fatigue in the unaffected knee joint and its influence on postural control and lower limb kinematics in stroke patients. *Neural Regen Res*. 2017;12(5):765-9.

171. Paulsen G, Cumming KT, Hamarsland H, Borsheim E, Berntsen S, Raastad T. Can supplementation with vitamin C and E alter physiological adaptations to strength training? *BMC Sports Sci Med Rehabil*. 2014;6:28.

172. Pedrinelli A, Ejnisman L, Fagotti L, Dvorak J, Tscholl PM. Medications and nutritional supplements in athletes during the 2000, 2004, 2008, and 2012 FIFA Futsal World Cups. *Biomed Res Int*. 2015;2015:870308.

173. Perrier ET. Shifting focus: From hydration for performance to hydration for health. *Ann Nutr Metab*. 2017;70(Suppl 1):4-12.

174. Phillips SM, Van Loon LJ. Dietary protein for athletes: From requirements to optimum adaptation. *J Sports Sci*. 2011;29(Suppl 1):S29-38.

175. Picard M, Hepple RT, Burelle Y. Mitochondrial functional specialization in glycolytic and oxidative muscle fibers: Tailoring the organelle for optimal function. *Am J Physiol Cell Physiol*. 2012;302(4):C629-41.

176. Plews DJ, Laursen PB, Stanley J, Kilding AE, Buchheit M. Training adaptation and heart rate variability in elite endurance athletes: Opening the door to effective monitoring. *Sports Med*. 2013;43(9):773-81.

177. Plunkett BA, Callister R, Watson TA, Garg ML. Dietary antioxidant restriction affects the inflammatory response in athletes. *Br J Nutr*. 2010;103(8):1179-84.

178. Powers HJ. Riboflavin (vitamin B-2) and health. *Am J Clin Nutr*. 2003;77(6):1352-60.

179. Pravenec M, Kozich V, Krijt J, Sokolova J, Zidek V, Landa V, et al. Folate deficiency is associated with oxidative stress, increased blood pressure, and insulin resistance in spontaneously hypertensive rats. *Am J Hypertens*. 2013;26(1):135-40.

180. Providencia R, Teixeira C, Segal OR, Ullstein A, Lambiase PD. Call for joint informed consent in athletes with inherited cardiac conditions. *Open Heart*. 2017;4(1):e000516.

181. Quail SL, Morris RW, Balleine BW. Stress associated changes in Pavlovian-instrumental transfer in humans. *Q J Exp Psychol (Hove)*. 2017;70(4):675-85.

182. Raasch WG, Hergan DJ. Treatment of stress fractures: The fundamentals. *Clin Sports Med*. 2006;25(1):29-36, vii.

183. Rapoport BI. Metabolic factors limiting performance in marathon runners. *PLoS Comput Biol.* 2010;6(10):e1000960.

184. Robson-Ansley PJ, Gleeson M, Ansley L. Fatigue management in the preparation of Olympic athletes. *J Sports Sci.* 2009;27(13):1409-20.

185. Rossi FE, Landreth A, Beam S, Jones T, Norton L, Cholewa JM. The Effects of a sports nutrition education intervention on nutritional status, sport nutrition knowledge, body composition, and performance during off season training in NCAA Division I baseball players. *J Sports Sci Med.* 2017;16(1):60-8.

186. Ruiz-Nunez B, Pruimboom L, Dijck-Brouwer DA, Muskiet FA. Lifestyle and nutritional imbalances associated with Western diseases: Causes and consequences of chronic systemic low-grade inflammation in an evolutionary context. *J Nutr Biochem.* 2013;24(7):1183-201.

187. Samuels C. Sleep, recovery, and performance: The new frontier in high-performance athletics. *Phys Med Rehabil Clin N Am.* 2009;20(1):149-59, ix.

188. Sandlin MI, Rosenbaum AJ, Taghavi CE, Charlton TP, O'Malley MJ. High-risk stress fractures in elite athletes. *Instr Course Lect.* 2017;66:281-92.

189. Savoie FA, Dion T, Asselin A, Goulet ED. Sodium-induced hyperhydration decreases urine output and improves fluid balance compared with glycerol- and water-induced hyperhydration. *Appl Physiol Nutr Metab.* 2015;40(1):51-8.

190. Savva SC, Tornaritis M, Savva ME, Kourides Y, Panagi A, Silikiotou N, et al. Waist circumference and waist-to-height ratio are better predictors of cardiovascular disease risk factors in children than body mass index. *Int J Obes Relat Metab Disord.* 2000;24(11):1453-8.

191. Saw AE, Main LC, Gastin PB. Monitoring the athlete training response: Subjective self-reported measures trump commonly used objective measures: A systematic review. *Br J Sports Med.* 2016;50(5):281-91.

192. Sawka MN, Burke LM, Eichner ER, Maughan RJ, Montain SJ, Stachenfeld NS. American College of Sports Medicine position stand. Exercise and fluid replacement. *Med Sci Sports Exerc.* 2007;39(2):377-90.

193. Schoenfeld BJ. The use of nonsteroidal anti-inflammatory drugs for exercise-induced muscle damage: Implications for skeletal muscle development. *Sports Med.* 2012;42(12):1017-28.

194. Schwartz RS, Merkel-Kraus S, Schwarz JG, Wickstrom KK, Peichel G, Garberich RF, et al. Increased coronary artery plaque volume among male marathon runners. *Missouri Medicine.* 2014;111(2):85.

195. Seiler S, Haugen O, Kuffel E. Autonomic recovery after exercise in trained athletes: Intensity and duration effects. *Med Sci Sports Exerc.* 2007;39(8):1366-73.

196. Selye H. Forty years of stress research: Principal remaining problems and misconceptions. *Can Med Assoc J.* 1976;115(1):53-6.

197. Selye H. A syndrome produced by diverse nocuous agents. 1936. *J Neuropsychiatry Clin Neurosci.* 1998;10(2):230-1.

198. Shahidi F. Nutraceuticals and functional foods: Whole versus processed foods. *Food Sci Technol.* 2009;20:376-87.

199. Sharwood KA, Collins M, Goedecke JH, Wilson G, Noakes TD. Weight changes, medical complications, and performance during an Ironman triathlon. *Br J Sports Med.* 2004;38(6):718-24.

200. Shirreffs SM, Sawka MN. Fluid and electrolyte needs for training, competition, and recovery. *J Sports Sci.* 2011;29(Suppl 1):S39-46.

201. Shuler FD, Wingate MK, Moore GH, Giangarra C. Sports health benefits of vitamin D. *Sports Health.* 2012;4(6):496-501.

202. Siegl A, E MK, Tam N, Koschnick S, Langerak NG, Skorski S, et al. Submaximal markers of fatigue and overreaching: Implications for monitoring athletes. *Int J Sports Med.* 2017;38(9):675-82.

203. Siems W, Wiswedel I, Salerno C, Crifo C, Augustin W, Schild L, et al. Beta-carotene breakdown products may impair mitochondrial functions—potential side effects of high-dose beta-carotene supplementation. *J Nutr Biochem.* 2005;16(7):385-97.

204. Simpson NS, Gibbs EL, Matheson GO. Optimizing sleep to maximize performance: implications and recommendations for elite athletes. *Scand J Med Sci Sports.* 2017;27(3):266-74.

205. Skaug A, Sveen O, Raastad T. An antioxidant and multivitamin supplement reduced improvements in VO(2)max. *J Sports Med Phys Fitness.* 2014;54(1):63-9.

206. Slyper AH. The influence of carbohydrate quality on cardiovascular disease, the metabolic syndrome, type 2 diabetes, and obesity - an overview. *J Pediatr Endocrinol Metab.* 2013;26(7-8):617-29.

207. Spargoli G. The acute effects of concentric versus eccentric muscle fatigue on shoulder active repositioning sense. *Int J Sports Phys Ther.* 2017;12(2):219-26.

208. Spiegel K, Leproult R, Van Cauter E. Impact of sleep debt on metabolic and endocrine function. *Lancet.* 1999;354(9188):1435-9.

209. Spiegel K, Tasali E, Penev P, Van Cauter E. Brief communication: Sleep curtailment in healthy young men is associated with decreased leptin levels, elevated ghrelin levels, and increased hunger and appetite. *Ann Intern Med.* 2004;141(11):846-50.

210. Spiegel K, Knutson K, Leproult R, Tasali E, Van Cauter E. Sleep loss: A novel risk factor for insulin resistance and Type 2 diabetes. *J Appl Physiol (1985).* 2005;99(5):2008-19.

211. Sripetchwandee J, Pipatpiboon N, Chattipakorn N, Chattipakorn S. Combined therapy of iron chelator and antioxidant completely restores brain dysfunction induced by iron toxicity. *PLoS One.* 2014;9(1):e85115.

212. Stanhope KL, Schwarz JM, Havel PJ. Adverse metabolic effects of dietary fructose: Results from the recent epidemiological, clinical, and mechanistic studies. *Curr Opin Lipidol.* 2013;24(3):198-206.

213. Stanley J, Peake JM, Buchheit M. Cardiac parasympathetic reactivation following exercise: Implications for training prescription. *Sports Med.* 2013;43(12):1259-77.

214. Sundgot-Borgen J, Meyer NL, Lohman TG, Ackland TR, Maughan RJ, Stewart AD, et al. How to minimise the health risks to athletes who compete in weight-sensitive sports review and position statement on behalf of the Ad Hoc Research Working Group on Body Composition, Health and Performance, under the auspices of the IOC Medical Commission. *Br J Sports Med.* 2013;47(16):1012-22.

215. Suzuki K, Nakaji S, Yamada M, Totsuka M, Sato K, Sugawara K. Systemic inflammatory response to exhaustive exercise. Cytokine kinetics. *Exerc Immunol Rev.* 2002;8:6-48.

216. Teixeira V, Valente H, Casal S, Marques F, Moreira P. Antioxidant status, oxidative stress, and damage in elite trained kayakers and canoeists and sedentary controls. *Int J Sport Nutr Exerc Metab.* 2009;19(5):443-56.

217. Temme KE, Hoch AZ. Recognition and rehabilitation of the female athlete triad/tetrad: A multidisciplinary approach. *Curr Sports Med Rep.* 2013;12(3):190-9.

218. Ten Haaf T, van Staveren S, Oudenhoven E, Piacentini MF, Meeusen R, Roelands B, et al. Prediction of functional overreaching from subjective fatigue and readiness to train after only 3 days of cycling. *Int J Sports Physiol Perform.* 2017;12(Suppl 2):S287–S94.

219. Thein-Nissenbaum J, Hammer E. Treatment strategies for the female athlete triad in the adolescent athlete: Current perspectives. *Open Access J Sports Med.* 2017;8:85-95.

220. Theodorou AA, Nikolaidis MG, Paschalis V, Koutsias S, Panayiotou G, Fatouros IG, et al. No effect of antioxidant supplementation on muscle performance and blood redox status adaptations to eccentric training. *Am J Clin Nutr.* 2011;93(6):1373-83.

221. Thomas DT, Erdman KA, Burke LM. Position of the Academy of Nutrition and Dietetics, Dietitians of Canada, and the American College of Sports Medicine: Nutrition and athletic performance. *J Acad Nutr Diet.* 2016;116(3):501-28.

222. Thompson PD, Funk EJ, Carleton RA, Sturner WQ. Incidence of death during jogging in Rhode Island from 1975 through 1980. *JAMA.* 1982;247(18):2535-8.

223. Thunenkotter T, Schmied C, Grimm K, Dvorak J, Kindermann W. Precompetition cardiac assessment of football players participating in the 2006 FIFA World Cup Germany. *Clin J Sport Med.* 2009;19(4):322-5.

224. Tidball JG. Inflammatory processes in muscle injury and repair. *Am J Physiol Regul Integr Comp Physiol.* 2005;288(2):R345-53.

225. Trappe S, Costill D, Thomas R. Effect of swim taper on whole muscle and single muscle fiber

contractile properties. *Med Sci Sports Exerc.* 2000;32(12):48-56.

226. Tscholl P, Feddermann N, Junge A, Dvorak J. The use and abuse of painkillers in international soccer: Data from 6 FIFA tournaments for female and youth players. *Am J Sports Med.* 2009;37(2):260-5.

227. Tscholl PM, Vaso M, Weber A, Dvorak J. High prevalence of medication use in professional football tournaments including the World Cups between 2002 and 2014: A narrative review with a focus on NSAIDs. *Br J Sports Med.* 2015;49(9):580-2.

228. Ulrich-Lai YM, Herman JP. Neural regulation of endocrine and autonomic stress responses. *Nat Rev Neurosci.* 2009;10(6):397-409.

229. Urhausen A, Gabriel H, Kindermann W. Blood hormones as markers of training stress and overtraining. *Sports Med.* 1995;20(4):251-76.

230. Van Cauter E, Spiegel K, Tasali E, Leproult R. Metabolic consequences of sleep and sleep loss. *Sleep Med.* 2008;9(Suppl 1):S23-8.

231. Van Wijck K, Lenaerts K, Van Bijnen AA, Boonen B, Van Loon LJ, Dejong CH, et al. Aggravation of exercise-induced intestinal injury by ibuprofen in athletes. *Med Sci Sports Exerc.* 2012;44(12):2257-62.

232. Virchenko O, Skoglund B, Aspenberg P. Parecoxib impairs early tendon repair but improves later remodeling. *Am J Sports Med.* 2004;32(7):1743-7.

233. Volek JS, Noakes T, Phinney SD. Rethinking fat as a fuel for endurance exercise. *Eur J Sport Sci.* 2015;15(1):13-20.

234. Volek JS, Freidenreich DJ, Saenz C, Kunces LJ, Creighton BC, Bartley JM, et al. Metabolic characteristics of keto-adapted ultra-endurance runners. *Metabolism.* 2016;65(3):100-10.

235. Wall BA, Watson G, Peiffer JJ, Abbiss CR, Siegel R, Laursen PB. Current hydration guidelines are erroneous: Dehydration does not impair exercise performance in the heat. *Br J Sports Med.* 2015;49(16):1077-83.

236. Wardenaar F, Brinkmans N, Ceelen I, Van Rooij B, Mensink M, Witkamp R, et al. Micronutrient intakes in 553 Dutch elite and sub-elite athletes: Prevalence of low and high intakes in users and non-users of nutritional supplements. *Nutrients.* 2017;9(2).

237. Warner DC, Schnepf G, Barrett MS, Dian D, Swigonski NL. Prevalence, attitudes, and behaviors related to the use of nonsteroidal anti-inflammatory drugs (NSAIDs) in student athletes. *J Adolesc Health.* 2002;30(3):150-3.

238. Watanabe S, Aizawa J, Shimoda M, Enomoto M, Nakamura T, Okawa A, et al. Effect of short-term fatigue, induced by high-intensity exercise, on the profile of the ground reaction force during single-leg anterior drop-jumps. *J Phys Ther Sci.* 2016;28(12):3371-5.

239. Watson TA, Callister R, Taylor RD, Sibbritt DW, MacDonald-Wicks LK, Garg ML. Antioxidant restriction and oxidative stress in short-duration exhaustive exercise. *Med Sci Sports Exerc.* 2005;37(1):63-71.

240. Webster CC, Noakes TD, Chacko SK, Swart J, Kohn TA, Smith JA. Gluconeogenesis during endurance exercise in cyclists habituated to a long-term low carbohydrate high fat diet. *J Physiol.* 2016;594(15):4389-405.

241. Weidner TG, Gehlsen G, Dwyer GB, Schurr T. Effects of viral upper respiratory illness on running gait. *J Athl Train.* 1997;32(4):309-14.

242. Westman EC. Is dietary carbohydrate essential for human nutrition? *Am J Clin Nutr.* 2002;75(5):951-3; author reply 3-4.

243. Wojtys EM, Wylie BB, Huston LJ. The effects of muscle fatigue on neuromuscular function and anterior tibial translation in healthy knees. *Am J Sports Med.* 1996;24(5):615-21.

244. Wright CJ, Abbey EL, Brandon BA, Reisman EJ, Kirkpatrick CM. Cardiovascular disease risk profile of NCAA Division III intercollegiate football athletes: A pilot study. *Phys Sportsmed.* 2017;45(3):280-5.

245. Wright M, Chesterton P, Wijnbergen M, O'Rourke A, Macpherson T. The Effect of a simulated soccer match on anterior cruciate ligament injury risk factors. *Int J Sports Med.* 2017;38(8):620-6.

246. Yamamoto JB, Yamamoto BE, Yamamoto PP, Yamamoto LG. Epidemiology of college athlete sizes, 1950s to current. *Res Sports Med.* 2008;16(2):111-27.

247. Yashiro H, Takagahara S, Tamura YO, Miyahisa I, Matsui J, Suzuki H, et al. A novel selective inhibitor of delta-5 desaturase lowers Insulin resistance and reduces body weight in diet-

induced obese C57BL/6J mice. *PLoS One.* 2016;11(11):e0166198.

248. Young AJ, Lowe GM. Antioxidant and prooxidant properties of carotenoids. *Arch Biochem Biophys.* 2001;385(1):20-7.

249. Zajac A, Poprzecki S, Maszczyk A, Czuba M, Michalczyk M, Zydek G. The effects of a ketogenic diet on exercise metabolism and physical performance in off-road cyclists. *Nutrients.* 2014;6(7):2493-508.

250. Zappacosta B, Mastroiacovo P, Persichilli S, Pounis G, Ruggeri S, Minucci A, et al. Homocysteine lowering by folate-rich diet or pharmacological supplementations in subjects with moderate hyperhomocysteinemia. *Nutrients.* 2013;5(5):1531-43.

251. Zhang Q, Zheng J, Qiu J, Wu X, Xu Y, Shen W, et al. ALDH2 restores exhaustive exercise-induced mitochondrial dysfunction in skeletal muscle. *Biochem Biophys Res Commun.* 2017;485(4):753-60.

Chapter 8

1. Abbiss CR, Quod MJ, Levin G, Martin DT, Laursen PB. Accuracy of the Velotron ergometer and SRM power meter. *Int J Sports Med.* 2009;30(2):107-12.

2. Abotel K. The Crippling Cost of Sports Injuries. https://wwwforbescom/sites/sap/2015/08/11/the -crippling-cost-of-sports-injuries /#d25f5db4d1f7. 2015.

3. Abt G, Lovell R. The use of individualized speed and intensity thresholds for determining the distance run at high-intensity in professional soccer. *J Sports Sci.* 2009;27(9):893-8.

4. Akenhead R, Nassis GP. Training load and player monitoring in high-level football: Current practice and perceptions. *Int J Sports Physiol Perform.* 2016;11(5):587-93.

5. Akenhead R, French D, Thompson KG, Hayes PR. The acceleration dependent validity and reliability of 10 Hz GPS. *J Sci Med Sport.* 2014;17(5):562-6.

6. Banister EW. Modeling elite athletic performance. In MacDougall JD, Wenger HA, Green HJ, eds. *Physiological Testing of Elite Athletes.* Champaign, IL: Human Kinetics; 1991.

7. Beneke R, von Duvillard SP. Determination of maximal lactate steady state response in selected sports events. *Med Sci Sports Exerc.* 1996;28(2):241-6.

8. Beneke R, Leithauser RM, Hutler M. Dependence of the maximal lactate steady state on the motor pattern of exercise. *Br J Sports Med.* 2001;35(3):192-6.

9. Billat LV. Interval training for performance: A scientific and empirical practice. Special recommendations for middle- and long-distance running. Part I: Aerobic interval training. *Sports Med* 2001;1(31):13-31.

10. Billat LV. Interval training for performance: A scientific and empirical practice. Special recommendations for middle- and long-distance running. Part II: Anaerobic interval training. *Sports Med.* 2001;31(2):75-90.

11. Billat V, Sirvent P, Py G, Koralsztein JP, Mercier J. The concept of maximal lactate steady state: A bridge between biochemistry, physiology and sport science. *Sports Med.* 2003;33(6):407-26.

12. Bishop PA, Smith JF, Kime JC, Mayo JM, Tin YH. Comparison of a manual and an automated enzymatic technique for determining blood lactate concentrations. *Int J Sports Med.* 1992;13(1):36-9.

13. Borg GA. Psychophysical bases of perceived exertion. *Med Sci Sports Exerc.* 1982;14(5):377-81.

14. Bowen L, Gross AS, Gimpel M, Li FX. Accumulated workloads and the acute:chronic workload ratio relate to injury risk in elite youth football players. *Br J Sports Med.* 2017;51(5):452-9.

15. Brooks GA. The lactate shuttle during exercise and recovery. *Med Sci Sports Exerc.* 1986;18(3):360-8.

16. Brown DM, Dwyer DB, Robertson SJ, Gastin PB. Metabolic power method underestimates energy expenditure in field sport movements using a GPS tracking system. *Int J Sports Physiol Perform.* 2016;11(8):1067-73.

17. Buchheit M. Monitoring training status with HR measures: Do all roads lead to Rome? *Front Physiol.* 2014;27(5):73.

18. Buchheit M. Player tracking technology: What if we were all wrong? Monitoring Athlete Training Loads - The Hows and Whys; 23-25/02/2016; Doha, Qatar: 2nd Aspire Sport Science Conference, https://vimeo.com/159904163; 2016.

19. Buchheit M. The numbers will love you back in return-I promise. *Int J Sports Physiol Perform.* 2016;11(4):551-4.

20. Buchheit M, Simpson BM. Player tracking technology: Half-full or half-empty glass? *Int J Sports Physiol Perform.* 2017;12(Suppl 2):S235–S41.

21. Buchheit M, Gray A, Morin JB. Assessing stride variables and vertical stiffness with GPS-embedded accelerometers: Preliminary insights for the monitoring of neuromuscular fatigue on the field. *J Sports Sci Med.* 2015;14(4):698-701.

22. Buchheit M, Manouvrier C, Cassirame J, Morin JB. Monitoring locomotor load in soccer: Is metabolic power, powerful? *Int J Sports Med.* 2015;36(14):1149-55.

23. Buchheit M, Allen A, Poon TK, Modonutti M, Gregson W, Di Salvo V. Integrating different tracking systems in football: Multiple camera semi-automatic system, local position measurement and GPS technologies. *J Sports Sci.* 2014;32(20)(20):1844-57.

24. Buchheit M, Al Haddad H, Simpson BM, Palazzi D, Bourdon PC, Di Salvo V, et al. Monitoring accelerations with GPS in football: Time to slow down? *Int J Sports Physiol Perform.* 2014;9(3):442-5.

25. Buchheit M, Hammond K, Bourdon PC, Simpson BM, Garvican-Lewis LA, Schmidt WF, et al. Relative match intensities at high altitude in highly-trained young soccer players (ISA3600). *J Sports Sci Med.* 2015;14(1):98-102.

26. Cardinale M, Varley MC. Wearable training-monitoring technology: Applications, challenges, and opportunities. *Int J Sports Physiol Perform.* 2017;12(Suppl 2):S255–s62.

27. Cerretelli P, Di Prampero PE. Kinetics of respiratory gas exchange and cardiac output at the onset of exercise. *Scand J Respir Dis.* 1971;Suppl (77):35a-g.

28. Cobbaert C, Morales C, van Fessem M, Kemperman H. Precision, accuracy and linearity of radiometer EML 105 whole blood metabolite biosensors. *Ann Clin Biochem.* 1999;36(Pt 6):730-8.

29. Coutts AJ. In the age of technology, Occam's razor still applies. *Int J Sports Physiol Perform.* 2014;9(5):741.

30. Coutts AJ, Rampinini E, Marcora SM, Castagna C, Impellizzeri FM. Heart rate and blood lactate correlates of perceived exertion during small-sided soccer games. *J Sci Med Sport.* 2009;12(1):79-84.

31. Coyle EF, Martin WH, Ehsani AA, Hagberg JM, Bloomfield SA, Sinacore DR, et al. Blood lactate threshold in some well-trained ischemic heart disease patients. *J Appl Physiol.* 1983;54(1):18-23.

32. Coyle EF, Feltner ME, Kautz SA, Hamilton MT, Montain SJ, Baylor AM, et al. Physiological and biomechanical factors associated with elite endurance cycling performance. *Med Sci Sports Exerc.* 1991;23(1):93-107.

33. Dascombe BJ, Reaburn PR, Sirotic AC, Coutts AJ. The reliability of the i-STAT clinical portable analyser. *J Sci Med Sport/Sports Med Aust.* 2007;10(3):135-40.

34. di Prampero PE, Fusi S, Sepulcri L, Morin JB, Belli A, Antonutto G. Sprint running: A new energetic approach. *J Exp Biol.* 2005;208(Pt 14):2809-16.

35. Duhig S, Shield AJ, Opar D, Gabbett TJ, Ferguson C, Williams M. Effect of high-speed running on hamstring strain injury risk. *Br J Sports Med.* 2016;50(24):1536-40.

36. Fell JW, Rayfield JM, Gulbin JP, Gaffney PT. Evaluation of the Accusport Lactate Analyser. *Int J Sports Med.* 1998;19(3):199-204.

37. Foster C, Hector LL, Welsh R, Schrager M, Green MA, Snyder AC. Effects of specific versus cross-training on running performance. *Eur J Appl Physiol Occup Physiol.* 1995;70(4):367-72.

38. Hader K, Mendez-Villanueva A, Palazzi D, Ahmaidi S, Buchheit M. Metabolic power requirement of change of direction speed in young soccer players: Not all is what it seems. *PLoS One.* 2016;11(3):e0149839.

39. Hagglund M, Walden M, Magnusson H, Kristenson K, Bengtsson H, Ekstrand J. Injuries affect team performance negatively in professional football: An 11-year follow-up of the UEFA Champions League injury study. *Br J Sports Med.* 2013;47(12):738-42.

40. Harris NK, Cronin J, Taylor KL, Boris J, Sheppard J. Understanding position transducer technology for strength and conditioning practitioners. *Strength Cond J.* 2010;32(4):66-79.

41. Haugen T, Buchheit M. Sprint running performance monitoring: Methodological and practical considerations. *Sports Med*. 2016;46(5):641-56.

42. Highton J, Mullen T, Norris J, Oxendale C, Twist C. Energy expenditure derived from micro-technology is not suitable for assessing internal load in collision-based activities. *Int J Sports Physiol Perform*. 2017;12(2):264-7.

43. Hill-Haas S, Coutts A, Rowsell G, Dawson B. Variability of acute physiological responses and performance profiles of youth soccer players in small-sided games. *J Sci Med Sport*. 2008;11(5):487-90.

44. Impellizzeri FM, Rampinini E, Coutts AJ, Sassi A, Marcora SM. Use of RPE-based training load in soccer. *Med Sci Sports Exerc*. 2004;36(6):1042-7.

45. Laursen PB, Jenkins DG. The scientific basis for high-intensity interval training: Optimising training programmes and maximising performance in highly trained endurance athletes. *Sports Med*. 2002;32(1):53-73.

46. Malone JJ, Lovell R, Varley MC, Coutts AJ. Unpacking the black box: Applications and considerations for using GPS devices in sport. *Int J Sports Physiol Perform*. 2017;12(Suppl 2):S218–s26.

47. Manzi V, Bovenzi A, Franco Impellizzeri M, Carminati I, Castagna C. Individual training-load and aerobic-fitness variables in premiership soccer players during the precompetitive season. *J Strength Cond Res*. 2013;27(3):631-6.

48. Marsland F, Mackintosh C, Anson J, Lyons K, Waddington G, Chapman DW. Using micro-sensor data to quantify macro kinematics of classical cross-country skiing during on-snow training. *Sports Biomech*. 2015;14(4):435-47.

49. Marsland F, Mackintosh C, Holmberg HC, Anson J, Waddington G, Lyons K, et al. Full course macro-kinematic analysis of a 10 km classical cross-country skiing competition. *PLoS One*. 2017;12(8):e0182262.

50. Mendez-Villanueva A, Buchheit M, Simpson BM, Bourdon PC. Match play intensity distribution in youth soccer. *Int J Sport Med*. 2013;34(2):101-10.

51. Michael JS, Rooney KB, Smith RM. The dynamics of elite paddling on a kayak simulator. *J Sports Sci*. 2012;30(7):661-8.

52. Midgley AW, McNaughton LR, Carroll S. Reproducibility of time at or near VO2max during intermittent treadmill running. *Int J Sports Med*. 2007;28(1):40-7.

53. Nielsen OB, de Paoli F, Overgaard K. Protective effects of lactic acid on force production in rat skeletal muscle. *J Physiol*. 2001;536(Pt 1):161-6.

54. Osgnach C, Poser S, Bernardini R, Rinaldo R, di Prampero PE. Energy cost and metabolic power in elite soccer: A new match analysis approach. *Med Sci Sports Exerc*. 2010;42(1):170-8.

55. Quod MJ, Martin DT, Martin JC, Laursen PB. The power profile predicts road cycling MMP. *Int J Sports Med*. 2010;31(6):397-401.

56. Ritchie D, Hopkins WG, Buchheit M, Cordy J, Bartlett JD. Quantification of training load during return to play after upper- and lower-body injury in Australian Rules Football. *Int J Sports Physiol Perform*. 2017;12(5):634-41.

57. Robergs RA, Ghiasvand F, Parker D. Biochemistry of exercise-induced metabolic acidosis. *Am J Physiol Regul Integr Comp Physiol*. 2004;287(3):R502-16.

58. Scott TJ, Black CR, Quinn J, Coutts AJ. Validity and reliability of the session-RPE method for quantifying training in Australian football: A comparison of the CR10 and CR100 scales. *J Strength Cond Res*. 2013;27(1):270-6.

59. Scott TJ, Thornton HR, Scott MTU, Dascombe BJ, Duthie GM. Differences between relative and absolute speed and metabolic thresholds in Rugby League. *Int J Sports Physiol Perform*. 2017:1-21.

60. Seiler S. What is best practice for training intensity and duration distribution in endurance athletes? *Int J Sports Physiol Perform*. 2010;5(3):276-91.

61. Seiler S, Hetlelid KJ. The impact of rest duration on work intensity and RPE during interval training. *Med Sci Sports Exerc*. 2005;37(9):1601-7.

62. Smith TB, Hopkins WG. Measures of rowing performance. *Sports Med*. 2012;42(4):343-58.

63. Stevens TG, de Ruiter CJ, van Maurik D, van Lierop CJ, Savelsbergh GJ, Beek PJ. Measured and estimated energy cost of constant and shuttle running in soccer players. *Med Sci Sports Exerc*. 2015;47(6):1219-24.

64. van Someren KA, Howatson G, Nunan D, Thatcher R, Shave R. Comparison of the Lactate Pro and Analox GM7 blood lactate analysers. *Int J Sports Med.* 2005;26(8):657-61.

Chapter 9

1. Achten J, Jeukendrup AE. Heart rate monitoring: Applications and limitations. *Sports Med.* 2003;33(7):517-38.

2. Akenhead R, Nassis GP. Training load and player monitoring in high-level football: Current practice and perceptions. *Int J Sports Physiol Perform.* 2016;11(5):587-93.

3. Akubat I, Patel E, Barrett S, Abt G. Methods of monitoring the training and match load and their relationship to changes in fitness in professional youth soccer players. *J Sports Sci.* 2012;30(14):1473-80.

4. Al Haddad H, Parouty J, Buchheit M. Effect of daily cold water immersion on heart rate variability and subjective ratings of well-being in highly trained swimmers. *Int J Sports Physiol Perform.* 2012;7(1):33-8.

5. Al Haddad H, Laursen PB, Chollet D, Ahmaidi S, Buchheit M. Reliability of resting and postexercise heart rate measures. *Int J Sports Med.* 2011;32(8):598-605.

6. Aughey RJ. Applications of GPS technologies to field sports. *Int J Sports Physiol Perform.* 2011;6(3):295-310.

7. Barnes KR, Hopkins WG, McGuigan MR, Kilding AE. Effects of different uphill interval-training programs on running economy and performance. *Int J Sports Physiol Perform.* 2013;8(6):639-47.

8. Barrett S, Midgley A, Lovell R. PlayerLoad: Reliability, convergent validity, and influence of unit position during treadmill running. *Int J Sports Physiol Perform.* 2014;9(6):945-52.

9. Bartlett JD, O'Connor F, Pitchford N, Torres-Ronda L, Robertson SJ. Relationships between internal and external training load in team-sport athletes: Evidence for an individualized approach. *Int J Sports Physiol Perform.* 2017;12(2):230-4.

10. Batterham AM, Hopkins WG. Making meaningful inferences about magnitudes. *Int J Sports Physiol Perform.* 2006;1(1):50-7.

11. Beneke R, Leithauser RM, Ochentel O. Blood lactate diagnostics in exercise testing and training. *Int J Sports Physiol Perform.* 2011;6(1):8-24.

12. Berglund B, Safstrom H. Psychological monitoring and modulation of training load of world-class canoeists. *Med Sci Sports Exerc.* 1994;26(8):1036-40.

13. Billman GE, Hoskins RS. Time-series analysis of heart rate variability during submaximal exercise. Evidence for reduced cardiac vagal tone in animals susceptible to ventricular fibrillation. *Circulation.* 1989;80(1):146-57.

14. Borresen J, Lambert MI. Changes in heart rate recovery in response to acute changes in training load. *Eur J Appl Physiol.* 2007;101(4):503-11.

15. Borresen J, Lambert MI. Autonomic control of heart rate during and after exercise: Measurements and implications for monitoring training status. *Sports Med.* 2008;38(8):633-46.

16. Borresen J, Lambert MI. The quantification of training load, the training response and the effect on performance. *Sports Med.* 2009;39(9):779-95.

17. Bosquet L, Gamelin FX, Berthoin S. Is aerobic endurance a determinant of cardiac autonomic regulation? *Eur J Appl Physiol.* 2007;100(3):363-9.

18. Bosquet L, Gamelin FX, Berthoin S. Reliability of postexercise heart rate recovery. *Int J Sports Med.* 2008;29(3):238-43.

19. Bosquet L, Merkari S, Arvisais D, Aubert AE. Is heart rate a convenient tool to monitor over-reaching? A systematic review of the literature. *Br J Sports Med.* 2008;42(9):709-14.

20. Bouchard C, Rankinen T. Individual differences in response to regular physical activity. *Med Sci Sports Exerc.* 2001;33:S446-51.

21. Brandenberger G, Buchheit M, Ehrhart J, Simon C, Piquard F. Is slow wave sleep an appropriate recording condition for heart rate variability analysis? *Auton Neurosci.* 2005;121(1-2):81-6.

22. Brenner IK, Thomas S, Shephard RJ. Autonomic regulation of the circulation during exercise and heat exposure. Inferences from heart rate variability. *Sports Med.* 1998;26(2):85-99.

23. Brink MS, Visscher C, Coutts AJ, Lemmink KA. Changes in perceived stress and recovery in overreached young elite soccer players. *Scand J Med Sci Sports.* 2010:[Epub ahead of print] Oct 7.

24. Buchheit M. Monitoring training status with HR measures: Do all roads lead to Rome? *Front Physiol.* 2014;27(5):73.

25. Buchheit M. The numbers will love you back in return–I promise. *Int J Sports Physiol Perform.* 2016;11(4):551-4.

26. Buchheit M. Applying the acute:chronic workload ratio in elite football: Worth the effort? *Br J Sports Med.* 2017;51(18):1325-7.

27. Buchheit M. Want to see my report, coach? *Aspetar Journal.* 2017(6):34-43. http://www .aspetar.com/journal/upload/PDF/2017216161135 .pdf.

28. Buchheit M. Trivial effects are clearly important. *Sport Perform Sci Rep.* Jan 5, 2018;1.

29. Buchheit M. Magnitudes matter more than beetroot juice. *Sport Perform Sci Rep.* Jan 15, 2018;1.

30. Buchheit M, Gindre C. Cardiac parasympathetic regulation: Respective associations with cardio-respiratory fitness and training load. *Am J Physiol Heart Circ Physiol.* 2006;291(1):H451-H8.

31. Buchheit M, Laursen PB. High-intensity interval training, solutions to the programming puzzle. Part II: Anaerobic energy, neuromuscular load and practical applications. *Sports Med.* 2013;43(10):927-54.

32. Buchheit M, Rabbani A. 30-15 Intermittent Fitness Test vs. Yo-Yo Intermittent Recovery Test Level 1: Relationship and sensitivity to training. *Int J Sports Physiol Perform.* 2014;9(3):522-4.

33. Buchheit M, Simpson BM. Player tracking technology: Half-full or half-empty glass? *Int J Sports Physiol Perform.* 2017;12(Suppl 2):S235–S41.

34. Buchheit M, Gray A, Morin JB. Assessing stride variables and vertical stiffness with GPS-embedded accelerometers: Preliminary insights for the monitoring of neuromuscular fatigue on the field. *J Sports Sci Med.* 2015;14(4):698-701.

35. Buchheit M, Cholley Y, Lambert P. Psychometric and physiological responses to a preseason competitive camp in the heat with a 6-hour time difference in elite soccer players. *Int J Sports Physiol Perform.* 2016;11(2):176-81.

36. Buchheit M, Papelier Y, Laursen PB, Ahmaidi S. Noninvasive assessment of cardiac parasympathetic function: Post-exercise heart rate recovery or heart rate variability? *Am J Physiol Heart Circ Physiol.* 2007;293(1):H8-H10.

37. Buchheit M, Laursen PB, Al Haddad H, Ahmaidi S. Exercise-induced plasma volume expansion and post-exercise parasympathetic reactivation. *Eur J Appl Physiol.* 2009;105(3):471-81.

38. Buchheit M, Mendez-Villanueva A, Quod M, Bourdon P. Determinants of the variability of heart rate measures during a competitive period in young soccer players. *Eur J Appl Physiol.* 2010;109:869-78.

39. Buchheit M, Lacome M, Cholley Y, Simpson BM. Neuromuscular responses to conditioned soccer sessions assessed via GPS-embedded accelerometers: Insights into tactical periodization. *Int J Sports Physiol Perform.* Sep 2017;5:1-21.

40. Buchheit M, Simon C, Piquard F, Ehrhart J, Brandenberger G. Effect of increased training load on vagal-related indexes of heart rate variability: A novel sleep approach. *Am J Physiol Heart Circ Physiol.* 2004;287:H2813-H8.

41. Buchheit M, Voss SC, Nybo L, Mohr M, Racinais S. Physiological and performance adaptations to an in-season soccer camp in the heat: Associations with heart rate and heart rate variability. *Scand J Med Sci Sports.* 2011;21(6):e477-85.

42. Buchheit M, Al Haddad H, Mendez-Villanueva A, Quod MJ, Bourdon PC. Effect of maturation on hemodynamic and autonomic control recovery following maximal running exercise in highly trained young soccer players. *Front Physiol.* 2011;2:69.

43. Buchheit M, Simpson MB, Al Haddad H, Bourdon PC, Mendez-Villanueva A. Monitoring changes in physical performance with heart rate measures in young soccer players. *Eur J Appl Physiol.* 2012;112(2):711-23.

44. Buchheit M, Simon C, Charloux A, Doutreleau S, Piquard F, Brandenberger G. Relationship between very high physical activity energy expenditure, heart rate variability and self-estimate of health status in middle-aged individuals. *Int J Sports Med.* 2006;27(9):697-701.

45. Buchheit M, Millet GP, Parisy A, Pourchez S, Laursen PB, Ahmaidi S. Supramaximal training and post-exercise parasympathetic reactivation in adolescents. *Med Sci Sports Exerc.* 2008;40(2):362-71.

46. Buchheit M, Chivot A, Parouty J, Mercier D, Al Haddad H, Laursen PB, et al. Monitoring endurance running performance using cardiac parasympathetic function. *Eur J Appl Physiol.* 2010;108:1153-67.

47. Buchheit M, Racinais S, Bilsborough JC, Bourdon PC, Voss SC, Hocking J, et al. Monitoring fitness, fatigue and running performance during a pre-season training camp in elite football players. *J Sci Med Sport.* 2013;16(6):550-5.

48. Buchheit M, Simpson BM, Schmidt W, Aughey RJ, Soria R, Hunt R, et al. Predicting sickness during a 2-week soccer camp at 3600 m (ISA3600). *Br J Sports Med.* 2013;47(Suppl 1):i124-i7.

49. Buchheit M, Simpson BM, Garvican-Lewis LA, Hammond K, Kley M, Schmidt WF, et al. Wellness, fatigue and physical performance acclimatisation to a 2-week soccer camp at 3600 m (ISA3600). *Br J Sports Med.* 2013;(47 Suppl):i100-i6.

50. Burgess DJ. The research doesn't always apply: Practical solutions to evidence-based training-load monitoring in elite team sports. *Int J Sports Physiol Perform.* 2017;12 (Suppl 2):S2136–s41.

51. Burton AR, Rahman K, Kadota Y, Lloyd A, Vollmer-Conna U. Reduced heart rate variability predicts poor sleep quality in a case-control study of chronic fatigue syndrome. *Exp Brain Res.* 2010;204(1):71-8.

52. Carey DL, Blanch P, Ong KL, Crossley KM, Crow J, Morris ME. Training loads and injury risk in Australian football-differing acute:chronic workload ratios influence match injury risk. *Br J Sports Med.* 2017;51(16):1215-20.

53. Carling C. Interpreting physical performance in professional soccer match-play: Should we be more pragmatic in our approach? *Sports Med.* 2013;43(8):655-63.

54. Cassirame J, Stuckey MI, Sheppard F, Tordi N. Accuracy of the Minicardio system for heart rate variability analysis compared to ECG. *J Sports Med Phys Fitness.* 2013;53(3):248-54.

55. Castagna C, Impellizzeri FM, Chaouachi A, Bordon C, Manzi V. Effect of training intensity distribution on aerobic fitness variables in elite soccer players: A case study. *J Strength Cond Res.* 2011;25(1):66-71.

56. Cerretelli P, Di Prampero PE. Kinetics of respiratory gas exchange and cardiac output at the onset of exercise. *Scand J Respir Dis.* 1971;(Suppl 77):35a-g.

57. Chen JL, Yeh DP, Lee JP, Chen CY, Huang CY, Lee SD, et al. Parasympathetic nervous activity mirrors recovery status in weightlifting perfor-

mance after training. *J Strength Cond Res.* 2011;25(6):1546-52.

58. Cormack SJ, Newton RU, McGuigan MR, Cormie P. Neuromuscular and endocrine responses of elite players during an Australian rules football season. *Int J Sports Physiol Perform.* 2008;3(4):439-53.

59. Daanen HA, Lamberts RP, Kallen VL, Jin A, Van Meeteren NL. A systematic review on heart-rate recovery to monitor changes in training status in athletes. *Int J Sports Physiol Perform.* 2012;7(3):251-60.

60. Dellaserra CL, Gao Y, Ransdell L. Use of integrated technology in team sports: A review of opportunities, challenges, and future directions for athletes. *J Strength Cond Res.* 2014;28(2):556-73.

61. Drew MK, Finch CF. The relationship between training load and injury, illness and soreness: A systematic and literature review. *Sports Med.* 2016;46(6):861-83.

62. Dupuy O, Mekary S, Berryman N, Bherer L, Audiffren M, Bosquet L. Reliability of heart rate measures used to assess post-exercise parasympathetic reactivation. *Clin Physiol Funct Imaging.* 2012;32(4):296-304.

63. Ekkekakis P. *The Measurement of Affect, Mood, and Emotion: A Guide for Health-Behavioral Research.* New York: Cambridge University Press; 2013.

64. Esco MR, Flatt AA. Ultra-short-term heart rate variability indexes at rest and post-exercise in athletes: Evaluating the agreement with accepted recommendations. *J Sports Sci Med.* 2014;13(3):535-41.

65. Fanchini M, Rampinini E, Riggio M, Coutts A, Pecci C, McCall A. Despite association, the acute:chronic work load ratio does not predict non-contact injury in elite footballers. *Science and Medicine in Football.* 2018: In press.

66. Flatt AA, Esco MR. Validity of the ithleteTM smart phone application for determining ultra-short-term heart rate variability. *Journal of Human Kinetics.* 2013;39:85-92.

67. Fowler PM, Murray A, Farooq A, Lumley N, Taylor L. Subjective and objective responses to two Rugby 7's World Series competitions. *Journal of Strength and Conditioning Research.* [Ahead of print.]

68. Gamelin FX, Berthoin S, Bosquet L. Validity of the polar S810 heart rate monitor to measure R-R intervals at rest. *Med Sci Sports Exerc.* 2006;38(5):887-93.

69. Garet M, Tournaire N, Roche F, Laurent R, Lacour JR, Barthelemy JC, et al. Individual interdependence between nocturnal ANS activity and performance in swimmers. *Med Sci Sports Exerc.* 2004;36(12):2112-8.

70. Garvican LA, Hammond K, Varley M, Gore CJ, Billaut F, Aughey RJ. Lower running performance and exacerbated fatigue in soccer played at 1600 m. *Int J Sports Physiol Perform.* May 22, 2013. [Epub ahead of print].

71. Green HJ, Thomson JA, Ball ME, Hughson RL, Houston ME, Sharratt MT. Alterations in blood volume following short-term supramaximal exercise. *J Appl Physiol.* 1984;56(1):145-9.

72. Halson SL. Monitoring training load to understand fatigue in athletes. *Sports Med.* 2014;44(Suppl 2):S139-47.

73. Hamilton DK. Explosive performance in young soccer players during several games in succession: a tournament scenario. *J Aust Strength Cond.* 2009;17(2):3-10.

74. Hamilton RM, McKechnie PS, Macfarlane PW. Can cardiac vagal tone be estimated from the 10-second ECG? *Int J Cardiol.* 2004;95(1):109-15.

75. Hampson R, Jowett S. Effects of coach leadership and coach–athlete relationship on collective efficacy. *Scand J Med Sci Sports.* 2014;24(2):454-60.

76. Hautala AJ, Kiviniemi AM, Tulppo MP. Individual responses to aerobic exercise: The role of the autonomic nervous system. *Neurosci Biobehav Rev.* 2009;33(2):107-15.

77. Hautala AJ, Tulppo MP, Makikallio TH, Laukkanen R, Nissila S, Huikuri HV. Changes in cardiac autonomic regulation after prolonged maximal exercise. *Clin Physiol.* 2001;21(2):238-45.

78. Hautala AJ, Kiviniemi AM, Makikallio TH, Kinnunen H, Nissila S, Huikuri HV, et al. Individual differences in the responses to endurance and resistance training. *Eur J Appl Physiol.* 2006;96(5):535-42.

79. Hedelin R, Bjerle P, Henriksson-Larsen K. Heart rate variability in athletes: Relationship with central and peripheral performance. *Med Sci Sports Exerc.* 2001;33(8):1394-8.

80. Hedman AE, Hartikainen JE, Tahvanainen KU, Hakumaki MO. The high frequency component of heart rate variability reflects cardiac parasympathetic modulation rather than parasympathetic "tone." *Acta Physiol Scand.* 1995;155(3):267-73.

81. Heisterberg MF, Fahrenkrug J, Andersen JL. Multiple blood samples in elite soccer players. Is it worthwhile? *J Sports Sci.* 2014;32(13):1324-7.

82. Heisterberg MF, Fahrenkrug J, Krustrup P, Storskov A, Kjaer M, Andersen JL. Extensive monitoring through multiple blood samples in professional soccer players. *J Strength Cond Res.* 2013;27(5):1260-71.

83. Hooper SL, Mackinnon LT. Monitoring overtraining in athletes. Recommendations. *Sports Med.* 1995;20(5):321-7.

84. Hopkins W. Spreadsheets for analysis of controlled trials, with adjustment for a subject characteristic. *Sportscience.* 2006;10:46-50. Accessed July 4, 2009. Available at http://sportsci .org/6/wghcontrial.htm.

85. Hopkins WG. Measures of reliability in sports medicine and science. *Sports Med.* 2000;30(1):1-15.

86. Hopkins WG. Precision of the estimate of a subject's true value (Excel spreadsheet) (2000). In Internet Society for Sport Science: www .sportsci.org/resource/stats/xprecisionsubject .xls2000 (April 25, 2014).

87. Hopkins WG. Statistical vs clinical or practical significance. *Sportscience* 2002;6. http://www .sportsci.org/jour/0201/Statistical_vs_clinical .ppt.

88. Hopkins WG. How to interpret changes in an athletic performance test. *Sportscience.* 2004; 8:1-7.

89. Hopkins WG, Hawley JA, Burke LM. Design and analysis of research on sport performance enhancement. *Med Sci Sports Exerc.* 1999;31(3):472-85.

90. Hopkins WG, Marshall SW, Batterham AM, Hanin J. Progressive statistics for studies in sports medicine and exercise science. *Med Sci Sports Exerc.* 2009;41(1):3-13.

91. Hug B, Heyer L, Naef N, Buchheit M, Werhrlin JP, Millet GP. Tapering for marathon and cardiac autonomic function. Jul 2014;35(8):676-83.

92. Hulin BT, Gabbett TJ, Lawson DW, Caputi P, Sampson JA. The acute:chronic workload ratio

predicts injury: High chronic workload may decrease injury risk in elite rugby league players. *Br J Sports Med.* 2016;50(4):231-6.

93. Iellamo F, Legramante JM, Pigozzi F, Spataro A, Norbiato G, Lucini D, et al. Conversion from vagal to sympathetic predominance with strenuous training in high-performance world class athletes. *Circulation.* 2002;105(23):2719-24.

94. Impellizzeri FM, Rampinini E, Coutts AJ, Sassi A, Marcora SM. Use of RPE-based training load in soccer. *Med Sci Sports Exerc.* 2004;36(6):1042-7.

95. Iwasaki K, Zhang R, Zuckerman JH, Levine BD. Dose-response relationship of the cardiovascular adaptation to endurance training in healthy adults: How much training for what benefit? *J Appl Physiol.* 2003;95(4):1575-83.

96. Kellmann M, Kallus K. *Recovery-Stress Questionnaire for Athletes: User manual.* Champaign, IL: Human Kinetics; 2001.

97. Kiely J. Periodization paradigms in the 21st century: Evidence-led or tradition-driven? *Int J Sports Physiol Perform.* 2012;7(3):242-50.

98. Kiviniemi AM, Hautala AJ, Kinnunen H, Tulppo MP. Endurance training guided individually by daily heart rate variability measurements. *Eur J Appl Physiol.* 2007;101(6):743-51.

99. Kiviniemi AM, Hautala AJ, Seppanen T, Makikallio TH, Huikuri HV, Tulppo MP. Saturation of high-frequency oscillations of R-R intervals in healthy subjects and patients after acute myocardial infarction during ambulatory conditions. *Am J Physiol Heart Circ Physiol.* 2004;287(5):H1921-H7.

100. Kiviniemi AM, Hautala AJ, Kinnunen H, Nissila J, Virtanen P, Karjalainen J, et al. Daily Exercise prescription based on heart rate variability among men and women. *Med Sci Sports Exerc.* Jul 2010;42(7):1355-63.

101. Kukielka M, Seals DR, Billman GE. Cardiac vagal modulation of heart rate during prolonged submaximal exercise in animals with healed myocardial infarctions: Effects of training. *Am J Physiol Heart Circ Physiol.* 2006;290(4):H1680-5.

102. Lacome M, Simpson BM, Buchheit M. Monitoring training status with player-tracking technology. Still on the way to Rome. *Aspetar Journal.* 2018: In Press.

103. Ladell WS. Assessment of group acclimatization to heat and humidity. *J Physiol.* 1951;115(3):296-312.

104. Lamberts RP, Lemmink KA, Durandt JJ, Lambert MI. Variation in heart rate during submaximal exercise: Implications for monitoring training. *J Strength Cond Res.* 2004;18(3):641-5.

105. Lamberts RP, Swart J, Noakes TD, Lambert MI. Changes in heart rate recovery after high-intensity training in well-trained cyclists. *Eur J Appl Physiol.* 2009;105(5):705-13.

106. Lamberts RP, Maskell S, Borresen J, Lambert MI. Adapting workload improves the measurement of heart rate recovery. *Int J Sports Med.* 2011;32(9):698-702.

107. Laursen PB. Training for intense exercise performance: High-intensity or high-volume training? *Scand J Med Sci Sports.* 2010;20(Suppl 2):1-10.

108. Le Meur Y, Buchheit M, Aubry A, Coutts AJ, Hausswirth C. Assessing overreaching with heart-rate recovery: What is the minimal exercise intensity required? *Int J Sports Physiol Perform.* 2017;12(4):569-73.

109. Le Meur Y, Hausswirth C, Natta F, Couturier A, Bignet F, Vidal PP. A multidisciplinary approach to overreaching detection in endurance trained athletes. *J Appl Physiol (1985).* 2013;114(3):411-20.

110. Le Meur Y, Pichon A, Schaal K, Schmitt L, Louis J, Gueneron J, et al. Evidence of parasympathetic hyperactivity in functionally overreached athletes. *Med Sci Sports Exerc.* 2013;45(11):2061-71.

111. Leicht AS, Allen GD. Moderate-term reproducibility of heart rate variability during rest and light to moderate exercise in children. *Braz J Med Biol Res.* 2008;41(7):627-33.

112. Malik M, Camm AJ, Amaral LA, Goldberger AL, Ivanov P, Stanley HE, et al. Components of heart rate variability—what they really mean and what we really measure. *Am J Cardiol.* 1993;72(11):821-2.

113. Malone S, Owen A, Newton M, Mendes B, Collins KD, Gabbett TJ. The acute:chronic workload ratio in relation to injury risk in professional soccer. *J Sci Med Sport.* 2017;20(6):561-5.

114. Mann T, Lamberts RP, Lambert MI. Methods of prescribing relative exercise intensity: Physiological and practical considerations. *Sports Med*. 2013;43(7):613-25.

115. Manzi V, Iellamo F, Impellizzeri F, D'Ottavio S, Castagna C. Relation between individualized training impulses and performance in distance runners. *Med Sci Sports Exerc*. 2009;41(11):2090-6.

116. Manzi V, Bovenzi A, Franco Impellizzeri M, Carminati I, Castagna C. Individual training-load and aerobic-fitness variables in premiership soccer players during the precompetitive season. *J Strength Cond Res*. 2013;27(3):631-6.

117. Manzi V, Castagna C, Padua E, Lombardo M, D'Ottavio S, Massaro M, et al. Dose-response relationship of autonomic nervous system responses to individualized training impulse in marathon runners. *Am J Physiol Heart Circ Physiol*. 2009;296(6):H1733-40.

118. Mateo M, Blasco-Lafarga C, Martinez-Navarro I, Guzman JF, Zabala M. Heart rate variability and pre-competitive anxiety in BMX discipline. *Eur J Appl Physiol*. 2012;112(1):113-23.

119. McLean BD, Coutts AJ, Kelly V, McGuigan MR, Cormack SJ. Neuromuscular, endocrine, and perceptual fatigue responses during different length between-match microcycles in professional rugby league players. *Int J Sports Physiol Perform*. 2010;5(3):367-83.

120. McNarry MA, Lewis MJ. Heart rate variability reproducibility during exercise. *Physiol Meas*. 2012;33(7):1123-33.

121. Meeusen R, Duclos M, Gleeson M, Rietjens G, Steinacker J, Urhausen A. Prevention, diagnosis and treatment of the overtraining syndrome. *Eur J Sport Sci*. 2006;6:1-14.

122. Meeusen R, Duclos M, Foster C, Fry A, Gleeson M, Nieman D, et al. Prevention, diagnosis and treatment of the overtraining syndrome: Joint consensus statement of the European College of Sport Science (ECSS) and the American College of Sports Medicine (ACSM). *Eur J Sport Sci*. 2013;13(1):1-24.

123. Meister S, Aus der Funten K, Meyer T. Repeated monitoring of blood parameters for evaluating strain and overload in elite football players: Is it justified? *J Sports Sci*. 2014;32(13):1328-31.

124. Morales J, Garcia V, Garcia-Masso X, Salva P, Escobar R, Busca B. The use of heart rate variability in assessing precompetitive stress in high-standard judo athletes. *Int J Sports Med*. 2013;34(2):144-51.

125. Morin JB, Jeannin T, Chevallier B, Belli A. Spring-mass model characteristics during sprint running: Correlation with performance and fatigue-induced changes. *Int J Sports Med*. 2006;27(2):158-65.

126. Murray NB, Gabbett TJ, Townshend AD, Blanch P. Calculating acute:chronic workload ratios using exponentially weighted moving averages provides a more sensitive indicator of injury likelihood than rolling averages. *Br J Sports Med*. 2017;51(9):749-54.

127. Myllymaki T, Kyrolainen H, Savolainen K, Hokka L, Jakonen R, Juuti T, et al. Effects of vigorous late-night exercise on sleep quality and cardiac autonomic activity. *J Sleep Res*. 2011;20(1 Pt 2):146-53.

128. Nakamura FY, Flatt AA, Pereira LA, Ramirez-Campillo R, Loturco I, Esco MR. Ultra-short-term heart rate variability is sensitive to training effects in team sports players. *J Sports Sci Med*. 2015;14(3):602-5.

129. Norris SR, Smith DJ. Planning, periodization, and sequencing of training and competition: The rationale for a competently planned, optimally executed training and competition program, supported by a multidisciplinary team. In Kellmann M, ed. *Enhancing Recovery: Preventing Underperformance in Athletes*. Champaign, IL: Human Kinetics; 2002: 121-41.

130. Nussinovitch U, Elishkevitz KP, Katz K, Nussinovitch M, Segev S, Volovitz B, et al. Reliability of ultra-short ECG indices for heart rate variability. *Ann Noninvasive Electrocardiol*. 2011;16(2):117-22.

131. Nussinovitch U, Elishkevitz KP, Kaminer K, Nussinovitch M, Segev S, Volovitz B, et al. The efficiency of 10-second resting heart rate for the evaluation of short-term heart rate variability indices. *Pacing Clin Electrophysiol*. 2011;34(11):1498-502.

132. Otzenberger H, Gronfier C, Simon C, Charloux A, Ehrhart J, Piquard F, et al. Dynamic heart rate variability: A tool for exploring sympathovagal balance continuously during sleep in men. *Am J Physiol*. 1998;275:H946-H50.

133. Pagani M, Lucini D. Can autonomic monitoring predict results in distance runners? *Am J Physiol Heart Circ Physiol*. 2009;296(6):H1721-2.

134. Parouty J, Al Haddad H, Quod MJ, Leprêtre PM, Ahmaidi S, Buchheit M. Effect of cold water immersion on 100-m sprint performance in well-trained swimmers. *Eur J Appl Physiol.* 2010;109(3):483-90.

135. Parrado E, Garcia MA, Ramos J, Cervantes JC, Rodas G, Capdevila L. Comparison of Omega Wave System and Polar S810i to detect R-R intervals at rest. *Int J Sports Med.* 2010;31(5):336-41.

136. Penttila J, Helminen A, Jartti T, Kuusela T, Huikuri HV, Tulppo MP, et al. Time domain, geometrical and frequency domain analysis of cardiac vagal outflow: Effects of various respiratory patterns. *Clin Physiol.* 2001;21(3):365-76.

137. Pichot V, Busso T, Roche F, Garet M, Costes F, Duverney D, et al. Autonomic adaptations to intensive and overload training periods: A laboratory study. *Med Sci Sports Exerc.* 2002;34(10):1660-6.

138. Pichot V, Roche F, Gaspoz JM, Enjolras F, Antoniadis A, Minini P, et al. Relation between heart rate variability and training load in middle-distance runners. *Med Sci Sports Exerc.* 2000;32(10):1729-36.

139. Plews DJ, Laursen PB, Kilding AE, Buchheit M. Heart rate variability in elite triathletes, is variation in variability the key to effective training? A case comparison. *Eur J Appl Physiol.* 2012;112(11):3729-41.

140. Plews DJ, Laursen PB, Kilding AE, Buchheit M. Heart rate variability and training intensity distribution in elite rowers. *Int J Sports Physiol Perform.* 2014;9(6):1026-32.

141. Plews DJ, Laursen PB, Kilding AE, Buchheit M. Evaluating training adaptation with heart rate measures: A methodological comparison. *Int J Sports Physiol Perform.* 2013;8(6):688-91.

142. Plews DJ, Laursen PB, Kilding AE, Buchheit M. Training adaptation and heart rate variability in elite endurance athletes - opening the door to effective monitoring. *Sports Med.* 2013;43(9):773-81.

143. Plews DJ, Laursen PB, Kilding AE, Buchheit M. Heart rate variability and training intensity distribution in elite rowers. *Int J Sports Physiol Perform.* 2014: Apr 3 [Epub ahead of print].

144. Plews DJ, Laursen PB, Le Meur Y, Hausswirth C, Kilding AE, Buchheit M. Monitoring training with heart rate variability: How much compliance is needed for valid assessment? *Int J Sports Physiol Perform.* 2014: In press.

145. Plews DJ, Scott B, Altini M, Wood M, Kilding AE, Laursen PB. Comparison of heart-rate-variability recording with smartphone photoplethysmography, Polar H7 Chest Strap, and electrocardiography. *Int J Sports Physiol Perform.* 2017;12(10):1324-8.

146. Portier H, Louisy F, Laude D, Berthelot, Guezennec CY. Intense endurance training on heart rate and blood pressure variability in runners. *Med Sci Sports Exerc.* 2001;33(7):1120-5.

147. Rowsell GJ, Coutts AJ, Reaburn P, Hill-Haas S. Effects of cold-water immersion on physical performance between successive matches in high-performance junior male soccer players. *J Sports Sci.* 2009;27(6):565-73.

148. Saboul D, Pialoux V, Hautier C. The impact of breathing on HRV measurements: Implications for the longitudinal follow-up of athletes. *Eur J Sport Science.* 2013: Feb 8 [Epub ahead of print].

149. Sandercock GR, Bromley PD, Brodie DA. The reliability of short-term measurements of heart rate variability. *Int J Cardiol.* 2005;103(3):238-47.

150. Saw A, Main L, Robertson S, Gastin P. Athlete self-report measure use and associated psychological alterations. *Sports.* 2017;5(3):54.

151. Saw AE, Main LC, Gastin PB. Role of a self-report measure in athlete preparation. *Journal of Strength and Conditioning Research.* 2015;29(3):685-91.

152. Saw AE, Main LC, Gastin PB. Monitoring athletes through self-report: Factors influencing implementation. *J Sports Sci Med.* 2015;14:137-46.

153. Saw AE, Main LC, Gastin PB. Monitoring the athlete training response: Subjective self-reported measures trump commonly used objective measures: A systematic review. *Br J Sports Med.* 2016;50(5):281-91.

154. Saw AE, Kellmann M, Main LC, Gastin PB. Athlete self-report measures in research and practice: Considerations for the discerning reader and fastidious practitioner. *Int J Sports Physiol Perform.* 2017;12(S2):127-35.

155. Scharhag-Rosenberger F, Meyer T, Walitzek S, Kindermann W. Time course of changes in

endurance capacity: A 1-yr training study. *Med Sci Sports Exerc.* 2009;41(5):1130-7.

156. Schmitt L, Regnard J, Desmarets M, Mauny F, Mourot L, Fouillot JP, et al. Fatigue shifts and scatters heart rate variability in elite endurance athletes. *PLoS One.* 2013;8(8):e71588.

157. Silva JR, Rumpf MC, Hertzog M, Castagna C, Farooq A, Girard O, et al. Acute and residual soccer match-related fatigue: A systematic review and meta-analysis. *Sports Med.* 2018;48(3):539-83.

158. Spinelli L, Petretta M, Marciano F, Testa G, Rao MA, Volpe M, et al. Cardiac autonomic responses to volume overload in normal subjects and in patients with dilated cardiomyopathy. *Am J Physiol.* 1999;277(4 Pt 2):H1361-8.

159. Stanley J, Peake JM, Buchheit M. Cardiac parasympathetic reactivation following exercise: Implications for training prescription. *Sports Med.* 2013;43(12):1259-77.

160. Stanley J, Peake JM, Buchheit M. Consecutive days of cold water immersion: Effects on cycling performance and heart rate variability. *Eur J Appl Physiol.* 2013;113(2):371-84.

161. Task Force. Heart rate variability: Standards of measurement, physiological interpretation and clinical use. Task Force of the European Society of Cardiology and the North American Society of Pacing and Electrophysiology. *Circulation.* 1996;93(5):1043-65.

162. Taylor K, Chapman D, Cronin J, Newton M, Gill N. Fatigue monitoring in high performance sport: A survey of current trends. *Journal of Australian Strength and Conditioning.* 2012;20(1):12-23.

163. ten Haaf T, van Staveren S, Oudenhoven E, Piacentini MF, Meeusen R, Roelands B, et al. Prediction of functional overreaching from subjective fatigue and readiness to train after only 3 days of cycling. *Int J Sports Physiol Perform.* 2017;12(S2):87-94.

164. Thorpe RT, Strudwick AJ, Buchheit M, Atkinson G, Drust B, Gregson W. Tracking morning fatigue status across in-season training weeks in elite soccer players. *Int J Sports Physiol Perform.* 2016;11(7):947-52.

165. Tulppo MP, Makikallio TH, Seppanen T, Airaksinen JK, Huikuri HV. Heart rate dynamics during accentuated sympathovagal interaction. *Am J Physiol.* 1998;274(3 Pt 2):H810-6.

166. Twist C, Highton J. Monitoring fatigue and recovery in rugby league players. *Int J Sports Physiol Perform.* 2013;8(5):467-74.

167. Wallen MB, Hasson D, Theorell T, Canlon B, Osika W. Possibilities and limitations of the Polar RS800 in measuring heart rate variability at rest. *Eur J Appl Physiol.* 2012;112(3):1153-65.

168. Weippert M, Kumar M, Kreuzfeld S, Arndt D, Rieger A, Stoll R. Comparison of three mobile devices for measuring R-R intervals and heart rate variability: Polar S810i, Suunto t6 and an ambulatory ECG system. *Eur J Appl Physiol.* 2010;109(4):779-86.

169. Wikipedia. http://en.wikipedia.org/wiki/Nick_Broad. Accessed June 2, 2018.

170. Winsley RJ, Armstrong N, Bywater K, Fawkner SG. Reliability of heart rate variability measures at rest and during light exercise in children. *Br J Sports Med.* 2003;37(6):550-2.

171. Yamamoto K, Miyachi M, Saitoh T, Yoshioka A, Onodera S. Effects of endurance training on resting and post-exercise cardiac autonomic control. *Med Sci Sports Exerc.* 2001;33(9):1496-502.

172. Cohen S, Kamarck T, Mermelstein R. A global measure of perceived stress. *Journal of Health and Social Behavior.* 1983;24:385-96.

173. Dean J, Whelan J, Meyers A. An incredibly quick way to assess mood states: The incredibly short POMS. Presented at Annual Conference of the Association for the Advancement of Applied Sport Psychology, 1990.

174. Grove JR, Main LC, Partridge K, Bishop DJ, Russell S, Shepherdson A, Ferguson L. Training distress and performance readiness: Laboratory and field validation of a brief self-report measure. *Scand J Med Sci Sports.* 2014;24:e483-90.

175. Grove JR, Prapavessis H. Preliminary evidence for the reliability and validity of an abbreviated Profile of Mood States. *International Journal of Sport Psychology.* 1992;23:93-109.

176. Hitzschke B, Holst T, Ferrauti A, Meyer T, Pfeiffer M, Kellmann M. Entwicklung des Akutmaßes zur Erfassung von Erholung und Beanspruchung im Sport [Development of the Acute Recovery and Stress Scale]. *Diagnostica.* 2016.

177. Hitzschke B, Kölling S, Ferrauti A, Meyer T, Pfeiffer M, Kellmann M. Entwicklung der Kurzskala zur Erfassung von Erholung und Beanspruchung im Sport (KEB) [Development

of the Short Recovery and Stress Scale for Sports (SSRS)]. *Zeitschrift für Sportpsychologie.* 2015;22:146-61.

178. James DV, Barnes AJ, Lopes P, Wood DM. Heart rate variability: Response following a single bout of interval training. *Int J Sports Med.* 2002;23:247-51.

179. Kellmann M, Kallus KW. Recovery-stress questionnaire for athletes. In Kallus, KW, Kellman, M, eds. *The Recovery-Stress Questionnaires: User manual.* Frankfurt am Main: Pearson Assessment & Information GmbH; 2016:86-131.

180. Kellmann M, Kölling S, Hitzschke B. *Das Akutmaß und die Kurzskala zur Erfassung von Erholung und Beanspruchung im Sport: Manual [The Acute Measure and the Short Scale of Recovery and Stress for Sports: Manual].* Köln: Sportverlag Strauß; 2016.

181. Kellmann M, Patrick T, Botterill C, Wilson C. The Recovery-Cue and its use in applied settings: Practical suggestions regarding assessment and monitoring of recovery. In Kellmann, M, ed. *Enhancing Recovery: Preventing Underperformance in Athletes.* Champaign, IL: Human Kinetics; 2002:219-29.

182. Kenttä G, Hassmén P, Raglin JS. Mood state monitoring of training and recovery in elite kayakers. *European Journal of Sport Science.* 2006;6:245–53.

183. Laurent CM, Green JM, Bishop PA, Sjokvist J, Schumacker RE, Richardson MT, Curtner-Smith M. A practical approach to monitoring recovery: Development of a perceived recovery status scale. *Journal of Strength and Conditioning Research.* 2011;25:620-28.

184. Lundqvist C, Kenttä G. Positive emotions are not simply the absence of the negative ones: Development and validation of the Emotional Recovery Questionnaire (EmRecQ). *Sport Psychologist.* 2010;24:468-88.

185. Main L, Grove JR. A multi-component assessment model for monitoring training distress among athletes. *European Journal of Sport Science.* 2009;9:195-202.

186. McNair P, Lorr M, Droppleman L. *POMS Manual.* San Diego, CA: Education and Industrial Testing Service; 1981.

187. Micklewright D, Gibson ASC, Gladwell V, Al Salman A. Development and validity of the Rating-of-Fatigue Scale. *Sports Medicine.* 2017;47:2375-93.

188. Mourot L, Bouhaddi M, Tordi N, Rouillon JD, Regnard J. Short- and long-term effects of a single bout of exercise on heart rate variability: Comparison between constant and interval training exercises. *Eur J Appl Physiol.* 2004;92:508-17.

189. Niewiadomski W, Gasiorowska A, Krauss B, Mroz A, Cybulski G. Suppression of heart rate variability after supramaximal exertion. *Clin Physiol Funct Imaging.* 2007;27:309-19.

190. Raglin JS, Morgan WP. Development of a scale for use in monitoring training-induced distress in athletes. *International Journal of Sports Medicine.* 1994;15:84-8.

191. Rushall BS. A tool for measuring stress tolerance in elite athletes. *Journal of Applied Sport Psychology.* 1990;2:51-66.

192. Shacham S. A shortened version of the Profile of Mood States. *Journal of Personality Assessment.* 1983;47:305-306.

193. Terry P, Lane A, Fogarty G. Construct validity of the Profile of Mood States-Adolescents for use with adults. *Psychology of Sport and Exercise.* 2003;4:125-39.

194. Terry PC, Lane AM, Lane HJ, Keohane L. Development and validation of a mood measure for adolescents. *Journal of Sports Sciences.* 1999;17:861-72.

Chapter 10

1. Benjamin DJ, Berger OJ, Johannesson M, Nosek AB, Wagenmakers EJ, Berk R, et al. Redefine statistical significance. *Nature Human Behaviour* [Internet]. 2017 (September 1, 2017).

2. Buchheit M. The numbers will love you back in return—I promise. *Int J Sports Physiol Perform.* 2016;11(4):551-4.

3. Buchheit M. Houston, we still have a problem. *Int J Sports Physiol Perform.* 2017;12(8):1111-14.

4. Buchheit M. Outside the Box. *Int J Sports Physiol Perform.* 2017;12(8):1001-2.

5. Buchheit M, Laursen PB. High-intensity interval training, solutions to the programming puzzle. Part II: Anaerobic energy, neuromuscular load and practical applications. *Sports Med.* 2013;43(10):927-54.

6. Buchheit M, Laursen PB. High-intensity interval training, solutions to the programming puzzle: Part I: Cardiopulmonary emphasis. *Sports Med.* 2013;43(5):313-38.

7. Close GL. Close Nutrition [Internet] 2017. (September 22) Available from: http://www .closenutrition.com/?p=619.

8. Cohen J. Things I have learned (so far). *American Psychologist*. 1990;45:1304-12.

9. Cressey E. Eric Cressey [Internet] 2017. (September, 22) Available from: https://ericcressey.com /the-success-is-in-the-struggle.

10. Ericsson KA, Pool E. *Peak: Secrets From the New Science of Expertise*. Boston: Houghton Mifflin Harcourt; 2016.

11. MacInnis MJ, Gibala MJ. Physiological adaptations to interval training and the role of exercise intensity. *J Physiol*. 2017;595(9):2915-30.

12. Maxwell JC. *Thinking for a Change: 11 Ways Highly Successful People Approach Life and Work*. New York: Warner Books Inc,; 2005.

13. McCaw A. *7 Keys to Being a Great Coach: Become Your Best and They Will Too*. Whyte K, ed. PrintShopCentral.com; 2016.

14. Nuzzo R. Scientific method: Statistical errors. *Nature*. 2014;506(7487):150-2.

15. Thompson WR. Worldwide Survey of Fitness Trends for 2018: The CREP Edition. *ACSM's Health & Fitness Journal*. 2017;21(6):10-19.

Chapter 11

1. Alm P, Yu J-G. Physiological characters in mixed martial arts. *Am J Sports Sci*. 2013;1(2):12-7.

2. Amtmann J, Amtmann K, Spath W. Lactate and rate of perceived exertion responses of athletes training for and competing in a mixed martial arts event. *J Strength Cond Res*. 2008;22:645-7.

3. Andreato LV, Moraes SFd, Gomes TLdM, Esteves JDC, Andreato TV, Franchini E. Estimated aerobic power, muscle strength and flexibility in elite Brazilian jiu-jitsu athletes. *Science & Sports*. 2011;26(6):329-37.

4. Atha J, Yeadon M, Sandover J, Parsons K. The damaging punch. *Br Med J*. 1985;291:1756-7.

5. Beneke R, Beyer T, Jachner C, Erasmus J, Hutler M. Energetics of karate kumite. *Eur J Appl Physiol*. 2004;92:518-23.

6. Brandao F, Fernandes H, Vilaca Alves J, Fonseca S, Machado Reis V. Hematological and biochemical markers after a Brazilian jiu-jitsu tournament in world-class athletes. *Rev Bras Cineantropom Desempenho Hum*. 2014;16(2):144-51.

7. Bridge C, Ferreira da Silva Santos J, Chaabene H, Pieter W, Franchini E. Physical and physiological profiles of taekwondo athletes. *Sports Med*. 2014;44(6):713-33.

8. Buchheit M. Monitoring training status with HR measures: Do all roads lead to Rome? *Front Physiol*. 2014;27(5):73.

9. Buchheit M, Laursen P. High-intensity interval training, solutions to the programming puzzle. Part I: cardiopulmonary emphasis. *Sports Med*. 2013;43(5):313-38.

10. Buchheit M, Laursen P. High-intensity interval training, solutions to the programming puzzle. Part II: anaerobic energy, neuromuscular load and practical applications. *Sports Med*. 2013;43(10):927-54.

11. Buse G. No holds barred sport fighting: A 10 year review of mixed martial arts competition. *Br J Sports Med*. 2006;40:169-72.

12. Callister R, Callister RJ, Staron R, Fleck S, Tesch P, Dudley G. Physiological characteristics of elite judo athletes. *Sports Med*. 1991;12(2):196-203.

13. Chaabene H, Hachana Y, Franchini E, Mkaouer B, Chamari K. Physical and physiological profile of elite karate athletes. *Sports Med*. 2012;42(10):829-43.

14. Chaabene H, Tabben M, Mkaouer B, Franchini E, Negra Y, Hammami M, et al. Amature boxing: Physical and physiological attributes. *Sports Med*. 2015;45:337-52.

15. Christen J, Foster C, Porcari J, Mikat R. Temporal robustness of the session ration of percieved exertion. *Int J Sport Phys Perf*. 2016;11(8):1088-93.

16. Claudino J, Cronin J, Mezencio B, McMaster D, McGuigan M, Tricoli V, et al. The countermovement jump to monitor neuromuscular status: A meta-analysis. *J Sci Med Sport*. 2017;20(4):397-402.

17. Davis P, Leithauser R, Beneke P. The energetics of semicontact 3×2-min amature boxing. *Int J Sports Physiol Perform*. 2014;9(2):233-9.

18. Del Vecchio F, Hirata S, Franchini E. A review of the time-motion analysis and combat development in mixed martial arts matches at regional level tournaments. *Perceptual & Motor Skills*. 2011;112:639-48.

19. Estevan I, Alvarez O, Falco C, Molina-Garcia J, Castillo I. Impact force and time analysis influenced by execution distance in a roundhouse kick to the head in taekwondo. *J Strength Cond Res*. 2011;25(10):2851-6.

20. Franchini E, Takito M, Kiss M, Sterkowicz S. Physical fitness and anthropometrical differences between elite and non-elite judo players. *Biol Sport*. 2005;22(4):315-28.

21. Gastin P. Energy system interaction and relative contribution during maximal exercise. *Sports Med*. 2001;31(10):725-41.

22. Gathercole R, Sporer B, Stellingwerff T, Sleivert G. Comparison of the capacity of different jump and sprint field tests to detect neuromuscular fatigue. *J Strength Cond Res*. 2015;29(9):2522-31.

23. Haff G, Nimphius S. Training principles for power. *Strength Cond J*. 2012;34(6):2-12.

24. Hayes P, Quinn M. A mathmatical model for quantifying training. *Eur J Appl Physiol*. 2009;106(6):839-47.

25. Heller J, Peric T, Dlouha R, Kohlikova E, Melichna J, Novakova H. Physiological profiles of male and female taekwondo (ITF) black belts. *J Sport Sci*. 1998;16:243-9.

26. Horswill C. Physiology of wrestling. In Garrett W, Kirkendall D, eds. *Exercise and Sport Science*. Philadelphia: Lippincott, Williams & Wilkins; 2000:955-64.

27. Horswill C, Scott J, Galea P. Comparison of maximum aerobic power, maximum anaerobic power, and skinfold thickness of elite and nonelite junior wrestlers. *Int J Sports Med*. 1989;10:165-8.

28. Hulin B, Gabbett T, Caputi P, Lawson D, Sampson J. Low chronic workload and the acute:chronic workload ratio are more predictive of injury than between-match recovery time: A two-season prospective cohort study in elite rugby league players. *Br J Sports Med*. 2016;50(16):1008-12.

29. Issurin V. Block periodization versus traditional training theory: A review. *J Sports Med Phys Fitness*. 2008;48(1):65-75.

30. James L, Haff G, Kelly V, Beckman E. Towards a determination of the physiological characteristics distinguishing succesful mixed martial arts athletes: A systematic review of combat sport literature. *Sports Med*. 2016;46:1525-51.

31. James L, Beckman E, Kelly V, Haff G. The neuromuscular qualities of higher and lower-level mixed martial arts competitors. *Int J Sport Phys Perf*. 2016;12(5):612-20.

32. James L, Robertson S, Haff G, Beckman E, Kelly V. Identifying the performance characteristics of a winning outcome in elite mixed martial arts competition. *J Sci Med Sport*. 2017;20(3):296-301.

33. Jamieson J. *Ultimate MMA Conditioning*. Kirkland, WA: Performance Sports, Inc.; 2009.

34. Khanna G, Manna I. Study of the physiological profile of Indian boxers. *J Sports Sci Med*. 2006;5:90-8.

35. Kraemer W, Fry A, Rubin M, Triplett-McBride T, Gordon S, Koziris L, et al. Physiological and performance responses to tournament wrestling. *Med Sci Sports Exerc*. 2001;33(8):1367-78.

36. Laursen P, Jenkins D. The scientific basis for high-intensity interval training. *Sports Med*. 2002;32(1):53-73.

37. Lellamo F, Pigozzi F, Spataro A, Lucini D, Pagani M. T-wave and heart rate variability changes to assess training in world-class athletes. *Med Sci Sports Exerc*. 2004;36(8):1342-6.

38. MacDougall D, Sale D. *The Physiology of Training for High Performance*. Oxford: Oxford University Press; 2014.

39. Mack J, Stojsih S, Sherman S, Dau N, Bir C, eds. Amateur boxer biomechanics and punch force. In Jensen R, Ebben W. Petushek E, Richter C, Roemer K, eds. *Proceedings of the 28th Conference of the International Society of Biomechanics in Sports*. Marquette, MI: n.p., 2010:453-56.

40. Matsushigue K, Hartmann K, Franchini E. Taekwondo: Physiological responses and match analysis. *J Strength Cond Res*. 2009;23:1112-7.

41. Miarka B, Coswig V, Vecchio F, Brito C, Amtmann J. Comparisons of time-motion analysis of mixed martial arts rounds by weight division. *Int J Perf Analy Sport*. 2015;15:1189-201.

42. Murray N, Gabbett T, Townsend A, Blanch P. Calculating acute:chronic workload ratios using exponentially weighted moving averages provides a more sensitve indicator of injury likelihood than rolling averages. *Br J Sports Med*. 2016;51(9):749-54.

43. Nilsson J, Csergo S, Gullstrand L, Tveit P, Refsnes P. Work-time profile, blood lactate concentration, and rating of perceived exertion in the 1998 Greco-Roman wrestling World Championship. *J Sport Sci*. 2002;20:939-45.

44. Oliveira M, Moreira D, Godoy J, Cambraia A. Avaliacao da forca de preensao palmar em atletas

de jiu-jitsu de nivel competitivo. *Rev Bras Ciencia e Movi*. 2006;14(3):63-70.

45. Pedzich W, Mastalera A, Urbanik C. The comparison of the dynamics of selected leg strokes in taekwondo WTF. *Acta Bioeng Biomech*. 2006;8(1):1-9.

46. Saw A, Main L, Gastin P. Monitoring the athlete training response: Subjective self-reported measures trump commonly used objective measures: A systematic review. *Sports Med*. 2016;50(5):281-91.

47. Schick M, Brown L, Coburn J, Beam W, Schick E, Dabbs N. Physiological profile of mixed martial artists. *Med Sport*. 2010;14(4):182-7.

48. Smith M. Physiological profile of senior and junior England international amateur boxers. *J Sports Sci Med*. 2006;5:74-89.

49. Song T, Garvie G. Anthropometric, flexibility, strength and physiological measures of Canadian wrestlers and comparison of Canadian and Japanese Olympic wrestlers. *Can J Appl Sport Sci*. 1980;5:1-8.

50. Tabata I, Irisawa K, Kouzaki M, Nishimura K, Ogita F, Miyachi M. Metabolic profile of high intensity intermittent exercise. *Med Sci Sports Exerc*. 1997;29(3):390-5.

51. Vecchio FD, Bianchi S, Hirata S, Chacon-Mikahil M. Analise morfo-funcional de praticantes de brazilian jiu-jitsu e estudo da temporalidade e da quantificação das ações motoras na modalidade. *Movimento e Percepção*. 2007;7:263-81.

52. Walilko T, Viano D, Bir C. Biomechanics of the head for Olympic boxer punches to the face. *Br J Sports Med*. 2005;39(10):710-9.

53. Yoon J. Physiological profiles of elite senior wrestlers. *Sports Med*. 2002;32(4):225-33.

54. Yoon J, Bang D, Jun H. The development of sparring types for elite Korean national wrestlers. *Korean J Sport Sci*. 1994;5(2):15-24.

Chapter 12

1. Abbiss CR, Laursen PB. Describing and understanding pacing strategies during athletic competition. *Sports Med*. 2008;38(3):239-52.

2. Ainegren M, Carlsson P, Tinnsten M, Laaksonen MS. Skiing economy and efficiency in recreational and elite cross-country skiers. *J Strength Cond Res*. 2013;27(5):1239-52.

3. Andersson E, Holmberg HC, Ortenblad N, Bjorklund G. Metabolic responses and pacing strategies during successive sprint skiing time trials. *Med Sci Sports Exerc*. 2016.

4. Andersson E, Pellegrini B, Sandbakk O, Stuggl T, Holmberg HC. The effects of skiing velocity on mechanical aspects of diagonal cross-country skiing. *Sports Biomech*. 2014;13(3):267-84.

5. Andersson E, Supej M, Sandbakk O, Sperlich B, Stoggl T, Holmberg HC. Analysis of sprint cross-country skiing using a differential global navigation satellite system. *Eur J Appl Physiol*. 2010;110(3):585-95.

6. Bolger CM, Kocbach J, Hegge AM, Sandbakk O. Speed and heart-rate profiles in skating and classical cross-country skiing competitions. *Int J Sports Physiol Perform*. 2015;10(7):873-80.

7. Helgerud J, Hoydal K, Wang E, Karlsen T, Berg P, Bjerkaas M, et al. Aerobic high-intensity intervals improve VO2max more than moderate training. *Med Sci Sports Exerc*. 2007;39(4):665-71.

8. Holmberg HC. The elite cross-country skier provides unique insights into human exercise physiology. *Scand J Med Sci Sports*. 2015;25 Suppl 4:100-9.

9. Holmberg HC, Rosdahl H, Svedenhag J. Lung function, arterial saturation and oxygen uptake in elite cross country skiers: influence of exercise mode. *Scand J Med Sci Sports*. 2007;17(4):437-44.

10. Lindinger SJ, Stoggl T, Muller E, Holmberg HC. Control of speed during the double poling technique performed by elite cross-country skiers. *Med Sci Sports Exerc*. 2009;41(1):210-20.

11. Losnegard T, Hallen J. Physiological differences between sprint- and distance-specialized cross-country skiers. *Int J Sports Physiol Perform*. 2014;9(1):25-31.

12. Losnegard T, Myklebust H, Hallen J. Anaerobic capacity as a determinant of performance in sprint skiing. *Med Sci Sports Exerc*. 2012;44(4):673-81.

13. Losnegard T, Kjeldsen K, Skattebo O. An analysis of the pacing strategies adopted by elite cross-country skiers. *J Strength Cond Res*. 2016.

14. Losnegard T, Myklebust H, Spencer M, Hallen J. Seasonal variations in VO2max, O2-cost, O2-deficit, and performance in elite cross-country skiers. *J Strength Cond Res*. 2013;27(7):1780-90.

15. Norman RW, Ounpuu S, Fraser M, Mitchell R. Mechanical power output and estimated metabolic rates of Nordic skiers during Olympic competition. *Int J Sport Biomech*. 1989;5:169-84.

16. Ortenblad N, Westerblad H, Nielsen J. Muscle glycogen stores and fatigue. *J Physiol*. 2013;591(18):4405-13.

17. Sandbakk O, Holmberg HC. A reappraisal of success factors for Olympic cross-country skiing. *Int J Sports Physiol Perform*. 2014;9(1):117-21.

18. Sandbakk O, Holmberg HC. Physiological capacity and training routines of elite cross-country skiers: Approaching the upper limits of human endurance. *Int J Sports Physiol Perform*. 2017:1-26.

19. Sandbakk O, Ettema G, Holmberg HC. The influence of incline and speed on work rate, gross efficiency and kinematics of roller ski skating. *Eur J Appl Physiol*. 2012;112(8):2829-38.

20. Sandbakk O, Hegge AM, Ettema G. The role of incline, performance level, and gender on the gross mechanical efficiency of roller ski skating. *Front Physiol*. 2013;4:293.

21. Sandbakk O, Holmberg HC, Leirdal S, Ettema G. Metabolic rate and gross efficiency at high work rates in world class and national level sprint skiers. *Eur J Appl Physiol*. 2010;109(3):473-81.

22. Sandbakk O, Holmberg HC, Leirdal S, Ettema G. The physiology of world-class sprint skiers. *Scand J Med Sci Sports*. 2011;21(6):e9-16.

23. Sandbakk O, Sandbakk SB, Ettema G, Welde B. Effects of intensity and duration in aerobic high-intensity interval training in highly trained junior cross-country skiers. *J Strength Cond Res*. 2013;27(7):1974-80.

24. Sandbakk O, Ettema G, Leirdal S, Jakobsen V, Holmberg HC. Analysis of a sprint ski race and associated laboratory determinants of world-class performance. *Eur J Appl Physiol*. 2011;111(6):947-57.

25. Sandbakk O, Hegge AM, Losnegard T, Skattebo O, Tonnessen E, Holmberg HC. The physiological capacity of the world's highest ranked female cross-country skiers. *Med Sci Sports Exerc*. 2016;48(6):1091-100.

26. Sandbakk O, Losnegard T, Skattebo O, Hegge AM, Tonnessen E, Kocbach J. Analysis of classical time-trial performance and technique-specific physiological determinants in elite female cross-country skiers. *Front Physiol*. 2016;7:326.

27. Stoggl T, Holmberg HC. Double-poling biomechanics of elite cross-country skiers: Flat versus uphill terrain. *Med Sci Sports Exerc*. 2016.

28. Stoggl T, Lindinger S, Muller E. Evaluation of an upper-body strength test for the cross-country skiing sprint. *Med Sci Sports Exerc*. 2007;39(7):1160-9.

29. Stoggl T, Muller E, Ainegren M, Holmberg HC. General strength and kinetics: Fundamental to sprinting faster in cross country skiing? *Scand J Med Sci Sports*. 2011;21(6):791-803.

30. Sylta O, Tonnessen E, Seiler S. Do elite endurance athletes report their training accurately? *Int J Sports Physiol Perform*. 2014;9(1):85-92.

31. Sylta O, Tonnessen E, Sandbakk O, Hammarstrom D, Danielsen J, Skovereng K, et al. Effects of HIIT on physiological and hormonal adaptions in well-trained cyclists. *Med Sci Sports Exerc*. 2017;49(6):1137-46.

32. Tonnessen E, Haugen TA, Hem E, Leirstein S, Seiler S. Maximal aerobic capacity in the winter-Olympics endurance disciplines: Olympic-medal benchmarks for the time period 1990-2013. *Int J Sports Physiol Perform*. 2015;10(7):835-9.

33. Vandbakk K, Welde B, Kruken AH, Baumgart J, Ettema G, Karlsen T, et al. Effects of upper-body sprint-interval training on strength and endurance capacities in female cross-country skiers. *PLoS One*. 2017;12(2):e0172706.

Chapter 13

1. Arrese AL, Izquierdo DM, Urdiales DM. A review of the maximal oxygen uptake values necessary for different running performance levels. *New Studies in Athletic*. 2005;20(3):7-20.

2. Boileau RA, Mayhew JL, Riner WF, Lussier L. Physiological characteristics of elite middle and long distance runners. *Can J Appl Sport Sci*. 1982;7(3):167-72.

3. Brandon LJ. Physiological factors associated with middle distance running performance. *Sports Med*. 1995;19(4):268-77.

4. Coe P. *Winning Running: Successful 800m & 1500m Racing and Training*: The Crowood Press, Ramsbury, Marlborough, Wiltshire; 1996.

5. Duffield R, Dawson B, Goodman C. Energy system contribution to 1500- and 3000-metre

track running. *J Sports Sci.* 2005;23(10):993-1002.

6. Hanon C, Lehenaff D, Gajer B, Mathieu C, Vollmer JC. Analyse comparée de différentes séances de développement de VO2max. *Il èmes journées internationales des sciences du sport: Expertise et sport de haut-niveau,* November 12-15, 2002.

7. Hanon C, Thomas C. Effects of optimal pacing strategies for 400-, 800-, and 1500-m races on the VO2 response. *J Sports Sci.* 2011;29(9):905-12.

8. Hanon C, Leveque JM, Thomas C, Vivier L. Pacing strategy and VO2 kinetics during a 1500-m race. *Int J Sports Med.* 2008;29(3):206-11.

9. Houmard JA, Costill DL, Mitchell JB, Park SH, Chenier TC. The role of anaerobic ability in middle distance running performance. *Eur J Appl Physiol Occup Physiol.* 1991;62(1):40-3.

10. Ingham SA, Whyte GP, Pedlar C, Bailey DM, Dunman N, Nevill AM. Determinants of 800-m and 1500-m running performance using allometric models. *Med Sci Sports Exerc.* 2008;40(2):345-50.

11. Keul J. Die Bedeutung des aeroben und anaeroben Leistungsvermögens für Mittel und Langstreckenläufer *Die Lehre der Leichtathletik* 1975;7-18.

12. Noakes TD, Lambert MI, Hauman R. Which lap is the slowest? An analysis of 32 world mile record performances. *Br J Sports Med.* 2009;43(10):760-4.

13. Rabadan M, Diaz V, Calderon FJ, Benito PJ, Peinado AB, Maffulli N. Physiological determinants of specialty of elite middle- and long-distance runners. *J Sports Sci.* 2011;29(9):975-82.

14. Spencer MR, Gastin PB. Energy system contribution during 200- to 1500-m running in highly trained athletes. *Med Sci Sports Exerc.* 2001;33(1):157-62.

15. Svedenhag J, Sjodin B. Maximal and submaximal oxygen uptakes and blood lactate levels in elite male middle- and long-distance runners. *Int J Sports Med.* 1984;5(5):255-61.

16. Thiel C, Foster C, Banzer W, De Koning J. Pacing in Olympic track races: Competitive tactics versus best performance strategy. *J Sports Sci.* 2012;30(11):1107-15.

17. Tjelta LI. Physiological factors affecting performance in elite distance runners. *Acta Kinesiologiae Universitatis Tartuensis.* 2016;22:7-19.

18. Weyand PG, Davis JA. Running performance has a structural basis. *J Exp Biol.* 2005;208(Pt 14):2625-31.

19. Wilson H. *Running My Way*: N.p.: Sackville Books; 1998.

Chapter 14

1. Banister EW, Calvert TW. Planning for future performance: Implications for long term training. *Canadian Journal of Applied Sport Sciences Journal Canadien des Sciences Appliquees au Sport.* 1980;5(3):170-6.

2. Barnes K, Hopkins W, McGuigan M, Kilding A. Effects of different uphill interval-training programs on running economy and performance. *Int J Sports Physiol Perform.* 2013;8(6):639-47.

3. Barnes KR, Kilding AE. Strategies to improve running economy. *Sports Med.* 2015;45(1):37-56.

4. Bartlett JD, Hawley JA, Morton JP. Carbohydrate availability and exercise training adaptation: Too much of a good thing? *Eur J Sport Sci.* 2015;15(1):3-12.

5. Billat V. Interval training for performance: A scientific and empirical practice. Special recommendations for middle- and long-distance running. Part II: Anaerobic interval training. *Sports Med.* 2001;31(2):75-90.

6. Billat V. Interval training for performance: A scientific and empirical practice. Special recommendations for middle- and long-distance running. Part I: Aerobic interval training. *Sports Med.* 2001;31(1):13-31.

7. Billat V, Lepretre PM, Heugas AM, Laurence MH, Salim D, Koralsztein JP. Training and bioenergetic characteristics in elite male and female Kenyan runners. *Med Sci Sports Exerc.* 2003;35(2):297-304; discussion 5-6.

8. Billat VL, Demarle A, Slawinski J, Paiva M, Koralsztein JP. Physical and training characteristics of top-class marathon runners. *Med Sci Sports Exerc.* 2001;33(12):2089-97.

9. Bonetti DL, Hopkins WG. Sea-level exercise performance following adaptation to hypoxia: A meta-analysis. *Sports Med.* 2009;39(2):107-27.

10. Buchheit M. Monitoring training status with HR measures: Do all roads lead to Rome? *Frontiers in Physiology.* 2014;5:73.

11. Buchheit M, Laursen PB. High-intensity interval training, solutions to the programming puzzle.

Part I: Cardiopulmonary emphasis. *Sports Med.* 2013;43(5):313-38.

12. Buchheit M, Laursen PB. High-intensity interval training, solutions to the programming puzzle. Part II: Anaerobic energy, neuromuscular load and practical applications. *Sports Med.* 2013;43(10):927-54.

13. Burke LM, Read RS. Dietary supplements in sport. *Sports Medicine.* 1993;15(1):43-65.

14. Casadio JR, Kilding AE, Cotter JD, Laursen PB. From lab to real world: Heat acclimation considerations for elite athletes. *Sports Med.* 2016.

15. Chapman DW, Sharma AP, Saunders AG. The effect of brief downhill running training on running economy and lower body strength and power. *J Strength Cond Res.* 2017;31(Suppl 1):S115-16.

16. Close GL, Hamilton DL, Philp A, Burke LM, Morton JP. New strategies in sport nutrition to increase exercise performance. *Free Radic Biol Med.* 2016;98:144-58.

17. Esteve-Lanao J, Foster C, Seiler S, Lucia A. Impact of training intensity distribution on performance in endurance athletes. *J Strength Cond Res.* 2007;21(3):943-9.

18. Esteve-Lanao J, San Juan AF, Earnest CP, Foster C, Lucia A. How do endurance runners actually train? Relationship with competition performance. *Med Sci Sports Exerc.* 2005;37(3):496-504.

19. Foster C, Rodriguez-Marroyo JA, de Koning JJ. Monitoring training loads: The past, the present, and the future. *Int J Sports Physiol Perform.* 2017;12(Suppl 2):S22-S8.

20. Foster C, Florhaug JA, Franklin J, Gottschall L, Hrovatin LA, Parker S, et al. A new approach to monitoring exercise training. *J Strength Cond Res.* 2001;15(1):109-15.

21. Franch J, Madsen K, Djurhuus MS, Pedersen PK. Improved running economy following intensified training correlates with reduced ventilatory demands. *Med Sci Sports Exerc.* 1998;30(8):1250-6.

22. Gabbett TJ. The training-injury prevention paradox: Should athletes be training smarter and harder? *Br J Sports Med.* 2016;50(5):273-80.

23. Gabbett TJ, Ullah S. Relationship between running loads and soft-tissue injury in elite team sport athletes. *J Strength Cond Res.* 2012;26(4):953-60.

24. Garrett A, Creasy R, Rehrer N, Patterson M, Cotter J. Effectiveness of short-term heat acclimation for highly trained athletes. *Eur J Appl Physiol.* 2012;112(5):1827-37.

25. Gore CJ, Clark SA, Saunders PU. Nonhematological mechanisms of improved sea-level performance after hypoxic exposure. *Med Sci Sports Exerc.* 2007;39(9):1600-9.

26. Gore CJ, Sharpe K, Garvican-Lewis LA, Saunders PU, Humberstone CE, Robertson EY, et al. Altitude training and haemoglobin mass from the optimised carbon monoxide rebreathing method determined by a meta-analysis. *Br J Sports Med.* 2013;47 Suppl 1:i31-9.

27. Hetlelid KJ, Plews DJ, Herold E, Laursen PB, Seiler S. Rethinking the role of fat oxidation: Substrate utilisation during high-intensity interval training in well-trained and recreationally trained runners. *BMJ Open Sport & Exercise Medicine.* 2015;1(1).

28. Issurin V. New horizons for the methodology and physiology of training periodization. *Sports Med.* 2010;1(40):189-206.

29. Jeukendrup AE. Periodized nutrition for athletes. *Sports Med.* 2017:1-13.

30. Kruse TN, Carter RE, Rosedahl JK, Joyner MJ. Speed trends in male distance running. *PLoS ONE.* 2014;9(11):e112978.

31. Larsen HB, Sheel AW. The Kenyan runners. *Scand J Med Sci Sports.* 2015;25 Suppl 4:110-8.

32. Laursen P, Jenkins D. The scientific basis for high-intensity interval training: Optimising training programmes and maximising performance in highly trained endurance athletes. *Sports Med.* 2002;32(1):53-73.

33. Laursen PB. Training for intense exercise performance: High-intensity or high-volume training? *Scand J Med Sci Sports.* 2010;20:1-10.

34. Le Meur Y, Hausswirth C, Natta F, Couturier A, Bignet F, Vidal PP. A multidisciplinary approach to overreaching detection in endurance trained athletes. *J Appl Physiol (1985).* 2013;114(3):411-20.

35. Lobigs LM, Sharpe K, Garvican-Lewis LA, Gore CJ, Peeling P, Dawson B, et al. The athlete's hematological response to hypoxia: A meta-analysis on the influence of altitude exposure on key biomarkers of erythropoiesis. *Am J Hematol.* 2018;93(1):74-83.

36. Lundby C, Robach P. Does 'altitude training' increase exercise performance in elite athletes? *Exp Physiol.* 2016;101(7):783-88.

37. Maffetone PB, Malcata R, Rivera I, Laursen PB. The Boston Marathon versus the World Marathon Majors. *PLoS ONE.* 2017;12(9):e0184024.

38. Marquet LA, Brisswalter J, Louis J, Tiollier E, Burke LM, Hawley JA, et al. Enhanced endurance performance by periodization of CHO intake: "Sleep low" strategy. *Med Sci Sports Exerc.* 2016;48(4):663-72.

39. McMahon NF, Leveritt MD, Pavey TG. The effect of dietary nitrate supplementation on endurance exercise performance in healthy adults: A systematic review and meta-analysis. *Sports Med.* 2017;47(4):735-56.

40. Mytton GJ, Archer DT, Turner L, Skorski S, Renfree A, Thompson KG, et al. Increased variability of lap speeds: Differentiating medalists and nonmedalists in middle-distance running and swimming events. *Int J Sports Physiol Perform.* 2015;10(3):369-73.

41. Paluska S. Caffeine and exercise. *Curr Sports Med Rep.* 2003;2(4):213-9.

42. Periard JD, Racinais S, Sawka MN. Adaptations and mechanisms of human heat acclimation: Applications for competitive athletes and sports. *Scand J Med Sci Sports.* 2015;25 Suppl 1:20-38.

43. Racinais S, Alonso JM, Coutts AJ, Flouris AD, Girard O, Gonzalez-Alonso J, et al. Consensus recommendations on training and competing in the heat. *Scand J Med Sci Sports.* 2015;25 Suppl 1:6-19.

44. Robinson N, Sottas PE, Schumacher YO. The athlete biological passport: How to personalize anti-doping testing across an athlete's career? *Med Sport Sci.* 2017;62:107-18.

45. Ronnestad BR, Hansen J. A scientific approach to improve physiological capacity of an elite cyclist. *Int J Sports Physiol Perform.* 2017:1-11.

46. Ronnestad BR, Hansen J, Ellefsen S. Block periodization of high-intensity aerobic intervals provides superior training effects in trained cyclists. *Scand J Med Sci Sports.* 2014;24(1):34-42.

47. Ronnestad BR, Hansen J, Thyli V, Bakken TA, Sandbakk O. 5-week block periodization increases aerobic power in elite cross-country skiers. *Scand J Med Sci Sports.* 2016;26(2):140-46.

48. Sandford GN, Pearson S, Allen SV, Malcata RM, Kilding AE, Ross A, et al. Tactical behaviors in men's 800m Olympic and World Championship medalists: A changing of the guard. *Int J Sports Physiol Perform.* 2018;13(2):246-49.

49. Saw AE, Main LC, Gastin PB. Monitoring the athlete training response: Subjective self-reported measures trump commonly used objective measures: A systematic review. *Br J Sports Med.* 2016;50(5):281-91.

50. Seiler KS. What is best practice for training intensity and duration distribution in endurance athletes? *Int J Sports Physiol Perform.* 2010;5(3):276-91.

51. Seiler KS. Seiler's hierarchy of endurance training needs. *European Endurance Conference, European Athletics Coaching Summit Series.* 2016. Available online at: www.researchgate.net /publication/310725768_Seiler's_Hierarchy_of _Endurance_Training_Needs (accessed September 9, 2017).

52. Sharma AP, Garvican-Lewis LA, Clark B, Stanley J, Robertson EY, Saunders PU, et al. Training at 2100 m altitude affects running speed and session RPE at different intensities in elite middle-distance runners. *Int J Sports Physiol Perform.* 2017;12(Suppl 2): S2147-S2152.

53. Sjodin B, Svedenhag J. Applied physiology of marathon running. *Sports Med.* 1985;2(2):83-99.

54. Skiba PF. Calculation of Power Output and Quantification of Training Stress in Distance Runners: The Development of the GOVSS Algorithm. 2006. Available online at: http:// runscribe.com/wp-content/uploads/power /GOVSS.pdf (accessed September 9, 2017).

55. Stanley J, Peake J, Buchheit M. Cardiac parasympathetic reactivation following exercise: Implications for training prescription. *Sports Med.* 2013;43(12):1259-77.

56. Stanley J, D'Auria S, Buchheit M. Cardiac parasympathetic activity and race performance: an elite triathlete case study. *Int J Sports Physiol Perform.* 2015;10(4):528-34.

57. Stanley J, Halliday A, D'Auria S, Buchheit M, Leicht A. Effect of sauna-based heat acclimation on plasma volume and heart rate variability. *Eur J Appl Physiol.* 2015;115(4):785-94.

58. Stellingwerff T. Case study: Nutrition and training periodization in three elite marathon runners. *Int J Sport Nutr Exerc Metab.* 2012;22(5):392-400.

59. Tonnessen E, Sylta O, Haugen TA, Hem E, Svendsen IS, Seiler S. The road to gold: training and peaking characteristics in the year prior to a gold medal endurance performance. *PLoS One.* 2014;9(7):e101796.

60. Tonnessen E, Svendsen IS, Ronnestad BR, Hisdal J, Haugen TA, Seiler S. The annual training periodization of 8 world champions in orienteering. *Int J Sports Physiol Perform.* 2015;10(1):29-38.

61. Wilber RL, Pitsiladis YP. Kenyan and Ethiopian distance runners: What makes them so good? *Int J Sports Physiol Perform.* 2012;7(2):92-102.

Chapter 15

1. Abbiss CR, Quod MJ, Levin G, Martin DT, Laursen PB. Accuracy of the Velotron ergometer and SRM power meter. *Int J Sports Med.* 2009;30(2):107-12.

2. Abbiss CR, Straker L, Quod MJ, Martin DT, Laursen PB. Examining pacing profiles in elite female road cyclists using exposure variation analysis. *Br J Sports Med.* 2010;44(6):437-42.

3. Allen H, Coggan A. *Training and Racing With a Power Meter*: Boulder, CO: VeloPress; 2010.

4. Bell PG, Furber MJ, KA VANS, Anton-Solanas A, Swart J. The physiological profile of a multiple Tour de France winning cyclist. *Med Sci Sports Exerc.* 2017;49(1):115-23.

5. Burke LM. Nutritional practices of male and female endurance cyclists. *Sports Med.* 2001;31(7):521-32.

6. Close GL, Hamilton DL, Philp A, Burke LM, Morton JP. New strategies in sport nutrition to increase exercise performance. *Free Radic Biol Med.* 2016;98:144-58.

7. Ebert TR, Martin DT, Stephens B, Withers RT. Power output during a professional men's road-cycling tour. *Int J Sports Physiol Perform.* 2006;1(4):324-35.

8. Gardner AS, Stephens S, Martin DT, Lawton E, Lee H, Jenkins D. Accuracy of SRM and power tap power monitoring systems for bicycling. *Med Sci Sports Exerc.* 2004;36(7):1252-8.

9. Hansen EA, Jorgensen LV, Jensen K, Fregly BJ, Sjogaard G. Crank inertial load affects freely chosen pedal rate during cycling. *J Biomech.* 2002;35(2):277-85.

10. Hawley JA, Stepto NK. Adaptations to training in endurance cyclists: implications for performance. *Sports Med.* 2001;31(7):511-20.

11. Impey SG, Hearris MA, Hammond KM, Bartlett JD, Louis J, Close GL, et al. Fuel for the work required: A theoretical framework for carbohydrate periodization and the glycogen threshold hypothesis. *Sports Med.* 2018; 48(5):1031-48.

12. Laursen PB. Training for intense exercise performance: High-intensity or high-volume training? *Scan J Med Sci Sports.* 2010;20 Suppl 2:1-10.

13. Lucia A, Hoyos J, Chicharro JL. Physiology of professional road cycling. *Sports Med.* 2001;31(5):325-37.

14. Lucia A, Pardo J, Durantez A, Hoyos J, Chicharro JL. Physiological differences between professional and elite road cyclists. *Int J Sports Med.* 1998;19(5):342-8.

15. Matveyev L. *Fundamentals of Sports Training.* Moscow: Progress; 1981.

16. Menaspa P, Sias M, Bates G, La Torre A. Demands of World Cup competitions in elite women's road cycling. *Int J Sports Physiol Perform.* 2017;12(10):1293-6.

17. Menaspa P, Quod M, Martin DT, Peiffer JJ, Abbiss CR. Physical demands of sprinting in professional road cycling. *Int J Sports Med.* 2015;36(13):1058-62.

18. Padilla S, Mujika I, Orbananos J, Santisteban J, Angulo F, Jose Goiriena J. Exercise intensity and load during mass-start stage races in professional road cycling. *Med Sci Sports Exerc.* 2001;33(5):796-802.

19. Passfield L, Hopker JG, Jobson S, Friel D, Zabala M. Knowledge is power: Issues of measuring training and performance in cycling. *J Sports Sci.* 2017;35(14):1426-34.

20. Quod MJ, Martin DT, Martin JC, Laursen PB. The power profile predicts road cycling MMP. *Int J Sports Med.* 2010;31(6):397-401.

21. Stone MH, Stone, M., Sands, W.A. *Principles and Practice of Resistance Training.* Champaign, IL: Human Kinetics; 2007.

22. Tschien P. A necessary direction in training: The integration of biological adaptation in the training program. *Coaching and Sport Science Journal.* 1995;1:2-14.

Chapter 16

1. Banister EW, editor. *Modeling Elite Athletic Performance*: Champaign, IL: Human Kinetics; 1991.

2. Foster C, Florhaug JA, Franklin J, Gottschall L, Hrovatin LA, Parker S, et al. A new approach to monitoring exercise training. *J Strength Cond Res.* 2001;15(1):109-15.

3. Hagerman FC. Applied physiology of rowing. *Sports Med.* 1984;1(4):303-26.

4. Holt AC, Plews D, Oberlin-Brown K, Merien F, Kilding AE. Autonomic and performance recovery after high intensity exercise in rowers. *Int J Sport Physiol Perform.* 2017;In Press.

5. Ingham SA, Whyte GP, Jones K, Nevill AM. Determinants of 2,000 m rowing ergometer performance in elite rowers. *Eur J Appl Physiol.* 2002;88(3):243-6.

6. Issurin V. Block periodization versus traditional training theory: A review. *J Sports Med Phys Fitness.* 2008;48(1):65-75.

7. Kerr DA, Ross WD, Norton K, Hume P, Kagawa M, Ackland TR. Olympic lightweight and open-class rowers possess distinctive physical and proportionality characteristics. *J Sports Sci.* 2007;25(1):43-53.

8. Kleshnev V, ed. *The Biomechanics of Rowing.* United Kingdom: The Crowood Press; 2016.

9. Laursen PB, Jenkins DG. The scientific basis for high-intensity interval training: Optimising training programmes and maximising performance in highly trained endurance athletes. *Sports Med.* 2002;32(1):53-73.

10. Lawton TW, Cronin JB, McGuigan MR. Strength testing and training of rowers: A review. *Sports Med.* 2011;41(5):413-32.

11. Lawton TW, Cronin JB, McGuigan MR. Strength, power, and muscular endurance exercise and elite rowing ergometer performance. *J Strength Cond Res.* 2013;27(7):1928-35.

12. Maestu J, Jurimae J, Jurimae T. Monitoring of performance and training in rowing. *Sports Med.* 2005;35(7):597-617.

13. Marcolin G, Lentola A, Paoli A, and Petrone N. Rowing on a boat versus rowing on an ergometer: A biomechanical and electro-myographycal preliminary study. *Procedia Engineering* 2015:112 461-6.

14. Neal CM, Hunter AM, Galloway SD. A 6-month analysis of training-intensity distribution and physiological adaptation in Ironman triathletes. *J Sports Sci.* 2011;29(14):1515-23.

15. Neal CM, Hunter AM, Brennan L, O'Sullivan A, Hamilton DL, De Vito G, et al. Six weeks of a polarized training-intensity distribution leads to greater physiological and performance adaptations than a threshold model in trained cyclists. *J Appl Physiol (1985).* 2013;114(4):461-71.

16. Plews DJ, Laursen PB. Training intensity distribution over a four-year cycle in Olympic champion rowers: Different roads lead to Rio. *Int J Sport Physiol.* 2017;27(9):1-24.

17. Plews DJ, Laursen PB, Stanley J, Kilding AE, Buchheit M. Training adaptation and heart rate variability in elite endurance athletes: Opening the door to effective monitoring. *Sports Med.* 2013;43(9):773-81.

18. Samuels CH. Jet lag and travel fatigue: A comprehensive management plan for sport medicine physicians and high-performance support teams. *Clin J Sport Med.* 2012;22(3):268-73.

19. Seiler S. What is best practice for training intensity and duration distribution in endurance athletes? *Int J Sports Physiol Perform.* 2010;5(3):276-91.

20. Stanley J, Peake JM, Buchheit M. Cardiac parasympathetic reactivation following exercise: Implication for training prescription. *Sport Med.* 2013; 43(12):1259-77.

21. Steinacker JM. Physiological aspects of training in rowing. *Int J Sports Med.* 1993;14 Suppl 1:S3-10.

22. Stoggl TL, Sperlich B. The training intensity distribution among well-trained and elite endurance athletes. *Front Physiol.* 2015;6:295.

Chapter 17

1. Achten J, Jeukendrup AE. Heart rate monitoring. *Sports Med.* 2003;33(7):517-38.

2. Anderson M, Hopkins W, Roberts A, Pyne D. Ability of test measures to predict competitive performance in elite swimmers. *J Sports Sci.* 2008;26(2):123-30.

3. Anderson ME, Hopkins WG, Roberts AD, Pyne DB. Monitoring seasonal and long-term changes in test performance in elite swimmers. *Eur J Sport Sci.* 2006;6(3):145-54.

4. Bex T, Baguet A, Achten E, Aerts P, De Clercq D, Derave W. Cyclic movement frequency is associated with muscle typology in athletes. *Scand J Med Sci Sports.* 2017;27(2):223-9.

5. Borg GA. Psychophysical bases of perceived exertion. *Med Sci Sports Exerc.* 1982;14(5):377-81.

6. Buchheit M. Outside the box. *Int J Sports Physiol Perform.* 2017;12:1001-2.

7. Carlile F. *Forbes Carlile on Swimming.* London: Pelham Books; 1963.

8. Chatard J-C, Wilson B. Effect of fastskin suits on performance, drag, and energy cost of swimming. *Med Sci Sports Exerc.* 2008;40(6):1149.

9. Costill D, Thomas R, Robergs R, Pascoe D, Lambert C, Barr S, et al. Adaptations to swimming training: Influence of training volume. *Med Sci Sports Exerc.* 1991;23(3):371-7.

10. Counsilman JE. *The Science of Swimming.* Englewood Cliffs, NJ: Prentice Hall; 1968.

11. de Koning JJ, Noordhof DA, Uitslag TP, Galiart RE, Dodge C, Foster C. An approach to estimating gross efficiency during high-intensity exercise. *Int J Sports Physiol Perform.* 2013;8(6):682-4.

12. Di Prampero P. The energy cost of human locomotion on land and in water. *Int J Sports Med.* 1986;7(2):55-72.

13. Dunbar CC, Robertson RJ, Baun R, Blandin MF, Metz K, Burdett R, et al. The validity of regulating exercise intensity by ratings of perceived exertion. *Med Sci Sports Exerc.* 1992; 24(1):94-9.

14. Foley R, Lahr MM. The role of "the aquatic" in human evolution: Constraining the aquatic ape hypothesis. *Evolutionary Anthropology: Issues, News, and Reviews.* 2014;23(2):56-9.

15. Halson SL. Monitoring training load to understand fatigue in athletes. *Sports Med.* 2014;44(2):139-47.

16. Hawley J, Burke L. *Peak Performance: Training and Nutritional Strategies for Sport.* Sydney, Australia: Allen & Unwin; 1998.

17. Hellard P, Weber S, Rodriguez F, Mader A, editors. Influence of oxidative and glycolytic capacities on the muscular energy metabolism and performance in 200-m freestyle swimming: a case study. 4th FINA World Aquatics Convention; 2016; Windsor, Canada.

18. Hellard P, Scordia C, Avalos M, Mujika I, Pyne DB. Modelling of optimal training load patterns during the 11 weeks preceding major competition in elite swimmers. *Applied Physiology, Nutrition, and Metabolism.* 2017;42(10):1106-17.

19. Hellard P, Pla R, Rodríguez FA, Simbana D, Pyne DB. Dynamics of the metabolic response during a competitive 100-m freestyle in elite male swimmers. *Int J Sports Physiol Perform.* 2018:1-28.

20. Hellard P, Avalos M, Lacoste L, Barale F, Chatard J-C, Millet GP. Assessing the limitations of the Banister model in monitoring training. *J Sports Sci.* 2006;24(5):509-20.

21. Hellard P, Avalos M, Hausswirth C, Pyne D, Toussaint J-F, Mujika I. Identifying optimal overload and taper in elite swimmers over time. *J Sports Sci Med.* 2013;12(4):668.

22. Hellard P, Rodríguez FA, Dupont C, Pyne DB, Mader A, Weber S. *Simulated Metabolic Responses During High-Intensity Interval Training Based on a Mathematical Model in Elite Swimmers.* NOVA; 2018.

23. Holmer I, Astrand P. Swimming training and maximal oxygen uptake. *J Appl Physiol.* 1972;33(4):510-3.

24. Hopkins WG. Quantification of training in competitive sports. *Sports Med.* 1991;12(3):161-83.

25. Huot-Marchand F, Nesi X, Sidney M, Alberty M, Pelayo P. Swimming: Variations of stroking parameters associated with 200 m competitive performance improvement in top-standard front crawl swimmers. *Sports Biomechanics.* 2005;4(1):89-100.

26. Laughlin M, Roseguini B. Mechanisms for exercise training-induced increases in skeletal muscle blood flow capacity: differences with interval sprint training versus aerobic endurance training. *Journal of Physiology and Pharmacology: An Official Journal of the Polish Physiological Society.* 2008;59(Suppl 7):71.

27. Laursen P. Training for intense exercise performance: High-intensity or high-volume training? *Scand J Med Sci Sports.* 2010;20(s2):1-10.

28. Maglischo EW. *Swimming Fastest.* Champaign, IL: Human Kinetics; 2003.

29. Mauger A, Neuloh J, Castle P. Analysis of pacing strategy selection in elite 400-m freestyle swimming. *Med Sci Sports Exerc.* 2012;44(11):2205-12.

30. McGibbon K, Pyne D, Shephard M, Thompson K. Pacing in swimming: A systematic review. Submitted for peer review. 2018.

31. Mujika I. *Tapering and Peaking for Optimal Performance.* Champaign, IL: Human Kinetics 1; 2009.

32. Mujika I, Chatard J-C, Busso T, Geyssant A, Barale F, Lacoste L. Effects of training on performance in competitive swimming. *Can J Appl Physiol.* 1995;20(4):395-406.

33. Olbrecht J. *The Science of Winning: Planning, Periodizing and Optimizing Swim Training.* Tienen, Belgium: F&G Partners; 2015.

34. Paton CD, Hopkins WG. Effects of high-intensity training on performance and physiology of endurance athletes. *Sportscience.* 2004;8:25-41.

35. Pyne D, Touretski G. An analysis of the training of Olympic sprint champion Alexandre Popov. *Australian Swim Coach.* 1993;10(5):5-14.

36. Pyne D, Maw G, Goldsmith W. Protocols for the physiological assessment of swimmers. In: *Physiological Tests for Elite Athletes Australian Sports Commission.* Champaign, IL: Human Kinetics. 2000:372-82.

37. Pyne DB, Sharp RL. Physical and energy requirements of competitive swimming events. *International Journal of Sport Nutrition and Exercise Metabolism.* 2014;24(4):351-9.

38. Robertson E, Pyne D, Hopkins W, Anson J. Analysis of lap times in international swimming competitions. *J Sports Sci.* 2009;27(4):387-95.

39. Rodríguez FA, Mader A. Energy systems in swimming. In: *World Book of Swimming From Science to Performance.* New York: Nova. 2011:225-40.

40. Rushall BS. Swimming energy training in the 21st century: The justification for radical changes. *Swimming Science Bulletin* 2014;(39).

41. Saw AE, Main LC, Gastin PB. Monitoring the athlete training response: Subjective self-reported measures trump commonly used objective measures: A systematic review. *Br J Sports Med.* 2015:bjsports-2015-094758.

42. Secher NH, Volianitis S. Are the arms and legs in competition for cardiac output? *Med Sci Sports Exerc.* 2006;38(10):1797-803.

43. Seiler S, Tønnessen E. SPORTSCIENCE· sportsci. org. *Sportscience.* 2009;13:32-53.

44. Sousa A, Figueiredo P, Oliveira N, Oliveira J, Silva A, Keskinen K, et al. VO2 kinetics in 200-m race-pace front crawl swimming. *Int J Sports Med.* 2011;32(10):765-70.

45. Toussaint HM, Hollander AP. Energetics of competitive swimming. *Sports Med.* 1994;18(6):384-405.

Chapter 18

1. Balsalobre-Fernandez C, Glaister M, Lockey RA. The validity and reliability of an iPhone app for measuring vertical jump performance. *J Sports Sci.* 2015;33(15):1574-9.

2. Baquet G, Berthoin S, Dupont G, Blondel N, Fabre C, Van Praagh E. Effects of high intensity intermittent training on peak $\dot{V}O_2$ in prepubertal children. *Int J Sports Med.* 2002;23(6):439-44.

3. Bosco C, Mognoni P, Luhtanen P. Relationship between isokinetic performance and ballistic movement. *European Journal of Applied Physiology and Occupational Physiology.* 1983;51(3):357-64.

4. Buchheit M. The 30-15 intermittent fitness test: Accuracy for individualizing interval training of young intermittent sport players. *Journal of Strength & Conditioning Research.* 2008;22(2):365-74.

5. Buchheit M, Laursen PB. High-intensity interval training, solutions to the programming puzzle: Part I: Cardiopulmonary emphasis. *Sports Med.* 2013;43(5):313-38.

6. Buchheit M, Morgan W, Wallace J, Bode M, Poulos N. Physiological, psychometric, and performance effects of the Christmas break in Australian football. *Int J Sports Physiol Perform.* 2015;10(1):120-3.

7. Buchheit M, Laursen P, Kuhnle J, Ruch D, Renaud C, Ahmaidi S. Game-based training in young elite handball players. *Int J Sports Med.* 2009;30(4):251.

8. Christensen PM, Krustrup P, Gunnarsson TP, Kiilerich K, Nybo L, Bangsbo J. VO2 kinetics and performance in soccer players after intense training and inactivity. *Medicine and Science in Sports and Exercise.* 2011;43(9):1716-24.

9. Coutts AJ, Gomes RV, Viveiros L, Aoki MS. Monitoring training loads in elite tennis. *Revista Brasileira de Cineantropometria & Desempenho Humano.* 2010;12(3):217-20.

10. DiFiori JP, Benjamin HJ, Brenner JS, Gregory A, Jayanthi N, Landry GL, et al. Overuse injuries and burnout in youth sports: A position statement from the American Medical Society for Sports Medicine. *Br J Sports Med.* 2014;48(4):287-8.

11. Duffield R, Murphy A, Kellett A, Reid M. Recovery from repeated on-court tennis sessions: Combining cold water immersion, compression and sleep recovery interventions. *Int J Sports Physiol Perform*. 2014;9(2):273-82.

12. Fernandez-Fernandez J, Sanz-Rivas D, Mendez-Villanueva A. A review of the activity profile and physiological demands of tennis match play. *Strength Cond J*. 2009;31(4):15-26.

13. Fernandez-Fernandez J, Ulbricht A, Ferrauti A. Fitness testing of tennis players: How valuable is it? *Br J Sports Med*. 2014;48(Suppl 1):i22-31.

14. Fernandez-Fernandez J, Sanz-Rivas D, Fernandez-Garcia B, Mendez-Villanueva A. Match activity and physiological load during a clay-court tennis tournament in elite female players. *J Sports Sci*. 2008;26(14):1589-95.

15. Fernandez-Fernandez J, Zimek R, Wiewelhove T, Ferrauti A. High-intensity interval training vs. repeated-sprint training in tennis. *J Strength Cond Res*. 2012;26(1):53-62.

16. Fernandez-Fernandez J, Sanz-Rivas D, Kovacs MS, Moya M. In-season effect of a combined repeated sprint and explosive strength training program on elite junior tennis players. *J Strength Cond Res*. 2015;29(2):351-7.

17. Fernandez-Fernandez J, Sanz-Rivas D, Sarabia JM, Moya M. Preseason training: The effects of a 17-day high-intensity shock microcycle in elite tennis players. *J Sports Sci Med*. 2015;14(4):783-91.

18. Fernandez-Fernandez J, Sanz D, Sarabia JM, Moya M. The effects of sport-specific drills training or high-intensity interval training in young tennis players. *Int J Sports Physiol Perform*. 2017;12(1):90-8.

19. Fernandez-Fernandez J, Sanz-Rivas D, Sanchez-Munoz C, de la Aleja Tellez JG, Buchheit M, Mendez-Villanueva A. Physiological responses to on-court vs running interval training in competitive tennis players. *J Sports Sci Med*. 2011;10(3):540-5.

20. Fernandez-Fernandez J, Boullosa DA, Sanz-Rivas D, Abreu L, Filaire E, Mendez-Villanueva A. Psychophysiological stress responses during training and competition in young female competitive tennis players. *Int J Sports Med*. 2015;36(1):22-8.

21. Fernandez J, Mendez-Villanueva A, Pluim B. Intensity of tennis match play. *Br J Sports Med*. 2006;40(5):387-91.

22. Ferrauti A, Kinner V, Fernandez-Fernandez J. The Hit & Turn Tennis Test: An acoustically controlled endurance test for tennis players. *J Sports Sci*. 2011;29(5):485-94.

23. Foster C, Florhaug JA, Franklin J, Gottschall L, Hrovatin LA, Parker S, et al. A new approach to monitoring exercise training. *J Strength Cond Res*. 2001;15(1):109-15.

24. Gallo-Salazar C, Del Coso J, Barbado D, Lopez-Valenciano A, Santos-Rosa FJ, Sanz-Rivas D, et al. Impact of a competition with two consecutive matches in a day on physical performance in young tennis players. *Appl Physiol Nutr Metab*. 2017;42(7):750-6.

25. Gibala MJ, McGee SL. Metabolic adaptations to short-term high-intensity interval training: A little pain for a lot of gain? *Exerc Sport Sci Rev*. 2008;36(2):58-63.

26. Girard O, Millet GP. Physical determinants of tennis performance in competitive teenage players. *J Strength Cond Res*. 2009;23(6):1867-72.

27. Girard O, Lattier G, Maffiuletti NA, Micallef J-P, Millet GP. Neuromuscular fatigue during a prolonged intermittent exercise: Application to tennis. *Journal of Electromyography and Kinesiology*. 2008;18(6):1038-46.

28. Gomes RV, Moreira A, Lodo L, Nosaka K, Coutts AJ, Aoki MS. Monitoring training loads, stress, immune-endocrine responses and performance in tennis players. *Biol Sport*. 2013;30(3):173-80.

29. Harrison CB, Gill ND, Kinugasa T, Kilding AE. Development of aerobic fitness in young team sport athletes. *Sports Med*. 2015;45(7):969-83.

30. Haydar B, Al Haddad H, Ahmaidi S, Buchheit M. Assessing inter-effort recovery and change of direction ability with the 30-15 Intermittent Fitness Test. *J Sports Sci Med*. 2011;10(2):346.

31. Hill-Haas S, Coutts A, Rowsell G, Dawson B. Generic versus small-sided game training in soccer. *Int J Sports Med*. 2009;30(9):636-42.

32. Jayanthi N, Feller E, Smith A. Junior competitive tennis: Ideal training and tournament recommendations. *J Med Sci Tennis*. 2013;18:30-6.

33. Kovacs MS. Tennis physiology: Training the competitive athlete. *Sports Med.* 2007;37(3):189-98.

34. Laursen PB, Jenkins DG. The scientific basis for high-intensity interval training: Optimising training programmes and maximising performance in highly trained endurance athletes. *Sports Med.* 2002;32(1):53-73.

35. Mendez-Villanueva A, Fernandez-Fernandez J, Bishop D. Exercise-induced homeostatic perturbations provoked by singles tennis match play with reference to development of fatigue. *Br J Sports Med.* 2007;41(11):717-22; discussion 22.

36. Mendez-Villanueva A, Fernandez-Fernandez J, Bishop D, Fernandez-Garcia B, Terrados N. Activity patterns, blood lactate concentrations and ratings of perceived exertion during a professional singles tennis tournament. *Br J Sports Med.* 2007;41(5):296-300.

37. Moreno-Pérez V, Ayala F, Fernandez-Fernandez J, Vera-Garcia FJ. Descriptive profile of hip range of motion in elite tennis players. *Physical Therapy in Sport.* 2016;19:43-8.

38. Murphy A, Duffield R, Kellett A, Reid M. The relationship of training load to physical capacity changes during international tours in high performance junior tennis players. *Int J Sports Physiol Perform.* 2015;10(2):253-60.

39. Murphy A, Duffield R, Kellett A, Reid M. A descriptive analysis of internal and external loads for elite-level tennis drills. *Int J Sports Physiol Perform.* 2014;9(5):863-70.

40. Murphy AP, Duffield R, Kellett A, Reid M. A descriptive analysis of internal and external loads for elite-level tennis drills. *Int J Sports Physiol Perform.* 2014;9(5):863-70.

41. Pluim BM, Staal JB, Windler GE, Jayanthi N. Tennis injuries: Occurrence, aetiology, and prevention. *Br J Sports Med.* 2006;40(5):415-23.

42. Reid M, Duffield R, Dawson B, Baker J, Crespo M. Quantification of the physiological and performance characteristics of on-court tennis drills. *Br J Sports Med.* 2008;42(2):146-51.

43. Reid MM, Duffield R, Minett GM, Sibte N, Murphy AP, Baker J. Physiological, perceptual, and technical responses to on-court tennis training on hard and clay courts. *J Strength Cond Res.* 2013;27(6):1487-95.

44. Smekal G, von Duvillard SP, Rihacek C, Pokan R, Hofmann P, Baron R, et al. A physiological profile of tennis match play. *Med Sci Sports Exerc.* 2001;33(6):999-1005.

45. Sperlich B, De Marées M, Koehler K, Linville J, Holmberg H-C, Mester J. Effects of 5 weeks' high-intensity interval training vs. volume training in 14-year-old soccer players. *J Strength Cond Res.* 2011;25(5):1271-8.

46. Ulbricht A, Fernandez-Fernandez J, Mendez-Villanueva A, Ferrauti A. Impact of fitness characteristics on tennis performance in elite junior tennis players. *J Strength Cond Res.* 2016;30(4):989-98.

47. Wiewelhove T, Fernandez-Fernandez J, Raeder C, Kappenstein J, Meyer T, Kellmann M, et al. Acute responses and muscle damage in different high-intensity interval running protocols. *J Sports Med Phys Fitness.* 2016;56(5):606-15.

Chapter 19

1. Abbiss CR, Laursen PB. Describing and understanding pacing strategies during athletic competition. *Sports Medicine.* 2008;38(3):239-52.

2. Allen H, Coggan A. *Training and Racing With a Power Meter.* Boulder, CO: VeloPress; 2010.

3. Banister EW. Modeling elite athletic performance. In: MacDougall JD, Wenger HA, Green HJ, eds. *Physiological Testing of Elite Athletes.* Champaign, IL: Human Kinetics; 1991.

4. Banister EW, Calvert TW. Planning for future performance: Implications for long-term training. *Can J Appl Sport Sci.* 1980;5(3):170-6.

5. Barnes KR, Kilding AE. Strategies to improve running economy. *Sports Med.* 2015;45(1):37-56.

6. Bentley DJ, Millet GP, Vleck VE, McNaughton LR. Specific aspects of contemporary triathlon: Implications for physiological analysis and performance. *Sports Med.* 2002;32(6):345-59.

7. Bentley DJ, McNaughton LR, Lamyman R, Roberts SP. The effects of prior incremental cycle exercise on the physiological responses during incremental running to exhaustion: Relevance for sprint triathlon performance. *J Sports Sci.* 2003;21(1):29-38.

8. Bentley DJ, Cox GR, Green D, Laursen PB. Maximising performance in triathlon: applied physiological and nutritional aspects of elite and non-elite competitions. *J Sci and Med Sport / Sports Med Australia.* 2008;11(4):407-16.

9. Burke LM. Fueling strategies to optimize performance: Training high or training low? *Scandinavian J Med Sci Sports.* 2010;20 (Suppl 2):48-58.

10. Burke LM, Hawley JA, Wong SH, Jeukendrup AE. Carbohydrates for training and competition. *J Sports Sci.* 2011;29 (Suppl 1):S17-27.

11. Frandsen J, Vest SD, Larsen S, Dela F, Helge JW. Maximal fat oxidation is related to performance in an Ironman triathlon. *Int J Sports Med.* 2017;38(13):975-82.

12. Hausswirth C, Bigard AX, Guezennec CY. Relationships between running mechanics and energy cost of running at the end of a triathlon and a marathon. *Int J Sports Med.* 1997;18(5):330-9.

13. Hooper SL, Mackinnon LT, Howard A, Gordon RD, Bachmann AW. Markers for monitoring overtraining and recovery. *Med Sci Sports Exerc.* 1995;27(1):106-12.

14. Issurin VB. New horizons for the methodology and physiology of training periodization. *Sports Med.* 2010;40(3):189-206.

15. Laursen PB. Long distance triathlon: Demands, preparation and performance. *J Hum Sport Exerc.* 2011;6(2):247-63.

16. Laursen PB, Rhodes EC. Factors affecting performance in an ultraendurance triathlon. *Sports Med.* 2001;31(3):195-209.

17. Laursen PB, Rhodes EC, Langill RH, McKenzie DC, Taunton JE. The effect of the cycle phase on run performance in an ultraendurance triathlon. *Adv Exerc Sports Physiol.* 2001;7(3):81-6.

18. Laursen PB, Knez WL, Shing CM, Langill RH, Rhodes EC, Jenkins DG. Relationship between laboratory-measured variables and heart rate during an ultra-endurance triathlon. *Journal of Sports Sciences.* 2005;23(10):1111-20.

19. Laursen PB, Knez WL, Shing CM, Langill RH, Rhodes EC, Jenkins DG. Relationship between laboratory-measured variables and heart rate during an ultra-endurance triathlon. *J Sports Sci.* 2005;23(10):1111-20.

20. Marquet LA, Brisswalter J, Louis J, Tiollier E, Burke LM, Hawley JA, et al. Enhanced endurance performance by periodization of carbohydrate intake: "Sleep low" strategy. *Med Sci Sports Exerc.* 2016;48(4):663-72.

21. Morton RH, Fitz-Clarke JR, Banister EW. Modeling human performance in running. *J Appl Physiol (1985).* 1990;69(3):1171-7.

22. Mujika I. Olympic preparation of a world-class female triathlete. *Int J Sports Physiol Perform.* 2014;9(4):727-31.

23. Nimmerichter A, Eston R, Bachl N, Williams C. Effects of low and high cadence interval training on power output in flat and uphill cycling time-trials. *Eur J Appl Physiol.* 2012;112(1):69-78.

24. Plews DJ, Laursen PB, Kilding AE, Buchheit M. Heart rate variability in elite triathletes, is variation in variability the key to effective training? A case comparison. *Eur J Appl Physiol.* 2012;112(11):3729-41.

25. Plews DJ, Laursen PB, Stanley J, Kilding AE, Buchheit M. Training adaptation and heart rate variability in elite endurance athletes: Opening the door to effective monitoring. *Sports Med.* 2013;43(9):773-81.

26. Plews DJ, Scott B, Altini M, Wood M, Kilding AE, Laursen PB. Comparison of heart-rate-variability recording with smartphone photoplethysmographic, Polar H7 chest strap, and electrocardiogram methods. *Int J Sports Physiol Perform.* 2017:1-17.

27. Sedgwick PE, Wortley GC, Wright JM, Asplund C, Roberts WO, Usman S. Medical clearance for desert and land sports, adventure, and endurance events. *Clin J Sport Med.* 2015;25(5):418-24.

28. Telles T, Barroso R, Figueiredo P, Salgueiro DF, Vilas-Boas JP, Junior OA. Effect of hand paddles and parachute on backstroke coordination and stroke parameters. *J Sports Sci.* 2017;35(9):906-11.

29. Volek JS, Freidenreich DJ, Saenz C, Kunces LJ, Creighton BC, Bartley JM, et al. Metabolic characteristics of keto-adapted ultra-endurance runners. *Metabolism.* 2016;65(3):100-10.

30. Wakayoshi K, Ikuta K, Yoshida T, Udo M, Moritani T, Mutoh Y, et al. Determination and validity of critical velocity as an index of swimming performance in the competitive swimmer. *Eur J Appl Physiol Occup Physiol.* 1992;64(2):153-7.

31. Webster CC, Swart J, Noakes TD, Smith JA. A carbohydrate ingestion intervention in an elite athlete who follows a LCHF diet. *Int J Sports Physiol Perform.* 2017:1-12.

32. Wood T. Lost metabolic machinery during ketosis? Depends where you are looking. *Strength Cond J.* 2017;39(5):94-5.

33. Yeo WK, Lessard SJ, Chen ZP, Garnham AP, Burke LM, Rivas DA, et al. Fat adaptation followed by carbohydrate restoration increases AMPK activity in skeletal muscle from trained humans. *J Appl Physiol.* 2008;105(5):1519-26.

Chapter 20

1. Bosch TA, Burruss TP, Weir NL, Fielding KA, Engel BE, Weston TD, et al. Abdominal body composition differences in NFL football players. *J Strength Cond Res.* 2014;28(12):3313-9.

2. Brophy RH, Wright RW, Powell JW, Matava MJ. Injuries to kickers in American football: The National Football League experience. *Am J Sports Med.* 2010;38(6):1166-73.

3. Brophy RH, Lyman S, Chehab EL, Barnes RP, Rodeo SA, Warren RF. Predictive value of prior injury on career in professional American football is affected by player position. *Am J Sports Med.* 2009;37(4):768-75.

4. Buchheit M, Laursen PB. High-intensity interval training, solutions to the programming puzzle. Part II: Anaerobic energy, neuromuscular load and practical applications. *Sports Med.* 2013;43(10):927-54.

5. Buchheit M, Laursen PB. High-intensity interval training, solutions to the programming puzzle: Part I: Cardiopulmonary emphasis. *Sports Med.* 2013;43(5):313-38.

6. Cormack SJ, Newton RU, McGuigan MR. Neuro-muscular and endocrine responses of elite players to an Australian rules football match. *Int J Sports Physiol Perform.* 2008;3(3):359-74.

7. Dyreson M. The Super Bowl as a television spectacle: Global designs, global niches, and parochial patterns. *International Journal of the History of Sport.* 2017;34(1-2):139-56.

8. Edwards T, Spiteri T, Piggott B, Haff GG, Joyce C. A narrative review of the physical demands and injury incidence in American football: Application of current knowledge and practices in workload management. *Sports Med.* 2017:1-11.

9. Fry AC, Kraemer WJ. Physical performance characteristics of American collegiate football players. *J Strength Cond Res.* 1991;5(3):126-38.

10. Fullagar HH, McCunn R, Murray A. An updated review of the applied physiology of American collegiate football: The physical demands, strength/conditioning, nutritional considerations and injury characteristics of America's favourite game. *Int J Sports Physiol Perform.* 2017;12(10):1396-1403.

11. Gabbett TJ. The training–injury prevention paradox: Should athletes be training smarter and harder? *Br J Sports Med.* 2016;50(5):273-80.

12. Gallo TF, Cormack SJ, Gabbett TJ, Lorenzen CH. Pre-training perceived wellness impacts training output in Australian football players. *J Sports Sci.* 2016;34(15):1445-51.

13. Govus AD, Coutts A, Duffield R, Murray A, Fullagar H. Relationship between pre-training subjective wellness measures, player load and rating of perceived exertion training load in American college football. *Int J Sports Physiol Perform.* 2018;13(1):95-101.

14. Hoffman J. Physiological demands of American football. *Sports Science Exchange.* 2015;28(143):1-6.

15. Hoffman JR. The applied physiology of American football. *Int J Sports Physiol Perform.* 2008;3(3):387-92.

16. Hoffman JR, Kang J, Ratamess NA, Faigenbaum AD. Biochemical and hormonal responses during an intercollegiate football season. *Med Sci Sports Exerc.* 2005;37(7):1237-41.

17. Hoffman JR, Maresh CM, Newton RU, Rubin MR, French DN, Volek JS, et al. Performance, biochemical, and endocrine changes during a competitive football game. *Med Sci Sports Exerc.* 2002;34(11):1845-53.

18. Hopsicker P, Dyreson M. Super Bowl Sunday: A national holiday and a global curiosity. *International Journal of the History of Sport.* 2017;34(1-2):1-6.

19. Impellizzeri FM, Rampinini E, Coutts AJ, Sassi A, Marcora SM. Use of RPE-based training load in soccer. *Med Sci Sports Exerc.* 2004;36(6):1042-7.

20. Iosia MF, Bishop PA. Analysis of exercise-to-rest ratios during division IA televised football competition. *J Strength Cond Res.* 2008;22(2):332-40.

21. Jacobson BH, Conchola EG, Glass RG, Thompson BJ. Longitudinal morphological and performance profiles for American, NCAA Division I

football players. *J Strength Cond Res.* 2013;27(9):2347-54.

22. Kraemer W, Gotshalk L. *Physiology of American Football.* Baltimore, MD: Lippincott, Williams & Wilkins; 2000:795-813.

23. Kraemer WJ, Torine JC, Dudley J, Martin GJ. Nonlinear periodization: Insights for use in collegiate and professional American football resistance training programs. *Strength Cond J.* 2015;37(6):17-36.

24. Kraemer WJ, Torine JC, Silvestre R, French DN, Ratamess NA, Spiering BA, et al. Body size and composition of National Football League players. *J Strength Cond Res.* 2005;19(3):485-9.

25. MacLean SA, Basch CH, Garcia P. Alcohol and violence in 2017 National Football League Super Bowl commercials. *Health Promotion Perspectives.* 2017;7(3):163-7.

26. Malone S, Roe M, Doran DA, Gabbett TJ, Collins K. High chronic training loads and exposure to bouts of maximal velocity running reduce injury risk in elite Gaelic football. *J Sci Med Sport.* 2017;20(3):250-4.

27. Malone S, Owen A, Newton M, Mendes B, Tiernan L, Hughes B, et al. Wellbeing perception and the impact on external training output among elite soccer players. *J Sci Med Sport.* 2018;21(1):29-34.

28. McCall A, Ardern C, Delecroix B, Abaidia A-e, Dunlop G, Dupont G. Adding a quick and simple psychological measure of player readiness into the return to play mix: A single player case study from professional football (soccer). *Sport Performance & Science Reports.* Nov. 2017;1:1-3. https://sportperfsci.com/wp-content/uploads /2017/11/SPSR8_McCall-et-al._171110_8v1_final .pdf.

29. National Football League Seasonal Statistics 2017. Available from http://www.nfl.com/stats/.

30. Pincivero DM, Bompa TO. A physiological review of American football. *Sports Med.* 1997;23(4):247-60.

31. Pryor JL, Huggins RA, Casa DJ, Palmieri GA, Kraemer WJ, Maresh CM. A Profile of a National Football League team. *J Strength Cond Res.* 2014;28(1):7-13.

32. Robbins DW. The National Football League (NFL) Combine: Does normalized data better predict performance in the NFL draft? *J Strength Cond Res.* 2010;24(11):2888-99.

33. Robbins DW. Positional physical characteristics of players drafted into the National Football League. *J Strength Cond Res.* 2011;25(10):2661-7.

34. Rogalski B, Dawson B, Heasman J, Gabbett TJ. Training and game loads and injury risk in elite Australian footballers. *J Sci Med Sport.* 2013;16(6):499-503.

35. Sierer SP, Battaglini CL, Mihalik JP, Shields EW, Tomasini NT. The National Football League Combine: Performance differences between drafted and nondrafted players entering the 2004 and 2005 drafts. *J Strength Cond Res.* 2008;22(1):6-12.

36. Stone J, Kreutzer A, Mata J, Nystrom M, Jagim A, Jones M, et al. Changes in creatine kinase and hormones over the course of an American football season. *J Strength Cond Res.* 2017.

37. Trexler ET, Smith-Ryan AE, Mann JB, Ivey PA, Hirsch KR, Mock MG. Longitudinal body composition changes in NCAA Division I college football players. *J Strength Cond Res.* 2017;31(1):1-8.

38. Ward PA, Ramsden S, Coutts AJ, Hulton AT, Drust B. Positional differences in running and non-running activities during elite American football training. *J Strength Cond Res.* 2018;32(7):2072-84.

39. Wellman AD, Coad SC, Goulet GC, McLellan CP. Quantification of accelerometer derived impacts associated with competitive games in National Collegiate Athletic Association Division I college football players. *J Strength Cond Res.* 2017;31(2):330-8.

40. Wellman AD, Coad SC, Flynn PJ, Climstein M, McLellan CP. Movement demands and perceived wellness associated with preseason training camp in NCAA Division I college football players. *J Strength Cond Res.* 2017;31(10):2704-18.

41. Wellman AD, Coad SC, Flynn PJ, Siam TK, McLellan CP. A comparison of pre-season and in-season practice and game loads in NCAA Division I football players. *J Strength Cond Res.* Jul 2017.

42. Yamashita D, Asakura M, Ito Y, Yamada S, Yamada Y. Physical characteristics and perfor-

mance of Japanese top-level American football players. *J Strength Cond Res.* 2017;31(9):2455-61.

Chapter 21

1. Aughey RJ. Widening margin in activity profile between elite- and sub-elite Australian football: A case study. *J Sci Med Sport.* 2013;16(4):382-6.

2. Austin DJ, Gabbett TJ, Jenkins DJ. Repeated high-intensity exercise in a professional rugby league. *J Strength Cond Res.* 2011;25(7):1898-904.

3. Bilsborough JC, Greenway K, Opar D, Livingstone S, Cordy J, Coutts AJ. Changes in body composition during the competition season: Relationships with training, physical performance and team selection in Australian Football players. *Int J Sports Physiol Perf.* 2014:In review.

4. Bilsborough JC, Greenway K, Opar D, Livingstone S, Cordy JT, Bird S, et al. Comparison of anthropometry, upper body strength and lower body power characteristics in different levels of Australian Football players. *J Strength Cond Res.* 2014;29(3):826-34.

5. Buchheit M. Monitoring training status with HR measures: Do all roads lead to Rome? *Frontiers in Physiology.* 2014;5(73).

6. Buchheit M, Laursen PB. High-intensity interval training, solutions to the programming puzzle: Part I: Cardiopulmonary emphasis. *Sports Med.* 2013;43(5):313-38.

7. Buchheit M, Laursen PB. High-intensity interval training, solutions to the programming puzzle. Part II: Anaerobic energy, neuromuscular load and practical applications. *Sports Med.* 2013;43(10):927-54.

8. Buchheit M, Racinais S, Bilsborough JC, Bourdon PC, Voss SC, Hocking J, et al. Monitoring fitness, fatigue and running performance during a pre-season training camp in elite football players. *J Sci Med Sport.* 2013;16(6):550-5.

9. Burgess D, Naughton G, Norton K. Quantifying the gap between under 18 and senior AFL football: 2003-2009. *Int J Sports Physiol Perf.* 2012;7(1):53-8.

10. Corbett DM, Sweeting AJ, Robertson S. Weak relationships between stint duration, physical and skilled match performance in Australian Football. *Frontiers in Physiology.* 2017;8:820.

11. Corbett DM, Bartlett JD, O'Connor F, Back N, Torres-Ronda L, Robertson S. Development of physical and skill training drill prescription systems for elite Australian Rules football. *Science and Medicine in Football.* 2017:1-7.

12. Coutts AJ. In the age of technology, Occam's razor still applies. *Int J Sports Physiol Perf.* 2014;9(5):741.

13. Coutts AJ. Challenges in developing evidence-based practice in high-performance sport. *Int J Sports Physiol Perf.* 2017;12(6):717-8.

14. Coutts AJ, Crowcroft S, Kempton T. Developing athlete monitoring systems: Theoretical basis and practical applications. In: Kellmann M, Beckmann J, eds. *Sport, Recovery and Performance: Interdisciplinary Insights.* Abingdon: Routledge; 2018.

15. Coutts AJ, Quinn J, Hocking J, Castagna C, Rampinini E. Match running performance in elite Australian Rules Football. *J Sci Med Sport.* 2010;13(5):543-8.

16. Delaney JA, Thornton HR, Burgess DJ, Dascombe BJ, Duthie GM. Duration-specific running intensities of Australian Football match-play. *J Sci Med Sport.* 2017;20(7):689-94.

17. Duhig S, Shield AJ, Opar D, Gabbett TJ, Ferguson C, Williams M. Effect of high-speed running on hamstring strain injury risk. *Brit J Sport Med.* 2016;50(24):1536-40.

18. Farrow D, Pyne D, Gabbett T. Skill and physiological demands of open and closed training drills in Australian Football. *International Journal of Sports Science & Coaching.* 2008;3(4):485-94.

19. Foster C, Florhaug JA, Franklin J, Gottschall L, Hrovatin LA, Parker S, et al. A new approach to monitoring exercise training. *J Strength Cond Res.* 2001;15(1):109-15.

20. Gabbett TJ. The training-injury prevention paradox: Should athletes be training smarter and harder? *Br J Sports Med.* 2016;50(5):273-80.

21. Gray AJ, Jenkins DG. Match analysis and the physiological demands of Australian football. *Sports Med.* 2010;40(4):347-60.

22. Hill-Haas SV, Dawson B, Impellizzeri FM, Coutts AJ. Physiology of small-sided games training in football: A systematic review. *Sports Med.* 2011;41(3):199-220.

23. Hiscock D, Dawson B, Heasman J, Peeling P. Game movements and player performance in the Australian Football League. *International Journal of Performance Analysis in Sport*. 2017;12(3):531-45.

24. Johnston RJ, Watsford ML, Pine MJ, Spurrs RW, Murphy A, Pruyn EC. Movement demands and match performance in professional Australian football. *Int J Sport Med*. 2012;33(2):89-93.

25. Kempton T, Sirotic AC, Coutts AJ. Metabolic power demands of rugby league match-play. *Int J Sports Physiol Perf*. 2015;10(1):23-8.

26. Kempton T, Sullivan CJ, Bilsborough JC, Cordy J, Coutts AJ. Match-to-match variation in physical activity and technical skill measures in professional Australian Football. *J Sci Med Sport*. 2015;18(1):109-13.

27. Loader J, Montgomery PG, Williams MD, Lorenzen C, Kemp JG. Classifying training drills based on movement demands in Australian Football. *Int J Sports Sci Coach*. 2012;7(1):57-68.

28. Malone S, Owen A, Mendes B, Hughes B, Collins K, Gabbett TJ. High-speed running and sprinting as an injury risk factor in soccer: Can well-developed physical qualities reduce the risk? *J Sci Med Sport*. 2018;21(3):257-62.

29. McLean BD, Coutts AJ, Kelly V, McGuigan MR, Cormack SJ. Neuromuscular, endocrine, and perceptual fatigue responses during different length between-match microcycles in professional rugby league players. *Int J Sports Physiol Perf*. 2010;5(3):367-83.

30. Moreira A, Kempton T, Aoki MS, Sirotic AC, Coutts AJ. The impact of three different length between-match microcycles on training loads in professional rugby league players. *Int J Sports Physiol Perf*. 2015;10(6):767-73.

31. Murray NB, Gabbett TJ, Townshend AD. Relationship between pre-season training load and in-season availability in elite Australian football players. *Int J Sports Physiol Perf*. 2017;12(6):749-55.

32. Racinais S, Buchheit M, Bilsborough J, Bourdon PC, Cordy J, Coutts AJ. Physiological and performance responses to a training camp in the heat in professional Australian football players. *Int J Sports Physiol Perf*. 2014;9(4):598-603.

33. Rampinini E, Impellizzeri F, Castagna C, Abt G, Chamari K, Sassi A, et al. Factors influencing physiological responses to small-sided soccer games. *J Sports Sci*. 2007;6(25):659-66.

34. Ritchie D, Hopkins WG, Buchheit M, Cordy J, Bartlett JD. Quantification of training and competition load across a season in an elite Australian Football club. *Int J Sports Physiol Perf*. 2016;11(4):474-9.

35. Ryan AS, Coutts AJ, Hocking J, Dillon P, Kempton TK. Factors affecting match running performance in professional Australian Football. *Int J Sports Physiol Perf*. 2017;12(9):1199-204.

36. Scott TJ, Black CR, Quinn J, Coutts AJ. Validity and reliability of the session-RPE method for quantifying training in Australian football: A comparison of the CR10 and CR100 scales. *J Strength Cond Res*. 2013;27(1):270-6.

37. Slattery KM, Wallace LK, Bentley DJ, Coutts AJ. Effect of training load on simulated team sport match performance. *Appl Physiol Nutr Metab*. 2012;37(2):315-22.

38. Spencer M, Lawrence S, Rechichi C, Bishop D, Dawson B, Goodman C. Time-motion analysis of elite field hockey, with special reference to repeated-sprint activity. *J Sports Sci*. 2004;22(9):843-50.

39. Sullivan C, Bilsborough JC, Cianciosi M, Hocking J, Cordy JT, Coutts AJ. Factors affecting match performance in professional Australian football. *Int J Sports Physiol Perf*. 2014;9(3):561-6.

40. Sullivan C, Bilsborough JC, Cianciosi M, Hocking J, Cordy J, Coutts AJ. Match score affects activity profile and skill performance in professional Australian Football players. *J Sci Med Sport*. 2014;17:326-31.

41. Varley MC, Gabbett T, Aughey RJ. Activity profiles of professional soccer, rugby league and Australian football match play. *J Sports Sci*. 2014;32(20):1858-66.

42. Young WB, Newton RU, Doyle TL, Chapman D, Cormack S, Stewart G, et al. Physiological and anthropometric characteristics of starters and non-starters and playing positions in elite Australian Rules Football: a case study. *J Sci Med Sport*. 2005;8(3):333-45.

Chapter 22

1. Camp CL, Zajac JM, Pearson DB, Sinatro AM, Spiker AM, Werner BC, et al. Decreased shoulder external rotation and flexion are greater predictors of injury than internal rotation deficits:

Analysis of 132 pitcher-seasons in professional baseball. *Arthroscopy*. 2017;33(9):1629-36.

2. Cornell, DJ, Paxson, JL, Caplinger, RA, Seligman, JR, Davis, NA, Flees, RJ, et al. In-game heart rate responses among professional baseball starting pitchers. *J Strength Cond Res*. 2017;31(1):24-9.

3. Gibala M, McGee S. Metabolic adaptations to short-term high-intensity interval training: A little pain for a lot of gain? *Exerc & Sorts Sci Reviews*. 2008;36(2):58-63.

4. Gillett J, Dawes J, Spaniol F, Rhea M, Rogowski J, Magrini M, et al. A description and comparison of cardiorespiratory fitness measures in relation to pitching performance among professional baseball pitchers. *J Strength Cond Res*. 2016;4(14):1-8.

5. Hoffman J, Vazquez J, Pichardo N, and Tenenbaum G. Anthropometric and performance comparisons in professional baseball players. *J Strength Cond Res*. 2009;23(8):2173-8.

6. Hughes L, Paton B, Rosenblatt B, Gissane C, Patterson SD. Blood flow restriction training in clinical musculoskeletal rehabilitation: A systematic review and meta-analysis. *Br J Sports Med*. 2107;51(13):1003-11.

7. Jones CM, Griffiths PC, Mellalieu SD. Training load and fatigue marker associations with injury and illness: A systematic review of longitudinal studies. *Sports Med*. 2017;47(5):943-74.

8. Mangine G, Hoffman J, Fragala M, Vazquez J, Krause M, Gillett J, et al. Effect of age on anthropometric and physical performance measures in professional baseball players. *J Strength Cond Res*. 2013;27(2):375-81.

9. Mangine G, Hoffman J, Vazquez J, Pichardo N, Fragala M, and Stout J. Predictors of fielding performance in professional baseball players. *Int J Sports Physiol Perf*. 2013;8:510-16.

10. Rhea M, Oliverson J, Marshall G, Peterson M, Kenn J, and Naclerio Ayllon F. Noncompatibility of power and endurance training among college baseball players. *J Strength Cond Res*. 2008;22(1):230-4.

11. Spaniol F. Body composition and baseball performance. *Perf Training J*. 2005;4(1):10-11.

12. Szymanksi DJ. Physiology of baseball pitching dictates specific exercise intensity for conditioning. *Strength Cond J*. 2009;31(2):41-7.

13. Wilk KE, Macrina LC, Fleisig GS, Aune KT, Porterfield RA, Harker P, et al. Deficits in glenohumeral passive range of motion increase risk of shoulder injury in professional baseball pitchers: A prospective study. *Am J Sports Med*. 2015;43(10):2379-85.

14. Yang SC, Wang CC, Lee SD, Lee YU, Chan KH, Chen YL, et al. Impact of 12-s rule on performance and muscle damage of baseball pitchers. *Med Sci Sports Exerc*. 2016;48(12):2512-16.

Chapter 23

1. Aglioti SM, Cesari P, Romani M, Urgesi C. Action anticipation and motor resonance in elite basketball players. *Nature Neuroscience*. 2008;11(9):1109-16.

2. Aguiar M, Botelho G, Lago C, Maças V, Sampaio J. A review on the effects of soccer small-sided games. *J Hum Kinet*. 2012;33:103-13.

3. Alexander J, Hopkinson T, Wundersitz D, Serpell B, Mara J, Ball N. Validity of a wearable accelerometer device to measure average acceleration values during high-speed running. *J Strength Cond Res*. 2016;30(11):3007-13.

4. Astorino TA, Allen RP, Roberson DW, Jurancich M. Effect of high-intensity interval training on cardiovascular function, VO2max, and muscular force. *J Strength Cond Res*. 2012;26(1):138-45.

5. Atl H, Köklü Y, Alemdaroğlu U, Koçak FU. A comparison of heart rate response and frequencies of technical actions between half-court and full-court 3-a-side games in high school female basketball players. *J Strength Cond Res*. 2013;27(2):352-6.

6. Bartlett JD, O'Connor F, Pitchford N, Torres-Ronda L, Robertson SJ. Relationships between internal and external training load in team-sport athletes: Evidence for an individualized approach. *Int J Sports Physiol Perform*. 2017;12(2):230-4.

7. Ben Abdelkrim N, El Fazaa S, El Ati J. Time-motion analysis and physiological data of elite under-19-year-old basketball players during competition. *Brit J Sport Med*. 2007;41(2):69-75.

8. Ben Abdelkrim N, Castagna C, Jabri I, Battikh T, El Fazaa S, El Ati J. Activity profile and physiological requirements of junior elite basketball players in relation to aerobic–anaerobic fitness. *J Strength Cond Res*. 2010;24(9):2330-42.

9. Buchheit M. Monitoring training status with HR measures: Do all roads lead to Rome? *Front Physiol.* Feb 2014;27(5):73.

10. Buchheit M, Laursen PB. High-intensity interval training, Solutions to the programming puzzle: Part I: Cardiopulmonary emphasis. *Sports Med.* 2013;43(5):313-38.

11. Burns AS, Lauder TD. Deep water running: an effective non-weightbearing exercise for the maintenance of land-based running performance. *Mil Med.* 2001;166(3):253-8.

12. Cardinale M, Varley MC. Wearable training monitoring technology: Applications, challenges and opportunities. *Int J Sports Physiol Perform.* 2017;12(Suppl 2):S255–S62.

13. Castagna C, Impellizzeri FM, Chaouachi A, Ben Abdelkrim N, Manzi V. Physiological responses to ball-drills in regional level male basketball players. *J Sports Sci.* 2011;29(12):1329-36.

14. Castagna C, Impellizzeri F, Chaouachi A, Ben Abdelkrim N, Manzi V. Physiological responses to ball-drills in regional level male basketball players. *J Sports Sci.* 2011;29(12):1329-36.

15. Castagna C, Manzi V, D'Ottavio S, Annino G, Padua E, Bishop D. Relation between maximal aerobic power and the ability to repeat sprints in young basketball players. *J Strength Cond Res.* 2007;21(4):1172-6.

16. Clark IE, West BM, Reynolds SK, Murray SR, Pettitt RW. Applying the critical velocity model for an off-season interval training program. *J Strength Cond Res.* 2013;27(12):3335-41.

17. Davids K, Araújo D, Correia V, Vilar L. How small-sided and conditioned games enhance acquisition of movement and decision-making skills. *Exerc Sport Sci Rev.* 2013;41(3):154-61.

18. Delextrat A, Kraiem S. Heart-rate responses by playing position during ball drills in basketball. *Int J Sports Physiol Perform.* 2013;8:410-8.

19. Delextrat A, Martinez A. small-sided game training improves aerobic capacity and technical skills in basketball players. *Int J Sports Med.* 2014;35(5):385-91.

20. Dellal A, Chamari K, Pintus A, Girard O, Cotte T, Keller D. Heart rate responses during small-sided games and short intermittent running training in elite soccer players: A comparative study. *J Strength Cond Res.* 2008;22(5):1449-57.

21. Gibson J. *The Ecological Approach to Visual Perception.* Boston: Houghton Mifflin; 1979. 332 p.

22. González-Badillo JJ, Ribas J. *Fundamentos del entrenamiento de fuerza.* Barcelona: INDE; 1999.

23. Hill-Haas SV, Coutts AJ, Rowsell GJ, Dawson BT. Generic versus small-sided game training in soccer. *Int J Sports Med.* 2009;30(9):636-42.

24. Impellizzeri FM, Rampinini E, Marcora SM. Physiological assessment of aerobic training in soccer. *J Sports Sci.* 2005;23(6):583-92.

25. Impellizzeri FM, Marcora SM, Castagna C, Reilly R, Sassi A, Iaia FM, et al. Physiological and performance effects of generic versus specific aerobic training in soccer players. *Int J Sports Med.* 2006;27:483-92.

26. Kauffman SA. *The Origins of Order: Self Organization and Selection in Evolution.* Oxford: Oxford University Press; 1993.

27. Klusemann MJ, Pyne DB, Foster C, Drinkwater EJ. Optimising technical skills and physical loading in small-sided basketball games. *J Sports Sci.* 2012;30(14):1463-71.

28. McInnes SE, Carlson JS, Jones CJ, McKenna MJ. The physiological load imposed on basketball players during competition. *J Sports Sci.* 1995;13(5):387-97.

29. Midgley AW, McNaughton LR, Wilkinson M. Is there an optimal training intensity for enhancing the maximal oxygen uptake of distance runners? Empirical research findings, current opinions, physiological rationale and practical recommendations. *Sports Med.* 2006;36(2):117-32.

30. Montgomery PG, Pyne DB, Minahan CL. The physical and physiological demands of basketball training and competition. *Int J Sports Physiol Perform.* 2010;5(1):75-86.

31. Moras G. *La preparación integral en el Voleibol.* Barcelona: Paidotribo; 1994.

32. Nassis GP, Hertzog M, Brito J. Workload assessment in soccer: An open-minded, critical thinking approach is needed. *J Strength Cond Res.* 2017;31(8):e77–e8.

33. Nicolella D, Torres-Ronda L, Saylor K, Schelling X. Validity and reliability of an accelerometer-based player tracking device. *PLoS One.* 2017;(Under Review).

34. Perše M, Kristan M, Kovačič S, Vučković G, Perš J. A trajectory-based analysis of coordinated team activity in a basketball game. *Computer Vision and Image Understanding.* 2009;113(5):612-21.

35. Rampinini E, Impellizzeri FM, Castagna C, Abt G, Chamari K, Sassi A, et al. Factors influencing physiological responses to small-sided soccer games. *J Sports Sci.* 2007;25(6):659-66.

36. Redford P. Which NBA Team Is The Tallest? : fivethirtyeight.com; 2016 [Available from: https://fivethirtyeight.com/features/which-nba-team-is-the-tallest/]

37. Reilly T, Morris T, Whyte G. The specificity of training prescription and physiological assessment: A review. *J Sports Sci.* 2009;27(6):575-89.

38. Remmert H. Analysis of group-tactical offensive behavior in elite basketball on the basis of a process orientated model. *Eur J Sport Sci.* 2003;3(3):1-12.

39. Sampaio J, Abrantes C, Leite N. Power, heart rate and perceived exertion to 3×3 and 4×4 basketball small-sided games. *Rev Psicol Deporte.* 2009;18:463-7.

40. Sampaio J, McGarry T, Calleja-Gonzalez J, Jimenez Saiz S, Schelling IDAX, Balciunas M. Exploring game performance in the National Basketball Association using player tracking data. *PLoS One.* 2015;10(7):e0132894.

41. Sandbakk O, Sandbakk SB, Ettema G, Welde B. Effects of intensity and duration in aerobic high-intensity interval training in highly-trained junior cross-country skiers. *J Strength Cond Res.* 2012;27(7):1974-80.

42. Scanlan AT, Wen N, Tucker PS, Borges NR, Dalbo VJ. Training mode influences the relationships between training load models during basketball conditioning. *Int J Sports Physiol Perform.* 2014;9(5):851-6.

43. Schelling X. Resistencia en baloncesto. Calidad vs Cantidad. *Minut ACEB.* 2011;9:6-8.

44. Schelling X, Torres-Ronda L. Conditioning for basketball: Quality and quantity of training. *Strength Cond J.* 2013;36(6):89-94.

45. Schelling X, Torres L. Accelerometer load profiles for basketball-specific drills in elite players. *J Sports Sci Med.* 2016;15(4):585-91.

46. Schelling X, Calleja-Gonzalez J, Torres-Ronda L, Terrados N. Using testosterone and cortisol as biomarker for training individualization in elite basketball: A 4-year follow-up study. *J Strength Cond Res.* 2015;29(2):368-78.

47. Seirul·lo F, ed. *Planificación a largo plazo en los deportes colectivos. Curso sobre Entrenamiento Deportivo en la Infancia y la Adolescencia.* 1998; Canarias, www.entrenamientodeportivo.com.

48. Stöckel T, Breslin G. The influence of visual contextual information on the emergence of the especial skill in basketball. *J Sport Exerc Psychol.* 2013;35(5):536-41.

49. Stone NM, Kilding AE. Aerobic conditioning for team sport athletes. *Sports Med.* 2009;39(8):615-42.

50. Tessitore A, Meeusen R, Cortis C, Capranica L. Effects of different recovery interventions on anaerobic performances following preseason soccer training. *J Strength Cond Res.* 2007;21(3):745-50.

51. Torres-Ronda L, Schelling X. Critical process for the implementation of technology in sport organizations. *Strength Cond J.* 2017;39(6):54-9.

52. Torres-Ronda L, Ric A, Llabres-Torres I, de Las Heras B, Schelling X. Position-dependent cardiovascular response and time-motion analysis during training drills and friendly matches in elite male basketball players. *J Strength Cond Res.* 2015;30(1):60-70.

53. Torres-Ronda L, Ric A, Llabres-Torres I, de Las Heras B, Schelling IDAX. Position-dependent cardiovascular response and time-motion analysis during training drills and friendly matches in elite male basketball players. *J Strength Cond Res.* 2016;30(1):60-70.

54. Varley MC, Aughey RJ. Acceleration profiles in elite Australian soccer. *Int J Sports Med.* 2013;34(1):34-9.

55. Weast JA, Shockley K, Riley MA. The influence of athletic experience and kinematic information on skill-relevant affordance perception. *Q J Exp Psychol.* 2011;64(4):689-706.

56. Wundersitz DW, Gastin PB, Robertson S, Davey PC, Netto KJ. Validation of a trunk-mounted accelerometer to measure peak impacts during team sport movements. *Int J Sports Med.* 2015;36(9):742-6.

57. Yarrow K, Brown P, Krakauer JW. Inside the brain of an elite athlete: The neural processes that support high achievement in sports. *Nature Rev.* 2009;10:585-96.

Chapter 24

1. Brandon R. *Investigations of the Neuromuscular Response During and Following Elite Maximum Strength and Power Type Resistance Exercise.* Scotland: University of Stirling; 2011.

2. Campbell FW, Rothwell SE, Perry MJ. Bad light stops play. *Ophthalmic and Physiological Optics.* 1987;7(2):165-7.

3. Douglas MJ, Tam N. Analysis of team performances at the ICC World Twenty20 Cup 2009. *International Journal of Performance Analysis in Sport.* 2010;10(1):47-53.

4. Genet R, Petersen C, eds. Cricket batting placement distribution analysed by bowling line and length at the 2013 ICC Champions Trophy. *World Congress of Performance Analysis of Sport X*; 2017, September 3-6: Opatija, Croatia.

5. Houghton L, Dawson B, Rubenson J. Performance in a simulated cricket batting innings (BATEX): Reliability and discrimination between playing standards. *J Sports Sci.* 2011;29(10):1097-103.

6. MacDonald DC. Performance analysis of fielding and wicket-keeping in cricket to inform strength and conditioning practice. PhD diss., Auckland University, 2015, https://aut.researchgateway.ac.nz /bitstream/handle/10292/8819/MacDonaldD.pdf ?sequence=3&isAllowed=y.

7. McLeod P. Visual reaction time and high-speed ball games. *Perception.* 1987;16(1):49-59.

8. Mehta R. http://www.espncricinfo.com/magazine /content/story/258645.html: ESPNcricinfo.com. 2006.

9. Najdan JM, Robins TM, Glazier SP. Determinants of success in English domestic Twenty20 cricket. *International Journal of Performance Analysis in Sport.* 2014;14(1):276-95.

10. Noakes TD, Durandt JJ. Physiological requirements of cricket. *J Sports Sci.* 2000;18(12):919-29.

11. Orchard JW, Kountouris A, Sims K. Incidence and prevalence of elite male cricket injuries using updated consensus definitions. *Open Access Journal of Sports Medicine.* 2016;7:187.

12. Orchard JW, James T, Portus M, Kountouris A, Dennis R. Fast bowlers in cricket demonstrate up to 3- to 4-week delay between high workloads and increased risk of injury. *Amer J Sports Med.* 2009;37(6):1186-92.

13. Petersen C, Genet R, eds. Captain and coaches playbook app: A practical display of fielding data. *5th World Congress of Science and Medicine in Cricket*; 2015, March 23-27: Sydney, Australia.

14. Petersen C, Pyne DB, Portus MJ, Dawson B. Analysis of Twenty/20 cricket performance during the 2008 Indian Premier League. *International Journal of Performance Analysis in Sport.* 2008;8(3):63-9.

15. Petersen C, Pyne DB, Portus MR, Dawson B. Quantifying positional movement patterns in Twenty20 cricket. *International Journal of Performance Analysis in Sport.* 2009;9(2):165-70.

16. Petersen CJ. Comparison of performance at the 2007 and 2015 Cricket World Cups. *Int J Sports Sci Coach.* 2017;12(3):404-10.

17. Petersen CJ, Pyne D, Dawson B, Portus M, Kellett A. Movement patterns in cricket vary by both position and game format. *J Sports Sci.* 2010;28(1):45-52.

18. Petersen CJ, Pyne DB, Dawson BT, Kellett AD, Portus MR. Comparison of training and game demands of national level cricketers. *J Strength Cond Res.* 2011;25(5):1306-11.

19. Petersen CJ, Portus MR, Pyne DB, Dawson BT, Cramer MN, Kellett AD. Partial heat acclimation in cricketers using a 4-day high intensity cycling protocol. *Int J Sports Physiol Perform.* 2010;5(4):535-45.

20. Portus M, Kellett A, Karppinen S, Timms S. Physiological tests for elite athletes, 2nd Edition. In: Tanner R, Gore C, eds. *Chapter 18 Cricket Players.* Champaign, IL: Human Kinetics; 2012: 289-97.

21. Pote L, Christie CJ. Physiological responses of batsmen during a simulated One Day International century. *South African Journal of Sports Medicine.* 2016;28(2):39-42.

22. Pyke F, Davis K. *Cutting Edge Cricket.* Champaign, IL: Human Kinetics; 2010.

23. Renshaw I, Fairweather MM. Cricket bowling deliveries and the discrimination ability of professional and amateur batters. *J Sports Sci.* 2000;18(12):951-7.

24. Tyndall N. Personal communication. 2017.

25. Vickery W, Dascombe B, Duffield R, Kellett A, Portus M. The influence of field size, player number and rule changes on the physiological responses and movement demands of small-sided games for cricket training. *J Sports Sci.* 2013;31(6):629-38.

26. Vickery W, Duffield R, Crowther R, Beakley D, Blanch P, Dascombe BJ. Comparison of the physical and technical demands of cricket players during training and match-play. *J Strength Cond Res.* 2018;32(3):821-29.

27. Wigmore T. Northants' T20 nous a tribute to moneyball approach. ESPNcricinfo.com. 2016. Available from: http://www.espncricinfo.com /county-cricket-2017/content/story/1070189.html.

28. Woolmer B, Noakes T, Moffett H. *Bob Woolmer's Art and Science of Cricket.* London: New Holland Publishers; 2008.

Chapter 25

1. Abbott HA. Positional and Match Action Profiles of Elite Women's Field Hockey Players in Relationship to the 2015 FIH Rule Changes. Electronic Theses and Dissertations. Paper 3092: University of Tennessee; 2016.

2. Buchheit M. The 30-15 Intermittent Fitness Test: 10 year review. *Myorobie Journal.* 2010;1(September):1-9.

3. Cormack SJ, Mooney MG, Morgan W, McGuigan MR. Influence of neuromuscular fatigue on accelerometer load in elite Australian football players. *Int J Sports Physiol Perform.* 2013;8(4):373-8.

4. Impellizzeri FM, Rampinini E, Coutts AJ, Sassi A, Marcora SM. Use of RPE-based training load in soccer. *Med Sci Sports Exerc.* 2004;36(6):1042-7.

5. Jennings D, Cormack SJ, Coutts AJ, Aughey RJ. GPS analysis of an international field hockey tournament. *Int J Sports Physiol Perform.* 2012;7(3):224-31.

6. Jones B, Hamilton DK, Cooper CE. Muscle oxygen changes following sprint interval cycling training in elite field hockey players. *PLoS One.* 2015;10(3):e0120338.

7. Lemmink KA, Visscher SH. Role of energy systems in two intermittent field tests in women field hockey players. *J Strength Cond Res.* 2006;20(3):682-8.

8. McGuigan MR, Doyle TL, Newton M, Edwards DJ, Nimphius S, Newton RU. Eccentric utilization ratio: Effect of sport and phase of training. *J Strength Cond Res.* 2006;20(4):992-5.

9. Spencer M, Bishop D, Lawrence S. Longitudinal assessment of the effects of field-hockey training on repeated sprint ability. *J Sci Med Sport.* 2004;7(3):323-34.

10. Spencer M, Lawrence S, Rechichi C, Bishop D, Dawson B, Goodman C. Time-motion analysis of elite field hockey, with special reference to repeated-sprint activity. *J Sports Sci.* 2004;22(9):843-50.

11. Sweet TW, Foster C, McGuigan MR, Brice G. Quantitation of resistance training using the session rating of perceived exertion method. *J Strength Cond Res.* 2004;18(4):796-802.

Chapter 26

1. Bell G, Game A, Bouchard J, Reid C, Gervais P, Snydmiller G. Near maximal heart rate responses during a varsity ice hockey game. *Applied Physiology, Nutrition and Metabolism.* 2011;36(S2).

2. Besson C, Buchheit M, Praz M, Deriaz O, Millet GP. Cardiorespiratory responses to the 30-15 intermittent ice test. *Int J Sports Physiol Perform.* 2013;8(2):173-80.

3. Bracko MR, Fellingham GW, Hall LT, Fisher AG, Cryer W. Performance skating characteristics of professional ice hockey forwards. *Sports Medicine, Training and Rehabilitation.* 1998;8(3):251-63.

4. Buchheit M, Lefebvre B, Laursen PB, Ahmaidi S. Reliability, usefulness, and validity of the 30-15 Intermittent Ice Test in young elite ice hockey players. *J Strength Cond Res.* 2011;25(5):1457-64.

5. Cox MH, Miles DS, Verde TJ, Rhodes EC. Applied physiology of ice hockey. *Sports Med.* 1995;19(3):184-201.

6. Girard O, Mendez-Villanueva A, Bishop D. Repeated-sprint ability–Part I: Factors contributing to fatigue. *Sports Med.* 2011;41(8):673-94.

7. Jackson JK. *Time-Motion Characteristics and Heart Rate Profiles Displayed by Female University Ice Hockey Players.* Edmonton, Canada: University of Alberta; 2015.

8. Janot JM, Beltz NM, Dalleck LD. Multiple off-ice performance variables predict on-ice skating performance in male and female Division III ice hockey players. *J Sports Sci Med.* 2015;14(3):522-9.

9. Manners TW. Sport-specific training for ice hockey. *Strength Cond J.* 2004;April.

10. Montgomery DL. Physiology of ice hockey. *Sports Med.* 1988;5(2):99-126.

11. Peterson BJ, Fitzgerald JS, Dietz CC, Ziegler KS, Baker SE, Snyder EM. Off-ice anaerobic power does not predict on-ice repeated shift performance in hockey. *J Strength Cond Res.* 2016;30(9):2375-81.

12. Quinney HA, Dewart R, Game A, Snydmiller G, Warburton D, Bell G. A 26 year physiological description of a National Hockey League team. *Appl Physiol Nutr Metab.* 2008;33(4):753-60.

Chapter 27

1. Al Haddad H, Laursen PB, Chollet D, Ahmaidi S, Buchheit M. Reliability of resting and postexercise heart rate measures. *Int J Sports Med.* 2011;32(8):598-605.

2. Bompa TO, Carrera M. *Periodization Training for Sports,* 2nd Edition. Champaign, IL: Human Kinetics; 2005.

3. Buchheit M. Individualizing high-intensity interval training in intermittent sport athletes with the 30-15 Intermittent Fitness Test. *NSCA Hot Topic Series wwwnsca-liftorg.* 2011; November.

4. Buchheit M. Should we be recommending repeated sprints to improve repeated-sprint performance? *Sports Med.* 2012;42(2):169-72.

5. Buchheit M. Programming high-intensity training in handball. *Aspetar–Sports Medicine Journal.* 2014;3(Targeted topic–sports medicine in handball):120-8.

6. Buchheit M. Monitoring training status with HR measures: Do all roads lead to Rome? *Front Physiol.* 2014;27(5):73.

7. Buchheit M, Laursen PB. High-intensity interval training, solutions to the programming puzzle: Part I: Cardiopulmonary emphasis. *Sports Med.* 2013;43(5):313-38.

8. Buchheit M, Laursen PB. High-intensity interval training, solutions to the programming puzzle. Part II: Anaerobic energy, neuromuscular load and practical applications. *Sports Med.* 2013;43(10):927-54.

9. Buchheit M, Lepretre PM, Behaegel AL, Millet GP, Ahmaidi S. Cardiorespiratory responses during running and sport-specific exercises in handball players. *J Sci Med Sport* 2008; 12(3):399-405.

10. Buchheit M, Mendez-Villanueva A, Quod MJ, Quesnel T, Ahmaidi S. Improving acceleration and repeated sprint ability in well-trained adolescent handball players: Speed vs. sprint interval training. *Int J Sports Physiol Perform.* 2010;5(2):152-64.

11. Buchheit M, Morgan W, Wallace J, Bode M, Poulos N. Physiological, psychometric, and performance effects of the Christmas break in Australian football. *Int J Sports Physiol Perform.* 2015;10(1):120-3.

12. Buchheit M, Millet GP, Parisy A, Pourchez S, Laursen PB, Ahmaidi S. Supramaximal training and post-exercise parasympathetic reactivation in adolescents. *Med Sci Sports Exerc.* 2008;40(2):362-71.

13. Buchheit M, Laursen PB, Kuhnle J, Ruch D, Renaud C, Ahmaidi S. Game-based training in young elite handball players. *Int J Sports Med.* 2009;30(4):251-8.

14. Buchheit M, Lepretre PM, Behaegel AL, Millet GP, Cuvelier G, Ahmaidi S. Cardiorespiratory responses during running and sport-specific exercises in handball players. *J Sci Med Sport.* 2009;12(3):399-405.

15. Buchheit M, Al Haddad H, Leprêtre PM, Millet G, Newton M, Ahmaidi S. Cardiorespiratory and cardiac autonomic responses to 30-15: Intermittent fitness test. *J Strength Cond Res.* 2009;23(1):93-100.

16. Cardinale M, Whiteley R, Hosny AA, Popovic N. Activity profiles and positional differences of handball players during the World Championships in Qatar 2015. *Int J Sports Physiol Perform.* 2017;12(7):908-15.

17. Corvino M, Tessitore A, Minganti C, Šibila M. Effect of court dimensions on players' external and internal load during small-sided handball games *J Sports Sci & Med.* 2014;13(2):297-303.

18. Delgado-Bordonau JL, Mendez-Villanueva A. The Tactical Periodization Model. In: Sum ME, ed. *Fitness in Soccer: The Science and Practical Application.* Groningen, The Netherlands: Moveo Ergo Sum; 2014.

19. Dello Iacono A, Martone D, Zagatto AM, Meckel Y, Sindiani M, Milic M, et al. Effect of contact and no-contact small-sided games on elite handball players. *J Sports Sci.* 2016;35(1):1-9.

20. Francis C. *Training for Speed.* Bellingham, WA: Faccioni Speed & Conditioning Consultants; 1997.

21. Gorostiaga EM, Granados C, Ibanez J, Izquierdo M. Differences in physical fitness and throwing velocity among elite and amateur male handball players. *Int J Sports Med.* 2005;26(3):225-32.

22. Hopkins WG, Marshall SW, Batterham AM, Hanin J. Progressive statistics for studies in sports medicine and exercise science. *Med Sci Sports Exerc.* 2009;41(1):3-13.

23. Impellizzeri FM, Rampinini E, Coutts AJ, Sassi A, Marcora SM. Use of RPE-based training load in soccer. *Med Sci Sports Exerc.* 2004;36(6):1042-7.

24. Karcher C, Buchheit M. On-court demands of elite handball, with special reference to playing positions. *Sports Med.* 2014;44(6):797-814.

25. Loftin M, Anderson P, Lytton L, Pittman P, Warren B. Heart rate response during handball singles match-play and selected physical fitness components of experienced male handball players. *J Sports Med Phys Fitness.* 1996;36(2):95-9.

26. Luteberget LS, Spencer M. High-intensity events in international women's team handball matches. *Int J Sports Physiol Perform.* 2017;12(1):56-61.

27. Rannou F, Prioux J, Zouhal H, Gratas-Delamarche A, Delamarche P. Physiological profile of handball players. *J Sports Med Phys Fitness.* 2001;41(3):349-53.

28. Saw AE, Main LC, Gastin PB. Monitoring the athlete training response: Subjective self-reported measures trump commonly used objective measures: A systematic review. *Br J Sports Med.* 2016;50(5):281-91.

29. Spencer M, Bishop D, Dawson B, Goodman C. Physiological and metabolic responses of repeated-sprint activities: Specific to field-based team sports. *Sports Med.* 2005;35(12):1025-44.

30. Stanley J, Peake JM, Buchheit M. Cardiac parasympathetic reactivation following exercise: Implications for training prescription. *Sports Med.* 2013;43(12):1259-77.

31. Ufland P, Ahmaidi S, Buchheit M. Repeated-sprint performance, locomotor profile and muscle oxygen uptake recovery. *Int J Sport Med.* 2013;34(10):924-30.

32. Wik EH, Luteberget LS, Spencer M. Activity profiles in international female team handball using PlayerLoad. *Int J Sports Physiol Perform.* 2017;12(7):934-42.

Chapter 28

1. Austin D, Gabbett T, Jenkins D. The physical demands of Super 14 Rugby Union. *J Sci Med Sport.* 2011;14(3):259-63.

2. Bishop D, Girard O, Mendez-Villanueva A. Repeated-sprint ability–Part II: Recommendations for training. *Sports Med.* 2011;41(9):741-56.

3. Clemente FM, Wong del P, Martins FM, Mendes RS. Acute effects of the number of players and scoring method on physiological, physical, and technical performance in small-sided soccer games. *Res Sports Med.* 2014;22(4):380-97.

4. Cunniffe B, Proctor W, Baker JS, Davies B. An evaluation of the physiological demands of elite Rugby Union using global positioning system tracking software. *J Strength Cond Res.* 2009;23(4):1195-203.

5. Cunningham DJ, Shearer DA, Drawer S, Pollard B, Eager R, Taylor N, et al. Movement demands of elite under-20s and senior international Rugby Union players. *PLoS One.* 2016;11(11):e0164990.

6. Deutsch MU, Kearney GA, Rehrer NJ. Time-motion analysis of professional Rugby Union players during match-play. *J Sports Sci.* 2007;25(4):461-72.

7. Duthie G, Pyne D, Hooper S. Time-motion analysis of 2001 and 2002 Super 12 rugby. *J Sports Sci.* 2005;23(5):523-30.

8. Duthie GM, Pyne DB, Hooper SL. Applied physiology and game analysis of Rugby Union. *Sports Med.* 2003;33(13):973-91.

9. Eaves S, Hughes M. Patterns of play of international Rugby Union teams before and after the introduction of professional status. *International Journal of Performance Analysis in Sport.* 2003;3(2):103-11.

10. Eaves SJ, Hughes MD, Lamb KL. The consequences of the introduction of professional playing status on game action variables in international Northern Hemisphere Rugby Union football. *International Journal of Performance Analysis in Sport.* 2005;5(2):58-86.

11. Fuller CW, Brooks JH, Cancea RJ, Hall J, Kemp SP. Contact events in Rugby Union and their propensity to cause injury. *Br J Sports Med.* 2007;41(12):862-7.

12. Gabbett TJ, Jenkins D, Abernethy B. Game-based training for improving skill and physical fitness in team sport athletes. *Int J Sports Sci Coach.* 2009;4(2):273-83.

13. Hogarth LW, Burkett BJ, McKean MR. Match demands of professional rugby football codes: A review from 2008 to 2015. *Int J Sports Sci Coach.* 2016;11(3):451-63.

14. James N, Mellalieu SD, Jones NM. The development of position-specific performance indicators in professional Rugby Union. *J Sports Sci.* 2005;23(1):63-72.

15. Jones MR, West DJ, Crewther BT, Cook CJ, Kilduff LP. Quantifying positional and temporal movement patterns in professional Rugby Union using global positioning system. *Eur J Sport Sci.* 2015;15(6):488-96.

16. Jones NMP, Mellalieu SD, James N. Team performance indicators as a function of winning and losing in Rugby Union. *International Journal of Performance Analysis in Sport.* 2004;4(1):61-71.

17. Jones RM, Cook CC, Kilduff LP, Milanovic Z, James N, Sporis G, et al. Relationship between repeated sprint ability and aerobic capacity in professional soccer players. *Scientific World Journal.* 2013;2013:952350.

18. Owen AL, Wong DP, Paul D, Dellal A. Physical and technical comparisons between various-sided games within professional soccer. *Int J Sports Med.* 2014;35(4):286-92.

19. Quarrie K, Handcock P, Waller AE, Chalmers DJ, Toomey MJ, Wilson BD. The New Zealand rugby injury and performance project. III. Anthropometric and physical performance characteristics of players. *Br J Sports Med.* 1995;29(4):263-70.

20. Quarrie KL, Hopkins WG. Changes in player characteristics and match activities in Bledisloe Cup Rugby Union from 1972 to 2004. *J Sports Sci.* 2007;25(8):895-903.

21. Quarrie KL, Hopkins WG, Anthony MJ, Gill ND. Positional demands of international Rugby Union: Evaluation of player actions and movements. *J Sci Med Sport.* 2013;16(4):353-9.

22. Roberts SP, Trewartha G, Higgitt RJ, El-Abd J, Stokes KA. The physical demands of elite English Rugby Union. *J Sports Sci.* 2008;26(8):825-33.

23. Smart D, Hopkins WG, Quarrie KL, Gill N. The relationship between physical fitness and game behaviours in Rugby Union players. *Eur J Sport Sci.* 2014;14(Suppl 1):S8–S17.

24. Smith TB, Hébert-Losier K, McClymont D. An examination of the jump-and-lift factors influencing the time to reach peak catch height during a Rugby Union lineout. *J Sports Sci.* 2017:1-7.

25. Swaby R, Jones PA, Comfort P. Relationship between maximum aerobic speed performance and distance covered in Rugby Union games. *J Strength Cond Res.* 2016;30(10):2788-93.

26. Tee JC, Lambert MI, Coopoo Y. GPS comparison of training activities and game demands of professional Rugby Union. *Int J Sports Sci Coach.* 2016;11(2):200-11.

27. Tomlin DL, Wenger HA. The relationship between aerobic fitness and recovery from high intensity intermittent exercise. *Sports Med.* 2001;31(1):1-11.

28. Twist C, Worsfold P. *The Science of Rugby.* London: Taylor & Francis; 2015.

Chapter 29

1. Bellenger C. Predicting maximal aerobic speed through set distance time-trials. *Eur J Appl Physiol.* 2015;115(12):2593-8.

2. Bompa TO, Carrera M. *Periodization Training for Sports,* 2nd Edition. Champlain, IL: Human Kinetics; 2005.

3. Buchheit M. Individualizing high-intensity interval training in intermittent sport athletes with the 30-15 Intermittent Fitness Test. *NSCA Hot Topic Series wwwnsca-liftorg.* 2011;November.

4. Buchheit M. Monitoring training status with HR measures: Do all roads lead to Rome? *Front Physiol.* 2014;27(5):73.

5. Buchheit M, Laursen PB. High-intensity interval training, solutions to the programming puzzle. Part II: Anaerobic energy, neuromuscular load and practical applications. *Sports Med.* 2013;43(10):927-54.

6. Buchheit M, Laursen PB. High-intensity interval training, solutions to the programming puzzle: Part I: Cardiopulmonary emphasis. *Sports Med.* 2013;43(5):313-38.

7. Buchheit M, Simpson B. Player tracking technology: Half-full or half-empty glass? *Int J Sports Physiol Perform.* 2017;12(Suppl 2):S235–S41.

8. Buchheit M, Mendez-Villanueva A, Quod MJ, Quesnel T, Ahmaidi S. Improving acceleration and repeated sprint ability in well-trained adolescent handball players: speed vs. sprint interval training. *Int J Sports Physiol Perform.* 2010;5(2):152-64.

9. Buchheit M, Morgan W, Wallace J, Bode M, Poulos N. Physiological, psychometric, and performance effects of the Christmas break in Australian Football. *Int J Sports Physiol Perform.* 2015;10(1):120-3.

10. Clarke AC, Anson J, Pyne D. Physiologically based GPS speed zones for evaluating running demands in Women's Rugby Sevens. *J Sports Sci.* 2015;33(11):1101-8.

11. Coughlan GF. Physical game demands in elite Rugby Union: A global positioning system analysis and possible implications for rehabilitation. *Journal of Orthopaedic and Sports Physical Therapy.* 2011;41(8):600-5.

12. Duthie GM. A framework for the physical development of elite Rugby Union players. *Int J Sports Physiol Perform.* 2006;1(1):2-13.

13. Francis C. *Training for Speed.* Bellingham, WA: Faccioni Speed & Conditioning Consultants; 1997.

14. Gabbett TJ. The training-injury prevention paradox: Should athletes be training smarter and harder? *Br J Sports Med.* 2016;50(5):273-80.

15. Higham DG, Pyne DB, Anson JM, Eddy A. Movement patterns in Rugby Sevens: Effects of tournament level, fatigue and substitute players. *J Sci Med Sport.* 2012;15(3):277-82.

16. Higham DG, Pyne DB, Anson JM, Eddy A. Physiological, anthropometric, and performance characteristics of Rugby Sevens players. *Int J Sports Physiol Perform.* 2013;8(1):19-27.

17. Higham DG, Pyne DB, Anson JM, Hopkins WG, Eddy A. Comparison of activity profiles and physiological demands between international Rugby Sevens matches and training. *J Strength Cond Res.* 2016;30(5):1287-94.

18. McLellan CP, Lovell DI. Performance analysis of professional, semiprofessional, and junior elite rugby league match-play using global positioning systems. *J Strength Cond Res.* 2013;27(12):3266-74.

19. Mitchell JA. Variable changes in body composition, strength and lower body power during an international sevens season *J Strength Cond Res.* 2016;30(4):1127-36.

20. Murray AM, Varley MC. Activity profile of International Rugby Sevens: Effect of score line, opponent, and substitutes. *Int J Sports Physiol Perform.* 2015;10(6):791-801.

21. Rienzi E. Investigation of anthropometric and work-rate profiles of Rugby Sevens players. *Journal of Sports Medicine and Physical Fitness.* 1999;39(2):160-4.

22. Robineau J, Lacome M, Piscione J, Bigard X, Babault N. Concurrent training in Rugby Sevens: Effects of high-intensity interval exercises. *Int J Sports Physiol Perform.* 2017;12(3):336-44.

23. Ross A, Gill N, Cronin J. Match analysis and player characteristics in Rugby Sevens. *Sports Med (Auckland, NZ).* 2014;44(3):357-67.

24. Ross A, Gill N, Cronin J. The match demands of international rugby sevens. *J Sports Sci.* 2015;33(10):1035-41.

25. Ross A, Gill ND, Cronin JB. A comparison of the match demands of international and provincial Rugby Sevens. *Int J Sports Physiol Perform.* 2015;10(6):786-90.

26. Ross A, Gill N, Cronin J, Malcata R. The relationship between physical characteristics and match performance in Rugby Sevens. *Eur J Sport Sci.* 2015;15(6):565-71.

27. Saw AE, Main LC, Gastin PB. Monitoring the athlete training response: Subjective self-reported measures trump commonly used objective measures: A systematic review. *Br J Sports Med.* 2016;50(5):281-91.

28. Schuster J, Howells D, Robineau J, Couderc A, Natera A, Lumley N, et al. Physical preparation recommendations for elite Rugby Sevens performance. *Int J Sports Physiol Perform.* 2017:1-42.

29. Suarez-Arrones L, Arenas C, López G, Requena B, Terrill O, Mendez-Villanueva A. Positional differences in match running performance and physical collisions in men Rugby Sevens. *Int J Sports Physiol Perform.* 2014;9(2):316-23.

30. Suarez-Arrones L, Núñez J, Sáez de Villareal E, Gálvez J, Suarez-Sanchez G, Munguía-Izquierdo D. Repeated-high-intensity-running activity and internal training load of elite Rugby Sevens players during international matches: A comparison between halves. *Int J Sports Physiol Perform.* 2016;11(4):495-9.

31. Suarez-Arrones LJ. Running demands and heart rate responses in men Rugby Sevens. *J Strength Cond Res.* 2012;26(11):3155-9.

32. Waldron M, Twist C, Highton J, Worsfold P, Daniels M. Movement and physiological match demands of elite rugby league using portable

global positioning systems. *J Sports Sci.* 2011;29(11):1223-30.

Chapter 30

1. Akenhead R, Nassis GP. Training load and player monitoring in high-level football: Current practice and perceptions. *Int J Sports Physiol Perform.* 2016;11(5):587-93.

2. Barnes C, Archer DT, Hogg B, Bush M, Bradley PS. The evolution of physical and technical performance parameters in the English Premier League. *Int J Sports Med.* 2014;35(13):1095-100.

3. Buchheit M. Individualizing high-intensity interval training in intermittent sport athletes with the 30-15 Intermittent Fitness Test. *NSCA Hot Topic Series wwwnsca-liftorg.* 2011;November.

4. Buchheit M. Monitoring training status with HR measures: Do all roads lead to Rome? *Front Physiol.* 2014;27(5):73.

5. Buchheit M, Laursen PB. High-intensity interval training, solutions to the programming puzzle: Part I: Cardiopulmonary emphasis. *Sports Med.* 2013;43(5):313-38.

6. Buchheit M, Laursen PB. High-intensity interval training, solutions to the programming puzzle. Part II: Anaerobic energy, neuromuscular load and practical applications. *Sports Med.* 2013;43(10):927-54.

7. Buchheit M, Simpson BM. Player tracking technology: Half-full or half-empty glass? *Int J Sports Physiol Perform.* 2017;12(Suppl 2):S235–S41.

8. Buchheit M, Haydar B, Ahmaidi S. Repeated sprints with directional changes: Do angles matter? *J Sports Sci.* 2012;30(6):555-62.

9. Buchheit M, Cholley Y, Lambert P. Psychometric and physiological responses to a preseason competitive camp in the heat with a 6-hour time difference in elite soccer players. *Int J Sports Physiol Perform.* 2016;11(2):176-81.

10. Buchheit M, Mendez-Villanueva A, Simpson BM, Bourdon PC. Match running performance and fitness in youth soccer. *Int J Sports Med.* 2010;31(11):818-25.

11. Buchheit M, Lacome M, Cholley Y, Simpson BM. Neuromuscular responses to conditioned soccer sessions assessed via GPS-embedded accelerometers: Insights into tactical periodization. *Int J Sports Physiol Perform.* Sept 2017;1-21.

12. Buchheit M, Morgan W, Wallace J, Bode M, Poulos N. Physiological, psychometric, and performance effects of the Christmas break in Australian football. *Int J Sports Physiol Perform.* 2015;10(1):120-3.

13. Carling C. Interpreting physical performance in professional soccer match-play: Should we be more pragmatic in our approach? *Sports Med.* 2013;43(8):655-63.

14. Carling C, Bloomfield J. The effect of an early dismissal on player work-rate in a professional soccer match. *J Sci Med Sport.* 2010;13(1):126-8.

15. Delgado-Bordonau JL, Mendez-Villanueva A. Tactical Periodization: Mourinho's best-kept secret? *Soccer Journal.* May/June 2015. http://growingthegame.ca/wp/wp-content/uploads/2015/07/Tactical-Periodization.pdf.

16. Dellal A, Lago-Penas C, Wong del P, Chamari K. Effect of the number of ball contacts within bouts of 4 vs. 4 small-sided soccer games. *Int J Sports Physiol Perform.* 2011;6(3):322-33.

17. Dellal A, Varliette C, Owen A, Chirico EN, Pialoux V. Small-sided games versus interval training in amateur soccer players: Effects on the aerobic capacity and the ability to perform intermittent exercises with changes of direction. *J Strength Cond Res.* 2012;26(10):2712-20.

18. Dellal A, Chamari K, Pintus A, Girard O, Cotte T, Keller D. Heart rate responses during small-sided games and short intermittent running training in elite soccer players: A comparative study. *J Strength Cond Res.* 2008;22(5):1449-57.

19. Fyfe JJ, Bishop DJ, Stepto NK. Interference between concurrent resistance and endurance exercise: molecular bases and the role of individual training variables. *Sports Med.* 2014;44(6):743-62.

20. Gabbett TJ. The training-injury prevention paradox: Should athletes be training smarter and harder? *Br J Sports Med.* 2016;50(5):273-80.

21. Hader K, Mendez-Villanueva A, Williams B, Ahmaidi S, Buchheit M. Changes of direction during high-intensity intermittent runs: Neuromuscular and metabolic responses. *BMC Sports Sci Med Rehabil.* 2014;6(1):2.

22. Hader K, Mendez-Villanueva A, Palazzi D, Ahmaidi S, Buchheit M. Metabolic power requirement of change of direction speed in

young soccer players: Not all is what it seems. *PLoS One.* 2016;11(3):e0149839.

23. Hill-Haas SV, Coutts AJ, Rowsell GJ, Dawson BT. Generic versus small-sided game training in soccer. *Int J Sports Med.* 2009;30(9):636-42.

24. Hill-Haas SV, Dawson B, Impellizzeri FM, Coutts AJ. Physiology of small-sided games training in football: A systematic review. *Sports Med.* 2011;41(3):199-220.

25. Impellizzeri FM, Rampinini E, Coutts AJ, Sassi A, Marcora SM. Use of RPE-based training load in soccer. *Med Sci Sports Exerc.* 2004;36(6):1042-7.

26. Impellizzeri FM, Marcora SM, Castagna C, Reilly T, Sassi A, Iaia FM, et al. Physiological and performance effects of generic versus specific aerobic training in soccer players. *Int J Sports Med.* 2006;27(6):483-92.

27. Lacome M, Simpson BM, Buchheit M. Locomotor and heart rate responses of floaters during small-sided games in elite soccer players: Effect of pitch size and goal keepers. *Int J Sports Physiol Perform.* Sept 2017;1-13.

28. Lacome M, Simpson BM, Cholley Y, Lambert P, Buchheit M. Small sided games in elite soccer: Does one size fit all? *Int J Sports Physiol Perform.* Jul 2017;1-24.

29. Mayer N, Bosquet L, Plaine F, Marles A, Jullien H, Lambert P, et al., eds. Reproducibility of physiological, neuromuscular and perceptual responses to small-sided games in highly-trained young soccer players. European College of Sport Science; 2013; Barcelona, June 26-29.

30. Mendez-Villanueva A, Buchheit M, Simpson BM, Bourdon PC. Match play intensity distribution in youth soccer. *Int J Sport Med.* 2013;34(2):101-10.

31. Mendez-Villanueva A, Buchheit M, Simpson B, Peltola E, Bourdon P. Does on-field sprinting performance in young soccer players depend on how fast they can run or how fast they do run? *J Strength Cond Res.* 2011;25(9):2634-8.

32. Morgans R, Di Michele R, Drust B. Soccer match-play represents an important component of the power training stimulus in premier league players. *Int J Sports Physiol Perform.* 2018;13(5):665-7.

33. Rabbani A, Buchheit M. Heart rate-based versus speed-based high-intensity interval training in young soccer players. In Favero T, Drust B, Dawson B, eds. *International Research in Science and Soccer II.* Abingdon, UK: Routledge; 2015.

34. Rampinini E, Impellizzeri F, Castagna C, Abt G, Chamari K, Sassi A, et al. Factors influencing physiological responses to small-sided soccer games. *J Sports Sci.* 2007;6(25):659-66.

35. Rebelo AN, Silva P, Rago V, Barreira D, Krustrup P. Differences in strength and speed demands between 4v4 and 8v8 small-sided football games. *J Sports Sci.* 2016;34(24): 2246-54.

36. Reilly T, Bangsbo J, Franks A. Anthropometric and physiological predispositions for elite soccer. *J Sports Sci.* 2000;18(9):669-83.

37. Saw AE, Main LC, Gastin PB. Monitoring the athlete training response: Subjective self-reported measures trump commonly used objective measures: A systematic review. *Br J Sports Med.* 2016;50(5):281-91.

38. Spencer M, Bishop D, Dawson B, Goodman C. Physiological and metabolic responses of repeated-sprint activities: Specific to field-based team sports. *Sports Med.* 2005;35(12):1025-44.

39. Ufland P, Ahmaidi S, Buchheit M. Repeated-sprint performance, locomotor profile and muscle oxygen uptake recovery. *Int J Sport Med.* 2013;34(10):924-30.

Index

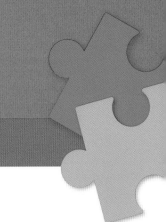

Note: The italicized *f* and *t* following page numbers refer to figures and tables, respectively.

About the Editors

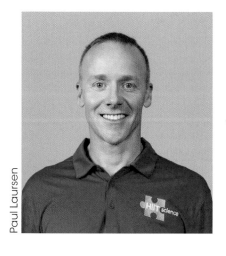

Paul Laursen

Paul Laursen, PhD, is an endurance coach, a sport scientist, and an adjunct professor for Auckland University of Technology in New Zealand. He earned his doctorate in exercise physiology from the University of Queensland, was formerly the physiology manager for High Performance Sport New Zealand, and now resides in British Columbia, Canada.

Laursen is well known throughout the international sport and strength and conditioning communities for his knowledge and research of high-intensity interval training. His other interests include heart rate variability, thermoregulation, health, and the application of artificial intelligence technologies to training. Laursen has published more than 125 peer-reviewed manuscripts in exercise and sport science journals; his publications with coauthor Martin Buchheit are among the most cited. Laursen is an active endurance athlete, having completed 18 Ironman triathlons.

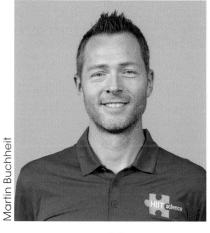

Martin Buchheit

Martin Buchheit, PhD, is a sport scientist, a strength and conditioning coach, and the head of performance for the Paris Saint-Germain Football (Soccer) Club. He is also an adjunct associate professor of exercise science for Victoria University in Australia. He previously worked as an exercise physiologist for ASPIRE Academy in Qatar, and he has served as a lecturer, consultant, and strength and conditioning coach for various organizations.

Buchheit received his doctorate in physiology from the University of Strasbourg in France. His main research focuses on assessing, improving, and monitoring the physiological determinants of team sport performance, with a greater emphasis on soccer and handball. Based on his field and research experiences, Buchheit developed the 30-15 intermittent fitness test (used to program high-intensity training; go to https://30-15ift.com for details) to improve high-intensity training prescription, and the 4'+3' running test to track changes in training status using heart rate (variability) and GPS/accelerometer data. He has also performed some research on the acute and chronic responses to hypoxic and heat exposure, and their possible ergogenic effects on physical performance in team sports.

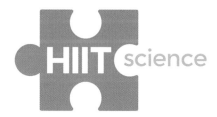

Buchheit has published more than 160 papers in peer-reviewed journals, with more than 100 as a first author. His overall scientific work has been cited more than 10,000 times, with the two-part review on high-intensity interval training coauthored with Paul Laursen being the most cited of all. Buchheit has been invited around the globe to share his experience in the fields of strength and conditioning and sport sciences, as well as to discuss his overall training approach in the elite setting. Further, he has been working on bridging the gap between science and practice and was involved in the launch of a new, open-access, reviewing-free web-platform aimed at improving research dissemination, *Sports Performance & Science Reports* (https://sportperfsci.com).

Buchheit is a former semi-pro handball player and is now an endurance athlete who has a personal best time of 2:54 in the marathon.

List of Contributors

Martyn Beaven
University of Waikato

Johann Bilsborough
Director of Performance, New England Patriots; High Performance Manager/Director of Sports Science, Boston Celtics

Robert Butler

Moses Cabrera
Head Strength and Conditioning Coach, New England Patriots

Carlos Alberto Cavalheiro

Aaron Coutts
University of Technology, Sydney, Australia

Wim Derave
Department of Movement and Sports Sciences, Ghent University, Belgium

Jaime Fernandez-Fernandez
Faculty of Physical Activity and Sports Sciences, University of León (Spain)

Duncan French, PhD
UFC Performance Institute

Jackson Fyfe
Centre for Sport Research (CSR), School of Exercise and Nutrition Sciences, Deakin University, Melbourne, Australia

Nic Gill
University of Waikato

Hani Al Haddad
Football Performance and Science Department, Aspire Academy

Dave Hamilton
Formerly Head Strength and Conditioning Coach for the GB Olympic Women's Field Hockey Team 2012, Director of Performance Science for the USA Olympic Field Hockey Team 2016

Philippe Hellard
French Swimming Federation

Joel Hocking

Aaron Kellett

Mathieu Lacome
Performance Department, Paris Saint-Germain, France

Matt Leonard

Philip Maffetone
https://philmaffetone.com/

Matt Nichol
www.MattNichol.com, www.biosteel.com

Carl Petersen
University of Canterbury, New Zealand

Daniel Plews
www.plewsandprof.com; Sports Performance Research Institute NZ, Auckland University of Technology, Auckland, New Zealand

Nick Poulos

Marc Quod

Øyvind Sandbakk, PhD
Professor and Managing Director, Centre for Elite Sports Research, Department of Neuromedicine and Movement Science, Norwegian University of Science and Technology

Anna Saw

Xavi Schelling
Institute of Sport, Exercise and Active Living, College of Sport and Exercise Science, Victoria University, Melbourne, VIC, Australia

Ben Simpson
Performance Department, Paris Saint-Germain, France

Jamie Stanley
South Australian Sports Institute, Australian Cycling Team, University of South Australia

Lorena Torres-Ronda
*Institute of Sport, Exercise and Active Living,
College of Sport and Exercise Science,
Victoria University, Melbourne, VIC, Australia*

Tom Vandenbogaerde
Swimming Australia

Jean Claude Vollmer

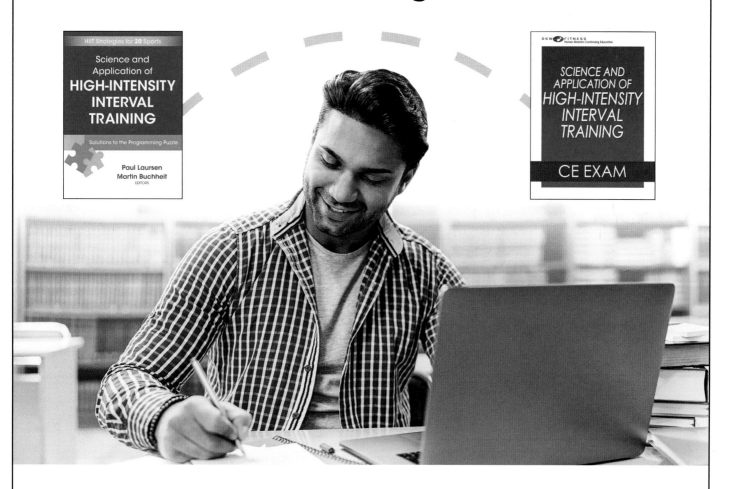
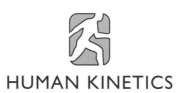